SECOND EDITION

The Cervical Spine

THE CERVICAL SPINE RESEARCH SOCIETY EDITORIAL COMMITTEE

80 Contributors

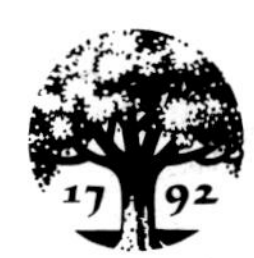

J. B. Lippincott Company
PHILADELPHIA
Cambridge / New York / St. Louis / San Francisco
London / Singapore / Sydney / Tokyo

Acquisitions Editor: Darlene Barela Cooke
Editorial Assistant: Robin Levin
Indexer: Nancy Weaver
Designer: Don Shenkle

Second Edition

1 3 5 6 4 2

Library of Congress Cataloging-in-Publication Data

The Cervical spine/the Cervical Spine Research Society, Editorial Committee.—2nd ed.
p. cm.
Bibliography: p.
Includes index.
ISBN 0-397-50827-1
1. Vertebrae, Cervical—Diseases. 2. Vertebrae—Abnormalities. 3. Vertebrae, Cervical—Wounds and injuries. I. Cervical Spine Research Society. Editorial Committee.
RD531.C47 1983a
616.7'3—dc19 88-13663
CIP

The authors and publisher have exerted every effort to ensure that drug selection and dosage set forth in this text are in accord with current recommendations and practice at the time of publication. However, in view of ongoing research, changes in government regulations, and the constant flow of information relatıng to drug therapy and drug reactions, the reader is urged to check the package inset for each drug for any change in indications and dosage and for added warnings and precautions. This is particularly important when the recommended agent is a new or infrequently employed drug.

This book is dedicated to the memory of
Robert W. Bailey

Contributors

John L. Alderman, Ph.D.

Associate Professor of Physiology
Chairman
Department of Physiology
University of Health Sciences
College of Osteopathic Medicine
Kansas City, Missouri

George Alker, M.D.

Professor and Chairman, Department of Radiology
SUNY/Buffalo School of Medicine and Biomedical Sciences
Director, Department of Radiology
Erie County Medical Center
Buffalo, New York

Ben L. Allen, Jr., M.D.

Professor of Surgery and Pediatrics
University of Texas Medical Branch Hospitals
Galveston, Texas

Lewis D. Anderson, M.D.

Professor and Chairman Orthopaedic Surgery
University of Southern Alabama College of Medicine
Vice President for Medical Affairs
University of South Alabama
Medical Director
University of South Alabama Medical Center
Mobile, Alabama

Joseph S. Barr, Jr., M.D.

Assistant Clinical Professor of Orthopaedic Surgery
Harvard Medical School
Visiting Orthopaedic Surgeon
Massachusetts General Hospital
Boston, Massachusetts

Enrique M. Boada, M.D.

Vice-Chairman
Traumatology and Orthopaedic Surgery Department
Guinta De Salud
La Alianza Hospital Central
Barcelona, Spain
Chief
Traumatology and Orthopaedic Surgery Services
Emergency Room
MUTUA Del Carmen Hospital
Granollers, Spain

Henry H. Bohlman, M.D.

Professor, Department of Orthopedic Surgery
Chief, Acute Spinal Cord Injury Service
Veterans Administration Medical Center
Professor, Orthopaedic Surgery
Case Western Reserve University School of Medicine
Chief, Reconstructive and Traumatic Spine Surgery Center
University Hospitals
Cleveland, Ohio

Alexander E. Brodsky, M.D.

Associate Clinical Professor, Orthopedic Surgery
Baylor College of Medicine and U.T.H.S.C.
Director, Orthopedic Pathology Laboratory
St. Luke's Episcopal Hospital
Medical Director, Texas Institute for Spinal Disorders
Director, Spinal Fellowship Program
Houston, Texas

Charles R. Clark, M.D.

Professor Orthopaedic Surgery
University of Iowa College of Medicine
Attending Physician
Department of Orthopaedic Surgery
University of Iowa Hospitals and Clinics
Iowa City, Iowa

Paul R. Cooper, M.D.

Associate Professor of Neurosurgery
New York University Medical Center
New York, New York

Robert Crowell, M.D.

Mount Carmel Medical Center
Columbus, Ohio

Joseph F. Cusick, M.D.

Professor of Neurosurgery
Medical College of Wisconsin
Milwaukee, Wisconsin

Robin I. Davidson, M.D.

Associate Professor of Neurosurgery
University of Massachusetts Medical School
Worcester, Massachusetts

Sanjay Desai, M.D.

Resident, Orthopaedic Surgery
University of Massachusetts Medical Center
Worcester, Massachusetts

Edward J. Dunn, M.D.

Chief of Orthopaedic Surgery
Worcester Memorial Hospital
Professor of Orthopaedic Surgery
University of Massachusetts Medical School
Worcester, Massachusetts

Thomas Edwards, Ph.D.

Associate Professor
Department of Orthopedic Surgery
Director, Orthopedic Research Laboratory
State University of New York
Health Science Center
Syracuse, New York

Frank J. Eismont, M.D.

Professor of Orthopedic Surgery
University of Miami School of Medicine
Co-Director of the Acute Spinal Cord Injury Unit
Jackson Memorial Hospital
Miami, Florida

Joseph A. Epstein, M.D., F.A.C.S.

Professor of Clinical Neurosurgery
State University of New York at Stony Brook
Stony Brook, New York
Attending Neurosurgeon
North Shore University Hospital-Cornell Medical Center
Manhasett, New York
Attending Neurosurgeon
Long Island Jewish Medical Center
New Hyde Park, New York

Nancy E. Epstein, M.D., F.A.C.S.

Assistant Professor of Clinical Neurosurgery
State University of New York at Stony Brook
Stony Brook, New York
Assistant Attending Neurosurgeon
North Shore University Hospital-Cornell Medical Center
Manhasset, New York
Staff Neurosurgeon
Long Island Jewish Medical Center
New Hyde Park, New York

J. William Fielding, M.D., F.R.C.S. (C)
Clinical Professor of Orthopaedic Surgery
College of Physicians and Surgeons of Columbia University
Director of the Department of Orthopaedic Surgery
St. Luke's-Roosevelt Hospital Center
New York, New York

Steven R. Garfin, M.D.
Associate Professor
University of California, San Diego
UCSD Medical Center
San Diego, California

Jacob J. Graham, M.D.
Associate Clinical Professor of Orthopaedic Surgery
Mount Sinai School of Medicine
Attending Orthopaedic Surgeon and Director
Emeritus Scoliosis Service
Orthopaedic Institute
Hospital for Joint Diseases
New York, New York

S. Ashby Grantham, M.D.
Professor of Clinical Orthopaedic Surgery
Columbia University College of Physicians and Surgeons
New York Orthopaedic Hospital
Columbia Presbyterian Medical Center
New York, New York

Robert W. Hensinger, M.D.
Professor of Surgery, Orthopaedics
University of Michigan
Chief, Pediatrics Orthopaedics
Mott Childrens Hospital
Ann Arbor, Michigan

Kiyoshi Harabayashi, M.D.
Associate Professor
Department of Orthopaedic Surgery
School of Medicine
Keio University
Tokyo, Japan

Martin D. Hoffman, M.D.
Assistant Professor
Department of Physical Medicine and Rehabilitation
The Medical College of Wisconsin
Milwaukee, Wisconsin

Mason Hohl, M.D.
Clinical Professor of Surgery/Orthopedics
UCLA Medical Center
Beverly Hills, California

Louis C.S. Hsu, M.B.B.S., F.R.C.S.E., F.A.C.S.
Reader in Orthopaedic Surgery
University of Hong Kong
Medical Director and Consultant Orthopaedic Surgeon
Duchess of Kent Children's Hospital at Sandy Bay
Honorary Orthopaedic Consultant
Queen Mary Hospital
Hong Kong

Michael H. Jofe, M.D.
Department of Orthopedic Surgery
Massachusetts General Hospital
Boston, Massachusetts

Rollin M. Johnson, M.D.
Associate Clinical Professor of Orthopaedic Surgery
Yale University School of Medicine
New Haven, Connecticut

Moe Khan, M.D., F.R.C.S.(C)
Professor and Head, Division of Neurosurgery
University of Saskatchewan
Professor and Head, Division of Neurosurgery
University Hospital
Saskatoon, Saskatchewan
Canada

Martin Hans Krag, M.D.
Assistant Professor
School of Medicine
University of Vermont
Department of Orthopaedics and Rehabilitation
Medical Center Hospital of Vermont
Burlington, Vermont

S. Henry LaRoca, M.D.
Clinical Professor of Orthopaedic Surgery
Tulane University
New Orleans, Louisiana

Sanford J. Larson, M.D., Ph.D.
Professor and Chairman
Department of Neurosurgery
Medical College of Wisconsin
Medical College of Wisconsin Affiliated Hospitals
Milwaukee, Wisconsin

Jonas V. Lieponis, M.D.
Assistant Clinical Professor
Orthopaedic Surgery
Yale University School of Medicine
Attending Physician, Spine Service
Yale-New Haven Hospital
New Haven, Connecticut

Stephen J. Lipson, M.D.
Department of Orthopedic Surgery
Harvard Medical School
Brigham and Women's Hospital
Boston, Massachusetts

Donlin M. Long, M.D., Ph.D.
Professor and Chairman
Department of Neurosurgery
Johns Hopkins University School of Medicine
Neurosurgeon-in-Chief, Johns Hopkins Hospital
Baltimore, Maryland

Dennis J. Maiman, M.D., Ph.D.
Associate Professor of Neurosurgery
Medical College of Wisconsin
Chief, Spinal Cord Injury Center
VA Medical Center
Medical Director, Spinal Cord Injury Center
Froedtert Memorial Lutheran Hospital
Milwaukee, Wisconsin

Christian Mazel
Service de Chirugie Orthoped
Groupe Hopitalier Pitie-Saltpetriere
Paris, France

Paul C. McAfee, M.D.
Chief, Spinal Reconstructive Surgery
Associate Professor of Orthopedics
Associate Professor of Neurosurgery
Johns Hopkins University School of Medicine
Johns Hopkins Hospital
Baltimore, Maryland

Ian McNab, M.D.
Emeritus Professor of Surgery
University of Toronto
Chief of Division of Orthopaedic Surgery
The Wellesley Hospital
Toronto, Canada

J. Donald McQueen, M.D., F.A.C.S., F.R.C.S.
Professor, Division of Neurosurgery
University of Saskatchewan
Saskatoon, Saskatchewan
Canada

Michael J. Murphy, M.D.
Assistant Clinical Professor of Orthopaedic Surgery
Yale University School of Medicine
Co-Director Spine Service
Yale New Haven Hospital
New Haven, Connecticut

Nathan E. Nachlas, M.D.
Clinical Instructor
Department of Otolaryngology, Head and Neck Surgery
University of Miami School of Medicine
Miami, Florida

Hiroshi Nakashima, M.D.
Department of Orthopaedic Surgery
Sumitomo Hospital
Osaka, Japan

Bruce E. Northrup, M.D.
Clinical Associate Professor of Neurosurgery
Thomas Jefferson University Medical School
Neurosurgeon, Thomas Jefferson University
Philadelphia, Pennsylvania

Kozo Okada, M.D.
Assistant Professor
Department of Orthopaedic Surgery
Kagawa Medical School
Kagawa, Japan

Keiro Ono, M.D.
Professor and Chairman
Department of Orthopaedic Surgery
Osaka University Medical School
Osaka, Japan

Manohar M. Panjabi, Ph.D., Dr. Tech.
Professor of Orthopaedic Surgery
Director of Biomechanics
Department of Orthopaedics and Rehabilitation
Yale Medical School
New Haven, Connecticut

Wesley W. Parke, Ph.D.
Professor of Anatomy
Chairman, Department of Anatomy
University of South Dakota School of Medicine
Vermillion, South Dakota

Lourens Penning, M.D.
Emeritus Professor of Neuroradiology
Department of Diagnostic Radiology
State University Hospital
Groningen, The Netherlands

Donald S. Pierce, A.B., M.D.
Associate Clinical Professor of Orthopaedic Surgery
Harvard Medical School
Visiting Orthopaedic Surgeon
Massachusetts General Hospital
Boston, Massachusetts

Peter D. Pizzutillo, M.D.
Associate Professor of Orthopaedic Surgery
Thomas Jefferson University
Director, Division of Pediatric Orthopaedics
Thomas Jefferson University Hospital
Philadelphia, Pennsylvania

Joseph Ransohoff, M.D.
Professor and Chairman
New York University Medical Center
New York, New York

Richard B. Raynor, M.D.
Clinical Professor of Neurosurgery
New York University Medical Center
Attending Neurosurgeon
St. Vincent's Hospital
New York, New York

Lee H. Riley, Jr., M.D.
Chairman of Orthopedic Surgery
Professor of Orthopedic Surgery
Johns Hopkins Hospital
Baltimore, Maryland

William Roberts, M.D.
Mercy Medical Center
St. Luke's Medical Center
Cedar Rapids, Iowa

Robert Robinson, M.D.
Professor Emeritus
Department of Orthopedic Surgery
Johns Hopkins Hospital
Baltimore, Maryland

Richard H. Rothman, M.D., Ph.D.
James Edwards Professor and Chairman
Department of Orthopaedic Surgery
Thomas Jefferson University
Chairman-Rothman Institute Pennsylvania Hospital
Philadelphia, Pennsylvania

Raymond Roy-Camille
Chef du Service de Chirugie Orthoped
Groupe Hospitalier, Pite-Saltpetriere
Paris, France

Gerard Saillant
Service de Chirugie Orthoped
Group Hospitalier Pitie-Saltpetriere
Paris, France

Tadashi Sasaki, M.D.
Director
Sasaki Orthopaedic Clinic
Tokyo, Japan

Kazuhiko Satomi, M.D.
Instructor
Department of Orthopaedic Surgery
School of Medicine
Keio University
Tokyo, Japan

Henry Sherk, M.D.
Professor of Surgery
Chief of Orthopedics and Rehabilitation
Medical College of Pennsylvania
Philadelphia, Pennsylvania

Edward H. Simmons, M.D., B.Sc.(Med.), F.R.C.S.(C), M.S.(Tor.), F.A.C.S.
Professor of Orthopaedic Surgery
The State University of New York at Buffalo
Head of the Department of Orthopaedic Hospital
The Buffalo General Hospital
Buffalo, New York

Wayne O. Southwick, M.D.
Professor of Orthopaedic Surgery
Yale University School of Medicine
Co-Director Spine Service
Yale New Haven Hospital
New Haven, Connecticut

E. Shannon Stauffer, M.D.
Professor and Chairman
Division of Orthopaedics and Rehabilitation
SIU School of Medicine
Director
Spinal Injury Center
Memorial Medical Center
Springfield, Illinois

Joseph S. Torg, M.D.
Professor of Orthopaedic Surgery
University of Pennsylvania School of Medicine
Director
University of Pennsylvania Sports Medicine Center
Philadelphia, Pennsylvania

Christopher G. Ullrich, M.D.
Clinical Assistant Professor of Radiology
Johns Hopkins University School of Medicine
Baltimore, Maryland
Section Chief
Magnetic Resonance Imaging
Charlotte Memorial Hospital and Medical Center
Charlotte, North Carolina

Henk Verbiest, M.D., Ph.D.
Professor of Neurosurgery
Emeritus Chairman
Utrecht University Neurosurgical Department
University Hospital
Utrecht, The Netherlands

Henry Wang, M.D.
Assistant Professor of Radiology
Johns Hopkins University
Johns Hopkins Hospital
Johns Hopkins Medical Institution
Baltimore, Maryland

Andreas Weidner, M.D., Priv.-Dozent
Paracelsus-Klinik
Am Natruber Holz 69
Federal Republic of Germany

Augustus A. White III, M.D., Dr.M.Sci.
Professor of Orthopedic Surgery
Harvard Medical School
Orthopedic Surgeon-in-Chief
Beth Israel Hospital
Boston, Massachusetts

Thomas S. Whitecloud III, M.D.
Professor of Orthopaedic Surgery
Department of Orthopaedics
Tulane University School of Medicine
Tulane University Hospital and Clinic
New Orleans, Louisiana

Thomas E. Whitesides, Jr., M.D.
Professor, Department of Orthopedic Surgery
Emory University School of Medicine
Emory Hospital
Atlanta, Georgia

Sam W. Wiesel
Professor of Orthopedic Surgery
George Washington University Medical Center
Washington, DC

John W. Wolf, Jr., M.D.
Assistant Clincial Professor
University of Cincinnati
Attending Staff Physician
Good Samaritan Hospital
Batavia, Ohio

Kazuo Yamashita, M.D.
Department of Orthopaedic Surgery
Osaka University Medical School
Osaka, Japan

Arthur C.M.C. Yau, M.D., F.R.C.S.E.
Former Professor of Orthopaedic Surgery
University of Hong Kong
Honorary Consultant Orthopaedic Surgeon
Duchess of Kent Children's Hospital at Sandy Bay
Hong Kong

Wise Young, M.D., Ph.D.
Associate Professor of Neurosurgery, Physiology, and Biophysics
New York University School of Medicine
Director
Neurosurgery Research Laboratories
New York University Medical Center
New York, New York

Preface

In Janury of 1973, Dr. J. William Fielding convened a group of nine physicians, who like him, had an interest in the cervical spine. The purpose of the meeting was to discuss the possible need for a cervical spine research society that would provide a forum in which the problems and challenges associated with the treatment of cervical spine disorders could be presented and discussed. It was the aim of the founders of the society to attract a multi-disciplinary and international group, and neurosurgeons, orthopedists, radiologists, anatomists, bioengineers, and others from North America, Europe, and Japan were invited to join. The first formal meeting was held in New York in December of 1973, and it was immediately apparent that the newly formed society would serve an important role in expanding and disseminating our knowledge of the cervical spine. Since then, the Cervical Spine Research Society has grown to a membership of 125, and new members who can make a real contribution are constantly being sought.

In addition to holding an annual meeting, the Society has published several symposia on such topics as the upper cervical spine, spondylotic myeloradiculopathy, and congenital malformations of the cervical spine. It has supported multicenter studies on the treatment of cervical spine tumors and odontoid fractures, and it has presented two Instructional Courses on the cervical spine. In 1983, a European section of the Cervical Spine Research Society was founded by the late Professor Mario Boni in Pavia, Italy, and since that year, annual meetings have also been held in Europe.

One of the Society's most significant achievements, however, was the first edition of *The Cervical Spine.* The idea for the book was presented to the Society by Dr. Robert Bailey in 1979. Dr. Bailey, who was President of the Society at that time, had already published his own book on the cervical spine and was considering revising his text as a second edition. He instead invited the Society to take over this project and publish the book under its own authorship. An editorial subcommittee was formed, and Dr. Bailey served as Chairman. Various members of the Society were asked to contribute chapters on their areas of interest as demonstrated by their work presented in the annual meetings, and the book was published in 1983. Dr. Bailey's interest, concern and guidance were critical factors in the success of that effort and in recognition of his contribution, the second edition is dedicated to his memory.

The second edition was thought necessary because of the advances and new developments that have occurred since the first edition was published. Magnetic resonance imaging and three dimensional C-T scanning, for example, are diagnostic techniques which were just appearing when the first edition was being prepared. Both these subjects are covered in the second edition. Internal fixation of the unstable cervical spine with plates and screws is a technique in wide use in countries other than the United States of America. The devices used in these techniques are not available here, however, because of requirements of the Food and Drug Administration. Despite the fact that these devices cannot be used in the United States at this time, it seemed appropriate to include descriptions of their application to cervical spine problems because they have had such extensive application elsewhere. Among subjects not covered in the first edition were sports injuries, laminoplasty for cervical myeloradiculopathy, nonoperative treatment for degenerative disorders, and a review of complications of cervical spine surgery. The section on biomechanics was greatly expanded to reflect the volume of work that has been done in this area, and a longer chapter on basic research in cord injury and regeneration was considered essential in the second edition to reflect the vital recent work also being done on these subjects. Several topics, such as thermography and discography, were not included in the second edition because their use and indications remain either controversial or not completely understood at this time. The second edition by necessity is a much longer book, but the information included in it should bring the reader up to date on recent developments in the basic science and clinical aspects of the diagnosis and treatment of the .cervical spine.

The Editorial Subcommittee has been privileged to work with the members of the Cervical Spine Research Society, who devoted their time and knowledge to this publication. Their contribution is gratefully acknowledged as is the backup and support of the members of the Society at large. They deserve special thanks and recognition for making this book possible.

Henry H. Sherk, M.D.

Founding Members of The Cervical Spine Research Society Present at First Meeting in New York, 1973

Robert W. Bailey
Henry Bohlman
Edward Dunn
J. William Fielding
Alice L. Garrett
Ashby Grantham
Robert Hensinger
Mason Hohl
Bernard Jacobs
Henry La Rocca
Donlin Long
Ian MacNab
Wesley Parke
Joseph Ransohoff
Lee H. Riley
Robert A. Robinson
Richard Rothman
Henry H. Sherk
Edward Simmons
Wayne O. Southwick
E. Shannon Stauffer
Augustus White
Thomas Whitesides

Contents

CHAPTER 1

Anatomy

Developmental Anatomy

HENRY H. SHERK AND WESLEY W. PARKE

The cervical spine develops through several phases as follows:

1. Embryologic phase
2. Fetal phase
3. Phases of infancy and early childhood and adolescence
4. Adult phase

EMBRYOLOGIC PHASE

After fertilization, the ovum migrates down the fallopian tube into the uterine cavity. During the 6 or 7 days it takes for this to occur, the ovum divides a number of times to form a solid cluster of cells called the morula. The morula becomes a hollow ball (the blastocyst) at 7 days after fertilization and implants itself into the endometrium. On one side of the blastocyst there develops a cluster of cells called the embryonic disc. The embryonic disc thickens and forms two distinct layers of cells called the endoderm and the ectoderm, and the embryo thus exists for a short time as a bilaminar structure.

In the third week of embryonic life, ectodermal cells sink into the dorsal surface of the caudal end of the embryo and push forward between the ectoderm and endoderm to form the mesoderm. In the midline, the mesoderm coalesces into an axial semirigid rod called the notochord. At the same time, the ectoderm has begun to form the neural plate on the dorsal surface of the embryo just above the notochord. The neural plate folds on itself to form the neural tube, which is the precursor to the spinal cord and brain. Coincident with the development of the notochord and neural tube, the mesoderm aggregates into somites on either side of the notochord, and at 4 weeks after fertilization the embryo is segmented and ready to undergo a fundamental metamorphosis into a vertebrated fetus.

Before resegmentation of the somites into the vertebrae, the mesoderm of the somites increases in size, and the somite mesoderm cells grow dorsally and laterally to become the myotomes and dermatomes (Fig. 1-1*A*). The cells that migrate me-

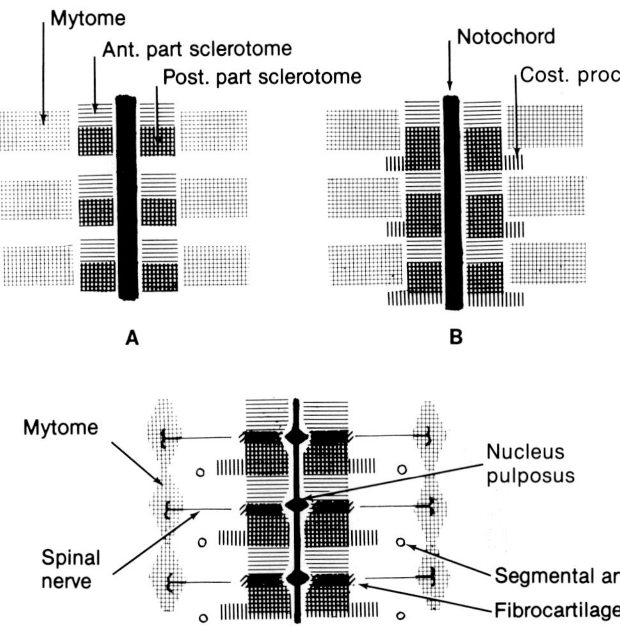

Fig. 1-1. A graphic schema of the resegmentation of the vertebral primordia and their eventual relationship with other segmental structures.

dially about the notochord and neural tube to become vertebrae are called, in aggregate at each level, the sclerotome. The intermediate mesoderm that migrates laterally away from the midline gives rise to such structures as the brachial arches, the pronephros, and the limb buds. At the height of the somite phase, the embryo has 41 segments and the somites can be easily seen distending the thin overlying ectoderm.

At 5 to 6 weeks, the embryo begins to resegment and the somites become vertebrae (Fig. 1-1*B*). Resegmentation occurs when the right and left somites at each level fuse across the midline, incorporating the notochord. Mesenchymal cells in the somite migrate toward the midportion of the somite where they aggregate as a densely staining cluster. This occurs about a cleft called the fissure of von Ebner. As the fissure of von Ebner widens, the clustered cells give rise to an intervertebral disc, and the caudal half of one somite fuses with the cranial half of the adjacent somite to form the primitive vertebral body (Fig. 1-1*C*). Cells migrate dorsally over the neural tube from the vertebral body to form the vertebral arches and ventrally to form the costal processes or ribs.

It has long been recognized that the craniocervical articulations had a complex evolution and developmental history. Most contemporary texts concede that the definitive mammalian axis has resulted from the fusion of centra derived from two upper cervical sclerotomes, but this concept has still failed to explain fully some segmental discrepancies and has been questioned on the basis of comparative evidence.[2] It is rather surprising that comparative embryologists previously described the existence of an obscure craniocervical hemisclerotome from studies of several mammalian groups, and its contributions to the upper cervical vertebrae have been recorded.[1] Yet its mention in most current anatomy and embryology texts is strangely lacking.

The more recent work of O'Rahilly, Müller, and Meyer[3] has reaffirmed the existence of a third centrum in the axis-odontoid complex of the human embryo. These authors designated the three axis centra X, Y, and Z, in descending order. The apical X component at first projects into the early foramen magnum and forms an occipitoaxial joint, which it retains as a syndesmosis by formation of the alar ligaments. The Y and Z components become the lower part of the odontoid process and the centrum of the axis. Each is related, respectively, to the first three cervical nerves, which explains the redundancy of cervical nerves in relation to the conventional numbering of the cervical vertebrae. Thus, the suboccipital (first cervical) nerve is the segmental nerve of the generally unrecognized sclerotomal precursor to the apical segment of the odontoid process.

Additional (noncentral) derivatives of this cryptic hemisclerotome may also explain other peculiarities in the metameric development of the craniocervical region. Cave[1] and Presley and Hallam[4] claim the mammalian apical odontoid element is the phylogenetic equivalent of the "proatlas" of reptiles. In most members of this vertebrate class this proatlas fuses to the occiput of the skull, whereas in mammals it fuses to the atlantal contribution to the odontoid. In the sphenodon, the only surviving member of a group of primitive reptiles, the proatlas exists as an independent vertebral element with its own neural arch. The confusion of this segment with the true atlantal derivatives in the sphenodon has fostered doubts concerning the multisegmental origin of the odontoid process.[2]

According to Cave[1] and Presley and Hallam,[4] all placental mammals also retain components of this

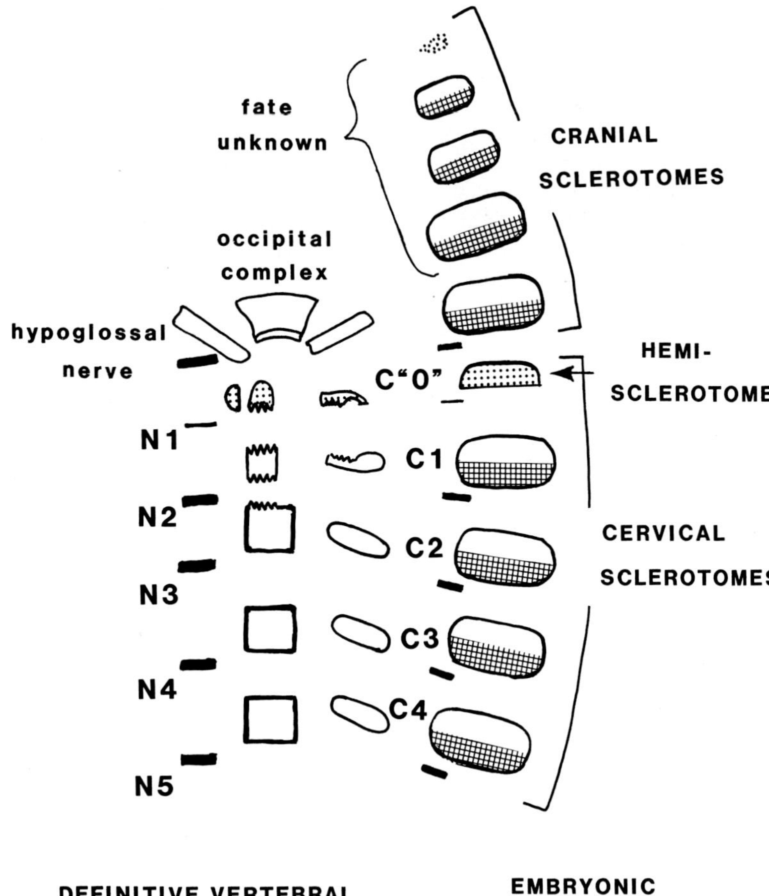

Fig. 1-2. This is a diagrammatic arrangement of the craniocervical sclerotomes and their segmentally related definitive vertebral elements and nerves. Note that the cranial and cervical sclerotomes form a continuum. In the early vertebrates, the lower two cranial sclerotomes were most likely committed to the cervical region, but expansion of the brain case in amniotes incorporated them into the skull, along with their related nerves (preamniotes have only ten cranial nerves). In mammals, the contributions of the cranial sclerotomes to the skull above the occiput have been lost or obscured, but the occipital complex, with its segmental hypoglossal nerve, is known to be of vertebral origin. With the simultaneous expansion of the skull and the requirements of increased craniocervical mobility, an "orphan" sclerotome, which is cranial in most reptiles and cervical in mammals, became the precursor to proatlas components; it is here designated the C"0" (zero) sclerotome. Its derivatives, being of only the cranial half of a sclerotome, would be primarily centrum and arch elements without disc primordia.

proatlas neural arch. In humans, these components are expressed as the dorsal part of the superior atlantal articular facet and the contiguous retroarticular ligament, which often ossifies to form a foramen for the vertebral artery. The atlas anterior arch is generally regarded as a retained and ossified hypochordal bow of an upper cervical vertebra. There is reason to believe that this arch, along with the superior part of the transverse ligament, is also a derivative of the cryptic hemisclerotome.

The existence of this hemisclerotome and its contribution to the cranial part of the odontoid also explains the segmental relationship of the os odontoidum. The fact that this anomaly is manifested as a spherule of bone suspended between the two alar ligaments was difficult to reconcile with a single-centrum origin of the odontoid process, which most likely would require the separation to occur caudal to the atlantal centrum rather than above it. Thus, regarding the os odontoidum as an isolated proatlas element is developmentally and phyletically consistent with the existence of a C"0" hemisclerotome and its derivatives (Figs. 1-2 and 1-3).

At the conclusion of the process of resegmentation, the embryo becomes a fetus (Figs. 1-4 and 1-5*A*).

FETAL PHASE

During the fetal phase, the mesenchymal anlagen of the vertebrae undergo the process of chondrogenesis and osteogenesis. Thus, the vertebrae do not change their shape or fundamental structure, but they do acquire a different tissue matrix and they do grow considerably in size. The process of chondrification begins at the cervicothoracic level and extends upward and downward along the vertebral column. Chondrification in the vertebral bodies usually begins in two centers on each side of the midline. The change in consistency of the vertebral body from soft mesenchymal tissue to hard cartilaginous tissue forces the notochordal tissue out of the vertebral body into the intervertebral disc space; the notochordal cells will remain there as the nucleus pulposus. Chondrification also occurs in each neural arch and in each costal process. The chondrification centers of the dorsal

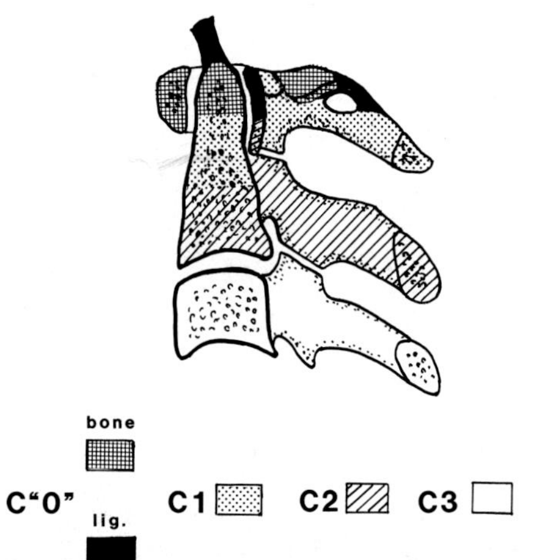

Fig. 1-3. This drawing shows the definitive contributions of the first three sclerotome segments to the atlantoaxial complex and its ligaments. The hemisclerotome C"0" provides the upper part of the odontoid process, the hypochordal anterior arch, and the dorsal part of the superior atlas facet as well as the alar, transverse (*upper part*), and retroarticular ligaments depicted in black. The conventionally designated C1 sclerotome then provides the remainder of the posterior arch and the inferior part of the odontoid process.

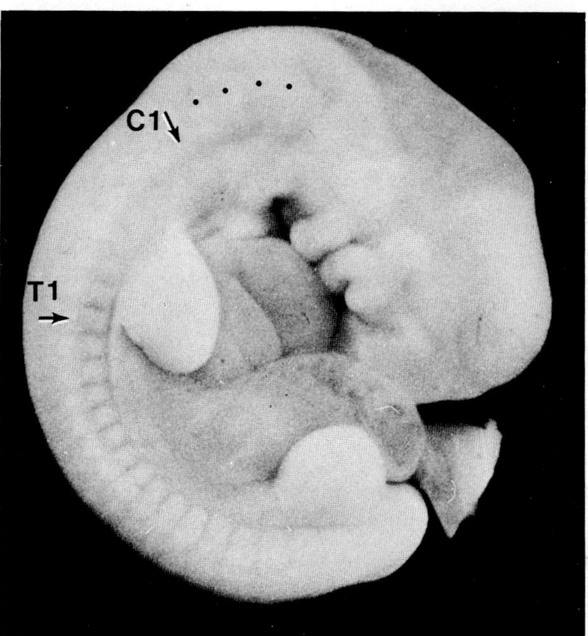

Fig. 1-4. A 5.5-mm human embryo showing the external manifestations of the somites. Note that the relationship of the cervical somites to the limb bud presages the nerves to be involved in the brachial plexus. The black dots rostral to the cervical somites indicate the position of the precervical somites that will form the basiocciput.

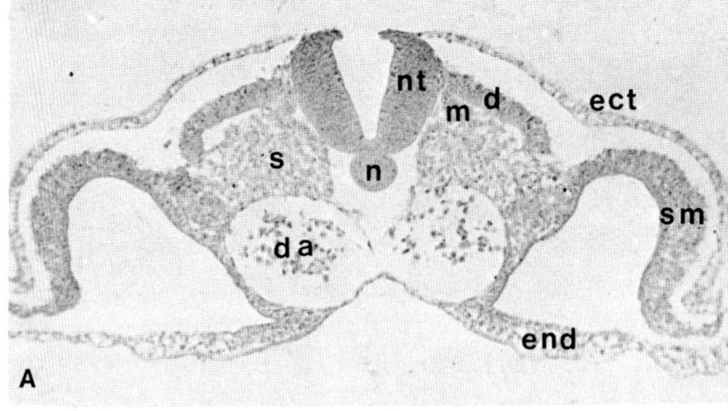

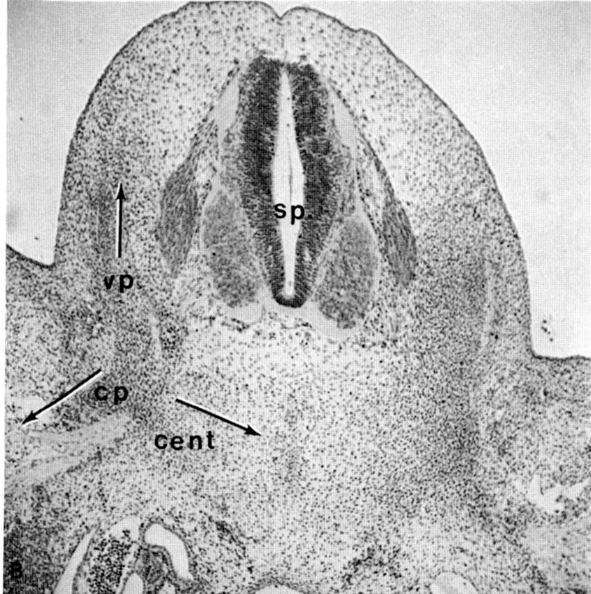

Fig. 1-5. (*A*) Thoracic somite cross section from a 20-somite chick embryo. The neural tube (*nt*) lies dorsal to the nonsegmental notochord, and the somite shows its differentiation into the dermatome (*d*), myotome (*m*), and sclerotome (*s*). The endoderm (*end*) and ectoderm (*ect*) enclose the somatic mesoderm (*sm*) in the lateral region. (*B*) Further development of the sclerotome into vertebral anlagen is indicated in the cross section of the mesenchymal (membranous) vertebra in a 9-mm pig embryo. The sclerotomal cell migration to preform the vertebra is indicated by a dorsal mass to form the vertebral process (*vp*), a ventral mass to form the centrum (*cent*) and a lateral mass to form the costal process (*cp*).

arches and costal processes soon merge, and chondrification proceeds up and down the arches to replace the mesenchymal tissue completely. The process of chondrification extends down the arches from these centers into the substance of the vertebral body, and by the end of the eighth week the cartilaginous arches have fused with the body (Figs. 1-5*B*, 1-6, and 1-7).

The occiput, atlas, and axis develop along slightly different lines. The first four somites in the embryo fuse to form the basiocciput into which the notochord extends rostrally to terminate at the fossa hypophysialis. The caudal portion of the fourth occipital somite fuses to the cranial portion of C1 to form the terminal portion of the basiocciput. The intervertebral disc at this level is represented by the apical and alar ligaments of the dens and the apical portion of the dens. The proatlas is a separate bony structure in some species, but in humans it appears to be represented only by the apical ossific nucleus of the odontoid process.

The vertebral body of C1 does not form a distinct centrum. The fusion of the caudal part of the C1 somite and the cranial part of the C2 somite forms the odontoid process, and the resultant mass of cells is incorporated into the vertebral body of C2. A dense band of tissue called the hypochordal bow extends ventrally around the vertebrae and at the C1 level gives rise to the anterior arch of the atlas. The hypochordal bow develops at each subsequent level but is much less pronounced cau-

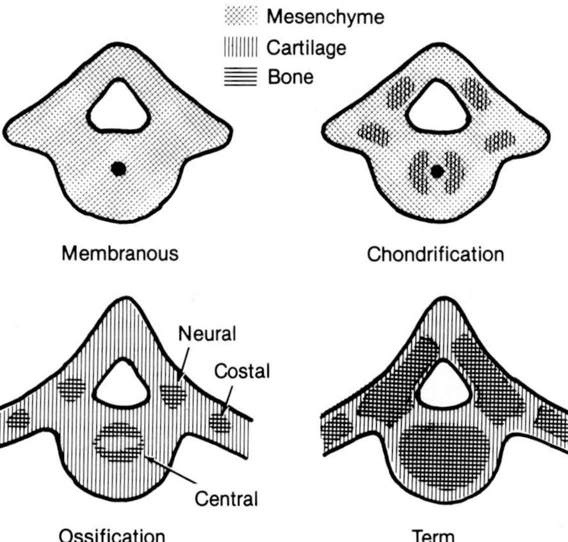

Fig. 1-6. A schema of the sequential changes in the development of a vertebral element. Note that the basic form of the vertebra preexists in two distinct types of tissue, that is, membranous mesenchyme and cartilage, before the definitive ossification from the indicated centers.

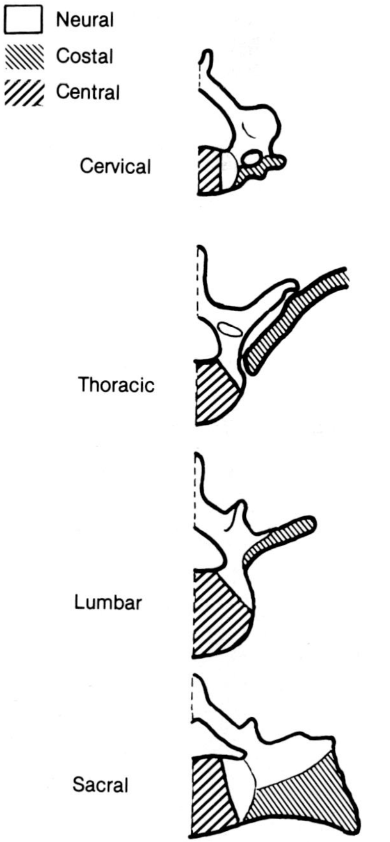

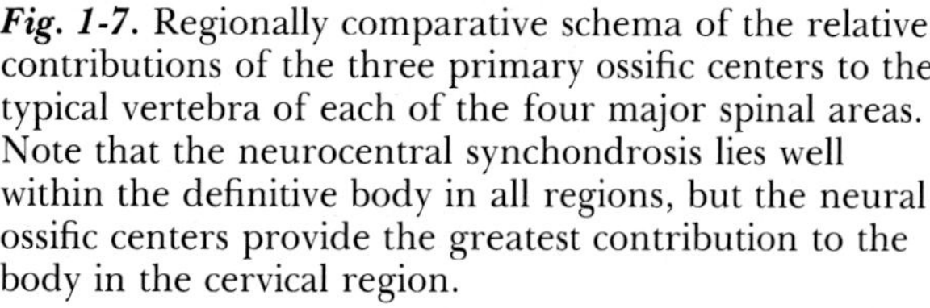
Fig. 1-7. Regionally comparative schema of the relative contributions of the three primary ossific centers to the typical vertebra of each of the four major spinal areas. Note that the neurocentral synchondrosis lies well within the definitive body in all regions, but the neural ossific centers provide the greatest contribution to the body in the cervical region.

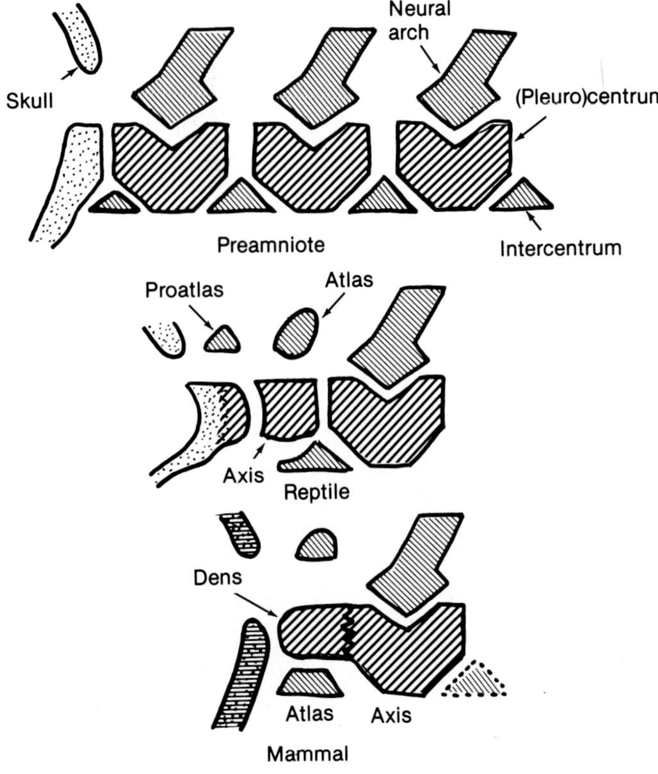

Fig. 1-8. Schematized concept of the evolution of the atlas–axis complex. The progressive reduction of the number of elements illustrated indicates that several segments eventually became incorporated in the skull, while the most cranial of the definitive cervical elements formed the craniocervical articulations. The intercentrum (hypochordal bar) is regarded as the antecedent of the anterior arch of the atlas, and the proatlas may become represented by the apical secondary center of ossification for the dens.

dally. It gives rise to the thick portion of the anterior longitudinal ligament, which overlies the anterior aspect of each vertebral body. The hypochordal bow is the analogue of the holocentrous vertebra in more primitive species, a structure that gives rise to a ventral hemal arch that covers and contains the aorta and vena cava in certain reptilian and amphibian species. The dorsal or neural arch containing the spinal cord persists in mammals, of course, and some mammals even manifest an accessory or intercentrous vertebra at each level. In humans, the anterior arch of the atlas is the only remnant of this phylogenetic progression (Fig. 1-8).

The process of ossification begins in the vertebrae from three ossific nuclei, one in the vertebral body and one in each neural arch. Ossific nuclei develop in the upper cervical spine at or about the second month of intrauterine life and gradually increase in size during later fetal life. The three primary ossific nuclei increase in size and occupy an increasing percentage of the substance of a vertebra. Where the ossific nuclei of the vertebral arches join the ossific nuclei of the vertebral body, a synchondrosis develops called the neurocentral joint. Thus, at birth, a typical lower cervical vertebra consists of three ossific components: a centrum and two neural arches that have not yet fused together posteriorly. In addition, the vertebral arches have not fused to the vertebral body itself. During the fetal period, the atlas ossifies from two centers in the upper cervical spine, one in each

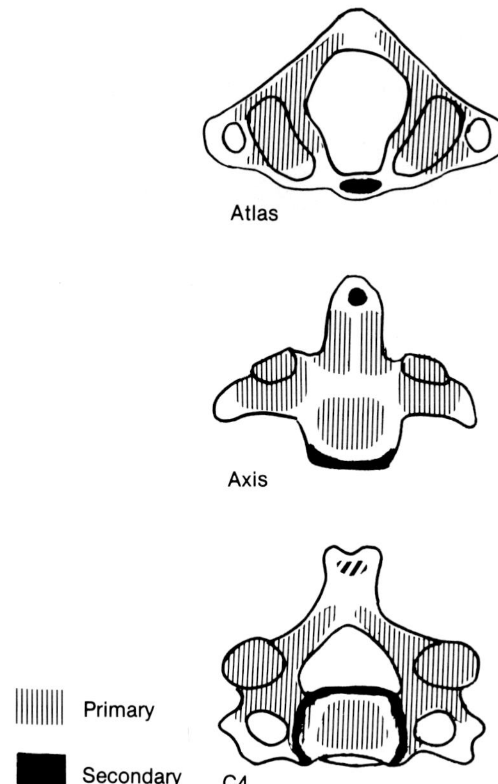

Fig. 1-9. Schematic representation of the ossification centers in the cervical vertebrae. The first two cervical vertebrae have atypical numbers of ossific centers. The atlas has but two primaries that correspond to the neural arch centers of the conventional elements. The secondary center that forms in the anterior arch is considered the phyletic remnant of the hypochordal bar (intercentrum) of lower vertebrates. The axis has five primary and two secondary centers. The dens ossifies from bilobed centers representing the original central center of C1. The apical secondary center may be a developmental representation of the original proatlas. The inferior secondary center of the axis forms the ring apophysis as in other vertebrae. The typical cervical vertebra as represented here by C4 arises from the conventional three primary and two secondary centers for the ring apophyses. A secondary center for the tip of the spinous process (*crosshatched*), although constant in more inferior elements, only appears sporadically in cervical vertebra, being more frequent in the lower (C6, C7) elements.

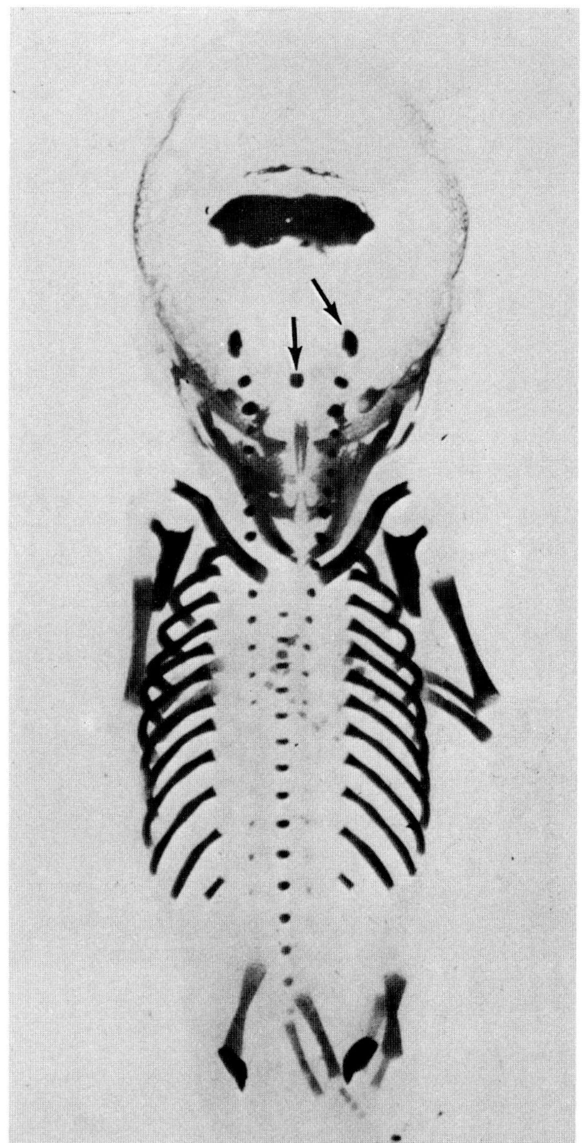

Fig. 1-10. A cleared alizarin-stained fetus of 54 mm (CRL). Differential commencement of ossification in various spinal regions is apparent. Note that the center for the centrum is first to appear in the lower thoracic and lumbar regions, whereas the two neural arch centers appear first in the cervical region. The arrows indicate the ossification centers for the occipital bone. The lateral two form the exoccipital contributions and the central one gives rise to the basioccipital center.

lateral mass. The axis ossifies from five nuclei early in fetal life. The odontoid process has paired ossific nuclei that fuse across the midline to become a single ossific structure at about the time of birth. The centrum of the vertebral body of the axis and the ossific nuclei of the neural arches of C2 develop in a manner similar to that described for the third through the seventh vertebrae (Figs. 1-9 and 1-10).

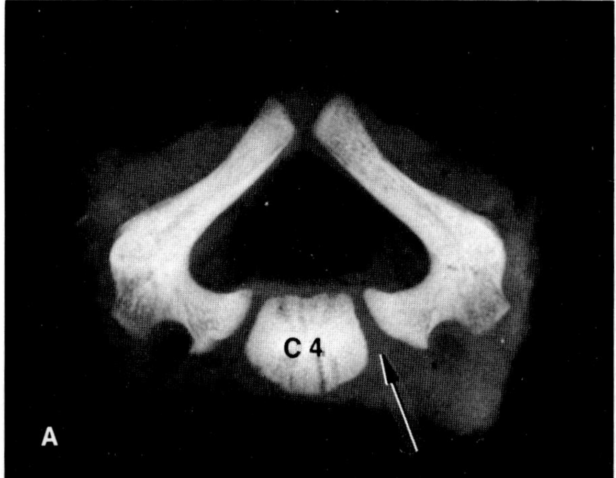

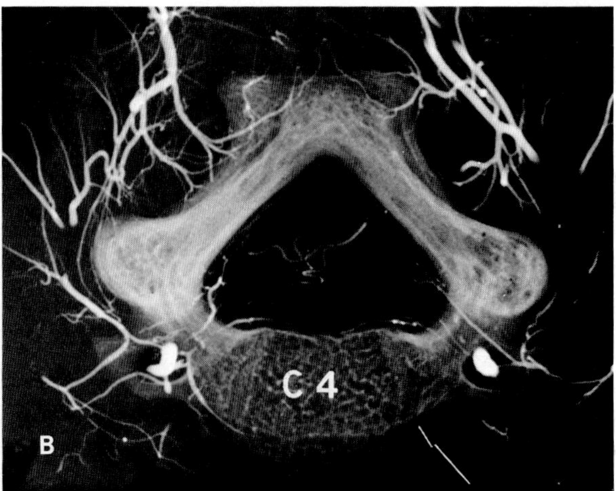

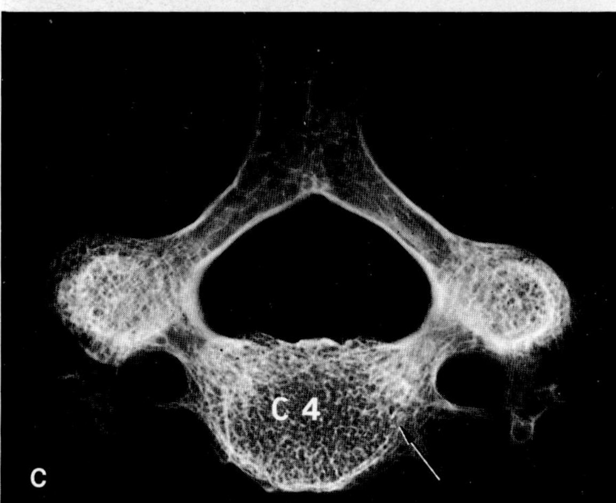

Fig. 1-11. Progressive ossification of cervical vertebrae as typified by C4. (*A*) The extent of ossification in a fetus of 34 weeks. Note that the costal contribution shows no evidence of ossification. The neurocentral synchondrosis is more medially situated in cervical vertebrae (*arrow*), allowing a greater contribution to the centrum from the neural arch than is found in more inferior segments. (*B*) A radiograph of C4 from a 6-year-old cadaver that had been arterially injected with barium sulfate. Note that the neurocentral synchondroses are still radiologically demonstrable (*arrow*) and the ossification of the costal contribution has completed the anterior part of the vertebral foramen. (*C*) A vertical radiograph of C4 from an adult. The arrow indicates the original position of the neurocentral synchondrosis that is no longer radiologically discernible. The definitive tuberosities of the spine have formed, and the anterior and posterior tuberosities of the transverse processes are fully ossified. Although these tuberosities may be from secondary centers in the thoracolumbar region, only an occasional secondary center appears in the tuberosity of the spine in cervical vertebrae.

INFANCY, EARLY CHILDHOOD, AND ADOLESCENCE

From the time a person is born until he reaches adult life, the vertebrae continue to ossify from the cartilaginous models that formed in the mesenchymal anlage. In the case of the first vertebra, the lateral masses have ossified at the time of birth, and ossification proceeds posteriorly into the posterior arches, usually completing the closure of the atlantal ring by the third year of life. An ossific nucleus also develops in the anterior arch at about 1 year of age, and this nucleus fuses with the lateral masses by 6 to 9 years of age.

The odontoid process develops an apical epiphysis when a child reaches the age of 2 years, and this fuses with the main portion of the odontoid by the 12th year. The odontoid itself begins to fuse with the ossific nucleus of the C2 vertebral body at the age of 4 years. The fusion begins circumferentially and is almost always complete by the age of 7 years. Almost one third of normal adults, however, have a remnant of cartilaginous tissue between the odontoid and the C2 vertebral body.

The second through seventh cervical vertebrae have similar patterns of ossification of the vertebral bodies and arches. The arch ossific nucleus at each level spreads from its point of origin at the base of the transverse process dorsally into the arch and ventrally into the pedicle. The arch ossific nucleus also extends down into the substance of the dorsolateral aspect of the vertebral body, and therefore, the neurocentral joint lies well within the vertebral body. A goodly portion of the vertebral body thus derives from the ossific nucleus of the arch on each side.

The secondary ossific nuclei usually appear by late childhood. These develop as a ring about the margins of the vertebral bodies and consist of hard cortical bone when they have formed completely. The secondary ring ossification centers fuse to the primary centers at about 15 to 16 years of age. The central portion of the cartilaginous end-plate remains unossified and is considered one of the components of the intervertebral disc.

Secondary centers also form at the tips of the spinous and transverse processes at early adolescence. These fuse to the underlying ossific nuclei at the end of the vertebral growth. Occasionally, the ventral part of the transverse process of the seventh cervical vertebra ossifies from a separate ossific nucleus, which manifests itself in the sixth month of fetal life and which fuses to the rest of the arch at about 5 years of age (Fig. 1-11).

ADULT PHASE

Histologic examination of developing cervical vertebrae in childhood and adolescence reveals an abrupt interface between bone and cartilage. The ossification fronts between the primary vertebral epiphyses and the cartilaginous end-plates, and the secondary ring epiphyses show little evidence of columnization. As a result, the cervical spine has limited longitudinal growth potential.

In the developing and immature cervical spine, the cartilaginous end-plate and the annular tissue of the intervertebral disc have less obvious and abrupt interfaces. The cartilaginous and ligamentous tissues merge into each other more gradually, and the junction between discal tissue and cartilaginous end-plate has considerably more mechanical strength than the junction of vertebral ossific nucleus and end-plate. Indeed, traumatic separations occur at the latter site, rather than at the former. In addition, capillaries, venioles, and arterioles make their way into the cartilaginous end-plate and secondary ring epiphysis as ossification advances, but the intervertebral disc consisting of cartilaginous end-plate, annulus, and nucleus pulposus remains avascular (Fig. 1-12).

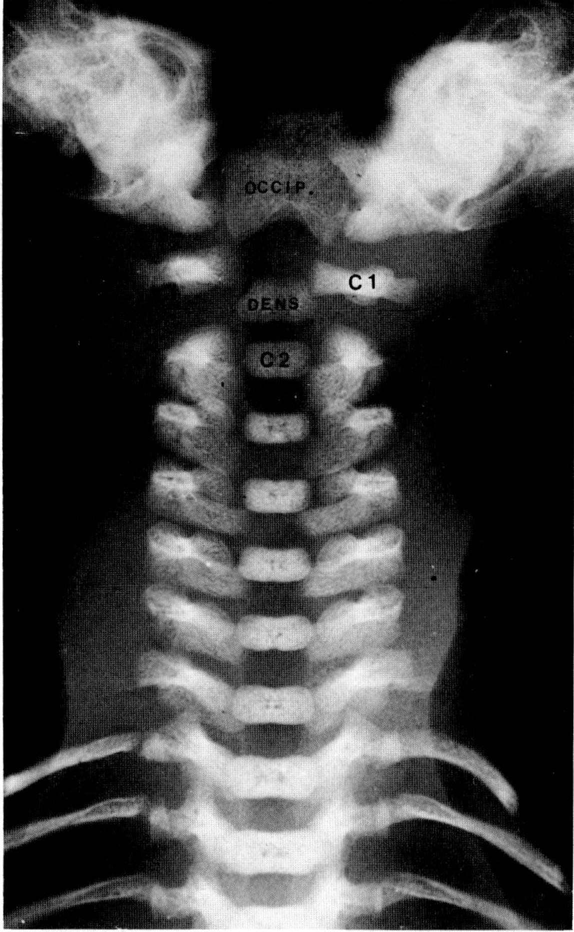

Fig. 1-12. A–P radiograph of a 30-week fetal cervical spine. The bilobed centers of ossification positioned above the central ossification of C2 constitute the dens. The intervening cartilage is the homologue of the first intervertebral disc, and its ossific replacement is frequently deficient in adults. No secondary centers are yet apparent, so the apex of the dens and the arches of the atlas are only represented in cartilage.

Histologic examination of the lateral and posterior margins of the intervertebral discs, however, even in very young subjects, reveals that loose fibrous and vascular tissue occupies the space between the uncus projecting upward from the superior surface of the caudal vertebra and the echancrure of the inferior surface of the more rostral vertebra. In children, this area begins to show fissuring, and as a person matures into adult life, the fissuring occupies a greater proportion of the intervertebral space. The cleft that develops in adults in this location, the joint of Luschka, has some of the characteristics of a synovial joint (a joint space containing synovial fluid between two bony surfaces and a fibrous and vascular matrix surrounding the joint space). At one time a con-

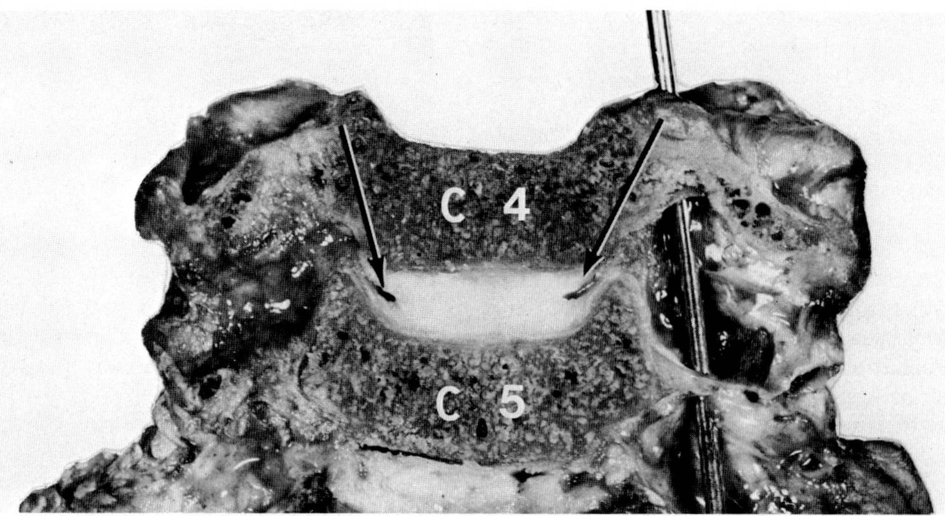

Fig. 1-13. Frontal section of a C4 disc with arrows indicating the uncovertebral "joints." These do not appear until the latter part of the first decade and are not uniform with regard to the level or side of their occurrence.

troversy evolved concerning the nature of this joint of Luschka: Was it a true joint or did it reflect adaptive changes only? It now appears that the cleft in the lateral margin of the cervical intervertebral discs develops normally in the process of maturation. The clefting, in fact, proceeds with continued alteration in the chemistry of the proteoglycans of the disc; as a result, most normal people have extensive fissuring in the disc spaces. With continued aging, these changes grow more evident. Accelerated by injury or disease, they may produce structural changes (Fig. 1-13).

REFERENCES

1. *CAVE AJE:* The morphologic constitution of the odontoid process. J Anat 72:621, 1938
2. *JENKINS FA:* The evolution and development of the dens of the mammalian axis. Anat Rec 164:173–184, 1969
3. *O'RAHILLY R, MÜLLER F, MEYER DB:* The human vertebral column at the end of the embryonic period proper: 2. The occipitocervical region. J Anat 136:181–195, 1983
4. *PRESLEY R, HALLAM LA:* A pro-atlas arch in mammals. J Anat 131:209, 1980

cular contents of the cervical spine, and (5) the related structures in the neck.

Normal Adult Anatomy

WESLEY W. PARKE AND HENRY H. SHERK

In this section we shall review the gross anatomy of the cervical spine as a basis for the broader discussion of diseases and injuries of the cervical spine in the chapters to follow. The cervical spine is a complex and vital region, and many critically important structures are in close proximity in a small area. Complete familiarity with the entire region is essential for the physician and surgeon attempting to treat disorders of the cervical spine, and the responsibility for evaluating patients with problems in this region should not be undertaken without thorough knowledge of its unique anatomy.

The components of the cervical spine are reviewed here in the following order: (1) the osseous components, (2) the ligaments and intervertebral discs, (3) the musculature, (4) the neural and vascular contents of the cervical spine, and (5) the related structures in the neck.

OSSEOUS COMPONENTS

The cervical spine consists of the first seven vertebrae in the spinal column. The fifth through the seventh vertebrae are similar in size and configuration, whereas the atlas (the first cervical vertebra) and the axis (the second cervical vertebra) have quite different structures (Figs. 1-14 and 1-15).

A typical lower cervical vertebra (third through seventh) has a small vertebral body that is concave on its superior surface and lipped by a raised edge of bone on its margin (Fig. 1-16). It is correspondingly convex on its inferior surface, although the anteroinferior portion of the vertebral body tends to project downward over the anterosuperior surface of the vertebra below it (Figs. 1-17, 1-18, 1-19, and 1-20). The lateral projections of the transverse processes are image features of the cervical vertebrae. Projecting laterally from the bodies and roots of the pedicles on each side is a bar of bone, which is, in fact, the rudimentary rib or costal process. This osseous structure fuses later-

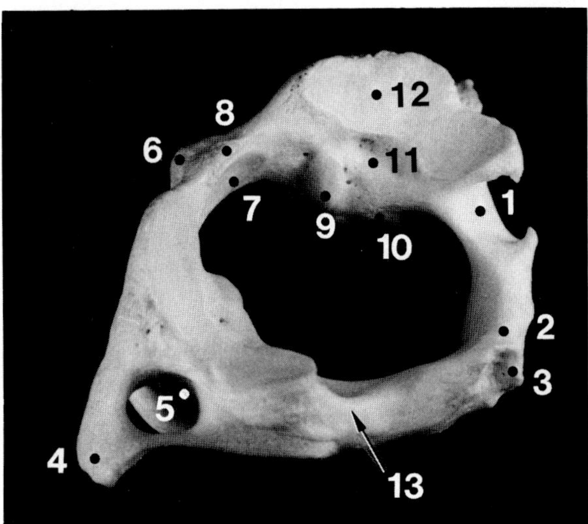

Fig. 1-14. The first cervical vertebra, or atlas. (*1*) Groove for vertebral artery. (*2*) Posterior arch of atlas. (*3*) Posterior tubercle. (*4*) Transverse process. (*5*) Transverse foramen. (*6*) Anterior tubercle. (*7*) Facet for dens. (*8*) Anterior arch of atlas. (*9*) Process for transverse ligament. (*10*) Inferior articular process. (*11*) Lateral mass. (*12*) Superior articular favea. (*13*) Strut of bone converting arterial groove into a foramen (occurs in 37% of cases).

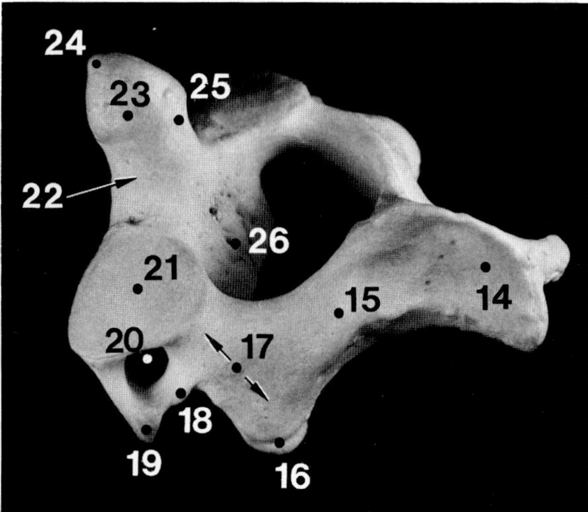

Fig. 1-15. The second cervical vertebra, or axis. (*15*) Lamina of neural arch. (*16*) Inferior articular process. (*17*) Pars interarticularis of neural arch. (*18*) Posterior tubercle of transverse process. (*19*) Anterior tubercle of transverse process. (*20*) Transverse foramen. (*21*) Articular facet of superior articular process. (22) Dens (neck area). (*23*) Attachment of alar ligament. (*24*) Apex (attachment of apical ligament). (*25*) Posterior articular surface of dens. (*26*) Vertebral body of axis.

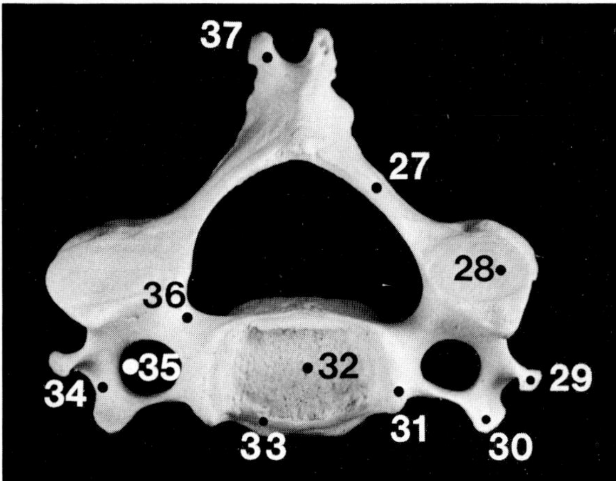

Fig. 1-16. Typical lower cervical vertebra. (*27*) Lamina of posterior arch. (*28*) Superior articular facet. (*29*) Posterior tubercle of transverse process (apex of transverse embryonic contribution to process). (*30*) Anterior tubercle of transverse process (apex of costal embryonic contribution to transverse process). (*31*) Uncinate process. (*32*) Vertebral body. (*33*) Annular epiphysis. (*34*) Spinal nerve sulcus (floored by costotransverse part of transverse process). (*35*) Transverse foramen. (*36*) Pedicle. (*37*) Bifid spinous process.

ally to the true transverse process through the costotransverse lamella. The rib element projects forward to end in the anterior tubercle of the transverse process, and the true transverse process projects slightly posteriorly to end in the posterior tubercle. The foramen transversarium (bounded by the rib element, true transverse process, costotransverse lamella, and vertebral body) transmits the vertebral artery, except at C7, where the foramen contains the accessory vertebral vein. The ventral ramus of each spinal nerve exits from the spinal column over the costotransverse lamella through a groove bounded posteriorly by the transverse process and posterior tubercle, and anteriorly by the vertebral artery and anterior tubercle. The groove is bounded by the vertebral body medially and by the facet joint and base of the lamina laterally. The floor and roof of the canal are made up of the superior and inferior pedicles, respectively.

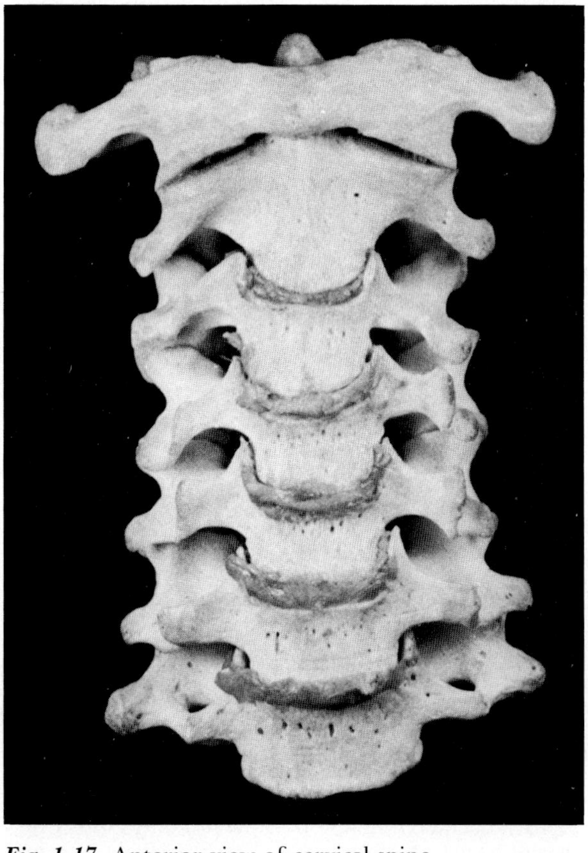

Fig. 1-17. Anterior view of cervical spine.

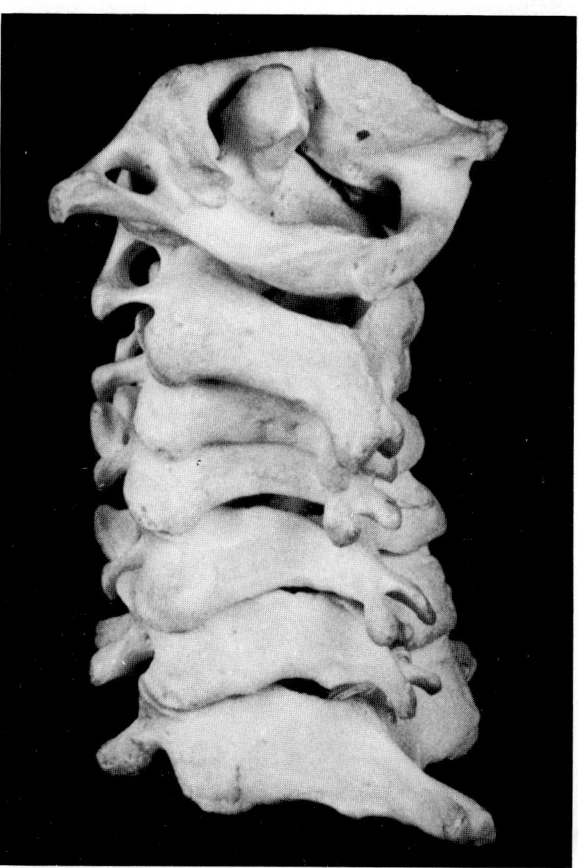

Fig. 1-18. Posterior lateral view of cervical spine in normal lordotic configuration.

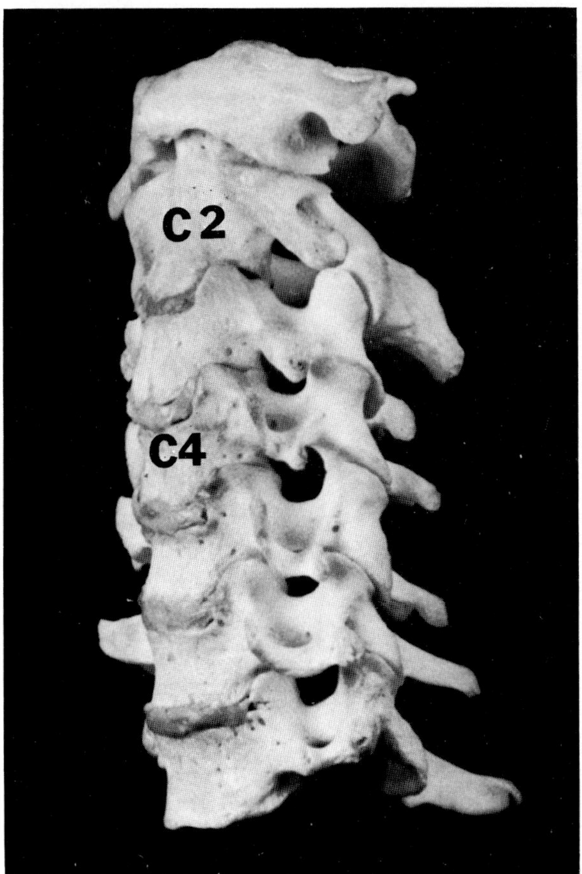

Fig. 1-19. Lateral oblique view of cervical spine showing anticular pillar collectively formed by anticular processes.

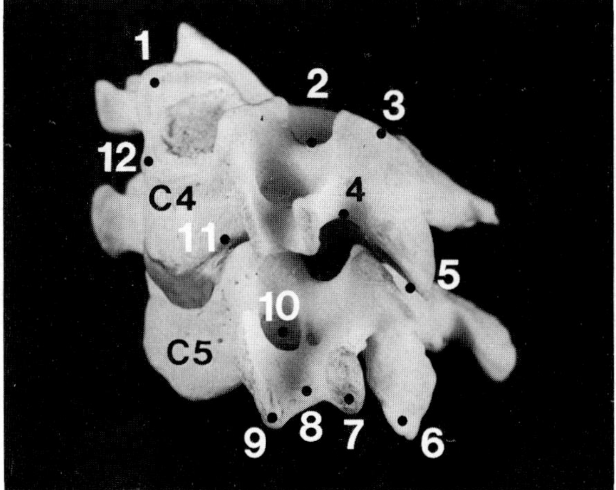

Fig. 1-20. Detailed superior oblique view of C4 and C5. (*1*) Uncinate process. (*2*) Superior intervertebral notch. (*3*) Superior articular process. (*4*) Inferior intervertebral notch. (*5*) Facet joint formed by opposing superior and inferior facets. (*6*) Inferior articular process. (*7*) Posterior tubercle of transverse process (C5). (*8*) Spinal nerve sulcus. (*9*) Anterior tubercle of transverse process. (*10*) Transverse foramen (note strut of bone that passed vein of periarterial venous plexus). (*11*) Echancrure (notch) of C4 that receives uncinate process of C5. (*12*) Annular epiphysis. Note discrepancy between width of neural sulcus of C4 and C5; the latter must accommodate the first root of the brachial plexus.

The spinous processes of the third, fourth, and fifth cervical vertebrae are usually bifid, whereas those of the sixth and seventh are longer and tapered at the ends. The large spinous process of C7 is called the vertebra prominens.

The axis vertebra is fused with the vertebral body of the first vertebra to form the odontoid process. The inferior surface of the axis vertebra resembles those of the vertebrae in the lower cervical spine. The laminae of C2 are heavy and strong, and the prominent spinous process is bifid.

The transverse process of the axis encloses a foramen transversarium for the vertebral artery but does not have the anterior tubercle derived from the costal element of the transverse process. The transverse process itself at C2 is thick and heavy, giving attachment to the longissimus cervicis, splenius cervicis, and other muscles.

The upper half of the axis vertebra has several distinctive features (Fig. 1-15). The superior articular facets are large and slightly convex, and face upward and outward to articulate with the inferior facets of the atlas vertebra. The axis extends upward into the odontoid process to reach the anterior lip of the foramen magnum. The odontoid process or dens originates somewhat below the shoulder of the axis and has a narrowed waist where it is compressed by the transverse ligament of the atlas. The dens widens out above this level and then tapers sharply to its apex.

The atlas is unique among vertebra in that it has no centrum, its vertebral body having been absorbed into the structure of the axis. The atlas, therefore, has a thick anterior arch that blends into the two bulky lateral masses (Fig. 1-14). On the superior aspect of the lateral masses are the kidney-shaped articulations for the occipital condyles. The occipital condyles face downward and outward while the superior atlantal joint facet faces upward and inward to support the occiput. The inferior atlantal facets are flatter and more circular than the superior facets and face downward and inward to transmit the weight of the skull onto the superior facet joints of the axis. The transverse processes of the atlas do not have a rib element and thus usually terminate in a single projection. The vertebral arteries continue upward from C2 through the foramen transversarium on each side and then loop posteriorly around the lateral masses to groove the bases of the rather thin posterior arches. The anatomy varies frequently: accessory foramina, incomplete atlantal arches, additional arches, and other malformations often manifest themselves.

An important anatomic feature of the atlas is the inward projection of a prominent tubercle of bone on each side. These structures give rise to the transverse ligament that keeps the odontoid process confined to the anterior third of the atlantal ring. This relationship permits free rotation of the atlas on the dens and C2, and provides for a stable configuration in flexion, extension, and lateral bending.

LIGAMENTS AND INTERVERTEBRAL DISCS

The skull and vertebrae are linked together by the ligaments and intervertebral discs to provide the neck with a stable yet flexible framework (Fig. 1-21). The lower cervical vertebrae from the caudal portion of the axis to T1 are similar in configuration. It is useful to consider the articulations of this part of the cervical spine in two parts: the articulations of the vertebral bodies and the articulations of the vertebral arches.

The anterior and posterior longitudinal ligaments extend over the entire length of the spine and act as the major stabilizers of the intervertebral joints. The anterior longitudinal ligament attaches to the anterior aspect of the axis vertebral body where it extends upward to merge into the anterior arch of the atlas and anterior atlantooccipital membrane. The anterior longitudinal ligament is closely attached to the intervertebral discs, but it is somewhat thicker over the concave part of the vertebral body from which it is slightly separated. The posterior longitudinal ligament is widest in the upper cervical spine and narrows caudally. Unlike the anterior longitudinal ligament, which has a ribbonlike structure, the posterior longitudinal ligament is waisted over the vertebral bodies and fans out over the intervertebral discs.

Each intervertebral disc has four components: the nucleus pulposus at the interior of the disc, the two cartilaginous end-plates on the facing vertebral surfaces, and the annulus fibrosus. The discs are contained more closely in the cervical spine than at other levels by the deeply concave structure of the superior surface of the caudal vertebra and the more convex inferior surface of the rostral vertebra. The upward projection on the superior

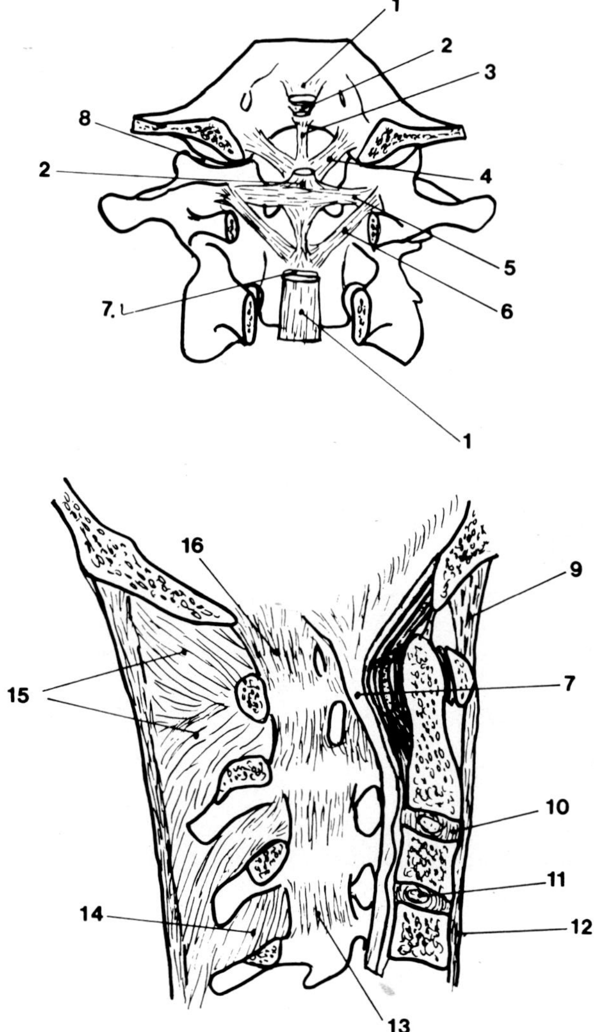

Fig. 1-21. Ligaments of the cervical spine. (*1*) Posterior longitudinal ligament. (*2*) Cruciform ligament (longitudinal band). (*3*) Apical ligament. (*4*) Alar ligament (check ligament). (*5*) Cruciform ligament (lateral band). (*6*) Accessory atlantoaxial ligament. (*7*) Tectorial membrane (anterior lamina of posterior longitudinal ligament). (*8*) Atlantooccipital joint. (*9*) Anterior atlantooccipital membrane. (*10*) Intervertebral disc (annulus). (*11*) Intervertebral disc (nucleus pulposus). (*12*) Anterior longitudinal ligament. (*13*) Ligamentum flavum. (*14*) Interspinal ligament. (*15*) Nuchal ligament. (*16*) Posterior atlantooccipital membrane.

surface of the caudal vertebra is called the uncus (or hook), and the edge of the rounded convex inferior surface on the more rostral vertebra is called the echancrure (or anvil). This area of contact between the cervical vertebra is closest and most obvious where the pedicle originates from the vertebral body. Early in life this area appears to have the same histologic appearance as the annulus fibrosus, but the degenerative and adaptive changes in this location lead to early fissuring in the annulus and the evolution of a false joint between the uncus and echancrure. These "uncovertebral joints" have also been referred to as the joints of Luschka since the publication of a monograph on their development by that author.

The articulations between the vertebral arches are maintained by (1) the supraspinous ligaments, which in the cervical spine have evolved into the ligamentum nuchae; (2) the interspinous ligaments; (3) the ligamentum flavum at each level; and (4) the synovial facet joints. In some quadrupeds, the ligamentum nuchae is an essential structure that maintains the head in an extended position; indeed, in some grazing animals, flexion of the neck requires voluntary action of the ventral musculature to pull the head downward against the resistance of the elastic ligamentum. This structure extends from the vertebra prominens to the external occipital protuberance in humans and, although considered rudimentary in comparison to its configuration in quadrupeds, it is probably a major stabilizer of the head and cervical spine. Its deeper fibers attach to the spinous process of each of the cervical vertebrae and reinforce the interspinous ligaments, which in the neck appear less developed than elsewhere in the spinal column. The ligamentum flavum in the cervical spine has considerable importance as a stabilizer in flexion because of its high content of elastic tissue. Flexion of the neck stretches and attenuates the ligamentum flavum, which, because of its high degree of elasticity, returns to its original configuration upon return of the neck to the neutral position. Thus, unless distal degeneration shortens the neck, the ligamentum flavum does not fold on itself to compress the dura in the neutral or extended position. The ligamentum flavum attaches to the anterior surface of the vertebral arch above and to the superior margin of the lamina of the vertebra below. There are two of these ligaments at each level, a right and a left, and they are separated by a small fissure. They merge with the interspinous ligaments posteriorly and with the fibrous capsule of the synovial facet joints anteriorly.

The facet joints in the lower cervical spine are diarthrodial joints with typical synovial membranes and fibrous capsules. The joints are distinctive in that the facets are more oblique than in the thoracic and lumbar spine, and the joint capsules are more lax than at other levels to permit gliding motion.

The articulation of the occiput, atlas, and axis differs considerably from that of the joints of the lower cervical spine and must be considered separately. The anterior longitudinal ligament extends upward to attach to the anterior arch of the atlas and onto the occipital membrane, and thence to the basiocciput anterior to the foramen magnum. The posterior longitudinal ligament extends upward to become the tectorial membrane. The tectorial membrane lies over the body of the axis and the odontoid and merges into the basiocciput at the level of the hypoglossal canals inside the skull.

Beneath the tectorial membrane lies the crural ligament. The most important component of this structure is the transverse ligament that extends across the ring of the atlas to enclose the odontoid process. The inferior and superior longitudinal bundles extend from the transverse ligament down to the body of the axis and up to the basiocciput, respectively. The accessory atlantoaxial ligaments extend from the bases of the lateral masses of the atlas to merge into the base of the dens and the body of the axis. These ligaments may be significant because of arteries they support, that is, branches of vertebral artery that provide the dens with a portion of its blood supply.

At the apex of the dens is the small apical ligament that attaches to the anterior rim of the foramen magnum. It is flanked by the two alar ligaments, which pass out to the lateral margin of the foramen magnum.

The joints between the dens and atlas, between the occipital condyles and atlas, and between the atlas and axis are synovial joints. The pivot joint between the odontoid process and the atlas and axis usually contains two small synovial cavities, one anteriorly between the anterior arch and the dens and the other between the dens and the transverse ligament.

MUSCULATURE OF THE NECK AND CERVICAL SPINE

Motion of the head and neck occurs by means of an extremely complex interaction between muscle groups working on the rigid osseous framework supported by the ligamentous system described previously (Figs. 1-22, 1-23, 1-24, and 1-25). It is

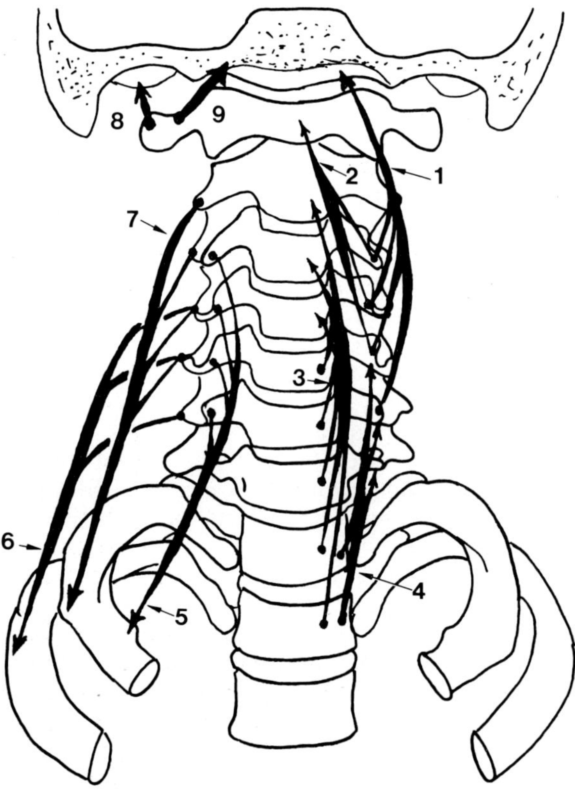

Fig. 1-22. Schema of the anterior muscles of cervical spine. (*1*) Longus capitis. (*2*) Longus colli (superior oblique part). (*3*) Longus colli (vertical part). (*4*) Longus colli (inferior oblique part). (*5*) Anterior scalene. (*6*) Posterior scalene. (*7*) Middle scalene. (*8*) Rectus capitis lateralis. (*9*) Rectus capitis medialis.

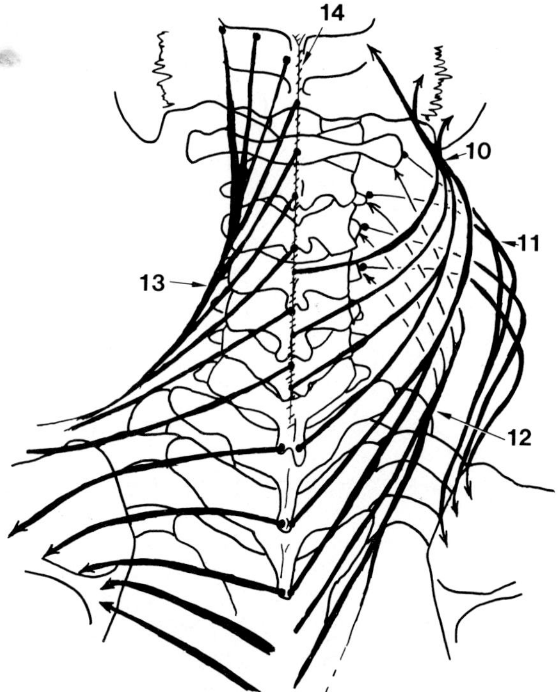

Fig. 1-23. Schema of the superficial muscles of posterior cervical region. (*10*) Splenius capitis. (*11*) Levator scapulae. (*12*) Splenius cervicis. (*13*) Trapezius (cervical part).

convenient to consider the muscles, therefore, in terms of the movements they produce and the ways in which their anatomic arrangement and structure accomplish this movement. The muscles involved in producing tension, flexion, rotation, and lateral bending of the neck and head are as follows.

EXTENSION

Splenius capitis
Splenius cervicis
Semispinalis capitis
Semispinalis cervicis
Longissimus capitis
Longissimus cervicis
Trapezius
Interspinalis
Rectus capitis posterior major
Rectus capitis posterior minor
Obliquus capitis superior
Sternocleidomastoid (posterior fibers)

FLEXION

Sternocleidomastoid (anterior fibers)
Longus colli
Longus capitis
Rectus capitis anterior

ROTATION AND LATERAL FLEXION

Sternocleidomastoid
Scalene group
Splenius capitis
Splenius cervicis
Longissimus capitis
Levator scapulae
Longus colli
Iliocostalis cervicis
Multifidi
Intertransversarii
Obliquus capitis inferior
Obliquus capitis superior
Rectus capitis lateralis

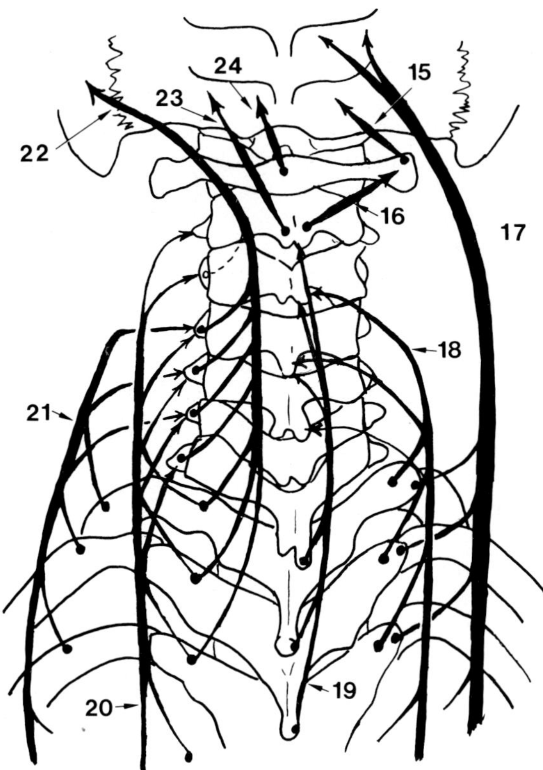

Fig. 1-24. Schema of the deeper spinal musculature of the cervical region. (*15*) Superior oblique muscle. (*16*) Inferior oblique muscle. (*17*) Semispinalis capitis. (*18*) Semispinalis cervicis. (*19*) Spinalis cervicis. (*20*) Longissimus cervicis. (*21*) Iliocostalis cervicis. (*22*) Longissimus capitis. (*23*) Rectus capitis posterior major. (*24*) Rectus capitis posterior minor.

Anatomically, these muscles can also be grouped according to their positional relationship to the spine, such as postvertebral, prevertebral, and lateral muscles of the neck.

The most superficial muscle of the postvertebral group is the trapezius, which originates on the medial part of the superior nuchal line and inserts on the spine of the scapula. Along with the levator scapulae, the trapezius extends the head when the upper limb and shoulder girdle remain fixed. It is innervated by the 11th cranial nerve. Most of the rest of the postvertebral muscles are innervated segmentally by the dorsal rami of the spinal nerves. Beneath the trapezius lies the splenius capitis and splenius cervicis, which take their origin from the spinous process of the lower cervical and upper thoracic spines. They insert on the transverse processes of the upper cervical spine and, in the case of the splenius capitis, on the mastoid process beneath the insertion of the sternocleidomastoid muscle.

Beneath the splenius lie the continuations of the erector spinal muscle into the cervical region: laterally on each side the iliocostalis cervicis, centrally the longissimus cervicis and longissimus capitis, and medially on each side the spinalis and semispinalis groups. The iliocostalis extends from the angles of the upper six ribs to the posterior tubercles of the transverse processes of the lower cervical vertebrae. The longissimus group extends from the transverse process of the upper thoracic vertebrae to the posterior tubercles of the transverse processes of the lower cervical vertebrae and thence up to the mastoid process as the longissimus capitis. The spinalis muscle in the neck is often not present but is replaced by the semispinalis groups

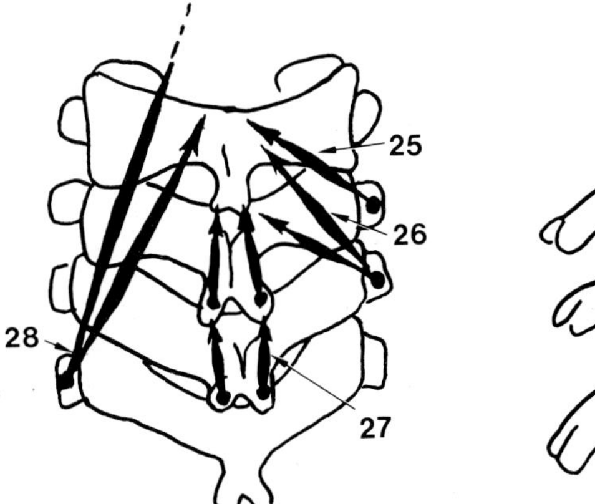

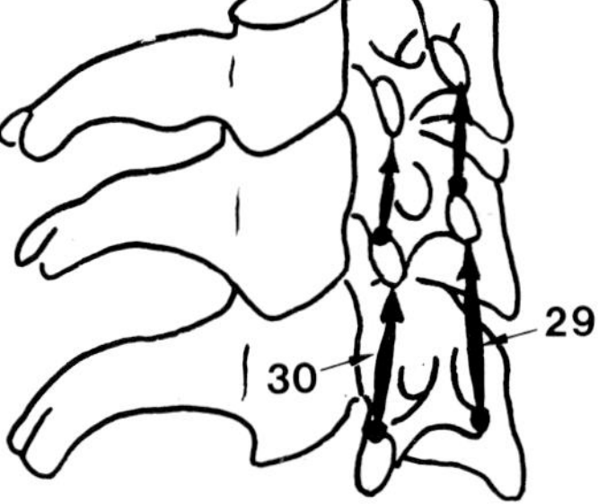

Fig. 1-25. Schema of the short muscles of the cervical spine. (*25*) Short rotator. (*26*) Long rotator. (*27*) Interspinales. (*28*) Multifidus. (*29*) Anterior intertransversarii. (*30*) Posterior intertransversarii.

of muscles that originate from tendinous slips arising on the posterior tubercles of the transverse processes of the upper thoracic and lower cervical vertebrae. These muscles insert into the spinous processes of the lower cervical spine and, in the case of the semispinalis capitis, into the area between the superior and inferior nuchal line of the occiput.

Beneath the semispinalis muscles lie the multifidi in the lower cervical spine. These extend from the transverse processes to the spinalis processes, crossing only one spinal segment. In the upper cervical spine, the deepest muscle layer consists of the rectus capitis posterior major and minor and the obliquus capitis inferior and superior. These muscles connect the spinous processes of the atlas and axis with the base of the skull, the spinous process of the axis with the transverse process of the atlas, and the transverse process of the atlas with the base of the skull. Their familiar configuration and relationship form the suboccipital triangle in which can be seen the vertebral artery, the dorsal ramus of the first cervical nerve, and the suboccipital plexus of veins.

The prevertebral muscles of the neck are the longus colli and longus capitis. The longus colli extends from C1 to T3 or T4, spanning the lateral portions of the vertebral bodies and having lateral attachment to the anterior tubercles of the lateral masses of C3, C4, C5, and C6. The longus capitis arises on the anterior tubercles of C3 through C6 and extends upward to the basiocciput; it is reinforced by the rectus capitis anterior and the rectus capitis lateralis.

The lateral muscles of the neck include, for purposes of this discussion, the sternocleidomastoid, the scalenes, and the levator scapulae. The first of these, the sternocleidomastoid, overlies the whole lateral and anterior aspect of the neck, covering the anterior and posterior tubercles of the transverse processes of C2 to C7. The attachment of the scalene muscles to the first and second ribs anterior to the vertebrae makes these muscles flexors when they act together and lateral benders or rotators when they act separately. They and the longus colli and capitis groups are innervated, apparently segmentally, by the ventral rami.

The levator scapulae is overlaid by the sternocleidomastoid in its upper third and by the trapezius in its lower third. It arises from the posterior tubercles of the upper three or four vertebrae and descends to the medial margin of the scapula.

The anterior muscles of the neck (*i.e.,* the hyoid muscles, the digastric muscles, the laryngeal muscles, and others) are not as related to the support and control of the cervical spine as are those already described. Some control of flexion may be maintained by the strap muscles anteriorly, but their primary function relates to positioning of the larynx and mandible, and they therefore are considered related structures.

The muscles of the neck are layered and almost interwoven in such a way that they have supporting and complementary actions. This is most apparent posteriorly where, for example, the vertically aligned trapezius overlies the splenius capitis, which is oblique from medially below to laterally above. The splenius in turn overlies the semispinalis cervicis, which is oblique from laterally below to medially above.

The muscles of the neck are also arranged in triangles, and many of the muscular components described as well as the important related structures can be located within their boundaries. The posterior triangle, formed by the sternocleidomastoid, clavicle, and trapezius muscles, has the semispinalis capitis, lavator scapulae, splenius capitis, scalenus medius, and scalenus anterior in the floor of its confines. Running obliquely across the floor of the posterior triangle is the omohyoid muscle, which subdivides it into the supraclavicular triangle and the occipital triangle. The anterior triangle is bounded by the midline of the neck anteriorly, the lower border of the mandible, and the anterior border of the sternocleidomastoid muscle. It is also subdivided by the submental triangle, the muscular triangle, the digastric triangle, and the carotid triangle. The carotid triangle bounded by the anterior border of the sternocleidomastoid, posterior belly of the digastric muscle, and the superior belly of the omohyoid contains the carotid sheath. It is an important landmark for surgeons making an anterior approach to the cervical spine.

NEURAL AND VASCULAR CONTENTS

The cervical portion of the spinal cord, of course, is the vital structure contained within the canal of the cervical spine. Running parallel with it on each side of the spinal column are the vertebral arteries that provide the cervical cord and the brain stem with their blood supply (Figs. 1-26, 1-27, 1-28, and 1-29).

The dura mater surrounding the cord is firmly attached to the rim of the foramen magnum. Within the cranium, the dura merges with the periosteum of the inside of the skull, but in the spinal cord it is separated from the vertebral arches and

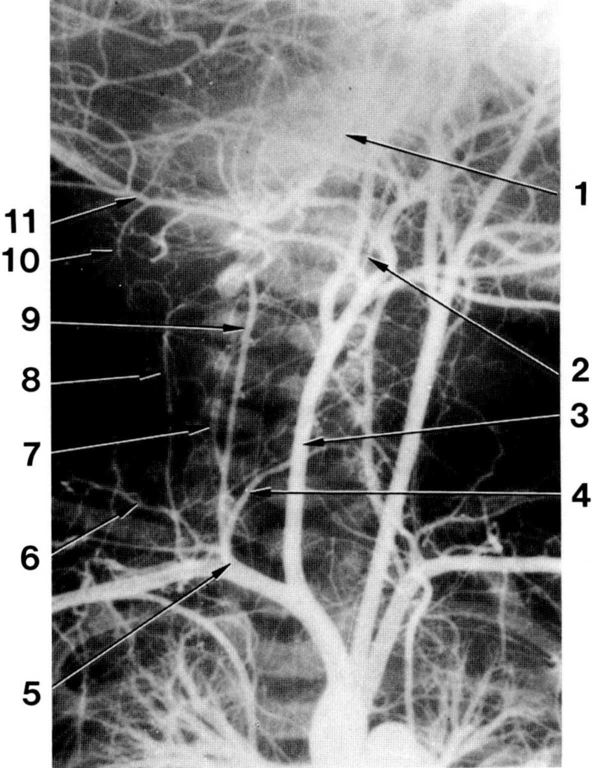

Fig. 1-26. Cervical arterial vasculature (30-week fetus); oblique view. (*1*) Basilar artery. (*2*) Ascending pharyngeal artery. (3) Right common carotid artery. (*4*) Inferior thyroid artery. (*5*) Subclavian origins of thyrocervical and costocervical trunks superimposed. (*6*) Transverse cervical artery. (7) Deep cervical artery. (*8*) Posterior cervical artery. (*9*) Right vertebral artery. (*10*) Descending branch of occipital artery. (*11*) Occipital artery.

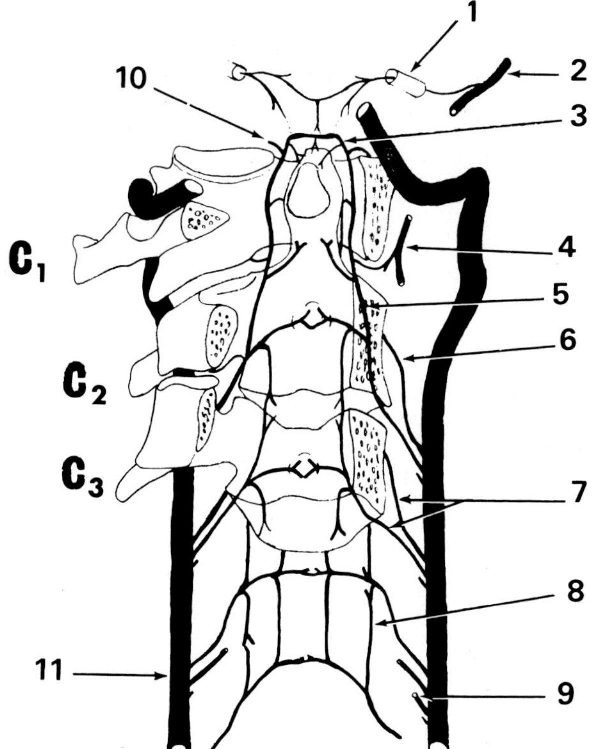

Fig. 1-27. Schema of arterial supply of upper cervical vertebrae. (*1*) Hypoglossal canal passing meningeal artery. (*2*) Occipital artery. (*3*) Apical arcade of odontoid process. (*4*) Ascending pharyngeal artery giving collateral branch beneath anterior arch of atlas. (*5*) Posterior ascending artery. (*6*) Anterior ascending artery. (*7*) Precentral and postcentral arteries to typical cervical vertebral body. (*8*) Anterior spinal plexus. (*9*) Medullary branch of vertebral artery. Radicular, prelaminary, and meningeal branches are also found at each level. (*10*) Collateral to ascending pharyngeal artery passing rostral to anterior arch of the atlas. (*11*) Left vertebral artery.

bodies by fat. The fatty protection is most pronounced dorsally. The arachnoid lines the dura, and the relatively wide subarachnoid space is filled with cerebral spinal fluid. The pia mater, closely attached to the spinal cord, laterally forms a linear fold that extends longitudinally the length of the spinal medulla. This fold gives rise to about 20 dentate ligaments on each side. These extend laterally between the ventral and dosal roots to attach to the dura and suspend the spinal medulla in the cerebral spinal fluid. Thus, the dentate ligament system further cushions and protects the cord in that it allows for considerable motion of the dura with relatively less motion of the spinal medulla.

The dorsal sensory rootlets enter the cord through the lateral longitudinal sulcus and the ventral motor rootlets exit the cord through the ventral lateral sulcus. The six or eight rootlets at each level leave the spinal medulla and are collected into a single bundle as they pass through the dura. Surrounded by the dura, they form a nerve root at each level. The nerve root is enlarged just outside the dura within the confines of the intervertebral foramina because of the spinal ganglion cells in the substance of the root. Distal to the intervertebral foramen, the root splits into the dorsal and ventral branches. In the cervical spine, of course, there are no white rami communicantes, but the gray rami from the sympathetic cervical

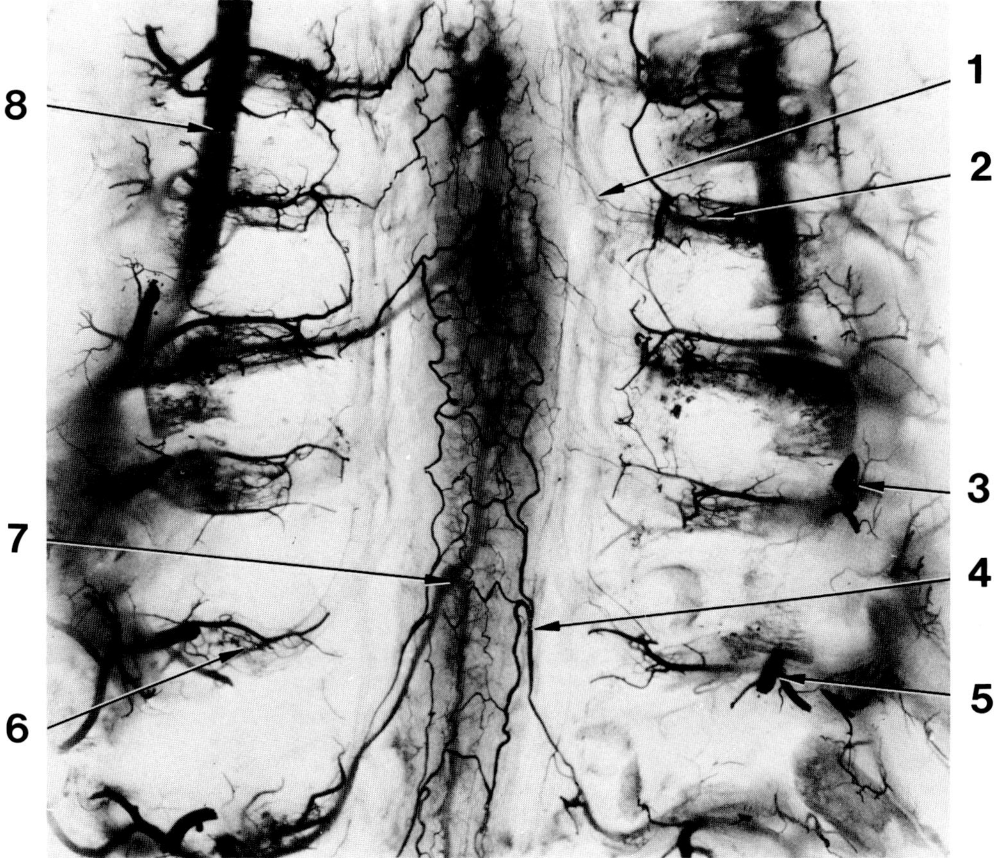

Fig. 1-28. Cleared and transilluminated dorsal aspect of the cervicothoracic section of the spinal cord from a fetus of 8 months' gestation after injection with latex and India ink. A dorsal medullary artery (*4*) can be seen supplying the left dorsolateral spinal artery, which, with its bilateral counterpart, runs an irregular and often interrupted course along the cord. An anterior medullary artery (*7*) can be seen supplying the single anterior spinal artery on the ventral aspect of the cord. A true radicular artery (*1*) supplies a dorsal ramus of the seventh cervical nerve and is derived from the plexus of the dorsal root ganglion (*2*). Segmental branches from the thyrocervical trunk (*3*) and costocervical trunk (*5*) are shown supplying the vasculature associated with the first and second thoracic nerves. A spinal branch of a second thoracic segmental artery (*6*) can be noted supplying meningeal and true radicular arteries by way of the dorsal root ganglion plexus of the left second thoracic nerve. The left vertebral artery (*8*) is shown supplying segmental branches to the sixth and seventh cervical nerves and the regionally associated structures. The caliber of the anterior medullary arteries and the anterior spinal artery are much greater than the dorsal counterparts because they supply approximately three fourths of the cord substance.

ganglion join the ventral primary divisions well outside the intervertebral foramina. The three sympathetic ganglia are usually in the connective tissue between the longus colli and longus capitis and the carotid sheath. The multiple branches of the cervical sympathetic chain include those ascending along the internal and external carotid arteries and those to the pharynx, cardiac plexus, and other areas, as well as those to the spinal nerves. The sympathetic chain is, therefore, not technically part of the spinal column but a related structure.

The nerve roots of the cervical spine pass almost directly laterally at each level to exit from the

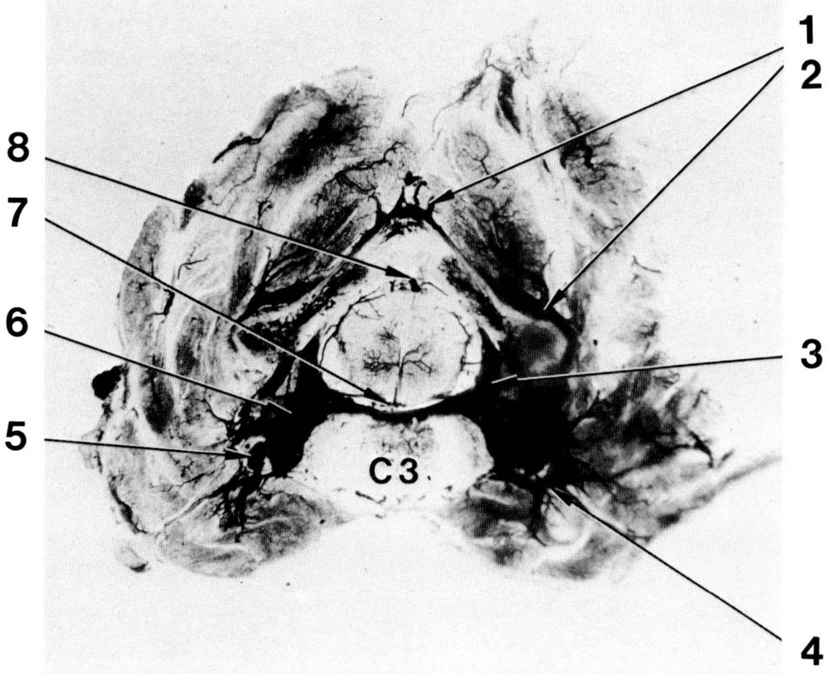

Fig. 1-29. Deep veins of the cervical spine. This cross section through C3 of a fetus injected with mixture of latex and India ink shows both veins and arteries. (*1 and 2*) External venous plexus of spine. (*3*) Epidural venous plexus. (*4*) Periarterial venous plexus of vertebral artery. (*5*) Vertebral artery. (*6*) Foraminal plexus forming major communication between external and internal (epidural) spinal plexuses. (*7*) Anterior spinal veins bracketing anterior spinal artery. (*8*) Dorsal spinal veins. Note arborization of the sulcal branches of the anterior spinal artery to supply most of the internal substance of cord. Also note venous communication running with the dentate ligament on the left side.

spinal canal at the same foraminal level from which the root originates from the cord. The horizontal direction of the cervical root is in contrast to the vertical passage of the lumbar roots caused by the ascent of the cord during growth.

The sinu-vertebral nerve originates from the dorsal root at each level and passes into each intervertebral foramina to supply sensation to the ligaments, meninges, and vascular structures within the spinal canal. It winds around the pedicle on each side and splits into ascending and descending branches to supply the structures noted with the various sensory modalities of position, pain, temperature, and so forth.

The familiar white and gray matter make up the internal structure of the spinal cord itself. The gray matter is centrally located and consists primarily of nerve cells; the white matter consists primarily of myelinated nerve fibers. The structure of the cervical cord varies at different levels and is markedly different overall from the structure of the thoracic and lumbar portions of the spinal cord.

The cervical cord enlarges at C3, expanding maximally to a 38-mm circumference at C6. It then tapers down into the third thoracic level. This enlargement is due to the increased nerve supply to the upper limbs and corresponds to the lumbar enlargement at the 12th thoracic level. The shape of the central gray matter differs from other levels in the spinal cord in that the dorsal horns are narrower than in the lumbar spine. The ventral horns are expanded; they are proportionally as large as the ventral horns at the lumbar levels and significantly larger than in the thoracic levels.

The white substance of the cervical cord has been divided into three columns or funiculi: dorsal, lateral, and ventral. The dorsal columns con-

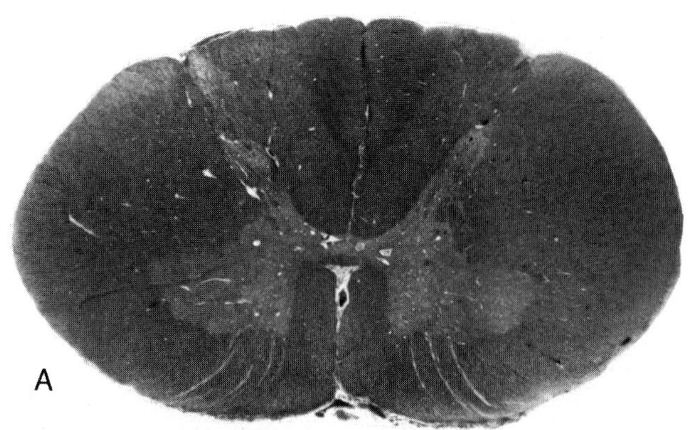
A

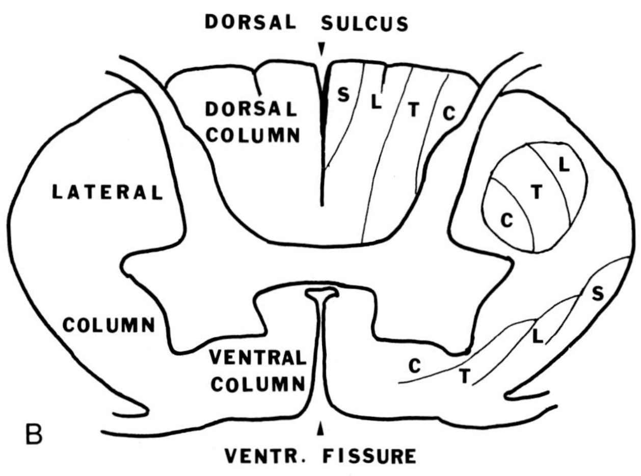
DORSAL SULCUS
DORSAL COLUMN
S
L
T
C
LATERAL
COLUMN
C
T
L
S
L
C
T
VENTRAL COLUMN
VENTR. FISSURE
B

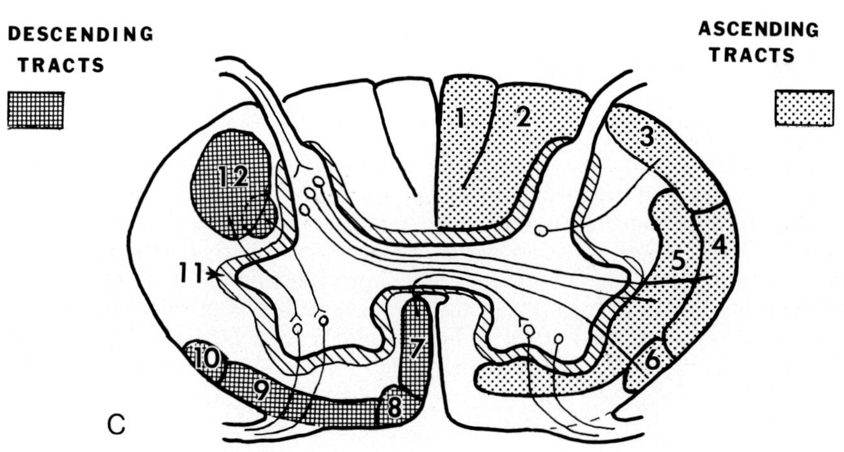
DESCENDING TRACTS
ASCENDING TRACTS
1
2
3
4
5
6
7
8
9
10
11
12
C

tain the fasciculus gracilis and fasciculus cuneatus, tracts that ascend in the cord mediating proprioceptive, vibratory, and tactile sensations. Large myelinated sensory nerves enter the cord through the medial portion of the dorsal roots, and these myelinated sensory fibers ascend in the dorsal columns. The fibers in the fasciculus gracilis and fasciculus cuneatus are laminated in a characteristic fashion. The fibers entering the columns from the lower portion of the body are more medially placed, and those entering the tracts from higher up in the body are more laterally placed. These fibers maintain their dorsal position, ending in the nucleus gracilis and nucleus cuneatus in the medulla (Fig. 1-30).

The lateral and ventral funiculi contain the corticospinal and spinothalamic tracts in addition to several other tracts to and from structures higher up in the central nervous system. The corticospinal tracts descend in the pyramidal tract by way of the cerebral peduncle from the motor cortex. In the caudal portion of the medulla and as far down the cord as C1, the pyramidal tracts decussate. In decussation, 70% of the pyramidal fibers cross over to the opposite side to become the lateral corticospinal tract of the lateral funiculus. Those fibers that do not decussate descend in the ventral funiculus as the ventral corticospinal tract. The corticospinal tracts mediate voluntary movement and synapse with anterior horn cells in the central gray matter from which arise the motor nerve fibers. The fibers of the corticospinal tract are layered in a manner similar to that noted in the dorsal funiculi, except that fibers ending the cervical cord are medially situated, whereas in the dorsal columns fibers originating in the cervical cord are laterally placed.

The spinothalamic tracts convey impulses for pain and temperature. Fine myelinated fibers enter the cord through the dorsal root laterally and terminate in the substantia gelatinosa of the dorsal horn of the gray matter. Axons leave this area and cross to the other side of the cord by way of the white matter ventral to the central canal. There these fibers ascend to the thalamus in either the ventral or lateral columns of the white matter as the ventral or lateral spinothalamic tracts, respectively. Axons from the dorsal root ganglion may ascend or descend one or two levels before crossing over to the contralateral side of the spinal cord.

Fig. 1-30. (*A*) Photomicrograph of a cross section of the cervical spinal cord at the level of C5: plastic-embedded section, 15 μ thick; Weigert stained. (*B*) A topographic arrangement of the cross-sectional anatomy of the cervical cord at the C5 level. Left side of column shows the arrangement of the major longitudinal columns (funiculi), while the right side depicts the approximate segmental arrangement of ascending and descending longitudinal tracts: sacral (S), lumbar (L), thoracic (T), and cervical (C). (*C*) A simplified schema of the arrangement of the main tracts of the cervical spinal cord at the C5 level. Ascending tracts on the left and descending tracts on the right are keyed as follows.

Ascending tracts: (*1*) Fasciculus gracilis; proprioception, vibration, pressure, and some tactile sensations from below the midthoracic region. (*2*) Fasciculus cuneatus; proprioception, vibration, pressure, and some tactile sensations from above the midthoracic level. (*3*) Dorsal and 4; ventral spinocerebellar tracts; carry exteroceptive and proprioceptive impulses from locomotor apparatus and skin for synergic control of voluntary movement. (*5*) Lateral spinothalamic tract; predominant pathway for somatic pain and thermal sensibilities. (*6*) Spinoolivary tract; conveys information from cutaneous receptors and muscle/tendon proprioceptive receptors.

Descending tracts: (*7*) Anterior corticospinal tract; uncrossed pyramidal motor fibers that cross at the level of segmental activation. (*8*) Tectospinal tract; fiber projections from tectum of midbrain, supposedly influenced by input of special sensations. (*9*) Vestibulospinal tract; fibers from lateral vestibular muscles that provide equilibrating control to anterior horn motor cells. (*10*) Olivospinal tract (bulbospinal) tract; (current information uncertain as to source and function). (*11*) Intersegmental (propriospinal) tracts; contain ascending and descending crossed and uncrossed fibers that provide intersegmental communications influencing both dorsal and ventral horn cells. (*12*) Lateral corticospinal tract; fibers from cortical motor cells that mostly have crossed in the pyramidal region and control motor activity of anterior horn cells at various segmental levels on the same side of the cord.

Thus there is some overlap of sensory innervation, and when a single dorsal root is sectioned, sensation is not completely lost in the distribution of that dorsal root.

The vertebral artery is the major source of blood supply for the cervical cord and cervical spine (Fig. 1-31). The vertebral arteries originate from the subclavian arteries on each side and are usually the first and largest branches of the subclavian artery. The arteries enter the foramen transversaria of C6 and ascend to the atlas, where they wind posteriorly around the lateral masses of the atlas and pass over the posterior arch of C1 just behind the lateral mass of that vertebra. The arteries pass through the posterior atlantooccipital membrane and thence anteriorly upward through the foramen magnum. The vertebral arteries come together just after passing through the foramen magnum to become the basilar artery. Just prior to their joining to form the basilar artery, one or both of the vertebral arteries give off a branch that joins with the branch from the opposite side and descends anteriorly on the spinal cord in the ventral median fissure of the spinal cord. This is called the anterior spinal artery, and its cervical portion lies beneath the pia and supplies the anterior part of the cord. The posterior spinal arteries also lie beneath the pia mater; they are paired and in this way differ from the anterior spinal artery, which is a single structure. The posterior spinal arteries descend from the vertebral arteries from which they originate and give rise to plexiform channels

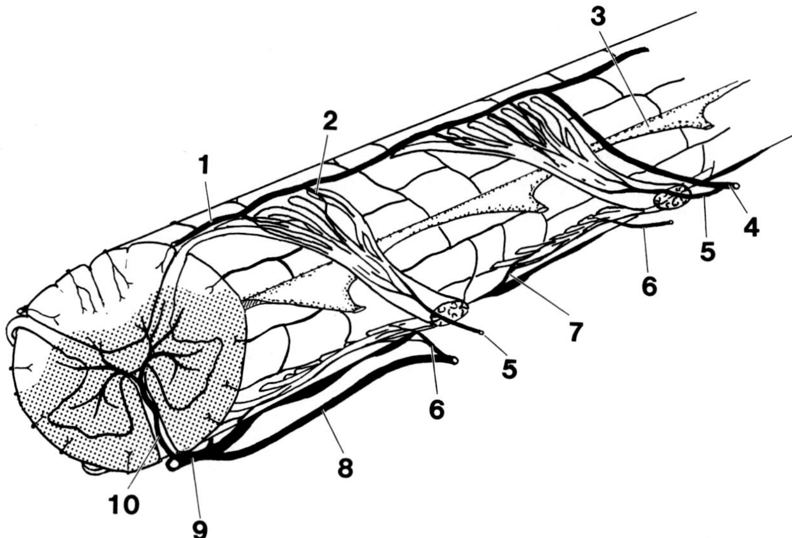

Fig. 1-31. Three-dimensional schema of the arterial supply of the cervical spinal cord and cervical spinal nerve roots. Stippled area on sectioned end of cord indicates the approximate quantity of cord tissue supplied by the anterior spinal artery via its central (internal) and coronal (external) branches. The remainder of the cord substance is supplied by the dorsolateral spinal arteries directly or through its coronal branches. Each spinal nerve root is supplied by a proximal and distal set of true radicular arteries that must be distinguished from the larger, irregularly located, medullary arteries that supply blood directly to the major longitudinal vessels of the cord. The proximal radicular arteries receive their flow from the longitudinal arteries or their coronal branches, and the distal radicular arteries are foramenal branches of segmental arteries or of the foramenal segment of a medullary artery. The medullary arteries do not supply midcourse branches to the root.

Legend key is as follows: (*1*) Dorsolateral spinal artery. (*2*) Proximal radicular artery of dorsal root. (*3*) Denticulate ligament. (*4*) Dorsal medullary artery. (*5*) Distal radicular artery to dorsal root. (*6*) Distal radicular artery for ventral root. (*7*) Proximal radicular artery for ventral root. (*8*) Ventral medullary artery. (*9*) Anterior spinal artery. (*10*) Central artery in anterior fissure. NB: The plexus of the vasa corona that ensheaths the cord is regionally supplied by the nearest longitudinal artery.

that are arranged transversely on the dorsum of the cord. The anterior and posterior spinal arteries also receive medullary feeders from the vertebral arteries as they ascend in the foramina transversaria. These vessels have a very variable distribution, but the medullary feeders or radicular arteries are more commonly seen and carry a greater blood flow in the cervical spine than in the thoracic spine. The medullary feeders, however, are inconstant branches of the segmental arteries that are evident at each level of the spine. The segmental branches supply the vertebrae themselves and form an anastomotic network with other arterial structures in this location. The segmental arteries, then, supply the vertebrae and surrounding tissues, usually at each level, but only a few segmental vessels give rise to radicular arteries or medullary feeders. The segmental vessels enter the intervertebral foramen at each level and branch extensively at a distribution point in this location.

The spinal cord has two major sources of blood supply: the anterior and posterior spinal arteries. These systems do not appear to anastomose with each other to a major degree. The anterior spinal artery, by means of a system of central branches, supplies the anterior column of the central gray cells and the ventral and lateral funiculi, that is, the corticospinal, spinal thalamic, and other ventral and lateral tracts. The posterior spinal system supplies the posterior columns (fasciculus cuneatus and gracilis) and the posterior horn of the central gray cells (Fig. 1-32).

Venous blood returns from the cord by way of a comparable system of anterior and posterior channels. The anterior system consists of three veins that run parallel to the longitudinal anterior spinal artery, and one of these accompanies the anterior artery in the median ventral fissure. There are three dorsal veins: one is central, lying along the dorsal median sulcus, and two are lateral, distributed dorsally in conjunction with the dorsal longitudinal arteries.

The bodies of the cervical vertebrae and most of the laminae are supplied segmentally by branches of the vertebral artery. At each segmental level, the vertebral arteries give off small branches that pass ventrally beneath the longus colli, usually to supply the colli muscles, the anterior aspect of the vertebral column, and the anterior longitudinal ligament. Also, at each segment the vertebral arteries give off branches that enter the intervertebral foramina, and at the distribution point branches pass caudally or rostrally to supply the posterior part of each vertebra and the posterior longitudinal ligament. Other branches pass dorsally from the distribution point and supply the lamina on the inside of the spinal canal, and still other variable branches supply the cord through the radicular vessels as described. Other branches pass from the vertebral artery dorsally at each level to supply the outer surface of the laminae and the posterior muscles of the neck. The deep cervical artery arising from the thyrocervical trunk from the subclavian artery also supplies these structures, and the dorsal segmental branches anastomose extensively with the deep cervical arteries at these levels. The blood supply of the odontoid process is also segmented. Branches from the ventral segmental artery to the body of the axis pass rostrally to supply the anterior aspect of the dens and anastomose with branches descending from the carotid artery along the alar ligaments. The posterior central arteries of the axis derive from branches of the vertebral arteries that pass into the intervertebral foramina from the vertebral arteries at the occipitoatlantal and atlantoaxial levels. There are extensive cross connections between these systems to supply the dens transverse ligament, the alar and apical ligaments, and the atlantal joints and arches.

The venous side of the circulation of the cervical vertebrae is classifiable into the broad groups of the internal and external systems of veins. The external system is arranged in the same distribution as the anterior central and posterior laminar arteries. The venous system within the spinal canal consists of a series of valveless sinuses in the epidural space. The plexiform sinuses are clustered at each level anteriorly in the canal just medial to the pedicles over the midportion of the vertebral bodies. They are thus thinnest and least apparent at the level of the intervertebral discs and most obvious at the narrowest portion of the posterior longitudinal ligament at each level. There they anastomose freely across the midline with the epidural veins on the opposite side. The epidural veins also anastomose with the basivertebral sinus, which is located in the space between the posterior longitudinal ligament and the posterior aspect of the vertebral body. This valveless complex of veins forms a continuous connection between the pelvis and the cerebral sinuses. The system exits from the spinal canal through the veins that pass out through the intervertebral foramina connecting the epidural complex with the caval and azygos systems.

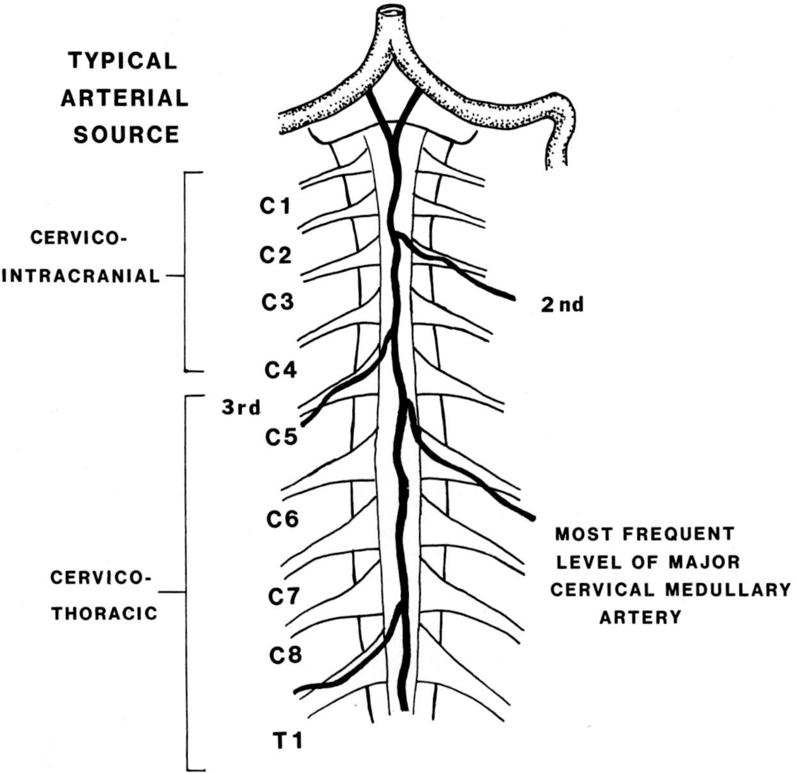

Fig. 1-32. Most frequent locations of cervical anterior medullary arteries according to the studies of Mannen,[1] with the relative consistency indicated for three segments. Although the cervical anterior spinal artery is anatomically continuous, the direction of blood flow in any section is dependent on its proximity to a medullary supply. As the flow is assisted from the regions adjacent to the cervical cord, the vascular domains may be divided into a cervicointracranial region, and a cervicothoracic region. The division was established at C4 since the postmortem injection studies by Taylor[2] indicated that the intracranial supply to the anterior spinal artery was effective only to this level. Although the medullary arteries showed no pronounced preference for either side, the pattern depicted here approximates the most frequently encountered arterial arrangement.

The cervicointracranial vascular region occupies the more capacious section of the spinal canal and is less likely to develop an anterior spinal artery (ASA) syndrome than the cervicothoracic section. It is significant that cervical spondylitic stenoses most frequently involve the C4 to C7 region, where the major medullary source to the ASA is most likely to be situated. The posterior medullary arteries are much smaller and more frequent in the segmental occurrence, but their supply to the cord is much less critical.

Note that the segmental levels indicated in the illustration take the same designation as their associated spinal nerves and therefore indicate one level in excess of the actual number of definitive cervical vertebrae.

Figures 1-33 through 1-37 are selected sectional views representative of the various regions related to the craniocervical junction and the cervical spine. Each plate consists of a CT scan that is matched to a photograph of a cross section prepared from a frozen cadaver. Owing to slightly different inclinations in the transverse planes of the sections and the variations in the degree of the cervical lordosis, the match can only be approximate. Since the intention here is to describe and illustrate the anatomy of the cervical spine, both the CT scans and the sections were enlarged and trimmed to enhance the detail of the vertebral structures and their most immediately related anatomy. All the sections are displayed with their ventral aspects in the superior position that is most consistent with the serial preparations viewed on scanner films. The photographs of the cadaver specimens are viewed from the inferior surface of each section and presented in superior-to-inferior order to follow the practices most frequently used in anatomic atlases.

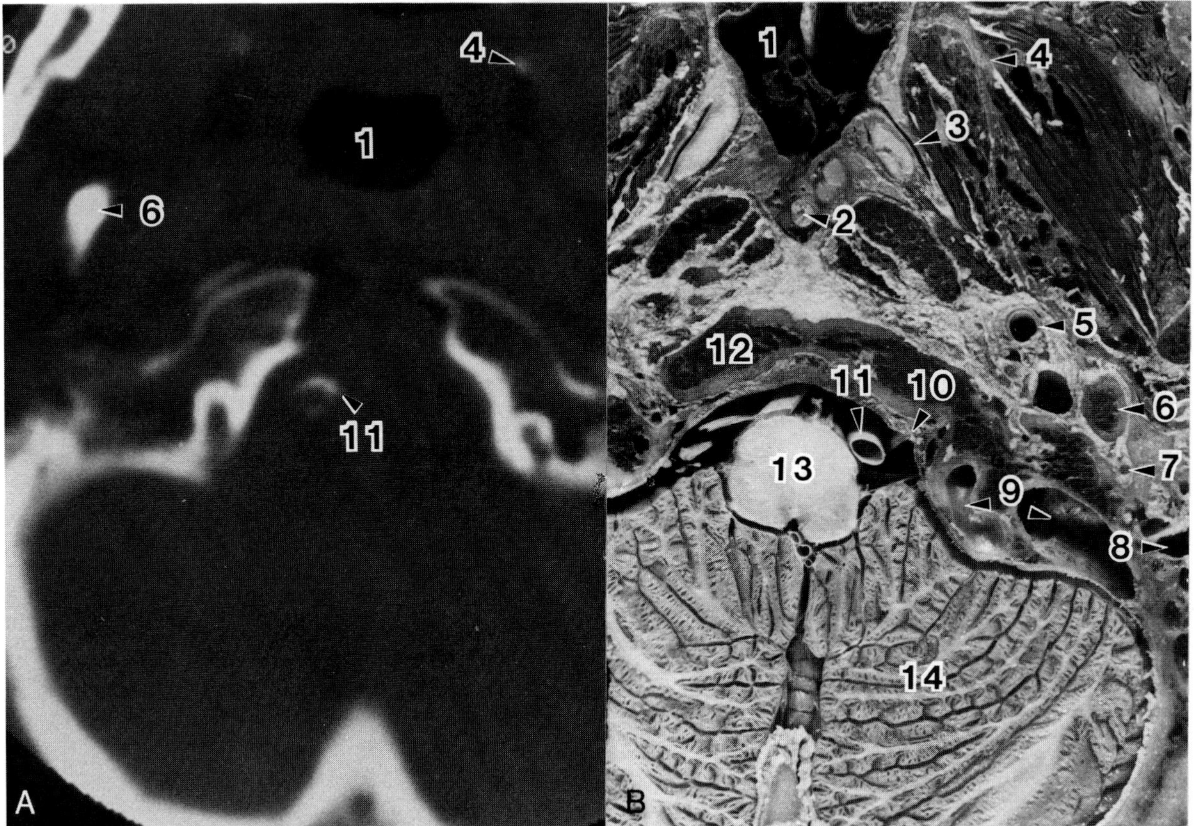

Fig. 1-33. Sectional view through the occipital bone and posterior cranial fossa, cerebellum, and medulla. Superiorly, the nasopharynx (*1*) is shown at the level where the pharyngeal raphe (*2*) is passing upward to attach to the pharyngeal tubercle of the basiocciput. Lateral to this may be seen the cartilages of the torus tubarium and opening (*3*) of the auditory tube. In the infratemporal fossa, the tip of the lateral pterygoid lamina (*2*) (also visible in scan) is seen giving rise to the lateral and medial pterygoid muscles. Posterolateral to the prevertebral muscle the internal carotid artery (*5*) brackets the retromandibular vein between it and the base of the styloid process (*6*). Just posterior to the process the seventh cranial nerve (facial nerve) (*7*) may be observed as it emerges from the stylomastoid foramen. The maxillary sinus (*4*) is indicated.

The section of the basiocciput and temporal bones has exposed the mastoid sinus (*8*) and the dome of the jugular fossa where the inferior petrosal sinus and sigmoid sinus (*9*) converge to form the bulb of the jugular vein. This section also has exposed the twelfth cranial nerve (hypoglossal nerve) as it exits through the opening of the hypoglossal canal (*10*). The left vertebral artery (*11*) is seen on the left side of the medulla and a "ghost" of the sclerotic right vertebral is visible on the scan. The basiocciput (*12*) shows a complete arch in the photograph, whereas in the scan it appears interrupted as the plane of section passed through the anterior rim of the foramen magnum. Between the lateral aspects of the medulla (*13*) and the cerebellum (*14*) the spinal part of the eleventh cranial nerve (accessory nerve) may be discerned.

RELATED STRUCTURES IN THE NECK

The important visceral, vascular, and neurologic structures in the neck can be related for practical purposes to the cervical spine in several ways (Figs. 1-33 through 1-37). It is useful, for example, to correlate a given anatomic structure in the neck to a vertebral level. The first cervical vertebra is behind the angle of the mandible, and the transverse process of the atlas is palpable between the angle

(*Text continues on p. 32*)

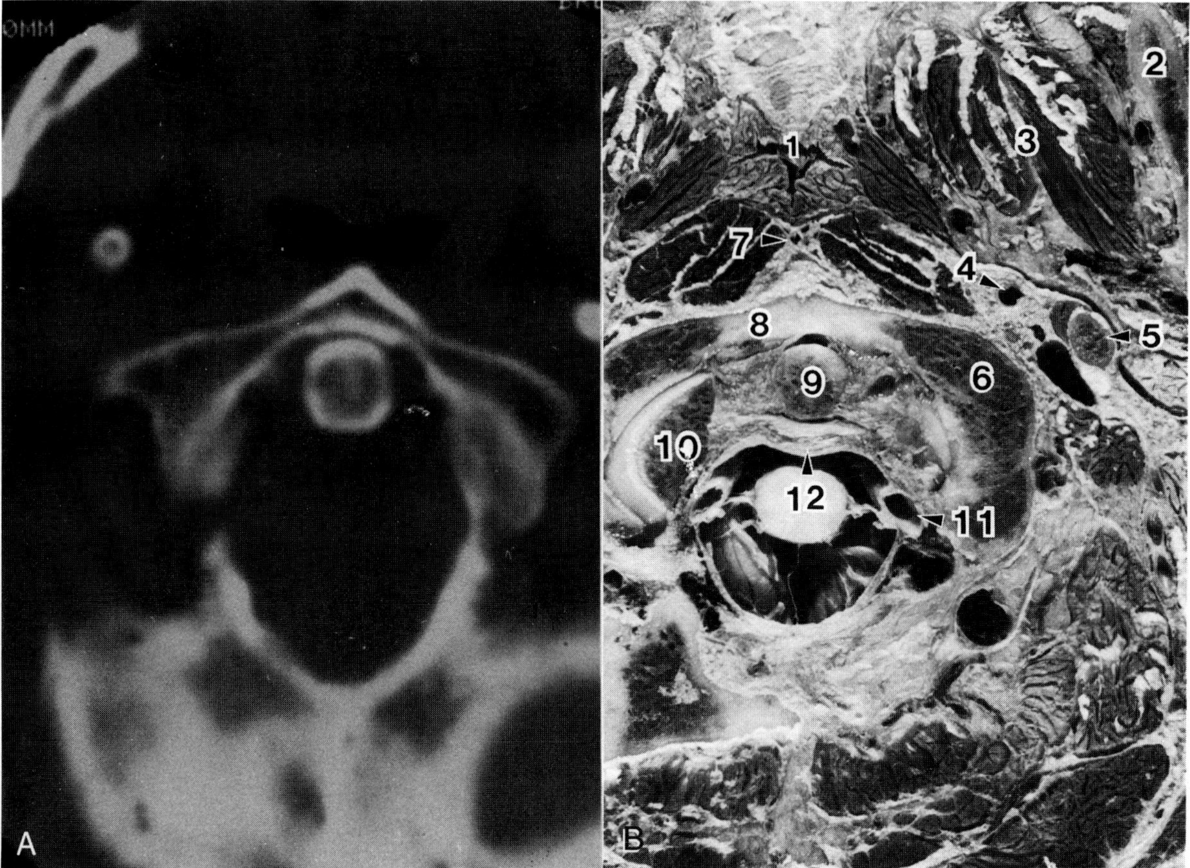

Fig. 1-34. Section through the superior half of the odontoid process, which is particularly revealing. The osseous components detected in the CT scan can only suggest the complexities of the lateral and median craniocervical articulations. In reading the scan, the viewer must mentally visualize the radiolucent elements that maintain the functional positions of the bone, and the derangements of these soft structures may then be inferred by unusual bone mobility or malposition.

In this view, both the scan and the cross section show the dorsosuperior extreme of the soft palate (*1*). On either side of pharyngeal slit, the levator veli palatini muscles are well defined. The ramus of the mandible (*2*) is related laterally to the median and lateral pterygoid muscles (*3*). Posterior to these, the internal carotid artery (*4*) lies anteromedial to the styloid process (*5*) whose anteromedial surface shows the origin of the stylohyoid muscle. The lateral mass of the atlas (*6*) has been sectioned. Between the prevertebral muscles is seen part of the venous plexus (*7*) that drains the upper posterior nasopharynx and communicates with the periodontoidal epidural veins by way of the pharyngovertebral veins carrying infective processes to the area of the spine. The anterior arch of the atlas (*8*) is partially sectioned, and the anterior median articular cavity between it and the odontoid process (*9*) is well illustrated. Lateral to the odontoid, the two robust alar ligaments are shown strongly fixed to the superior lateral aspect of this process. The left occipital condyle (*10*) is partially sectioned and shows the lateral craniovertebral articulation. Just medial to the anterior internal aspect of the condyle, the attachment of the right alar ligament to the alar tubercle of the skull is partially shown. The tubercle is suggested as a bony shadow on the same side of the CT scan.

Posterior to the odontoid process, the superior aspect of the transverse ligament of the atlas (*12*) is shown forming the posterior articular cavity of the median craniovertebral joint. The attachment of this ligament to the internal surface of the lateral mass of the atlas is best shown on the right side of the photograph (left side of specimen).

The structures passing through the foramen magnum are exceptionally well illustrated. The ample space allowed the lower medulla is evident and the spinal part of the accessory nerve (eleventh cranial nerve) is seen passing dorsal to the left vertebral artery (*11*). A sectioned layer of the intracranial dura partially obscures the true position of the posterior border of the foramen magnum and cerebellar tonsils in the photograph.

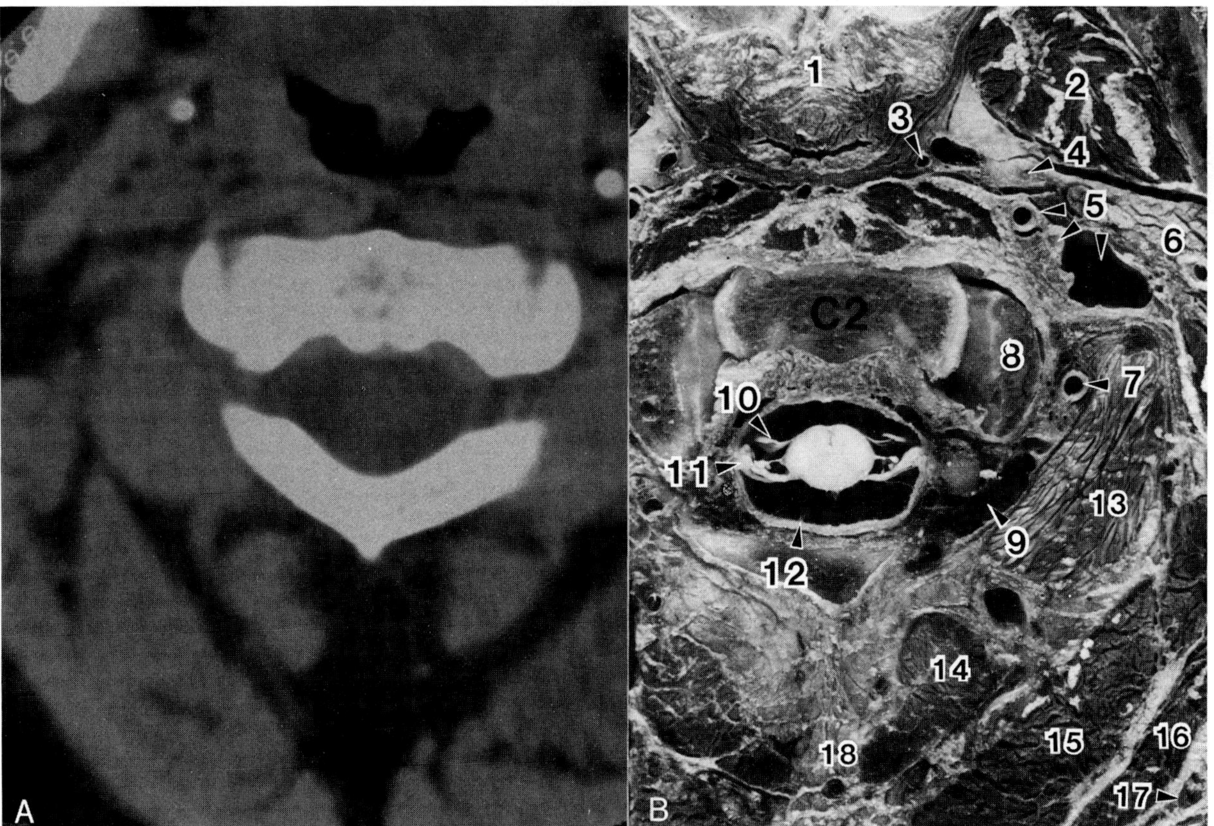

Fig. 1-35. Transverse section through the C1–C2 articulation showing the anatomic relations of the upper cervical vertebra. The uvular region of the palate marks the transition between the nasopharynx and the oropharynx (*1*). The internal pterygoid muscle (*2*) inserts on the medial surface of the body of the mandible. On the posterolateral surface of the superior pharyngeal constrictor, the ascending pharyngeal artery (*3*) is evident. The stylohyoid ligament (*4*) is often ossified, which is so indicated in the accompanying CT scan. Contents of the carotid sheath (*5*) are shown as the carotid artery, vagus nerve, and jugular vein by their respective arrows. Lateral to the sheath lies the deep lobe of the parotid gland (*6*). The vertebral artery (*7*) has assumed its most lateral position in its ascent to pass through the transverse foramen of the atlas. The lateral mass of the atlas (*8*) shows the sloping angulation of its inferior facet where it articulates with its complement on the body of C2. Dorsal to the body of C2, the thickening of the posterior longitudinal ligament indicates the formation of the inferior longitudinal bundle of the transverse ligament and tectorial membrane. Both the epidural and vertebral plexuses of veins (*9*) are most pronounced in the suboccipital region. The greater capacity of the upper cervical spinal canal is well illustrated here and is reflected in the greater volume of the intradural space. The cord is anchored centrally to this space by the ventral (*10*) and dorsal (*11*) roots of the second cervical nerve. Note that between these structures the lateral projection of the denticulate ligament encloses the ascending accessory nerve between it and the dorsal roots. Numerous dorsal arachnoid trabeculae (*12*) also help to hold the cord in its central position.

The dorsal nuchal musculature, well defined in both the scan and the cadaver specimen, is labeled as follows: obliquus capitis inferior (*13*), rectis capitis posterior major (*14*), semispinalis capitis (*15*), splenius capitis (*16*), and trapezius (*17*). The nuchal ligament (*18*) is indicated.

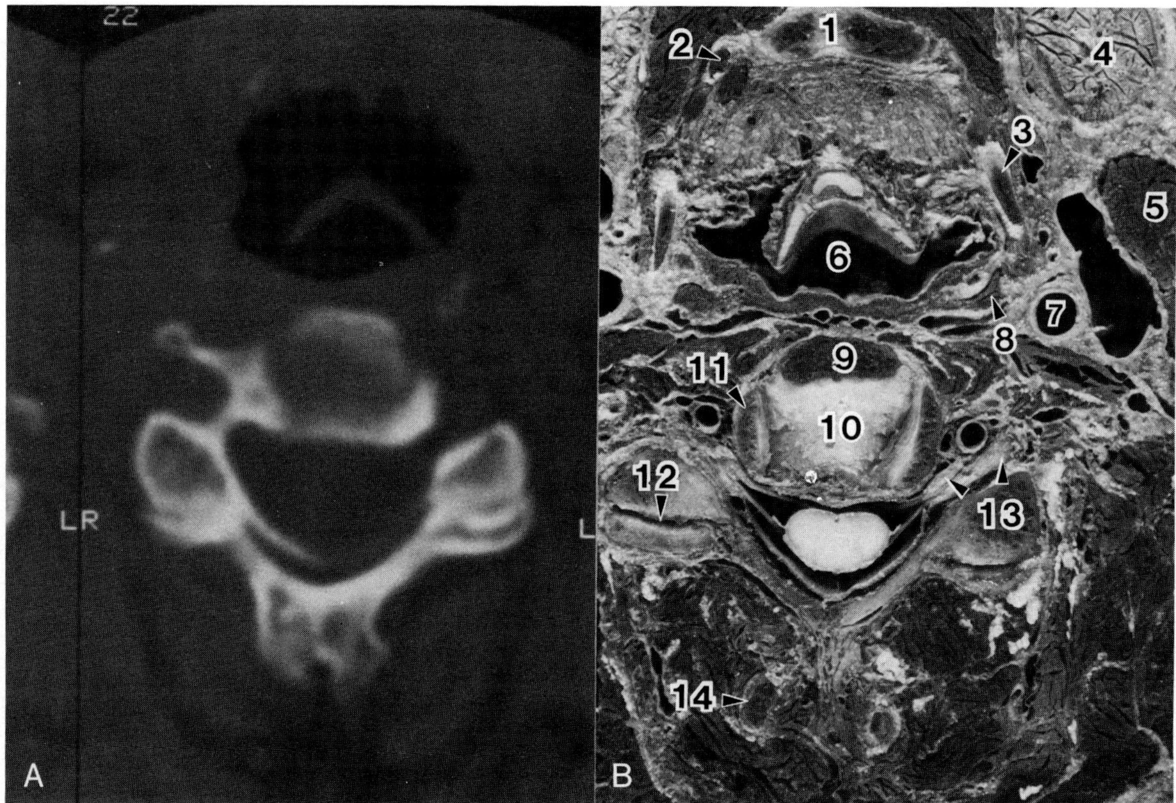

Fig. 1-36. Section through the C4–C5 intervertebral disc, characteristic of the midcervical spine and its immediately related anatomy. This disc is anteriorly related to the level of the hyoid bone, the body of which has been sectioned in the cadaver specimen (*1*) with the tip of the right lesser hyoid horn (*2*) shown in the upper left of the photograph and sections of the greater horns (*3*) evident on both sides. A slight shadow of the tips of the greater horns and right lesser horn may be detected in the attached scan.

Anterolateral to the hyoid bone and its anteriorly attached mylohyoid muscle lies the submandibular gland (*4*) that is posteriorly related to the sternocleidomastoid muscle (*5*).

The wide pharyngeal opening (*6*) is here transitional between the oral and laryngeal regions of the pharynx. Anterior to the center of the pharynx, the epiglottis and its cartilaginous core are seen as an inverted "V." The A–P angulation of the scan sections is about 5 ml more superior in the anterior aspects than the cadaver section. The internal carotid artery (*7*) readily defines the position of the carotid sheath and its associated structures. The middle pharyngeal constrictor (*8*) is attached anteriorly to the greater horns of the hyoid, and it lies posterior to the inferior part of the stylopharyngeus muscle.

In the region of the C4–C5 intervertebral disc (*10*), the projections characteristic of the midcervical vertebral bodies are evident. The downward projection of the anterior lip of the C4 body is readily discerned in both the scan and the cross section (*9*). At the same level, the plane of section also shows the upward projections of the uncinate processes of the C5 body (*11*). The same plane in both views also traverses the C4–C5 body (*11*) and the C4–C5 facet joints (*12*), the anterior elements of the joint belonging to C5, and the posterior elements to C4. Parts of the laminae of both arches are also shadowed in the scan.

The complex bony channel formed by the cervical intervertebral foramena is well indicated, with the relations of the dorsal and ventral roots (*13*) and the fifth cervical nerve shown. The relationship of the vertebral artery to the dorsal root ganglion (indicated by the lateral arrow of label [13]) may be discerned. Note that the vertebral artery is, at all levels, surrounded by the plexiform vertebral veins. Unlike the capacious spinal canal seen in superior levels, the cord in the middle and lower cervical regions becomes more confined and hence more subject to pressure from pathologic or traumatic alterations in canal diameter. Label *14* indicates the cordlike attachments of the semispinalis cervicis muscle.

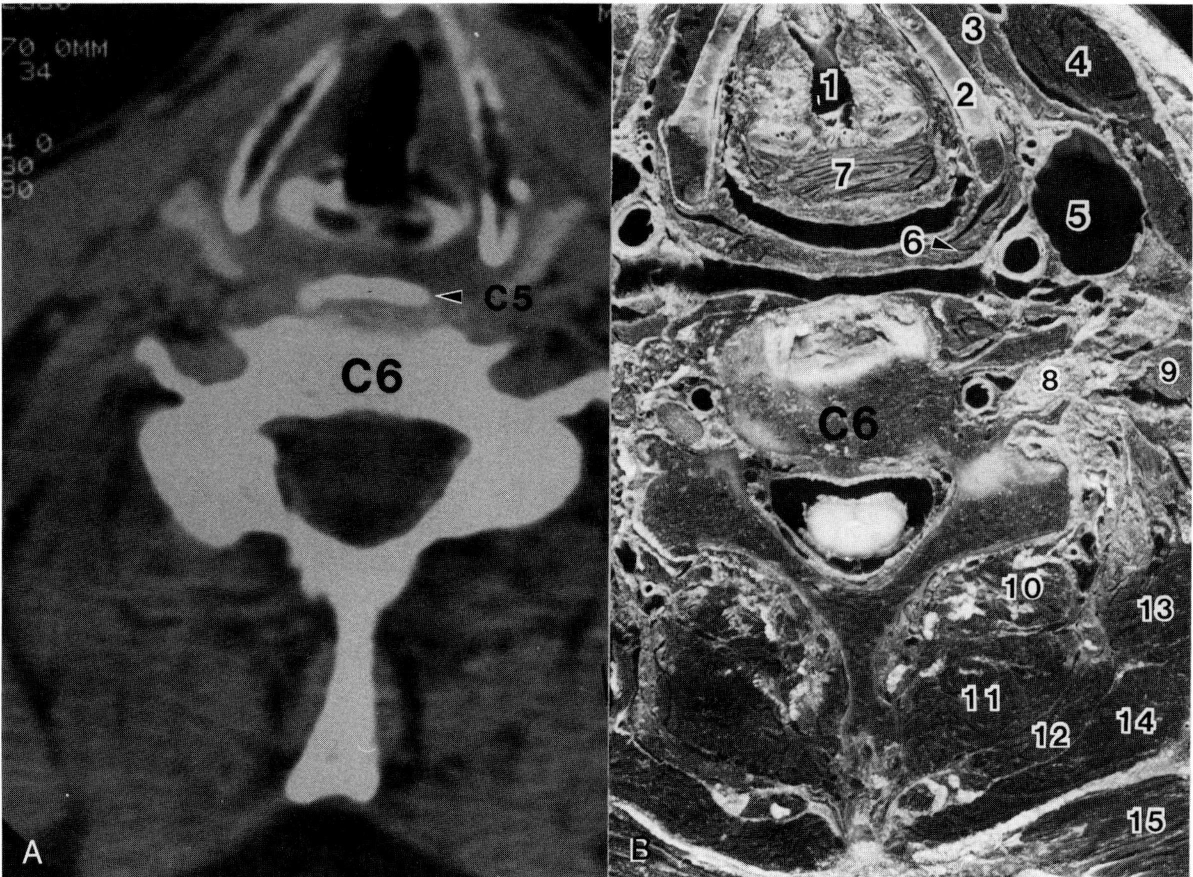

Fig. 1-37. Oblique cut section through the upper level of the C6 body, characteristic of the topographic relationships of the lower cervical spine. Anteriorly, the narrow opening in the larynx marks the level of the rima glottidis (*1*). The laminae of the thyroid cartilage (*2*) lie medial to the strap muscles (*3*) and sternocleidomastoid muscle (*4*). The much-enlarged internal jugular vein (*5*) is consistent with the fact that this specimen had a long-standing congestive right heart failure. The inferior pharyngeal constrictor muscle (*6*) separates the anterior laryngopharynx from the posterior retropharyngeal left. The transverse arytenoid muscles (*7*) are well depicted with their insertions into the muscular processes of the two arytenoid cartilages. (Owing to the cervical lordosis, both the scan and cross section show an oblique cut through the anterior rim of the C5–C6 disc with the bony lip of C5 showing in the scan.)

Lateral to the left vertebral artery (right side of photograph) the root of the sixth cervical nerve (*8*) is apparent. The middle scalene muscle (*9*) lies posterior to the root of the fifth cervical nerve, which in turn lies posterior to the anterior scalene. The posterior nuchal muscles are now characteristic of the thoracocervical region and are labeled as follows: multifidus muscle (*10*), semispinalis cervicis (*11*), semispinalis capitis (*12*), levator scapulae (*13*), splenius capitis (*14*), and trapezius (*15*).

of the mandible and the mastoid process. The hyoid bone is just anterior to the level of C3, the thyroid cartilage is anterior to C4, and the cricoid cartilage is opposite the sixth cervical vertebra.

The cervical triangles also provide a useful basis for relating these structures to the anatomy of the cervical spine. The boundaries of the triangles have already been described.

The anterior triangle (bounded by the lower border of the mandible, the anterior border of the sternocleidomastoid muscle, and the midline of the neck) is further subdivided. The carotid triangle is bounded by the anterior border of the sternocleidomastoid muscle, the anterior belly of the omohyoid muscle, and the posterior belly of the digastric muscle. The carotid triangle contains the carotid sheath in which the internal jugular vein, the common carotid artery, and the vagus nerve pass obliquely across the neck. The common carotid artery bifurcates into the internal and external carotid arteries within this triangle; the internal carotid artery gives rise to the superior thyroid artery and the ascending pharyngeal and lungal arteries within the limits of the carotid triangle. Also within this triangle are descending branches of the cervical plexus and several large venous communications with the internal jugular, including the common facial vein.

The muscular triangle is bounded by the anterior belly of the omohyoid muscle and the anterior branch of the sternocleidomastoid muscle; the midline of the anterior neck contains the "strap muscles" and the sternohyoid, sternothyroid, thyrohyoid, and omohyoid muscles. These muscles overlie the thyroid cartilage and larnyx, the trachea and esophagus, and the thyroid gland.

The digastric triangle bounded by the digastric muscle and the inferior border of the mandible contains salivary glands, branches of the facial nerve, and the hypoglossal nerve.

The posterior triangle contains the upper trunks of the branchial plexus and, in its lower part, the subclavian artery and vein arch over the first rib behind the clavicle. These vascular structures are just visible in the occipital triangle, the lower and smaller of the two subdivisions of the posterior triangle. The upper portion of the posterior triangle contains the spinal accessory nerve, which passes obliquely downward behind the sternocleidomastoid muscle to the trapezius. Cutaneous branches of the cervical plexus, the supraclavicular nerve, the great auricular nerve, the lesser occipital nerve, and the anterior cervical cutaneous nerve are also found in the posterior cervical triangle.

The fascia of the anterior part of the neck supports all of the foregoing structures and makes definition of the anatomic components relatively easy during dissection. The platysma muscle lies beneath the skin and on the most superficial layer of the deep fascia, also called the prebrachial fascia. This fascial layer extends from the trapezius muscle over the posterior triangle and splits to enclose the sternocleidomastoid muscle. It passes across the midline in front of the trachea to fuse with the same fascial layer of the opposite side. The middle layer of the deep cervical fascia covers and envelops the strap muscles and visceral structures and extends backward on each side to envelop the carotid sheath. It supports these structures by suspensory extensions to both the superficial or pretracheal layer of the deep fascia and the prevertebral fascia. The third layer of the deep fascia, then, is the prevertebral fascia, which covers the scalenus muscles, longus colli muscles, and longus capitis muscles on the anterior aspect of the cervical vertebrae and intervertebral discs. The prevertebral fascia almost merges into the anterior longitudinal ligament. Loose areolar tissue fills the space between the deep layer of the cervical fascia and the middle layer of the fascia covering the deep surface of the visceral components of the neck. This prevertebral space permits easy blunt dissection up and down the anterior aspect of the cervical spine on the deep fascial layer, providing for ready access to the front of the cervical spine.

REFERENCES

1. *Mannen T:* Vascular lesions in the spinal cord in the aged. Geriatrics 21:151–160, 1966.
2. *Taylor HR:* Vascular factors in the myelopathy associated with cervical spondylosis. Neurology, 14:62–68, 1964.

CHAPTER 2

Physiology and Biomechanics

Functional Anatomy of Joints and Discs

LOHRENS PENNING

REGION C2–C7

Movement Diagram and Center of Motion

This section is based primarily on data provided by radiographic motion studies. While visualization of the movement itself is best performed using fluoroscopy or cineradiography,[3] detailed analysis of the pattern and degree of motion requires a comparison of static radiographs of the spine in different positions. Superimposition is an accurate method of comparing radiographs. If the radiographic images of the cervical spine in two end-positions of a certain movement (*e.g.*, flexion–extension) are superimposed, a movement diagram can be obtained (Fig. 2-1). The term movement diagram (Bewegungsdiagramm) was introduced by Buetti-Bäuml[1] in 1954. He used the diagram mainly to demonstrate the degree of angular motion and of translation (Fig. 2-2). In a 1960 thesis[14] I defined a center of motion, relating both end-positions of the movement concerned (Fig. 2-3). This so-called "instantaneous" center assumes that the motion follows a circular path. Biomechanical studies of cadaver specimens of the spine[25,26] have shown that the center may change its position during motion, especially in the presence of degenerative disorders. Radiographic studies in subjects without signs of degeneration have convinced us that for motion from neutral position to flexion, and from neutral position to extension, the center of motion is about the same. For the study of normal anatomy related to motion, the supposition of a fixed center of motion therefore seems justified.

Pattern of Motion Determined by Apophyseal Joints

The elements primarily responsible for the mobility of the spine are the discs and the apophyseal joints. Each of these elements provides its relative contribution to degree and pattern of motion. The flexion–extension movement diagram suggests that the joints determine the pattern of motion. The joint spaces form part of a circle with the instantaneous center of motion as midpoint (Fig. 2-3).

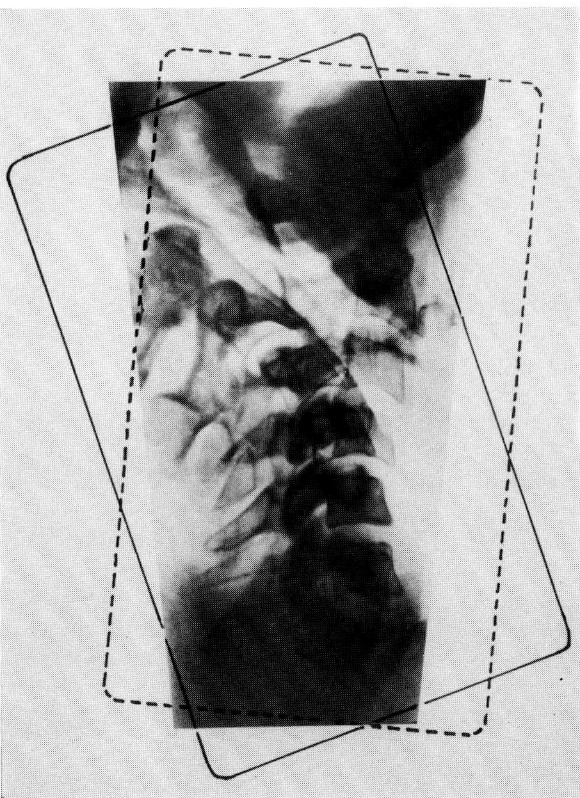

Fig. 2-1. Genesis of movement diagram. After superimposition of flexion and extension, radiographs of cervical spine bodies of C5 are made to match exactly. C4 is now shown in flexed and extended position with respect to "fixed" C5; we call this a movement diagram C4–C5, type I. C6 is also shown in flexed and extended position with respect to fixed C5; this we call movement diagram C5–C6, type II. As a rule, a movement diagram type I is used.

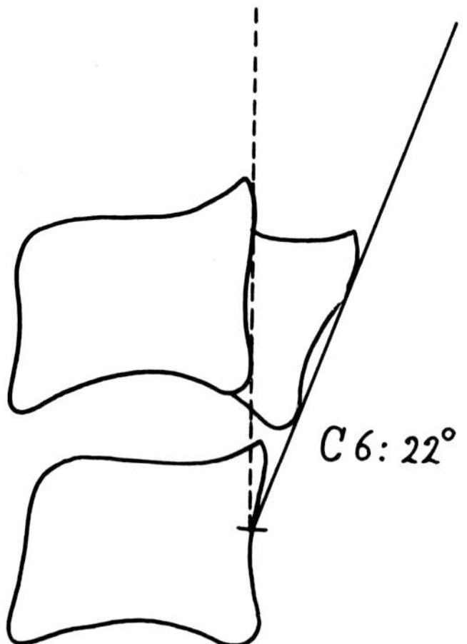

Fig. 2-2. Movement diagram of Buetti-Bäuml.[1] Redrawing of figure from monograph by Buetti-Bäuml represents body of C7 as "fixed," and C6 in flexed and extended positions. Angle between lines drawn along dorsal surface of vertebral bodies C6 represents degree of flexion–extension motion.

Comparison of the mean location of the flexion–extension center of motion in a group of subjects at different levels between C2 and T1 shows that at C2–C3 the mean location of the center is in the dorsocaudal part of the body of C3, and at C7–T1 about halfway to the cranial end-plate of T1. At the intermediate levels, the center gradually shifts from one extreme position to the other (Fig. 2-4). In 1960,[14] I demonstrated this in 20 cervical spines of young adults without radiographic signs of disc degeneration, and since then have always found the same type of regional difference of location of centers of motion between C2 and T1. This was confirmed in cadaver experiments by Lysell[10] in 1969.

The different location of flexion–extension centers is reflected by regional differences in anatomy of the articular processes. At C3 the articular processes rise far less above the level of the cranial vertebral end-plate than at C7 or T1 (Fig. 2-5). At intervening levels there is a gradual increase in rise between C3 and T1. This appears to correlate with the gradual cranial movement of the center of flexion–extension motion between C3 and T1, and thus seems to be another argument in favor of the apophyseal joints determining the pattern of motion.

It is evident that the more the center of motion is removed from the corresponding disc, the greater is the gliding motion of the cranial vertebra (Fig. 2-6). Therefore, the gliding motion is small at C7–T1 and large at C2–C3. If gliding motion is considered the expression of greater freedom of movement but less stability, one may understand that this motion has been limited at the caudal, fixed end of the cervical spine but is more liberally exercised at the cranial, free end.

Another argument supporting a decisive role for the apophyseal joints in determining the pattern of motion is the obligatory coupling of rotation and lateral flexion between C2 and T1. This coupling is explained by the oblique orientation of the apophyseal joints. For rotation, one articular process moves ventrally, and the contralateral process moves dorsally; however, ventral movement im-

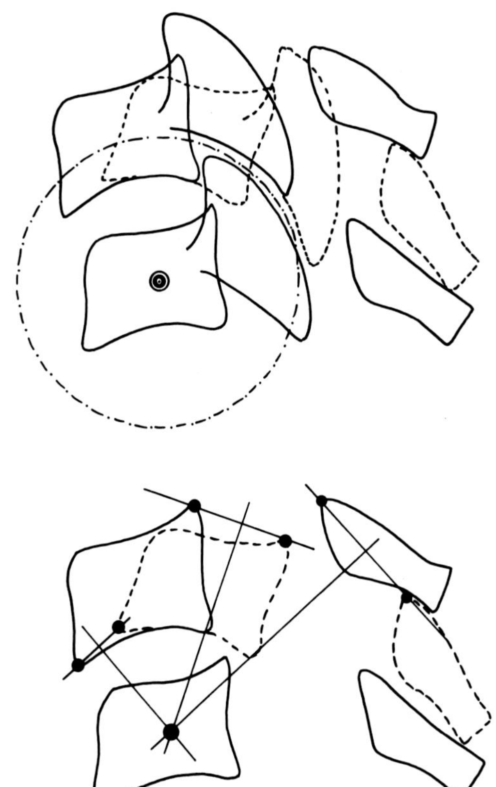

Fig. 2-3. Movement diagram of the author.[14] Upper movement diagram shows intervertebral joint space to coincide with arc of circle having center of motion as central point. Lower movement diagram illustrates construction of center of motion: indentical landmarks of "moving" vertebra are connected by lines; perpendicular lines constructed from their midpoints converge on center of motion (method ascribed to Euler. Another perhaps more accurate method is that of Pennal and coworkers[13]).

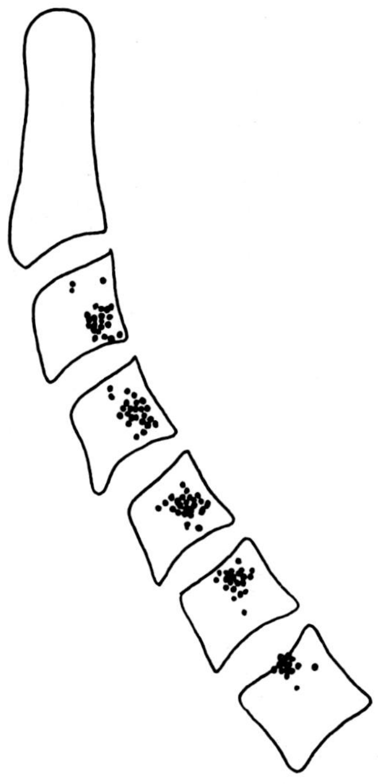

Fig. 2-4. Centers of flexion–extension motion C2–C7. Results of determination of flexion–extension centers of motion in 20 young adults without radiographic evidence of disc degeneration.[14] Regional differences in mean location of centers of motion are apparent.

plies cranial movement, and dorsal movement implies caudal movement. This combination of cranial movement on one side and caudal movement on the other constitutes lateral flexion (Fig. 2-7).

Study of movements of the lumbar spine also provides evidence in favor of the apophyseal joints prescribing the pattern of motion. It is known that rotation of the lumbar spine, at least from L1 to L5, is minimal. In a transverse section (Fig. 2-8), the joint spaces form part of a circle having its center at about the midpoint of the spinous process. For optimal rotation the center should be located at or near the center of the disc. The present location makes rotation virtually impossible, provided the disc is intact. Virchow[17,23] distinguished between radial orientation and tangential orientation of the articular facets. If rotation in anatomic specimens of vertebrae proved to be easily possible, he always found that the apophyseal joint surfaces were tangential to an arc around the center of the disc, and rotator muscles were present (see also Fig. 3-12).

In cadaver experiments Rolander[18] demonstrated that parallel displacement between the vertebral end-plates bordering a lumbar disc is severely limited. It never exceeded 2 mm, and only in a few instances exceeded 1 mm. The lumbar flexion–extension movement diagram shows that the orientation of the apophyseal joints is close to perpendicular to the plane of the vertebral endplates; thus, parallel displacement of these endplants is thwarted by the joints (Fig. 2-9).

Pattern of Motion Determined by Disc

Having established the ostensibly primary role of the joints in determining the pattern of motion, one will be surprised by the experimental finding of Rolander[18] that after removal of the articular

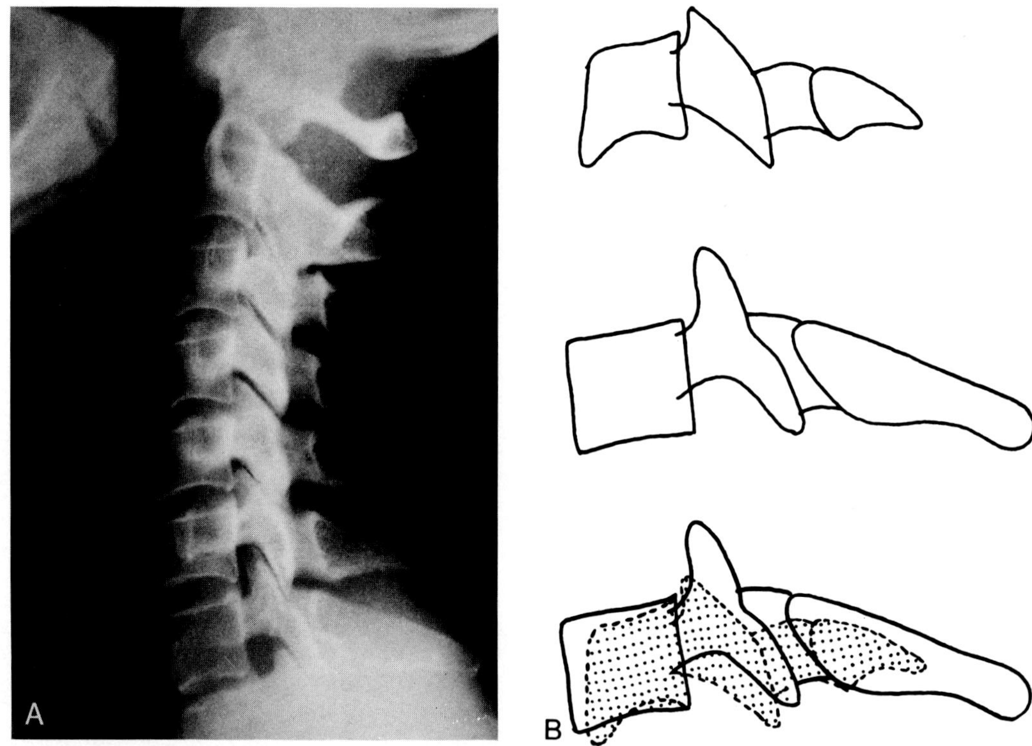

Fig. 2-5. Regional radiographic differences C2–T1. Lateral radiograph of cervical spine shows superior articular processes at C3 to rise to height above vertebral body that is lower than at C7. Separate drawings of these vertebrae also illustrate differences in the form of articular processes, spinous processes, and vertebral bodies. Note anteroinferior downward jutting of vertebral body C3 (Jackson[7]), which is absent at C7.

processes the pattern of motion of the (lumbar) vertebrae virtually remained the same. The degree of rotation increased somewhat, but it remained minimal (1° to 3° both sides together). The finding of Rolander seems to indicate that the disc plays a primary role in determining the pattern of motion, or at least is able to play this role independently of the apophyseal joints.

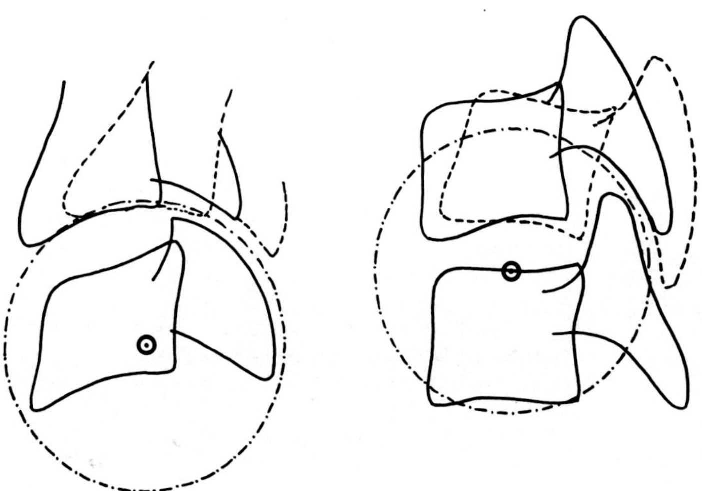

Fig. 2-6. Regional differences in gliding motion. (*Left*) A flexion–extension movement diagram, C2–C3, is shown. Gliding of C2 upon C3 is marked. Center of motion is far from disc C2–C3. (*Right*) A flexion–extension movement diagram C6–C7 shows minimal gliding of C6 upon C7. Center of motion near disc C6–C7. Note differences in shape between articular processes C2–C3 and C6–C7.

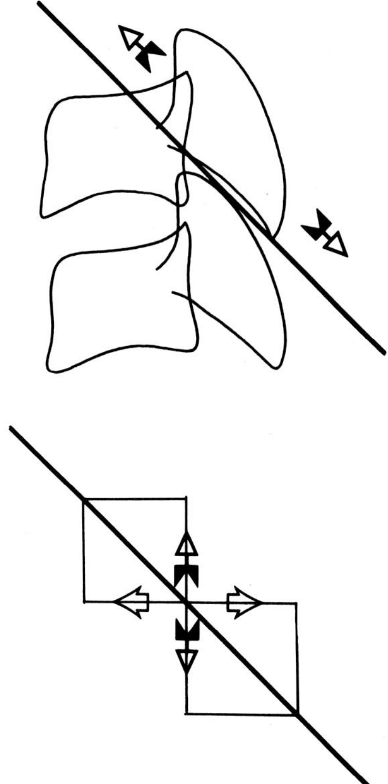

Fig. 2-7. Coupling of rotation and lateral flexion C2–T1. (*Top*) Owing to oblique orientation of intervertebral joint spaces (*drawn line*), articular facets must move obliquely upward or downward (*arrows*). (*Bottom*) These movements can be resolved into horizontal and vertical components. Vertical components correspond with lateral flexion, and horizontal components with rotation.

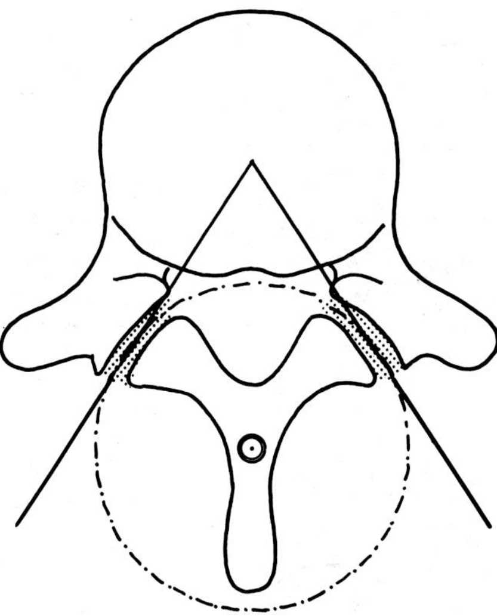

Fig. 2-8. Virtual impossibility of rotation in lumbar spine. Orientation of apophyseal joint spaces is radial with respect to center of disc (*drawn lines*). Joint spaces form part of circle with center point about midway on spinous process. Such orientation impedes rotation. For optimal rotation, joint spaces should form part of circle with its center point in center of disc (tangential orientation [Virchow[23]]).

It seems as if the role of the apophyseal joints consists of protecting the disc against abnormal patterns of motion, as may arise in the case of abnormal stress or overloading. Figure 2-10 attempts to clarify this. During lifting of loads with the lumbar spine bent forward, the lumbar vertebrae will be drawn ventrally, producing transverse shear forces within the disc. Such a shearing movement however is largely prevented by the arrangement of the articular processes, those of the cranial vertebra overlapping dorsally those of the caudal vertebra. A comparable arrangement is present in the cervical spine (Fig. 2-5).

If the disc plays an important role in determining the pattern of motion, its behavior in an isolated state is of interest. From the experiments of Rolander, and from other anatomic and biomechanical studies of normal lumbar discs,[18,19,26] it appears that tilting movements can easily be made, but rotation or horizontal translation (parallel displacement) of vertebral end-plates is severely

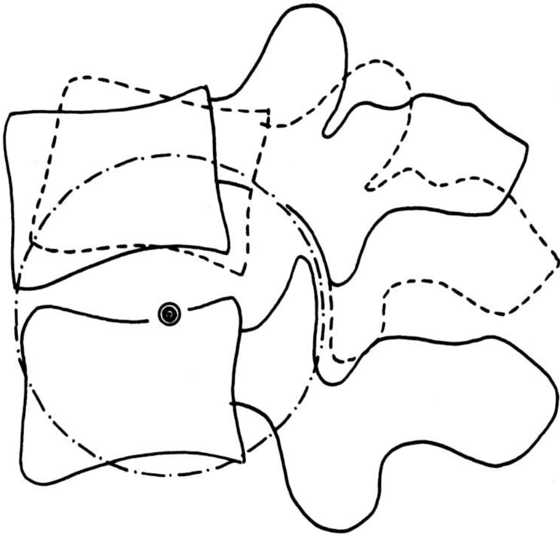

Fig. 2-9. Movement diagram L4–L5. Flexion–extension movement diagram of lumbar region L4–L5 with center of motion in mean location. Circle drawn through apophyseal joint spaces. Orientation of joints opposes horizontal motion (translation) of upper vertebra. In contrast to the gliding motion C2–C3, this is a tilting motion.

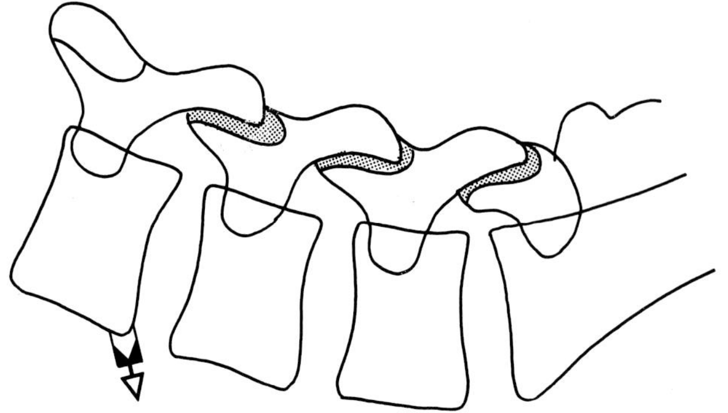

Fig. 2-10. Apophyseal joints protect discs against overloading. Lateral view shows lumbar spine in subject bending forward to lift load. Ventral gliding of cranial vertebrae on caudal vertebrae is impeded by roof-tile arrangement of articular processes.

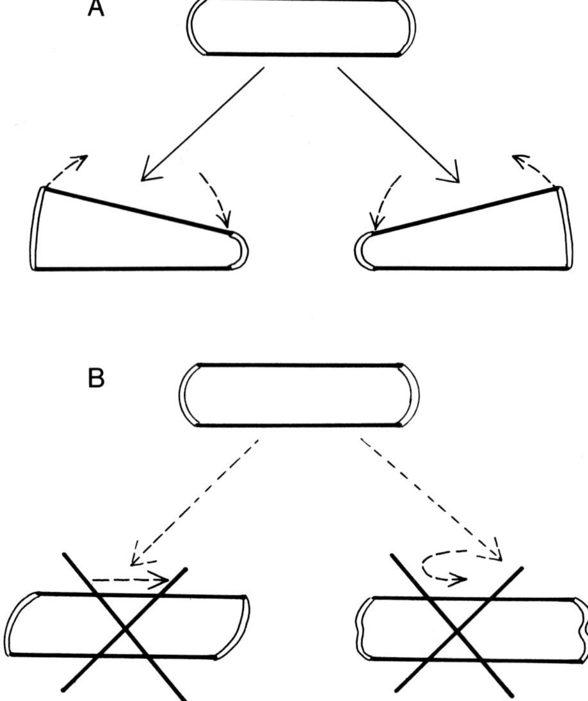

Fig. 2-11. Function of lumbar, or archetype, disc. (*A*) Schematic drawing of lumbar disc, which allows tilting (*i.e.*, flexion–extension in the sagittal plane, or lateral flexion in the frontal plane). Center of motion is in or close to the disc. (*B*) Translatory movement of vertebral end-plates (*left*) or rotation (*right*) is practically impossible (in cadaver experiments 1 to 2 mm, and 1° to 2°, respectively[18]).

limited, although not entirely prohibited. It should be stated here that research has concentrated mainly on lumbar discs and that in general the lumbar disc serves as a true representative of this anatomic structure. In fact, the lumbar disc most resembles the Greek athletic attribute it is named after.

Tilting of the normal (lumbar) disc is promoted by bulging of the fibrous anulus. Trying to obtain a workable model of a disc, I took two rounded and thin rigid plates, drew a rubber band around them, and filled the structure with water. It was virtually impossible to tilt one plate with respect to the other. This was ascribed to the absence of bulging of the rubber band, that is, the absence of overlength to allow unilateral increase in distance between the vertebral end-plates, which is essential for tilting motion. In a comparable model with a bulging band (Fig. 2-11), tilting was easily performed.

The severe limitation of rotation and translation is ascribed to the course of the anular fibers.[6] As soon as these movements occur, the fibers running in the direction of motion are stretched, preventing any further motion. Interestingly, Rolander[18] observed that as rotation occurs in the normal disc, the distance between the end-plates increases. It is tempting to speculate that this increase is due to stretching of anular fibers, which results in the decrease of anular bulge and hence in the decrease of the transverse diameter of the disc.

Archetype Disc and Its Pattern of Motion

If the lumbar disc, owing to its relatively simple gross-anatomic structure resembling the historical quoit, is considered the archetype of intervertebral body connection, its pattern of motion may likewise be considered the archetype of vertebral motion. Motion of the archetype disc is limited to the sagittal plane (flexion, extension) and the frontal plane (lateral flexion to the right and to the left). Rotation (in the axial transverse plane) is absent or minimal.

Comparative anatomic data support the conclusion that in the dog[12,15] and other quadrupeds both the movement of the cervical and the lumbar discs resembles that of the archetype disc. In an anesthetized dog the author measured a lateral flexion C2–C7 of 150°, both sides together. In the adult human spine this is about 70°.[14] Rotation from C2–C5 in the dog is absent (Fig. 2-12) and from C5 to C7 minimal.

According to the literature[10] and our own radiographic study,[16] rotation in the human cervical

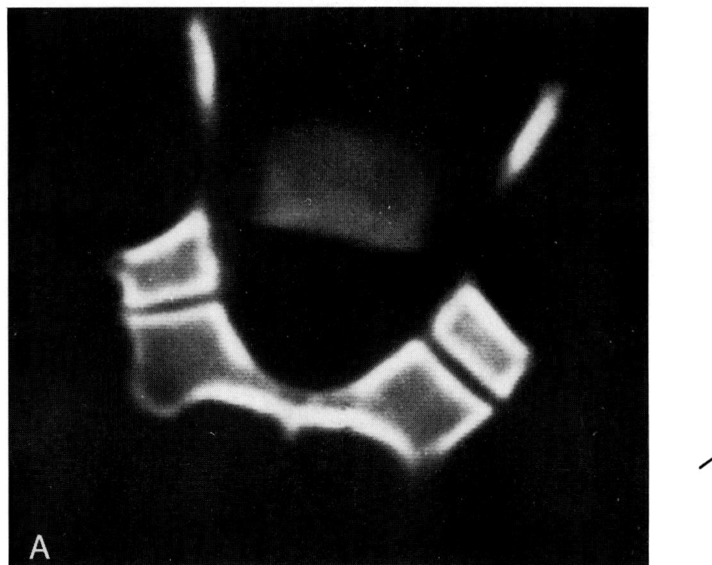

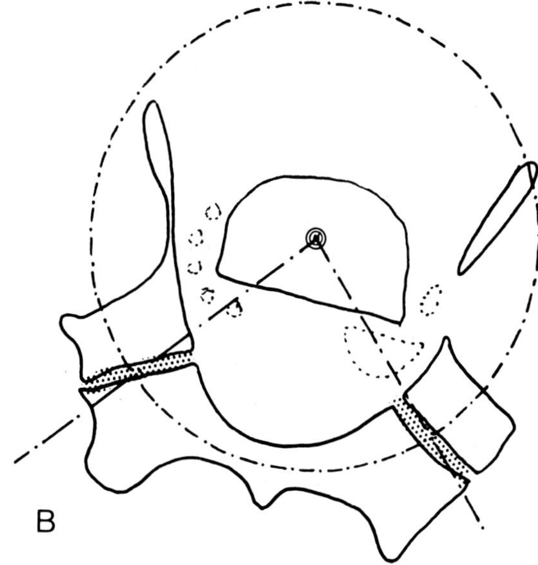

Fig. 2-12. Radial orientation of cervical joint spaces. (*A*) CT section shows C3–C4 region in cadaver dog spine. (*B*) Schematic drawing of CT section. Orientation of joint spaces (*shaded*) is radial with respect to center of disc. Circle through this center crosses joint spaces perpendicularly.

spine C2–C7 is considerable (Table 2-1). Compared with the archetype cervical disc of the dog, the human cervical disc has a markedly reduced faculty of lateral flexion, which at the same time has obligatorily been coupled with rotation.

If the disc plays an important role in determining the pattern of motion, it is to be expected that the human cervical disc will differ markedly in anatomic structure from the human lumbar disc, or from the archetype disc in general.

Cervical Disc, Uncovertebral Joints, and Rotation

In 1858 Luschka[9] described the jointlike formations lateral to the cervical discs, bordered laterally by the uncinate processes of the caudal vertebral bodies, and medially by the corresponding hollowings (*échancrures*) in the caudolateral aspects of the cranial vertebral bodies (Fig. 2-13). He suggested that these joints (here to be called uncovertebral joints) allowed the cervical disc a larger amount of freedom of movement.

Table 2-1. Mobility of Cervical Spine of Young Adults without Disc Degeneration

	Flexion–Extension[1]		Lateral Flexion[2]	Rotation[3]	
	Average	Range		Average	Range
Occiput–C1	15°	4° to 23°	5° (Occiput–C1 and C1–C2)	1°	−2° to 5°
C1–C2	13°	7° to 20°		41°	29° to 46°
C2–C3	12°	5° to 16°	35° (C2–C7)	3°	0° to 10°
C3–C4	18°	13° to 26°		6°	3° to 10°
C4–C5	20°	15° to 29°		7°	1° to 12°
C5–C6	20°	16° to 29°		7°	2° to 12°
C6–C7	15°	6° to 25°		5°	2° to 10°

[1] 20 subjects
[2] 5 subjects
[3] 26 subjects

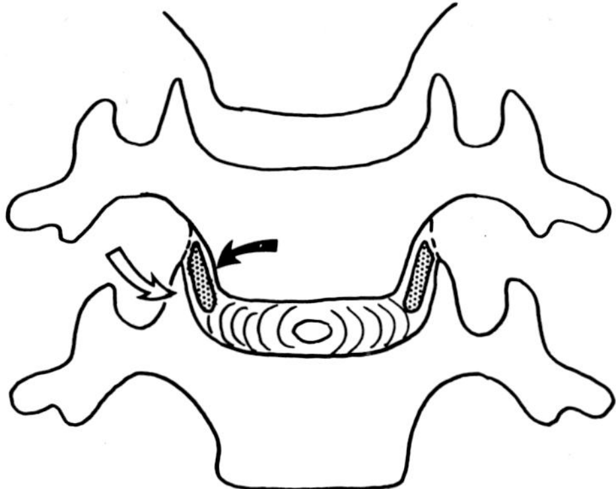

Fig. 2-13. Luschka's joints. Drawing after original illustration of Luschka.[9] Joints (film) are bordered caudolaterally by uncinate processes (*open arrow*) and craniomedially by their hollowed counterparts (échancrures, *dark arrow*). Caudomedially, joints are bordered by cervical disc.

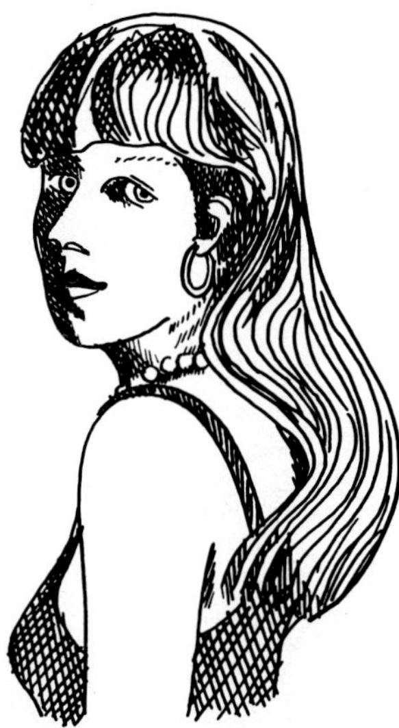

Fig. 2-15. Biped looking backward. To look backward biped rotates neck along longitudinal axis.

In a monograph dealing with Luschka's joints Hall[4] suggests that these joints in the human neck serve especially the purpose of rotation. In quadrupeds such rotation is not necessary because to look about them these mammals use lateral flexion of the neck (Fig. 2-14). Looking about takes place in the horizontal plane, and in quadrupeds this corresponds more or less to the frontal plane, or plane of lateral flexion, of their more or less horizontally oriented necks. In the human upright position the horizontal plane corresponds with the transverse plane, or plane of rotation, of the more or less vertically oriented cervical spine (Fig. 2-15).

In a comparative anatomic investigation of dried cervical vertebrae Hall established that uncinate processes are not only present in humans, but also in other primates, as well as in rodents and marsupials. All these species are obligatory or facultative bipeds, needing rotation of their necks to look about when in an upright position. I agree with Hall that, although in dried specimens the presence of uncovertebral joints cannot be verified, it is reasonable to assume their presence when uncinate processes are found.

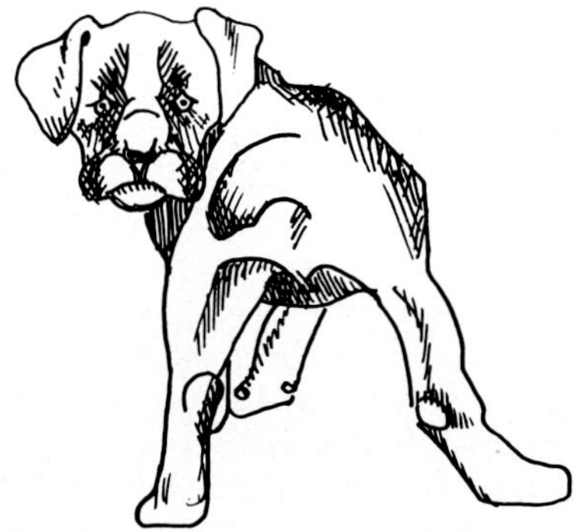

Fig. 2-14. Quadruped looking backward. To look backward, quadruped flexes neck laterally.

Speculating on the relationship between uncinate processes and uncovertebral joints on one hand, and rotation on the other hand, Hall suggests that the cervical disc in bipeds is in the process of developing back into a ball-and-socket joint, as is found in the cervical spines of birds.

Functional Anatomy of Apophyseal Joint Plane

We reasoned that the coupled motions of rotation and lateral flexion in the human spine are difficult to study in the conventional frontal and transverse planes. However, in the plane of apophyseal joints, the coupled motion is reduced to one motion around an axis more or less perpendicular to this plane (Fig. 2-16). Sections in this plane should best reflect anatomic morphology related to rotation, and possibly vizualize ball-and-socket joint–like configurations. Such sections are presented in Figure 2-17.

These sections indeed show some interesting anatomic details. More dorsally, the disc actually approximates the form of a ball-and-socket joint, the uncinate processes acting as rims of an *acetabulum,* into which the rounded shape of the cranial vertebral body fits. The height of the dorsal part of the disc between the uncovertebral joints is rather

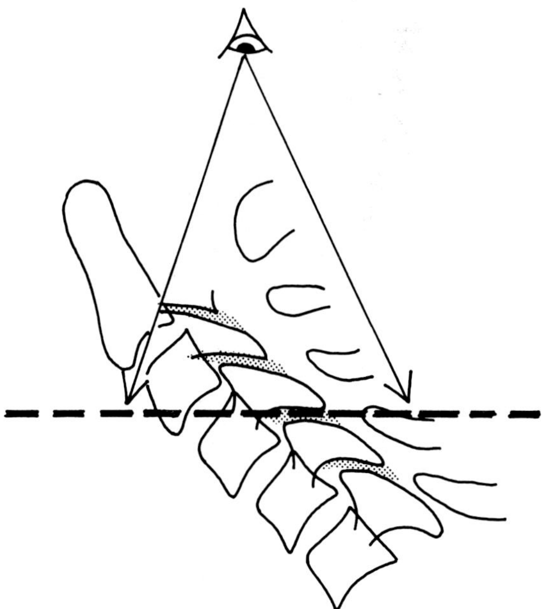

Fig. 2-16. Joint-plane view. Schematic drawing of lateral radiograph shows cervical spine with plane of section parallel to plane of apophyseal joints (*interrupted line*). Direction of observation is perpendicular to these planes (*arrows*). In the joint plane, rotation between cervical vertebrae is theoretically maximal.

small, adding to the suggestion of a complete diarthrotic joint. More ventrally, the disc assumes normal height. At the most ventral end the disc resembles the archetype disc, vertebral end-plates having become flat and unciform processes having nearly completely disappeared.

In sections perpendicular to the apophyseal joint plane (Fig. 2-18) rotation, theoretically, will be nil, which is reflected by the anatomic morphology (Fig. 2-19). The apophyseal joint spaces are more or less in line, opposing any rotation in this plane.

Axis of Rotation in Apophyseal Joint Plane: Coupling of Lateral Flexion and Rotation

In an attempt to define an axis of rotation for the apophyseal joint plane we obtained consecutive CT sections of human subjects in this plane (Fig. 2-20). In each of these sections, circles were drawn through the uncovertebral joint spaces in such a way that motion around the center points of these circles would guarantee parallel displacement of the uncovertebral joint planes, as in diarthrotic joints. Subsequently, the midpoints of these circles were transferred to the corresponding sections projected on a schematic drawing of a lateral radiograph of the cervical spine. The line connecting these points represents the axis of motion. Although the method used is not very accurate (drawing of the circles is, within limits, somewhat arbitrary), it gives an idea of the location and direction of such an axis. From the drawing it is evident that the axis runs more or less perpendicular with respect to the plane of the apophyseal joints, which is to be expected.

Although only one type of motion is permitted by this axis (rotation in the apophyseal joint plane), this motion is manifested in the frontal plane as lateral flexion, and in the transverse plane as rotation. It is interesting that from this point of view, coupling of lateral flexion and rotation results not from the oblique orientation of the apophyseal joints but from the oblique orientation of the axis of motion, which in turn is determined by the orientation of the uncovertebral joints. This supports the assumption that the disc determines the pattern of motion independently of the apophyseal joints. Because the unciform processes are not derived from the vertebral body, but from the vertebral arch,[21] the notion of *disc* should be enlarged to *disc and adjoining structures.*

In Figure 2-21 another method is shown to construct an axis of rotation. A CT section through the intervertebral joint plane was made with the subject supine and the head maximally rotated to the left. By superimposition of this image on a mirrored image (simulating rotation to the right) centers of rotation motion were determined and transferred to a schematic drawing of a lateral radiograph of the cervical spine. The result is comparable to that of Figure 2-20. Of course, these are incidental observations that are not very accurate and not related to any specific segment between C2 and T1, but that provide more insight into patterns of motion of the cervical spine.

Lysell[10] defined a center (not an axis) of motion which virtually did not move during rotation or lateral flexion of the cervical spine. It was located in the anterior contour of the vertebral body, where his radiographic landmarks were placed. The other landmarks, placed in the articular processes and spinous processes, moved around this center during lateral flexion or rotation (Fig. 2-22). It is understandable that Lysell could not define an axis of motion, because only the anterior landmarks were in the path of this axis. The importance of his finding is that in rotation of the head, rotation of the cervical spine C2–T1 is larger than the coupled lateral flexion, and, conversely, that upon lateral flexion of the head, lateral flexion C2–T1 is larger than the coupled rotation. This

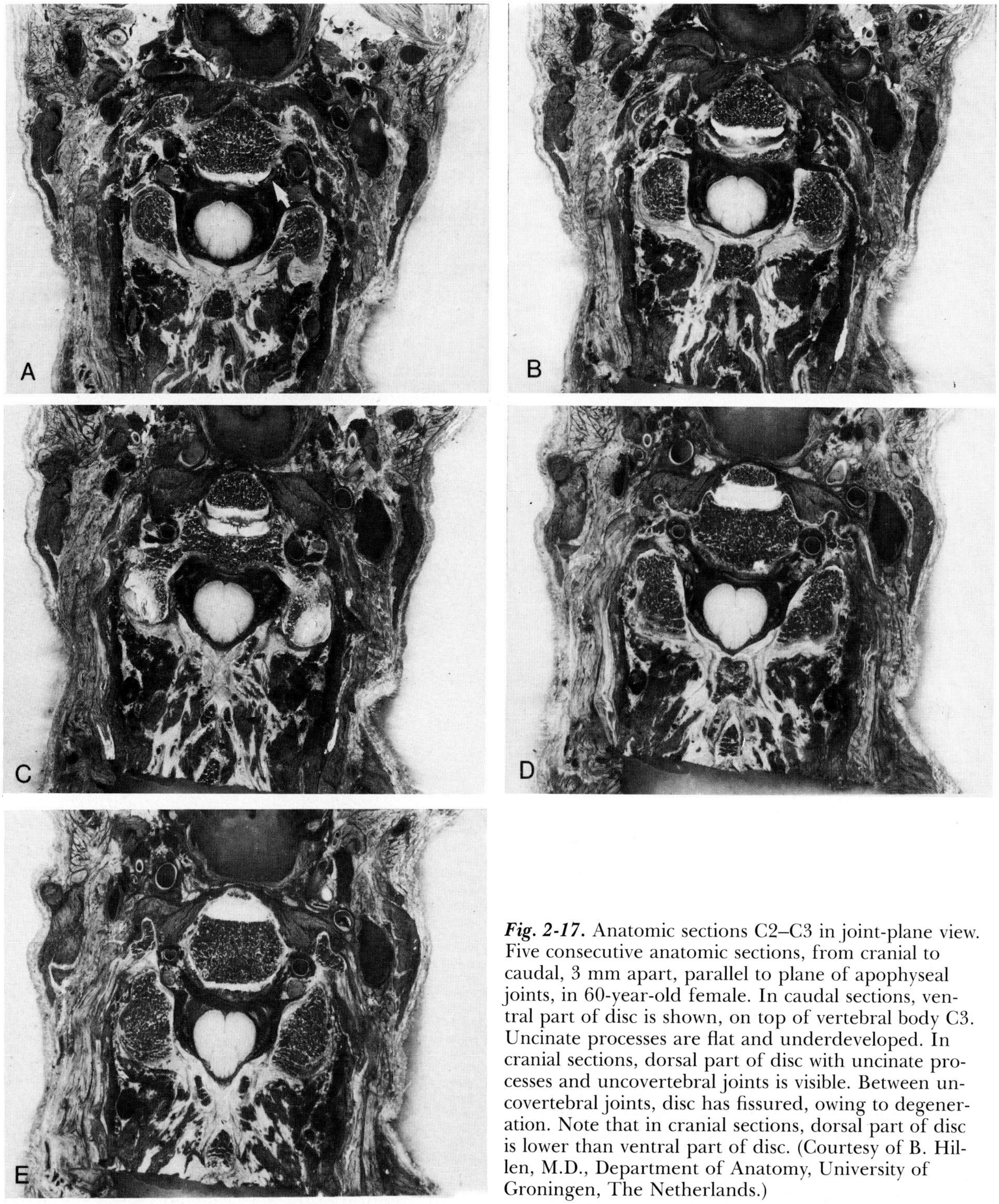

A

B

C

D

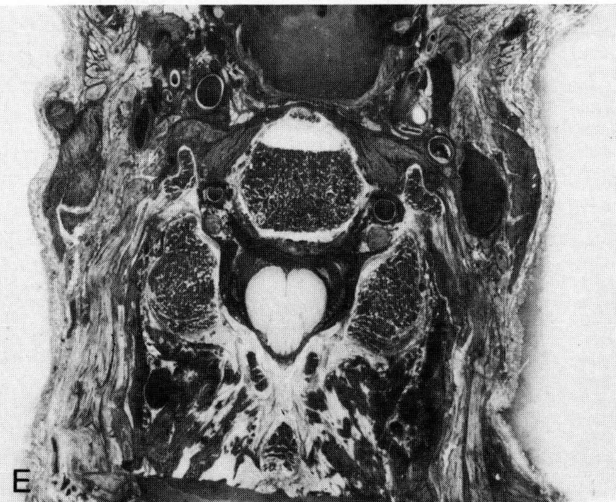

Fig. 2-17. Anatomic sections C2–C3 in joint-plane view. Five consecutive anatomic sections, from cranial to caudal, 3 mm apart, parallel to plane of apophyseal joints, in 60-year-old female. In caudal sections, ventral part of disc is shown, on top of vertebral body C3. Uncinate processes are flat and underdeveloped. In cranial sections, dorsal part of disc with uncinate processes and uncovertebral joints is visible. Between uncovertebral joints, disc has fissured, owing to degeneration. Note that in cranial sections, dorsal part of disc is lower than ventral part of disc. (Courtesy of B. Hillen, M.D., Department of Anatomy, University of Groningen, The Netherlands.)

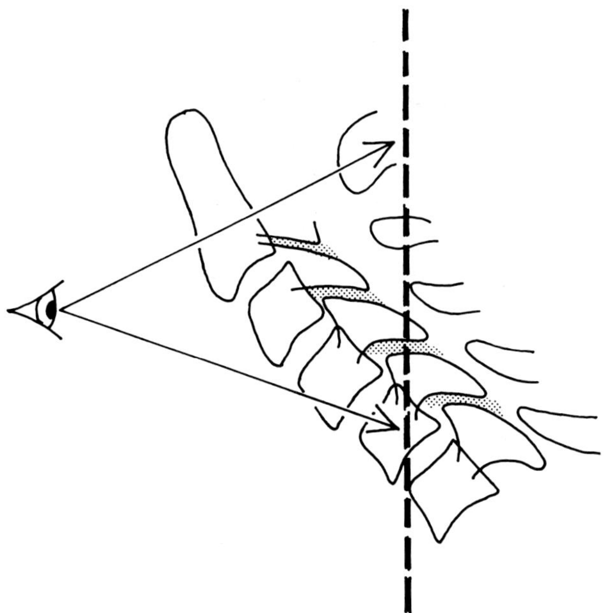

Fig. 2-18. Joint-space view. Plane of section (*interrupted line*) is perpendicular to plane of apophyseal joints. If viewed from the front (*arrows*) joint spaces will be visible. Theoretically, rotation between cervical vertebrae in this plane is nil.

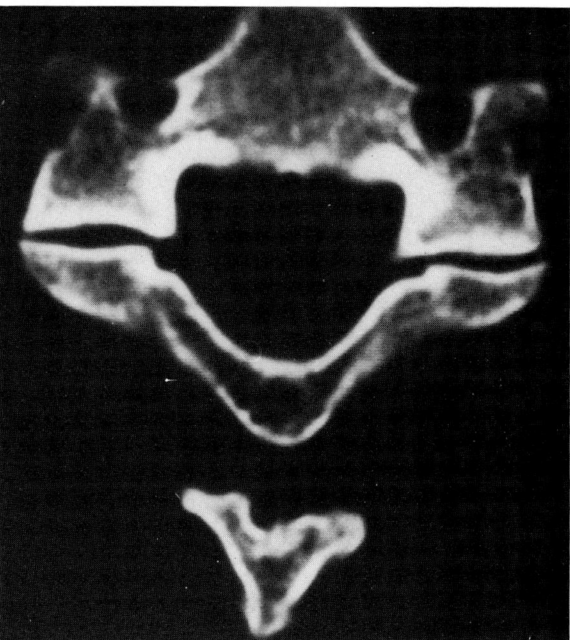

Fig. 2-19. CT section C4–C5 in joint-space view. CT section perpendicular to plane of apophyseal joints. Apophyseal joint spaces are approximately in line, indicating that rotation between vertebral bodies in this plane is impossible.

indicates that the axis for rotation/lateral flexion may assume different angulations with respect to Lysell's center of motion: in lateral flexion of the head it is toward the transverse plane, and in rotation, toward the frontal plane (Fig. 2-22).

Uncinate Processes and Rotation

As shown in Figure 2-17, the uncinate processes rise relatively high above the vertebral body dorsally but are rather flat, or absent, ventrally. The ventral part of the cervical disc thus resembles the archetype disc. This is reflected by the location of the center of rotation and lateral flexion motion in the sections presented in Figure 2-20: near the disc in the ventral sections, far from the disc in the more dorsal sections.

Figure 2-23 presents another method of clarifying the role of the uncinate processes in producing coupling of rotation and lateral flexion. In the archetype disc, lateral flexion produces some lateral translation into the direction of motion. If this type of motion is attempted in the presence of uncinate processes, the cranial vertebra abuts against the uncinate process of the caudal vertebra. To avoid this, the cranial vertebra must translate contralaterally to the direction of lateral flexion. As a result, lateral translation occurs in opposite directions ventrally and dorsally, which means rotation takes place. The primary function of lateral flexion in the archetype disc is therefore transformed into lateral flexion coupled with rotation, owing to the presence of uncinate processes on the dorsal half of the lateral aspects of the cervical disc.

Figure 2-24 represents the archetype disc and the cervical disc, with their two main axes of motion, in three-dimensional form. In the ideal archetype disc, the two axes of motion intersect at the level of the disc and are situated in the transverse plane (Spalteholz[19]). The cervical disc is saddle-shaped with the flexion–extension axis caudal to the disc, and the oblique rotation–lateral flexion axis is cranial to the disc.

Comparing these types, we see that in the cervical disc the axis of lateral flexion has been tilted obliquely with the hinge at the anterior aspect of the disc. The axis of flexion–extension has not changed its direction, but it is displaced caudally. Typical of the saddle-shaped joint (to which the cervical disc may be better compared than a ball-and-socket joint) is that the two axes of motion

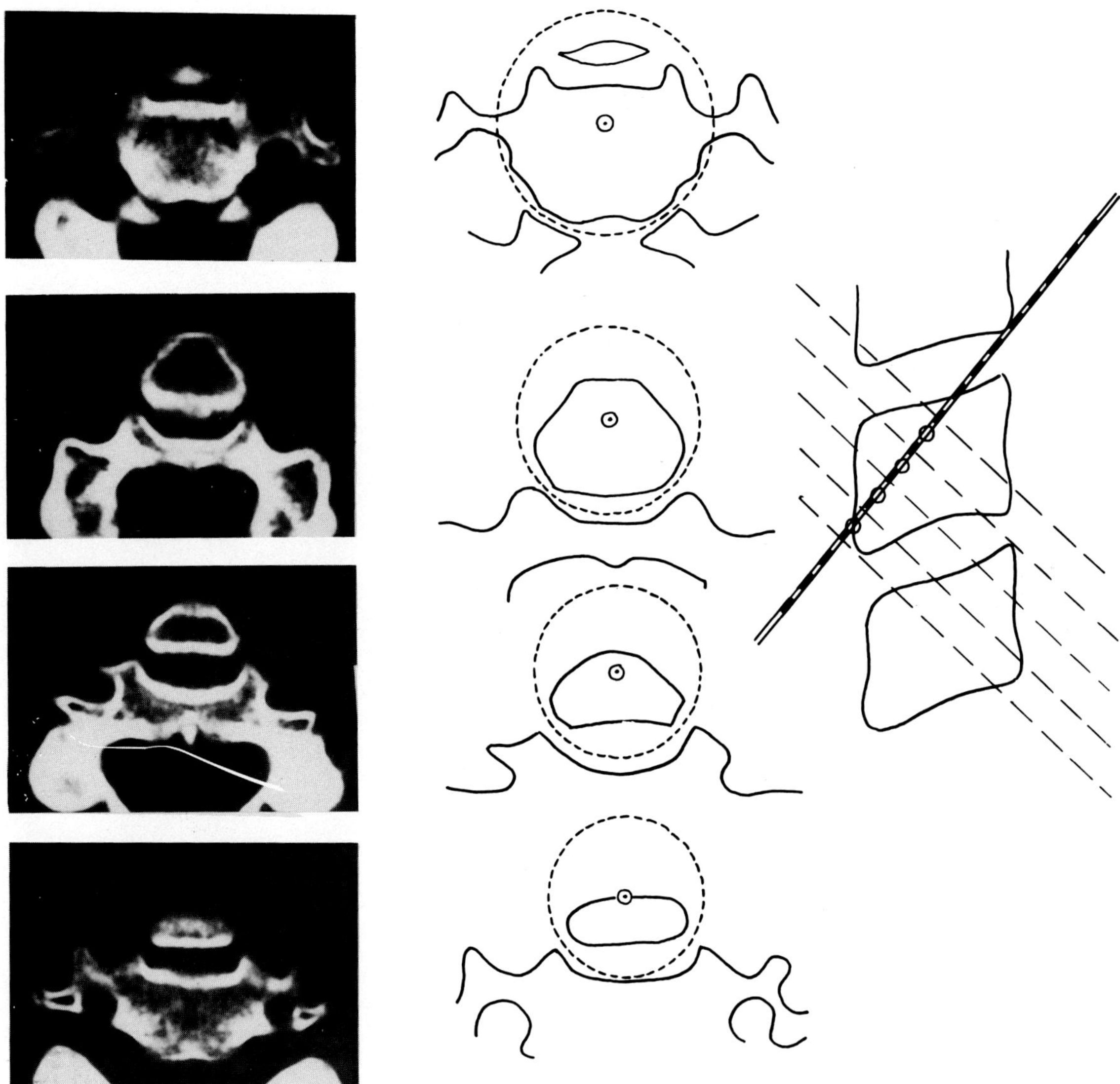

Fig. 2-20. Construction of axis for rotation/lateral flexion. (*Left row*) Images of CT slices are parallel to plane of intervertebral joints. (*Middle row*) Schematic drawings of the images. Circles have been drawn through uncovertebral joints. Centers of these circles are considered to correspond to centers of motion for uncovertebral joints. Centers are transferred to lateral radiograph showing corresponding CT levels, and are connected by line that is considered instantaneous axis of rotational motion, in this case between C2 and C3.

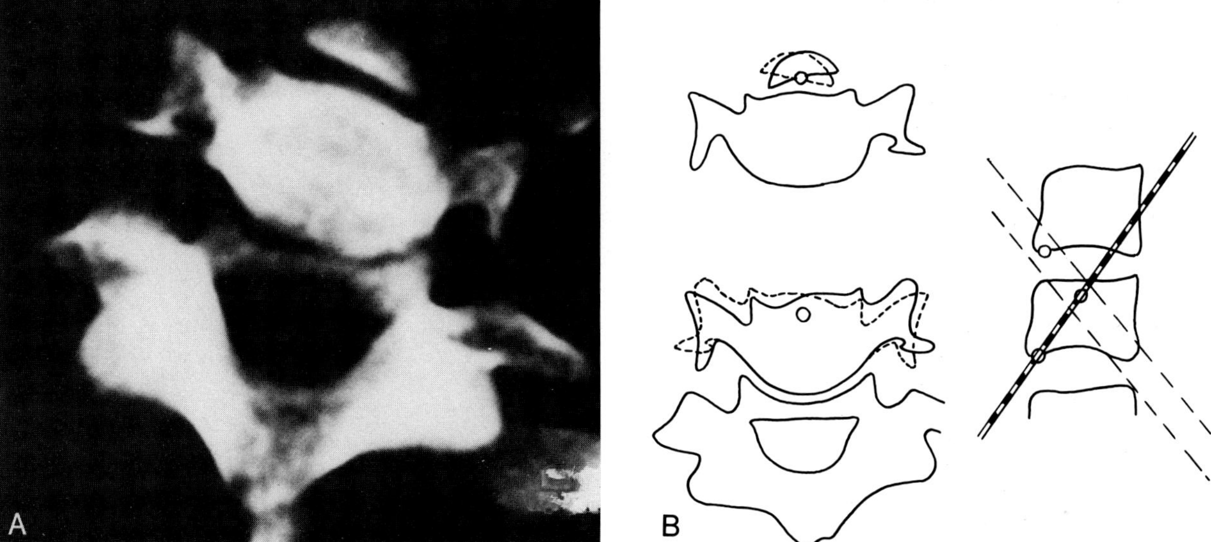

Fig. 2-21. Another construction of axis for rotation/lateral flexion. (*A*) CT section through plane of apophyseal joints is at level C5–C7. Subject has turned head maximally to left. Uppermost vertebra is C5, middle vertebra is C6 and lower vertebra is C7. B, *left,* Schematic drawing of C5 (*interrupted line*) and C6. Image of C5 has also been mirrored (*drawn line*) to allow construction of center of motion. B, *right,* Schematic drawing of C6 and C7, C6 also in mirrored position. Construction of center of motion. Centers of motion are transferred to right row: drawing of lateral radiograph of cervical spine C5–C7 with levels of CT sections. Centers are connected by line that represents axis of motion C6–C7 (center of C5–C6 motion has been transferred to C6–C7).

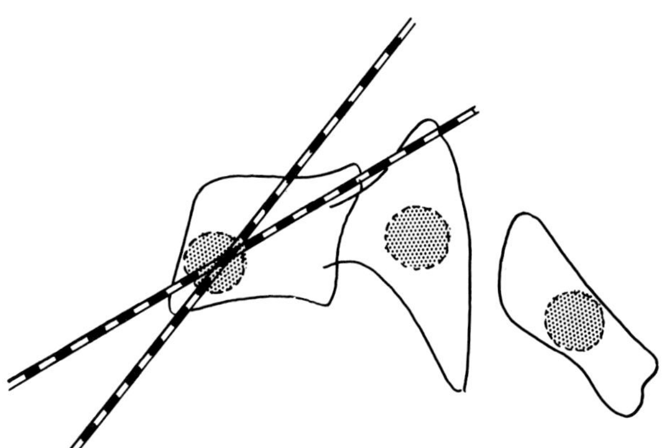

Fig. 2-22. Lysell's center of rotation and lateral flexion. In his radiographic method to study motion, Lysell placed metal balls in vertebrae of cadaver specimens: in anterior contour of vertebral body, in articular processes and in spinous processes. Shaded areas indicate sites of placement. Interrupted lines are axes of rotation and lateral flexion, as constructed in Figures 2-20 and 2-21. On basis of findings of Lysell one may expect axis to run more vertically in rotation of head, and more horizontally in lateral flexion, as indicated in this figure.

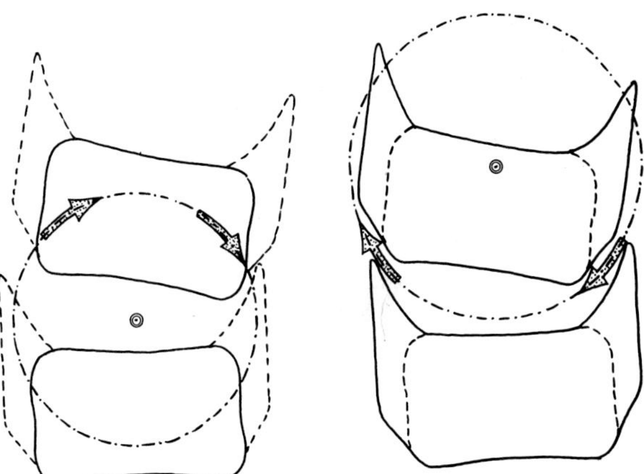

Fig. 2-23. Uncinate process and rotation. (*Left*) Lateral flexion in prototype disc is shown. Center of motion is in disc. If uncinate processes were present (*interrupted lines*) they would abut against each other. (*Right*) Lateral flexion in presence of uncinate processes is shown. To obtain smooth gliding motion at uncovertebral joints, center of motion is displaced cranially.

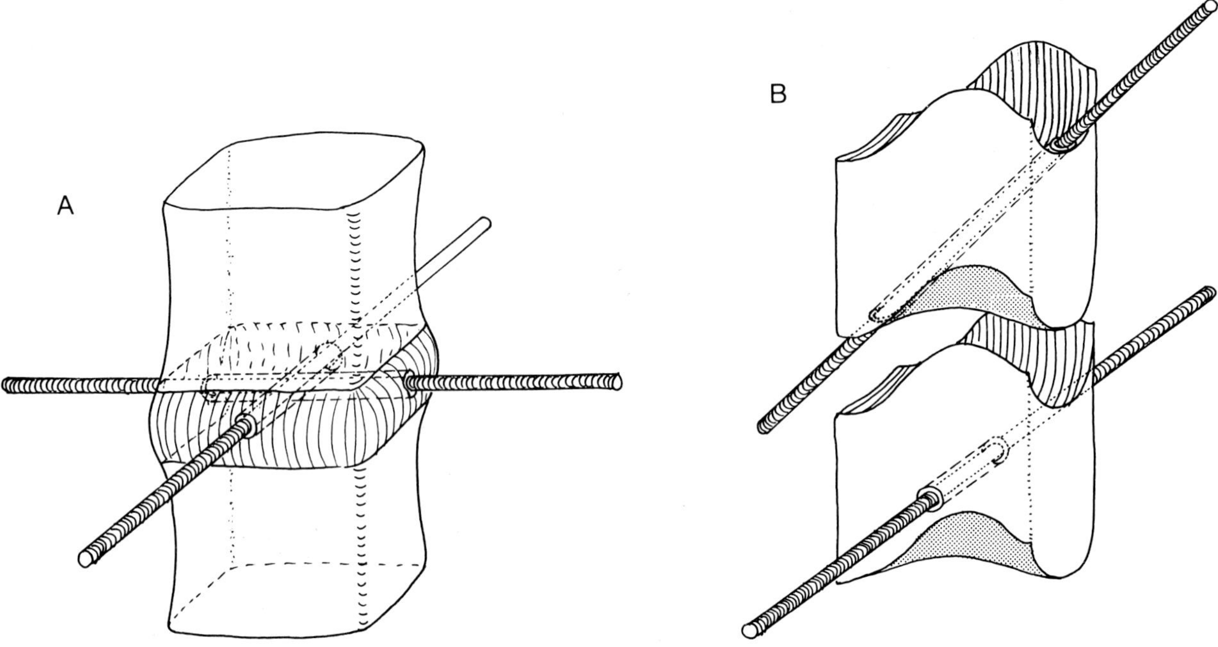

Fig. 2-24. Axes of motion in archetype disc and in human cervical disc. (*A*) Archetype disc with axes of flexion–extension and lateral flexion motion, which intersect at center of disc.[19] (*B*) Human cervical disc. The upper axis is for rotation/lateral flexion, the lower axis for flexion–extension (left lateral and slightly dorsal views).

have a perpendicular course and are situated on opposite sides of the joint[5] (compare the ellipsoid atlantooccipital joint in Fig. 2-28).

Functional Anatomic Adaptation of the Disc During Childhood

Töndury[21] has shown that at birth the uncinate processes are flat, and uncovertebral joint spaces are absent. In the course of childhood the processes are erected, and the uncovertebral joints are gradually formed by tissue-splitting. The adult cervical disc, with its faculty of rotation, thus develops from a more archetypical disc that, at least in the adult, cannot rotate. However, there are no indications that the patterns of motion of the neck in children differ from those in adults. The orientation of the apophyseal joint spaces in both is the same. Inspection of anatomic specimens of three fetuses (8 months old), three newborns and two children (2.5 years old), revealed a mean value of orientation of the apophyseal joints with respect to the transverse plane of 39°, as compared with the radiologically measured mean value of 38° in 38 adults, aged 15 to 75 years. Gliding movements of the cervical vertebrae during flexion–extension, especially at C2–C3 and C3–C4, are a normal phenomenon in the infant spine.[11] Coupling of lateral flexion with rotation is likewise expected as the result of the orientation of the apophyseal joints, although experimental evidence is lacking.

How can it be explained that the cervical disc in the young child, despite its more archetypical anatomy, follows the same pattern of motion as the adult cervical disc? Why does the adult cervical disc have such a different anatomic shape? According to anatomic textbooks,[20] the disc in children is highly elastic and compressible. With increasing age, its elasticity gradually diminishes. Due to its high elasticity the young cervical disc will be able to follow the pattern of motion prescribed by the apophyseal joints, that is, gliding movements of midcervical vertebrae during flexion–extension, and coupling of lateral flexion with rotation. With age, as elasticity of the disc decreases and loading of the spine increases, it is increasingly difficult for the disc to meet the demands of the apophyseal joints. To protect the disc, and preserve the patterns of motion, the uncinate processes are erected and the uncovertebral joints formed. They serve as guides helping the vertebral bodies to follow the motions prescribed by the apophyseal joints. This process of anatomic remodeling of the structures adjoining the cervical disc Töndbury calls "functional adaptation."[21]

Once the functional adaptation is completed, the disc and adjoining structures will be capable of performing the patterns of motion prescribed by the apophyseal joints independently of these joints. However, experimental work is necessary for further evidence that in the cervical spine, as in the lumbar spine (Rolander[18]), removal of the apophyseal joints will not affect the pattern of motion of the (normal) disc.

Analogy Between Uncovertebral and Costovertebral Joints

Luschka drew attention to resemblance between the uncovertebral and costovertebral joints. Because he considered the uncinate process the analogon of a costal head, he called this process eminentia costaria. Trolard[22] noted the absence of a joint cavity in the costovertebral joints at birth, and for an indefinite time thereafter. Commenting on this observation, Hall[4] refers to this delayed conversion of an amphiarthrosis (fibrocartilaginous joint) to a diarthrosis (synovial joint) as being strikingly similar to the postnatal development of the uncovertebral joints. In his own anatomic investigations, he noted that the costovertebral joints are created by fissuring in an already differentiated fibrous tissue. Hall speculates that the movements of the ribs are responsible for this fissuring.

Anatomically, the comparison is not entirely correct. In studying ossification centers Töndury[21] noted that those of the uncinate processes, present in the two upper thoracic vertebrae, are different from those of the first and second costal heads. Testud and Latarjet[20] pointed out that the comparison between uncovertebral and costovertebral joints is only valid for the superior parts of the costovertebral joints (Fig. 2-25). However, these anatomic differences need not detract from the assumption that the strikingly similar developments in the final creation of both the diarthrotic uncovertebral and costovertebral joints are the expression of functional adaptation to the patterns of motion prescribed by the apophyseal joints. As in the cervical spine, rotation in the thoracic spine is considerable (about 8° per segment between T1 and T8, both sides together[24–26]). It is not surprising, therefore, that in the thoracic spine, comparable, although not anatomically identical, adaptations of the disc and surrounding tissues are found to maintain specific motion after childhood.

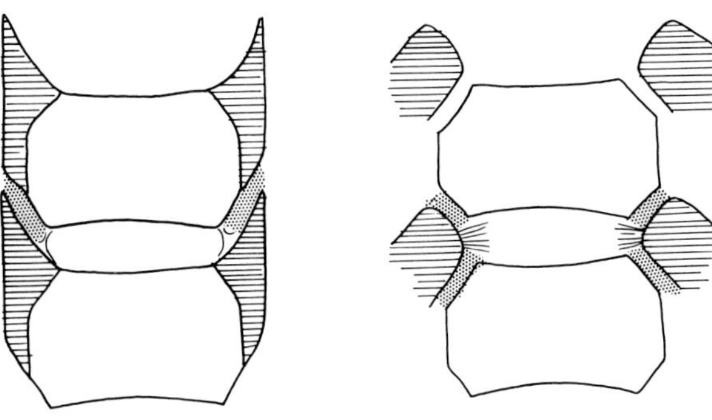

Fig. 2-25. Analogy between uncovertebral and costovertebral joints. (*Left*) A–P view of two cervical vertebrae with disc and uncovertebral joints. It is evident that analogy with uncovertebral joints is limited to cranial parts of costovertebral joints (*right*).

CRANIOVERTEBRAL REGION

Characteristic Anatomic Features

Characteristic anatomic features of the craniovertebral region are as follows: (1) absence of discs with instead synostosis between bodies of C1 and C2, and ligamentous connection between body of C1 (odontoid process) and basiocciput (alar and apical dental ligaments, tectorial membrane); (2) presence of atlas, articulating with occiput (atlantooccipital joints), axis (atlantoaxial joints) and odontoid process (in ring formed by anterior arch of atlas and transverse ligament).

Owing to the absence of a disc and the presence of a purely ligamentous connection between axis and occiput, the axis would have very large freedom of movement in all directions if the atlas were removed. The function of the atlas, it seems, is to stabilize the axis and control its movements with respect to the occiput (Fig. 2-26).

Atlantooccipital Joints

The atlantooccipital joints are relatively stable joints due to the marked rounding and congruence of their joint surfaces. They allow flexion and extension, and to a far lesser degree lateral flexion, but virtually no rotation (Table 2-1). The centers of flexion–extension and lateral flexion motion are shown in Figure 2-27.

The virtual absence of rotation is explained by anatomists[19] by the ellipsoid form of the joints. Comparative anatomy reveals that the faculty of rotation between atlas and occiput likewise is virtually absent in the dog and other mammals. The function of the atlantooccipital connection perhaps is best demonstrated in a schematic drawing of Werne[27] (Fig. 2-28). It clearly shows that the two

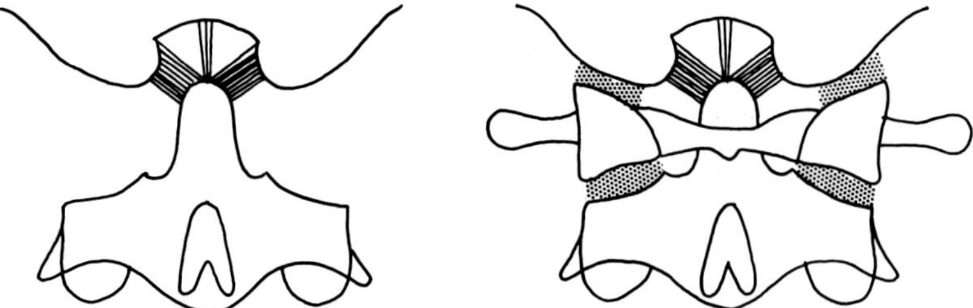

Fig. 2-26. Atlas as interposed bearing between occiput and axis vertebra. (*Left*) A–P projection of occiput and axis with alar ligaments and apical dental ligament. Without atlas, axis vertebra has large freedom of movement with respect to occiput. (*Right*) Atlas interposed to control motion between occiput and axis vertebra. Shaded areas indicate atlantooccipital and atlantoaxial joints.

axes of motion are on the same side of the atlantooccipital joints, whereas in a saddle joint they are on opposite sides (Fig. 2-24).

Atlantoaxial Joints

The atlantoaxial joints are unstable joints due to their opposed convexity with small contact area between the joint surfaces. This is necessary in order for the joint to perform movements in all directions: flexion–extension, lateral flexion, and rotation (Table 2-1). Stability between atlas and axis is dependent upon the transverse ligament. Its rupture or slackening causes atlantoaxial luxation with approximation of odontoid process and posterior atlantal arch. In practice, this approximation is halted half way, because on one hand the odontoid process is tethered by the alar ligaments, and on the other hand the atlas is kept in place by the atlantooccipital joints.

Lateral Flexion

Lateral flexion in the occipitoatlantoaxial complex is best studied by following the movement of the atlas with respect to the occiput during lateral flexion of the axis. The atlas moves laterally into the direction of lateral flexion (Fig. 2-29), which is understandable considering the triangular shape of the lateral atlantal masses. Conversely, if the atlas is pushed laterally, the head will incline into the same direction with respect to the axis.

Lateral flexion of the head is uncommon in daily life. However, it plays an important role in rotation of the head (Fig. 2-30). Because during C2–T1 rotation the axis vertebra is laterally flexed, the head is kept erect by contralateral flexion of the occipitoatlantoaxial complex. If, for instance, the head is maximally turned to the left (Fig. 2-29, top), the axis is laterally flexed to the left and the head must flex laterally to the right to remain in the horizontal plane. At the same time, the head rotates upon the axis to the left (or the axis rotates to the right with respect to the head). If the head is flexed laterally, for example, to the left, contrarotation of the occiput on the axis (to the right) compensates the rotation of the axis (to the left) caused by C2–T1 lateral flexion.

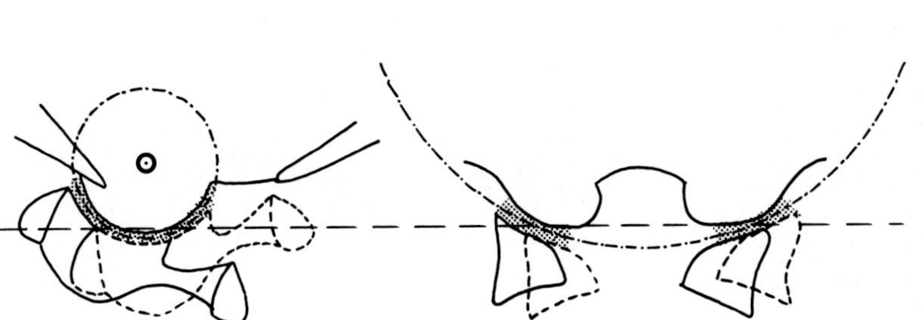

Fig. 2-27. Atlantooccipital movement diagrams. (*Left*) Flexion–extension diagram (*drawn line:* flexion; *interrupted line:* extension) with center of motion, forming circle passing through atlantooccipital joints (*shaded area*). (*Right*) Lateral flexion diagram with center of motion forming circle passing through atlantooccipital joints.

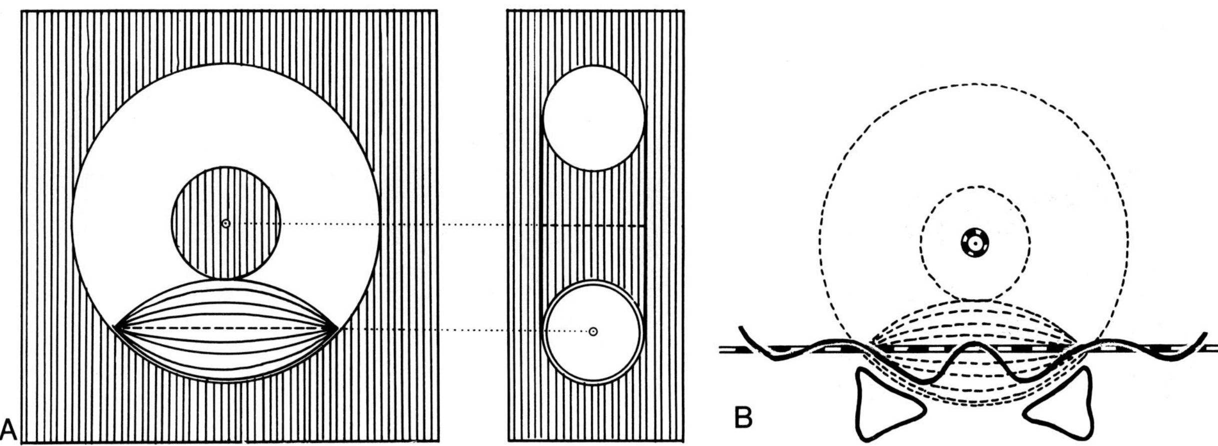

Fig. 2-28. Conceptual structure of Werne to demonstrate movement at atlantooccipital joints. (*A*) Werne[27] compared possibilities of movement in atlantooccipital joints with those of fusiform body within anular tube. Such movement cannot be directed by ligaments and is consequently function of shape of joints. Model (*left,* frontal view; *right,* lateral view) shows that rotation at atlantooccipital joints is impossible. (*B*) Simplified scheme of model of Werne shows atlantooccipital joints (in A–P projection) superimposed. To understand motion, assume occiput is fixed to fusiform body, and atlas to anular tube.

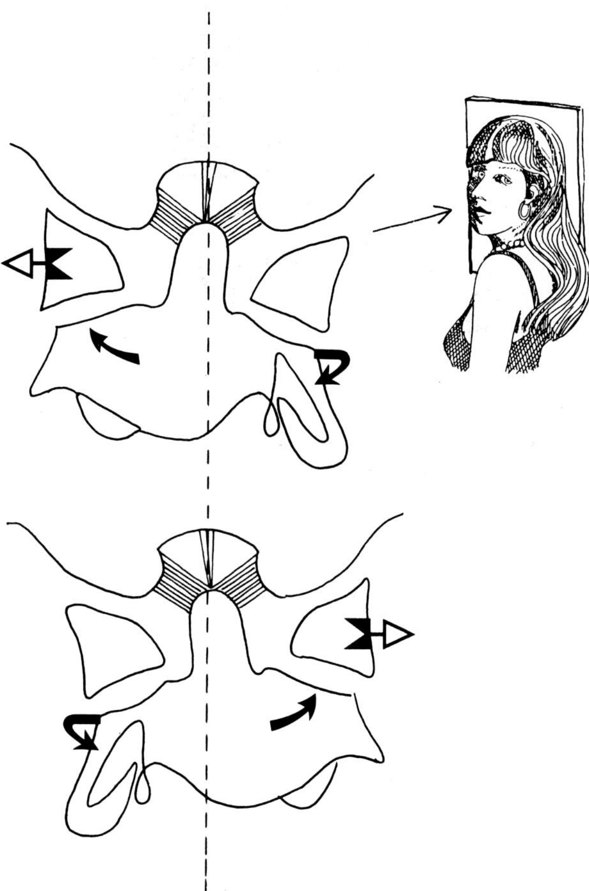

Fig. 2-29. Lateral flexion, occiput-axis. Atlas and occiput are shown in A–P projection. Axis vertebra is laterally flexed and rotated. (*Top*) Lateral flexion to right. This motion is produced by rotation of head maximally to left (direction of x-rays and position of film indicated). With respect to head, axis is rotated to right (*small arrows*). Owing to lateral flexion of axis, atlas moves to right (*large arrow*). (*Bottom*) Lateral flexion between occiput and axis to left. Motion is produced by rotation of head maximally to right. With respect to head, axis is rotated to left. Atlas moves to left.

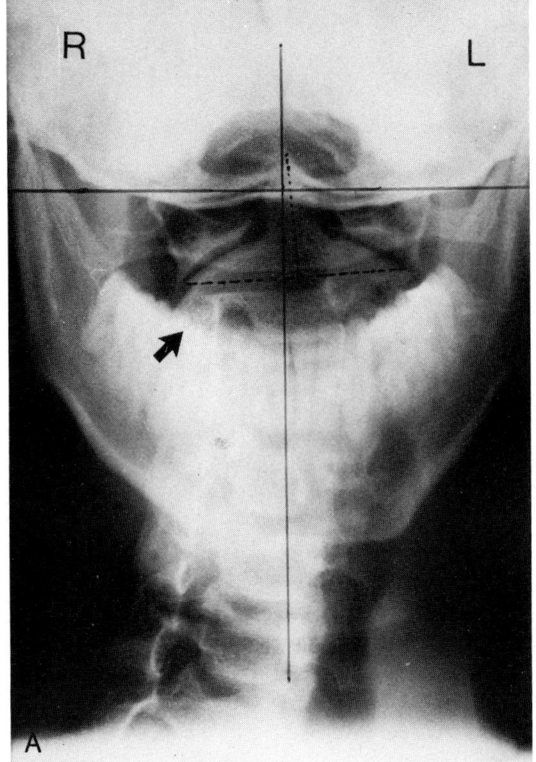

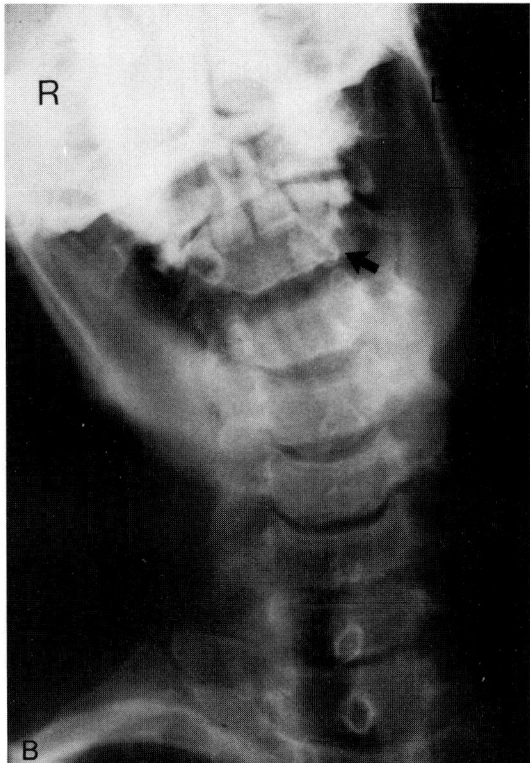

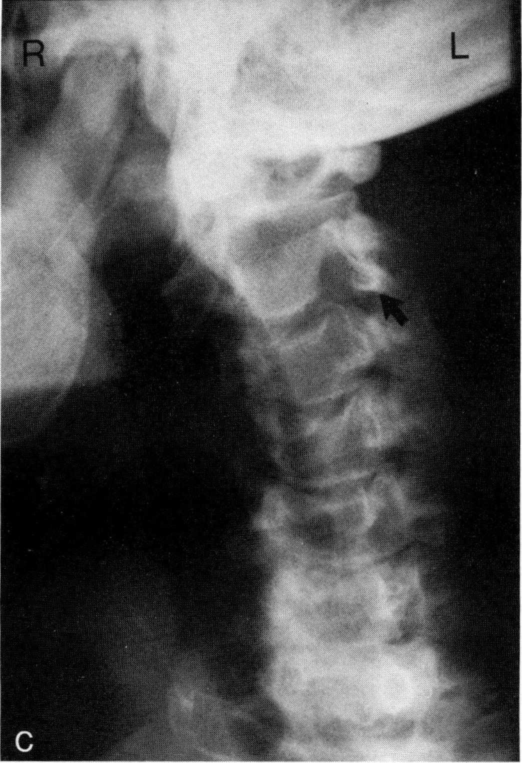

Fig. 2-30. Radiographic aspects of occipitoatlantoaxial rotation and lateral flexion. (*A*) A–P projection of head shows body rotated to left (or head rotated to right). Position corresponds with that of Figure 2-29, bottom. Drawn lines represent transverse and midsagittal plane of head, interrupted lines represent transverse plane and vertical axis of C2. Arrow points to spinous process of C2. (*B*) A–P projection shows head laterally flexed to right. Arrow points to spinous process C2 (axis vertebra is rotated and laterally flexed to right side). (*C*) A–P projection of body shows head turned to right. Arrow points to spinous process C2. C2 is rotated to right and laterally flexed to right.

As is evident from Figure 2-29 lateral flexion between head and axis is always a coupled motion in the atlantooccipital and atlantoaxial joints.

Rotation

Although precise data seem to be lacking, it is generally accepted that in the initial stages of head rotation only the atlantoaxial joints take part and are followed by gradually increasing rotation in the segments between axis and thoracic spine. This is explained by the lower resistance to rotation in the diarthrotic atlantoaxial joints, as compared with the resistance of the fibrocartilaginous discs in the lower cervical spine.

According to classical anatomic textbooks[2,19] atlantoaxial rotation occurs around an axis of motion, passing vertically through the odontoid process. This is in accordance with our observations[16] that the center of the odontoid process is found halfway between the lateral masses of the atlas, both in neutral position and in maximal rotation. The odontoid process remains in contact with the anterior arch of the atlas.

As is shown in Figure 2-31 the odontoid process projects itself in the center of the infraorbitomeatal, or horizontal plane. Rotation of the head thus takes place around a centrally placed vertical axis, passing through the odontoid process.

According to our investigations,[16] in young adults mean atlantoaxial rotation to the right or left is about 41°, with a maximum of 46°. In maximal rotation the joint surfaces articulate over only little area. Sudden overrotation of the head may cause interlocking of the atlantoaxial joint facets with impossibility to rotate the head back. An example is shown on page 67, Fig. 2-48.

To prevent overstretching the vertebral arteries possess overlength in the form of a loop between atlas and axis. The slack is taken up during atlantoaxial rotation (Fig. 2-32). The loop between atlas and occiput is not required to adapt to rotation (being virtually absent here) and perhaps may be regarded as a device for damping arterial pulse waves, comparable to the carotid syphon (Dörfler and Spatz, 1935, cited by Kunert[8]).

Flexion–Extension

Coupling between flexion–extension in the atlantooccipital and atlantoaxial joints is less strict than the coupling between lateral flexion in these joints. As a rule the posterior arch of the atlas keeps a more or less intermediate position between the occipital squama and the spinous process of the axis (Fig. 2-33 *top*). However, in the last stages of flexion of the head and neck, a paradox movement of extension may set in in the atlantooccipital joints. The result may be that in flexion the atlantooccipital joints are less flexed than in midposition. The following explanation is offered.

Horizontal translation of the head with respect to the axis-vertebra results in flexion–extension movements of the atlas (Fig. 2-33 *bottom*). This is due to the markedly curved contours of the atlantooccipital joints. Translation of the head in forward direction thus extends the atlantooccipital joint, and translation in backward direction flexes the atlantooccipital joint. During the initial stages of flexion of the head the atlantooccipital joint will likewise go into flexion. However, when the chin reaches the chest further flexion of the head is not possible. An attempt at further flexion of the neck will result in parallel movement of the head downward along the chest. This movement, comparable to the forward translation of the head of Figure 2-33 (*bottom, left*), will extend the atlantooccipital joint.

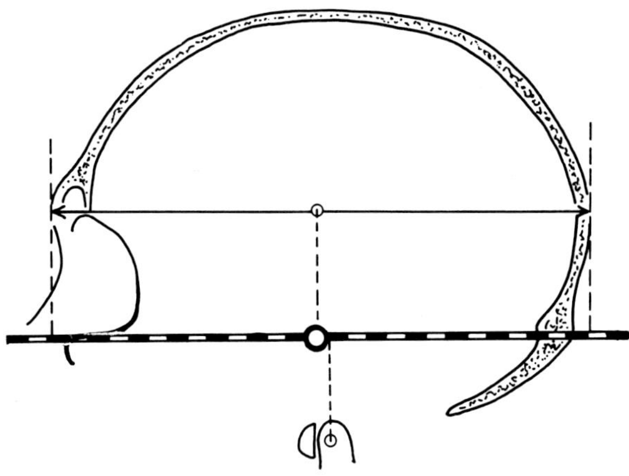

Fig. 2-31. Relationship between axis vertebra and skull. Schematic drawing of lateral projection of skull with infraorbitomeatal (or "horizontal") plane (*interrupted line*). Location of meatus is indicated by circle. On 52 radiographically normal skulls of male and female adults, the following measurements were made. Mean length of A–P diameter of skull (*drawn line*) is 20.5 cm. Point at half of this diameter projects 0.3 mm behind center of meatus (spread, 10 mm behind and 7 mm in front). Center of odontoid process projects 1.7 mm behind center of meatus (spread, 10 mm behind and 6 mm in front). Mean distance of center of odontoid process to infraorbitomeatal plane is 35 mm (spread 22 to 47 mm). No correction for radiologic magnification of about 12%.

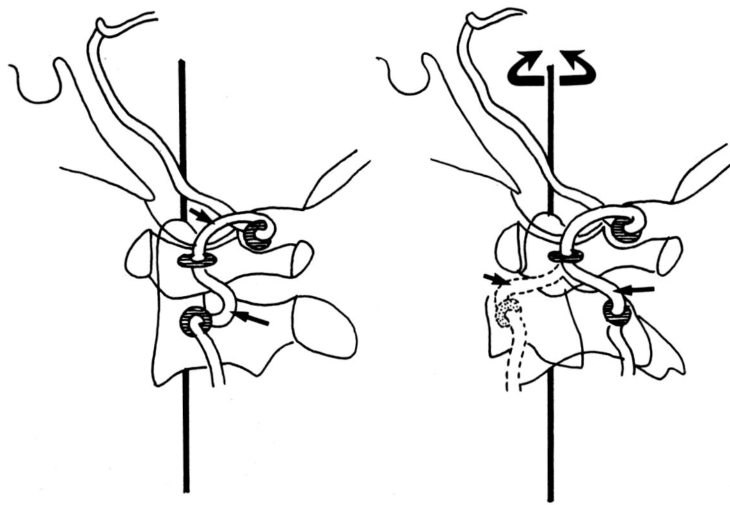

Fig. 2-32. Adaptation of vertebral artery to atlantoaxial rotation. (*Left*) Lateral projection of craniovertebral region shows left vertebral (and basilar) artery and axis of rotation (*vertical line*). Atlantoaxial and atlantooccipital loops of vertebral artery indicated by long and short arrow, respectively. (*Right*) Left vertebral artery is seen in rotation of axis vertebra to left (*long arrow*) and to right (*short arrow*). Slack of atlantoaxial loop is taken up in these positions of rotation. Atlantooccipital loop does not change its configuration.

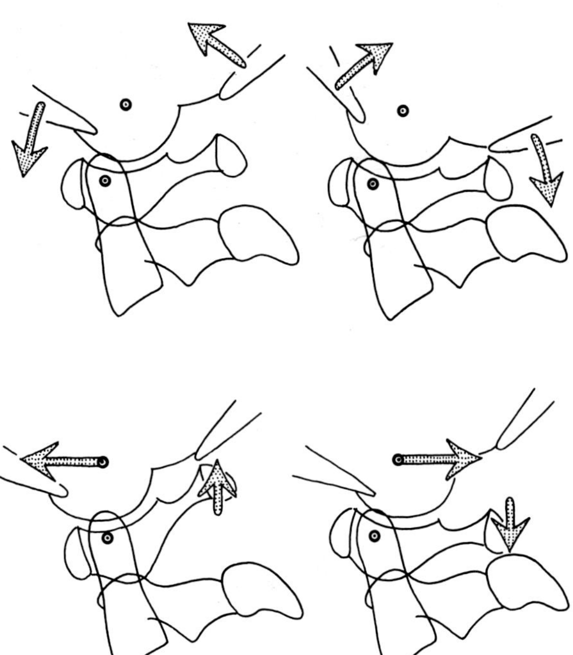

Fig. 2-33. Occipitoatlantoaxial motion in the sagittal plane. (*Top*) Flexion (*left*) and extension (*right*) are shown. Centers of motion between atlas and occiput, and between atlas and axis (in the odontoid process), are indicated. During flexion–extension, posterior arch of atlas tends to assume intermediate position between occipital squama and spinous process of axis. (*Bottom*) Horizontal translatory movement of head with respect to axis (assumed to be fixed) leads to atlantooccipital and atlantoaxial flexion–extension movements in opposite directions. (*Left*) Forward translation of head with extension of atlantooccipital joint and flexion of atlantoaxial joint is shown. (*Right*) Backward translation of head shows flexion of atlantooccipital joint and extension of atlantoaxial joint.

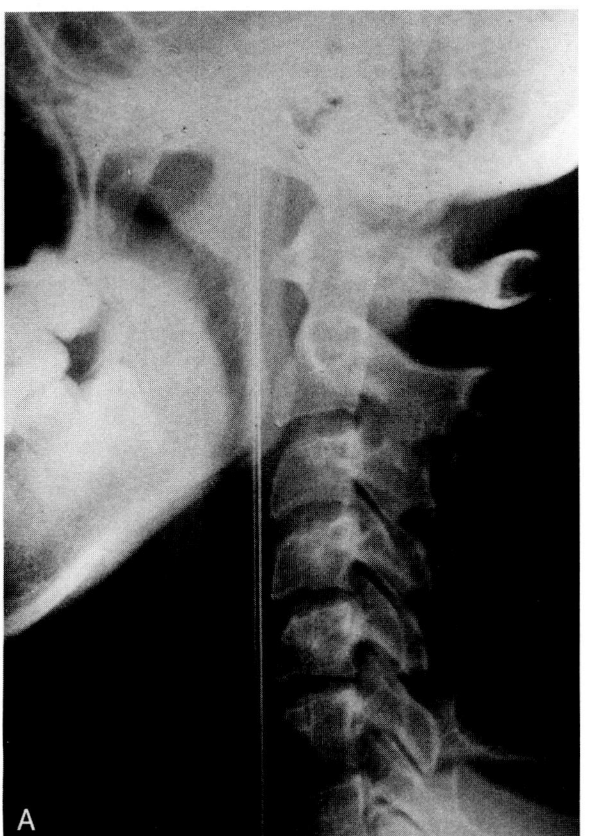

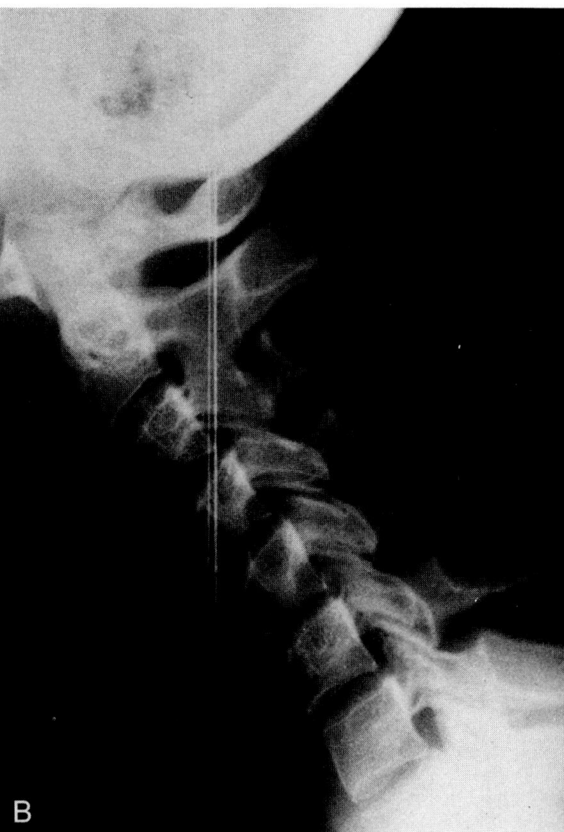

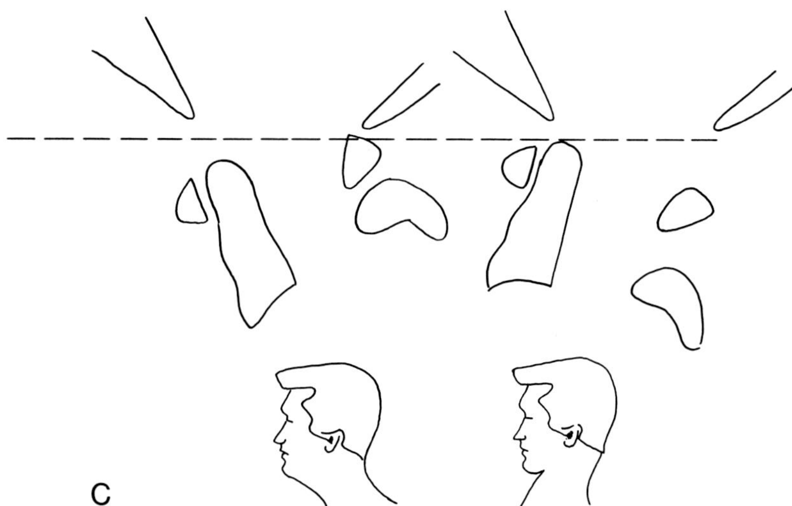

Fig. 2-34. Occipitoatlantoaxial motion during chin-in chin-out maneuver. Radiographs of cervical spine in chin-out (*A*) and chin-in (*B*) position. Vertical lines indicate direction of gravity. (*C, left*) Chin-out position with head remaining horizontal shows maximal extension of craniovertebral region. (*C, right*) Chin-in position shows maximal flexion between occiput and axis; 40° of motion. Adult is without radiologic signs of disc degeneration. (Courtesy of B. Vortman, M.D.).

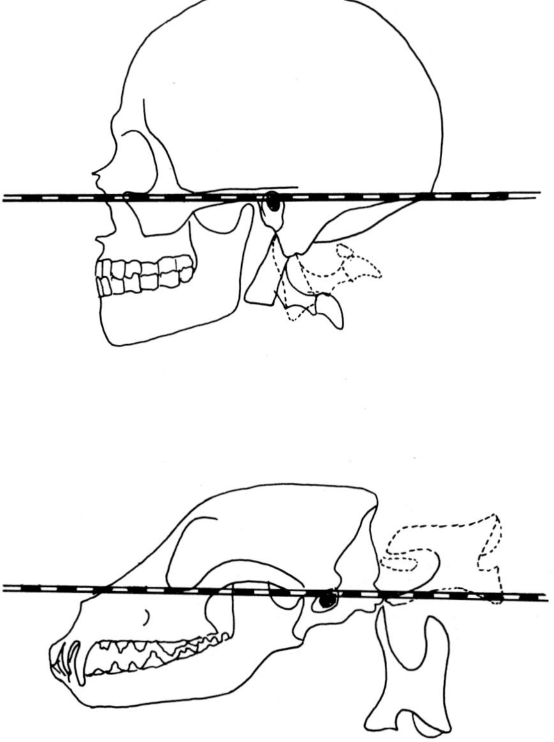

Fig. 2-35. Comparison between maximal occipitoaxial flexion–extension in humans and dogs. (*Top*) Lateral view is of human skull with horizontal plane. Axis is shown in maximal flexion (*drawn line*) and extension (*interrupted line*). (*Bottom*) Lateral view is of dog skull with horizontal plane and axis in flexion and extension. It is evident that extension is far greater in dog.

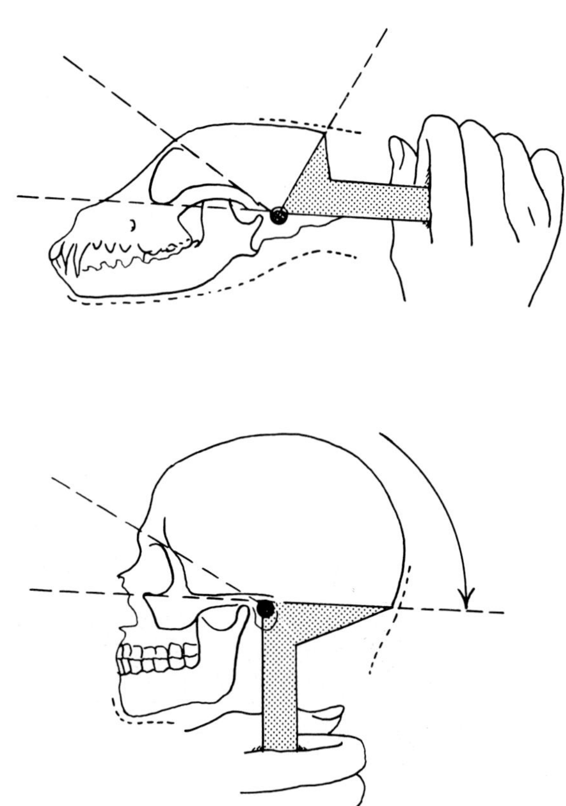

Fig. 2-36. "Handle of evolution." (*Top*) In dogs, nuchal plane is oriented more or less vertically, and neck, horizontally. Cranial cavity is small. (*Bottom*) In humans, nuchal plane has descended and neck has become more vertical ("pulled down"). It is obvious that this change markedly enlarges intracranial space.

During maximal chin-in and chin-out movements of the head (Fig. 2-34) flexion and extension, respectively, of the upper cervical spine are more extensive than during flexion and extension of the head and neck. A paradox motion in the atlantooccipital joint during flexion by chin-in maneuver has not been observed.

Comparison with Flexion–Extension in the Dog and Other Quadrupeds

Radiographic studies of motion of the cervical spine in dogs[15] revealed that the degree of extension in the occipitoatlantoaxial region far exceeds that of man (Fig. 2-35). Related to the horizontal plane (passing through the inferior orbital rims and upper parts of the external auditory meatus) the position of the axis vertebra in flexion is about the same, but differs markedly in extension. In man extension is limited by the more or less horizontal position of the nuchal plane of the occipital squama. In the dog such a limitation does not exist as the nuchal plane is more or less vertically orientated. The orientation of the nuchal plane (insertion site of nuchal muscles) is directly related to the orientation of the cervical spine: in man more vertical, in the dog more horizontal (Fig. 2-36).

The need for such extreme extension of the craniovertebral region in quadrupeds is especially obvious in grazing cattle: to bring the head and neck down maximal flexion at the cervicothoracic region is necessary, but to align the head with the neck maximal extension at the craniovertebral region must occur (Fig. 2-37). In this position, the animals can look ahead and about. A man in this position is unable to look ahead, owing to the very

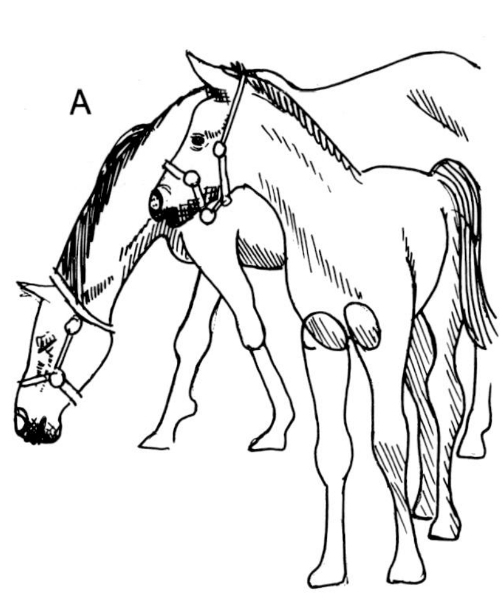

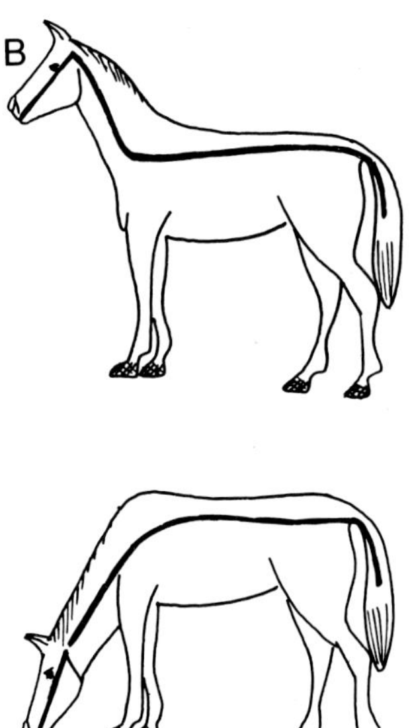

Fig. 2-37. Behavior of head and neck in grazing horses. (*A*) Grazing horse and foal standing alert. (*B*) During grazing, cervicothoracic junction is maximally flexed, but craniovertebral junction is maximally extended.

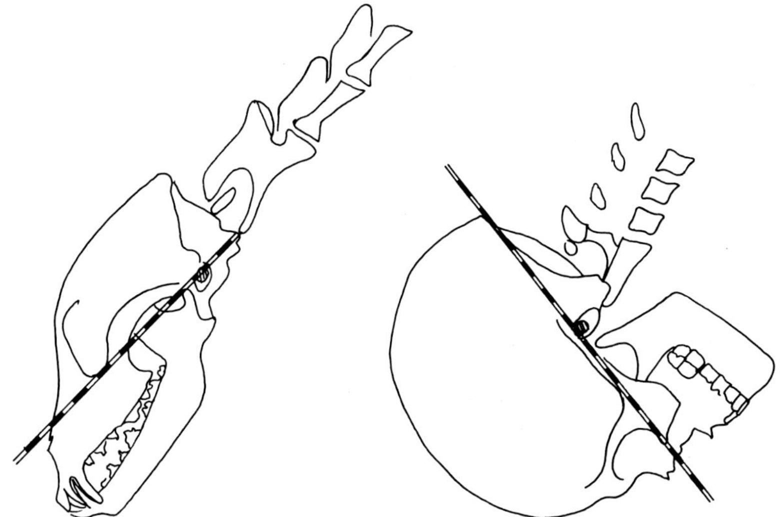

Fig. 2-38. Comparison between dog and man in head-down position. If humans on all fours took the same position as grazing cattle or sniffing dogs (*left*), they would be unable to look ahead (*right*).

limited possibility of extension of the craniovertebral region (Fig. 2-38).

REFERENCES

1. *Buetti-Baüml C:* Funktionelle Röntgendiagnostik der Halswirbelsäule Stuttgart, Thieme, 1954, pp 21–22
2. *Fick R:* Handbuch der Anatomie und Mechanik der Gelenke. Jena, S. Fischer Verlag, 1904
3. *Fielding JW:* Normal and selected abnormal motion of the cervical spine from the second cervical vertebra to the seventh cervical vertebra based on cineroentgenography. J Bone Joint Surg 46a:1779, 1964
4. *Hall MC:* Luschka's Joint. Springfield, IL, Charles C Thomas, 1965, pp. 1–141

5. *Hillen B:* Personal communication.
6. *Horton WG:* Further observations on the elastic mechanism of the intervertebral disc. J Bone Joint Surg 40B:552, 1958
7. *Jackson R:* The Cervical Syndrome. Springfield, IL, Charles C Thomas, 1956
8. *Kunert W:* Arteria vertebralis und Halswirbelsäule. Die Wirbelsäule in Forschung und Praxis, Band 20. Stuttgart, Hippokrates, 1961
9. *Luschka H:* Die Halbgelenke des Menschlichen Körpers. Berlin, Reimer, 1858
10. *Lysell E:* Motion in the cervical spine. An experimental study on autopsy specimens. Acta Orthop Scand (Suppl) 123:54, 1969
11. *Markuske H:* Untersuchungen zur Statik und Dynamik der kindlichen Halswirbelsäule: Der Aussagewert seitlicher Roentgenaufnahmen. Stuttgart, Hippokrates Verlag, 1971
12. *Miller ME, Christensen DVM, Evans HE:* Anatomy of the Dog. Philadelphia, WB Saunders Company, 1964
13. *Pennal GF, Conn GS, McDonald G, Dale G, Garside H:* Motion studies of the lumbar spine. A preliminary report. J Bone Joint Surg 54B:442–452, 1972
14. *Penning L:* Functioneel röntgenonderzoek bij degeneratieve en traumatische aandoeningen der laag-cervicale bewegingssegmenten. Thesis, Groningen, 1960, pp 3–13
15. *Penning L, Badoux DM:* Radiological study of the movements of the cervical spine on the dog compared with those in man. Anat Histol Embryol 15, 1986
16. *Penning L, Wilmink JT:* Rotation in the cervical spine. A CT study in normals (in press). Spine, 1987
17. *Reuter M:* Über die Eigenform die Bewegungsmöglichkeiten und einige Messungen an der Hundewirbelsäule. ZF Anat u Entw Gesch 99:117, 1933
18. *Rolander SD:* Motion of the lumbar spine with special reference to the stabilizing effect of posterior fusion. An experimental study on autopsy specimens. Acta Orthop Scand (Suppl) 90:83, 1966
19. *Spalteholz W:* Handatlas und Lehrbuch der Anatomie des Menschen, 15th ed. S. Hirzel Verlag, Zurich, Stuttgart, 1953
20. *Testud L, Latarjet A:* Traité d'anatomie humaine Tome 1: ostéologie, arthrologie, myologie. Paris, Doin & Cie, 1948, p 502
21. *Töndury G:* Entwicklungsgeschichte und Fehlbildungen der Halswirbelsäule. Stuttgart, Hippokrates, 1958: pp 87–100
22. *Trolard A:* Quelques articulations de la colonne vertébrale. Int Monatschr Anatom Physiol 10:3, 1893
23. *Virchow H:* Über die Bewegungsmöglichkeiten an der Wirbelsäule und am Thorax des wilden Kaninchens. Arch Anatomie, 1915, p 225. (For more references on Virchow, see biliography for Reuter.)
24. *White AA III:* Analysis of the mechanics of the thoracic spine in man. An experimental study of autopsy specimens. Acta Orthop Scand (Suppl) 127, 1969
25. *White AA III, Panjabi MM:* The basic kinematics of the human spine. A review of past and current knowledge. Spine 3:12, 1978
26. *White AA III, Panjabi MM:* Clinical Biomechanics of the Spine. Philadelphia, JB Lippincott, 1978, pp 61–90
27. *Werne S:* The possibilities of movements in the craniovertebral joints. Acta Orthop Scand 28:165, 1957

Clinically Relevant Kinematics of the Cervical Spine

MICHAEL H. JOFE, AUGUSTUS A. WHITE, AND MANOHAR M. PANJABI

Kinematics is that branch of mechanics that examines the motion of bodies without consideration of influencing forces. The two elements that determine the kinematics of skeletal body motion are the geometry of the articulating surfaces and the mechanical properties of the connecting structures. In the case of bodies that are able to roll and slide on each other, the geometry of the contracting surfaces determines the relative motion. In the case of bodies that are connected by deformable elements, the mechanical properties and the geometry of these elements influence the motion. In the spine, as in other articulating structures of the human body, both mechanisms come into play. For instance, in the cervical spine, relative motion between C1 and C2 is controlled by the geometry of the articular surfaces and by the geometry and elastic properties of the ligaments.[21]

Terms and Definitions

Coordinate System. The right-handed orthogonal (90° angle) coordinate system is an easy and efficient method for accurately describing cervical spine kinematics. Its conventions and its orientation for the spine are shown in Figure 2-39.
Rotation. Rotation is movement about an axis. An object (vertebral body) is said to be in rotation when its motion is such that all particles along a straight line in the object, or a hypothetical extension of this line, remain motionless relative to a fixed point. Using the right-handed orthogonal coordinate system, flexion–extension motion is rotation about the x axis. Rotation is measured in degrees or radians. (2π radians = 360°)
Translation. Translation is movement along an axis. An object is said to be in translation when motion is such that a straight line through the object always remains parallel to itself. Translation is measured in inches or centimeters.
Range of Motion. Range of motion is the distance or angle between two physiological extremes of translation or rotation.
Coupling. Coupling refers to motion when translation or rotation occurs simultaneously along and about their respective axes, or when rotation about one axis is associated with rotation about a second axis.
Instantaneous Axis of Rotation. At every moment in time, a rigid body in plane motion has a certain point within it or within some hypothetical extension of it that does not move. A line perpendicular to the plane of motion, and passing through this point, is called the instantaneous axis of rotation (IAR). Plane motion can be fully defined by the position of the IAR and the magnitude of rotation about it (Fig. 2-40).
Functional Spinal Unit. A functional spinal unit (also referred to as a motion segment) is the traditional unit of study in spinal kinematics. It consists of two adjacent vertebrae and their intervening soft tissues.

Supported in part by NIH grants #GM 07806 and #AM25601

A thorough knowledge of spinal kinematics is helpful in understanding all aspects of the diagnosis and management of spinal pathology. This is especially true of the cervical spine, for it is the most mobile portion of the spine. Because the functions and anatomic designs of the occipitoatlantoaxial complex and the lower cervical spine (C2–C7) are dissimilar, it is advantageous to study the kinematics of each region separately. Based on new information, new hypotheses, and clinical findings, some changes in the subdivisions of the spine are offered. The C0–C1–C2 (occipitoatlantoaxial) complex is grouped and labeled the upper cervical spine. Because of kinematic,[24] kinetic,[5] and clinical uniqueness,[32a] the cervical repair is divided into the middle cervical (C2–C5) and the lower cervical (C5-T1). See the list on this page for key terms and definitions.[36,37]

The study of cervical spine kinematics is ongoing. Much of the research presented here requires further confirmation and suggests new avenues for investigation. Attempts have been made to distill fact from postulate, and to integrate biomechanical research with clinical applications.

There are, as with any research field, numerous problems to overcome. The kinematics of interest is that of the *in vivo* cervical spine. The experimental techniques for precise, no-risk, *in vivo* measurements are yet to be developed. Physiologic muscle forces have not yet been simulated. The characteristics of the muscle forces that result in *in vivo* physiologic motions are not known. *In vitro* studies have been done to simulate vertebral motion, but it is not known whether the motions produced experimentally are the same as those produced *in vivo*. Obviously, these problems must be addressed. The purpose of this chapter is to present the state of the art in regard to cervical spine kinematics. Useful areas of clinical relevance are indicated.

OCCIPITOATLANTOAXIAL COMPLEX (C0–C1–C2)

The occipitoatlantoaxial complex is the most complicated series of articulations in the human body. It serves as a transition zone between the standard vertebral joint structures and the radically different skull. The joint complex functions to support

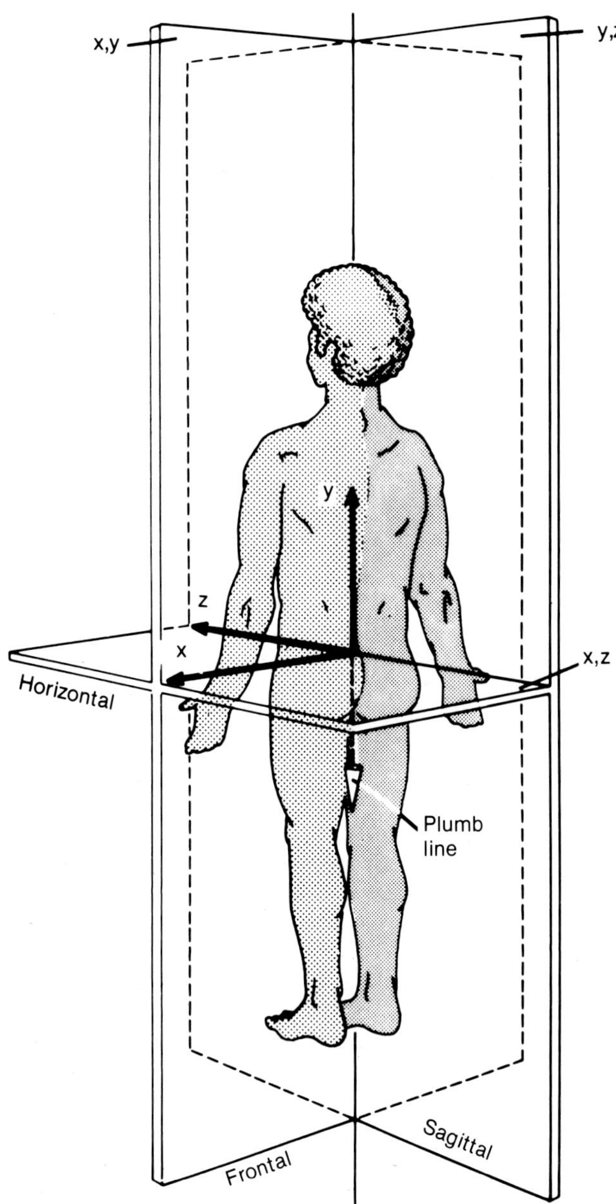

Fig. 2-39. The suggested central coordinate system with its origin between the cornua of the sacrum. Its orientation is as follows: The −y axis is described by the plumb line dropped from the origin, and the +x axis points to the left at a 90° angle to the y axis. The +z axis points forward at a 90° angle to both the y axis and x axis. The human body is shown in the anatomic position. There are some basic conventions that are observed that make this a useful system. The planes are as shown: the sagittal plane is the y, z plane; the frontal plane is the y, x plane; the horizontal plane is the x, z plane. Movements are described in relation to the origin of the coordinate system. The arrows indicate the positive direction of each axis. The origin is the zero point, and the direction opposite to the arrows is negative. Thus, direct forward translation is +z; up is +y; to the left is +x, and to the right is −x; down is −y; and backward is −z. The convention for rotations is determined by imagining oneself at the origin of the coordinate system looking in the positive direction of the axis. Clockwise rotations are $+\theta$ and counterclockwise rotations are $-\theta$. Thus, $+\theta x$ is roughly analogous to flexion; $+\theta z$ is analogous to right lateral bending; $+\theta y$ is axial rotation toward the left. A coordinate system may be set up at any defined point parallel to the master system described above. The location of the coordinate system should be clearly indicated for precise, accurate communications. In spinal kinematics, the motion is usually described in relation to the subjacent vertebra. The secondary coordinate system may be established in the body of the subjacent vertebrae. For *in vivo* measurements, the tip of its spinous process may be used. (Panjabi MM, White AA, Brand RA: A note on defining body parts configurations. J Biomech 7:385, 1974)

the head while allowing the necessary ranges of motion. In addition, it protects the spinal cord and adjacent vital structures during movement.[7]

One of the earliest studies on the kinematics of the occipitoatlantoaxial area was done by Weber and Weber in 1836.[5] More recently, cadaveric studies, plane radiographs, cineradiographs, and stereoradiographs have been used to investigate movement in this region.[10,27,34,35] Although each method has its inherent problems, together they provide an accurate description of motion within the area. One of the most detailed and convincing studies on the kinematics of this region was done by Werne.[34] Much of the work presented in this section is based upon his findings.

Range of Motion

Both the occipito–C1 and the C1–C2 articulations are involved in flexion–extension motion. Originally, it was thought that there was no significant flexion–extension at the C1–C2 joint.[9] However, Werne,[34] using radiographic studies, demon-

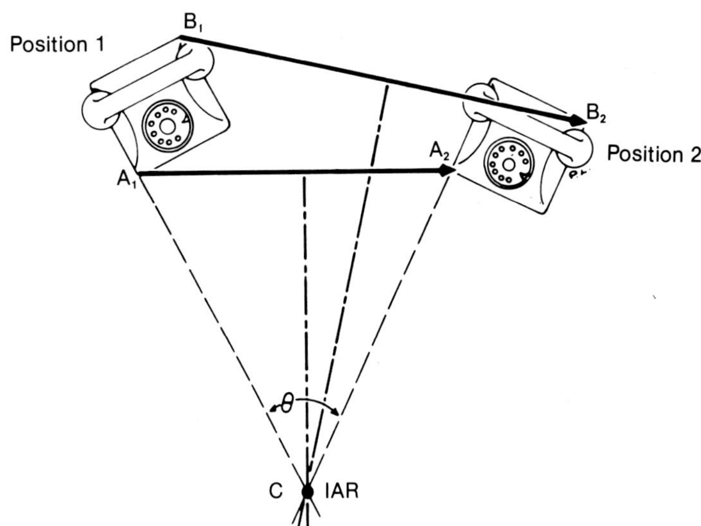

Fig. 2-40. The concept and the actual method of determining the instantaneous axis of rotation (IAR) in uniplanar motion. The IAR is determined by the intersection of the perpendicular bisectors of the two lines A_1A_2 and B_1B_2 (the translation vectors of the two points A and B on the telephone). The angle θ formed at the IAR by points A_1, A_2 or B_1, B_2 is the angle of rotation. (White AA III, Panjabi MM: Spinal kinematics. In The Research Status of Spinal Manipulative Therapy, NINCDS Monograph No 15, p 93. Washington, DC, US Department of Health, Education and Welfare, 1975)

strated that flexion–extension is present at both joints in the complex. He studied the region in 104 cases and found the occipitoatlantal joint to have an average range of motion in flexion–extension of 13.4°. The axis articulation was found to have an average range of 10° of motion (Fig. 2-41). Combined, this allows an average flexion–extension range of motion at the occipitoatlantoaxial complex of 23.4°. Werne's studies have been confirmed by other investigators.[15,16]

Recent evidence has shown that, along with flexion–extension, axial rotation occurs at both the occipitoatlantal and atlantoaxial joints. This contradicts prior evidence that rotation was not present between occiput and C1. Clark and coworkers[4] found there was 4.8° of axial rotation at the C0–C1 articulation. This is confirmed by Worth[38] and Depreux and Mestdagh.[6] Dvorak and coworkers[8] in a computerized axial tomography study of the *in vitro* cervical spine demonstrated a mean axial rotation of 4.3° at occiput–C1.

Most axial rotations (y-axis rotation) in the upper cervical spine take place at the atlantoaxial articulation.[27] The articular surfaces are convex with a horizontal orientation, a geometric design that allows maximum mobility. A representative figure for C1–C2 joint axis rotation is 47°. This encompasses 40% to 50% of the axial rotation in the neck, with the lower cervical spine contributing 50% to 60%.

The large rotation that occurs at the C1–C2 articulation can cause clinical problems. Selecki studied the effects of this rotation on the vertebral arteries that ascend vertically in the foramina transversarium and pass through both the C1–C2 and occipitoatlantal articulation before entering the skull.[31] He found that after 30° of rotation there is kinking of the contralateral vertebral artery. This kinking, which is also accompanied by stretching, first occurs as the vertebral artery exits from the transverse foramina and becomes more marked as the angle of rotation is increased. At 45° of rotation the ipsilateral artery also begins to kink (Fig. 2-42). If the flow in both arteries is compromised, symptoms related to decreased flow in the posterior fossa may be elicited.[2] Situations

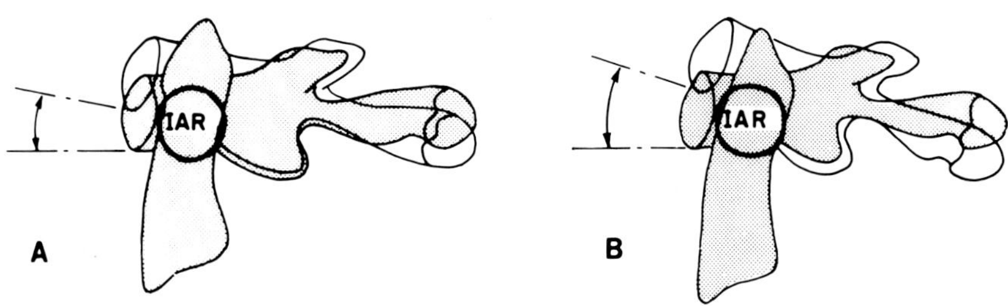

Fig. 2-41. (*A*) Representation of sagittal plane motion of C1 on C2, with the approximate IAR also indicated. Rotation is usually 10° to 15°. (*B*) The anterior curvature of the dens may permit some degree of additional sagittal plane motion in both rotation and translation.

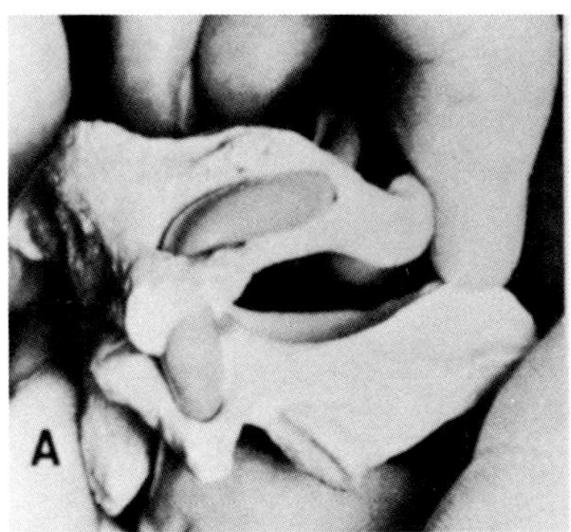

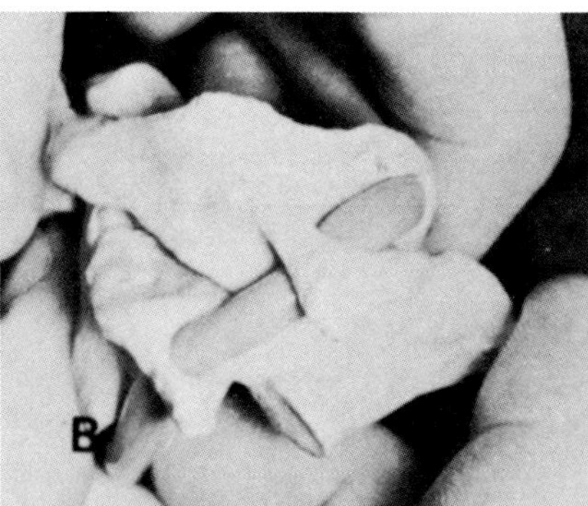

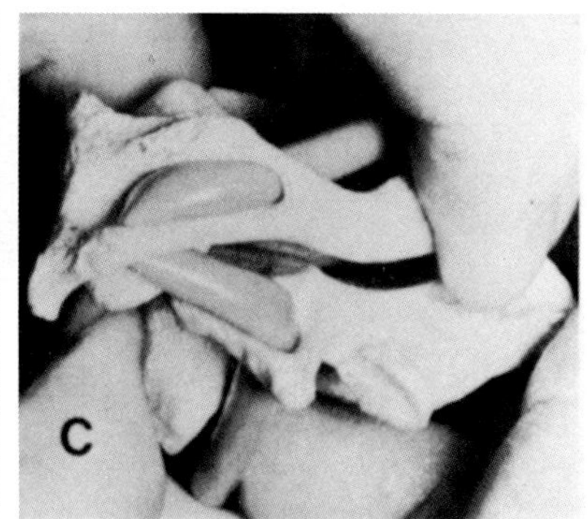

Fig. 2-42. The vertebral artery is represented by a piece of rubber tubing. (*A*) The atlas and axis are in neutral position. (*B*) The atlas is rotated to the left (+0y). (*C*) The atlas is rotated to the right (−0y). There is considerable excursion of the vertebral artery when rotary displacement takes place between the vertebrae. (Fielding JW: Cineroent-genography of the normal cervical spine. J Bone Joint Surg 39A:1280, 1957)

in which this phenomenon may occur include yoga, calisthenics, overhead work and cervical traction.[28] Similarly, cases of stroke have been reported following chiropractic manipulation of the neck and head.[2,25] Schelluas and coworkers reported angiographically confirmed vertebrobasilar injuries following chiropractic manipulation.[28] Other authors have reported similar complications in patients with no medical problems.[2,25] Evidentally, these accidents may occur in the absence of clinically apparent vascular or cervical spine disease.

According to Miller and Burton, there are usually premonitory symptoms, including nausea, visual disturbance, vomiting, and vertigo, during the preliminary treatments.[25] If chiropractic treatments are stopped at this stage, further irreversible damage can usually be avoided. In all instances, patients with cervical spondylosis or symptoms of vertebral vascular insufficiency should be warned against undergoing manipulation of the cervical spine. Cervical spine fusion may alleviate this symptom complex; however, further clinical studies are needed to verify this supposition.

Dvorak and coworkers,[8] in an *in vitro* study demonstrated increased rotation at both the occipitoatlantal and atlantoaxial articulation following severing the contralateral alar ligament. The alar ligaments are symmetrically placed on both sides of the dens with one portion connecting the dens to the occiput, and the remaining ligament connecting the dens to the atlas (Fig. 2-43*A*). *Left* axial rotation (+y-axis rotation), as in turning the head to look to one's left, is checked by the *right* alar ligament (Fig. 2-43*B*). The opposite is true for rotation to the right. The mechanism for lateral bending is more complex. This motion occurs only between the occiput and C1, and is controlled by both components of the alar ligaments (Fig. 2-43*C*). During left lateral bending (−z-axis rotation), the right upper portions of the alar ligament, connected to the occiput, and the left lower component, connected to the ring of C1, check the motion. The corollary is true for right lateral bending.

Following transection of the *left* alar ligament, axial rotation to the *right* at the occiput–C1 articulation increased from 4.35° to 9.4°, and at the atlantoaxial joint from 31.4° to 37.4°. This is a mean increase of 30% at the occipitoatlantalaxial complex. Dvorak and coworkers[8] postulate that damage to the alar ligament, *in vivo,* could occur following a motor vehicle accident, where a flexion-rotation force is applied to the occiput–C1–C2 complex. The resultant *hypermobility* could cause stretching and irritation of the vertebral artery and nerve, as well as the mechanoceptors and nociceptors of the apophyseal joint capsules. This may lead to the symptom complex of neck pain, headache, and dizziness that is associated with "whiplash injuries."

It should be noted that other authors disagree[38] and assert that *hypomobility* of the C0–C1 articulation is the problem in patients with neck pain following whiplash injuries. This is still a highly controversial area and more study is necessary.

In cadaver studies, Werne found an average of 11.9° of lateral bending at the occipito–C1 joint.[34] However, upon radiographic examination, he found the representative figure to be 7.8°. In retrospect, Werne believed that this discrepancy was

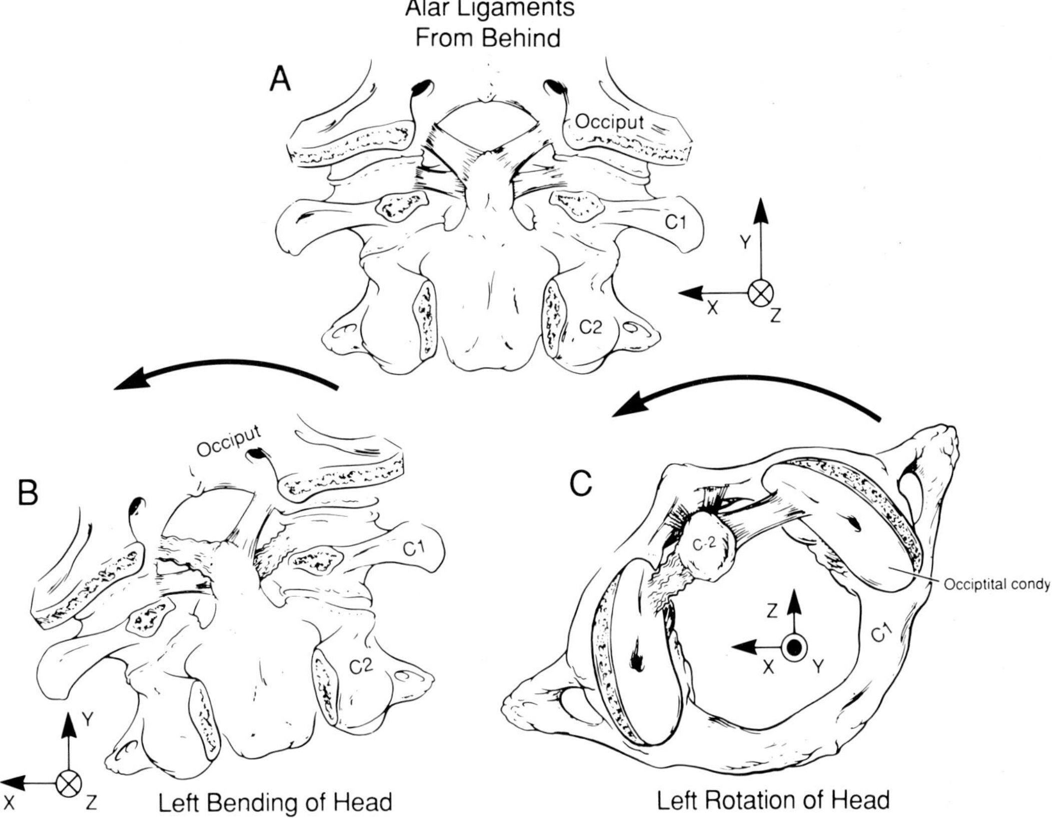

Fig. 2-43. Effects of alar ligament on motion at the C0-C1-C2 complex; (*A*) Normal anatomy; (*B*) Left bending of head; (*C*) Left rotation of the head.

caused by unavoidable experimental error in using cadavers. He concluded that the radiographic measurements were accurate. Although the latter figure is the most prevalent in the literature, other authors have arrived at very different values. Fick, for instance, reported as much as 30° to 40° of lateral bending.[9] Further work needs to be done in order to resolve this controversy and to provide an accurate value for lateral bending.

Jirout and others have concluded that in lateral bending of the neck, rotation occurs at the C1–C2 joint.[11,16,19,20] Jirout divided this rotation into two phases.[14] The initial phase involves a symmetrical rotation of C2 around the longitudinal axis of the cervical spine. In the second phase there is further rotation, which, in contrast, is asymmetrical and sometimes associated with a more pronounced lateral translation of the axis against the atlas. Jirout concluded that the atlas serves a role in the occipitoatlantoaxial complex similar to the role of a meniscus in other regions of the body.

Translatory movements in the occiput–C1–C2 complex are small. Werne, using cadavers, found the normal range of the axis translation at the occiput–C1 to be 1 mm.[34] This value was confirmed by Fielding using cineradiographic techniques.[10] Worth, also using cadavers, studied the posterior translation of the atlas relative to the occiput as the joints moved into extension from full flexion.[38] He concluded that there is an average of 5.5 mm of z-axis translation in this situation. This finding is in sharp contrast to the studies by Werne and Fielding as well as a study by Weisel.[10,33,34] Weisel studied flexion–extension films on army recruits complaining of neck pain. He concluded that the range of z-axis translation in the normal person is 0 mm to 1 mm, and anything greater than 1 mm should be considered clinically significant. Although more clinical and experimental data are needed to resolve this controversy, it is reasonable to consider movement greater than 1 mm to be probably abnormal.

In general, it is believed that there is little if any translation along the x and y axes at the occiput–C1 articulation.[11,34] In contrast, the atlas–axis articulation is believed to have significant translatory motion. Jackson carried out radiologic studies of 50 adults and 25 children in which the distance between the posterior inferior margin of the anterior arch of the atlas and the anterior surface of the dens was measured.[18] This measurement is equivalent to z-axis translation. Jackson found a maximum of 2.5 mm in adults and 4 mm in children. These results are in agreement with those of Fielding, who measured the z-axis translation in 20 fresh adult cadavers and concluded that z-axis translation does not exceed 3 mm in the normal person.[11] Fielding suggested that any value greater than 3 mm would lead to rupture of the transverse ligament.

Lateral (x-axis) translation of the C1–C2 joint is also a controversial subject. Some authors contend that there is only apparent translation due to axial rotation between C1 and C2.[36,37] They state that roentgenographically observed translation is due to radiographic distortions of the lateral masses of C1 relative to the dens.[32] However, Hohl and Baker, in radiologic studies, found that a lateral displacement of the atlas on the axis does occur when there is coupling of lateral bending and axial rotation.[16] They concluded that, under these circumstances, there may be up to 4 mm of x-axis translation. Jirout's findings are in agreement with this.[19] Although there is still controversy and a need for more investigation, most of the literature suggests that lateral displacement of C1–C2 greater than 4 mm is abnormal.

In summary, the representative figures for the ranges of motion for the units of the occipitoatlantoaxial complex are shown in Table 2-2. It should be emphasized that these values represent the best available information. However, as is evident from the previous discussion, there is still controversy concerning some of the basic biomechanical and kinematic characteristics.

Coupling Characteristics

Coupling, as defined previously, refers to motion when translation and rotation occur simultaneously along and about their respective axes, or when rotation about one axis is associated with rotation about a second axis. Each of the physiologic motions of the cervical spine, such as translation and rotation, has been described separately for the sake of simplicity; however, they are inherently linked. Coupling is primarily due to the geometry of the regional facet articulations. The connecting ligaments as well as the curvature of the spine play a secondary role. It is generally accepted that there is a strong coupling pattern at the atlantoaxial joint (Fig. 2-44). The axial (±y-axis) rotation of C1 is associated with vertical (y-axis) translation. However, there is some disagreement. Henke described a "double-threaded screw" mechanism due, he explained, to the biconvexity of the articulations between C1 and C2.[14] This analysis was criticized by Hultkrantz, who studied sagittal sections of the C1 and C2 articulations.[17] He found that some of the surfaces are slightly biconvex and that others are slightly biconcave. It has been observed that, although the actual bony configuration may be concave, the configuration of the cartilage is such that the complete articulation has a biconvex design. This design is thought to account for the screw motion. Hultkrantz reasoned that this screw movement (y-axis translation) is not characteristic of normal turning of the head but

Table 2-2. Representative Values of the Range of Rotation of the Occipitoatlantoaxial Complex

UNIT OF COMPLEX	TYPE OF MOTION	DEGREES OF MOTION
Occipitoatlantal joint (occiput–C1)	Flexion–extension (±θx)	13° (Moderate)
	Lateral bending (±θz)	8° (Moderate)
	Axial rotation (±θy)	10° (Moderate)
Atlantoaxial joint (C1–C2)	Flexion–extension (±θx)	10° (Moderate)
	Lateral bending (±θz)	0° (Negligible)
	Axial rotation (±θy)	65° (Extensive)

Based on review of literature and authors' analysis

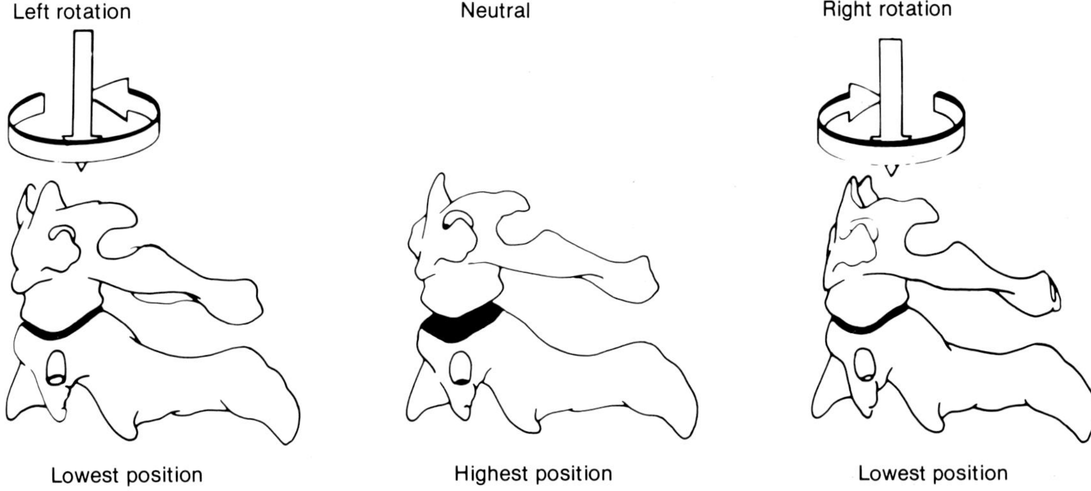

Fig. 2-44. Because of the anatomic design of the lateral articulations, C1 is highest in the middle position and lowest with the extremes of axial rotation to the right or the left.

probably occurs only at the extremes of the range of motion.

Hohl and Baker[16] described coupling of vertical translation of C1 with axial rotation of C1 on C2 using cineradiographics. Similarly, Werne concluded that the vertical displacement depends on the extent to which the longitudinal axis of the dens correlates with the imaginary longitudinal axis of the body.[34] The more "parallel" the two are, the more distinctive is the vertical displacement. Figure 2-45 demonstrates how the parallel alignment of the vertical axis of the coordinate system and the longitudinal axis of the dens can vary. In the example shown, there is an angle of approximately 45°. One can readily appreciate that the translation along the longitudinal axis of the dens can carry the atlas posteriorly or vertically, depending on the orientation of the dens.

Instantaneous Axes of Rotation

Henke identified the instantaneous axes of rotation (IAR) for occipitoatlantal motion by determining the center of each arch formed by the outline of the joints in the sagittal and frontal planes.[14] He found that the sagittal axis is located 2 cm to 3 cm above the apex of the dens. Although these measurements were made more than a century ago, they remain the only approximation of the motion of the occipitoatlantal articulation; however, the methods used do not necessarily give accurate results. In order to locate the axes accurately, experimental investigation must be carried out to analyze plane motion in carefully controlled situations.

For the atlantoaxial joint, the instantaneous axes of rotation can be estimated from the cineradiographic studies of Werne.[34] Sagittal plane motion locates the instantaneous axis of rotation for flexion–extension within the middle third of the dens. For axial (theta-y) rotation, the instantaneous axis of rotation may be assumed to lie in the central portion of the axis.

MIDDLE (C2–C5) AND LOWER (C5–T1) CERVICAL SPINE

The joints of the lower cervical spine (C2–T1) are anatomically distinct. Thus, the kinematics of this region are also unique. The most detailed work on the kinematics of this region of the cervical spine was done by Lysell, who carried out meticulous three-dimensional examinations on fresh autopsy specimens using radiographic techniques.[24] Much of the information presented in this section is based on his work.

Range of Motion

Studies of cervical spine mobility have looked at biomechanical, etiologic, and pathologic factors that affect the range of motion. Age is one such factor. Blanchard and Kottke, who studied a group of male students between the ages of 15 and 29,

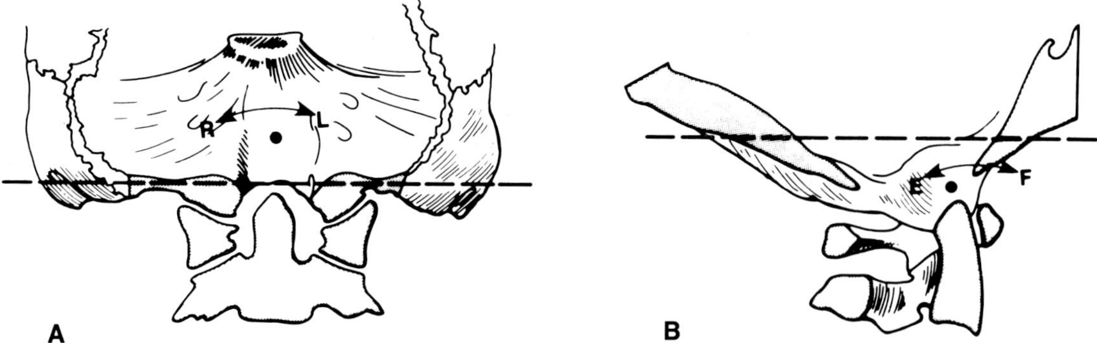

Fig. 2-45. (*A*) The approximate location of the IAR for the occipitoatlantal joint in the frontal plane. Lateral bending (R, L) of the occiput on C1 is thought to take place around the indicated dot. The broken line indicates the approximate location of the IAR for the flexion–extension (F, E) motion in the sagittal plane. (*B*) The converse is shown in the sagittal plane. The broken line localized the IAR for lateral bending and the dot shows the axes for flexion–extension.

discovered an inverse relationship between age and range of motion, that is, as age increases, mobility decreases.[3] The reason for this decrease in mobility is not clear. One would not expect subjects in this age group to have degenerative changes. Schoening and Hannan performed an *in vivo* study using goniometers to determine factors that affect cervical mobility.[30] They too found that age is an important consideration. They also found that pain in the neck, arm, and upper trunk; tenderness over the articular masses and spinal processes; pain with passive neck motion; and increased muscularity are all associated with a reduction in the range of motion. Curiously, they found that severity of interspace narrowing at one level has no effect on mobility; only, when narrowing exists at several levels is there an association between disc-space narrowing and decreased mobility.

Recently, Coffee and coworkers,[5] using a newly developed planar testing apparatus, examined the motion in three degrees of freedom in the upper half (C2–C5) and lower half (C5–T1) of the lower cervical spine. They found that the C2–C4 region exhibits greater stiffness for posterior motion, compared with anterior motion, as well as greater axial and shear stiffness than did the C5–C7 region. This information may have some relation to the different patterns of injury seen in the two regions as described by Torg and associates.[32a]

Lysell examined the relationship between disc degeneration and mobility.[24] Initially, using radiographs, he measured the range of motion of a functional spinal unit. Following this, he removed the intervertebral disc of that particular unit and graded it for degeneration. He found that there was no correlation between degree of disc degeneration and loss of mobility. This result applied to all directions of motion at all interfaces. Hadley and Fielding both reported similar findings,[11,13] yet other investigators have disagreed. Ball and Meijers studied the motion of 21 fresh postmortem cervical spines and concluded that there is decreased angular mobility when radiologic signs of disc degeneration are present.[1]

Raynor and colleagues[26] studied the effects of bilateral facet excision on the lower cervical spine. Little change was noted in z-axis motion, either to a direct anterior–posterior force, or as a result of a coupled motion. There was, however, a marked reduction in both primary and coupled motions in response to laterally applied forces. This decreased movement to lateral force could result in a lower threshold for injury potential in association with laterally applied forces. Conversely, flexion–extension forces would not be expected to lead to a greater risk of injury. These findings suggest the need for additional studies to better delineate the influence of the facet joints on the kinematics and kinetics of the cervical spine.

Rotation ranges for the lower cervical spine are shown in Table 2-3 and Figure 2-46. In flexion–extension, motion is concentrated in the central region. The C5–C6 interspace is generally considered to have the greatest range of motion, especially in the sagittal plane.[1,7,24] Kottke and Mondale, however, contend that the range of motion at C4–C5 and C6–C7 is not much different from the range of C5–C6.[23] For lateral bending and

Table 2-3. Limits and Representative Values of Range of Rotation of the Lower Cervical Spine

	FLEXION/EXTENSION (X-AXIS ROTATION)		LATERAL BENDING (Z-AXIS ROTATION)		AXIAL ROTATION (Y-AXIS ROTATION)	
INTERSPACE	LIMITS OF RANGES (DEGREES)	REPRESENTATIVE ANGLE (DEGREES)	LIMITS OF RANGES (DEGREES)	REPRESENTATIVE ANGLE (DEGREES)	LIMITS OF RANGES (DEGREES)	REPRESENTATIVE ANGLE (DEGREES)
C2–C3	5–23	8	11–20	10	6–28	9
C3–C4	7–38	13	9–15	11	10–28	11
C4–C5	8–39	12	0–16	11	10–26	12
C5–C6	4–34	17	0–16	8	8–34	10
C6–C7	1–29	16	0–17	7	6–15	9
C7–T1	4–17	9	0–17	4	5–13	8

(White AA III, Panjabi MM: The basic kinematics of the human spine. Spine 3:12, 1978)

axial rotation, the range of motion is smaller at the more caudal segments.

Range of motion in the lower cervical spine can be used in making clinical decisions concerning stability. The maximum sagittal plane translation (z-axis) occurring in the lower cervical spine under physiologic loads simulating flexion–extension has been measured. Direct measurements indicate that the upper limit of normal is 2.7 mm. The same measurements on radiographic examination would vary with the technique employed and the subsequent degree of magnification. White and coworkers suggest 3.5 mm as a guide for the upper limits of normal, taking into account radiographic magnification (a 182-mm tube-to-film, and a 36-cm spine-to-film, distance).[35] Thus, one may consider the adult cervical spine to be probably unstable when there is more than 3.5 mm of horizontal displacement of one vertebra in relation to an adjacent vertebra, measured on lateral radiographs.

In an effort to determine the values for y-axis translation, White and coworkers developed a method of clinical evaluation termed the *stretch test.*[37] Their procedure for the stretch test is outlined in Figure 2-47. The test measures the dis-

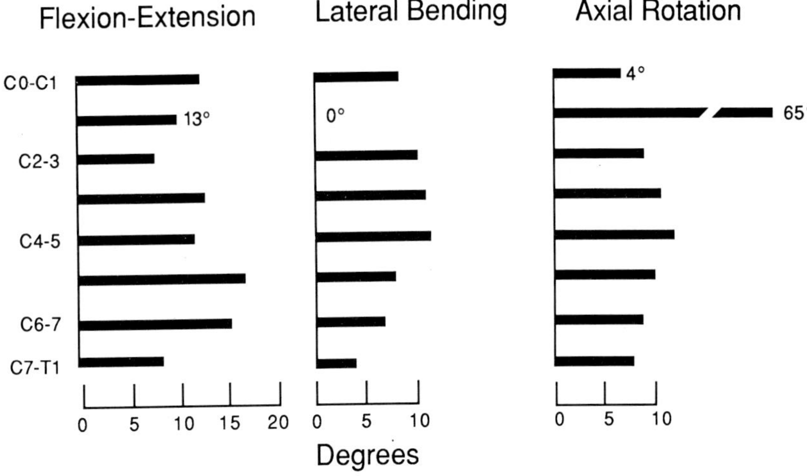

Fig. 2-46. A composite of the representative values for rotation at the different levels of the cervical spine in the traditional planes of motion. It is designed to allow a ready comparison of the motion in the various regions of the cervical spine, as well as the different types of movement in each region. (White AA III, Panjabi MM: The basic kinematics of the human spine: A review of past and current knowledge. Spine 3:12, 1978)

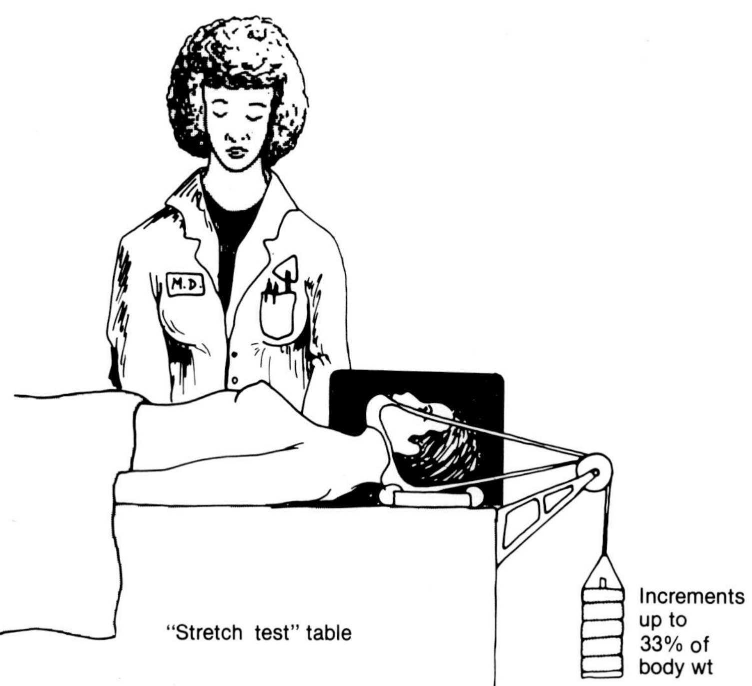

Fig. 2-47. Diagrammatic synopsis of stretch test. A physician who is knowledgeable about the test is in attendance. The neurologic status is monitored by following signs and symptoms. Incremental loads up to 33% of body weight or 65 lb are applied. Each lateral radiograph is checked prior to augmentation of the axial load. Note the neurologic hammer to symbolize neurologic exam and the roller platform under the head to reduce friction.

placement pattern of the cervical spine under carefully controlled conditions and identifies any abnormality in these patterns, which may be indicative of instability. Biomechanically, the spinal cord can tolerate considerable displacement in the axial (y-axis) direction.[29] Thus, in the acute clinical situation, a *carefully monitored* test employing displacement in the axial direction is safer than the potentially hazardous horizontal displacement. Based on a study of eight normal subjects, an abnormal stretch test is indicated by an interspace separation of greater than 1.7 mm. Similarly, any excessive relative axial displacement at the interspace in question should make one suspicious of structural damage. The investigators have developed a set of criteria for evaluation of clinical instability in the lower cervical spine. These criteria are presented in the form of a checklist shown in Table 2-4. More information on this system is available.[35,37]

Patterns of Motion

As a vertebra goes through its ranges of motion, its patterns of motion are determined by the geometric design of the structure and the physical properties of the soft-tissue attachments. The positions of the vertebra from full flexion to full extension have certain characteristic similarities and regional differences throughout the spine. In flexion, a cervical vertebra tilts and slides over its inferior vertebra. The intervertebral joint surface of the caudal vertebra slides upward and forward over the cranial joint surface. This movement is a combination of translation and rotation. At the same time the spinous processes separate. The joint space assumes a wedge shape with the base oriented posteriorly.[24]

Lysell used the term *top angle* to describe the steepness of the arch formed by the cervical vertebra going from full flexion to full extension.[24] The patterns of motion in the sagittal plane are shown diagrammatically in Figure 2-48. It is clear that the top angle lowers as the pattern of motion flattens. The steepest top angle is at C6, followed by C7. C2 is the flattest. The arcuity of the arch decreases in association with disc degeneration. This overall pattern is a statistically significant variation.[24]

Table 2-4. Checklist for the Diagnosis of Clinical Instability in the Lower Cervical Spine

ELEMENT	POINT VALUE
Anterior elements destroyed or unable to function	2
Posterior elements destroyed or unable to function	2
Relative sagittal plane translation >3.5 mm	2
Relative sagittal plane rotation >11°	2
Positive stretch test	2
Spinal cord damage	2
Nerve root damage	1
Abnormal disc narrowing	1
Dangerous loading anticipated	1
Total of 5 or more = unstable	

(White AA, Southwick WO, Panjabi MM: Clinical instability in the lower cervical spine: A review of past and current concepts. Spine 1:15, 1976)

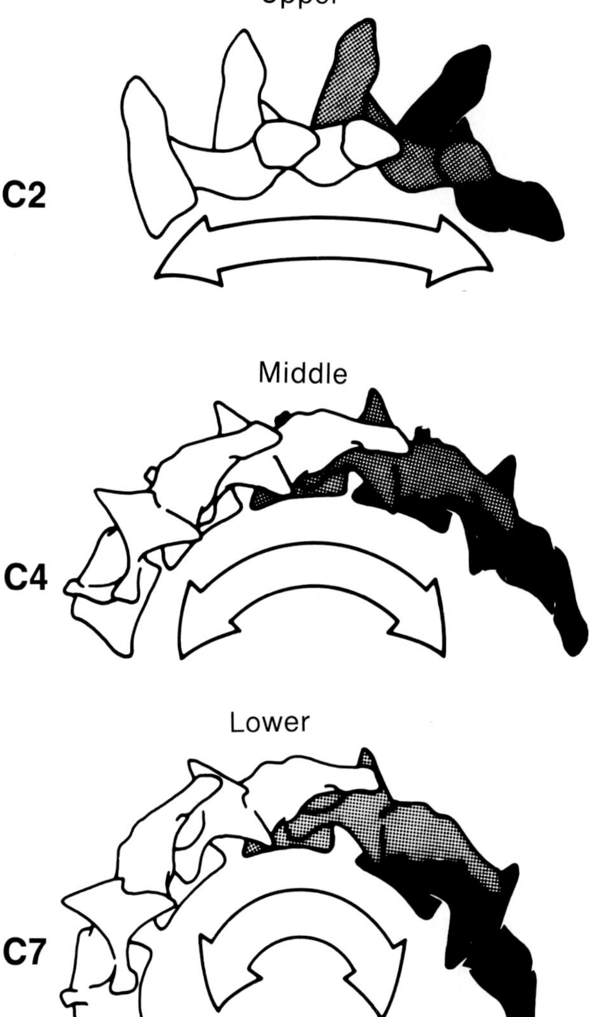

Fig. 2-48. A diagrammatic approximation of the relative cephalocaudal variations in radii of curvature of the arches, defined by the cervical vertebrae as they rotate and translate in the sagittal plane. The diagram depicts the patterns of motion of C2, C4, and C7, moving back and forth between full flexion and full extension.

Coupling Characteristics

The coupling pattern in the lower cervical spine is such that with lateral bending the spinous processes go toward the convexity of the curve.[24] Therefore, in lateral bending to the left the spinous processes go to the right, and in lateral bending to the right they go to the left (Fig. 2-10). (In the coordinate system, a positive θ z is coupled with negative θ y, negative θ z is coupled with positive θ y). This coupling pattern is marked and clinically significant in understanding cervical spine facet dislocations. For example, a facet dislocation may result when a traumatic force carries a joint beyond its normal range of motion. In this instance, there is exaggeration of the physiologic coupling between lateral bending and axial rotation. As a result, the facet on one side goes too far caudad, and the one on the opposite side goes too far cephalad and dislocates. A careful analysis and comprehension of this coupling pattern are useful in the manipulative reduction of a unilateral facet dislocation.

The amount of axial rotation that is coupled with lateral bending at various levels of the spine has also been described.[24] At the second cervical vertebra, there are 2° of coupled axial rotation for every 3° of lateral bending, a ratio of 2:3 (0.67). At the seventh cervical vertebra, there is 1° of coupled axial rotation for every 7.5° of lateral bending, a ratio of 1:7.5 (0.13). Between C2 and C7 there is a gradual cephalocaudal decrease in the amount of axial rotation that is associated with lateral bending. This phenomenon of gradual change in the coupling ratio may be related to a change in incline of the facet joints. Although this has not been measured or proven, it is generally believed that the incline of the facet joints in the sagittal plane increases cephalocaudally, a fact that may partially explain the relative frequency of unilateral facet location at C5 and below.

Instantaneous Axis of Rotation

The instantaneous axis of rotation for the cervical spine motion segments has been placed in different locations by various research workers.[36] This is partially due to methodological variations among investigators. Suggested locations include the body of the subadjacent vertebra, in the center of the vertebral body, in the disc, and also, specifically, the nucleus pulposus. An additional theory contends that the instantaneous axis of rotation for C2 lies in the posterior caudal portions of the subadjacent vertebra. However, there is a progression in which the instantaneous axis of rotation moves anterior and cephalad, such that C6 is located at the anterior cephalad portion of the adjacent vertebra.

For sagittal and horizontal plane motion, the instantaneous centers are thought to lie in the anterior portions of the subadjacent vertebra. This more anterior location is suggested by Lysell, who observed very little movement of his anterior measuring point. For lateral bending, the IAR is entirely speculative.

ACKNOWLEDGEMENT

The authors wish to express their sincere gratitude to Ms. Anya S. Vronsky for her patient and precise aid, and to Dr. Wilson C. Hayes for his insightful suggestions.

REFERENCES

1. *BALL J, MEIJERS KAE:* On cervical mobility. Ann Rheum Dis 23:429, 1964
2. *BARTON JW, MARGOLIS MT:* Rotational obstruction of the vertebral artery at the atlantoaxial joint. Neuroradiology 9:117, 1975
3. *BLANCHARD RS, KOTTKE FJ:* The study of degenerative changes of the cervical spine in relation to age. Bulletin University of Minnesota Hospital 24:470, 1953
4. *CLARK CR, GOEL VK, GALLES K, LIU YK:* Kinematics of the occipito-atlanto-axial complex. Transaction, Cervical Spine Research Society, 1986
5. *COFFEE MS, EDWARDS WT, HAYES WC, WHITE AA:* Mechanical response and strength of the human cervical spine. Transaction, Cervical Spine Research Society, 1986
6. *DEPREUX R, MESTDAGH H:* Anatomie functionelle de l'articulation sous occipatale. Lille Med 19:122, 1974
7. *DUNSKER SB, COLLEY DP, MAYFIELD FH:* Kinematics of the cervical spine. Clin Neurosurg 25:174, 1977
8. *DVORAK J, PANJABI MM, GERBER M:* Ct–functional diagnostics of the rotatory instability of the upper cervical spine (in press, 1987)
9. *FICK R:* Handbuch der Anatomie and Mechanik der Gelenke. Jena, S Fischer Verlag, 1904
10. *FIELDING JW:* Cineroentgenography of the normal cervical spine. J Bone Joint Surg 39A:1280, 1957
11. *FIELDING JW:* Normal and selected abnormal motion of the cervical spine from the second cervical vertebra to the seventh cervical vertebra based on cineroentgenography. J Bone Joint Surg 46A:1779, 1964
12. *FORD FR:* Syncope, vertigo and disturbances of vision resulting from intermittent obstruction of the vertebral arteries due to defect in the odontoid process and excessive mobility of the second cervical vertebra. Bulletin Johns Hopkins Hospital 91:168, 1952
13. *HADLEY LH:* Anatomicroradiographic studies: Development and the cervical region. In The Spine. Springfield, Illinois, Charles C Thomas, 1956
14. *HENKE W:* Hanbuch der Anatomie and Mechanik der Gelenke. Leipszig and Heidelberg, 1863
15. *HOHL M:* Normal motion in the upper portion of the cervical spine. J Bone Joint Surg 46A:1777, 1964
16. *HOHL M, BAKER HR:* The atlanto-axial joint. J Bone Joint Surg 46A:1739, 1964
17. *HULTKRANTZ JW:* Zur Mechanik der Kopfbewegungen beim Menschen. Kurgl Sv Vet Akad Handl 49(8):1912
18. *JACKSON H:* The diagnosis of minimal atlanto-axial subluxation. Br J Radiol 23:672, 1950
19. *JIROUT J:* Changes in the atlas–axis relations on lateral flexion of the head and neck. Neuroradiology 6:215, 1973
20. *JIROUT J:* The rotational component in the dynamics of the C2–3 spinal segment. Neuroradiology, 17:177, 1979
21. *JOHNSON RM, CRELIN ES, WHITE AA, PANJABI MM, SOUTHWICK WO:* Some new observations on the functional anatomy of the lower cervical spine. Clin Orthop 111:192, 1975
22. *JONES MD:* Cineradiographic studies of the normal cervical spine. California Medicine 93:293, 1960
23. *KOTTKE FJ, MONDALE MO:* Range of mobility of the cervical spine. Arch Phys Med 40:379, 1959
24. *LYSELL E:* Motion in the cervical spine. Acta Orthop Scand (Suppl) 123, 1969
25. *MILLER RG, BURTON R:* Stroke following chiropractic manipulation of the spine. JAMA 229:189, 1974
26. *RAYNOR R, MOSKOUICH R, ZIDEL P, PUGH J:* Alteration in primary and coupled neck motions following facetectomies. Presentation Cervical Spine Research Society, December 1986

27. *Penning L:* Normal movements of the cervical spine. Am J Roentgenol 130:317, 1979
28. *Schellaus KP, Latchaw RE, Wendling LR, Gold LHA:* Vertebrobasilar injuries following cervical manipulation. JAMA 244:1450, 1980
29. *Scher AT:* Anterior cervical subluxation: An unstable position. Am J Roentgenol 133:275, 1979
30. *Schoening HA, Hannan V:* Factors related to cervical spine mobility, Part I. Arch Phys Med Rehabil 45:602, 1964
31. *Selecki BR:* The effects of rotation of the atlas on the axis: Experimental work. Med J Aust 1:1012, 1969
32. *Shapiro R, Youngberg AS, Rothman SLG:* The differential diagnosis of traumatic lesions of the occipito-atlanto-axial segment. Radiol Clin North Am 11:505, 1973

32a. *Torg JS, Sennett B, Vegso JJ, Pavlov H, Lehman R:* Axial loading injuries to the middle cervical spine segment: An analysis and classification of twenty-five cases. Cervical Spine Research Society, December 1986

33. *Weisel SW, Rothman RH:* Occipitoatlantal hypermobility. Spine 4:187, 1979
34. *Werne S:* Studies in spontaneous atlas dislocation. Acta Orthop Scand (Suppl) 23, 1957
35. *White AA III, Johnson RM, Panjabi MM, Southwick WO:* Biomechanical analysis of clinical stability in the cervical spine. Clin Orthop 109:85, 1975
36. *White AA III, Panjabi MM:* Spinal Kinematics in the Research Status of Spinal Manipulative Therapy. NINCDS Monograph No. 15. Washington, DC, U.S. Department of Health, Education, and Welfare, 1975
37. *White AA III, Panjabi MM:* Clinical Biomechanics of the Spine. Philadelphia, JB Lippincott, 1978
38. *Worth D:* Kinematics of the Cranio-Vertebral Joints. Ph.D. Dissertation, Victoria Institute of Colleges, 1980

BIBLIOGRAPHY

Brattstrom H, Granholm L: Atlanto-axial fusion in rheumatoid arthritis. Acta Orthop Scand 47:619, 1976

Colachis SC, Strohm BR: Radiographic studies of cervical spine motion in normal subjects: Flexion and hyperextension. Arch Phys Med Rehabil 46:753, 1965

McSweeny T: Traumatic atlanto-axial fracture dislocation in a child. Paraplegia 17:372, 1979–1980

Panjabi MM, White AA, Keller D, Southwick WO, Friedlander G: Stability of the cervical spine under tension. J Biomech 111:189, 1978

Park WM, O'Neill M, McCall I: The radiology of rheumatoid involvement of the cervical spine. Skeletal Radiol 4:1, 1979

Penning L: Functional Pathology of the Cervical Spine. Excerpta Medica Amsterdam, 1968

White AA III, Panjabi MM: The basic kinematics of the human spine: A review of past and current knowledge. Spine 3:12, 1978

White AA III, Panjabi MM: The clinical biomechanics of the occipito-atlantoaxial complex. Orthop Clin North Am 9:867, 1978

Mechanisms of Injury in the Cervical Spine: Experimental Evidence and Biomechanical Modeling

ROBERT R. CROWELL, W. THOMAS EDWARDS, AND AUGUSTUS A. WHITE, III

The purpose of this chapter is to review the cogent clinical and experimental data regarding injury to the cervical spine and to describe the development and the relevance of biomechanical models of the cervical spine. The goal is to improve basic science and clinical understanding of the mechanisms of injury (MOI) in the cervical spine.

Research designed to improve understanding of the MOI in the cervical spine has employed clinical observation, experimental laboratory investigations, or biomechanical models. We submit that the biomechanical study of MOI in the spine should include the following four steps:

1. Clinical observation
2. Experimental investigation
3. Analytic study (modeling)
4. Validation

The successful completion of these four steps should result in a better understanding of MOI, and criteria for cervical spine injury may be established. We will proceed according to this sequence. Clinical observations lead to hypotheses to explain the mechanism of injury, based on descriptions of cervical spine fractures and dislocations. Classification of these injuries may refine our ability to discriminate and help us to understand the underlying biomechanics. Experimental investigations test hypotheses by simulating the conditions believed to produce injury. Although experimental studies provide quantitative data on vertebrae, ligaments, and the interconnecting structures, the results generally display the wide range of variation characteristic of biological testing. Analytic models developed in conjunction with experimental studies can provide more detailed descriptions of the internal biomechanical response of the tissues of the spine than can be obtained through experiment or clinical observation alone. Because biomechanical models are built from assumptions about the actual physical properties and interactions of the spine, they must be carefully validated by experimental data. Few studies address all four steps. This leaves the clinician and other interested readers with the task of gathering and interpreting findings scattered through the scientific literature.

Significant bodies of experimental and biomechanical data on the cervical spine appear in the orthopedic biomechanics literature and in publications of the transportation and aerospace industries. The authors have reviewed this literature and selected the information that was considered the most cogent, valid, and useful for an up-to-date understanding of MOI in the cervical spine.

CLINICAL EVALUATIONS OF CERVICAL SPINE INJURIES

Clinical estimations of MOI for the cervical spine have generally been based on plausible conceptualizations of the forces and displacements necessary to produce fractures and ligament injuries presumed from interpretations of radiographs. This section reports clinical descriptions of cervical spine injuries and the presumed MOI based primarily on such interpretations.

Spinal injuries have been classified according to the suspected mechanisms and level of injury. Mechanisms of injury have focused on the mechanical conditions at each cervical vertebra. The major injuring vector (MIV) concept presented by White and Panjabi[68] is such an example of a mechanical analysis of injury at the cervical spine segment level. However, studies of whole spines and cadavers reviewed in this chapter indicate that external mechanical conditions (*i.e.*, forces and moments applied at the head) do not always reflect the segmental conditions and patterns of injury at the level of the individual cervical vertebra. In the cervical spine, the upper region comprising of atlantooccipital and the atlantoaxial joints is subject to quite different injuries than those observed in the middle (C2–C5) and lower (C5–C7) cervical regions, owing to unique anatomic and mechanical characteristics. These groups of injuries are described separately in the following sections. The segmental patterns of injury for the middle and lower regions have not been separated in this section. However, there is evidence that different patterns of injury occur in those regions. This will also be discussed later in this section.

Injuries of the Upper Cervical Spine (C1–C2)

Dislocations in this region are generally fatal. Fractures of the atlas commonly involve two or more breaks in the ring and have been clinically presumed to be caused by axial compression. Fractures of the dens are commonly associated with an anterior or a posterior displacement of the atlas. Anterior displacement of the atlas on the axis is thought to be associated with flexion and anterior shear injuries whereas posterior displacement injuries are considered to be due to hyperextension moments and posterior shear forces.[68] Injury to the axis commonly occurs through the region of its pedicles (isthmus) with separation of the body of the axis from the C3 vertebra below, such as with traumatic spondylolisthesis or "hangman's fracture."[68]

Injuries of the Middle (C2–C5) and Lower (C5–C7) Cervical Spine

Extreme cervical compression may occur during a wide variety of activities. Similar external loading patterns occur in diving injuries, American football, trampoline injuries, auto crashes and emergency aircraft egress (ejection seat injuries). Compression forces are responsible for a number of nonfatal fractures in egress injury. These fractures have been classified by Kazarian[29] (1978) as (1) fractures of the vertebral body margins, (2) anterior wedge fractures, (3) lateral wedge fractures, and (4) cleavage fractures of the centrum. The anterior and lateral wedge fractures occur when flexion forces are combined with compression forces. The anterior wedge fracture is the most common nonfatal egress injury. It is considered to be clinically benign and complete recovery is possible. Pain and discomfort, however, may be significant and may cause two or more months of disability. This injury is characterized by collapse of the anterior part of the vertebral body. It is typically found in the regions C5–T1.[29]

Teardrop fractures are readily identified on lateral radiographs as the apparent anterior fracture of the vertebral body with an anterior-inferior fragment adjacent to the endplate, resembling "a drop of water dripping from the vertebral body."[60] The term "teardrop" reflected the sadness often associated with the neurologic sequelae. The mechanism of this injury has been described as hyperflexion[60] and as combined flexion and compression loading.[18] It is also important to recognize another more important fracture plane oriented in the sagittal plane, which often splits the vertical body into left and right halves (Fig. 2-49). These halves may rotate with backward displacement and neural canal encroachment. This often unappreciated component of vertebral injury, which frequently accompanies the teardrop fracture, has been described by Torg[66] and Fuentes and associates.[18]

Flexion injuries are presumed to result when the head and neck are forced forward on the trunk beyond the normal limits. Braakman and Penning (1971) have classified flexion injuries into compressive hyperflexion and distractive hyperflexion. Compressive hyperflexion mechanisms are those caused by forces that produce flexion of the neck combined with axial compression forces. Flexion of the head may accompany the flexion of regions of vertebral segments, but this head rotation is not necessary.[22] During this combination of forces and moments, various types of fractures may occur. Wedge compression fracture, as described above, is assumed to occur under relatively mild compressive forces. It can occur with disruption of the posterior elements, if the flexion moment is large enough.

Distractive hyperflexion may occur during deceleration where the flexion moments tend to separate the vertebral segments. Three types of injury result: hyperflexion sprain and unilateral and bilateral facet dislocations. Hyperflexion sprain is defined as a temporary or partial luxation of the intervertebral joints following traumatic hyperflexion under moderate forces, with rupture of the posterior ligaments and joint capsules, but without dislocation. This type of injury is assumed to be relatively rare because major forces are required to rupture the posterior ligaments. These major forces would likely result in interlocking of the facets and facet dislocation. Only rarely would the hyperflexion movement stop prior to interlocking (Braakman and Penning, 1968).[5a]

The definitive etiology of bilateral facet dislocation has not been well established. This injury involves the caudal facets of the superior vertebra being displaced anterior to the cephalic articular facets of the inferior vertebra. Extensive ligamentous disruption is produced, including tearing of the interspinous, intertransverse and capsular ligaments, the ligamenta flava, and a variable portion of the annulus (Fig. 2-50).[3] The flexion injury mechanism has been assumed,[2,45,68] although other authors have advocated extension (Taylor and Blackwood, 1948),[62a] vertical compression[2] and axial rotation mechanisms.[55] The experimental production of these injuries will be discussed in the following section.

Unilateral facet dislocation is assumed to occur from axial rotation moments as well as flexion moments and distraction forces. In this injury the caudal articular surface of one facet of the supe-

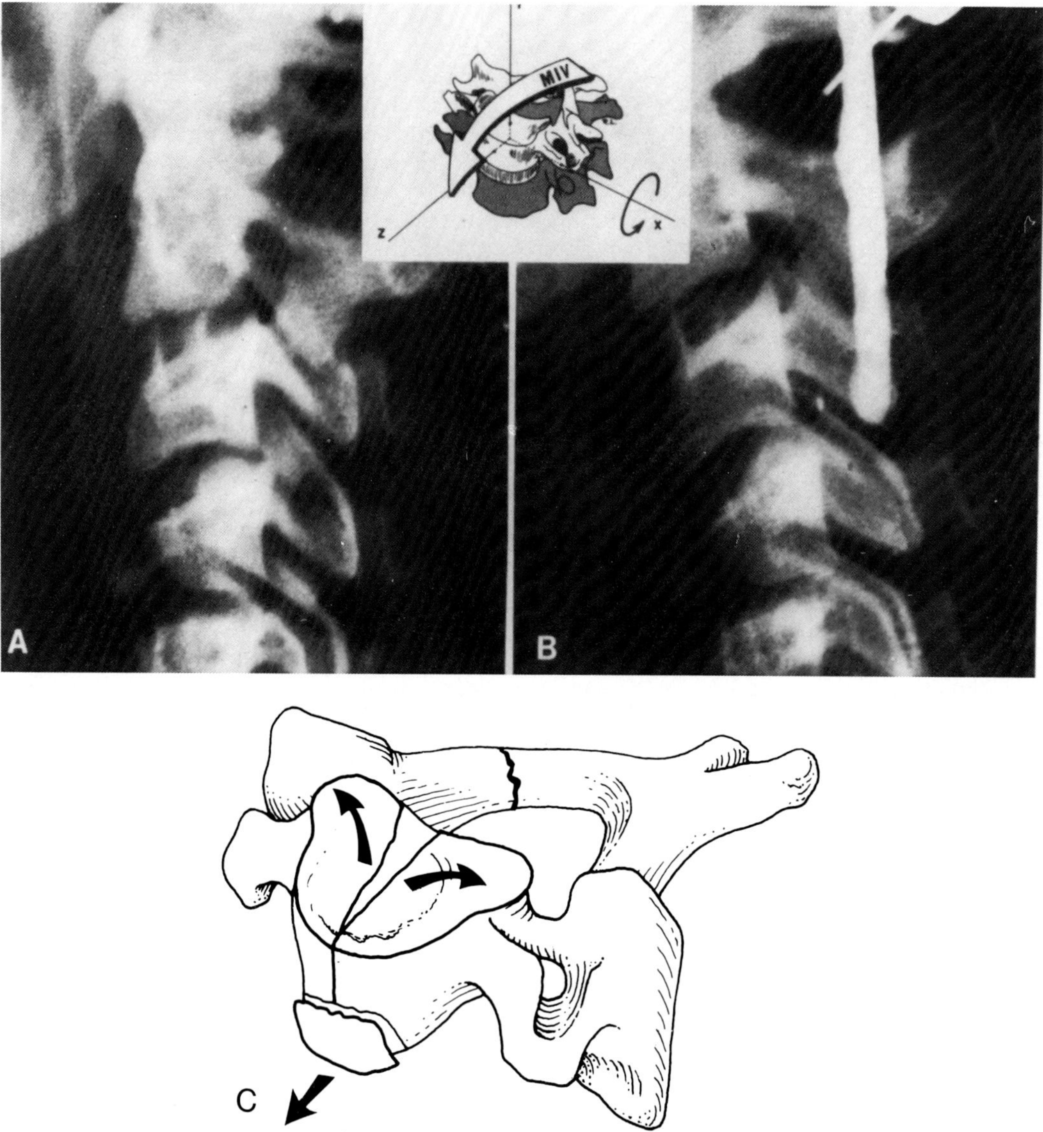

Fig. 2-49. The "teardrop" fracture. (*A*) In this lateral radiograph of a tetraplegic patient following a diving injury, a triangular anteroinferior fragment from the body of C4 is readily appreciated. (*B*) A complete myelographic block is demonstrated. (*C*) Orientation of common fracture planes, and directions of fragment displacement commonly occurring in this injury. (White AA III, Panjabi MM: Clinical Biomechanics of the Spine, 2nd ed. Copyright © 1988, JB Lippincott Company [in press])

rior vertebra is fixed too far anterior to the cephalic articular facet of the inferior vertebra. Depending on the presence of other associated forces, this may or may not be associated with a fracture of the involved superior articular facet or lamina (Fig. 2-51).[68] Tearing of the interspinous ligaments, a variable amount of the ligamenta flava, and the capsule of one facet joint occurs, and the facet dislocates.[3]

The key information from these studies is as follows: many fracture patterns demonstrate axial compression as a component of their mechanisms of injury, including the more severe cleavage fractures; clearly, wedge fractures also have a signifi-

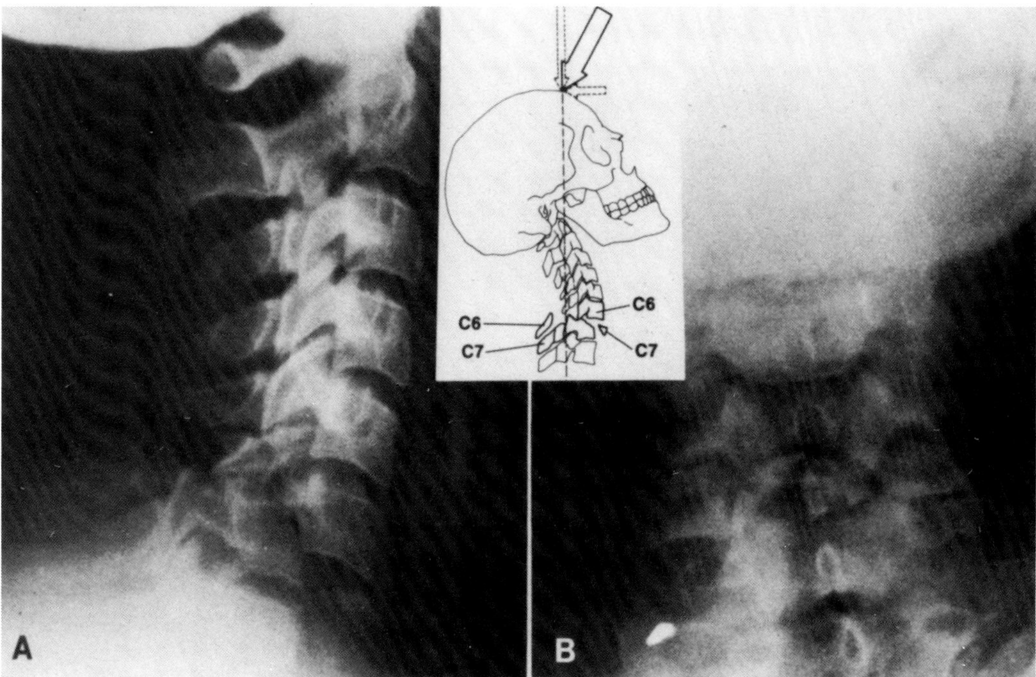

Fig. 2-50. Dislocation in lower cervical region. Complete ligamentous disruption must be present for such displacement to occur. (White AA III, Panjabi MM: Clinical Biomechanics of the Spine, 2nd ed. Copyright © 1988, JB Lippincott Company [in press])

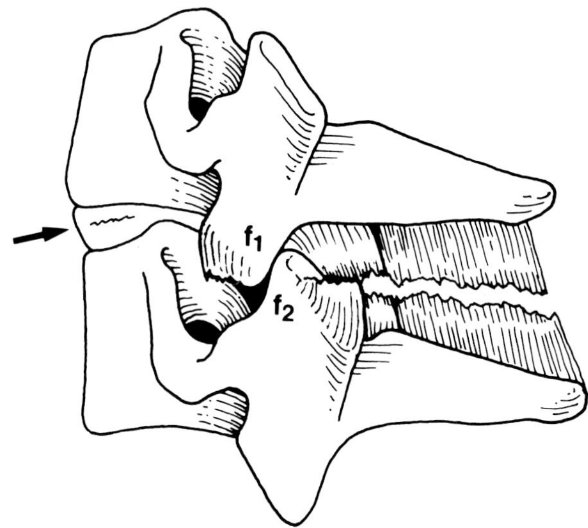

Fig. 2-51. Unilateral facet dislocation. The inferior facet (*f.1*) of the superior vertebra is displaced and "locked" anterior to the superior facet (*f.2*) of the vertebra below. The arrow points to a small tear in the annulus. (After Beatson TR: Fractures and dislocations of the cervical spine. J Bone Joint Surg 45B:21, 1963)

cant flexion component; flexion mechanisms may include anterior vertebral compression with posterior ligamentous structures loaded in tension; the mechanism of dislocations remains controversial and nonmidsagittal motions, such as axial rotation, may play an important role.

EXPERIMENTAL EVALUATION OF CERVICAL SPINE INJURIES

Based on consideration of the biomechanics of the cervical spine, we propose the following hypothesis. A given injured functional spinal unit may be subjected to various combinations of vertical forces, horizontal shear forces, and bending moments that correspond to certain patterns of reproducible fractures and associated ligamentous injuries. The authors also hypothesize that there exists a set of critical conditions of external loading characteristics and initial head-neck-thorax positions that determines the vertebral stresses and presence and severity of injury (Figs. 2-52 and 2-53). To investigate and interpret this hypothesis, quantitative descriptions of vertebral loads and dis-

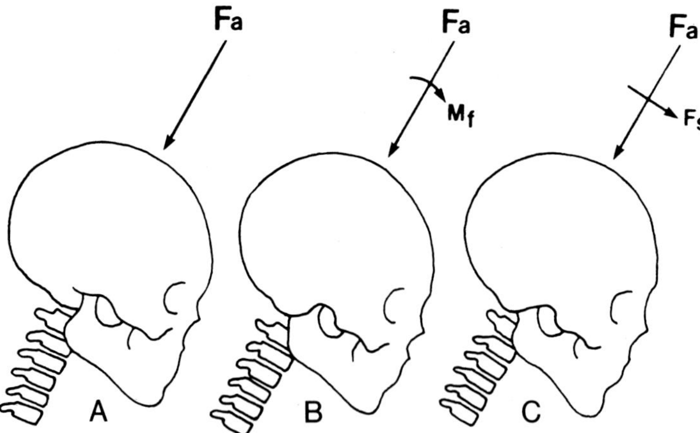

Fig. 2-52. Variation in external loading and influence on pattern of failure for the straightened cervical spine. (*A*) Axial loading will produce a sudden buckling at failure. (*B*) Eccentric axial impacts, which create an applied axial force and bending moment, will produce bending of the spine interposed in the load path prior to failure. (*C*) Nonaxial net forces may result in deflection of the head and neck out of the load path.

placement, and point and rate of load application are required.

As White and Panjabi have indicated, six components of displacement (translations and rotations) and the corresponding six components of load (forces and moments) at the level(s) of injury are needed to describe the biomechanical environment (Fig. 2-54). The major injuring vector(s) causing a specific cervical spine injury may be regarded as that net force vector and/or moment vector resulting from these components. Differing coordinate labeling systems have evolved in the medical, automotive, and aeronautical engineering literatures (Fig. 2-55). These differences should be noted in interpreting experimental descriptions (*e.g.*, acceleration in the z direction) from various sources. Fortunately, most systems utilize the vertebral body center for the origin, enabling direct comparison of results. We are optimistic that eventually some common labeling of the coordinate system will be practiced.[50,69]

Most frequently, compression, in combination with flexion or extension, is present during severe cervical injury.[66] The magnitudes of each compo-

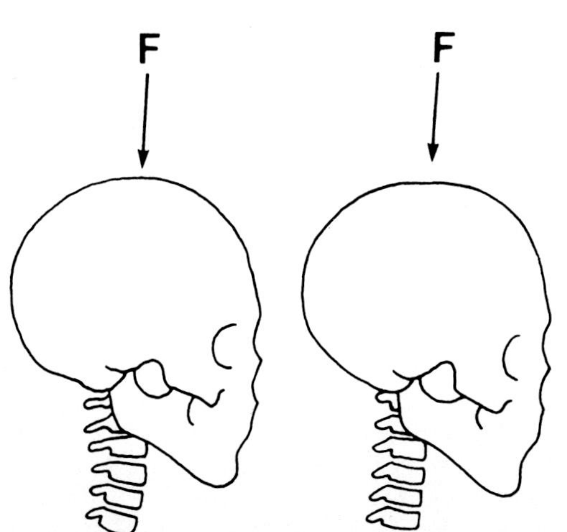

Fig. 2-53. Influence of initial cervical spine position on pattern of failure. *Left,* Axial loading of the initially bent cervical spine will produce bending prior to failure. *Right,* Axial loading along the straightened cervical spine will result in a buckling mode of failure.

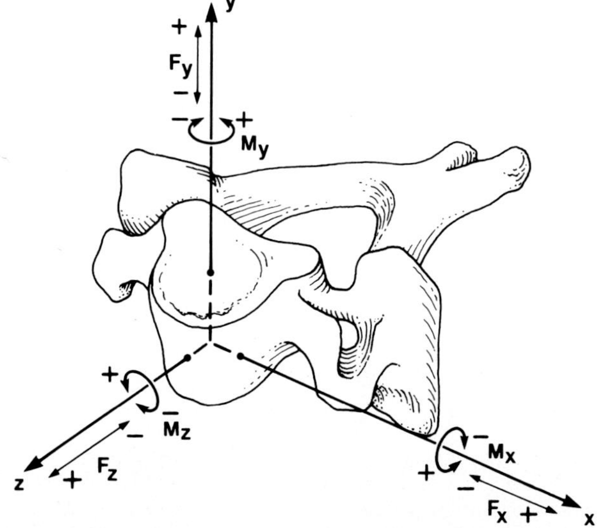

Fig. 2-54. Possible forces and moments acting at the segmental level. Any force or moment vector may be resolved into components acting along orthogonal (mutually perpendicular) axes. Stiffnesses may be different in the positive and negative directions.

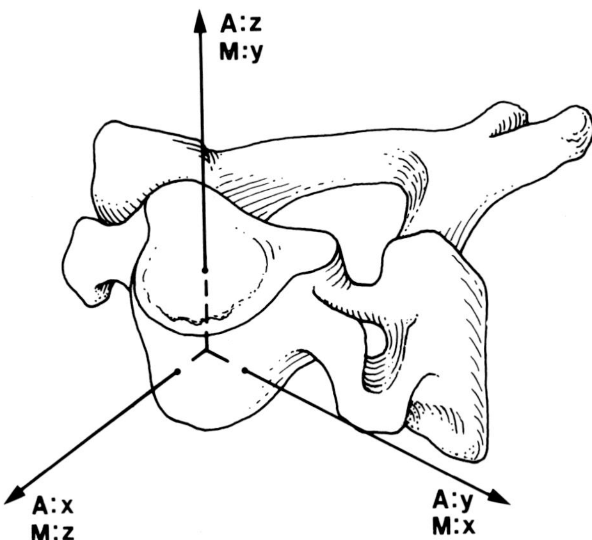

Fig. 2-55. Differing systems of coordinate labeling are in common use within the medical (*M*) literature and automotive and aeronautical (*A*) engineering literature.

nent of load and displacement for the specific injuries presumed to result from compressive loading have not been well quantified. It is also important to note that even though midsagittal plane analysis is a useful investigative concept and methodology, the mechanism of injury is much more complex and truly three-dimensional.

Experimental Studies

Much of the experimental work reporting specific cervical spine injuries with specific loading patterns exists within the automotive engineering literature. A number of studies of whole-body cadaveric testing and isolated spine segment testing have been reported in the Proceedings of the STAPP Car Crash Conferences.[1,22,36,46] Generally, compressive loadings of the cervical spine in varying degrees of forward and lateral flexion and extension have been performed. Marked variability in the load sustained to failure has been noted within and among the studies (see Table 2-5). Although a one-to-one correspondence between major injuring vectors at cervical segments and external patterns of loading has not been established, important observations can be made. The load magnitude, the rate and duration of load application (the time history), the point of load application, the direction of loading, and the initial cervical spine position and relative positions of the head and thorax, all determine the individual cervical spine injury.

During extreme compression, the entire cervical spine may bend or buckle in a manner not consistent with the patterns and range of normal coupled physiologic motion. The initial position of the head, neck and thorax is most important in determining the mechanical response to a given load combination.

Alem and coworkers,[1] in cadaver drop and pendulum impact studies (Fig. 2-56), noted that "buckling" of the cervical spine occurred with axial loading when the neck was positioned to simulate the natural attitude of normal sitting or standing persons. In virtually all tests, cervical spine damage was noted when the neck "buckled" under the impact load. In contrast, with similar impact loading no cervical spine damage was apparent when the spine was aligned along the line of action of the impact force. However, autopsies were not performed, and time histories are not reported for this group. It should be noted that these investigators used the term "buckling" to describe the displacements of the spine from an initial curved position, rather than displacements from a straight segmented column.[66]

Table 2-5. Vertical Loads Sustained to Failure

CADAVER SEGMENTS			
Author	Failure Load (N)	Load Velocity (m/s)	No. Cadavers
Bauze and Ardran	1420 (maximum)	slow hand pump	14
McElhaney and associates	960 to 6840	0.64	14
Maiman and associates	645 to 7440	0.0025 to 1.52	13
WHOLE CADAVERS			
Author	Load to Failure (N)	Load Velocity (m/s)	No. Cadavers
Yoganandan and associates	3000 to 14,700	4.2 to 5.4	15
Nusholtz and associates	3200 to 10,800	4.0 to 5.9	8
Alem and associates	3000 to 17,000	7 to 11	10

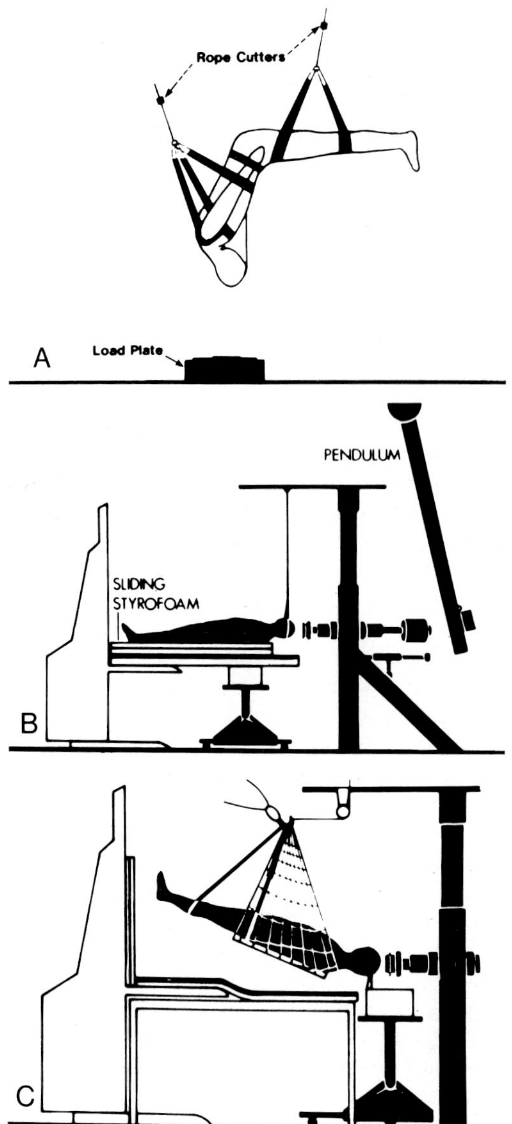

Fig. 2-56. Various techniques of cadaver impact testing. (Huelke DF, Nusholtz GS: Cervical spine biomechanics: A review of the literature. J Orthop Res 4:232. Copyright © 1986 by the Orthopaedic Research Society)

Maiman and coworkers[35] studied the relationship between cervical flexion/extension and its relation to failure load magnitude and cervical damage. Cadaver head-to-torso segments and cervical spine segments were subjected to axial loading either in a neutral upright position or prepositioned in 25° of flexion or extension. The point of load application for the neutral position was at the vertex, except for two specimens with loads applied 2 cm posterior or 2 cm anterior to the vertex. All specimens prepositioned in flexion or extension failed in an apparent flexion or extension mode, respectively. The cadavers with posteriorly applied loads failed in extension, and those with anteriorly applied loads failed in flexion. Of the neutral specimens loaded directly at the vertex, only two failed in apparent direct axial compression, one failed in extension, and two failed in flexion. The cadavers that were axially loaded sustained much greater loads to failure (mean 3567 N = 802 lb.) than those prepositioned in flexion or extension (mean 1823 and 1089 N = 417 and 245 lb., respectively).

The significance of the initial cervical spine position at the time of axial impact loadings was also studied by Hodgson and Thomas[22] in their cadaver impact tests. Cervical spine strains measured at the C3, C5, and C7 vertebral bodies were evaluated for various neck and thorax positions and also for differing directions of loading (Fig. 2-57). The highest vertebral body strains were seen as a result of axial loading at the crown of the head with relative flexion of the neck and chest, which will straighten the lower cervical lordosis.[66] Of the varying positions of load application, axial loading at the vertex with the cervical spine being neutral demonstrated the highest vertebral body strains, in comparison to positions of more anterior force application and more cervical extension. In comparing these results with those of Alem and coworkers,[1] it seems probable that the positions with the highest strain (*i.e.*, mild cervical-thoracic flexion with axial load carefully positioned along the axis of a straightened cervical spine) seen in the Hodgson and Thomas studies would be the positions that sustain the highest loads to failure. Had these strain studies (2450 N maximum impact load = 551 lb) been conducted at higher loads (such as the 3000 to 17,000 N impacts of the studies of Alem and coworkers), the low-strain positions may have exhibited greater damage.

Results from the above three studies suggest that the straightened cervical spine (as with mild forward flexion) can *withstand* the highest axial load magnitudes; but, perhaps even more importantly, the straightened cervical spine will *sustain* the highest load (and strain) magnitudes on external axial impacts, of all positions studied.

Yoganandan and colleagues[72] measured peak forces produced by vertical impact of restrained and unrestrained cadavers. Eight of 15 heads were restrained to simulate muscle forces supporting the head in a neutral position. The unrestrained cadavers demonstrated more rapid cervical flexion upon impact than did the restrained cadavers. Peak forces measured at the head were higher in the restrained (9800 to 14,700 N) than in the unrestrained (3000 to 7100 N) cadavers. Somewhat greater numbers of injuries occurred in the restrained cadaver cervical spines than in the unrestrained spines, although the restrained were dropped from a greater mean height (1.31 m versus 1.16 m). A predominance of anterior ligamentous and posterior bony injuries occurred in the restrained group, and posterior ligamentous and anterior bony injuries in the unrestrained group, corresponding to the flexion motion observed. This study suggests that there may be relatively decreased axial loading in spines that are allowed to flex immediately on impact. It also illustrates another potential response to external impacts, namely that of deflection of the head and cervical spine out of the load path.

Nusholtz and coworkers[46] suggest that cervical spine "flexion-type" damage from vertical impact from axial compression of the mildly flexed spine positioned in the midsagittal plane is unlikely. However, in these studies flexion type injuries, that is vertebral body compression and posterior ligamentous disruption, were readily produced in axially rotated or laterally flexed spines. Upper thoracic spine injuries were also seen frequently in these experiments. Thus this study emphasizes the importance of these nonmidsagittal plane forces and the importance of the thoracic response in vertical loading injuries.

The importance of nonmidsagittal motions was also emphasized by Roaf.[55] He was unable to produce purely ligamentous injury, by flexion or extension alone, in cadaver spine segments. With forced flexion, vertebral body fracture occurred prior to posterior ligamentous failure. With axial rotation and flexion, posterior ligamentous injuries were readily produced, and vertebral body fracture was dependent upon applied compression. Quantitative data regarding force and moment magnitude, and the technique of load application were not reported.

In contrast to the above studies, Crowell and associates[7] noted both posterior ligament injuries and compression fractures in cadaveric spine segments from the middle and lower regions that were subjected to pure flexion loads. Such failures occurred in six of seven middle segment specimens and in two of seven lower segment specimens subjected to flexion from 21° to 33° over two motion segments. Much more extensive ligament injuries, including posterior longitudinal ligament tears, occurred in two other specimens which were axially rotated 16° prior to flexion. This further emphasizes the importance of nonmidsagittal positions, such as axial rotation, in lowering the threshold of injury in flexion loading.

One purely ligamentous injury, the bilateral facet dislocation, was consistently produced by Bauze and Ardran[2] at relatively low load levels. Axial load was applied to a forward flexed cervical spine segment with the end below the dislocation stiffened by insertion of a rod into the neural canal. The combination of axial loading of the forward flexed cervical spine and stiffening of the segment below the level of injury created a sufficient local forward flexion moment and forward shear force component of the applied force to consistently produce this injury. The clinical significance of these specialized loading conditions remains unknown, and the relative necessity of nonmidsagittal plane loads in the production of purely ligamentous lesions in the clinical setting remains unproven by these studies. The degrees of stress concentration produced in this experiment limit considerably its simulation of the clinical setting, except for the partial arthrodesis of the cervical spine. Bilateral facet dislocation was produced in vertical unrestrained cadaver drop by Yoganandan and colleagues,[72] although nonmidsagittal position data are not reported.

Mechanisms creating other specific spine injuries have been demonstrated by McElhaney and associates[36] in cadaver spine segment loading studies. In these tests, a very small anterior-to-posterior distance variation from neutral (1 cm) in the point of application of axial spine loading, produced great variation in the type of fracture produced. The following fracture patterns were associated with specific loading conditions:

1. Extension fractures: Buckling of the straightened cervical spine in extension was noted with only 1 cm of posterior eccentricity of axial loading.
2. Jefferson fractures: These were experimentally produced with direct axial loading of the generally straight cervical spine, with slight extension (magnitude not reported) of the specimens noted on review of pretest and post-test x-rays.
3. Burst fractures: These fractures were produced by direct axial load of the straightened cervical spine segments, which were found to be slightly flexed on x-ray review. These specimens required larger loads and strain ener-

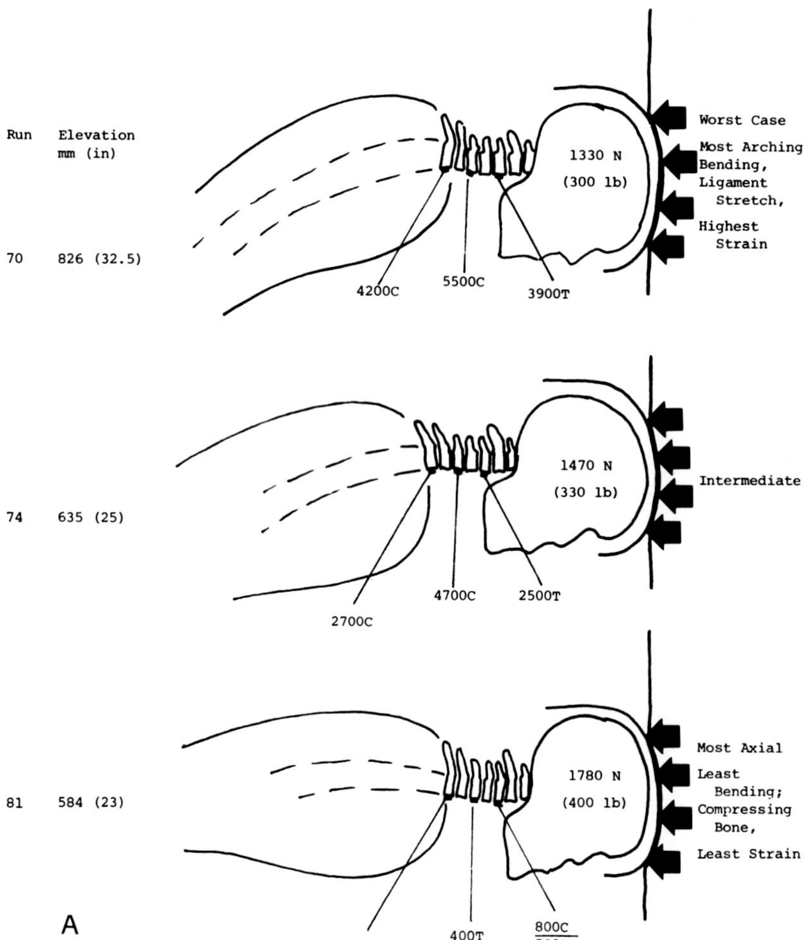

Fig. 2-57. Variation in cervical vertebral strain in (*A*) differing head-neck-thorax positions and (*B*) differing directions of impact load. (Hodgson VR, Thomas LM: Mechanisms of cervical spine injury during impact to the protected head, Proc 24th STAPP Car Crash Conference. Society of Automotive Engineers, Warrendale. Copyright © 1980, Society of Automotive Engineers)

gies prior to fracture than did the Jefferson fractures.

4. Anterior wedge fractures: Application of the axial load less than 1 cm anterior to neutral produced compression of the anterior vertebral body. Axial loads applied at a distance greater than 1 cm forward produced buckling rearward and subsequent disc and endplate failure.
5. The "teardrop" fracture[60]: This fracture has been experimentally produced by axial compression of the neutral and minimally flexed cervical spine.[1,35] The presence of a sagittal fracture plane, in addition to the more horizontal plane, is demonstrated in careful analyses of clinical injuries of this type.[18,66]
6. Disc ruptures: These injuries have been produced in many specimens subjected to axial impacts in various degrees of cervical flexion/extension.[1,72] Disc ruptures were most common in tests that also subjected the specimens to axial rotation and lateral flexion at the time of impact,[46] occurring in six of eight specimens.

Experimental Overview

These studies demonstrate that the initial head-neck-thorax position and loading conditions dictate the cervical spine response to impact. There appear to be three patterns of response: bending of the curved spine under axial load, buckling of the straightened spine under axial load, and deflection of the spine out of the load path. Varying the initial position alters the type of response, maximum load at failure, and extent of injury. Thus, in potentially subinjurious impacts the initial position may determine the presence or absence of

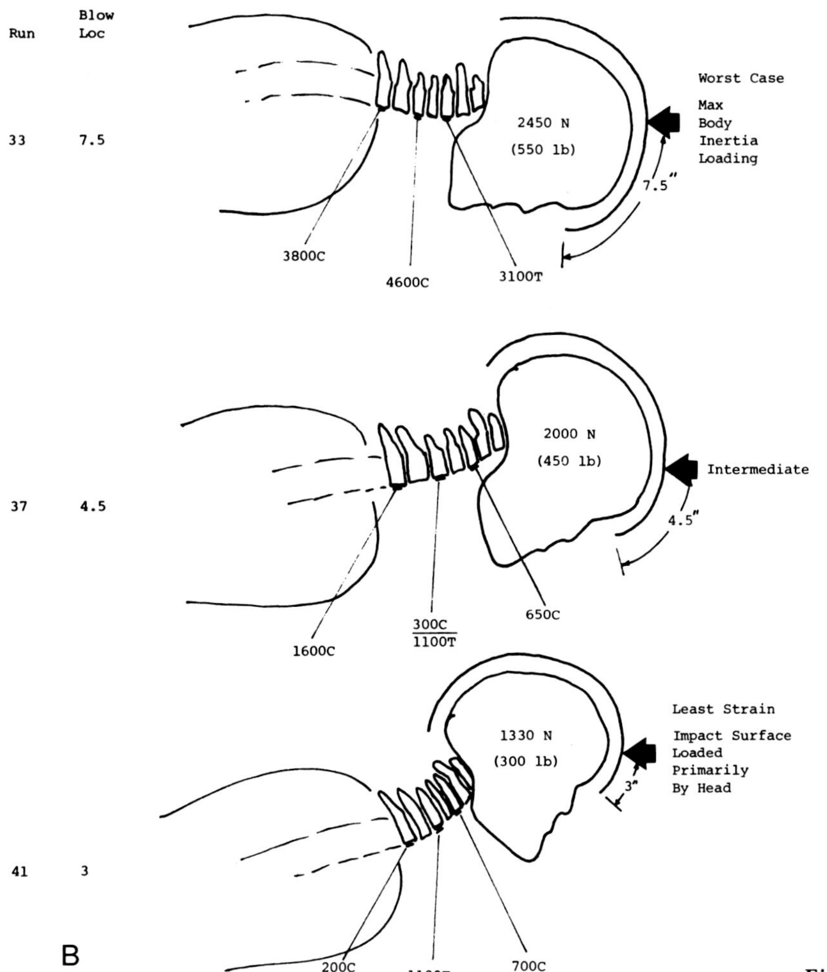

Fig. 2-57, B.

cervical spine damage. In addition, nonmidsagittal loads will lower the injury threshold.

For the cervical spine interposed in the load path, the presence of straightening will likely determine the maximum load magnitude borne prior to failure and also the axial displacement allowed, and hence the time duration of impact prior to failure. The moving body or pendulum possesses kinetic energy. The total kinetic energy absorbed by the cervical spine, may be conceptualized as work performed on the spine by the decelerating torso or pendulum. This work may be represented as the area beneath the force-displacement curve (Fig. 2-58). This work may be performed by relatively large forces applied for short distances prior to failure (*e.g.*, the straightened spine) or by smaller forces applied over longer distances (*e.g.*, the axial loading of the initially curved spine). The position of flexion/extension that maximizes the work performed prior to failure is not well established (Fig. 2-59). Studies that introduced the additional variables of axial rotation and lateral bending positions prior to impact suggested that cervical spines with such nonmidsagittal initial positions absorb less energy prior to failure.[46]

MATHEMATICAL MODELING OF THE CERVICAL SPINE

The parameters used to develop models of the spine that define its mechanical response include the following key factors:

1. Mechanical properties of bone and the interconnecting ligamentous structures
2. Vertebral, disc, and ligament geometry

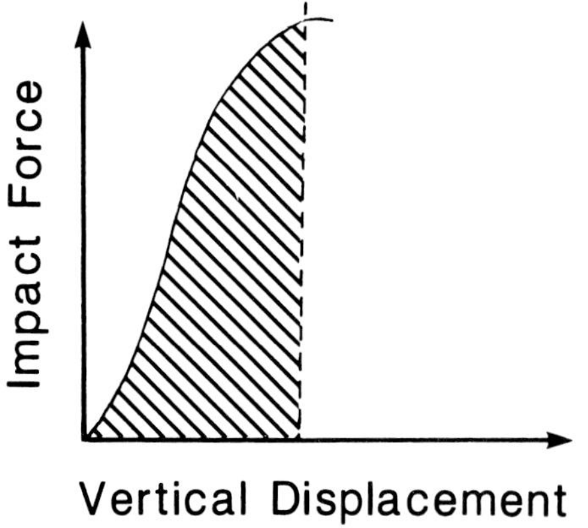

Fig. 2-58. Area beneath the force-displacement curve reflects the kinetic energy absorbed on impact.

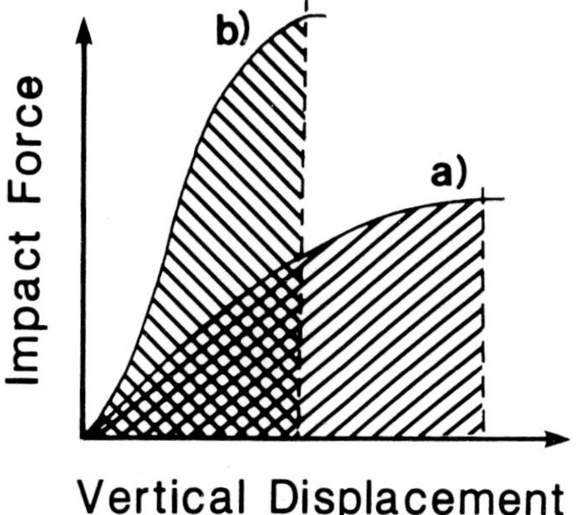

Fig. 2-59. Differing force-displacement relations possible on impact for differing initial head-neck-thorax positions. Peak force prior to failure appears to be higher with the cervical spine in a straightened position, although the position that maximizes kinetic energy absorbed prior to failure (area A versus area B) is not well established.

3. Load-displacement history
4. Boundary conditions for the region of interest
5. Mass of the vertebral components
6. Time-dependent properties

The method of modeling describes the way in which these inputs are treated and to a large extent defines limitations that can be placed on results. A brief review of the status of mathematical modeling will follow. The purpose is to provide the reader with a sense of the state of development of the science as well as its level of reliable applicability to clinical and medical-legal issues.

Anthropometric Models

The most fundamental aspect of a biomechanical model of the spine is the representation of the geometric relationships between the interconnecting components. Anthropometric data have been collected to describe the cervical spine. Virtually all biomechanical analyses of the spine begin with an appropriate geometric description of the region to be studied. Belytschko and colleagues,[5] Panjabi,[48] and others have advocated the refinement of geometric data.

Anthropometric data were recently published by Nissan and Gilad for the midsagittal plane of the cervical and lumbar regions of the spine for normal healthy men. Vertebral body height, overall size, and the intervertebral spacing were among the ten parameters obtained by lateral x-ray (Fig. 2-60 and Tables 2-6, 2-7, 2-8). All subjects were young (mean age 26.8 years) Caucasian males with normal spines. However, errors in the measurement of the vertebral bodies in the cervical region were as high as an estimated 10 percent. The error for the intervertebral spacing was greater, an es-

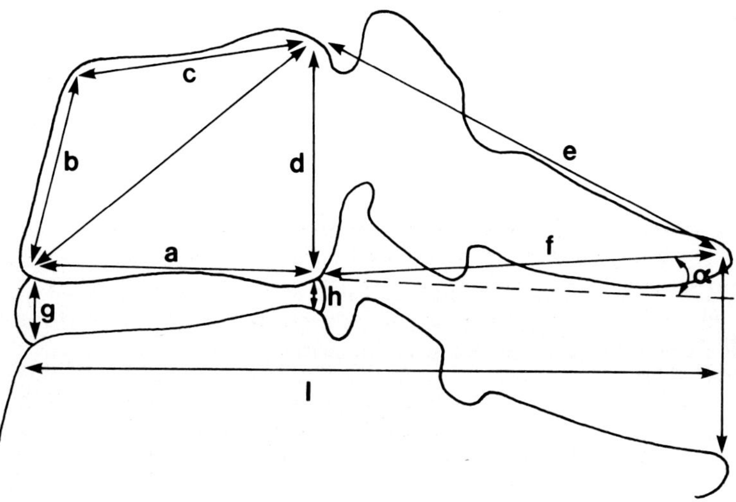

Fig. 2-60. Anthropometric measurements. These lateral radiographic geometric measurements are described for a group of young men as reported by Nissan and Gilad.[44] A standardized film-to-source distance of 1.5 m was used for these radiographs.

Table 2-6. Aeometric Parameters a–k for the Various Vertebra Measured (in mm) ($\bar{x}$ SD)

	N	a	b	c	d	e	f	g	h	i	k
C2	130	15.3±1.6	19.0±3.2	12.6±2.1	16.6±2.5	40.0±3.5	36.6±2.6	4.8±1.0	3.4±1.0	20.5±3.9	24.7±2.4
C3	141	15.6±1.5	14.1±1.3	14.8±1.5	14.5±1.4	34.4±3.1	30.6±3.0	5.3±0.9	3.3±0.9	17.5±3.5	23.4±1.9
C4	141	15.8±1.5	13.4±1.3	15.5±1.7	13.9±1.2	33.6±2.8	30.4±2.6	5.5±1.0	3.0±1.0	13.1±3.6	23.0±1.9
C5	141	16.1±1.5	12.7±1.3	15.5±1.7	13.8±1.4	35.4±3.1	33.0±3.2	5.4±1.0	3.0±0.9	11.4±3.5	22.6±1.8
C6	140	16.6±1.4	13.0±1.3	16.0±1.7	13.9±1.6	41.5±4.6	39.7±5.0	5.2±1.0	3.3±1.0	18.8±3.6	22.6±1.7
C7	126	16.3±1.4	14.6±1.4	16.4±1.4	14.9±1.4	49.6±3.5	46.4±3.3	4.7±1.2	3.5±1.2	17.4±3.2	22.8±1.6

Table 2-7. Angle of Inclination, α, and the Total Length, l, of the Cervical and Lumbar Vertebra, Calculated Values

		α		l
Vertebra	N	Radii	Degree	(mm)
C2	130	0.19	10.7	51.3
C3	141	0.25	14.4	45.2
C4	141	0.21	12.1	45.5
C5	141	0.11	6.1	48.9
C6	140	0.07	3.8	56.2
C7	126	0.13	7.3	62.3

timated 35 percent. The data are further limited by inclusion of sagittal plane dimensions only. Expansion of the anthropometric database to three dimensions and to other subjects will be a useful step for improved modeling accuracy.

Physical Models

A number of anthropomorphic physical models have been developed, which have progressively increased in complexity and accuracy of representation of the human neck to loading.[11,17,38] These test devices ("crash dummies") are generally used to predict the dynamic human response to impact testing of magnitudes unacceptable for human volunteers. Such data obtained may be validated by cadaveric testing and dynamic human testing under lower impact conditions. Newer physical models[11] estimate head accelerations, cervical disc pressures, and muscle strains. The accurate simulation of such parameters for a wide range of injurious and subinjurious conditions through such models is appealing, although further validation of the current models will be required before we can be confident of clinical conclusions drawn from these simulated structures.

Mathematical Models

Over the last 30 years mathematical models have been used to investigate head-neck kinematics and the biomechanics of cervical injury. The complexity and degree of sophistication of the models has increased steadily. Summaries of the investigations of the load-displacement response of the cervical spine have been presented by King and Chou,[30] McElhaney and Associates,[37] and Goldsmith.[19] Comparisons of analytic results with experimental data have been presented by Prasad and coworkers,[52] Landkof and coworkers,[31] Huston and associates.[25,26] Such comparisons are important as a means of establishing the validity of analytic models.

Early continuum models, which provided closed-form solutions, were obtained by Liu and Murray[34] and Shirazi.[61] These models represent the cervical spine as a continuous simplified structure with solutions satisfying equations of equilibrium for stresses derived from estimated loading conditions.

Finite difference solutions of the load-displacement response of the cervical spine were obtained

Table 2-8. Relationship Between the Vertebral Body Height Parameters b and d and the Respective Intervertebral Heights Parameters g and h

	g/b		h/d		(g+h)(b+d)	
	Mean	SD	Mean	SD	Mean	SD
C3	0.347	0.84	0.242	0.081	0.291	0.066
C4	0.399	0.078	0.239	0.073	0.317	0.058
C5	0.439	0.101	0.223	0.083	0.325	0.071
C6	0.420	0.088	0.229	0.086	0.310	0.064
C7	0.364	0.083	0.225	0.082	0.292	0.061

by Terry and Roberts,[63] Rybicki and Hopper,[57] Li and coworkers,[32] and Landkof and associates.[31] Such solutions are numerical procedures that fit experimental gross motion data with modeling constants describing the cervical response characteristics. These early models are limited by their depiction of the cervical spine as a simplified structure, such as a viscoelastic beam, which does not consider individual segmental motion or loads (Fig. 2-61).

"Lumped parameter" and "discrete parameter" model systems subjected to forward accelerations have been developed by Toth,[65] Hopkins,[23] Kaleps and coworkers,[27] Orne and Liu,[47] Prasad and King,[53] and Huston and coworkers.[25,26] These models have been extended to three dimensions by Merrill (1981),[38a] Williams and Belytschko,[70] and Deng and Goldsmith.[11] Parameters such as lumped masses, massless springs and hysteretic elements are estimated for components of models of varying complexity and anatomic accuracy. The accuracy of the models may be expected to depend largely on the accuracy of the modeling parameters. The advancement of model complexity with continued refinement of "lumped parameters" into increasingly anatomically accurate, and increasingly mechanically discrete, elements continues (Fig. 2-62). The potential uses of accurate mathematical models are many. Applications may include continued improvement in the design of protective devices for injurious conditions, modification of activity techniques, prediction of injurious activities for the normal and pathologic spine and prediction of dynamic response to therapeutic interventions.

Biomechanical Modeling Parameters

The development of mathematical models that describe the influences and responses of individual anatomic components of the neck requires a description of the mechanical properties of such components (the modeling parameters). A limited amount of strength data for individual components of the neck can be found in the literature (Table 2–9). Messerer[40] reported a series of compression tests on human vertebral bodies from all levels of spines of cadavers ranging in age from 25 to 80 years. For the cervical region the maximum compressive breaking load of the vertebral bodies is 2800 to 4200 N (Table 2-9) for the 20 to

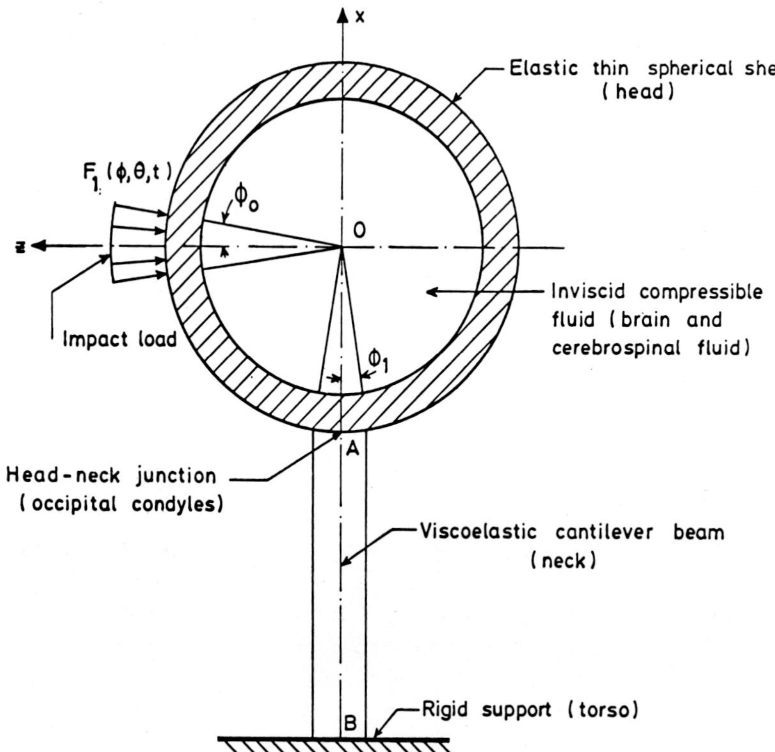

Fig. 2-61. Schematic diagram of mathematical model of cervical spine is used in estimation of dynamic responses to loading. (Landkof B, Goldsmith W, Sackman JL: Impact on a head-neck structure, J Biomech 9:141, 1976. Copyright © 1976, Pergamon Journals, Ltd)

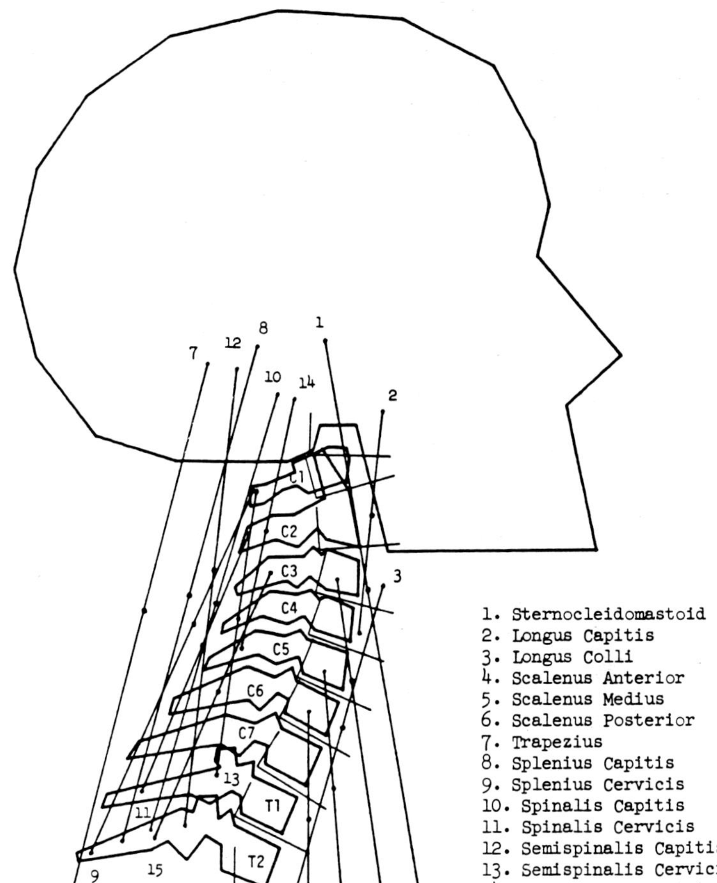

Fig. 2-62. Diagram shows parametric model of Deng and Goldsmith. (Deng YC, Goldsmith W: Response of a human head/neck/upper torso replica to dynamic loading—II. Analytic/numerical model. J Biomech 20:487, 1987. Copyright © 1987, Pergamon Journals Ltd)

40 year old.[40,62] Yamada[71] lists the compressive breaking load as 3089 N. The tensile strength of the ligaments in the neck is about 10 to 20 MPa, as determined for the ligamentum flavum[64] and longitudinal ligaments (Nachemson and Evans, 1968).[43a] In terms of maximum tensile breaking load, the ligament of the atlas appears to be the strongest with a breaking load of 1000 N,[16] followed by the anterior longitudinal ligament with a breaking load of 340 N and the posterior longitudinal ligament with a breaking load of 180 N.[64] The ultimate tensile strength of human muscle has been estimated to lie between 0.2 and 0.6 MPa for stretching of the passive muscle.[28] The estimated strength of active contracting muscle ranges from 0.4 to 1.0 MPa.[15,20,43]

The intervertebral disc and its interactions with the vertebral bodies play an important role in determining the strength of the motion segment. Sonoda[62] reported strength tests on human vertebral discs and vertebral bodies from all major regions of the spine in compression, tension, and torsion. For the cervical disc the compressive breaking load is reported for the 40 to 59 year old as 3200 N by Sonoda[62] and 3138 by Yamada.[71] The tensile breaking loads of the cervical discs are

Table 2-9. Cervical Component Properties

STRUCTURE	BREAKING LOAD
Cervical vertebral body	2800 to 4200 N
Transverse ligament of the atlas	1000 N
Anterior longitudinal ligament	3400 N
Posterior longitudinal ligament	1800 N
Cervical disc (compression)	3200 N
Cervical disc (tension)	1000 N
Cervical disc (torsion)	6 N-m

about equal (1000 N[62]), as are the torsional breaking moments (6 N-m[62]). Roaf[55] studied the interaction of the vertebrae and the intervertebral discs under vertical compression. He found that, although there is a very slight bulge of the annulus, there is no alteration in the shape of the nucleus pulposus, and the major distortion is a bulge of the vertebral end-plate. Direct measurements of vertebral end-plate deformation in the lumbar spine were made by means of suspended extensometers, without reference to points outside the motion segment, by Rolander and Blair.[56] At small loads they found that only the disc was deformed, but at larger loads the vertebra deflected at a greater rate than the disc. Bulging of the end-plates caused blood to be squeezed out of cancellous bone of the vertebral body into the perivertebral sinuses. This was considered by Roaf to be an important shock-absorbing mechanism in the spine. Upon further loading the end-plate bulged further and finally cracked. The efficacy of this mechanism is probably highly dependent on the loading rate.

Although Roaf made no quantitative studies, he claimed on the basis of radiographic studies of dye-injected nuclei pulposi that prior to end-plate fracture there is no distortion of the normal nucleus pulposus. Such evidence seems to indicate that some sort of hydraulic shock absorbing mechanism[21,55] and strengthening mechanism[29] exists in the vertebral body.

Biomechanical properties of the intervertebral joint have been measured by groups of researchers for each of the three mobile areas of the spine. All these studies have been conducted at low levels of load, far below conditions associated with vertebral fracture and ligamentous injury. Measurements of the load-displacement response of spine segments at larger load magnitudes by Panjabi and coworkers,[51] Miller and coworkers,[41] and Edwards and associates[12] have shown that the properties of the spine vary significantly as load magnitudes increase.

Experimental stiffness data for the cervical spine have been reported by Liu and Kreiger,[33] Moroney,[42] Panjabi and coworkers,[49] and Coffee and associates[6] (Table 2-10). The stiffness values reported by Panjabi and coworkers were measured at a relatively low-load magnitude (25 N), below the higher stiffnesses encountered prior to failure (Fig. 2-63). The Moroney stiffness data, used in the Deng and Goldsmith mathematical model, does not represent variation in segment stiffnesses at different cervical loads. In this model, individual segmental stiffnesses were assumed to be proportionate to the disc cross-sectional area for the cervical spine. The stiffness data of Liu and Kreiger, used for the Williams and Belytschko model, is reported for differing levels, although for only two specimens.

The stiffness data of Coffee and associates[6] suggest a marked difference in cervical spine stiffness between the middle (C2–C5) and lower (C5–T1) cervical spine (Table 2-9). Similar differences between the middle and lower segment rotational stiffnesses were reported by Liu and Krieger,[33] although in their two specimens translational stiffnesses were similar between the two segments. Consideration of such individual segmental variations and recognition of the three mechanically distinct regions of the cervical spine (the upper occiput–C1–C2) region plus the other two) may be important in accurate cervical spine modeling and understanding of injuries.

Coupling of cervical spine motions and coupled force-displacement data have been reported by

Table 2-10. Cervical Motion Segment Stiffnesses

		Translational Stiffness ($\times 10^5$ N/m)					Rotational Stiffnesses ($\times$ 10 N-m/radian)			
Author	Region	Compr	Tension	+Shear	−Shear	Lateral Shear	Flexion	Extension	Lateral Bend	Axial Rotation
Liu	Middle	36.9	5.9	—	—	—	2.9	7.1	15.8	17.6
	Lower	41.2	5.8	—	—	—	16.9	14.8	21.9	22.5
Coffee	Middle	51.8	9.0	5.8	2.2	—	8.6	—	—	—
	Lower	13.6	2.0	1.04	1.3	—	16.6	19.1	—	—
Moroney	All	10.8	3.9	1.4	0.5	1.2	15.2*	18.6*	17.2*	14.9*
Panjabi	All	1.4†	0.52†	0.34†	0.52†	0.52†	—	—	—	—

* Data modified by Deng and Goldsmith
† Measured at 25-N force

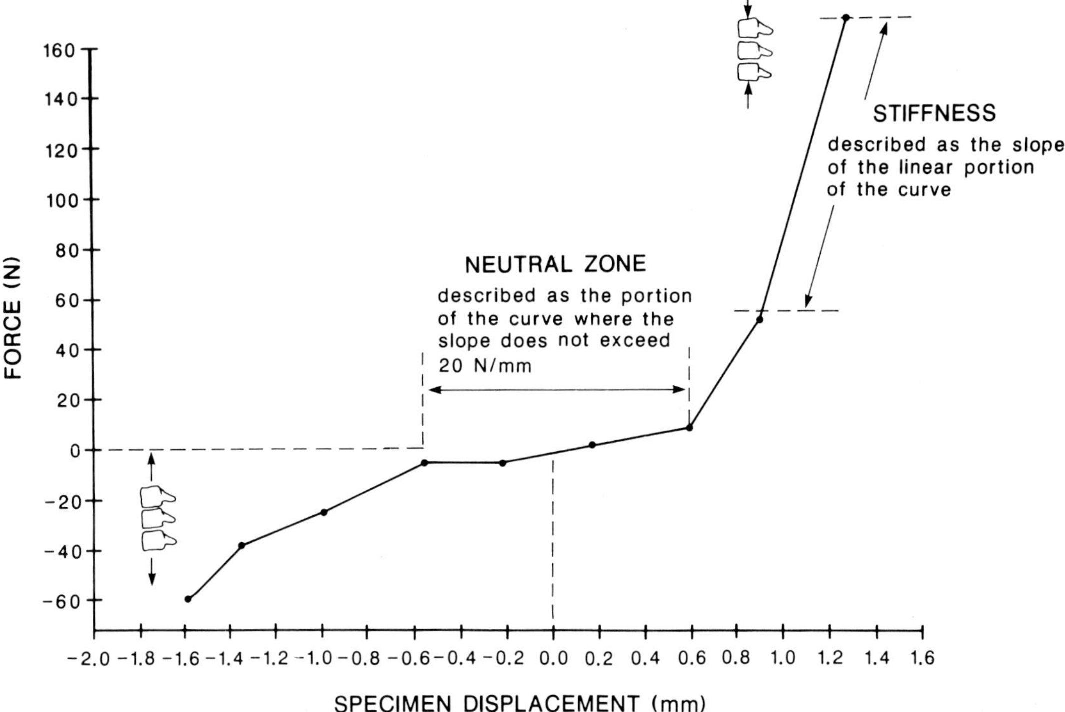

Fig. 2-63. Load-displacement curve for cervical spine segment. If the stiffness is measured below the steep portion of the curve, reported values will be substantially lower than other estimates.

Panjabi and associates.[49] These force-displacement data, which take three-dimensional coupled motion into consideration, enable formulation of stiffness matrices for each cervical level. These matrices predict three-dimensional responses to forces and moments of various directions and magnitudes. Recent sophisticated mathematical models[11] attempt prediction of such coupled responses. Incorporation of accurately coupled response estimates into models which predict complex three-dimensional load-displacement relations may significantly improve the accuracy of the models.

The accuracy of mathematical models will depend on both the sophistication of the modeling techniques and the accuracy of the mechanical property estimates of their components. Work continues in the characterization of the mechanical behavior of vertebral motion segments. Differences in segmental stiffnesses of cervical motion segments for 6 degrees of freedom have become progressively better defined, revealing differences between the middle and lower cervical motion segments, previously lumped together as the lower cervical spine.

VALIDATION OF MATHEMATICAL MODELS

Validation of these models has been performed by comparison of load responses predicted by the models with the experimentally determined responses of instrumented humans, other primates, and cadavers to those loads. Studied performed by Ewing and colleagues[13,14] have quantified the human head and neck response to forward and lateral impact accelerations using accelerometers and high-speed cameras. These results have been compared with recent modeling predictions of the responses to such impacts[10,11,70] with improving agreement in these later studies.

Cervical spine responses and injuries predicted by modeling techniques may also be validated by comparison with clinically observed phenomena. Modeling estimates of the response to impact may be compared with careful analysis of automobile accidents, including comparison of the vehicle paths, and internal and external automobile damage with soft-tissue and bony injuries. Similar comparisons may be possible for sports injury mechanisms, for which preimpact velocities and positional data may be obtained from game films, such as in the work of Torg.[66]

PROPOSED INJURY CRITERIA FOR THE NECK

A reliable quantitative load to failure criterion has not been established in these studies. A wide range of failure loads was observed within tests utilizing a consistent methodology, and an even wider range was observed among methodologies (Table 2-5).

A proposed injury criterion in extension and flexion of the neck is the equivalent moment at the occipital condyles. This equivalent moment consists of the moments produced by neck forces and chin-chest contact forces (if chin-chest contact occurs), taken with respect to the occipital condyles.[39] The following forces act on the head: the force of gravity, an axial force produced by the neck structure directed along the axis of the vertebral column parallel to the dens, a shear force that produces a distributed bending moment along the cervical spine, and a chin-chest contact force. Mertz and Patrick conducted volunteer tests on a 50th-percentile male for horizontal deceleration at various G levels, including a maximum of 9.6 G. These tests were used to determine the effects produced by varying the mass, center of gravity, and mass moment of inertia of the head by the addition of a helmet. The center of mass was varied from above the center of mass of the head to below.

In static tests on volunteers, maximum torque levels of 35.4 N-m in flexion and 23.8 N-m extension were obtained.[39] There is no contribution from the chin-chest contact in the static tests. In dynamic voluntary tests a maximum value of 47.6 N-m was reached in extension. In hyperflexion the chin-chest reaction resulted in a maximum equivalent moment of the condyles of 88.4 N-m sustained without injury. This exposure produced a pain extending from the posterior neck to the posterior midthorax and resulted in a stiff neck that lasted for several days.[39]

According to Mertz and Patrick[39] the maximum voluntary static neck reaction is about 1130 N in tension and 1110 N in compression. Under shear loads, the neck can withstand about 845 N. These static strength values apply to low-G conditions, where the viscous resisting forces produced by the muscles are not a large part of the resisting torque. In high-G situations the viscous contribution of the muscle reaction is comparable to the static strength, resulting in a higher resisting moment than predicted by a static strength analysis. In other words, the static values quoted may be a low estimate of the neck strength in the high-acceleration environment.

In cadavers tested in the horizontal direction, maximum torque levels of 177 and 190 N-m were achieved without apparent damage, as determined by x-ray analysis. A maximum anterior-posterior force of 2100 N was developed at the occipital condyles of one cadaver without producing any apparent neck trauma. However, these values for the Mertz and Patrick cadaver studies should be viewed with caution. Not all fractures are visible on x-rays, and it is not possible to identify ligamentous damage on radiographic examinations alone.

Alem,[1] as other investigators, noted a wide range of forces producing cervical spine damage and found force to be a poor predictor of injury. However, they found the impulse, the integral of force over time, to be a useful predictor of cervical spine injury in their cadaver study. In their series of 14 cadaver axial impacts for which impulse values are given, no cervical spine injuries were noted in 5 with applied impulses of 24 to 35 N-s, and cervical spine injuries were noted in 9 cadavers with applied impulses of 35 to 49 N-s.

In addition to structural bony or ligamentous force-to-injury criteria, forces producing neurologic sequelae have been studied. The association of increased risk of neurologic injury in association with greater vertebral injury has been recognized in clinical evaluations.[54] The possibility of neurologic deficit resulting from cervical spine injury is an area of research that is difficult to investigate using models, but that can be studied experimentally. Studies of nonhuman primates have identified the neural and physiologic effects of axially applied tension loads. Studies using male macaca mulatta monkeys conducted by Sances and associates[58] have shown that axial loads of 556 N to 1555 N produced immediate reduction of the somatosensory-evoked potential amplitude. When these loads were maintained, these changes were followed by changes in heart rate, blood pressure, and perfusion. It is clear that the concept of force magnitude and time dependency of injury is valid for quantifiable neurologic changes as well as for bony and ligamentous injuries. Such improved quantitation of time, cervical spine position, force and moment direction, and biologic variables, will improve the accuracy of injury prediction.

SUMMARY AND CONCLUSIONS

From these experimental studies, it is apparent that there exists a set of injury producing conditions of impact magnitude, direction, and rate of application for each head-neck-thorax position beyond which cervical spine injury will likely occur. The rate dependency of the critical impact load magnitude is reflected in the increased load to failure, with increased rate of load application seen in study comparisons and reflected in the injury prediction value of the impulse. Additional research is needed to confirm the impulse as the optimal load magnitude and time relation for the prediction of injury.

The qualitative types of impact responses possible for differing directions and points of load application will largely be determined by the critical initial conditions of head-neck-thorax positions. Certain responses will only occur for a limited range of cervical spine positions. For example, buckling, according to the true mechanical definition, will occur only for a straightened cervical spine under an axial load. Thus, the potential responses to impact—straight compression (failure by buckling), bending of the curved spine between the impact load and thorax inertial load, and deflection of the head and cervical spine out of the load path—will be determined by loading conditions and initial body position. Nonmidsagittal plane positions and loads may influence the directions and types of such responses, or lower the threshold of injury.

Direction for Future Research and Analysis

Additional cadaveric testing will help define the critical initial conditions and critical loading associated with spine injury. However, the supply of cadavers is limited and experimental cadaver testing is costly and cumbersome. Further, from the experimental studies it is apparent that there are several independent variables that determine the load magnitude and the type of kinematic and time response to impact loading. A prohibitively large number of cadavers would be required to evaluate the multiple combinations of independent variables needed to define the response to all such combinations of impact. Thus, accurate modeling analyses may play a significant role in defining such responses, with cadaver testing useful for validation of modeling results.

The continued improvement in three-dimensional descriptions of mechanical characteristics of cervical spine components, which identify level specific differences and define the range of variation within the population, will refine the accuracy of models. Such models, mathematical and physical, will then be able to improve response prediction for the wide range of physiologic and injury-producing loads encountered in life.

Clinical studies that identify and clarify injury patterns, and the associated biologic responses, define the utility of modeling studies. The expansion of modeling and experimental mechanical studies to pathologic mechanical states and their operative and nonoperative treatments will enable more accurate assessments of the need for, and efficacy of such treatments.

Increased communication and collaboration among investigators from various disciplines and academic and industrial backgrounds will accelerate understanding of cervical spine biomechanics. The collaboration of those attempting to solve similar problems for diverse purposes will result in a more efficient approach for the mutual benefit of all.

REFERENCES

1. *ALEM NM, NUSHOLTZ GS, MELVIN JW:* Head and neck response to axial impacts. *Proc 28th STAPP Car Crash Conference.* Soc Automotive Engineers, Warrendale, PA, 1984
2. *BAUZE RJ, ARDRAN GM:* Experimental production of forward dislocation in the human cervical spine. J Bone Joint Surg 60B:239, 1978
3. *BEATSON TR:* Fractures and dislocations of the cervical spine. J Bone Joint Surg 45B:21, 1963
4. *BELYTSCHKO TL, SCHWER L, PRIVITZER E:* Theory and application of a three-dimensional model of the human spine. Aviation Space Envir Med 49:158, 1978
5. *BELYTSCHKO T, SCHWER L, SCHULTZ AB:* A model for analytic investigation of three dimensional head spine dynamics. WPAFB, Aerospace Med Div, AMRL-TR-76-10, 1976

5a. *BRAAKMAN R, PENNING L:* The Hyperflexion Sprain of the Cervical Spine. Radiol. Clin. Biol. 37:309, 1968

6. *COFFEE MS, EDWARDS WT, HAYES WC, WHITE AA III:* Mechanical responses and strength of the human cervical spine. Exhibit, Am Spinal Injury Assoc meeting, Boston, March 1987
7. *CROWELL RR, COFFEE, MS, EDWARDS WT, WHITE*

AA III: Cervical ligament injuries under three dimensional loading. Proc Cervical Spine Res Soc, 1987

8. *CULVER RH, BENDER M, MELVIN JS:* Mechanisms, tolerances, and responses obtained under dynamic superior-inferior head impact. Final Report UM-HSRI-78-21, NTIS Order No PB-299-292, May 1978
9. *DAVIS D, BOHLMAN H, WALKER AE, FISHER R, ROBINSON R:* The pathological findings in fatal craniospinal injuries. J Neurosurg 34:603, 1971
10. *DENG YC, GOLDSMITH W:* Response of a human head/neck/upper torso replica to dynamic loading—I Physical model. J Biomech 20:471, 1987
11. *DENG YC, GOLDSMITH W:* Response of a human head/neck/upper torso replica to dynamic landing—II Analytic/numercial model. J Biomech 20:487, 1987
12. *EDWARDS WT, HAYES WC, POSNER I, WHITE AA III, MANN RW:* Variation in lumbar spine stiffness with load. J Biomed Engl 109:35, 1987
13. *EWING C, THOMAS D:* Human head and neck response to impact acceleration. (Monograph #21) National Aerospace Medical Research Laboratory, Pensacola, 1972
14. *EWING CL, THOMAS DJ, LUSTIK L, WILLEMS GC, MUZZY WH III, BECKER EB, JESSOP ME:* Dynamic response of human and primate head and neck to $+G_y$ impact acceleration. Report DOT HS-803-058 Naval Aerospace Medical Research Laboratory, Pensacola, 1978
15. *FICK R:* Handbook der Anatomie and Mechanik der Gelenke. Jena, Verlag G. Fischer, 1910
16. *FIELDING JW, COCHRAN GVB, LAWSING JF, HOHL M:* Tears of the transverse ligament of the atlas: a clinical and biomechanical study. J Bone Joint Surg 56A:1683, 1974
17. *FOSTER JK, KORTGE JO, WOLANIN MJ:* Hybrid III—A biomechanically based car crash dummy. Proc 21st STAPP Car Crash Conference, Society of Automotive Engineers, Warrendale, 1977, p 974
18. *FUENTES JM, BLONCOURT J, VLAHOVITCH B, CASTAN P:* Tear drop fractures. Contribution to the study of its mechanism and of osteo-disco-ligamentous lesions. Neurochirurgie 29:129, 1983
19. *GOLDSMITH W:* Some aspects of head and neck injury and protection. *In* Akkas N (ed): Proc NATO Adv Study Inst Prog Biomech, Series E, Appl Sci 32: 333 Alphen aan den Rijn, Sijthoff and Noordhoff, 1979
20. *HAXTON HA:* Absolute muscle force in ankle flexors in man. J Physiol 103: 267, 1944
21. *HENZEL JH, MOHR GC, VON GIERKE HE:* Reappraisal of biodynamic implications of human ejection. Aerosp Med 39: 231, 1968
22. *HODGSON VR, THOMAS LM:* Mechanisms of cervical spine injury during impact to the protected head. Proc 24th STAPP Car Crash Conference, Society of Automotive Engineers, Warrendale, 1980, p 17
23. *HOPKINS GR:* Nonlinear lumped-parameter mathematical model of dynamic response of the human body. Symposium on Biodynamic Models and their Applications, Aerospace Medical Research Laboratory (AMRL-TR-71-29), WPAFB, Ohio, 1971, p 843
24. *HUELKE DF, NUSHOLTZ GS:* Cervical spine biomechanics. A review of the literature. J Orthop Res 4:232, 1986
25. *HUSTON RL, HUSTON JC, HARLOW MW:* Comprehensive three dimensional head-neck model for impact and high acceleration studies. Aviation Space Envir Med 49:205, 1978
26. *HUSTON, RL, PASSERELLO CE, HESSEL RE, HARLOW MW:* On human body mechanics. Ann Biomed Engin 4:25, 1976
27. *KALEPS I, VON GIERKE HE, WEIS EB:* A five degree of freedom mathematical model of the body. Symposium on Biodynamic Models and their Applications, Aerospace Medical Research Laboratory (AMRL-TR-71-29), WPAFB, Ohio, 1971, p 211
28. *KATAKE K:* Studies on the strength of human skeletal muscles. J Kyoto Med Univ 69:463, 1961
29. *KAZARIAN LE:* Identification and classification of vertebral fractures following emergency capsule egress from military aircraft. Aviation Space Envir Med 49:150, 1978
30. *KING AI, CHOU CC:* Mathematical modelling, simulation, and experimental testing of biomechanical system crash response, J Biomech 9:301, 1976
31. *LANDKOF B, GOLDSMITH W, SACKMAN JL:* Impact on a head-neck structure. J Biomech 9:141, 1976
32. *LI TF, ADVANI SH, LEE YC:* The effect of initial curvature on the dynamic response of the spine to axial accelerations. Symposium on Biomechanical Models and their Applications. Aerospace Medical Research Laboratory (AMRL-TR-71-29), WPAFB, Ohio, 1971, p 621
33. *LIU YK, KRIEGER KW, NJUS G, UENO K, WAKENO K:* Investigation of cervical spine dynamics. Aerospace Medical Research Laboratory (AMRL-TR-138), WPAFB, Ohio, 1981 (cited in Williams and Belytschko)
34. *LIU YK, MURRAY JD:* A theoretical study of the effect of impulses on the human torso. *In* Fung YC (ed): Proc ASME Symp Biomechan 1966, p 167
35. *MAIMAN DJ, SANCES A, MYKLEBUST JB, LARSON SJ, HOUTERMAN C, CHILBERT M, EL-GHATIT AZ:* Compression injuries of the cervical spine: A biomechanical analysis. Neurosurgery 13:254, 1983

36. *McElhaney JH, Paver JG, McCracklin HJ:* Cervical spine compression responses. Proc 27th STAPP Car Crash Conference, Society of Automotive Engineers, Warrendale, 1983, p 163

37. *McElhaney JH, Roberts VL, Hilyard J:* Biomechanics of Trauma. Durham, Duke University Press, 1976

38. *Melvin JW, McElhaney JH Roberts VL:* Improved neck simulation for anthropomorphic dummies. Proc 16th STAPP Car Crash Conference, Society of Automotive Engineers, Warrendale, 1972, p 45

38a. *Merrill J, Goldsmith W, Deng Y-C:* Three-dimensional response of a lumped parameter head-neck model due to impact and impulse loading. J Biomech 17:81, 1984

39. *Mertz HJ, Patrick LM:* Strength and response of the human neck. Proc 15th STAPP Car Crash Conference, Society of Automotive Engineers, Warrendale, 1971, p 207

40. *Messerer O:* Ueber elastizitaet und festigkeit der menschlich en knochen, Stuttgart, JG Cottaschen Buchhandling, 1880

41. *Miller JAA, Schultz AB, Warwick DN, Spencer DL:* Mechanical properties of lumbar motion segments under large loads. J Biomech 19:79–84 1986

42. *Moroney S:* Mechanical Properties and Muscle Force Analysis of the Lower Cervical Spine. PhD thesis, University of Illinois at Chicago, 1984 (reported in Deng and Goldsmith)

43. *Morris CB:* The measurement of the strength of muscle relative to the cross-section. Res Quart Am Assoc Health Phys Ed Recrn 19:295, 1948

43a. *Nachemson AL, Evans JH:* Some mechanical properties of the third human lumbar interlaminar ligament (ligamentum flavum), J Biomech, 1:211, 1968

44. *Nissan M, Gilad I:* The cervical and lumbar vertebrae—anthropometric model. Engin Med 13:111, 1984

45. *Norton JL:* Fractures and dislocations of the cervical spine. J Bone Joint Surg 44A:115, 1962

46. *Nusholtz GS, Huelke DS, Lux P, Alem NM, Montalvo F:* Cervical spine injury mechanisms. Proc 27th STAPP Car Crash Conference, Society of Automotive Engineers, Warrendale, 1983, p 275

47. *Orne D, Liu YK:* A mathematical model of spinal response to impact. J Biomechan 4:49 1971

48. *Panjabi MM:* Three dimensional mathematical model of the human spine structure. J Biomech 6:761, 1973

49. *Panjabi MM, Summers DJ, Pelker RR, Videman T, Friedlander GE, Southwick WO:* Three-dimensional load-displacement cruves due to forces on the cervical spine. J Orthop Res 4:152, 1986

50. *Panjabi MM, White AA III, Brand RA:* A note on defining body parts configurations. J Biomech 7:385, 1974

51. *Panjabi MM, White AA III, Southwick WO:* Effect of preload on load-displacement curves of the lumbar spine. OCNA 8:181, 1977

52. *Prasad P, King AI, Ewing CL:* The role of articular facets during $+G_z$ acceleration. J Appl Mech 41:321, 1974

53. *Prasad P, King AI:* An experimentally validated dynamic model of the spine. J Appl Mech 41:546, 1974

54. *Riggins RS, Kraus JR:* The risk of neurological damage with fractures of the vertebrae. J Trauma 17:126, 1977

55. *Roaf R:* A study of the mechanics of spinal injuries. J Bone Joint Surg 42B:810, 1960

56. *Rolander SD, Blair WE:* Deformation and fracture of the vertebral end-plate. OCNA 6:75, 1975

57. *Rybicki EF, Hopper AT:* A dynamic model of the spine using a porous elastic material. Symposium on Biodynamic Models and their Applications, Aerospace Medical Research Laboratory (AMRL-TR-71-29) WPAFB, Ohio, 1971, p 851

58. *Sances A Jr, Myklebust J, Houterman C, Weber R, Lepkowski J, Cusick J, Larson S, Ewing C, Thomas D, Weiss M, Berger M, Jessop ME, Saltzman B:* Head and spine injuries. AGARD Conference Proceedings on Impact Injury Caused by Linear Acceleration-Mechanism, Prevention, and Cost, 1982

59. *Sances A, Weber RC, Larson SJ, Cusick JS, Myklebust JB, Walsh PR:* Bioengineering analysis of head and spine injuries. CRC Crit Rev Bioengineer 5:79, 1981

60. *Schneider RC, Kahn EA:* Chronic neurologic sequelae of acute trauma to the spine and spinal cord. J Bone Joint Surg 38A:985, 1956

61. *Shirazi M:* Response of the spine in biodynamic environments. Symposium on Biodynamic Models and their Applications, Aerospace Medical Research Laboratory (AMRL-TR-71-29), WPAFB, Ohio, 1971, p 843

62. *Sonoda T,* Studies on the Strength for Compression, Tension, and Torsion of The Human Vertebral Column. J Kyoto Pref Med Univ, 71:659, 1962

62a. *Taylor AR, Blackwood W:* Paraplegia in hyperextension cervical injuries with normal radiographic appearances. J Bone Joint Surg 30–B:245, 1948

63. *Terry CT, Roberts VL:* A viscoelastic model of the human spine subjected to $+G_x$ accelerations. J Biomechanics 1:161, 1968

64. *TKACZUK H:* Tensile properties of the human lumbar longitudinal ligaments. Thesis, Acta Orthop Scand (Suppl):115, 1968

65. *TOTH R:* Multiplying degree of freedom, nonlinear spinal model. Proc 19th Annual Conference on Engineering in Medicine and Biology 8:102, 1966

66. *TORG J:* Athletic Injuries to the Head and Face, Philadelphia, Lea & Febiger, 1982.

67. *VELEANU C:* Vertebral structural peculiarities with a role in the cervical spine mechanics. Folia Morphologica 19:388, 1971

68. *WHITE* AA *III, PANJABI MM:* Clinical Biomechanics of the Spine, Philadelphia, JB Lippincott, 1978

69. *WHITE AA III, PANJABI MM, BRAND RA:* A system for defining position and motion of human body parts. J Fed Med Biol Eng, 1975, p 261

70. *WILLIAMS JL, BELYTSCHKO TB:* A three-dimensional model of the human cervical spine for impact simulation. J Biomech Eng 105:321 1983

71. *YAMADA H:* Strength of Biological Materials, Huntington, R. E. Krieger, 1973

72. *YOGANANDAN N, SANCES A, MAIMAN DJ, MYKLEBUST JB, PECH P, LARSON SJ:* Experimental spinal injuries with vertical impact. Spine 11: 855, 1986

Biomechanics of Nonacute Cervical Spinal Cord Trauma

MANOHAR PANJABI AND
AUGUSTUS A. WHITE, III

Cervical spondylotic myelopathy is a disease in which adverse mechanical pressure is applied to the cervical spinal cord over a period of time. Neurologic dysfunctions are a direct result of this impingement. There have been many clinical studies but only a limited number of experimental studies. Of these, even fewer studies precisely quantify the mechanical impingement and the neurologic dysfunction. Impingement of the spinal cord may produce complex patterns of stresses in the cord. These may consist of compressive, tensile, and shear stresses, the magnitude and distribution of which depend on the clinical situation. There have been some excellent biomechanical studies of the nervous structures and their interaction with the spinal column. However, the present biomechanical knowledge is not adequate to relate the spinal cord impingement with the pathology of the cord and with the neurologic dysfunction. New biomechanical experiments, both *in vitro* as well as *in vivo,* are needed to provide the basis for such an understanding.

INTRODUCTION

Key words: spinal cord cervical, compression, spondylotic myelopathy, spinal cord biomechanics.

For proper function of the spinal cord, a certain minimum space is needed, both in neutral position and during physiological movements of the spine. Cervical spondylotic myelopathy is caused by a compromised spinal canal that leaves less space than necessary for the cord to function. The compromise in the spinal canal size may be partially developmental or primarily due to disc degeneration and osteophytic formations. A narrowed spinal canal may produce mechanical pressure on the spinal cord at one or more levels. This pressure may cause direct neurologic damage or produce ischemic changes secondary to canal compromise, which in turn leads to spinal dysfunction.

The functional size of the spinal canal may be further reduced, owing to physiologic movements of the spinal column. In extension of the spinal column, the canal length decreases, thus, increasing the cord cross-sectional area. This is a manifestation of Poisson's effect, defined as an increase in the cross-sectional area with a decrease in length, or vice versa, the total volume remaining the same. In addition, the cord is compressed by posterior protrusion of the disc annulus and buckling of the ligamentum flavum. Another mechanism is active in flexion of the spine. In this physiologic spinal motion, the cord tends to stretch. It may be stretched further over an osteophytic spur, producing local compression and bending. In addition, the stretching of the spinal cord may directly reduce its cross-sectional area, in accordance with the principles of elasticity (Poisson's effect).

Although there have been extensive reports on the clinical aspects of cervical spondylotic myelopathy, there are relatively few experimental studies in which effects of chronic compression are studied. Using animal models, the output of these experiments is monitored by electrical potentials, histology of the cord, and/or sometimes motor functions. Biomechanical aspects are seldom studied.

Alf Brieg pioneered the biomechanical research of the spinal cord and nerve roots. Besides the many original research papers, he has written two books detailing his work and ideas concerning the biomechanical effects on the nervous system.[2,3] Bohlman and colleagues[1] conducted experiments using a canine model, in which controlled pressures to the spinal cord over a set of time intervals were applied and the functional output of the spinal cord over time was monitored. Unfortunately, the pressures applied to the cord were not quantified. Raynor and Koplik[7] published a biomechanical analysis of trauma of the spinal cord. They hypothesized that it is the shear stress in the spinal cord, produced by anterior or posterior compression, that results in spinal cord dysfunction. This conceptual engineering analysis correlated nicely to the findings observed clinically and experimentally by Schneider and associates.[8,9] Finally, Tencer and colleagues, in a series of three papers, presented *in vitro* experimental results concerning pressure applied to the spinal cord by simulating spinal deformity, canal occlusion, and functional postures as well as surgical procedures.[11,12,13] These papers have produced reliable, biomechanical, and clinically relevant data using modern techniques.

The purpose of this presentation is twofold: (1) to describe the above-mentioned biomechanics literature in some detail and (2) to present a new qualitative biomechanical analysis of stress patterns in the spinal cord relevant to cervical spondylotic myelopathy.

BIOMECHANICS OF THE SPINAL CORD AND CANAL

For an understanding of the biomechanics of the pathologic conditions of the spinal cord, it is important to analyze the normal functioning of the spinal cord and column. Brieg[2,3] pioneered this type of research in a series of experiments. He used fresh whole cadavers, appropriately prepared to show by direct visual observation the movements and deformations of the spinal cord and the nerve roots. Physiologic movements of the spinal column were produced by bending the spine at different regions and in different planes. Several important findings have resulted from these studies. Brieg's work showed that the spinal canal length changes are accompanied by spinal cord length changes, without producing any significant stresses in the spinal cord. The mechanism is that of unfolding and folding the spinal cord, much like an accordion (Fig. 2-64). In flexion, the spinal canal increases in length, as the centers of rotation of vertebrae are anterior to the canal. Stretching of the ligamentum flavum occurs. In extension, the spinal canal decreases in length. The disc protrudes posteriorly into the canal,[4] while the liga-

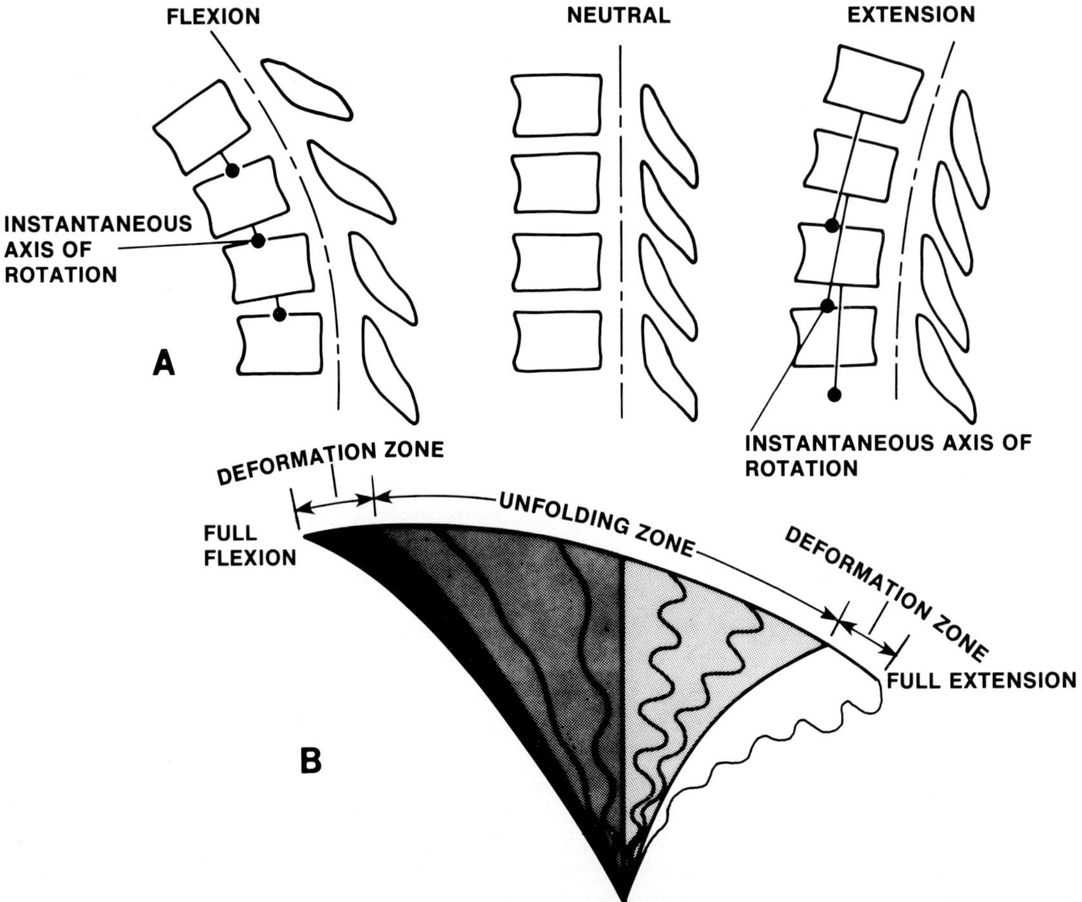

Fig. 2-64. The spinal canal and cord in flexion/extension. (*A*) In flexion, the length of the spinal canal increases, compared with that in neutral position. In extension, the length of the spinal canal decreases. This phenomenon is due to the location of the instantaneous axis of rotation anterior to the spinal canal. (*B*) The spinal cord is required to follow the changes in length of the spinal canal during physiologic motions. This occurs by means of the mechanisms of unfolding/folding and elastic deformation. (*B* is based on experimental findings of Breig.[2])

mentum flavum protrudes anteriorly.[6] Lesser changes take place during lateral bending and axial rotation. In normal anatomy, these physiologic movements of the spinal column do not produce any abnormal stresses and strains in the nervous tissue. In pathologic situations, however, such as hypertrophy of ligament flavum and abnormal disc bulge, osteophytic formations, ossification of posterior longitudinal ligament, and congenital narrow spinal canal, these same functional changes may result in abnormal stresses and strains in the spinal cord that lead to neurologic problems (Fig. 2-65).

An osteophyte, a bulging disc, and a hypertropic ligament flavum all apply direct compressive forces to the spinal cord in the transverse plane. This results in specific and well-defined patterns in the spinal cord. Although the stress patterns are three-dimensional and extremely complex, a simplified

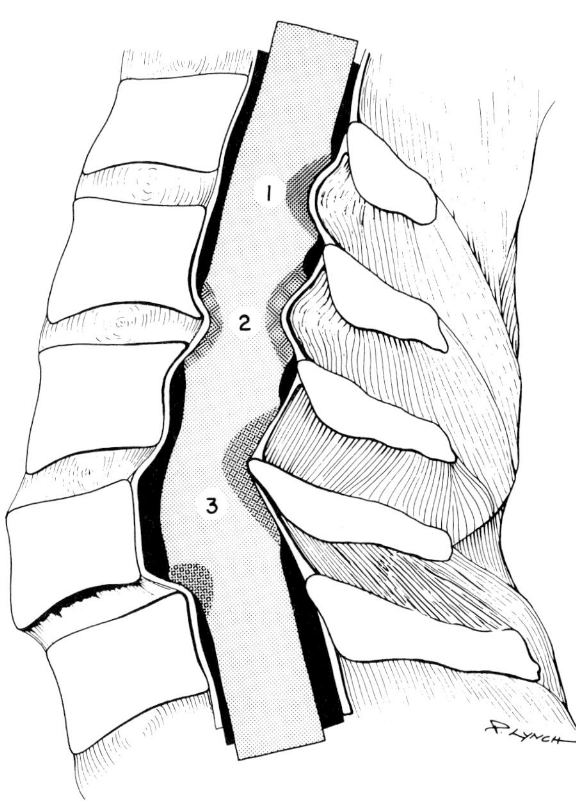

Fig. 2-65. In pathologic situations, well-coordinated physiologic movements of the spinal canal and the spinal cord may be disturbed, resulting in abnormal stresses and strains in the spinal cord that may lead to neurologic problems. Examples include 1) hypertrophy of ligantium flavium, 2) abnormal disk bulge, and 3) pathologic vertebral motion.

biomechanical analysis is helpful. Raynor and Koplik[7] conceptualized such a situation in biomechanical terms and provided a qualitative analysis of the stress patterns in the spinal cord due to a direct compression applied in the transverse plane.

It is known from engineering analysis of long structures with elliptic cross sections that when a transverse force, also called shear force, is applied to the structure on its flat side, well-defined stress patterns in the structure result (stress is defined as force per unit area). These stresses of the shear type are distributed with the maximum value in the center and zero along the periphery. Raynor and Koplik[7] applied this concept to the spinal cord. They argued that the stresses produced in the spinal cord by the application of transverse force adequately explain the neurologic dysfunction seen during trauma, in which the central areas of the spinal cord are preferentially damaged, compared with the peripheral areas. Although the analysis was conducted for trauma of the spinal cord, the results are equally valid for the application of a chronic transverse force (*e.g.,* due to an osteophyte). We will return to this subject in the next section.

There are several questions of practical and clinical importance concerning the treatment of myelopathy, in which biomechanics can be valuable. In a series of experiments, Tencer and coworkers[11,12,13] used fresh cadaveric spines from occiput to sacrum, including the spinal cord and dura. Although the spinal cord and dura were severed at the occiput level, the system was sutured closed and pressurized to provide normal CSF pressure. The basic set-up consisted of a specially constructed transverse load (force) applicator and displacement (translation) measurement transducer, designed to apply force to the spinal cord and to continuously monitor the displacement of the anterior and posterior walls of the dura. They studied the effects on the spinal cord of several parameters of the spinal column, for example, flexion angulation, shortening and distraction, and laminectomy. One of the interesting results of their study is shown in Figure 2-66*A*. The horizontal axis represents the canal occlusion, defined as the ratio of the canal instrusion (by the load applicator) to the canal diameter. On the vertical axis is shown the applied load. We see that the behavior is nonlinear, that is, increasing occlusion is accompanied by a relatively *greater* increase in the load. Simulating a kyphotic deformity by removing a 75% anterior body wedge or by performing a laminectomy did not alter the force-occlusion graph. Shown in Figure 2-28*B* is the displacement of the

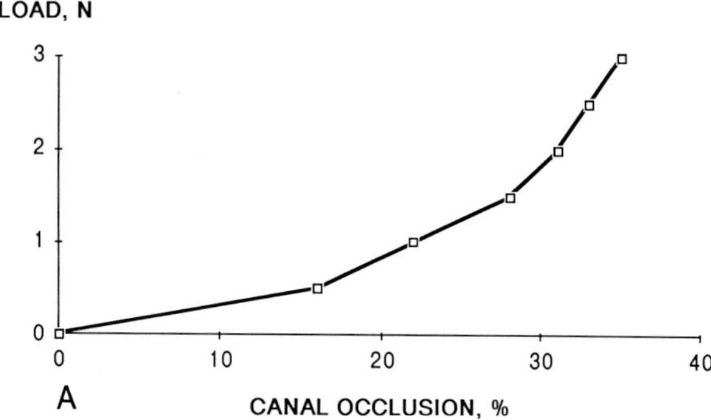

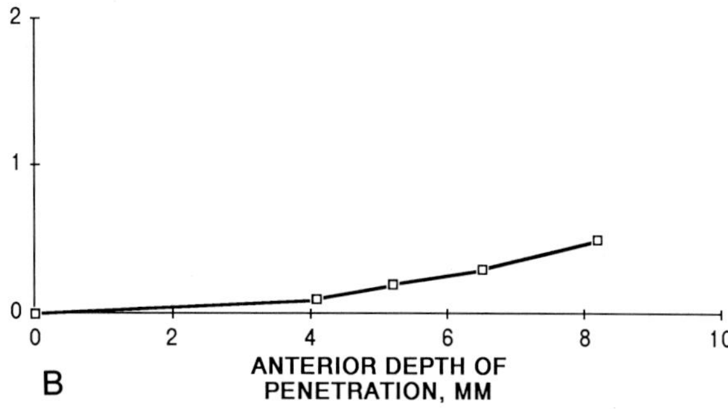

Fig. 2-66. (*A*) The relationship between the compression load applied and the occlusion of the canal is shown. (*B*) The relationship between the deflection of the posterior wall of the dura and the penetration of the spinal canal from the anterior is demonstrated. (*A* and *B* results are based on an experimental study by Tencer and associates.)[11,12,13]

posterior wall of the dura as a function of the displacement of the anterior wall of the dura. Notice that the posterior wall hardly moves when the anterior wall has been displaced up to 6, 8, or even 10 mm. This observation supports the view that the anterior impingement does not significantly affect the posterior wall of the dura. Therefore, posterior decompression, for example, laminectomy, will have little effect in decreasing the anterior pressure on the cord.

A QUALITATIVE BIOMECHANICAL ANALYSIS OF STRESSES IN THE SPINAL CORD

The purpose of this simple analysis of a complex phenomenon is to look at the qualitative stress patterns generated in the spinal cord as the result of a clinically relevant situation, for example, an impingement of the cord from the anterior, resulting in compression, stretching and bending of the cord (Fig. 2-67). The analysis builds on the earlier work of Brieg[2,3] and Raynor and Koplik.[7] For our biomechanical analysis, we consider the spinal cord to be a long structure made of a homogeneous material and having an elliptic cross section. Although we have used the term stress throughout this section, the term *strain* (percentage change in length) is equally valid. Because of the qualitative nature of the analysis, the terms are virtually equivalent.

The situation depicted in Figure 2-67 may be seen biomechanically as consisting of three simple loads applied simultaneously to the cord: (1) the compression load applied by osteophytic impingement, (2) the tensile load due to flexion of the spine, and (3) the bending load due to the change in the direction of the spinal cord over the osteophyte. We will analyze the stress patterns resulting from each of the three loads separately and then combine the results.

The first of the three loads considered is the direct compression (impingement) applied on the anterior surface of the cord and directed posteriorly. This force produces local compressive stresses that decrease in magnitude away from the point of contact (Fig. 2-68*A*). In addition, such a compression load produces shear stresses that have a value of zero at the point of load application and that increase toward the middle, being maximum in the center of the spinal cord (Fig. 2-68*B*). The compressive and shear stress patterns depicted are in the form of isostress contours, that is, each contour represents a single constant stress value. This convention is used throughout Figures 2-68, 2-69, and 2-70.

The second load studied is the tensile (tension) load. The tensile load applied to a long structure produces uniform tensile stress across the cross section (Fig. 2-69*A*).

The third load is the bending of the cord over an osteophyte. When a long structure is bent, there are differential stresses across the bent cross section. On the concave side of the bent structure, compressive stresses develop, while on the convex side tensile stresses occur (Fig. 2-69*B*). The magnitude of both stresses is highest on the outer surface of the structure. The stresses decrease toward the center and reach a zero value in the middle of the structure. The posterior region of the spinal cord is loaded in both tension and compression. The tensile forces are exerted during flexion, and the compression forces, from invagination of the

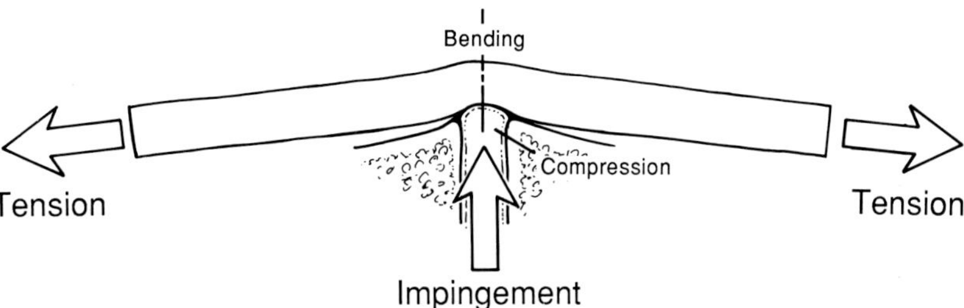

Fig. 2-67. Impingement of the spinal cord from the anterior results in compression, stretching (tension), and bending of the spinal cord.

yellow ligament, are exerted during extension. These biomechanical factors may account for the clinical observation of a predominance of posterior spinal cord dysfunction involved in patients with cervical spondylotic myelopathy.

Now we combine the effects of all the three loads acting on the spinal cord. This situation simulates a realistic one in which an osteophyte impinges on the spinal cord while the spinal column is flexed, resulting in combined compression, stretching, and bending of the spinal cord. The resulting stress patterns are summations of the stress patterns shown in Figures 2-68 and 2-69. The compressive and tensile stresses are normal stresses (*i.e.*, perpendicular to the cross section of the structure), and therefore together they provide a combined distribution of the normal stresses. The resulting pattern for the normal stresses is seen in Figure 2-70*A*. Starting from the anterior of the cord, we have high compressive stresses that decrease toward the center of the cord. A little beyond the center, the stresses may be nearly zero. Continuing toward the posterior, the stresses again increase but are now tensile in nature. It may be emphasized that our analysis is only qualitative, and, therefore, precise location of the point where the stresses are zero may vary. In addition, we have the shear stresses (Fig. 2-70*B*, originally shown in Fig. 2-68*B*). The shear stresses are maximum in the center of the cross section, and they decrease toward the periphery. It is interesting to note that the maximum shear stresses occur in the region where the central venulae are located. These venulae are thought to be the structures in the spinal cord least resistant to mechanical damage.[5]

DIRECT COMPRESSION LOAD

A Compressive Stress

B Shear Stress

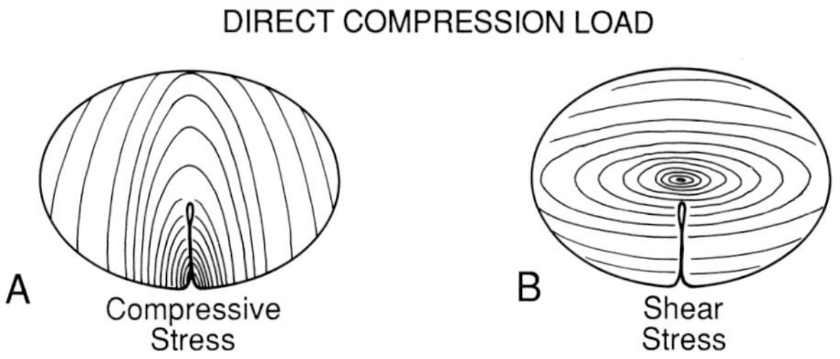

Fig. 2-68. (*A*) Direct compression force applied from the anterior produces local compressive stresses, which decrease in magnitude away from the point of contact. (*B*) In addition, anterior compression produces shear stresses in the cord that have the maximum value in its center.

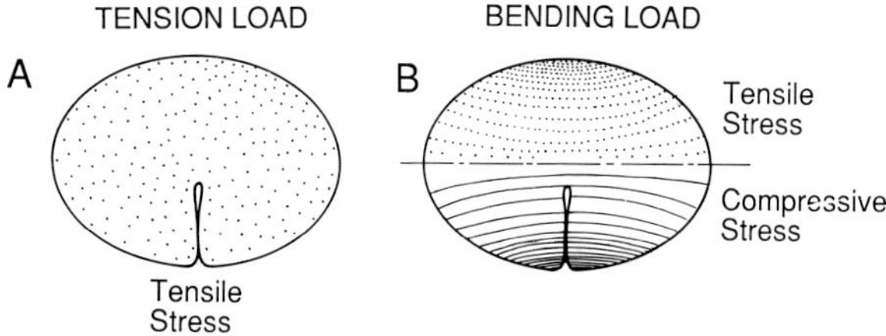

Fig. 2-69. (*A*) Tension load applied to the cord produces uniform tensile stresses in the entire cross section of the cord. (*B*) Bending of the spinal cord produces compressive stresses on the concave side and tensile stresses on the convex side of the bent spinal cord.

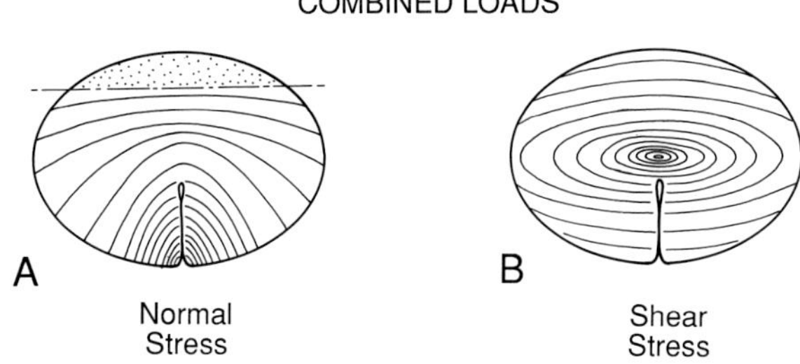

Fig. 2-70. The stresses due to the combined loads of compression, tension, and bending are shown. (*A*) Normal stresses, that is, stresses that are in the same direction as the length of the spinal cord, are compressive on the anterior side and tensile on the posterior side. (*B*) The shear stresses have a maximum value in the middle of the spinal cord and near-zero values on the anterior and posterior surfaces of the cord.

DISCUSSION

Biomechanics can be helpful in providing understanding of the cervical spondylotic myelopathy. When external forces are applied to the spinal cord they result in internal stresses and strains. To determine the basis of neurologic dysfunction due to loads applied to the cord, it is necessary to obtain precise relationships between the anatomic structures of the spinal cord (gray and white matters and blood supply) and the stresses produced. Two items are necessary to obtaining such relationships: detailed quantitative anatomy of the spinal cord and spinal column, and the specific stress patterns generated in the spinal cord. To determine the second item, it is necessary to know the physical properties of the spinal cord and dura and to develop mathematical models to simulate the spinal cord structures.

Although several studies provide descriptive anatomy of the spinal cord and column, a detailed quantitative anatomy is completely lacking. Concerning the mechanical properties of the spinal cord and dura, only a few studies are available, namely, those of Brieg,[2] Suderland,[10] and Tencer and coworkers.[11] All these biomechanical studies have been conducted by applying tensile forces to the spinal cord specimen. We have seen that the stresses produced in the spinal cord are of three types: shear, compressive, and tensile. Therefore, studies should be conducted to determine, in addition to the tensile properties, the shear and compressive properties of the spinal cord. Such data are presently not available. To our knowledge, no mathematical models exist that are suitable for relating the external loads applied to the cord to the internal stresses produced in it. However, it is feasible that such models could be developed by using modern techniques of finite elements.

Finally, experiments using animal models are needed to relate the computed stresses in the spinal cord to the neurologic dysfunction. Many *in vivo* experiments have been conducted in which mechanical pressure or certain compression was applied to the cord. However, the mechanical input was seldom quantified in precise biomechanical terms. These experiments have contributed significantly to our knowledge about the neurologic dysfunction caused by compression, but they are not suitable for relating the mechanical input to the neurologic dysfunction in a precise manner. New experiments must be designed and conducted. Specifically, it is necessary to precisely measure: (1) the mechanical input, in the form of the magnitude of cord compression or pressure, and its distribution on the spinal cord, and (2) the quantitative functional output of the animal.

Sometime in the future it may be possible, using biomechanical techniques, to relate specific bony pathology to internal stresses in the cord. The stresses, in turn, may be related to the neurologic dysfunction by the use of knowledge gained from quantitative animal experiments. Thus, a predictive algorithm may be developed to relate the spinal column pathology to neurologic dysfunction.

REFERENCES

1. *BOHLMAN HH, BAHNIUK E, FIELDS G, RASKULINECZ G:* Incomplete cervical spinal cord injury. 6:428–436,1981
2. *BREIG A:* Biomechanics of the central nervous system. Stockholm, Almquist & Wicksell, 1960
3. *BRIEG A:* Adverse mechanical tension in the central nervous system. Stockholm, Almquist & Wicksell, 1978
4. *BROWN T, HANSON R, YORRA A:* Some mechanical tests on the lumbo-sacral spine with particular reference to the intervertebral discs. J Bone Joint Surg 39A:1135, 1975
5. *DOHRMANN GJ:* Experimental cord trauma—a historical review. Arch Neurol 27:467, 1972
6. *PENNING L:* Functional pathology of cervical spine. Amsterdam, Excerpta Medica, 1968
7. *RAYNOR RB, KOPLIK B:* Cervical cord trauma: The relationship between clinical syndromes and force of injury. Spine 10:193–197, 1985
8. *SCHNEIDER RC:* The syndrome of acute anterior spinal cord injury. J Neurosurg 12:95–122, 1955
9. *SCHNEIDER RC, THOMPSON JM, BEBIN J:* The syndrome of acute central cervical cord injury. J Neurol Neurosurg Psychiat 21:216–227, 1958
10. *SUDERLAND S:* Nerve and nerve injuries. New York, Churchill Livingstone, 1978
11. *TENCER AF, ALLEN BL, FERGUSON RL:* A Biomechanical study of thoracolumbar spinal fractures with bone in the canal. Part III. Mechanical properties of the dura and its tethering ligaments. Spine 10:741–747, 1985
12. *TENCER AF, FERGUSON RL, ALLEN BL:* A biomechanical study of thoracolumbar spinal fractures with bone in the canal. Part II. The effect of flexion angulation, distraction, and shortening of the motion segment. Spine 10:586–589, 1985
13. *TENCER A, ALLEN B, FERGUSON RL:* A biomechanical study of thoracolumbar spinal fractures with bone in the canal. Part I. The effect of laminectomy. Spine 10:580–585, 1985

Cervical Orthoses

JOHN W. WOLF, JR. AND ROLLIN M. JOHNSON

Man's attempt to correct deformity and lessen pain through the use of braces is recorded from at least as early as the Fifth Egyptian Dynasty (2750–2625 B.C.).[17] The basic principles of many of our current orthoses can be traced directly to devices used by Hippocrates and his medical successors, through the armorers of the Middle Ages to the present (Fig. 2-71).

A multitude of cervical orthoses are available to the physician of today. They are often named after their inventors (*e.g.*, Thomas, Guilford), after the places where they were designed (*e.g.*, Philadelphia, Yale), or by descriptions (*e.g.*, "four-poster," SOMI). This system of nomenclature is somewhat provincial, however, and essentially identical orthoses may be known by several different names in different regions of the country. In 1973, a task force on standardization of prosthetic-orthotics terminology developed a systematic nomenclature and recommended that orthoses be described in terms of the joints they encompass and by an analysis of their control of joint motion.

Cervical orthoses can be divided into two basic types: skin contact orthoses and skeletal devices (halos). All cervical orthoses fall into one of the categories listed in order below, from least restrictive to most restrictive:

1. Cervical orthoses (CO)
   Soft
   Rigid
2. Head-cervical orthoses (HCO)
   Molded
   Poster type
3. Head-cervical-thoracic orthoses (HCTO)
   Molded
   Poster type
4. Halo devices

The head-cervical orthosis (HCO) is distinguished from a cervical orthosis (CO) by the presence of either a mandibular support or an occipital support, or both. A head-cervical-thoracic orthosis (HCTO) extends further distally than an HCO and utilizes the sternum, ribs and/or thoracic spine for additional points of support. Figure 2-34 illustrates orthoses from each of these four categories. Throughout this chapter, the nonhalo orthoses are referred to as conventional orthoses.

The goal of the physician in prescribing a cervical orthosis is to control the position of the cervical spine by the application of external forces. Control of the spine may be necessary for any combination of the following reasons:

1. Protection
2. Immobilization
3. Support
4. Correction of deformity

Paramount among these is protection of the spinal cord and nerve roots.

Because the cervical spine lies in close proximity to many vital structures in the neck that do not withstand direct pressure (*e.g.*, trachea, major vessels), a cervical orthosis must gain a purchase on the structures at each end of the neck, that is, the skull and the thorax, to function effectively. The success of any orthosis in immobilizing the cervical spine is directly related to the firmness of its attachment to these structures. Pathologic conditions or injuries that necessitate the unloading of the cervical spine or the maintenance of a traction force across the cervical vertebrae pose particularly difficult orthotic problems. Even the halo devices do not accomplish this goal reliably. Koch and Nickel have shown that the distracting forces imparted by the halo vest vary greatly with the position of the patient.[13]

There are a number of studies in the literature that document the range of motion of the normal cervical spine.[1-6, 15] There are only a few published studies that measure the motion of the cervical spine in an orthosis.[7-13, 19]

Johnson and coworkers have reported on the limitation of cervical motion produced by many types of cervical orthoses.[10] In this study, each subject served as his or her own control except in the cases of the halo vest. Results were reported as the percentage of normal motion allowed by the orthosis (Table 2-11).

Wolf and Jones have studied cervical immobilization imparted by halo casts and halo vests.[19] Their results are also summarized in Table 2-12. These data could not be presented as a percentage of normal motion allowed in the same subject, because all measurements were obtained from patients with injured spines. The data are compared, therefore, to published normal values for cervical spine motion.[15]

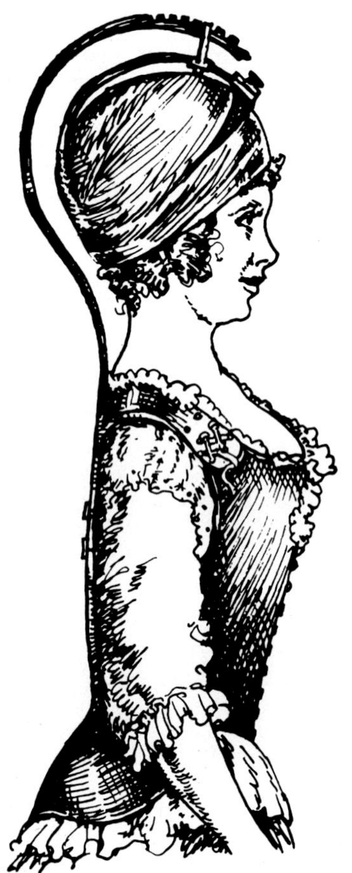

Fig. 2-71. Spinal brace with jury developed by Levancher in 1764. The same principle is used today. (Edwards JW: Orothopedic Appliances Atlas, Vol 1. Ann Arbor, American Academy of Orthopedic Surgeons, 1952)

Tables 2-11 and 2-12 list the effectiveness of these orthoses in limiting motion of the cervical spine taken as a whole. However, some braces are more effective in limiting particular motions or in limiting motion at specific intersegmental levels. A detailed discussion of specific cervical orthoses and our recommendations for their usage can be found later in this chapter.

CONTROL OF FLEXION–EXTENSION

When considering the control of flexion and extension at each intervertebral level, it can be seen that the most effective orthosis overall is unquestionably the halo vest or halo cast (Table 2-13).

When sagittal plane motion (flexion-extension) was measured at individual intervertebral levels in patients wearing halo vests, an interesting finding was noted. The cervical spine flexed at one level and simultaneously extended at other levels, similar to a plucked guitar string. This motion has been referred to as "paradoxical motion" by Hartman and coworkers and as "snaking" by Johnson and associates.[8,11] Measurement of these motions at each level created the impression that some levels moved more than the cervical spine as a whole.

Of the conventional orthoses, the SOMI orthosis appears to limit upper and midcervical flexion (between C1 and C5) most effectively, and the cervicothoracic brace is more effective at the lower levels (between C5 and T1). In extension, the molded cervicothoracic orthosis is consistently effective at nearly all intervertebral levels. Most orthoses are more effective in limiting flexion than they are in limiting extension. An important finding is that the SOMI brace is consistently less effective than the other braces in limiting extension at most segmental levels. This failure stems from the design of the occipital rest, which is not rigid and can be easily moved by the patient when the head or neck is extended (Fig. 2-72*E*).

CONTROL OF ROTATION

The control of rotation by the conventional orthoses is not as effective as control of flexion-extension. Here, again, the cervicothoracic orthosis is the most effective conventional orthosis but still allowed 18% of normal rotation in the study by Johnson and coworkers.[10] The halo vest is quite effective in controlling rotation owing to its excellent purchase on the skull. Both Wolf and Johnson found rotation limited to less than 5° in most cases.[10,19]

CONTROL OF LATERAL BENDING

None of the conventional orthoses controls lateral bending well. Although control of flexion and extension is aided by the ability to use the mandible and the occiput to increase the lever arm, no convenient purchase is available to help control lateral bending. The four-poster and the cervicothoracic orthoses, the two that are most effective, allowed 46% to 50% of normal motion, respectively. The halo vest, which does obtain a good purchase on

Table 2-11. Normal Cervical Motion Allowed from the Occiput to the First Thoracic Vertebra

	NUMBER OF SUBJECTS	MEAN AGE (YRS)	MEAN % OF NORMAL MOTION: FLEXION–EXTENSION	LATERAL BENDING	ROTATION
Normal	44	25.8	100	100	100
Soft collar	20	26.2	74.2	92.3	82.6
Philadelphia collar	17	25.8	28.9	66.4	43.7
Somi brace	22	25.0	27.7	65.6	33.6
Four-poster brace	27	25.9	20.6	45.9	27.1
Rigid cervico-thoracic brace	27	25.9	12.8	50.5	18.2
Halo vest	7	40.0	4	4	1

(After Johnson RM, Hart DL, Simmons EF, Ramsby GR, Southwick WO: Cervical orthoses: A study comparing their effectiveness in restricting cervical motion in normal subjects. J Bone Joint Surg 59A:332, 1977)

Table 2-12. Amount of Cervical Motion Between the Occiput and the First Thoracic Vertebra Allowed in Halo Devices

MOTION	NORMAL	HALO	% OF NORMAL
Flexion–extension	64°	7.5°	11.7%
Lateral bending	49°	4.1°	8.4%
Rotation	90°	2.2°	2.4%

(After Lysell E: Motion in the cervical spine: Thesis. Acta Orthop Scand 123 [Suppl], 1969; and Wolf JW, Jones HC: Comparison of cervical immobilization in halo-casts and halo-plastic jackets. Orthopaedic Transactions 5[1]:118, 1981)

the skull, effectively limited lateral bending to less than a 12° total arc in Wolf's study.

INDIVIDUAL ORTHOSES

Collars

SOFT COLLAR. Several published studies have documented the fact that a soft cervical collar does not effectively immobilize the cervical spine (Fig. 2-72A).[8,9,12] Hartman found "no evidence of restriction" of cervical motion in his cineradiography studies. This device is the lest effective of all orthoses listed in controlling cervical motion. It is,

Table 2-13. Flexion and Extension Allowed at Each Segmental Level (Mean Value in Degrees)

	MOTION	OCCIPUT–C1	C1–C2	C2–C3	C3–C4	C4–C5	C5–C6	C6–C7	C7–T1
Normal unrestricted	Flexion	0.7	7.7	7.2	9.8	10.3	11.4	12.5	9.0
	Extension	18.1	6.0	4.8	7.8	9.8	10.5	8.2	2.7
Soft collar	Flexion	1.3	5.1	4.5	7.4	8.4	9.9	9.7	7.7
	Extension	13.7	1.9	3.9	5.8	6.8	7.8	7.4	2.8
Philadelphia collar	Flexion	0.9	4.0	1.6	3.1	4.6	6.2	6.2	5.5
	Extension	6.8	4.5	1.8	3.4	5.8	5.9	5.8	1.3
Somi brace	Flexion	3.6	2.7	0.9	1.6	1.9	2.8	2.9	3.1
	Extension	9.1	5.4	4.4	6.3	6.0	6.0	5.6	2.1
Four-poster brace	Flexion	2.9	4.4	1.6	2.1	1.8	3.0	3.9	2.8
	Extension	9.3	3.2	2.0	3.2	3.4	2.9	3.1	1.6
Cervicothoracic brace	Flexion	1.3	5.0	1.8	2.9	2.8	1.6	0.7	2.4
	Extension	8.4	2.5	2.1	1.6	2.2	2.8	3.4	1.7
Halo	Total of Flexion and Extension		3.6	2.2	2.6	3.3	6.5	2.6	

(After Johnson RM, Hart DL, Simmons EF, Ramsby GR, Southwick WO: Cervical orthoses: A study comparing their effectiveness in restricting cervical motion in normal subjects. J Bone Joint Surg 59A:332, 1977; and Wolf JW, Jones HC: Comparison of cervical immobilization in halo-casts and halo-plastic jackets. Orthopaedic Transactions 5[1]:118, 1981)

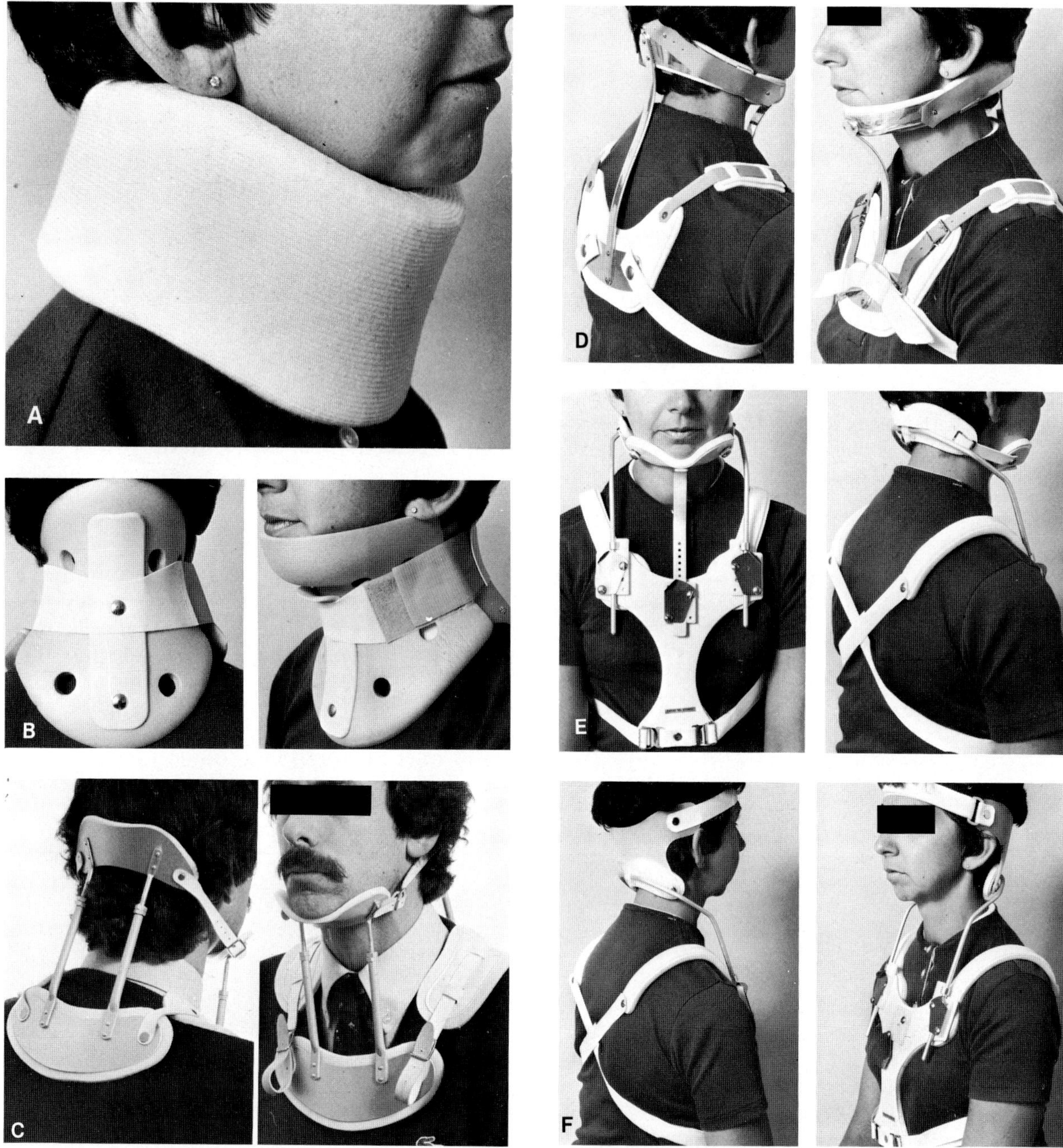
A
B
C
D
E
F

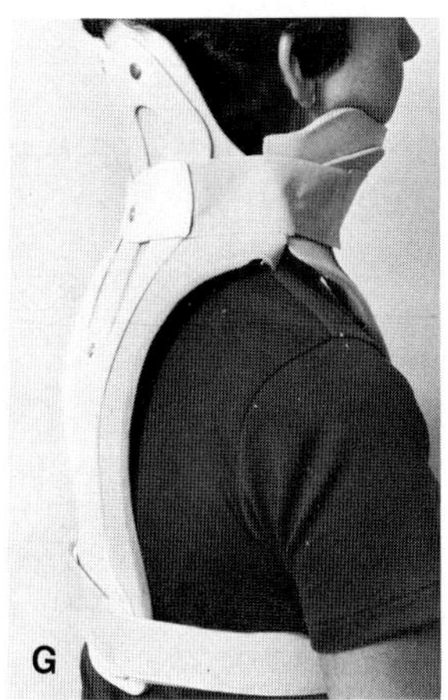

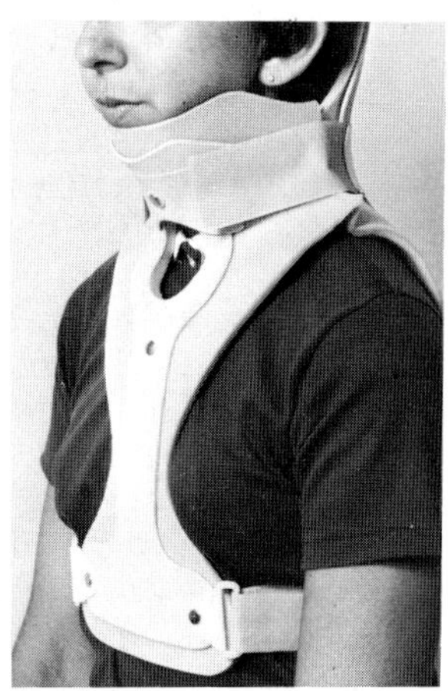

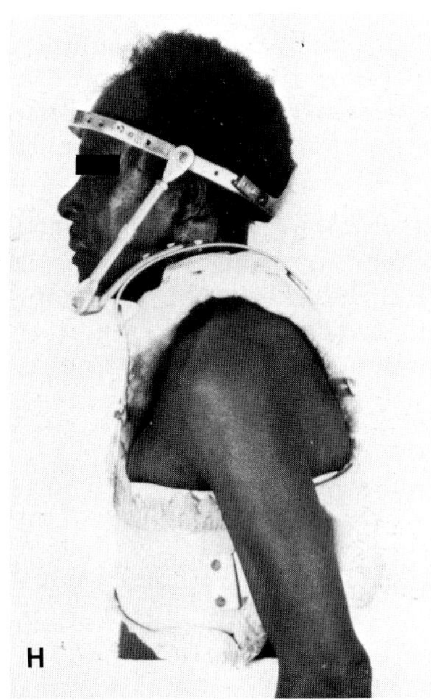

Fig. 2-72. (*A*) The soft cervical collar (CO) is made of stockinette filled with foam rubber. It is well tolerated by most patients but does not restrict cervical motion to any significant degree. (*B*) The Philadelphia collar (HCO) is made of Plastizote reinforced with anterior and posterior plastic struts. The front and rear halves fasten at the sides with Velcro. This orthosis has molded mandibular and occipital supports. (*C*) The four-poster brace (HCTO) has molded mandibular and occipital supports attached by adjustable struts to anterior and posterior padded thoracic plates. The front and back sections are connected to each other by leather straps below the ears and over the shoulders. There are no straps under the axillae. (*D*) The Guilford brace (HCTO) has padded mandibular and occipital supports rigidly connected to anterior and posterior thoracic plates. The front and back sections interlock to form a rigid metal ring below ear level. The thoracic plates are attached to each other both over the shoulders and by a strap under the axillae. (*E* and *F*) The SOMI orthosis (HCTO) has a rigid anterior plastic chest piece or yoke supported from the shoulder by curved rigid supports, which extend over the shoulders from anterior to posterior to the level of the scapular spines. The curved supports are connected to straps that cross in the back and attach to the bottom of the yoke in front after passing under the axillae. (*F*) Mandibular and occipital supports are attached to the anterior chest piece. (*E*) The advantage of this arrangement is that it allows the orthosis to be applied without moving the patient from the supine position. This orthosis is supplied with an optional head piece that snaps onto the occipital rest and passes around the patient's forehead. This arrangement allows the patient to remove the mandibular support while eating. (*G*) The molded cervicothoracic orthosis (HCTO) is similar to an extended Philadelphia collar. It is made of molded Plastizote anterior and posterior halves reinforced with plastic struts. The orthosis extends well down onto the thorax, and the two halves fasten there with straps passing beneath the axillae. Note the height of the occipital rest. (*H*) The halo vest (skeletal type HCTO) consists of a prefabricated plastic vest attached to a halo ring. The halo ring is rigidly affixed to the skull. The vest is lined with lamb's wool or Kodel. A plaster cast can be substituted for the plastic vest and attached to a similar superstructure. These orthoses provide the most rigid external restriction of cervical spine motion but require considerable experience to manage successfully.

however, quite comfortable and well accepted by most patients. A collar may serve as a reminder to the patient to restrict his activities and serves to assure him that he is under treatment.

PHILADELPHIA COLLAR. The Philadelphia collar is nearly as comfortable as a soft collar and significantly more effective in controlling neck motion (Fig. 2-72*B*). It is generally ineffective in controlling rotation and lateral bending.

Poster Braces

There are numerous poster-type orthoses available, all of which are essentially similar in principle (Fig. 2-72*C* and *D*). These orthoses are reasonably well tolerated by most patients and control cervical motion nearly as well as cervicothoracic braces. They are effective in controlling flexion, especially in the midcervical levels.

Cervicothoracic-Style Orthoses

SOMI BRACE. The name *SOMI* is an acronym for sterno-occipital-mandibular-immobilizer. It was found by Johnson and coworkers to be particularly effective in immobilizing the upper cervical spine (C1-C5) in flexion, but is less effective than the four-poster and rigid cervicothoracic orthoses in controlling every other motion. However, it has a unique feature that partially accounts for its widespread use: the SOMI is exceptionally easy to apply and adjust. It can be applied with the patient supine without the necessity of moving the cervical spine. It does have the failing, previously mentioned, of permitting more extension than most other orthoses and for this reason should not be employed for any injury that is unstable in extension. This orthosis is quite uncomfortable for patients confined to bed because the posterior portions of the plastic yoke are pressed into the scapulae by the mattress. It is reasonably well tol-

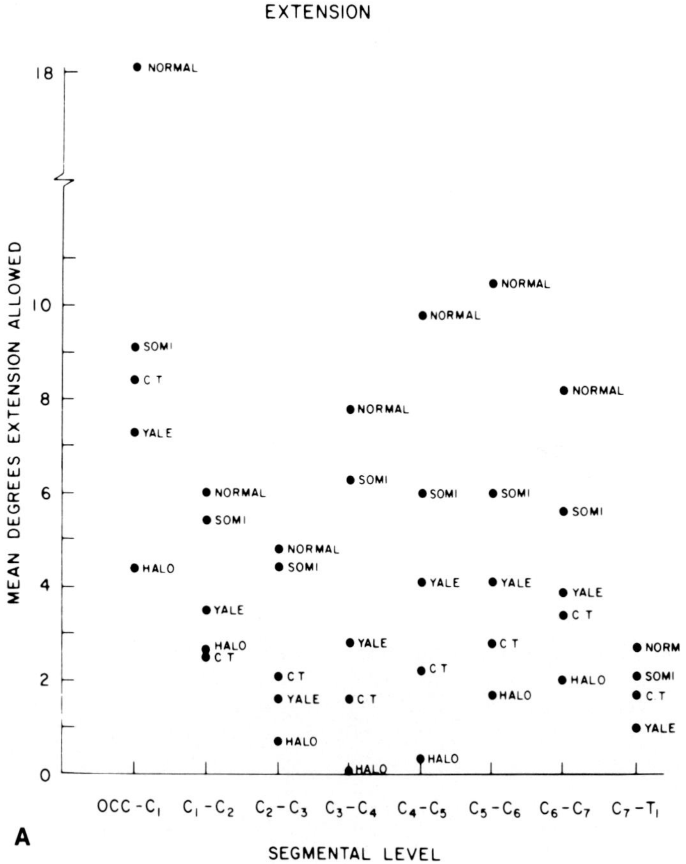

Fig. 2-73. Graphic representations of mean degrees of (*A*) extension and (*B*) flexion allowed at each intersegmental level of the cervical spine in normal unrestricted subjects compared to motion allowed in the most effective rigid orthoses. (Johnson RM, Owen JR, Hart DL et al: Cervical orthoses: A guide to their selection and use. Clin Orthop 145:1, 1981)

erated by ambulatory and wheelchair patients (Fig. 2-72*E*).

MOLDED CERVICOTHORACIC BRACES ("YALE" TYPE). Molded cervicothoracic devices are the most effective of the conventional (nonhalo) cervical orthoses in restricting neck motion (Fig. 2-72*F*). They are commercially available or can be fabricated.[20] They are most effective in controlling flexion–extension and reasonably effective in controlling rotation. These orthoses, however, only restrict lateral bending by approximately 50%.

Halo Devices

Two basic kinds of halo devices are currently used for control of neck motion: halo casts and halo vests. These devices afford the best control of all cervical motions. In his photographic and radiographic measurements of cervical motion in halo casts and halo vests, Wolf was not able to detect any significant differences between the two. Use of halo casts or vests, however, should be restricted to physicians with considerable experience in their application and complications.[14,16,18] As previously mentioned, even these orthoses will not maintain a distraction force across the cervical spine in an ambulatory patient.[13]

Mean Degrees of Flexion and Extension

Figure 2-73 summarizes the mean degrees of flexion and extension permitted by various orthoses.

CONCLUSIONS

Generally speaking, the better the purchase an orthosis has on the head and thorax, the more effectively it can limit motion of the cervical spine and support some of the weight of the head. It is equally true, however, that as the restriction of motion afforded by the orthosis and the area of skin contact increases, the patient's ability to tolerate the orthosis for an extended period of time

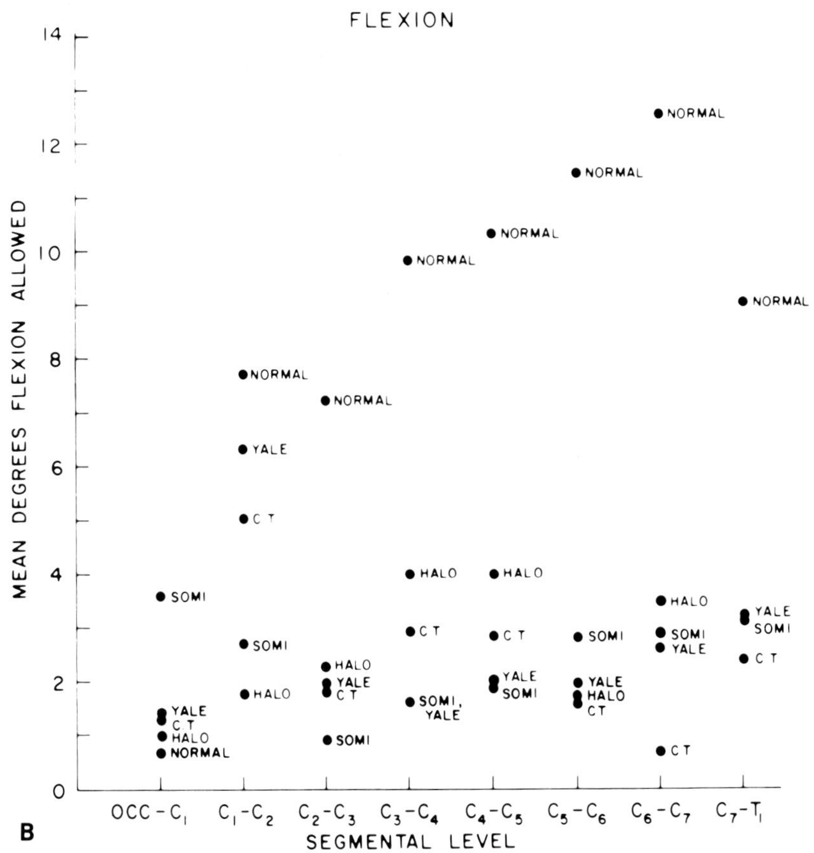

Fig. 2-73, B.

Table 2-14. Author's Recommendations of Orthoses for Use in Selected Clinical Conditions and Injuries.

CLINICAL CONDITION	PLANE OF INSTABILITY	RECOMMENDED ORTHOSIS
"Cervical Strain"	None	Philadelphia Collar
Ring of C1 (Jefferson's Fx)		
Stable	None	Cervicothoracic
Unstable	All	Halo
Odontoid Fx		
Type I	None	Cervicothoracic
Type II and III′	All	Halo
C_2 Neural Arch Fx (Hangman's Fx)		
Stable	Flexion	Somi
Unstable	All	Halo
Flexion Injuries		
Mid Cervical C_{3-5}	Flexion	Somi, Cervicothoracic
Low Cervical C_5–T_1	Flexion	Cervicothoracic
Extension Injuries		
Mid Cervical C_{3-5}	Extension	Halo, Cervicothoracic
Low Cervical C_5–T_1	Extension	Halo

decreases. Thus, a collar (CO) is better tolerated by most patients than is a halo-vest. The factor of patient acceptance must be considered whenever an orthosis is prescribed. Even an "ideal" orthosis does no good if it is not used.

The only orthosis that effectively controls motion between the occiput and C1 is the halo vest. Motion between the atlas and the axis, although somewhat easier to control, is also poorly restricted by most conventional (nonhalo) orthoses. Therefore, we recommend use of a halo device for most cases in which orthotic control of instability of the upper cervical spine (occiput–C2) is desired.

Instability of the cervical spine at lower levels can be controlled by several orthoses, as shown in Table 2-11. This is especially true for control of flexion. In nearly all cases, the halo allows the least motion, but the cervicothoracic, Yale, and SOMI devices are also effective, are generally better tolerated by the patient, and do not have the disadvantages of the halo devices. Table 2-14 lists our recommendations for orthoses for selected clinical conditions of the cervical spine. The goal of cervical bracing varies with the patient's problems. A cervical strain or minor ligamentous injury in which the stability of the spine has not been compromised and in which there is no neurologic injury can usually be treated with a less rigid orthosis. More serious injuries involving instability of the cervical spine, nerve root damage, or spinal cord damage usually are better treated by more restrictive orthoses. In these cases, an orthosis should be selected that provides restriction of motion at the proper intervertebral level and in the appropriate plane.

The criteria for selection of the best orthosis to use for an individual patient should take into account not only the nature of the injury and desired degree of immobilization but also orthosis availability, patient compliance, and physician-orthotist experience.

REFERENCES

1. *BHALLA SK, SIMMONS EH:* Normal ranges of intervertebral joint motion of the cervical spine. Can J Surg 12:181, 1969
2. *BUCK CA, DAMERON FB, DOW MJ, SKOWLAND HV:* Study of normal range of motion in the neck utilizing a bubble goniometer. Arch Phys Med Rehabil 40:390, 1959
3. *FERLIC D:* The range of motion of the "normal" cervical spine. John Hopkins Hospital Bulletin 110:59, 1962
4. *FIELDING JW:* Cineradiography of the normal cervical spine. NY State J Med 56:2984, 1956
5. *FIELDING JW:* Cineradiography of the normal cervical spine. J Bone Joint Surg 39A:1280, 1957

6. *Fielding JW:* Normal and selected abnormal motion of the cervical spine from the second cervical vertebra to the seventh cervical vertebra based on cineradiography. J Bone Joint Surg 46A:1779, 1964
7. *Fisher SV, Bowar JF, Awad EA:* Cervical orthoses' effect on cervical spine motion: Roentgenographic and goniometric method of study. Arch Phys Med Rehabil 58:109, 1977
8. *Hartman JT, Palumbo F, Hill BJ:* Cineradiography of the braced normal spine. Clin Orthop 109:97, 1975
9. *Johnson RM, Hart DL, Owen JR, Lerner E, Chapin W, Zeleznik R:* The Yale cervical orthosis: An evaluation of its effectiveness in restricting cervical motion in normal subjects and a comparison with other cervical orthoses. Phys Ther 58:865, 1978
10. *Johnson RM, Hart DL, Simmons EF, Ramsby GR, Southwick WO:* Cervical orthoses: A study comparing their effectiveness in restricting cervical motion in normal subjects. J Bone Joint Surg 59A:332, 1977
11. *Johnson RM, Owen JR, Hart DL, Callahan RA:* Cervical orthoses: A guide to their selection and use. Clin Orthop 154:34, 1981
12. *Jones MD:* Cineroentgenographic studies of the collar-immobilized cervical spine. J Neurosurg 17:633, 1960
13. *Koch RA, Nickel VL:* The halo vest: An evaluation of motion and forces across the neck. Spine 3(1), 1978
14. *Levine DB, Hankin S:* The halo yoke: A simplified device for attachment of the halo to a body cast. J Bone Joint Surg 54A:881, 1972
15. *Lysell E:* Motion in the cervical spine: Thesis. Acta Orthop Scand 123 (Suppl), 1969
16. *Perry J:* The halo in spinal abnormalities. Orthop Clin North Am 3:69, 1972
17. *Smith GE:* The most ancient splits. Br Med J 1:732, 1908
18. *Victor D, Bresnan M, Keller R:* Brain abscess complicating the use of halo traction. J Bone Joint Surg 55A:635, 1973
19. *Wolf JW, Jones HC:* Comparison of cervical immobilization in halo-casts and halo-plastic jackets. Orthopaedic Transactions 5(1):118, 1981
20. *Zeleznik R, Chapin W, Hart DL, Smith H, Southwick WO, Zito M:* Yale cervical orthosis. Phys Ther 58:861, 1978

BIBLIOGRAPHY

American Academy of Surgeons: Orthopedic Appliances Atlas, Vol I. Ann Arbor, JW Edwards, 1952

Anderson LD, D'Alonzo RT: Fractures of the odontoid process of the atlas. J Bone Joint Surg 56A:1663, 1974

Atlas of Orthotics, 2nd ed. St. Louis, CV Mosby Company, 1985

Bloomberg MH: Orthopaedic Braces. Philadelphia, JB Lippincott, 1964

Harris, EE: A new Orthotics terminology—a guide to its use for prescription and fee schedules, Orthot Prosthet 27(2):6, 1973

Harris, JD: In Redford JB (ed): Orthotics Et cetera, 3rd ed. Baltimore, Williams & Wilkins, 1986

Thompson H: The "halo" traction apparatus: A method of external splinting of the cervical spine after injury. J Bone Joint Surg 44B:665, 1962

White AA III, Panjabi MM: Clinical Biomechanics of the Spine. Philadelphia, JB Lippincott, 1978

CHAPTER 3

Roentgenographic Evaluation

Obtaining and Interpreting Plain Films in Cervical Spine Injury

LOURENS PENNING

INITIAL RADIOGRAPHY AND RADIOGRAPH EVALUATION

In radiography for cervical spine injury, the first aim is to obtain a lateral radiograph of the cervical spine. It should preferably be made with the patient still on the transportation stretcher, all handling being postponed until the results of the radiographic exmination are known. If handling is necessary, the patient should be lifted "as one piece" by at least four persons. Pressure sores are easily produced in patients with cord lesions and should be prevented by the use of a foam rubber mattress and pads of soft material between the knees and ankles and underneath the calves. Any source of harmful pressure—for example, hard objects in the pocket—should be removed. Suction, insertion of nasal or tracheal tubes, and so forth should be undertaken without moving the head or neck.

Care should be taken that the lower part of the cervical spine is depicted on the film; superimposition of shoulders must be overcome by traction on arms (Fig. 3-1).[22,27] If pulling on the arms proves unsuccessful, the flying angel projection may be tried (Fig. 3-2).[27] Experience has shown that most fractures and luxations are missed at the lower end of the cervical spine.[25]

If performed correctly, the lateral radiograph will disclose the great majority of lesions, including those causing dangerous instability.

In unconscious patients and patients with multiple injuries, fractures of the cervical spine are easily overlooked because they are not expected (Fig. 3-3). It is a good rule to examine the cervical spine radiologically in every case of head injury. Head injuries often produce abnormal movements of the cervical spine, which are capable of causing fractures or luxations. If the cervical spine injury is overlooked, endotracheal intubation, suction, and so forth may inflict irreparable damage upon the spinal cord.[17]

After it has been ascertained that all seven vertebrae are depicted on the radiograph, the outlines of the bony spinal canal are studied. They reflect

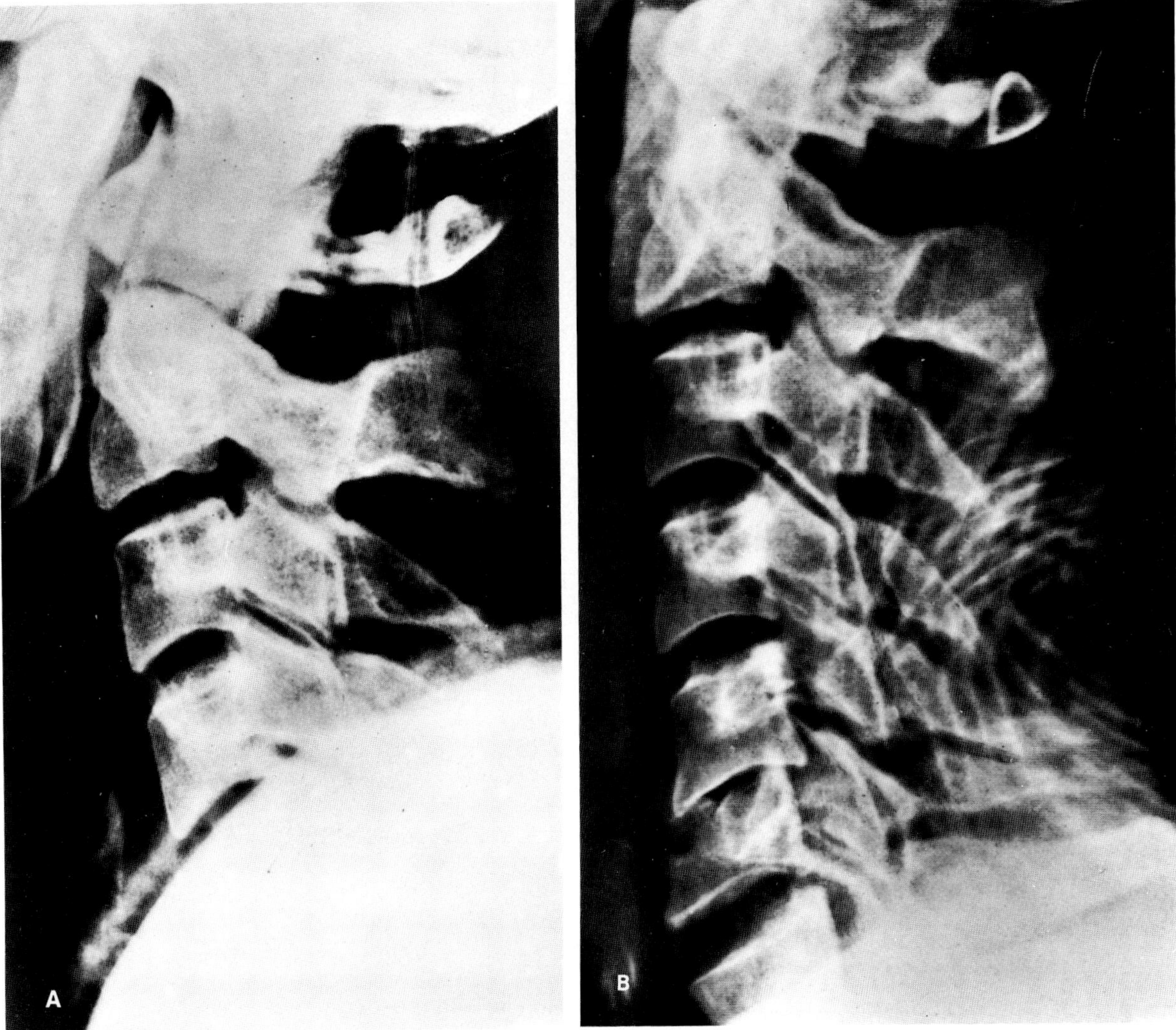

Fig. 3-1. Superimposition of the shoulders on fracture of C6 in a 44-year-old male who fell from a platform 7 m high. (Clinical examination revealed Brown-Séquard syndrome.) (*A*) Radiograph disclosing fracture of the posterior arch of atlas. The shoulders are superimposing the lower cervical vertebrae. (*B*) Downward traction on the arms reveals an additional compression fracture of vertebral body of C6. Artifacts overlying the spinous processes are due to support under the neck in order to maintain the lordotic curve.

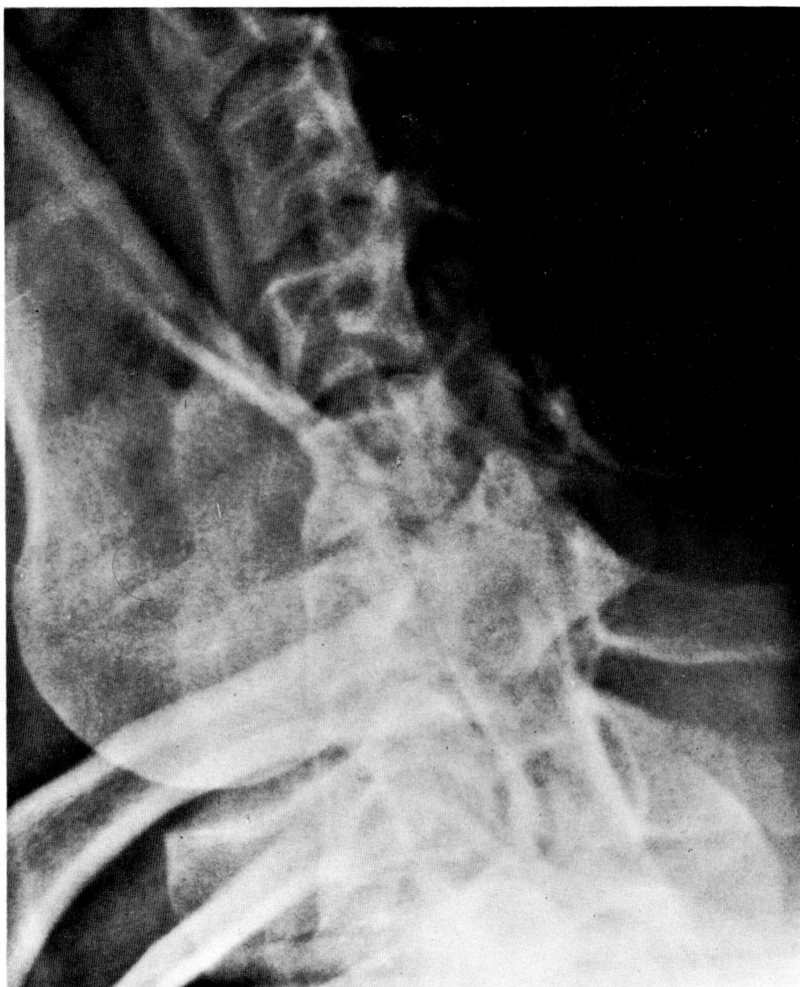

Fig. 3-2. Flying angel projection. The patient is supine with the cassette placed on the lateral aspect of the shoulder. The arm on the same side as the cassette is raised above the head while the opposite arm is pulled towards the feet in order to depress the shoulder. The tube is centered on the head of the humerus at the level of the acromion process. Care must be taken that the film and the tube are parallel. (Technique from Scher A, Vambeck V: An approach to the radiological examination of the cervicodorsal junction following injury. Clin Radiol 28:243–246, 1977)

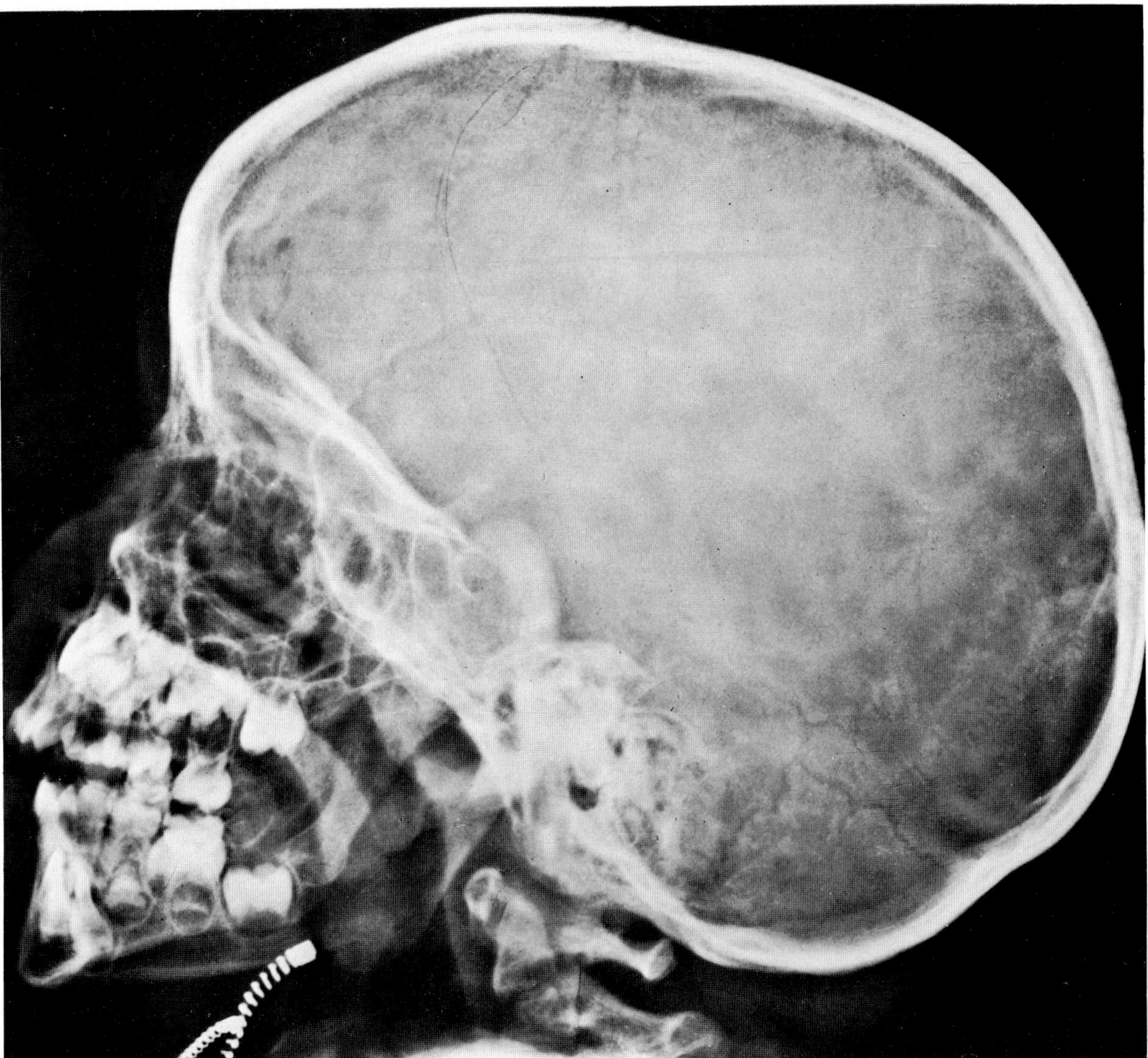

Fig. 3-3. The diagnosis of epiphysiolysis of the odontoid process was initially missed on this lateral skull film of 4-year-old boy knocked down by a car. After laparotomy, done because of a battered kidney and hematoma of the liver, respiration had to be maintained artificially; complete cord lesion below the level of C1–C2 was diagnosed. Cervical spine films then drew attention to the epiphysiolysis. Cord lesion proved to be permanent.

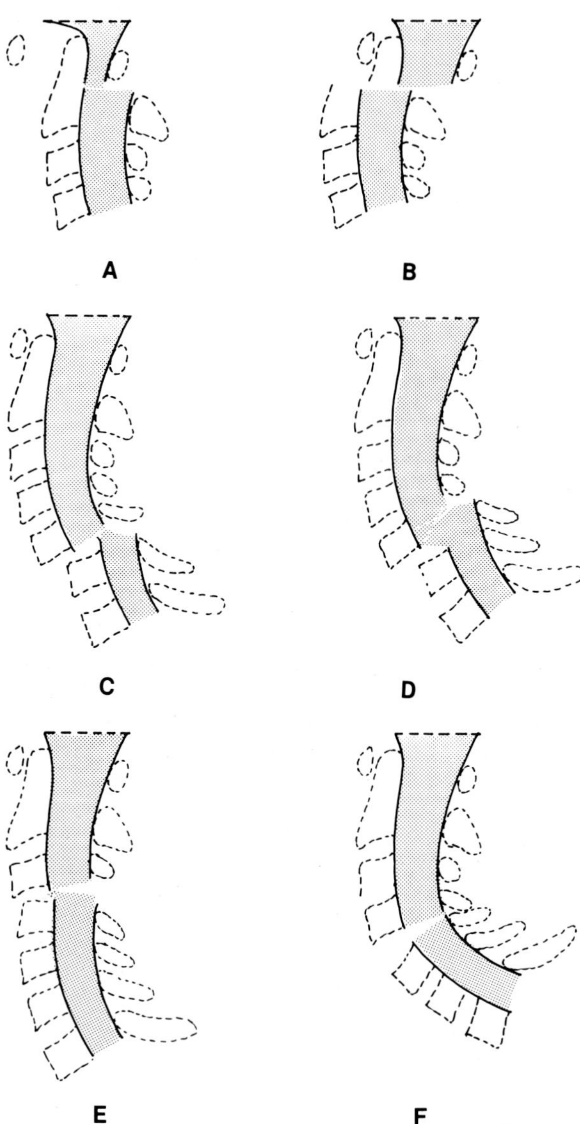

Fig. 3-4. Outlines of the spinal canal in several types of injury. Outlines of the bony canal are represented by lines drawn along the posterior borders of the vertebral bodies and the anterior margins of the spinous processes. The canal itself is accentuated by shading. (*A*) Anterior pure atlantoaxial luxation, with narrowing of the spinal canal between the odontoid process and the posterior arch of atlas. (*B*) Posterior atlantoaxial luxation due to odontoid fracture (or os odontoideum). Note the narrowing of the canal between the odontoid process and the posterior arch of the axis. (*C*) Hyperflexion luxation of C5–C6. There is no fracture of arch C5. Note the narrowing of the canal between arch C5 and body C6. (*D*) Hyperflexion luxation of C5–C6 with fracture of arch C5 ("cord-saving fracture"). There is no narrowing of the spinal canal. (*E*) Kyphotic angulation due to hyperflexion injury with disruption of the posterior ligaments. (*F*) Lordotic angulation due to hyperextension injury with disruption of the anterior longitudinal ligament and the intervertebral disc.

the topographic relationship between the vertebrae and indicate possible endangering of the spinal cord. Normally they form a funnellike figure with a smoothly curved spout. In cases of fractures or luxations, the figure may be deformed in several ways; examples are given in Figure 3-4. Any abnormality in the outlines of the bony spinal canal indicates a need for further examination to determine its cause, which could be interlocking of articular facets or a compression fracture of vertebral body, for example.

Next, the prevertebral space is evaluated. Widening (by hematoma) indicates injury to the cervical spine and may draw attention to the possibility of certain fractures that might otherwise be missed (Fig. 3-5 and Table 3-1). This is especially true for small anterior avulsions of vertebral bodies, cartilaginous rims, or spondylotic spurs due to distractive hyperextension, and for odontoid fracture without displacement. Demonstration of prevertebral swelling is useful to the anesthetist considering intubation. It also may help explain respiratory distress or difficulties in swallowing. Absence of prevertebral hematoma, however, does not exclude injury to the cervical spine.

An attempt should be made to explain the mech-

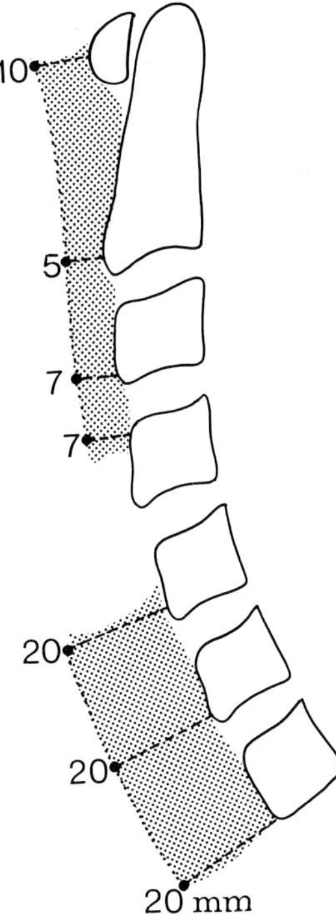

Fig. 3-5. Radiologic width of the prevertebral space: the upper limits of normal width (see Table 3-1 for the range of normal width). Measurements (in mm) are indicated along lines perpendicular to the air shadow of the pharynx and trachea. Larger measurements in injury are considered evidence of prevertebral widening due to hematoma. Note that normal retropharyngeal space is markedly smaller than retrotracheal space (the latter incorporates the esophagus).

anism of injury, which may give an idea of the localization and the extent of soft-tissue injury, reveal possible instability, and indicate therapeutic measures to be taken. A distinction can be made between compressive and distractive forces, which may act during hyperflexion or hyperextension (Figs. 3-6 and 3-7). Occasionally, compression and disruption may act together, the head moving through an arc as suggested by Whitley and Forsyth (Fig. 3-8).[33] Lateral flexion and rotational forces may play an additional role, especially in unilateral lesions. Hyperrotation is important in the production of atlantoaxial rotation luxation (Fig. 3-9).

Sometimes parallel displacement of the head with respect to the trunk, or vice versa, best explains the type of neck injury produced. This movement causes opposite motions at the upper and lower cervical spine, for example, hyperextension at the upper cervical region and hyperflexion at the lower cervical region, if the head moves forward with respect to the trunk (Fig. 3-10). It may explain the simultaneous occurrence of a hyperextension fracture of the posterior arch of the atlas and a hyperflexion luxation of the lower cervical spine, for example. Severe disruptive lesions at the craniovertebral junction have been described in parallel movement of the head in deceleration experiments.[29a] Fractures of the odontoid process are generally explained by sudden forward or backward movement of the head with respect to the trunk.[15a]

A somewhat controversial subject is the so-called whiplash injury; in our experience, plain radio-

Table 3-1. Normal Prevertebral Soft Tissue Width

LEVEL	FLEXION MM	MIDPOSITION MM	EXTENSION MM
C1	5.6 (2–11)	4.6 (1–10)	3.6 (1– 8)
C2	4.1 (2– 6)	3.2 (1– 5)	3.8 (2– 6)
C3	4.2 (3– 7)	3.4 (2– 7)	4.1 (3– 6)
C4	5.8 (4– 7)	5.1 (2– 7)	6.1 (4– 8)
C5	17.1 (11–22)	14.9 (8–20)	15.2 (10–20)
C6	16.3 (12–20)	15.1 (11–20)	13.9 (7–19)
C7	14.7 (9–20)	13.9 (9–20)	11.9 (7–21)

The midposition widths were measured on lateral radiographs of 50 noninjured patients, normal except for varying degrees of cervical spondylosis in some; their average age was 46 years, with a spread of 15 to 78 years. Widths in flexion and extension were measured in 20 patients with normal prevertebral widths in midposition; their average age was 31 years, with a spread of 16 to 67 years. The sites of measurement are indicated in Fig. 3-5. No correction has been made for radiologic magnification (about 1.3).

(Penning L: Prevertebral hematoma in cervical spine injury: Incidence and etiological significance. Neuroradio 1:557–565, 1980)

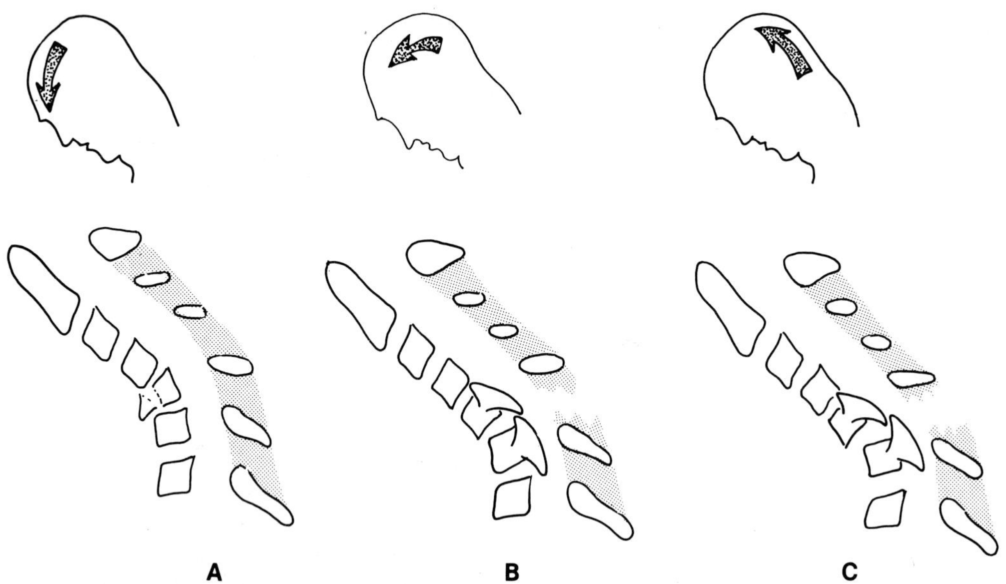

Fig. 3-6. Mechanisms in hyperflexion injury. (*A*) Hyperflexion injury with anterior compression. The arrow indicates movement of the head. Note the compression fracture of the vertebral body; the posterior ligaments have remained intact. (*B*) Hyperflexion injury with disruption of posterior ligaments (kyphotic angulation), not resulting in interlocking articular facets. This represents a transition between *A* and *C*. Sometimes additional slight compression of vertebral bodies is present. (*C*) Hyperflexion injury with disruption of posterior ligaments and interlocking of articular facets (hyperflexion luxation).

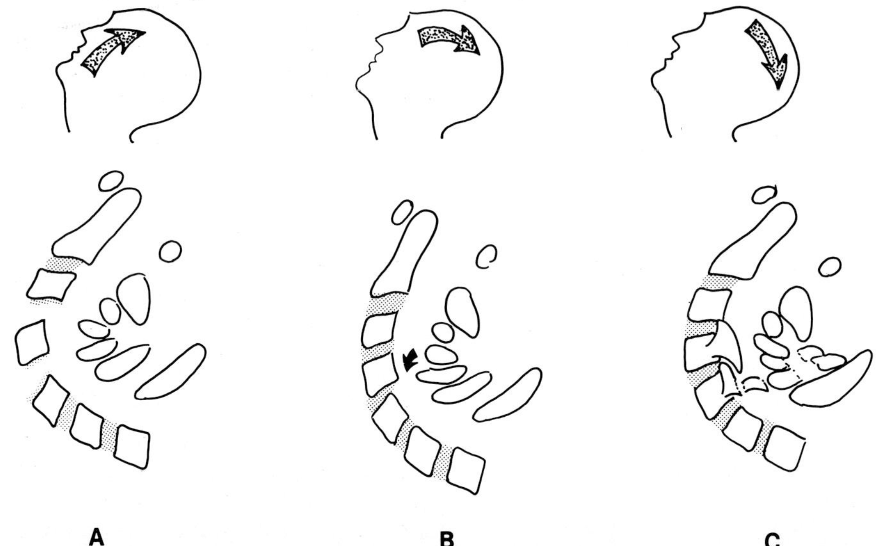

Fig. 3-7. Mechanisms in hyperextension injury. (*A*) Hyperextension injury with anterior distraction. The arrow indicates movement of the head. Note rupture of the discs and the anterior longitudinal ligament. Avulsions of anterior edges, apophyseal rims, or spondylotic spurs of vertebral bodies may be present. There are no compression fractures of posterior elements. After injury the spine may return to a normal position. (*B*) hyperextension injury with or without rupture of the anterior longitudinal ligament and no posterior compression. Preexisting retrolisthesis and stenosis of the spinal canal will result in pincers mechanism compressing the spinal cord, even in trivial injury (*small arrow*). (*C*) Hyperextension injury with posterior compression. The arrow indicates movement of the head. There are compression fractures of the posterior elements, but no disruption of anterior longitudinal ligament.

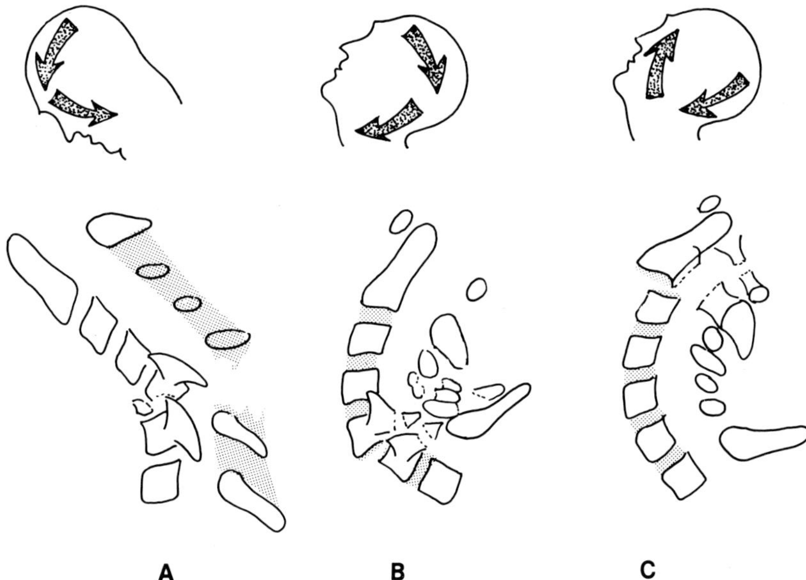

Fig. 3-8. Mechanisms of injury in movement of the head through an arc. (*A*) Hyperflexion fracture luxation with anterior compression and posterior distraction, resulting in a compression fracture of the vertebral body, and local disruption of articular joints and posterior ligaments. The head moves through an arc as indicated by the arrows. (*B*) Hyperextension fracture luxation with anterior disruption and posterior compression, resulting in local disc rupture with massive vertebral displacement, and fractures of articular and spinous processes. The head moves through an arc as indicated. (*C*) Hangman's fracture (through pedicles of axis with additional anterior displacement of axial body and fracture of posterior arch of atlas) due to hyperextension with anterior distraction and posterior compression. According to Whitley and Forsyth, the head moves through an arc as indicated by the arrows.

graphy is usually negative. The primary movement of the head in this type of injury is extension, followed by flexion.[1a] Demonstration of prevertebral hematoma is important in proving (hyperextensive) laceration of the anterior longitudinal ligament, but the sign will be missed if the first radiographs are not made within 1 or 2 weeks after the injury. Sometimes calcification of the anterior longitudinal ligament occurs weeks or months after a neck injury (Fig. 3-11).

Finally, assessment of spine instability should be undertaken. Instability in fresh injury cases may be defined as the chance of damage to the cord and roots by movements of the head and neck. Dangerous instability is especially to be expected in odontoid fractures, interlocking of articular facets, hyperflexion and hyperextenison fracture luxation, and lordotic angulation (distractive hyperextension).[15] In such cases, further radiographic examination is deferred until adequate immobilization (*e.g.*, by skull traction) is obtained. Dangerous instability is even more prevalent in elderly patients because of additional weakening of discs and ligaments by aging and spondylosis.

ADDITIONAL RADIOGRAPHY

The anteroposterior radiograph may provide some useful additional information. Normally, the spinous processes are projected in a vertical row at more or less equal distances. Local widening of the interspinous distance (more than 1½ times the interspinous distances above and below the widening) indicates the presence of interlocking of articular facets or hyperflexion sprain (Fig. 3-12).[24] The sign is especially useful if the corresponding region has remained obscured by the shoulders in the lateral projection. Scoliotic angulation is observed in unilateral interlocking or unilateral compression of articular facets (Fig. 3-13). Traumatic tilting of an articular process is well disclosed by anteroposterior radiography (Fig. 3-14). Open-

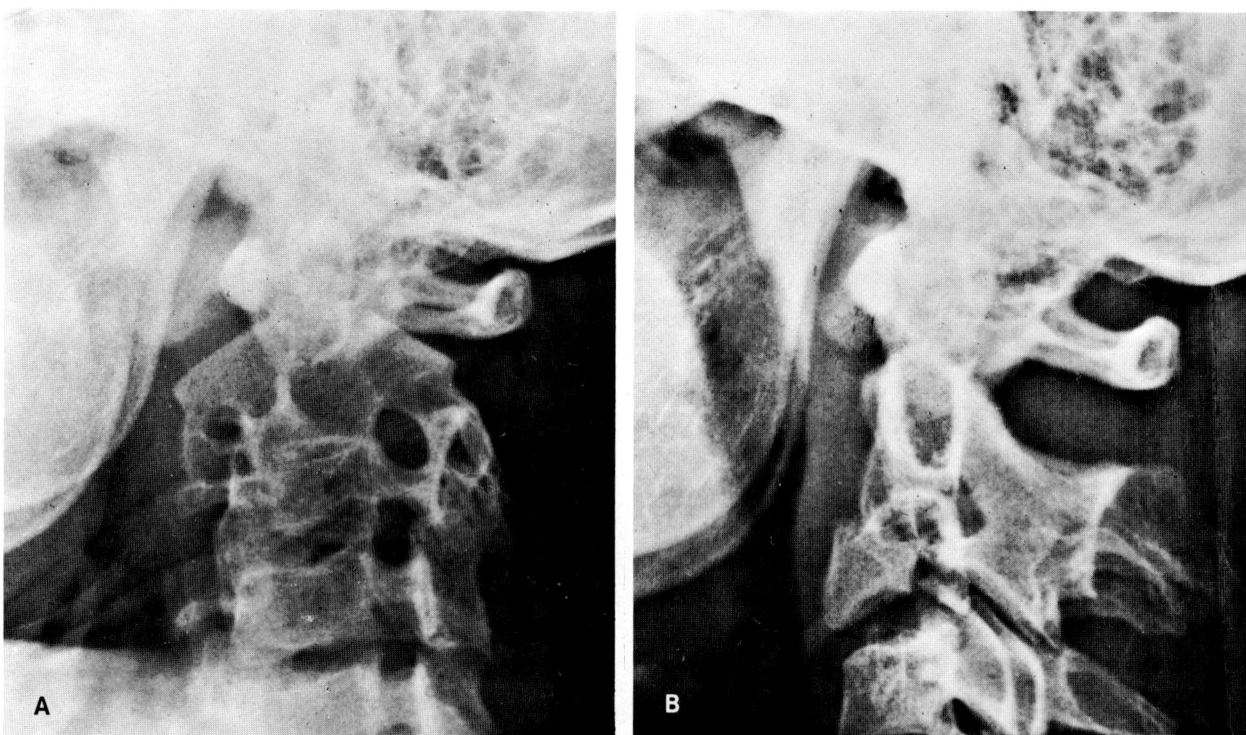

Fig. 3-9. Atlantoaxial rotation luxation in a 21-year-old woman who was in an automobile accident. Incomplete transverse lesion. The head was rotated to the right, and it was impossible to turn it to the normal position. (*A*) Radiograph with the head strictly lateral (super-imposition of both lower jaws), the atlas lateral, and the axis in an oblique projection; the estimated atlantoaxial rotation is about 50°. (*B*) After skull traction there was rapid reduction of the luxation. Note the block vertebrae C2–C3 with fracture of their anteroinferior part.

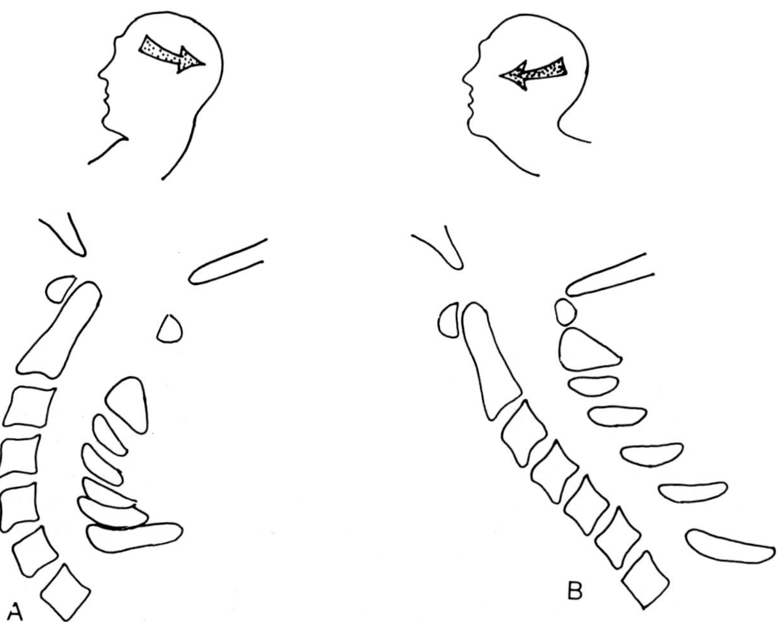

Fig. 3-10. (*A*) Mechanisms of injury in parallel movement of the head with respect to the trunk. (*B*) Forced forward movement of the head causes hyperextension of the upper cervical region and hyperflexion of the lower cervical region. Backward movement of the head causes hyperflexion of the upper cervical region and hyperextension of the lower cervical region.

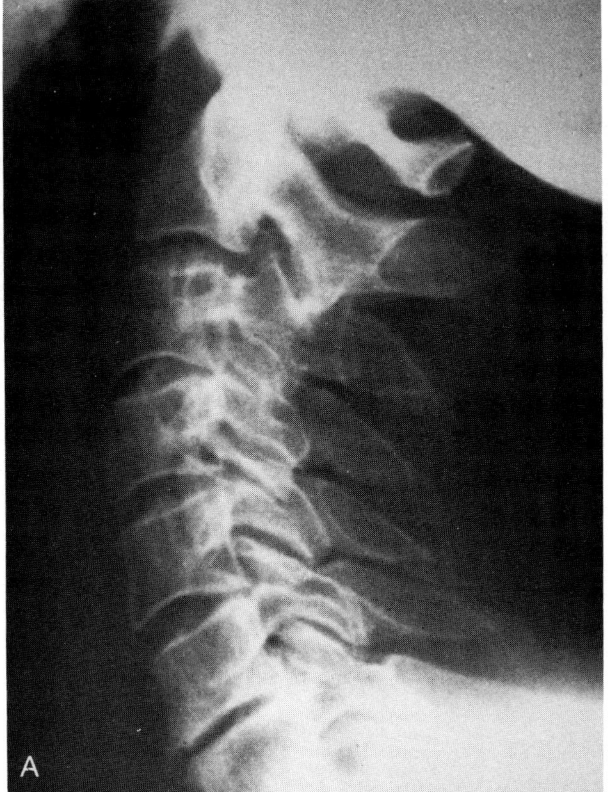

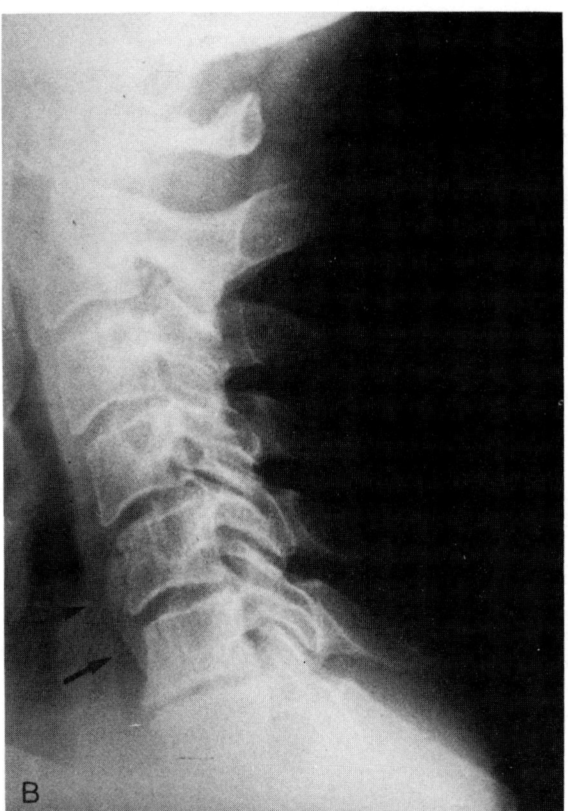

Fig. 3-11. This 50-year-old male had been involved in a head-on collision car accident, resulting in brain concussion and laceration of the top of the skull. During ambulation 10 days after the injury he began to complain of neck pain. Radiographs of the cervical spine were negative except for anterior spondylosis and degenerative disc narrowing C6–C7 (*A*). However, repeat radiography 9 months later revealed the presence of local calcification of the anterior longitudinal ligament at C5–C6. (*B*) This was considered evidence of laceration of this ligament at the time of injury (hyperextension injury most probable).

mouth views may provide additional information in fractures of the atlas, odontoid process, or lateral masses of the axis (Fig. 3-15).

As a rule, oblique views are made at an angle of about 45°, but less rotation (*e.g.*, 15° out of lateral projection) may provide a better view of the articular processes (a semi-oblique or off-lateral view, Fig. 3-16).[4] With a patient in skull traction, oblique views are best made with a transportable x-ray apparatus with a C-arch, the patient remaining supine (Fig. 3-17). In other cases, the patient is slightly rotated by raising one shoulder. Oblique views are essential in evaluation of the apophyseal joints (*e.g.*, to determine the side of the lesion in unilateral interlocking, see Fig. 3-15) or in radiographic checking of reposition of interlocking.

Tomography may be helpful in some cases, for example, in the case of odontoid fracture without displacement, and in the case of fracture of an articular process (Fig. 3-12). If tomography in lateral projection does not yield good results owing to superimposition of shoulders, the off-lateral view, as mentioned above, should be tried. The use of stereoscopic films is a matter of preference; the acquainted viewer may obtain a lot of information which, however, cannot be conveyed to the unacquainted. Computed tomography (CT) is discussed in the following section, Computed Tomography and Newer Techniques of Myelography. It may be stated here that CT is especially useful in demonstrating fractures running perpendicular to the (axial) plane of investigation. Fig.

(Text continues on p. 121)

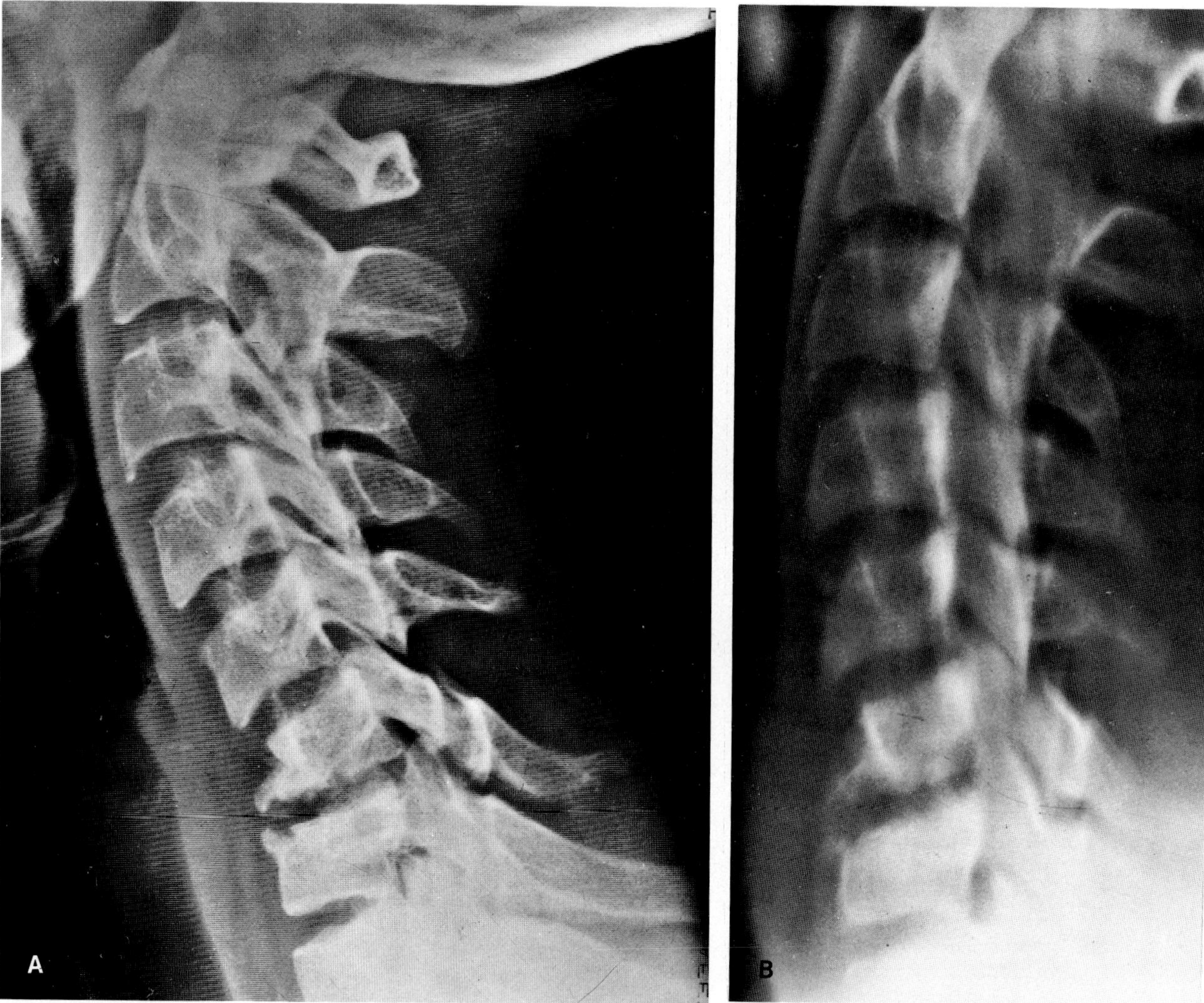

Fig. 3-12. Hyperflexion with anterior compression and posterior distraction. This 22-year-old man collided with a halting truck while riding on a moped, resulting in fracture of the arch through the articular processes, and incomplete and transient transverse lesion. (*A*) Lateral radiograph showing compression fractures of body C6 and, to a lesser degree, C7. Arch C6 is displaced downward. (*B* and *C*) Fractures of the articular processes analyzed by tomography: on the right side, note the fracture with diastasis (*B*), and on left side the fracture without diastasis (*C*). Note normal notching of articular process C7. (*D*) A–P radiograph showing diastasis of spinous processes C5 and C6, due to local rupture of interspinous ligaments. The probable mechanism of injury is hyperflexion with anterior compression and posterior distraction.

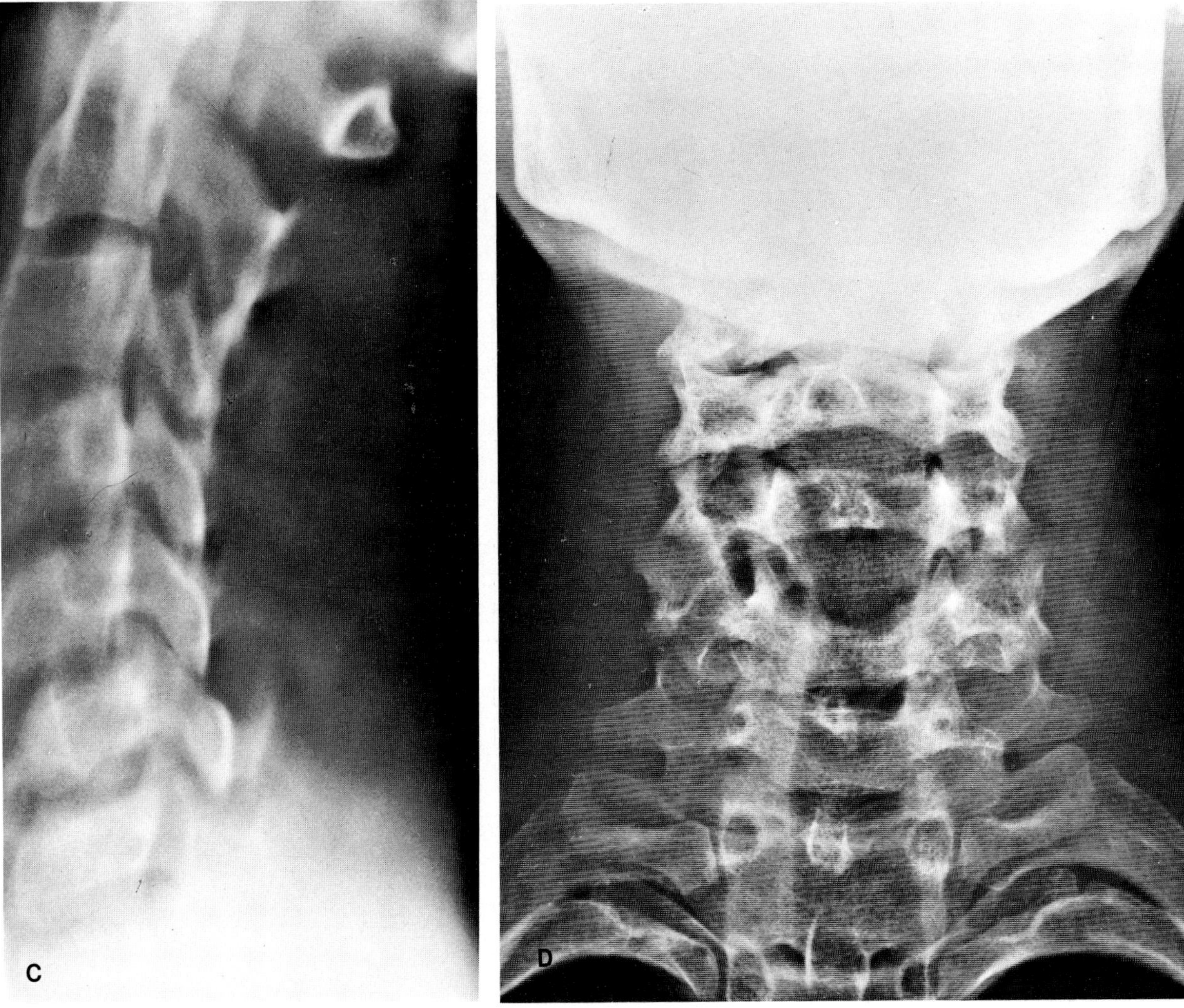

***Fig. 3-12,** cont'd*

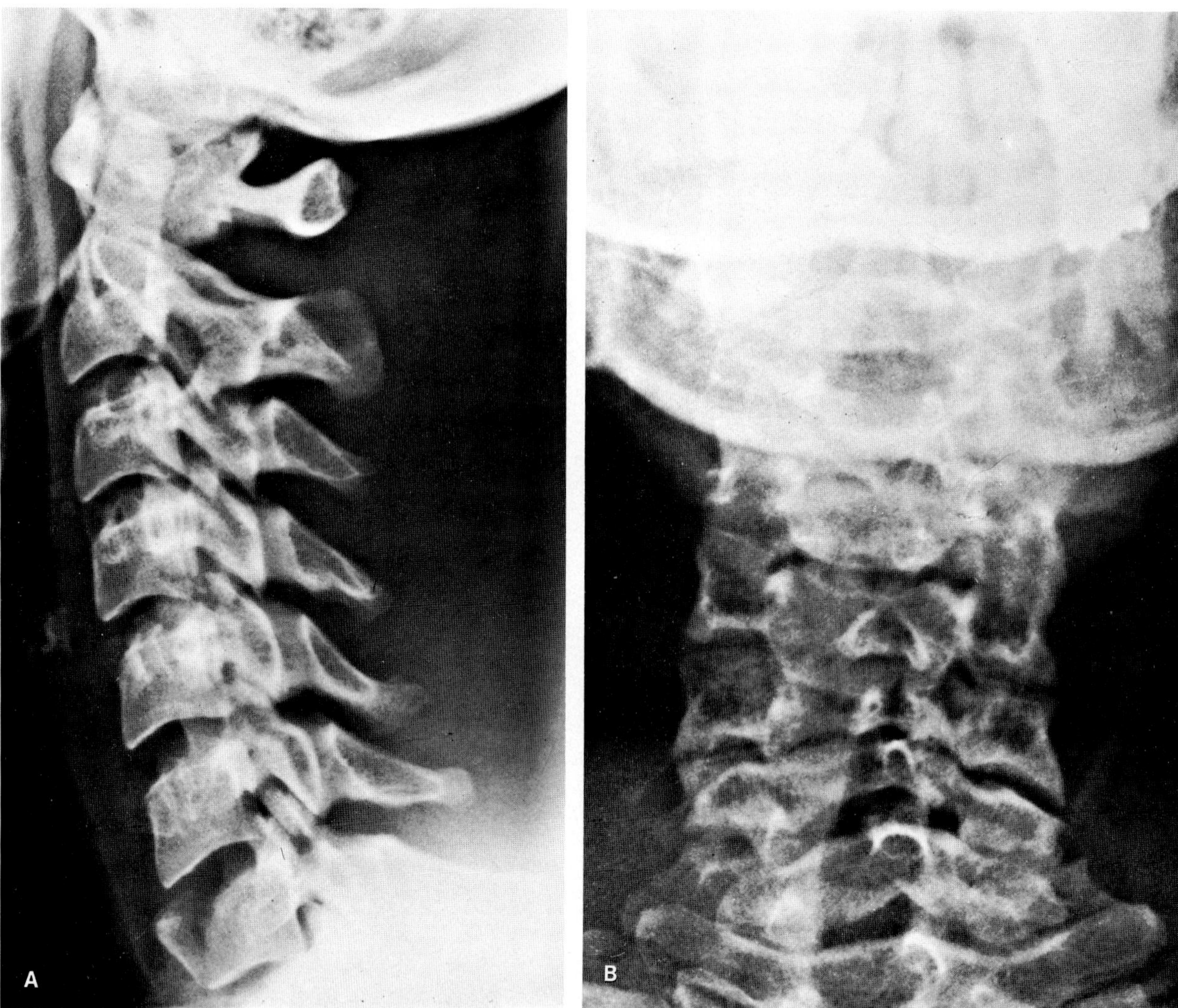

Fig. 3-13. This 24-year-old woman fell from the seventh floor of a building into a shallow pond. She had Brown-Séquard syndrome below C6. (*A*) Lateral projection: compression fracture of body C7. The situation of the articular processes and the apophyseal joints of C6–C7 is not clear. (*B*) AP projection: scoliotic angulation of the row of spinous processes at C6 or C7. (*C*) This oblique view reveals that there is interlocking of articular processes C6–C7 on the left side. (*D*) An oblique view of the right side reveals that the row of articular processes is more or less in line at C6–C7. A communitive fracture of articular process is at T3.

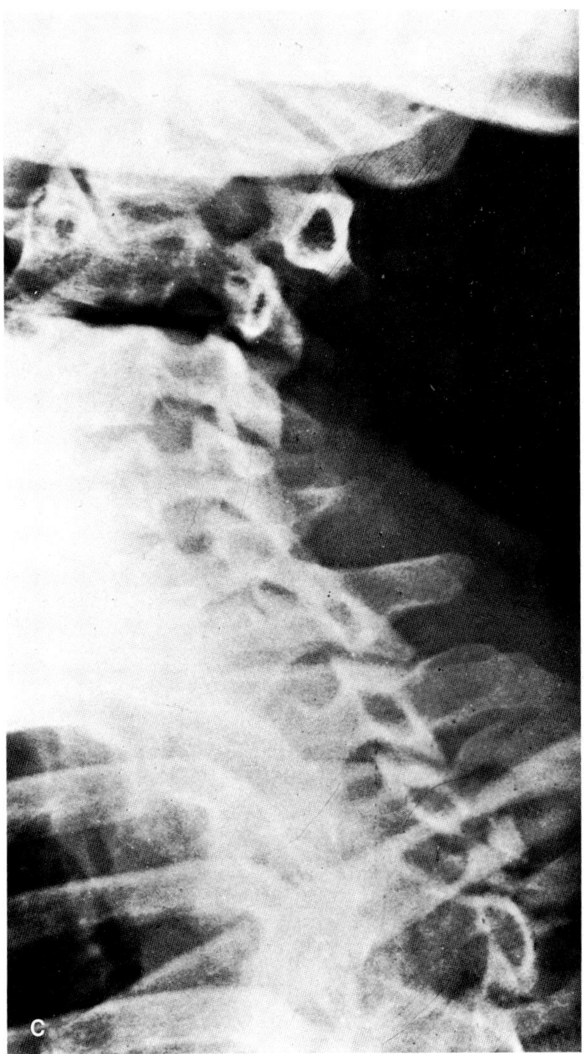

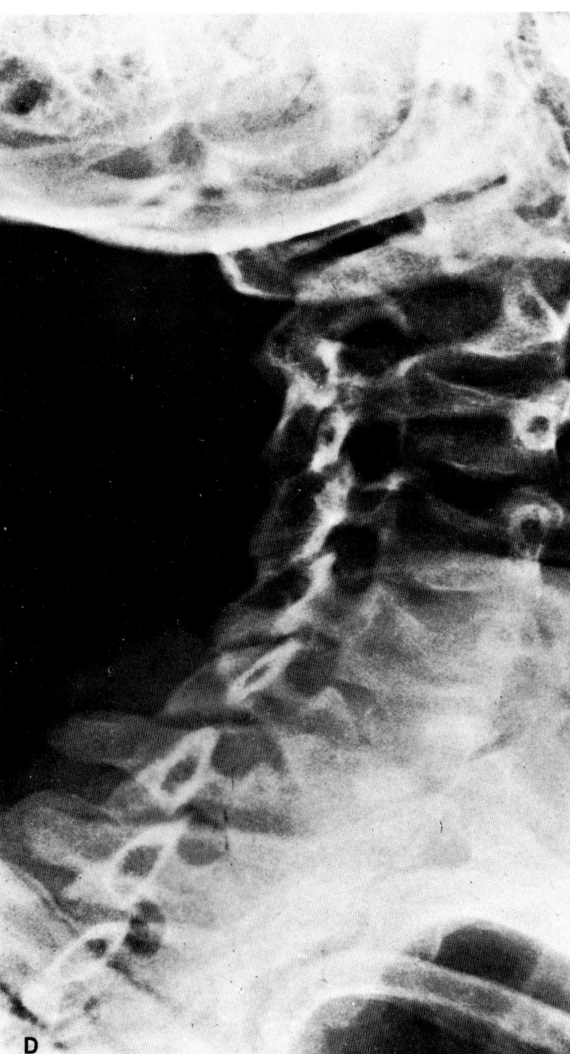

***Fig. 3-13**, cont'd*

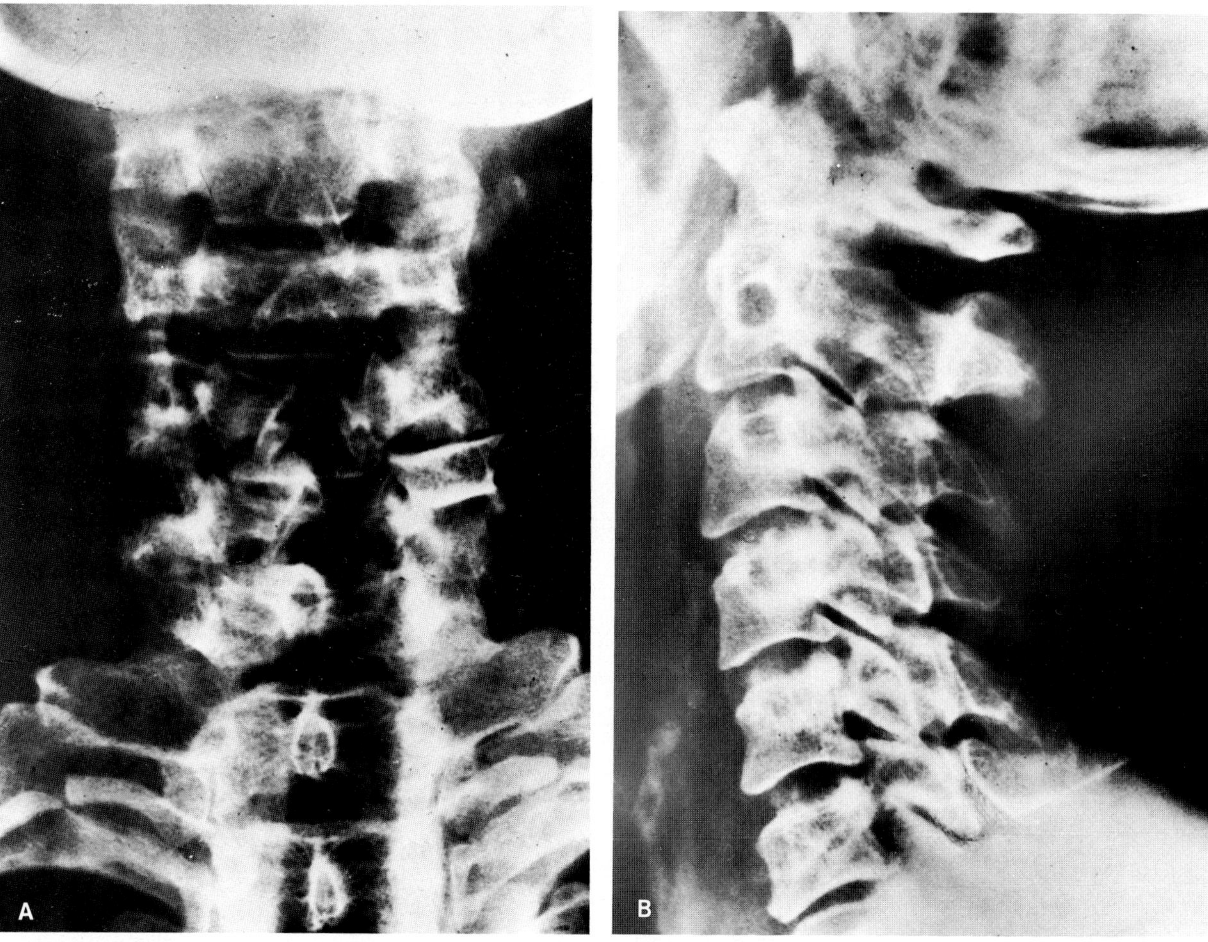

Fig. 3-14. Traumatic tilting of the articular process. (*A*) An A–P radiograph discloses end-on projection of joint surfaces of left-sided articular process of C6, due to traumatic tilting; this is not well visualized on the lateral radiograph (*B*). These are radiographs from a 37-year-old man who complained of neck pain and restricted movements after a car accident. Probable mechanism of injury: compressive hyperextension and lateral flexion to the left.

3-16 provides an example of fractures of the vertebral arch not visualized by plain radiography or conventional tomography. Although the fractures around the articular process C4 had already been made likely by the abnormalities found in plain radiography, the fractures around the articular process C3 came as a surprise.

PITFALLS IN RADIOGRAPH INTERPRETATION

Congenital or Developmental Anomalies

Anomalies in our context are important into two directions. They may cause difficulties in interpretation and lead to a false diagnosis of fracture or luxation. They also predispose to severe subjective or objective symptomatology after even minor injuries. This is due to the abnormal anatomical relationship with less "play" for the nervous system to escape traumatic occurrences.

CONGENITAL BASILAR IMPRESSION. A high position of the odontoid process above Chamberlain's line as a rule is due to congenital malformation of the base of the skull with occipitalization of the atlas or hypoplasty of the occipital bone (Fig. 3-18; for differential diagnosis, see Fig. 3-19). Conditions that predispose to neurologic damage after injury are a sharpened clivoaxial angle, atlantoaxial luxation, constriction of the foramen magnum, and the presence of tonsillar ectopy (Arnold-Chiari malformation). Trauma is the precipitating factor in the onset of chronic neurologic symptomatology in about half of the cases; as a rule it is not severe and does not always result in immediate onset of symptoms.[28]

OS ODONTOIDEUM. The clinical significance of os odontoideum is the great mobility between the ossicle and the body of the axis (Fig. 3-20). In acute trauma, it has to be differentiated from fracture of the odontoid process. This should not be difficult, because the os is rounded and does not match up with the body of the axis, as is true in an odontoid fracture.[23] In chronic cases, differentiation from pseudoarthrosis of the odontoid process may be difficult or impossible, especially because some consider os odontoideum always to be an aquired lesion.[10] Evidence in favor of os odontoideum as a congenital malformation includes shortening of the A–P diameter of the atlantal ring, overdevelopment or absence of the anterior arch of the atlas, and the presence of additional anomalies such as

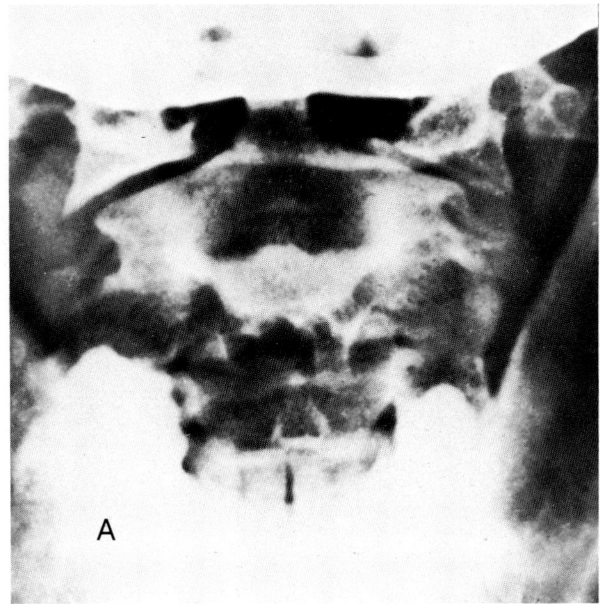

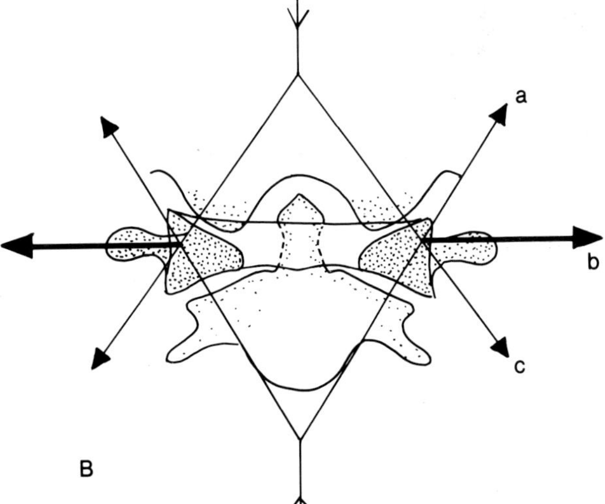

Fig. 3-15. Jefferson's type of atlantal fracture in a 36-year-old woman who complained of neck pain after a car accident. (*A*) A–P radiograph through the open mouth reveals an outward spread of both lateral atlantal masses. A diagnosis of bursting fracture of Jefferson was made. (*B*) Mechanism of injury as presented by Jefferson in 1920. (*a*) and (*c*) are the atlas, axis and vertebral column. The resultant of these forces (*b*) is more or less horizontal and "spreads" the atlas laterally.

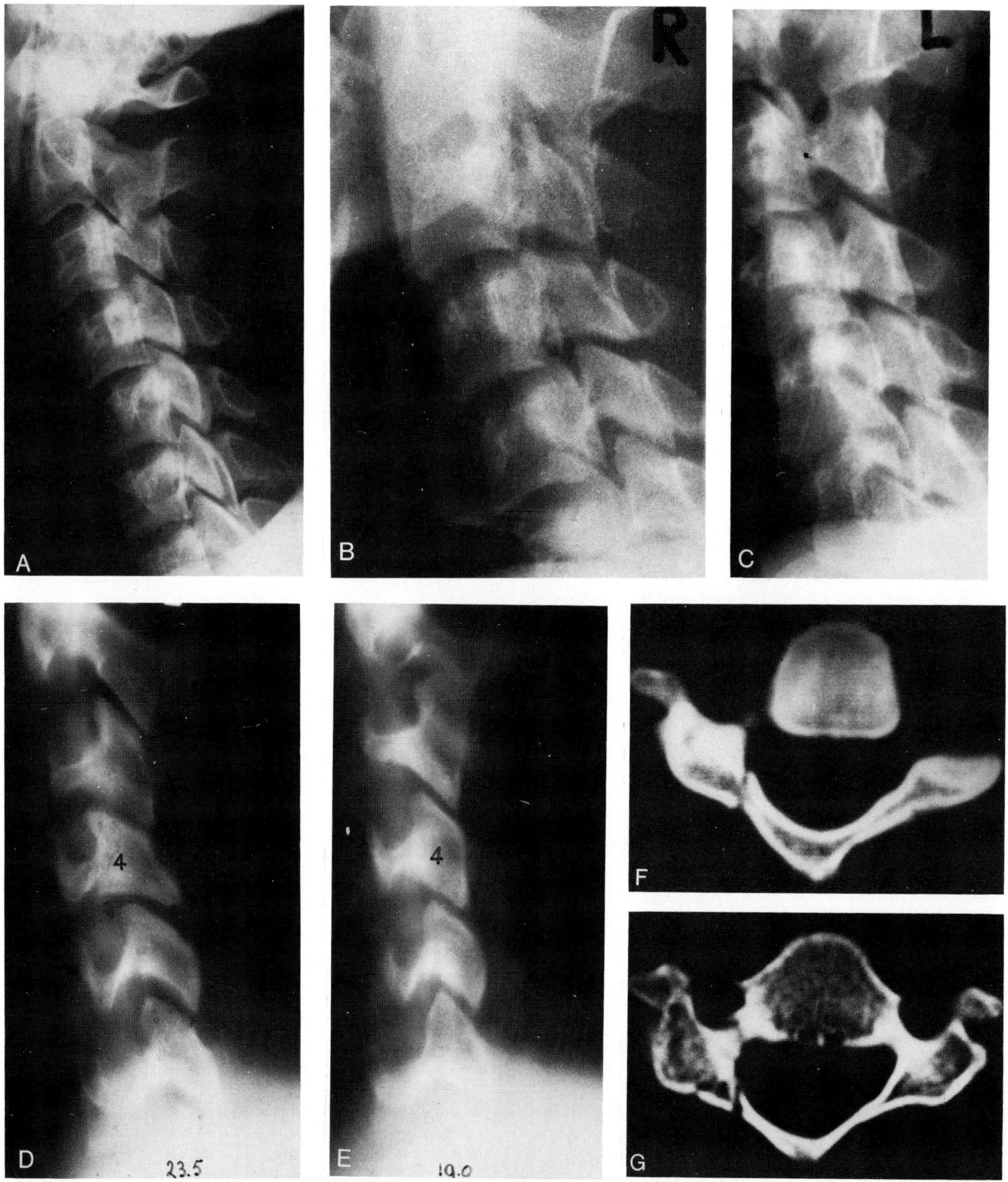
R
L
A
B
C
4
4
D
E
F
G
23.5
19.0

Fig. 3-16. Fracture of the right-sided articular process C4 (*A*). The lateral projection of the cervical spine of this 18-year-old man, who was thrown out of the car during a skid, is puzzling. Anterolisthesis C3–C4 draws attention to the articular processes, which are visualized by an off-lateral projection on the right (*B*) and left (*C*). The right-sided articular process C4 is tilted, the inferior articular surface having adopted a more horizontal course. The deformation of the articular process is also visible on a lateral tomogram (right side, *D*; left side, *E*). Additional CT investigation revealed the presence of fractures of the arch around the tilted articular process C4 (*F*). Surprisingly similar fractures were present around the right-sided articular process of C3 (*G*). Most probable mechanism of injury is lateral hyperflexion to the right.

the Klippel-Feil anomaly and partial fusions of the bodies of C1, C2, or C3.

There are numerous other anomalies in the occipitocervical region, most of which have no clinical significance.[31] Some of them may be mistaken for fractures, for example, partial absence of the arch of the atlas (Fig. 3-21).

SPONDYLOLISTHESIS OF THE CERVICAL SPINE. Mostly occurs at C6, but occasionally has been described at C2 and C4.[6] Spondylolisthesis of the axis should be differentiated from hangman's fracture (Fig. 3-22).[12] Criteria for differentiation are additional congenital anomalies, such as fusion of parts of C2 and C3, and difficulties in matching the parts of the ostensible fracture. As in odontoideum, the congenital origin of the defect is open for discussion; it is possible that, owing to the congenital fusion of the arches, abnormal stress on the pedicles of the axis has resulted in fracture.

An example of spondylolisthesis of C6 is given in Figure 3-23. Other defects of pedicles or arches do occur and should not be mistaken for fractures.[21]

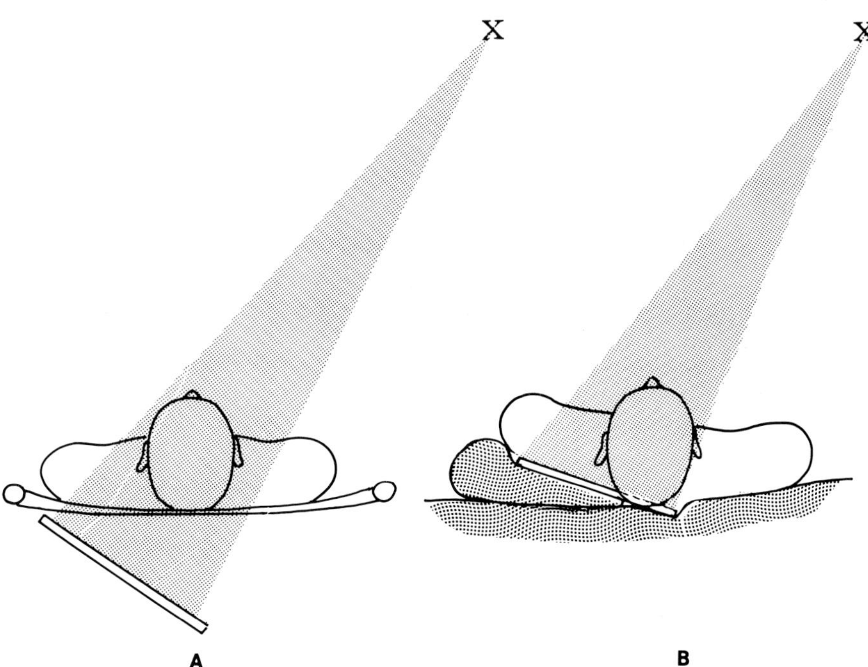

Fig. 3-17. Positioning for oblique views of the cervical spine in acute-injury patients. (*A*) Cassette (kept in place by appropriate holder) below the stretcher or frame. (*B*) Cassette underneath the neck and raised shoulder of a patient lying on a mattress.

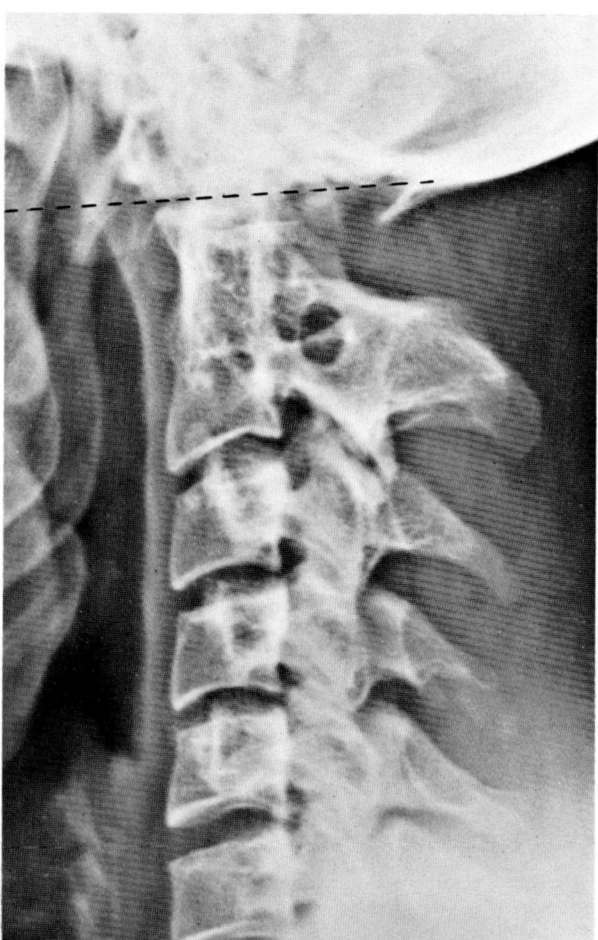

Fig. 3-18. Congenital basilar impression in a 31-year-old man who complained of unsteadiness of gait and suboccipital pain after a moped injury that resulted in brain contusion and fracture of the left clavicle. Neurologic investigation revealed nystagmus, ataxia, dysarthria, dysmetria, and some loss of appreciation of vibration in the legs. There were no pyramidal signs. Lateral radiograph of the cervical spine showed congenital atlantooccipital fusion, anterior atlantoaxial luxation (anterior atlantodental interspace 10 mm), rise of odontoid process 11 mm above Chamberlain's line, and block vertebrae C2–C3.

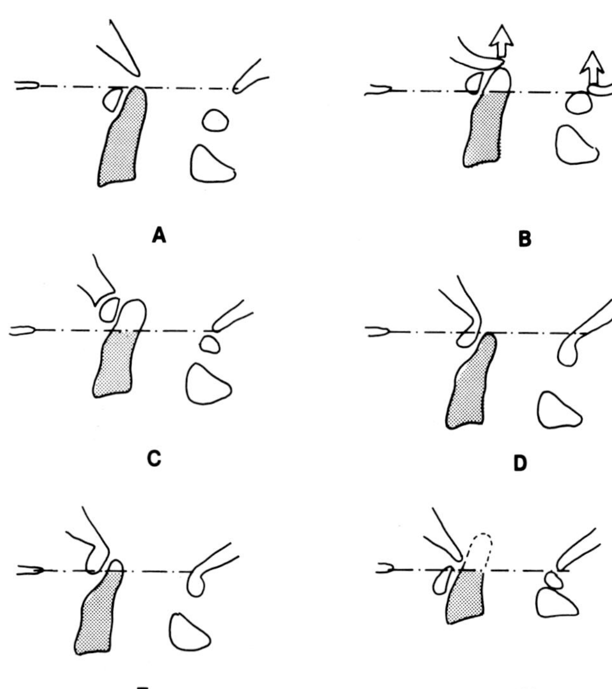

Fig. 3-19. Differential diagnosis of high position of the odontoid process above Chamberlain's line. (*A*) The tip of the odontoid process should rise not more than 5 mm above Chamberlain's line (between the dorsal rim of the foramen magnum and thc hard palate). The average height of the tip is 1 mm below Chamberlain's line. (*B*) Basilar impression is due to weakening of the skull base due to bone diseases (e.g., morbus Paget, osteomalacia). (*C*) Congenital basilar impression due to hypoplasia of the basiocciput. (*D*) Congenital atlantooccipital fusion without hypoplasia of the basiocciput, which need not result in abnormal position of the odontoid process. Anterior atlantoaxial luxation may be present. (*E*) Congenital basilar impression with hypoplasia of the occiput and atlantooccipital fusion. Hypoplasia of the odontoid process and anterior atlantoaxial luxation may be present. (*F*) Basilar erosion with destruction of the atlantooccipital and atlantoaxial joints, resulting in ascent of the odontoid process through the atlantal ring into the posterior fossa.

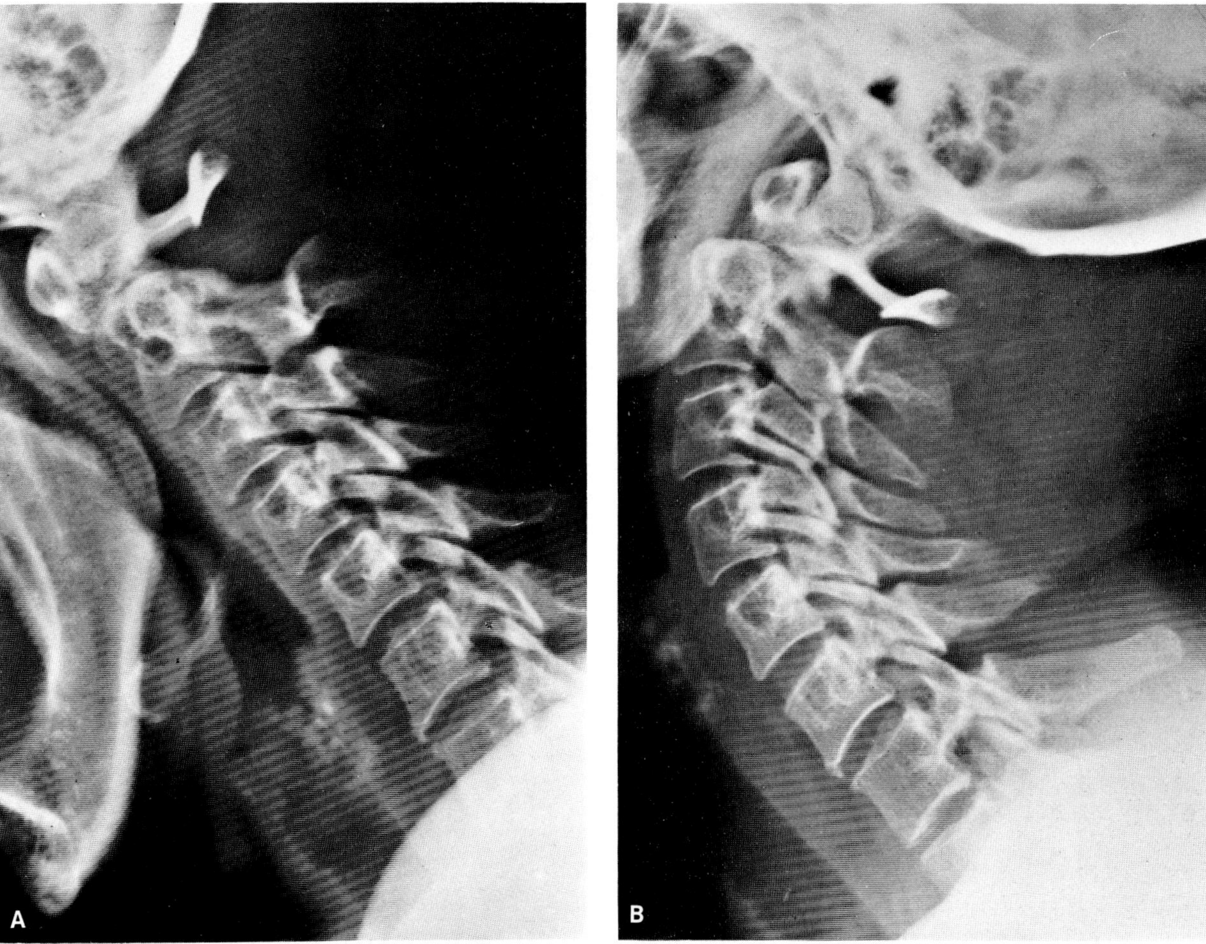

Fig. 3-20. Os odontoideum of a 41-year-old woman who experienced radiating pains and loss of strength in both arms for 1 year. Apart from a fall from a bicycle, there was no history of injury. Lateral radiographs in flexion (*A*) and extension (*B*) show marked atlantoaxial instability due to a mobile os odontoideum. Its congenital origin is suggested by a hypoplastic and stenotic atlantal arch. The diameter of the bony spinal canal between the os and the posterior arch of atlas was 11 mm (normal: 17–30 mm). In extension, the posterior arch of the atlas and the spinous process of C2 are aligned; in flexion, the os and the axial body are aligned, the spinal canal being narrowed between the axial body and the atlantal arch.

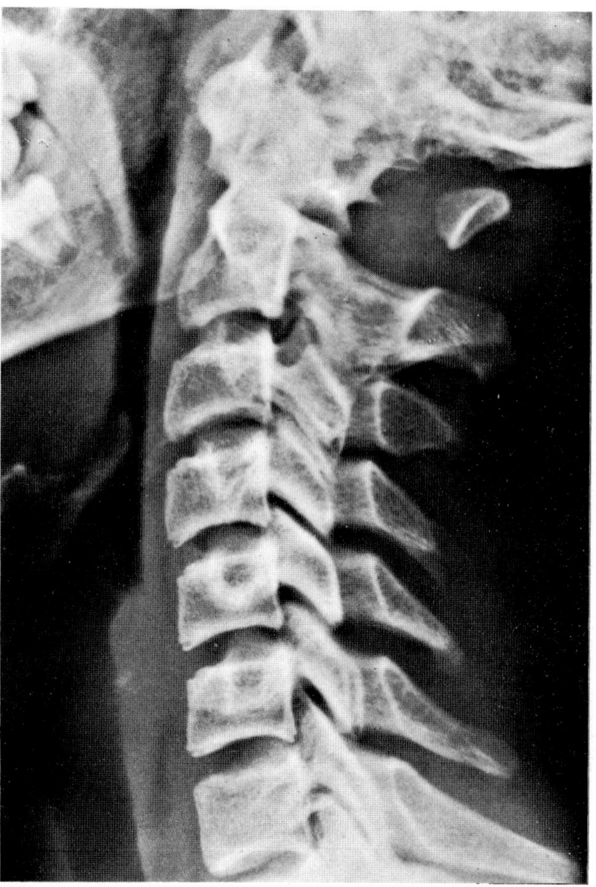

Fig. 3-21. Bilateral partial aplasia of the bony atlantal ring in a 17-year-old girl, accidentally discovered during radiography of her jaws for dental correction. Note the epiphyseal rims at the anteroinferior and anterosuperior edges of the vertebral bodies, which appear in the second decade of life and subsequently fuse with vertebral bodies (see also Fig. 3-30).

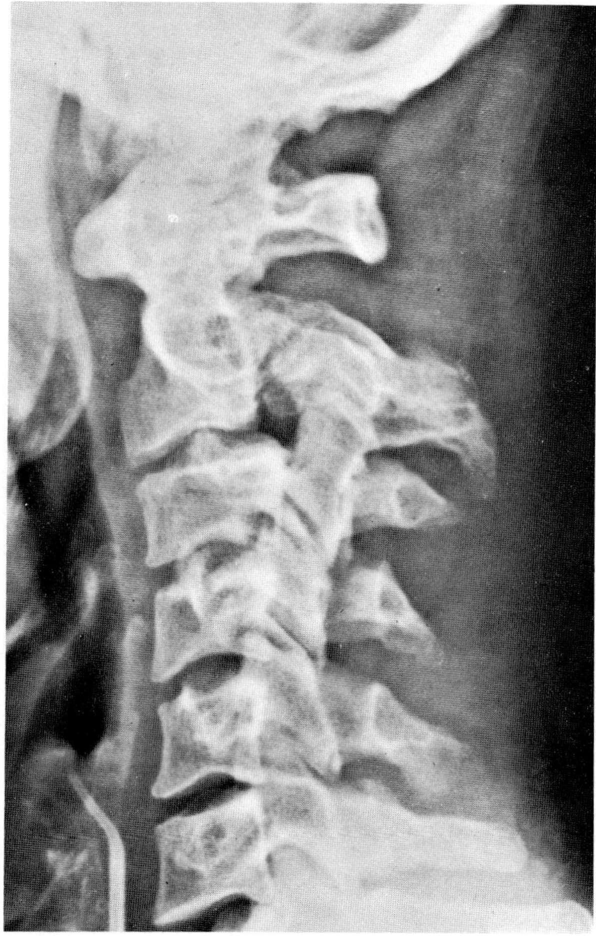

Fig. 3-22. Lateral radiograph of a 41-year-old man with a history of radiating pains in the left arm shows spondylolisthesis of C2 with linear defect (lysis) in the arch of axis. Apophyseal joints C2–C3 are placed far posteriorly. The posterior arch of the axis is open (no cortical delineation of the anterior margin of spinous process C2). Note platyspondylia of C3; the articular pillars of the vertebrae are unusually high. All deformities described are considered to be of developmental origin.

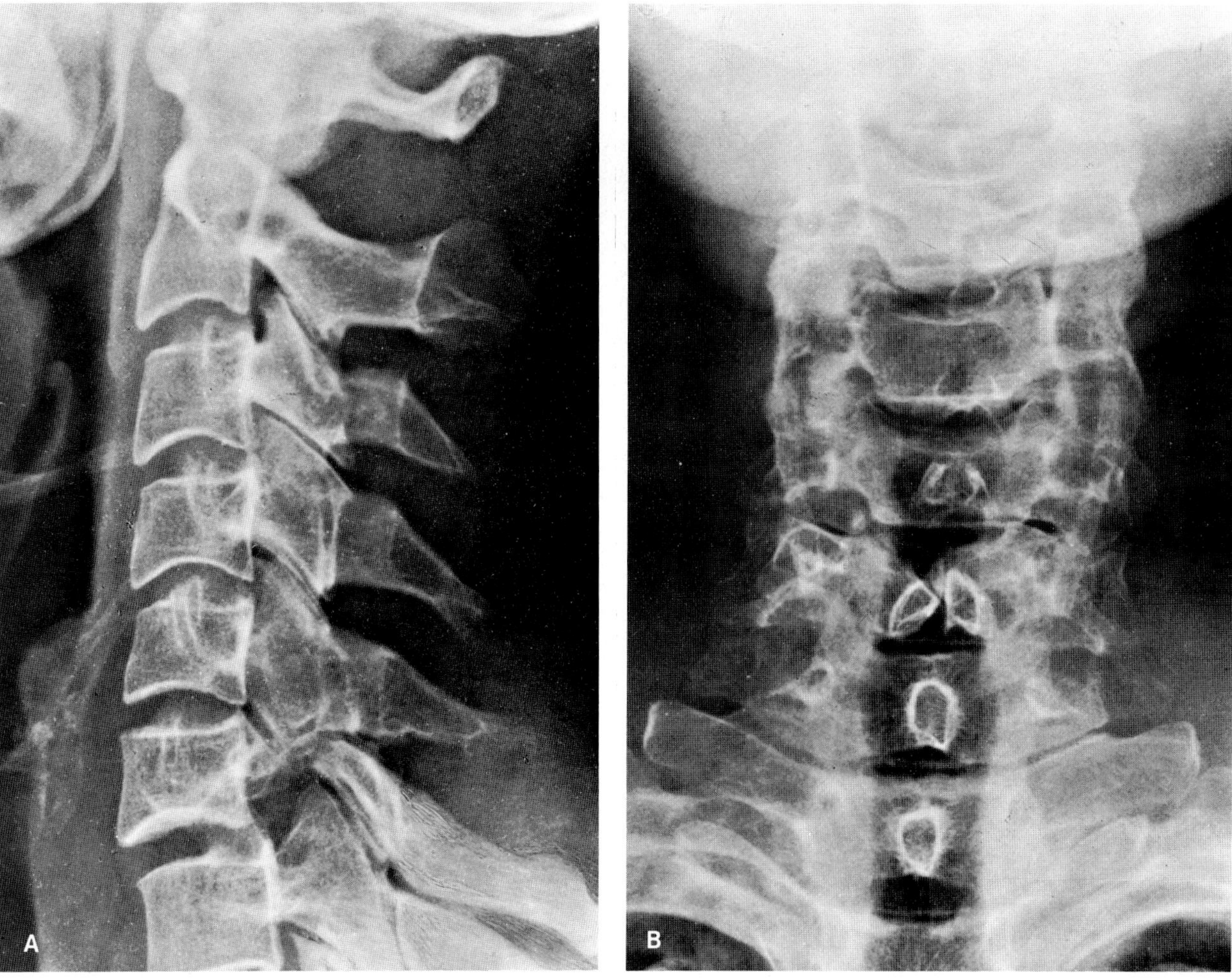

Fig. 3-23. Spondylolisthesis of C6 in a 40-year-old man without a history of injury and with vague complaints of dysphagia. (*A*) Lateral radiograph shows spondylolisthesis of C6 with separation of articular pillars at the interarticular portion. An additional developmental anomaly is bifid spinous process, best seen on A–P radiograph (*B*).

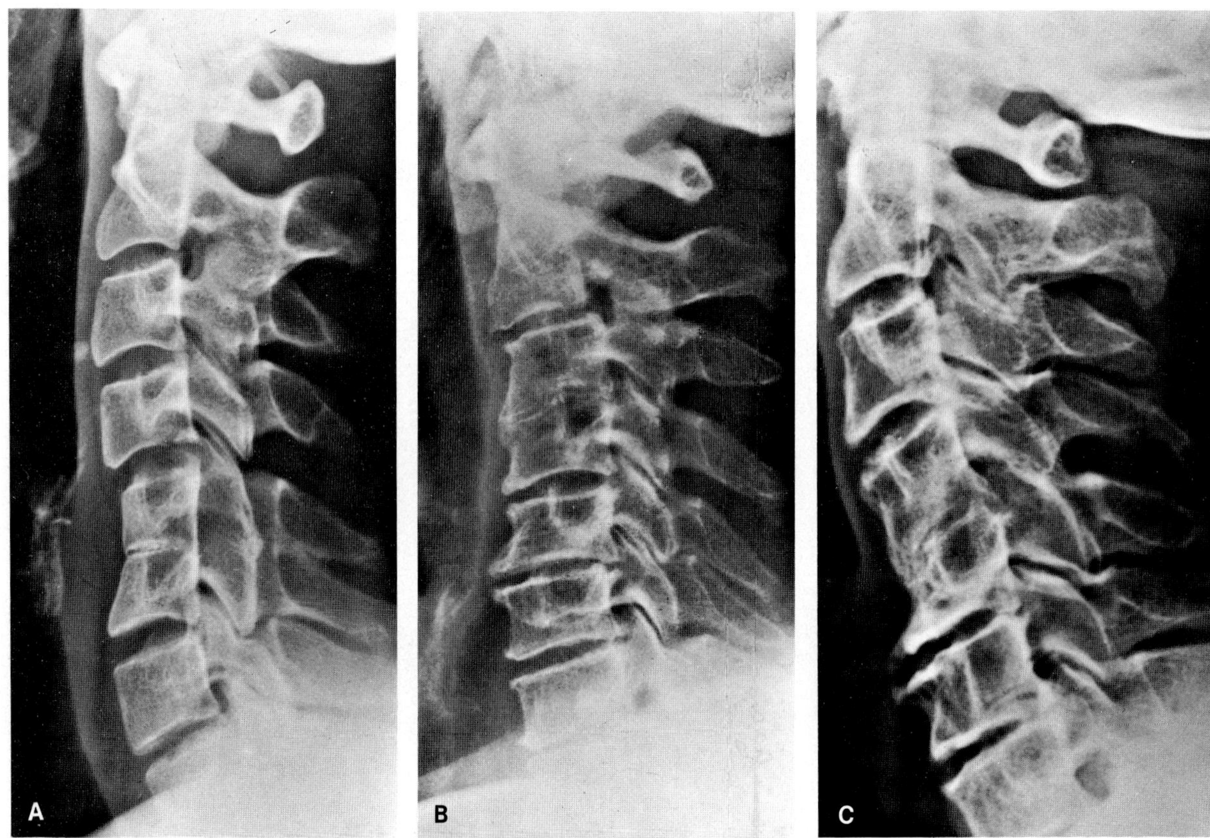

Fig. 3-24. Block vertebrae. (*A*) Congenital block vertebrae of C5–C6. The disc space C5–C6 is still visible in vestigial form, with local waisting of vertebral block. Note the fusion of articular pillars C5 and C6, with disappearance of joint space, and fusion of the posterior arches. Poor visibility of joint space C2–C3 is a normal fiding owing to inclination of joint surfaces. (*B*) Spondylotic block vertebrae of C3–C4, broadening at disc level. Note the normal apophyseal joints and arches. There is marked spondylarthrosis of other parts of the cervical spine. (*C*) Traumatic block vertebrae of C4–C5, 4 years after hyperflexion injury. Fusion occurred spontaneously. There is a kyphotic angulation of 15°.

CONGENITAL BLOCK VERTEBRAE. These, as do other anomalies, predispose to neurologic implications after even minor injuries. Block vertebrae C2–C3 may occur in association with congenital basilar impression (Fig. 3-18). Block vertebrae of congenital origin are characterized by waisting at the level of the fusion, the disc often remaining visible in vestigial form (Fig. 3-24). Such waisting is absent in secondary fusion due to spondylarthrosis, rheumatoid arthritis, or ankylosing spondylitis (Fig. 3-25). In congenital block vertebrae, part of arches or processes are also fused. Fusion secondary to trauma as a rule is associated with a marked degree of kyphotic angulation (Fig. 3-24*C*). Fusion may also be the result of anterior spondylodesis.[2]

Superimposition of Normal Structures

Mach bands are optical phenomena in which dark and light lines appear at the borders of structures of different radiodensity in radiographs.[7] They may be especially disturbing at the level of the odontoid or uncinate processes, producing the illusion of fractures (Figs. 3-26 and 3-27). In contrast to fractures, Mach bands do continue and may be followed outside the bony structure allegedly fractured.

Superimposition of teeth or air in the vocal fis-

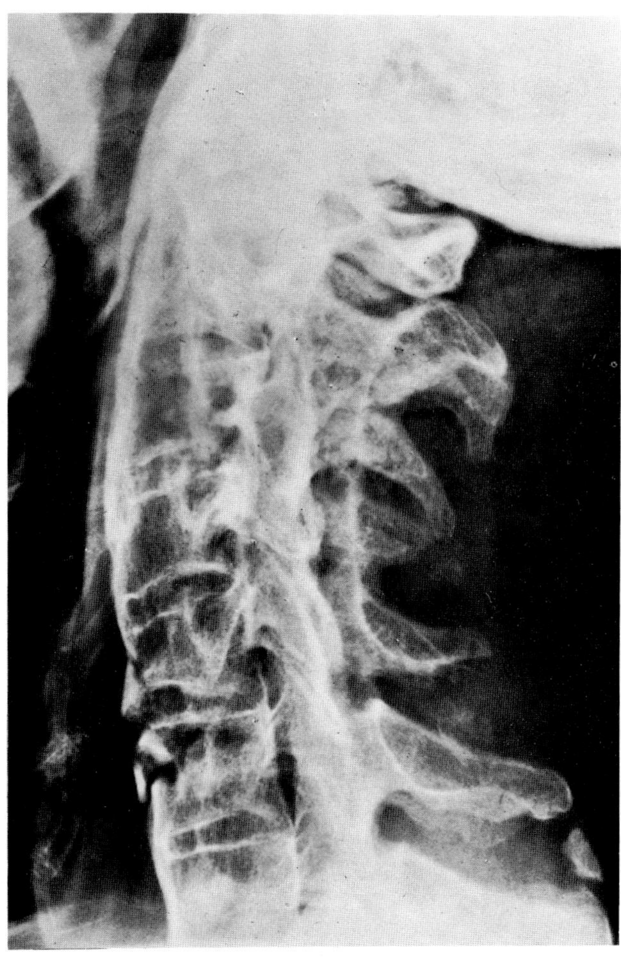

Fig. 3-25. Fracture in ankylosing spondylitis. This 66-year-old man, known to have ankylosing spondylitis for many years, fell from a bicycle. He experienced neck pain owing to a bilateral nerve root lesion of C6. Lateral radiograph shows a fracture of the calcified anterior longitudinal ligament at C5–C6 and wedge compression of body C5. There is partial ossification of the supraspinous ligament at C6–C7.

sure may suggest vertical fractures of the odontoid process or vertebral bodies (Fig. 3-28).

Degeneration of the uncovertebral joints causes a distinct horizontal lucent line over the vertebral body (Fig. 3-29).

Variations of Normal Anatomy

VERTEBRAL BODIES. A slight wedge shape may be incidentally found without a history of injury. Flattening of vertebral bodies is encountered in spondylarthrosis (Fig. 3-29). The end-on projection of uncovertebral joints or apophyseal joints on vertebral bodies in the lateral view should not be mistaken for fractures (Fig. 3-29). Ossifying epiphyseal end-plates of vertebral bodies are a normal finding during the second decade of life; they may be avulsed in hyperextension injury (Figs. 3-21 and 3-30).[1,19] Ossifications within the anterior longitudinal ligament may suggest broken spondylotic spurs (Fig. 3-31).

ARTICULAR PROCESSES AND APOPHYSEAL JOINTS. In the midcervical region, the articular processes as a rule do have a rhomboid form in lateral projection. However, the frequency of variation from the rhomboid form is rather high, especially at C6 and C7. The articular process of C7 often is notched on its back and elongated so that the posterior edge of the inferior process lies backward in relation to the posterior edges of the other cervical articular processes (Fig. 3-32).[18]

Arthrotic changes of the apophyseal joint may flatten and elongate the articular processes, giving a false impression of compression.

A high incidence of apparent compression is found if special projections are used, for example,

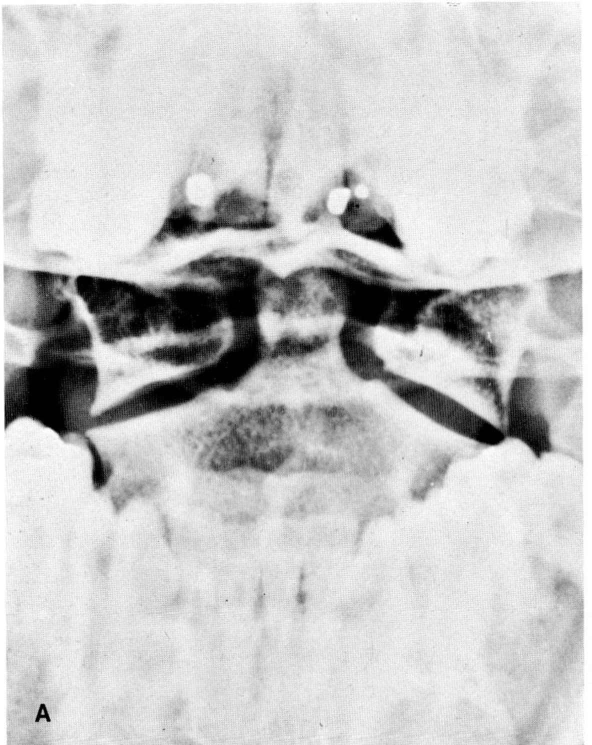

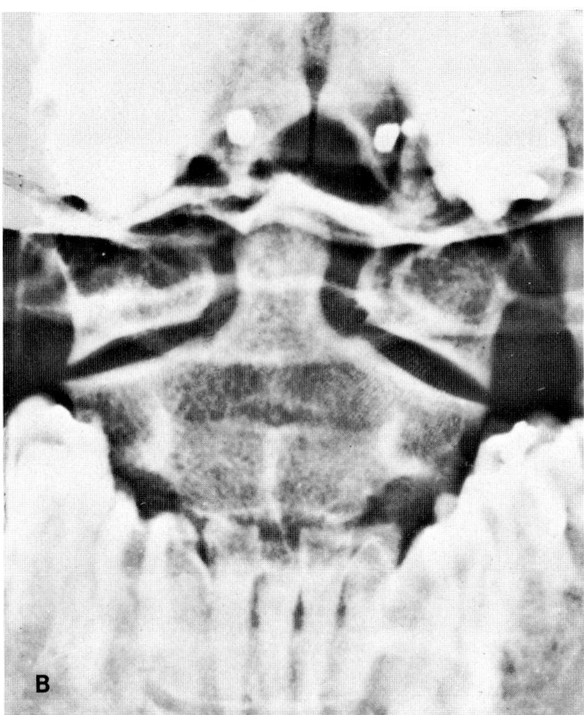

Fig. 3-26. Pseudofracture of the odontoid process. (*A*) Open-mouth view suggests a fracture of the odontoid process. (*B*) Repeat exposure at a slightly different angle shows a normal odontoid process. Pseudofracture must be due to a Mach line, probably produced by the posterior arch of atlas.

anteroposterior views with a 20° to 30° caudal direction of the central ray. In patients without a history of trauma, unilateral "compression" was noted in nearly half the cases.[30] To reduce the chance of a false-positive diagnosis in doubtful cases, tomography is preferred to these special projections.

In the lateral projection, all apophyseal joint spaces are clearly visible, except those between C2 and C3; this is due to slight inclination of the joints in lateral direction (Fig. 3-23).

Normal and Abnormal Relationships Between Vertebrae

VARIATIONS IN POSTURE, ANGULATIONS, AND TORTICOLLIS. Normally, in midposition with the patient sitting or standing, the cervical spine shows a slight lordotic curvature. However, there are many variations, including a straight spine and even a slightly kyphotic curvature.[1] Curvatures are partly influenced by posture as a whole. In a lying position, and especially in comatose patients, the spine may sag and assume a kyphotic position.

In kyphotic angulation, the cervical spine as a whole is in midposition with one segment more or less flexed. Slight kyphotic angulation is often encountered in spondylarthrosis, notably at the C5–C6 level. Marked kyphotic angulation after trauma is due to local disruption of the posterior ligaments as the result of hyperflexion injury, with or without interlocking of articular facets (see Fig. 3-33*B*).[20] Compression fractures of vertebral bodies may also produce local kyphosis, which has a tendency to progress. Scoliotic angulation is found in unilateral compression of an articular process or in unilateral interlocking at that level.

In torticollis, the spine may show a variable degree of kyphosis, scoliosis, or rotation. This causes puzzling radiographic images that may lead to misinterpretation. Projections should therefore be standardized as much as possible, for example, by using strictly lateral or A–P view of the trunk on

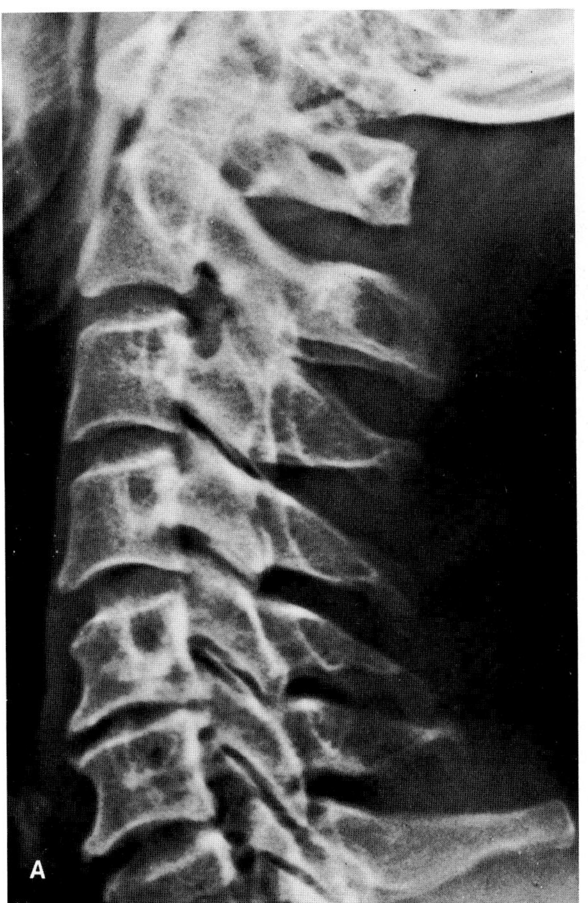

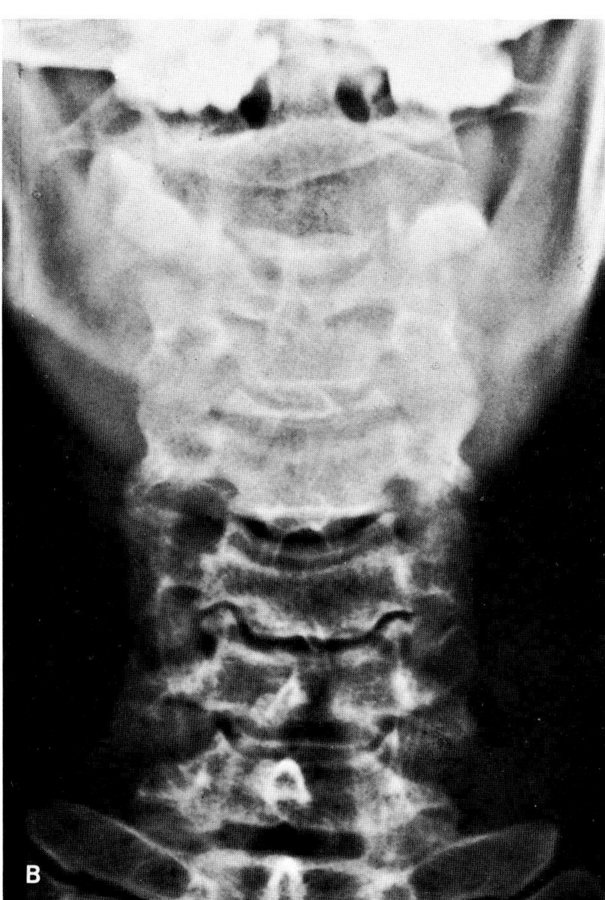

Fig. 3-27. Cervical spondylosis, retrolisthesis of C5–C6, and pseudofractures of uncinate processes of C6. This 41-year-old woman with neck pain had no history of injury but showed marked spondylarthrotic changes at C5–C7. (*A*) Lateral radiograph shows retrolisthesis of C5–C6 due to disc narrowing. (*B*) A–P radiograph shows marked uncarthrosis of C5–C6 producing a horizontal dark line on the body of C5 (*A*), which must not be taken for a fracture. Pseudofractures of uncinate processes of C6 (*B*) are due to the Mach effect caused by the inferior edge of the arch of C5. The apophyseal joint spaces of C2–C3 are poorly visible on the lateral radiograph (*A*) owing to normal inclination of the joint surfaces.

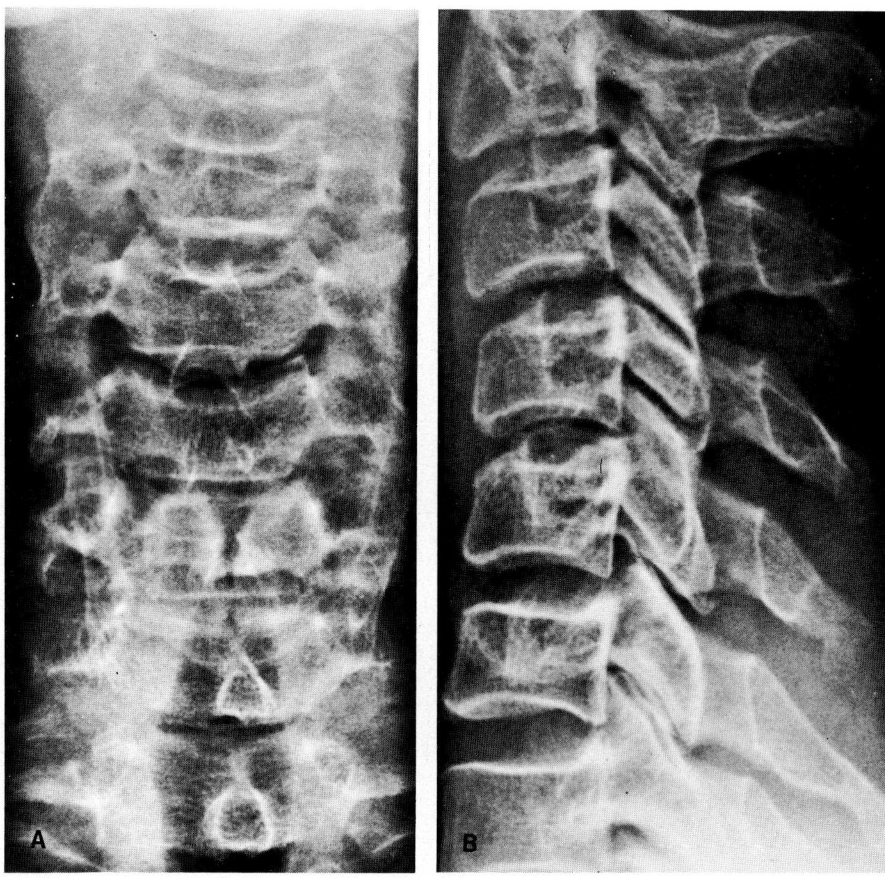

Fig. 3-28. Pseudofracture of C6. (*A*) A–P radiograph shows vertical lucency of body C6, which, although it suggests a fracture, is produced by vocal fissure. (*B*) lateral radiograph shows a normal body C6.

the head. Radiography should be repeated after the torticollis has subsided. Torticollis is most often observed in atlantoaxial lesions; it does not appear in fractures and luxations of the lower cervical spine. In young adults, torticollis may follow trivial injury, as a rule after a free interval of several hours. It is produced by reflex spasm of paraspinal muscles. Rotation is usually marked; attempts at correction meet with painful resistance. It is important to rule out anterior atlantoaxial luxation (widened anterior atlantodental interspace) due to infection of the upper respiratory tract. In this so-called spontaneous atlantoxial luxation, a variable degree of atlantoaxial rotation may be present (see Fig. 3-36*D*).[11,32]

LUXATION, SUBLUXATION, AND PSEUDOSUBLUXATION. A luxation may be defined as the complete and lasting disruption of the articular facets of a synovial joint. In the lower cervical spine (C2–C7) this applies to the apophyseal joints only, not to the intervertebral discs. The latter may slip, causing anterolisthesis or retrolisthesis of vertebral bodies (see following section, "Retrolisthesis and Anterolisthesis"). A luxation is present in the interlocking of articular facets and in marked diastasis (as in hyperflexion fracture luxation, see Figs. 3-8*A* and 3-33).

The designation *subluxation* should be avoided because it is often abused to express uncertainty about presence of pathology, and may wrongly suggest it. For example, the step formation along the posterior borders of the vertebral bodies in flexed or kyphotic spines in children, especially at the C2–C3 and C3–C4 levels, has repeatedly led to a diagnosis of subluxation (Fig. 3-34). It is now

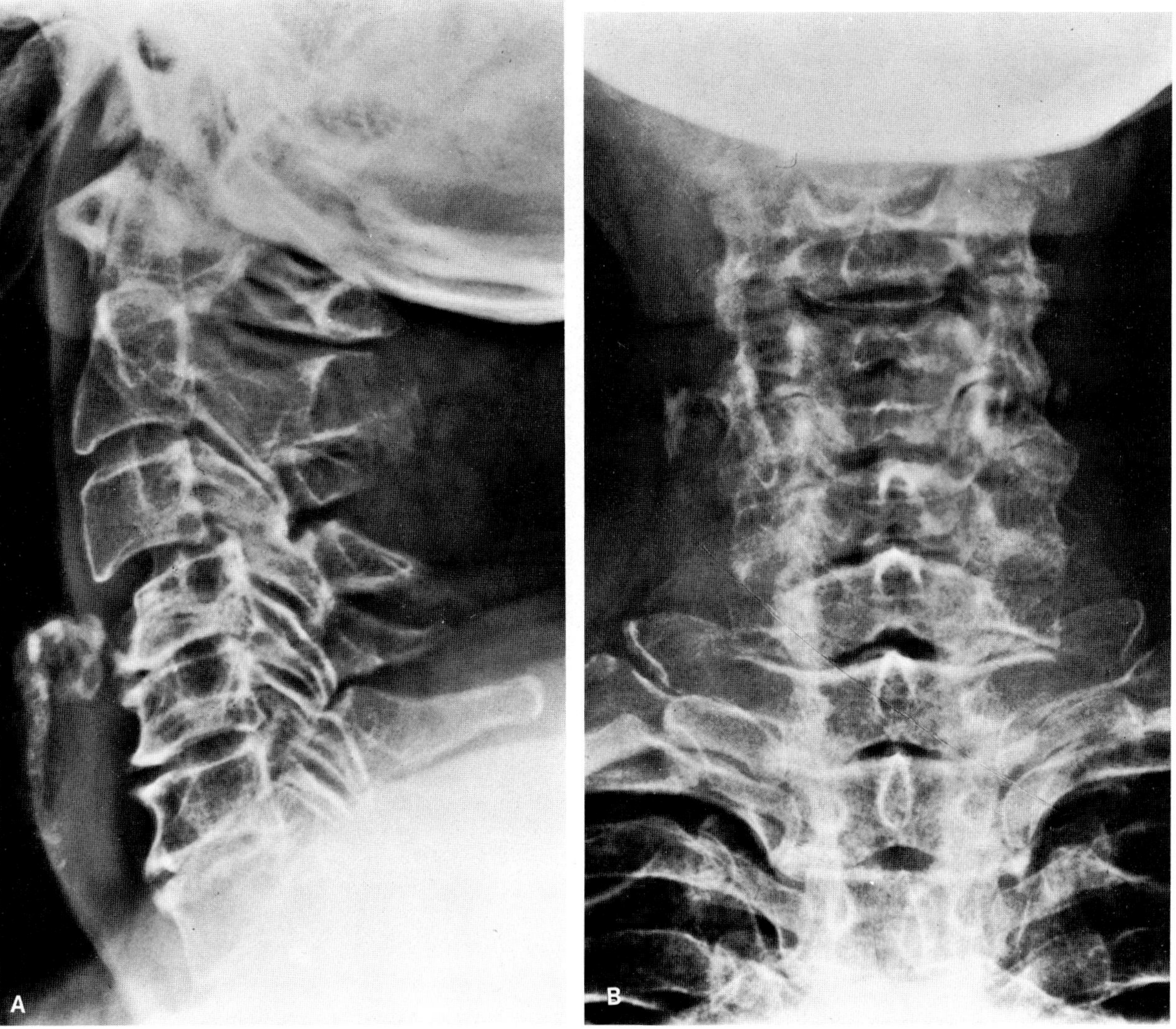

Fig. 3-29. Spondylarthrotic anterolisthesis, retrolisthesis, and platyspondylia. This 73-year-old woman with no history of injury showed marked spondylarthrotic changes of the cervical spine. Note the anterolisthesis of C3–C4, due to arthrosis of apophyseal joints (posterior spurring, disappearance of cartilaginous joint space). The retrolisthesis of C4–C5 is due to disc narrowing; the apophyseal joint spaces are normal. (*B*) A–P radiograph showing marked uncarthrosis at this level, producing a horizontal lucent line on the body of C5 in the lateral radiograph (*A*). The same holds true for C5–C6, although to a lesser extent. There is spondylarthrotic flattening (platyspondylia) of vertebral bodies C4, C5, and C6 (compare with C3 and C7).

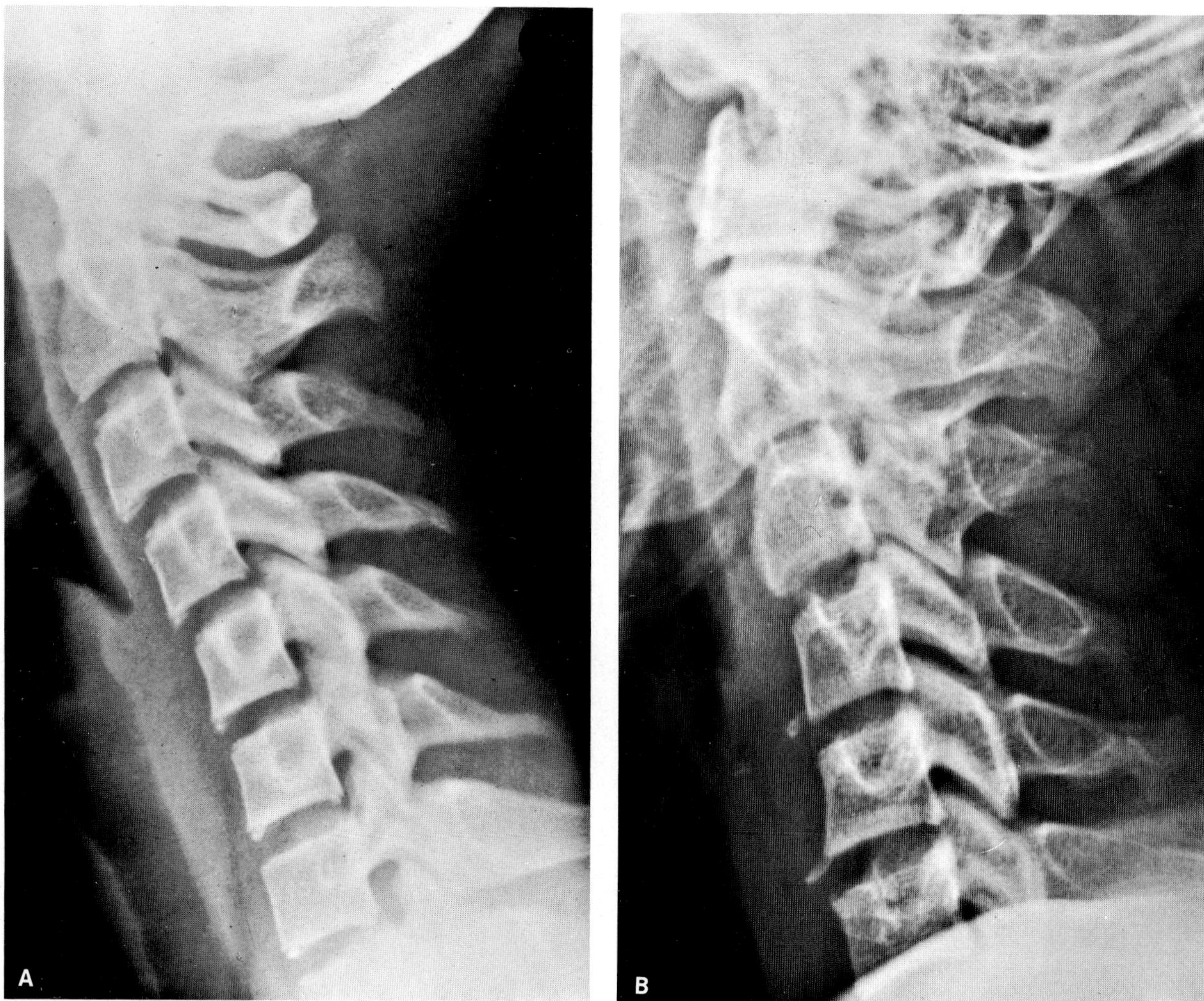

Fig. 3-30. Traumatic avulsion of the epiphyseal end-plates of the vertebral bodies ("vertebral rims"). (*A*) Normal epiphyseal end-plates in a girl aged 12. (*B*) Traumatic avulsion of epiphyseal end-plates at the lower borders of C4 and C5 in an 18-year-old man. Note the slight prevertebral widening at C4 (9 mm). This patient sustained a cerebral contusion, multiple facial fractures, and skin lacerations as a result of a frontal collision with a tractor. There were no signs of cervical cord lesion. Probable mechanism: hyperextension with anterior distraction.

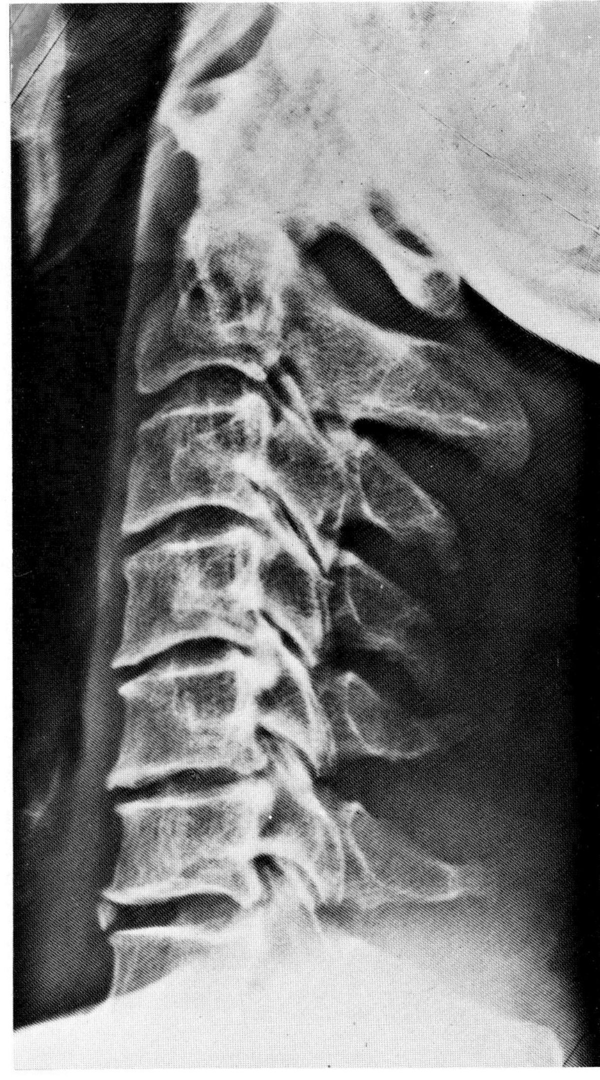

Fig. 3-31. Ossification of the anterior longitudinal ligament in a 69-year-old man with progressive myelopathy, most probably caused by stenosis of the cervical spinal canal. The bony diameter at C5 was 14 mm (normal: 12–21 mm); additional narrowing was caused by posterior spondylosis of vertebral bodies C4–C6. Incidental findings included ossification of the anterior longitudinal ligament at C6–C7 and persisting apophysis of spinous process C7.

recognized as a normal variation or pseudosubluxation. Telescoping subluxation is a nontraumatic condition caused by approximation of vertebrae due to disc degeneration, with concomitant telescoping of articular processes without disruption of joint surfaces (Fig. 3-35C).[13]

Atlantoaxial luxations are divided into anterior, posterior, and rotational types (Fig. 3-36). The luxation is called pure if the odontoid process has remained intact and if anterior displacement of more than 2 to 3 mm in adults and 4 to 5 mm in children is due to rupture of the transverse ligament. Such traumatic rupture may occur, but usually the odontoid fractures before the ligament tears.[8,9,34] In pure luxation, preexisting conditions such as congenital basilar impression, rheumatoid arthritis, or ankylosing spondylitis should be excluded. In children, spontaneous pure atlantoaxial luxation may be encountered in infections in the upper part of the neck.[11,32] In rheumatoid arthritis, there is often simultaneous erosion of the odontoid process; sometimes the odontoid process has moved upward owing to destruction of the lateral atlantoaxial and atlantooccipital joints (Fig. 3-37).

Traumatic pure atlantoaxial luxation in the posterior direction is extremely rare.[14,26]

Anterior or posterior luxation, possibly com-

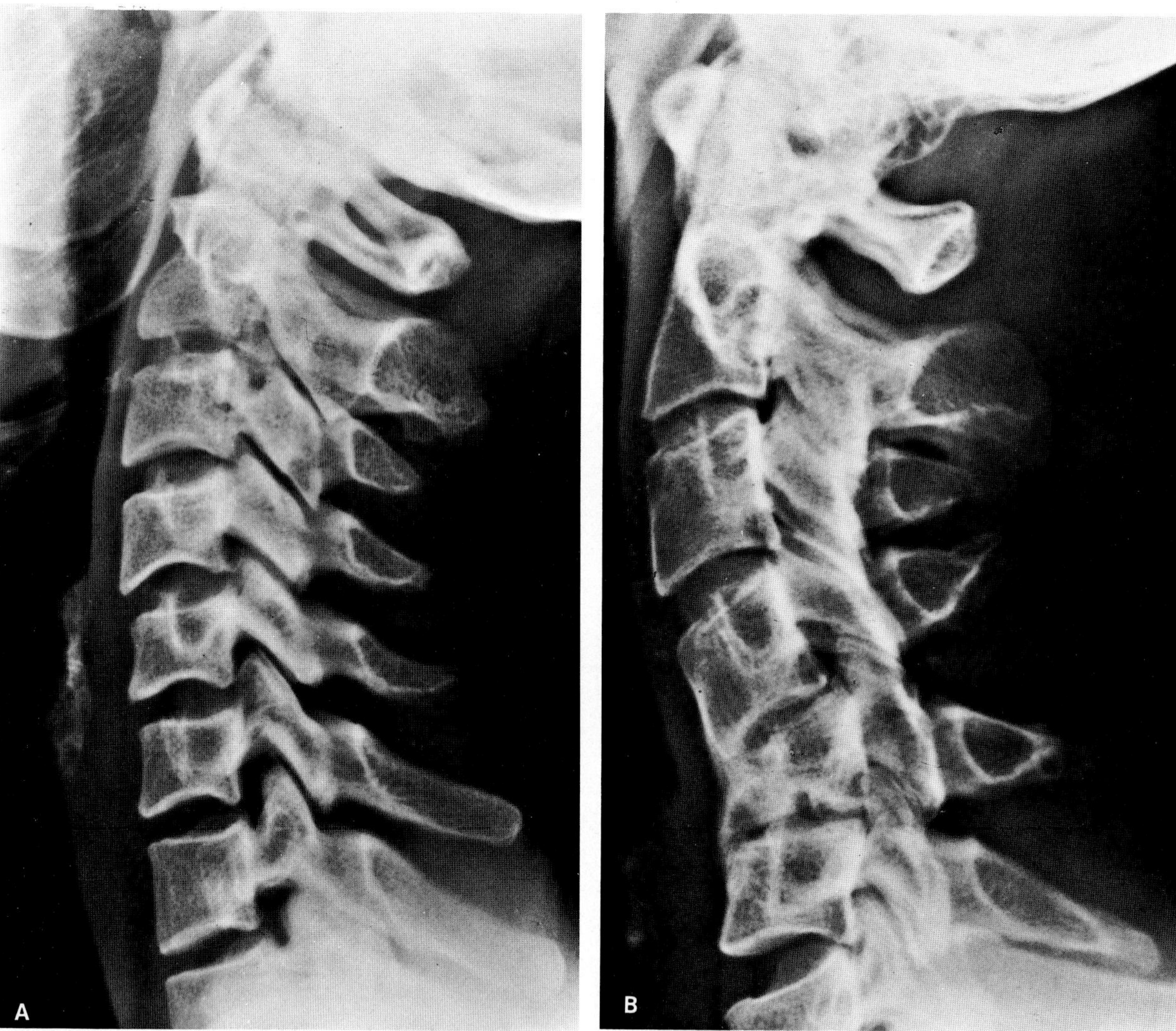

Fig. 3-32. Notching of the articular processes. (*A*) Notching of articular processes of C6 and C7 in a normal person. Note the lengthening of the articular pillars of C6 and C7 compared with C5 and C4. Apophyseal joint spaces C7–T1 are located more posteriorly than joint spaces C6–C7 or C5–C6. (*B*) Old compression fracture of C5 in a 21-year-old man, caused by a head-on dive into shallow water; no neurologic symptoms were evident. Note the fusion of C4, C5, and C6 in kyphotic angulation. Normal notching of the articular processes of C7 should not be taken as a sign of compression.

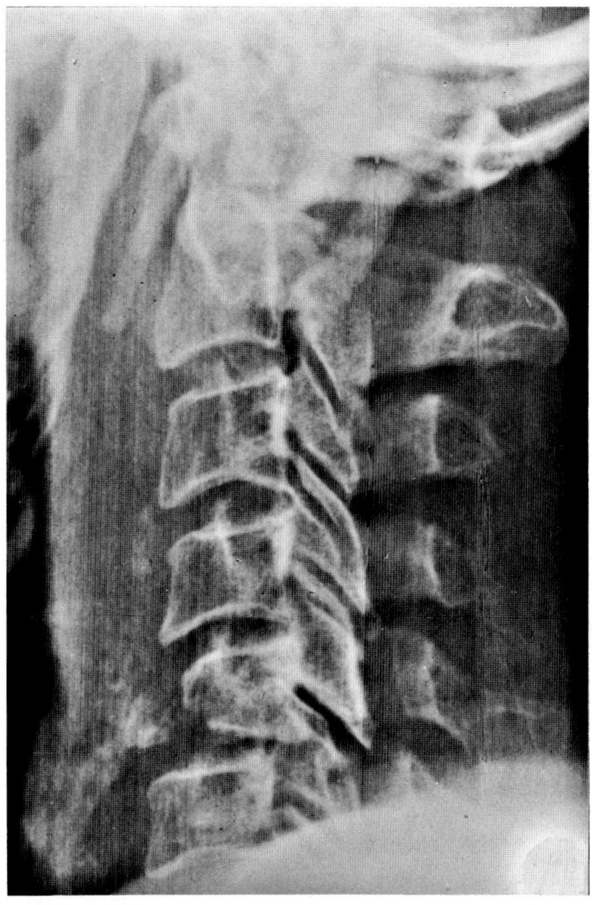

Fig. 3-33. Hyperflexion luxation fracture in a 57-year-old man due to a fall down a flight of stairs. Apart from tinglings in the fingers of both hands, no neurologic signs were evident. This lateral radiograph reveals a compression fracture of vertebral body C5 with marked retrolisthesis and diastasis of the apophyseal joint spaces of C5–C6. Note the prevertebral hematoma. Mechanism of injury: hyperflexion with anterior compression and posterior distraction.

bined with some degree of lateral luxation, is a common finding in fresh and old nonunited fractures of the odontoid process and in os odontoideum.

Rotatory luxation may be diagnosed if rotation exceeds 40° and the articular facets are shown to be interlocked on CT scans. Radiography with the head in the lateral position will reveal the atlas to be in the same lateral position, because rotation between occiput and atlas is virtually impossible. However, the axis and lower cervical spine will have rotated more than 45°, presenting themselves as in oblique projection (Fig. 3-10). Smaller degrees of atlantoaxial rotation (less than 40°) are within the physiologic range of movement and may not be called luxation or subluxation. Their occurrence is evident from the rotated position of the head during radiography (*e.g.*, as the result of muscle spasm). In the absence of head rotation, atlantoaxial (counter) rotation may be compensatory for rotation of the lower cervical spine in scoliosis or in unilateral interlocking or unilateral articular mass compression. In the lateral radiograph, C2 rotation is evidenced by projection of a lateral mass anterior to the axial body (Fig. 3-36).

Asymmetric position of the odontoid process between the lateral masses of the atlas in the A–P view, or lateral overriding (offset) of the atlantoaxial joint edges, is no sign *per se* of injury to the upper cervical region. In our opinion, the margins of normalcy should be rather wide in order to avoid pitfalls. However, bilateral atlantal overriding is an indication of atlantal burst fracture (Jefferson's fracture) with bilateral atlantal spread, or anterior atlantoaxial luxation, in which the ostensible atlantal spread is caused by relatively large radiologic magnification (Fig. 3-15).[16,29] It has also been described in simultaneous anterior and posterior spina bifida of the atlas.[3]

Differences in interspace between the posterior

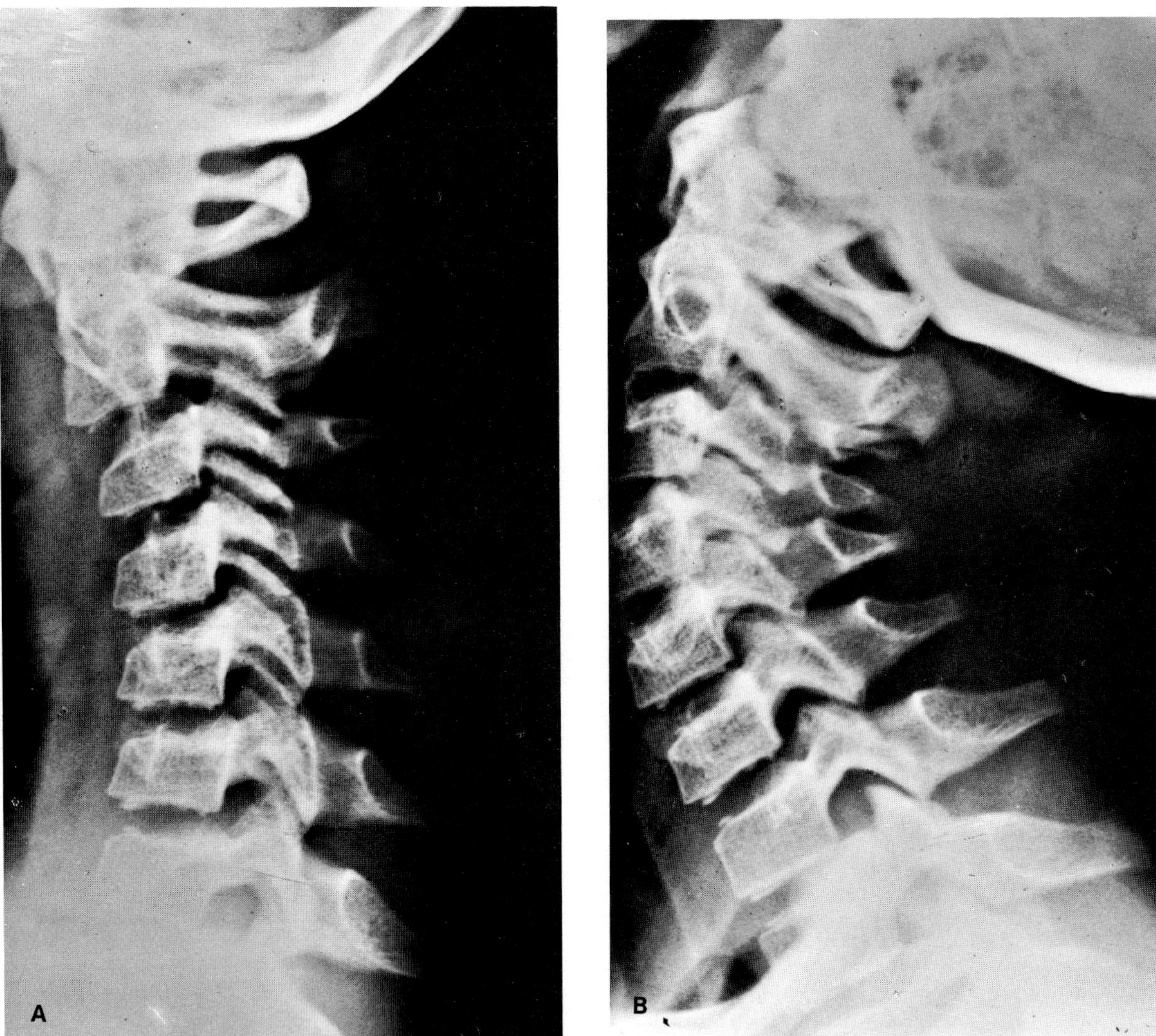

Fig. 3-34. This 9-year-old girl with no history of injury showed pseudosubluxations of the cervical spine in a flexed position. (*A*) In a flexed position the cervical spine shows marked step formation (anterolisthesis) of the posterior borders of the vertebral bodies. (*B*) In extension, reverse step formation is evident. These findings are normal in children and should not be diagnosed as subluxation. In adults, step formation is less obvious owing to the more vertical position of the apophyseal joints and less mobility, resulting in relatively less gliding movement of the vertebrae. (H. Scheier, Zürich)

Fig. 3-35. Relationships in apophyseal joints. (*A*) The normal vertebral relationship in lateral view. (*B*) Normal flexion–extension movement (*arrow* indicates instantaneous axis of movement). Note anterior gliding in flexion and posterior gliding in extension, not to be confused with retrolisthesis and anterolisthesis, which occur in midposition. (*C*) Retrolisthesis due to disc narrowing (*arrow*). The oblique course of the apophyseal joints forces the upper vertebra in posteroinferior direction (*open arrow*). The designation *telescoping subluxation of apophyseal joints* should not be used because it might wrongly suggest traumatic genesis. (*D*) Anterolisthesis due to disappearance of joint cartilage by arthrosis or arthritis (*arrow*). The upper vertebra slips anteriorly (*open arrow*). (*E*) Traumatic interlocking as the result of hyperflexion with posterior distraction. (*F*) Traumatic diastasis of apophyseal joint space in hyperflexion fracture luxation with anterior compression and posterior distraction.

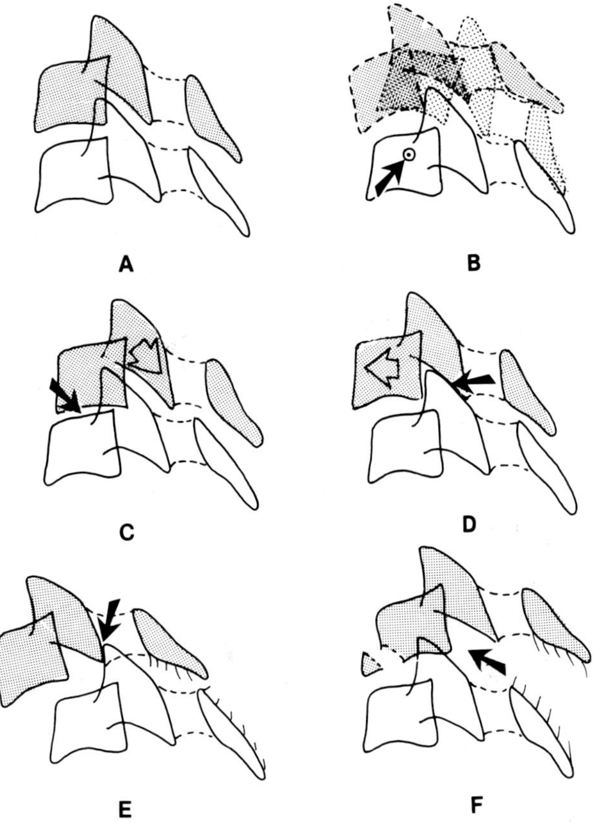

arch of the atlas and the occiput on one hand, and the spinous processes of the axis on the other hand, have no pathologic significance and do not indicate posterior ligament rupture as may be the case in the C2 to C7 region.

Retrolisthesis and Anterolisthesis. In retrolisthesis, a vertebral body slips posteriorly in relation to the vertebrae below. In spondylarthrosis, retrolisthesis is a common finding in disc narrowing in the midcervical region (C3–C6; Figs. 3-27 and 3-29). It is explained by the oblique position of the intervertebral joints, which forces the upper vertebral body slightly backward in approaching the vertebral body below. Retrolisthesis is often seen below block vertebrae, especially C2 and C3.

Retrolisthesis in disc narrowing without fracture of the corresponding vertebral body should not be considered the result of injury, but of preexisting spondylarthrosis. Retrolisthesis with fracture is a common finding in hyperflexion injury with compression (Fig. 3-33).

Retrolisthesis is the cause of extra narrowing of the spinal canal in retroflexion. In congenital or acquired stenosis of the canal, this may cause pinching of the cord even in mild hyperextension injuries.

Anterolisthesis (forward slipping of a vertebral body) is produced by arthrotic or arthritic changes of the intervertebral joints (Fig. 3-29). It is also encountered in spondylolisthesis (Figs. 3-22 and 3-23). Trauma may cause anterolisthesis through the interlocking of articular facets in hyperflexion injury or through compression of articular facets in hyperextension injury. At C2–C3, marked anterolisthesis may be encountered in hangman's fracture. Anterolisthesis in the presence of arthrotic or arthritic changes without evidence of fracture should not be considered the result of injury.

In a recent literature report[19a] an extensive review of false-positive interpretations of radiographs in cervical spine injury is presented. The

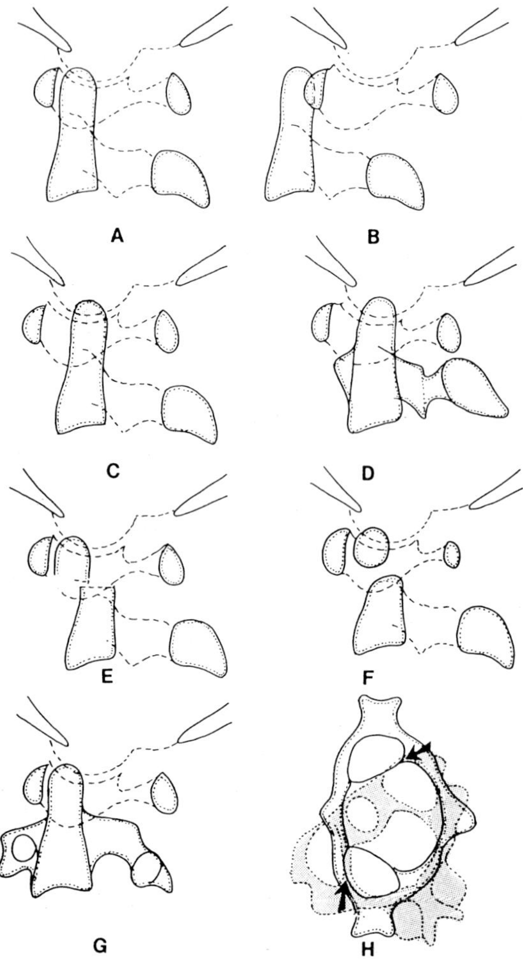

Fig. 3-36. Schematic representation of several types of atlantoaxial luxation. (*A*) Normal atlantoaxial relationship, that is, anterior atlantodental interspace not exceeding 2 mm in adults and 5 mm in children. (*B*) Pure posterior atlantoaxial luxation. (*C*) Pure anterior atlantoaxial luxation. Note the pathologically enlarged anterior atlantodental interspace. Further anterior luxation is counteracted by the checkrein effect of the alar ligaments (film). (*D*) Atlantoaxial luxation with rotation as it occurs spontaneously in infections of the upper respiratory tract. Atlantoaxial rotation remains within the normal limit of 30° to 40°. (*E*) Anterior atlantoaxial fracture luxation (odontoid fracture). Luxation may also occur in a posterior or lateral direction. Intermittent luxation may be the result of nearthrotic or pseudoarthrotic healing. (*F*) Anterior atlantoaxial luxation due to os odontoideum. Luxation may also occur in the posterior direction. Luxation, as a rule, is intermittent (atlantoaxial instability), depending on the position of the head. Note the shortening of the atlantal A–P diameter and deformation of the anterior and posterior arches. (*G, H*) Atlantoaxial rotation luxation. Rotation markedly exceeds the normal limit of 40° because of interlocking of the articular facets (*arrows*). There is no rotation between the atlas and the occiput.

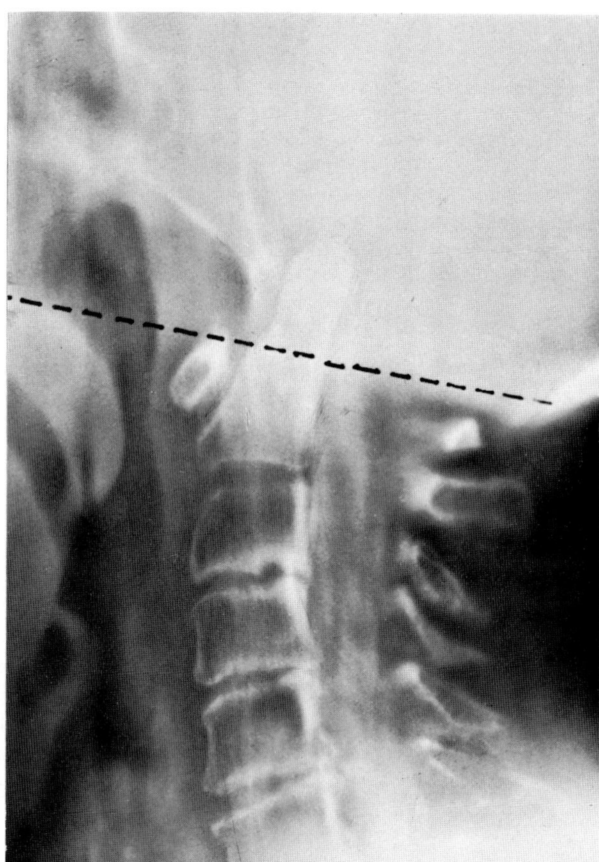

Fig. 3-37. Basilar erosion in rheumatoid arthritis in a 38-year-old woman with a history of rheumatoid arthritis for 20 years and complaints of headache. Neurologic examination revealed the presence of the extrapyramidal syndrome. This midline tomogram shows the ascent of the axial body through the atlantal ring due to rheumatoid destruction of atlantoaxial and atlantooccipital joints (probably old and long-standing). The interrupted line is Chamberlain's line. Note the rheumatoid changes of vertebral end-plates.

most common causes of error were degenerative disorders (retrolisthesis or anterolisthesis diagnosed as traumatic subluxation; uncovertebral joint degeneration; platyspondylia, ossification of the anterior longitudinal ligament) and congenital anomalies (block vertebrae, asymmetry at the base of the odontoid, os odontoideum).

REFERENCES

1. Bailey DK: The normal cervical spine in infants and children. Radiol Clin North Am 59:712, 1952

1a. Bogduk N: The anatomy and pathophysiology of whiplash. Review Paper. Clin Biomech 1:92–101, 1986

2. *Braunstein E, Hunter LY, Bailey RW:* Long-term radiographic changes following anterior cervical fusion. Clin Radiol 31:201, 1980
3. *Budin E, Sondheimer F:* Lateral spread of the atlas without fracture. Radiol 87:1095, 1966
4. *Buetti-Bäuml C:* Funktionelle Röntgendiagnostik der Halswirbelsäule. Stuttgart, Georg Thieme, 1964
5. *Cattel LHS, Filtzer DL:* Pseudosubluxation and other normal variations of the cervical spine in children. J Bone Joint Surg 47A:1295, 1965
6. *Charlton DP, Gehweiler JA, Morgan CL, Martinez S, Daffner RH:* Spondylolysis and spondylolisthesis of the cervical spine. Skeletal Radiol 3:79, 1978
7. *Daffner RH:* Pseudofracture of the dens: Mach bands. Am J Roentgenol 128:607, 1977
8. *Davis D, Bohlman H, Walker AE, Fisher R, Robinson R:* The pathological findings in fatal craniospinal injuries. J Neurosurg 5:603, 1971
9. *Fielding JW, Cochran GVB, Lawsing JF, Hohl M:* Tears of the transverse ligament of the atlas. J Bone Joint Surg 56A:1683, 1974
10. *Fielding JW, Griffin PP:* Os odontoideum: An acquired lesion. J Bone Joint Surg 59A:37, 1977
11. *Fielding JW, Hawkins RJ:* Atlantoaxial rotatory fixation. J Bone Joint Surg 59A:37, 1977
12. *Gehweiler JA, Martinez S, Clark WM, Miller MD, Stewart GC:* Spondylolisthesis of the axis vertebra. Am J Roentgenol 128:682, 1977
13. *Hadley LA:* The Spine: Anatomico-Radiographic Studies, Development and the Cervical Spine. Springfield, IL, Charles C Thomas, 1964
14. *Haralson RH, Boyd HB:* Posterior dislocation of the atlas on the axis without fracture. J Bone Joint Surg 51A:561, 1969
15. *Holdworth FW:* Fractures, dislocations, and fracture-dislocations of the spine. J Bone Joint Surg 52A:1534, 1970

15a. *Howorth MB, Petrie JG:* Injuries of the spine. Baltimore, Williams & Wilkins, 1964

16. *Jefferson G:* Fracture of atlas vertebra: Report of four cases and review of those previously reported. Br J Surg 7:407, 1920
17. *Kapp JP:* Endotracheal intubation in patients with fractures of the cervical spine. J Neurosurg 42:731, 1975
18. *Kattan KR:* The notched articular process of C7 (dorsalization of C7). Am J Roentgenol 126:612, 1976
19. *Keller RH:* Traumatic displacement of the cartilaginous vertebral rim: A sign of intervertebral disc prolapse. Radiology 110:21, 1974

19a. *Kim KS, Rogers LF, Regenbogen V:* Pitfalls in plain film diagnosis of cervical spine injuries: false positive interpretation. Surg Neurol 25:381–392, 1986

20. *Lidström A:* Injuries in the cervical spine. Acta Chir Scand 106:212, 1954
21. *Liliequist B:* Absent cervical pedicle. Acta Neurochir 38:125, 1977
22. *Lodge T, Higginbottom E:* Fractures and dislocations of the cervical spine. X-ray Focus 7:2, 1966
23. *Minderhoud JM, Braakman R, Penning L:* Os odontoideum: Clinical, radiological and therapeutic aspects. J Neurol Sci 8:521, 1969
24. *Naidich JB, Naidich TP, Garfein C, Leibeskind AL, Hyman RA:* The widened interspinous distance: A useful sign of anterior cervical dislocation in the supine frontal projection. Radiology 123:113, 1977
25. *Paakkala T, Keski-Nisula L, Lektinen E:* Fehlbefundung in der Röntgendiagnostik der Halswirbelsäulenverletzungen. Fortschr Röntgenstr 128:550, 1978
26. *Patzakis MJ, Knopf A, Elfering M, et al:* Posterior dislocation of the atlas on the axis: A case report. J Bone Joint Surg 56A:1260, 1974
27. *Scher A, Vambeck V:* An approach to the radiological examination of the cervicodorsal junction following injury. Clin Radiol 28:243, 1977
28. *Schmidt H, Sartor K, Heckl L:* Bone malformations of the cranio-vertebral region. In Handbook of Clinical Neurology, Vol 32, pp 1–98. Amsterdam, Excerpta Medica, 1977
29. *Spense KF, Decker S, Sell KW:* Bursting atlantal fracture associated with rupture of tranverse ligament. J Bone Joint Surg 52A:543, 1970

29a. *Unterharnscheidt F:* Neuropathology of rhesus monkeys undergoing -Gx impact acceleration. In Ewing CL, Thomas, DJ, Sances A, Larson SJ (eds): Impact Injury of the Head and Spine, pp 94–176. Springfield, IL, Charles C Thomas, 1983

30. *Vines FS:* The significance of "occult" fractures of the cervical spine. Am J Roentgenol 107:493, 1969
31. *Wackenheim A:* Roentgendiagnosis of the Craniovertebral Region. New York, Springer-Verlag, 1974.
32. *Watson JR:* Spontaneous hyperaemic dislocation of the atlas. Proc R Soc Med 25:586, 1932
33. *Whitley JR, Forsyth HF:* Classification of cervical spine injuries. Am J Roentgenol 83:633, 1960
34. *Zeitler E, Markuske H:* Roentgenolgische Bewegungsanalyse der Halswirbelsäule bei gesunden Kindern. Fortschr Roentgenstr 96:87, 1962

Computed Tomography with and without Myelography

GEORGE ALKER

The first computed tomography (CT) scanner became commercially available in 1972. It was capable of scanning the head only, although the craniovertebral junction and the upper two cervical segments could be examined in some patients. It revolutionized neuroradiology and has become an indispensable diagnostic modality for examination of the intracranial structures. Wide-aperature scanners designed to scan the entire body became available in 1974, making possible the examination of the spine. Since that time, ample evidence has accumulated in the literature to prove that CT scanning is an extremely important modality in the examination of the spinal column as well.

PROJECTION

CT scanners are capable of scanning only in the transverse axial plane. The cross-sectional images thereby produced are useful in complementing the standard A–P, lateral, and oblique radiographs. Most scanners offer a computer program that makes it possible to reformat images in the coronal and sagittal planes from transverse axial views. Thin overlapping sections are desirable for a reformatted image of high quality. Reformatting is extremely helpful in evaluating the cervical spine in a variety of diseases. It is indispensable for the evaluation of the injured spine. The procedure is somewhat time-consuming and may not be practical or necessary in every case. My technique for routine examination of the cervical spine consists of a 4-mm slice thickness and 3-mm longitudinal spacing of the slices, allowing for a 1-mm overlap. It provides good image quality and allows for subsequent reformatting, if in the judgment of the supervising physician that is desirable for a complete evaluation of the spine.

CONTRAST ENHANCEMENT

Currently available scanners provide excellent detail of the bony structures and of the paravertebral soft tissues. However, the contents of the spinal canal, especially the spinal cord, usually cannot be adequately examined without the injection of a contrast agent. Opacification of the subarachnoid space by intrathecal contrast material allows excellent visualization of the spinal cord and of nonosseous masses within the canal. Intrathecal contrast enhancement may be performed to augment the CT scan (CT myelography or CTM), or the CT scan may follow a conventional radiographic myelogram. Water soluble nonionic contrast agents are well suited for this purpose. Iohexol (Omnipaque) and iopamidol (Isovue) are equally suitable. If in the course of conventional myelography a finding makes desirable further investigation with the use of CT, the opacification of the subarachnoid space is sufficient to permit the scan for several hours. This provides the option of combining the two procedures, even if CT scanning was not originally planned. It is not possible if the oily contrast material iophendylate (Pantopaque) is used, which is too dense and tends to break up into globules.

The injection of contrast material into the spinal canal converts an otherwise noninvasive procedure to an invasive one, and it is not necessary if the examinaiton primarily concerns the bony structures. It is, however, useful when a soft-tissue lesion, such as disc herniation, vascular malformation, or soft-tissue neoplasm is suspected.

Generally, because of the much greater sensitivity of the scanner to small differences in density, a lower concentration of contrast material is required to achieve excellent visualization on CT than would be necessary for conventional radiographic myelography. I use a dose of 10 ml of iohexol 180 or of iopamidol 200 injected via the lumbar route if CT scanning only is desired. I employ a dose of 15 ml of iohexol 240 or of iopamidol 300 via the lumbar route for conventional radiographic myelography of the cervical spine. The concentration of contrast material in the spinal canal remains sufficient for a CT scan up to 4 or 5 hours after myelography. A delay of this magnitude is often necessary in a busy x-ray department where the scanner tends to be heavily scheduled.

CLINICAL APPLICATION

The major contribution of CT scanning to the radiographic evaluation of the cervical spine is the cross-sectional view. This is not available on conventional radiographic examinations, and it com-

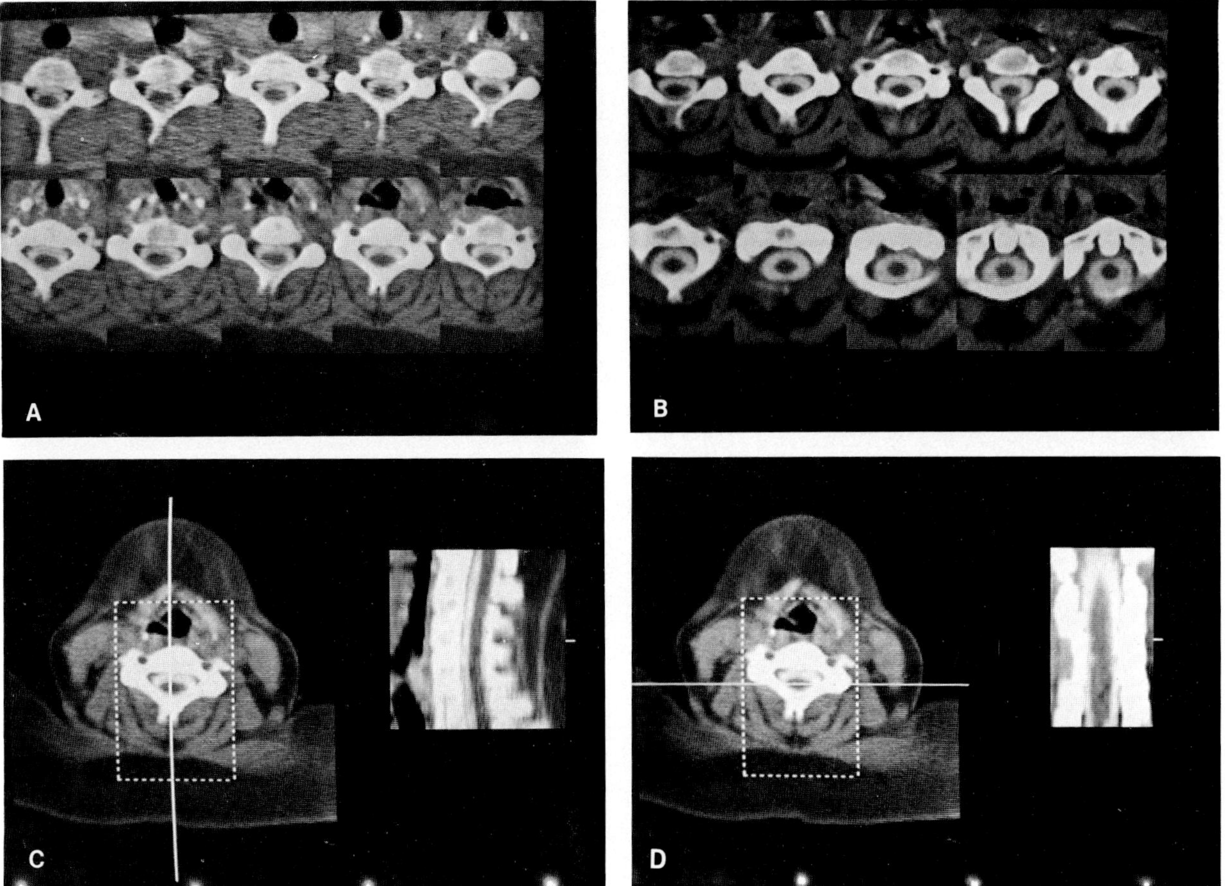

Fig. 3-38. (*A* and *B*) Normal series of cervical scans with intrathecal metrizamide. These are 8-mm-thick sections with 5-mm spacing (3-mm overlap). Computer reconstruction in (*C*) sagittal and (*D*) coronal planes complement the axial views. Because of the lordotic curve, the entire length of the cervical cord cannot be seen on any one coronal view.

plements the A–P, lateral, and oblique views. The availability of CT scanning greatly diminished the need for conventional radiographic tomography, including complex motion tomography. CT scanning involves significantly lower radiation exposure and provides more information, particularly regarding the soft tissues.

CT scanning is especially helpful in depicting the size and shape of the bony spinal canal and of the pedicles, laminae, and spinous processes, all of which are difficult to discern on conventional radiographs and even on tomograms (Fig. 3-38). At the upper cervical levels and the craniovertebral junction, the relationship of the atlas and the odontoid are well demonstrated, and at times the transverse ligament may be seen. In this area, the spinal cord is often visible, even without intrathecal contrast enhancement, because of the relatively small size of the cord compared with the osseous canal and the interposed spinal fluid, which is of lower density than the cord.

The CT scan must be evaluated along with at least an A–P and a lateral radiograph or with reconstruction in the coronal and sagittal planes. Findings that are not demonstrable on transverse axial views but are readily visible on conventional radiographic views include fusion of vertebral segments, changes in the height of the intervertebral space, and compression fracture and wedging of the vertebral body.

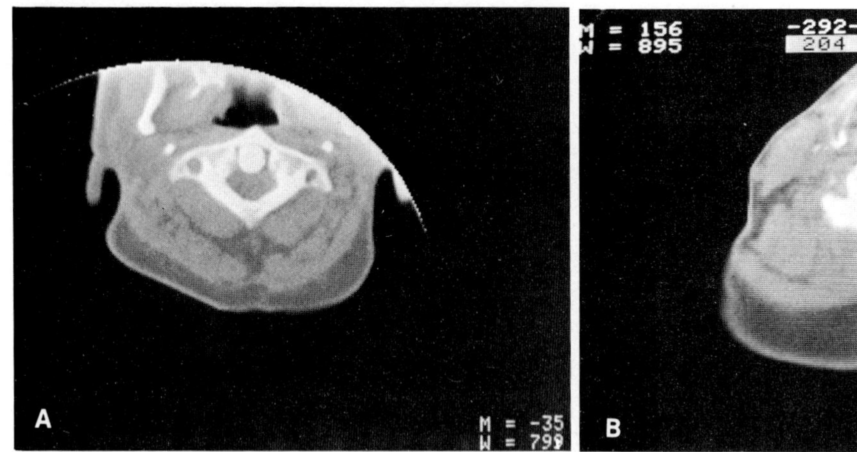

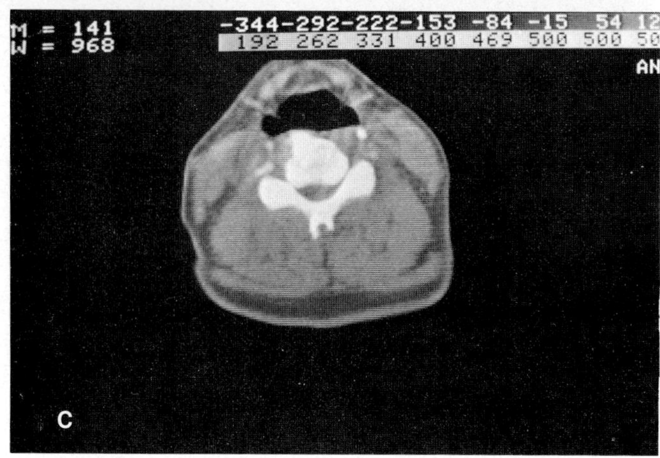

Fig. 3-39. Small spinal canal (spinal stenosis). This 57-year-old man has an unusually small spinal canal throughout its length. (*A*) Even at the level of the atlas it is barely larger than the spinal cord. (*B*) At the level of C3, spurring is largely anteriorly directed. The spinal cord is essentially unaffected at that level. (*C*) At C5 there is significant encroachment of the spinal canal and intervertebral foramina, by bony spurring resulting from disc degeneration.

CONGENITAL VARIATIONS AND MALFORMATIONS

The size and shape of the bony spinal canal varies from patient to patient. A congenitally small spinal canal is easily detected on the CT scan (Fig. 3-39). The use of the computer allows very accurate measurements of the dimensions of the spinal canal. In measuring the A–P diameter, however, one must keep in mind that there is a variation in this diameter depending on whether the measurement is made on a section at the middle of the vertebral body or near a disc space. Similarly, the transverse diameter of the canal shows great variations between adjacent slices. The significance of a smaller-than-average spinal canal can be better appreciated with the use of intrathecal contrast enhancement, through which the size and shape of the spinal cord becomes quite obvious. Spina bifida and absent pedicles are among the congenital malformations also depicted on the scan.

Patients with Down's syndrome are prone to congenital malformations of the odontoid process and atlantoaxial subluxation. CT scanning may be used in the examination of these patients to evaluate the integrity of the relationship between the anterior arch of the atlas and the odontoid process in flexion and in extension, and to evaluate the space available for the spinal cord in the case of subluxation. At the C1–C2 level, intrathecal contrast injection is usually not required to visualize the spinal cord; thus, CT scanning is a suitable noninvasive method for single examination or serial observation of patients with Down's syndrome.

INFLAMMATORY DISEASES

Rheumatoid arthritis of the craniovertebral junction is well demonstrated by CT scan. Disruption of the transverse ligament is evidenced by atlantoaxial subluxation and intrusion of the odontoid process into the foramen magnum (Fig. 3-40). The space available to the spinal cord is reduced, resulting in cord compression. Other inflammatory processes may cause destruction of any portion of the cervical vertebrae and present as a mass in the spinal canal. The latter requires intrathecal contrast enhancement for accurate visualization.

DEGENERATIVE DISEASES

The size and shape of the spinal canal is affected by cervical spondylosis, resulting in acquired spinal stenosis. Bony spurring occurs at the posterior aspect of the vertebral bodies at disc spaces, causing a decrease in the anteroposterior dimension of the spinal canal. In severe cases, the canal may be reduced to a crescentic shape. The spurs are usually bilateral, but they may predominate on one side (Figs. 3-41 and 3-42). Bony spurs originating from the uncovertebral joints intrude into the intervertebral foramina on one or both sides.

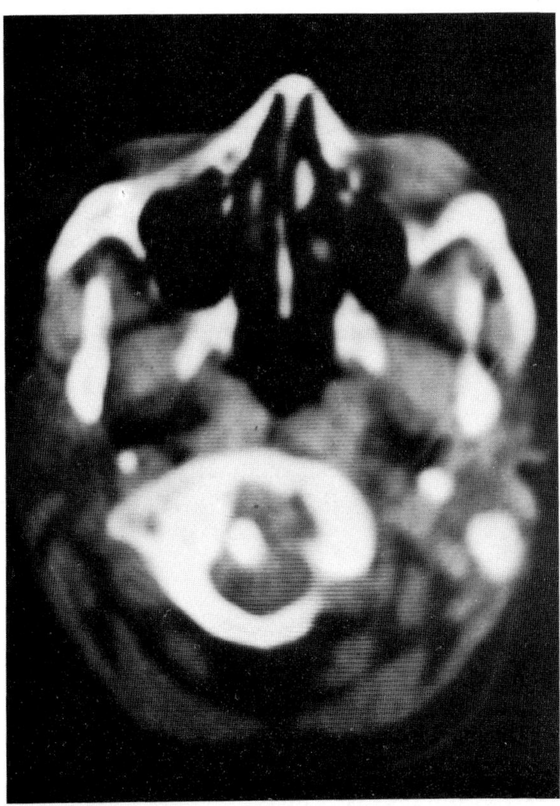

Fig. 3-40. Rheumatoid arthritis of the cranial vertebral junction. There is subluxation of the odontoid process toward the left and projection of its tip into the foramen magnum.

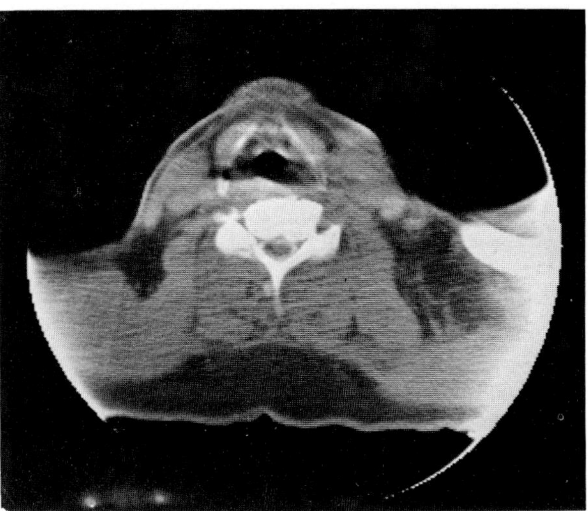

Fig. 3-41. Severe cervical spondylosis with intrathecal contrast enhancement. The relationship of the size of the spinal cord to the spinal canal, severely narrowed by large bony bars, is well demonstrated. Virtually the entire spinal canal is taken up by the spinal cord, which is somewhat compressed in its anteroposterior diameter.

Ankylosing spinal hyperostosis (Forestier's disease) results in thickening and ossification of the anterior spinal ligament, ultimately leading to immobilization of the cervical spine due to the anterior bony bridging between the segments. With mobility greatly reduced, few, if any, bony spurs project into the spinal canal (Fig. 3-43).

DISC HERNIATION

The detection of soft-disc herniation in the cervical area requires very thin sections (1.5 to 2 mm) and intravenous contrast enhancement, which helps to delineate the opacified epidural venous plexus from extruded disc material that does not opacify. The reason for this approach is the paucity of epidural fat in the cervical area compared with the lower lumbar region, where disc herniation is relatively easily detected. At times, intrathecal contrast enhancement (CTM) may be necessary (Fig. 3-44). Precise localization of disc herniation is extremely helpful to the operating surgeon.

TUMORS

CT scanning has a distinct advantage over conventional radiographs in the evaluation of primary or metastatic tumors of the cervical vertebrae. In-

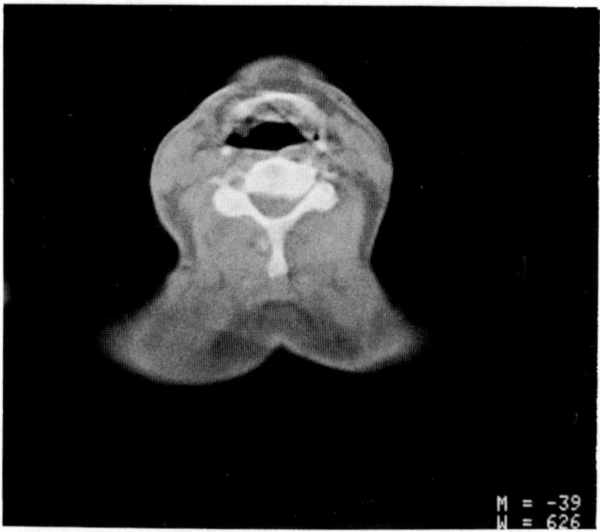

Fig. 3-42. Cervical spondylosis with predominantly unilateral involvement. Bony spurs projecting from the uncovertebral joints in this patient cause narrowing primarily of the left side of the spinal canal and of the left intervertebral foramen at C5–C6. The spinal cord is not seen without the use of intrathecal metrizamide.

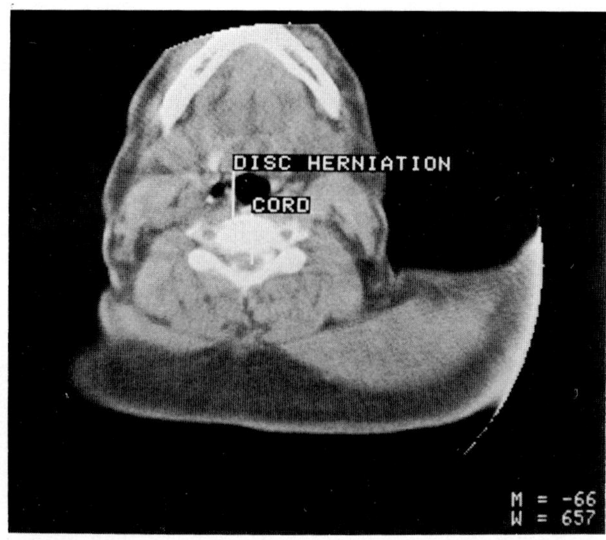

Fig. 3-44. Cervical disc herniation. Intrathecal metrizamide is essential in demonstrating this soft disc herniation at the C6–C7 level. It is eccentric in position, affecting primarily the right lateral aspect of the spinal canal and the right intervertebral foramen. The spinal cord is slightly rotated and displaced to the left.

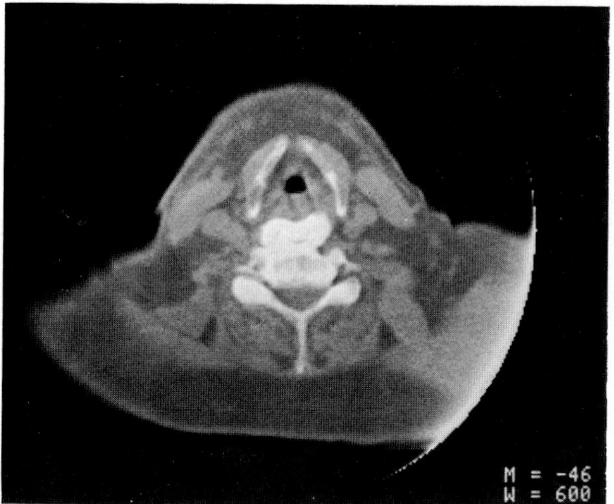

Fig. 3-43. Ankylosing spinal hyperostosis (Forestier's disease). In this condition, there is marked increase in the thickness of the anterior spinal ligament with calcification and ossification of that structure, resulting in anterior fusion between the vertebrae. The large anterior bony mass is well demonstrated in this patient who has only very slight bony spurring in the region of the spinal canal.

volvement of the pedicles, laminae, and spinous processes are usually difficult to appreciate on conventional radiographic views. The cross-sectional image provided by the CT scan provides accurate visualization of the posterior elements of the vertebrae, making it possible to delineate extension of tumor in these areas (Fig. 3-45). CT demonstrates not only the osseous involvement but also the extension of tumor into the paravertebral soft tissues (Fig. 3-46). Thus, a more complete assessment of the lesion is obtained and a suitable site for biopsy is chosen. The density of the lesion, however, is nonspecific, and the histologic diagnosis cannot be predicted on the basis of the scan alone.

TRAUMA

CT scanning has become virtually indispensable in the evaluation of the patient with spinal trauma. Here, again, the cross-sectional view is its main advantage, and it complements the conventional radiographic projections. In my experience in a large spinal cord injury unit, CT scanning has become an integral part of the evaluation of the patient with spinal injuries. In all but a few instances, it has replaced multidirectional tomography, which requires more patient handling and a larger radiation dose than does the CT scan. The scan is per-

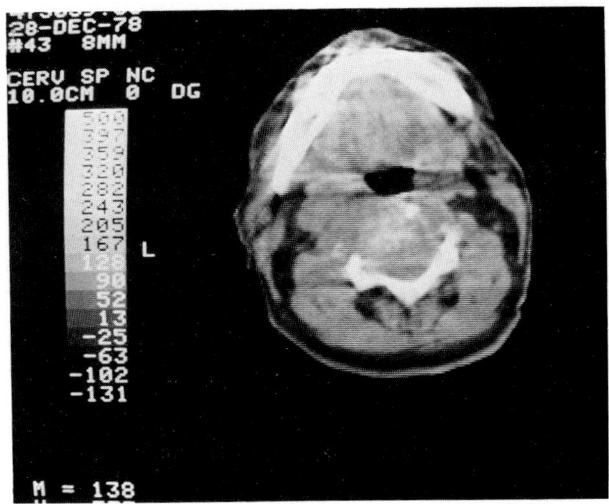

Fig. 3-45. Metastatic tumor involving C3. Metastatic hypernephroma destroyed the body of the C3 vertebra as well as the right pedicle and a portion of the lamina.

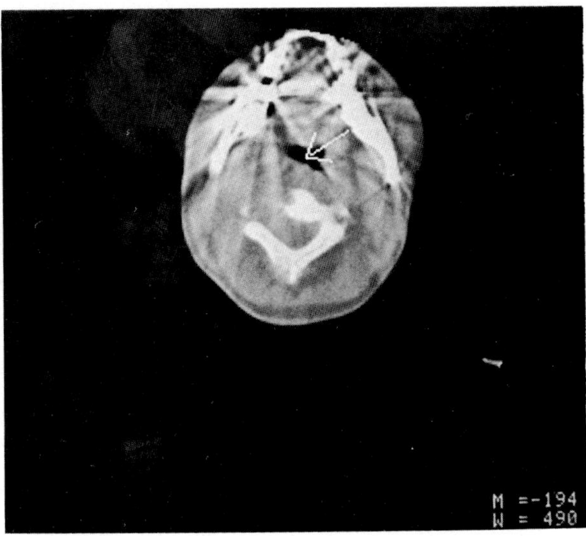

Fig. 3-46. Chordoma. This 19-year-old woman complained of severe neck pain for several months. The CT scan shows destruction of the right half of the body and of the right transverse process of C2. The asymmetry of the nasopharyngeal air shadow (*arrow*) indicates extension of the tumor into the soft tissues anteriorly and laterally.

formed early, shortly after arrival of the patient in the emergency room. The current protocol requires A–P, lateral, and open mouth odontoid views followed immediately by CT scanning, if the radiographs show spinal injury or if spinal injury is suspected on clinical examination. This protocol is used extensively by the team of physicians of the spinal cord injury unit in planning appropriate therapy.

Internal or external metallic fixation devices used in stabilizing the injured spine do cause some streaky artifacts. However, they do not significantly degrade the usefulness of the examination (Fig. 3-47).

Fractures of the pedicles and laminae, which are difficult to see on conventional radiographs, are well demonstrated on the CT scan. Nearly all patients with cervical spine injuries in the spinal cord injury unit have fractures of the vertebral arch or of transverse or articulating processes that are visible on the CT scan but not on conventional radiographs. Reconstruction in the coronal and sagittal planes supplies additional useful information, particularly in the lower cervical area where the shoulders and restricted mobility of the injured patient make evaluation on lateral radiographs difficult.

In many instances, intrusion of disc material and cartilage fragments into the spinal canal following trauma are also demonstrated on the CT scan. At times, however, injection of intrathecal contrast material is necessary to depict a soft-tissue mass,

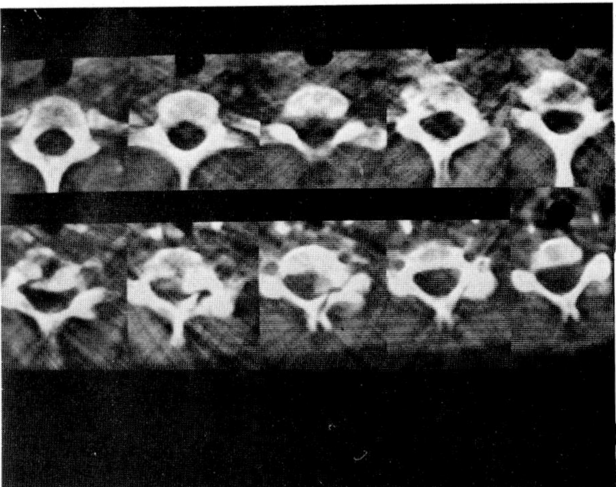

Fig. 3-47. Bone fragment intruding into the spinal canal. The compression fractue of C4 in this 38-year-old woman resulted in intrusion of the left half of the vertebral body into the spinal canal and intervertebral foramen. There is also a fracture of the lamina of C4 on the left side. The numerous small linear artifacts on the scan resulted from a halo jacket being in place during the examination. The presence of the metallic immobilization device does not significantly detract from the usefulness of the scan.

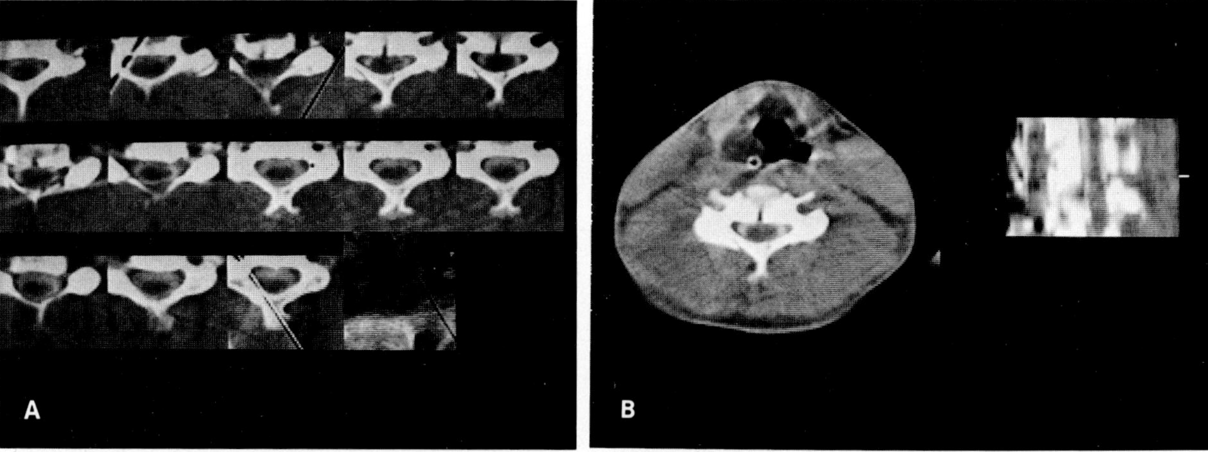

Fig. 3-48. Fractue of the C6 vertebra resulting from hyperflexion and axial loading in a 20-year-old man. (*A*) There is a midsagittal fracture of the body of C6 along with bilateral fractures of the laminae. There is expansion in the anterior-posterior dimensions of the vertebral body, resulting in compression of the spinal canal. The compression of the somewhat enlarged and edematous spinal cord is well demonstrated with the use of intrathecal metrizamide. (*B*) The enlargement of the spinal cord is especially evident on the midsagittal reconstruction.

such as disc herniation or hematoma that compresses the spinal cord. The demonstration of a displaced or enlarged spinal cord also requires intrathecal contrast enhancement (Fig. 3-48). The patient with acute spinal injury is usually not a suitable candidate for conventional radiographic myelography. Under those circumstances the patient is rolled on his side, 10 ml of iohexol 180 or iopamidol 200 is injected, and the patient is returned to the supine position. The radiographic table is tilted in the head-down (Trandelenburg) position for a few minutes, and the patient is transferred to the CT scanner. The entire examination is performed with far less patient handling than with conventional myelography.

Long-term sequelae of spinal cord injury are also shown on CT with the use of intrathecal contrast enhancement. The findings include atrophy, deformity, and displacement of the spinal cord by scarring (Fig. 3-49). Progressive posttraumatic cystic myelopathy was diagnosed with the help of intrathecal metrizamide and CT scanning by Edgar and coworkers. This complication of spinal cord injury may develop years later, with progressive loss of neurologic function after a post-injury plateau. The intramedullary cyst in this condition is best demonstrated on scans obtained several hours after myelography when the contrast material accumulates in the cystic cavity.

The availability of magnetic resonance imaging (MRI), has changed the indications for CT scanning. CT remains unquestionably the imaging procedure of choice in the area of the cervical spine, when evaluation of bony structures are of para-

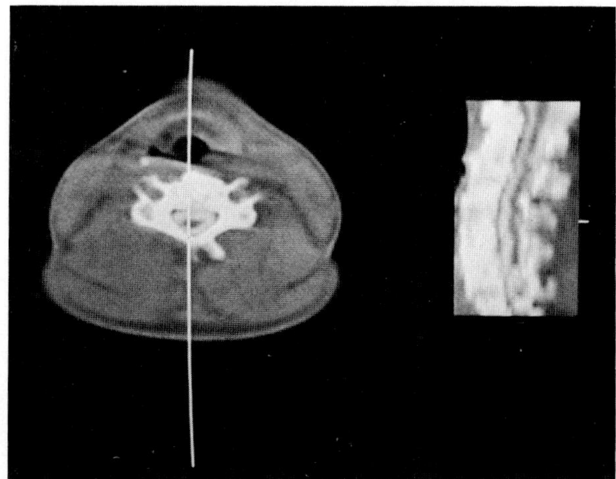

Fig. 3-49. Posttraumatic spinal cord atrophy. This 26-year-old quadraplegic underwent metrizamide myelography for progression of his neurologic deficit three years after the original injury. Severe spinal cord atrophy is seen with a small irregulate cord occupying the otherwise normal spinal canal.

mount interest (*e.g.,* for fractures, bone destruction, or bone proliferation). MRI is clearly superior for depicting the soft-tissue contents of the spinal canal (*e.g.,* the spinal cord or soft-tissue masses) without the injection of intravenous or intrathecal contrast material. The two imaging procedures are complementary.

BIBLIOGRAPHY

Coin GJ, Pennink M, Ahmad WD, Keranen VJ: Diving-type injury of the cervical spine: Contribution of computed tomography to management. J Comput Assist Tomogr 3:362, 1979

Lauten GJ, Wehunt WD: Computed tomography in absent cervical pedicle. Am J Neuroradiol 1:201, 1980

Miller EM, Norman D: The role of computed tomography in the evaluation of neck masses. Radiology 133:146, 1979

Post MJ (ed): Radiographic Evaluation of the Spine. New York, Masson Publications, 1980

Seibert CE, Dreisbach JN, Swanson WB, Edgar RE, Williams P, Hahn H: Progressive post-traumatic cystic myelopathy: Neuroradiologic evaluation. Am J Neuroradiol 2:115, 1981

Semine AA, Ertel AN, Godberg MJ, Bull MJ: Cervical spine instability in children with Down syndrome (trisomy 21). J Bone Joint Surg 60:649, 1978

Three-Dimensional CT of the Cervical Spine: Introduction and Clinical Applications

CHRISTOPHER G. ULLRICH

Multiplanar reconstruction computed tomographic (CT) images were initially introduced in the late 1970s. These two-dimensional (2-D) computer displays are produced by reprocessing axial CT image data into other tomographic projections, typically sagittal or coronal views. This technique has gained routine clinical acceptance and is readily available. Three-dimensional computed tomography (3-D CT) is a recently developed computer-generated graphics display that integrates a series of successive routine CT images into more lifelike pictures. This approach is directly related to the prior development of computer-aided design and computer-aided manufacturing (CAD/CAM) systems. This section reviews the basic concept of 2-D and 3-D computer graphics and demonstrates some of the current clinical applications of 3-D CT in the cervical spine. The 3-D CT illustrations in this chapter were prepared with a CEMAX 1500 image processor,* installed at the Charlotte Memorial Hospital and Medical Center, Charlotte, North Carolina. Axial CT images were produced with a General Electric CT 9800 Computed Tomography System.†

The axial CT image is defined by a cartesian coordinate system called the matrix. Values for *x* and *y* respectively denote the horizontal and vertical edges of the axial CT matrix. The *pixel* (picture element) is the basic unit of a matrix. The *voxel* (volume element) is the volume of tissue defined by the pixel and the CT image thickness. The matrix position of each voxel is mathematically described by *x* and *y* coordinate numbers. Based on the detected x-ray attenuation data, the CT scanner calculates and assigns an appropriate Hounsfield number to each voxel. By designating shades of gray for various Hounsfield number values, the familiar CT video image display is created.

* CEMAX Inc., Santa Clara, California, 95054, U.S.A.

† General Electric Medical Systems, Milwaukee, Wisconsin, 53201, U.S.A.

The *z* axis mathematically describes the movement of the CT scanner table, and therefore, defines the spatial relationships among successive axial CT images. A consecutive series of axial CT images may be considered a three-dimensional array of voxel or Hounsfield number data for which spatial locations are defined by the matrix, the CT image thickness, and the CT table increment between successive axial CT images. The computer precisely identifies the spatial location of each voxel by *x, y,* and *z* coordinate numbers.

Two-dimensional CT multiplanar reconstruction images are produced by selecting the appropriate voxel data from each successive axial CT image to create a "new" tomographic view. Selecting voxel data in the *yz* plane produces a sagittal view, while *xz* plane data represent a coronal view (Fig. 3-50). These images can be no better than the quality of the axial CT image data from which they are derived. "Targeted" algorithms produce the best axial CT images of the cervical spine. The 2D-CT reconstruction images have the same contrast resolution as the original axial CT images; they also retain the spatial resolution of the axial CT images along the *x* and *y* axes. However, spatial resolution along the *z* axis, which is only subtly evident on the axial CT images, is prominently displayed on the 2-D CT reconstruction images. The *z*-axis spatial resolution, which is directly related to the CT image thickness and the CT table incrementation, is usually inferior to the spatial resolution obtained along the *x* and *y* axes of the original axial CT image. As a general principle, the "quality" of a 2-D CT reconstruction image is dramatically improved by using thinner axial CT images and smaller CT table increments. If the CT gantry was angled for the axial images, a software correction must be used; otherwise the reconstruction image will be spatially distorted.

Currently, 3-D CT images are most commonly produced using a surface contour method. Simply described, the voxels in each CT image that define the edge of the structure to be displayed are identified. The computer does this by identifying all of the voxels that have Hounsfield numbers above a threshold value selected by the system operator. A line is drawn connecting each edge defining voxel, and the contour (outline) of the surface anatomy is thereby obtained. Since the relationship between successive axial CT images is also known, a spatial or 3-D array of data describing the anatomic outline is defined. If a reference light source is assumed, shading is introduced to the data, and the visual perception of three dimensions is created

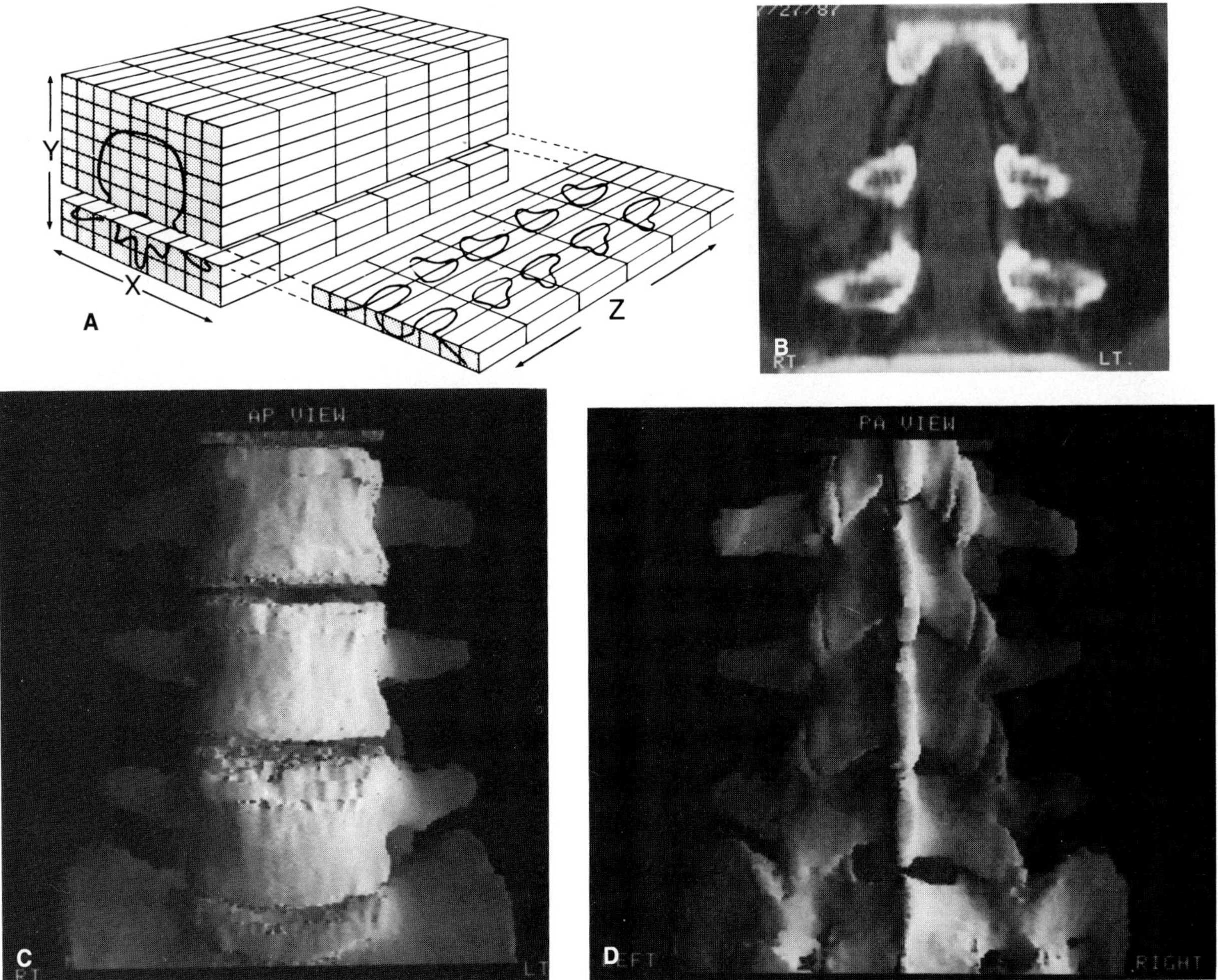

Fig. 3-50. The basic concept of 2-D and 3-D CT reconstruction images. (*A*) Six consecutive axial CT images of the lumbar spine are depicted in this schematic diagram. Each rectangular block represents a voxel. A consecutive series of axial CT images is a three-dimensional array of voxels or Hounsfield number data whose spatial locations are defined by the matrix, the CT image thickness, and the CT table movement. The computer selection of appropriate voxels to produce a 2-D CT coronal reconstruction image (*xz* plane of voxels) is illustrated. (*B*) This typical 2-D CT coronal reconstruction image of the lumbar spine from L3 to S1 through the midpedicle area clearly shows the nerve roots exiting into the neural foramina. This image retains the tissue-density discrimination of the original axial CT images. (*C*) The voxels defining the surface of the vertebral body are identified and a reference light source is assumed, and the same basic CT data is now a 3-D CT image. This A–P view clearly demonstrates the anatomic relationship between the vertebral bodies. Osteophytes are also identified, but all the adjacent soft-tissue structures are absent. (*D*) The P–A view (180° rotation) beautifully demonstrates the alignment of the facet joints in a fashion unobtainable with 2-D CT techniques and with a clarity seldom achieved with conventional radiography. The lifelike quality of these 3-D CT images is striking.

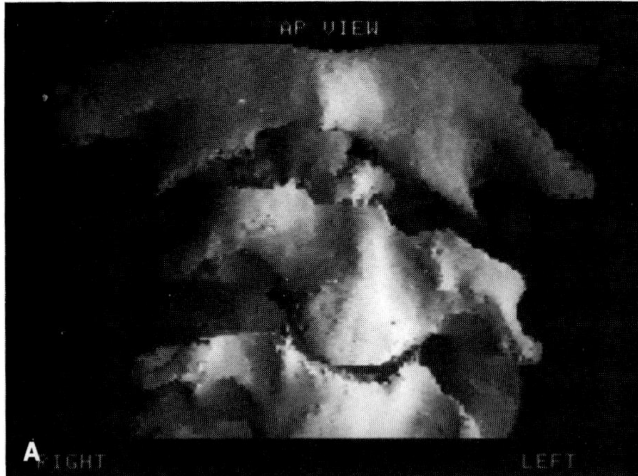

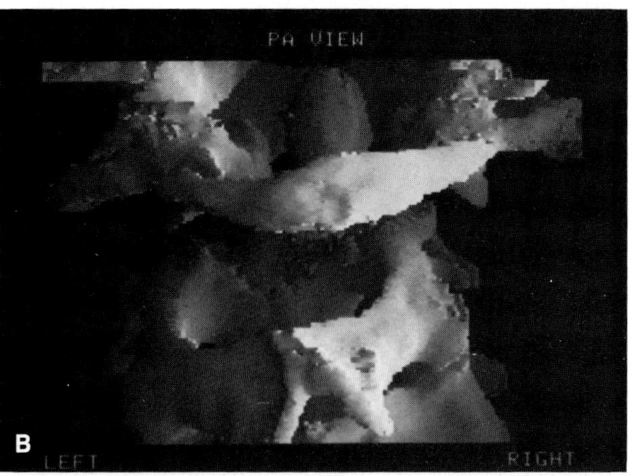

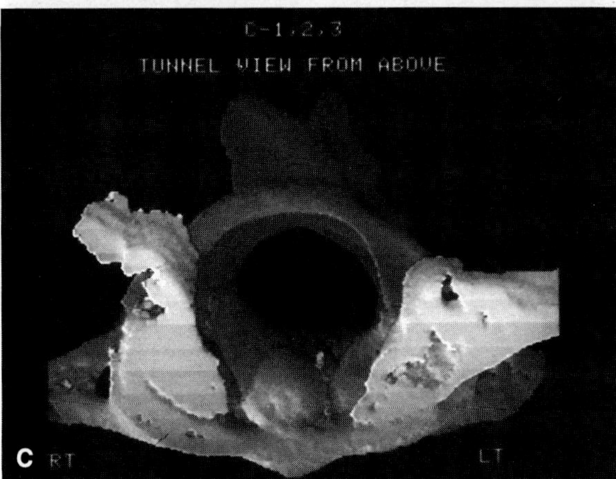

Fig. 3-51. C1–C2 Fracture/dislocation. This auto-accident victim was neurologically intact. (*A* and *B*) A–P and P–A 3-D CT views show a Type-II dens fracture with complete dislocation of C1 from C2. The facet joint capsules at C1–C2 must be disrupted. (*C*) Axial view shows a normal relationship between the odontoid and the anterior arch of C1. Mild spinal canal compromise on the right is due to a fracture fragment in the spinal canal.

(Fig. 3-50). Unlike 2-D CT, these contour 3-D CT images provide no density discrimination beyond locating the surface defining voxels based on the selected threshold Hounsfield number value. Once created, these 3-D CT images may be rotated to allow evaluation from many perspectives. The images may be sectioned or edited to reveal internal surface details. Color coding may be used to highlight anatomic relationships. The technical factors that improve 2-D CT reconstruction images have a similar impact on 3-D CT images. The 3-D images add no new information, but they do display certain aspects of the axial CT data to better advantage.

Three-dimensional CT using contour techniques most effectively displays the bony anatomy of the cervical spine, although soft tissues may also be visualized. Currently, fractures of the cervical spine are a leading application because of the complex structural relationships present in that area (see Fig. 3-51). 3-D CT is excellent for displaying the displacement of bone fragments and the subluxation of the facet joints. Bony compromise of the neural foramen and spinal canal is best demonstrated by sectioning and rotation of the 3-D whole-spine image. The "split sagittal view" (see Fig. 3-52) is commonly used for this purpose. All of these views are obtained from a single axial CT image series that may be acquired while the patient is still immobilized on the trauma board. Any view can then be produced without further direct patient examination. The risk of injury associated with repositioning the patient for different x-ray projections is largely eliminated. The actual patient examination time is relatively short. 3-D CT also facilitates the postsurgical assessment of reduction, decompression, and fusion.

The advantages of 3-D CT for evaluating frac-

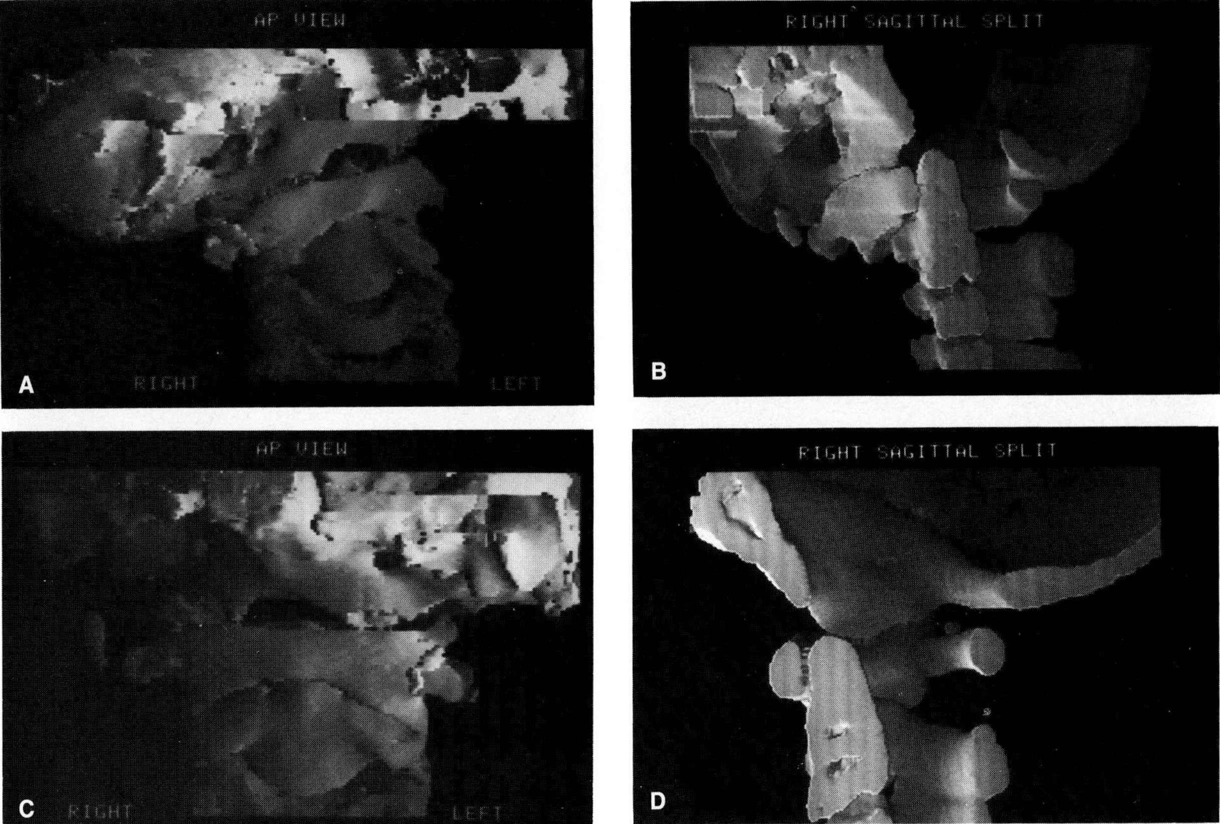

Fig. 3-52. C1–C2 Rotatory dislocation. This young child complained of persistent neck pain and torticollis after a fall. (*A*) A–P 3-D CT shows an anterior rotatory dislocation of the right lateral mass of C1. (*B*) A midline right "sagittal split" image rotated +20° shows the dislocation of C1 to better advantage and shows the A–P diameter of the spinal canal at C1 is compromised. No fracture is seen. The dislocation was reduced by traction and the patient placed in a minerva cast. Reexamination 3 weeks post-injury on A–P (*C*) and right sagittal split (*D*) images shows good approximation of normal alignment. Note the much larger A–P diameter of the spinal canal at C1 now.

tures also apply to cervical spondylosis (Fig. 3-53). However, except in patients with vertebral subluxation, the clinical utility of 3-D CT images for routine cervical spondylosis is less clearly established at this time. When image display capabilities allowing the simultaneous viewing of the spinal cord and nerve roots in relation to the bone are developed, the value of 3-D CT for patients with cervical spondylosis and myelopathy will be greatly enhanced.

In the craniocervical junction region, 3-D CT beautifully demonstrates rotatory subluxation and dislocation (Fig. 3-52). Rotatory abnormalities of the cervical spine are especially difficult to assess satisfactorily using axial and 2-D CT reconstruction images. 3-D CT also displays the erosions and subluxations associated with rheumatoid arthritis to advantage. Congenital spinal anomalies in children may be thoroughly studied with CT images using a very low x-ray dose, while maintaining excellent bony definition (Fig. 3-54). The relatively short examination time is a great advantage when sedation is required. Necessary follow-up examinations may also be produced with low patient x-ray exposure.

Surface contour 3-D CT images have several

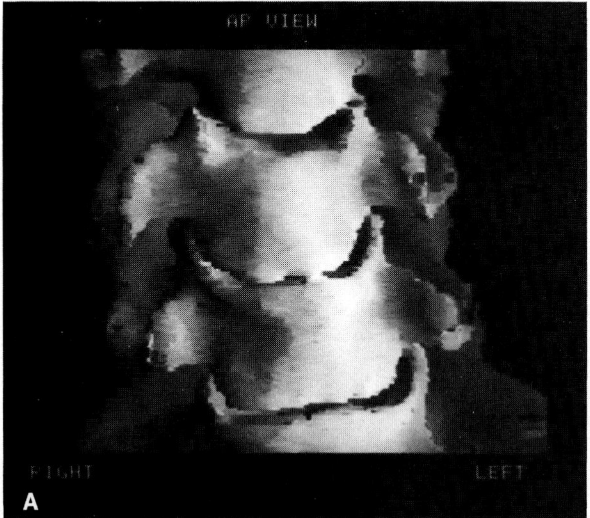

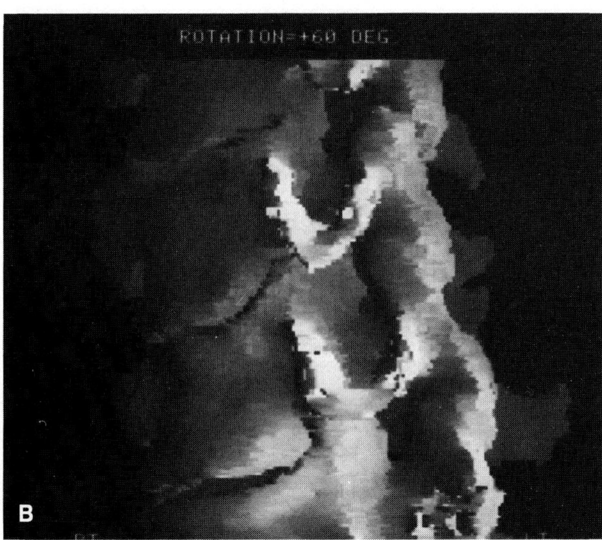

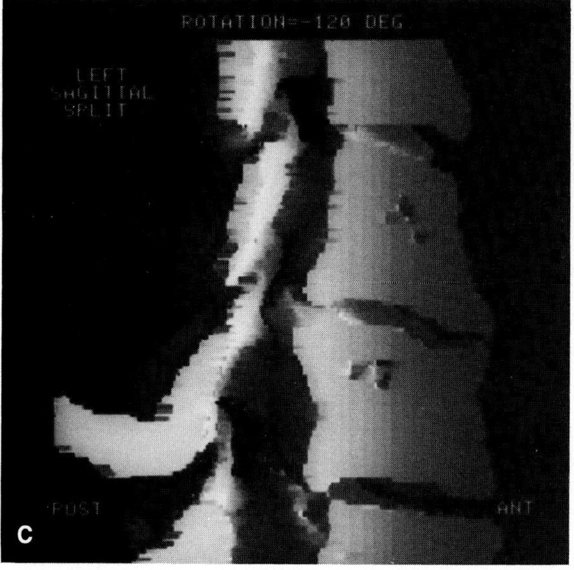

Fig. 3-53. Cervical spondylosis with neural foramen stenosis. (*A*) This A–P 3D-CT image from C4 to C7 shows disc space narrowing and uncovertebral spur formation that is most advanced at C5–C6. A minimal dextroscoliosis is present. (*B*) A +60° rotation view shows large uncovertebral spurs; the neural foramina are partially obscured by the transverse processes. (*C*) A left split sagittal view rotated −120° shows a marked neural foramen stenosis on the left at C5–C6, with C4–C5 and C6–C7 showing less advanced changes. This split sagittal view provides the best demonstration of the neural foramen.

important limitations. Spatial resolution greater than 1.5 to 3.0 mm along the z axis is difficult to achieve. Patient motion rapidly destroys the quality and value of these recalculated images. Contour techniques provide a surface display without the tissue density discrimination, or "see through" character, of routine CT images. Contour image processing times tend to be long, and technical costs are relatively expensive.

Adjacent soft-tissue structures tend to have very similar Hounsfield number values. Therefore, it is difficult for the computer to easily identify the soft-tissue surface of interest. Soft-tissue contours often require extensive operator editing, but they can be produced. Once achieved, they can be combined with bone contour data to produce composite displays. Similar composite images can clearly display the relationship between bone and bullet fragments (Fig. 3-55).

Medical applications of 3-D computer graphics technology are now being intensively researched. Rapid progress is being made in image processing, display, and analysis techniques. "Noncontour" data processing techniques show promise for bet-

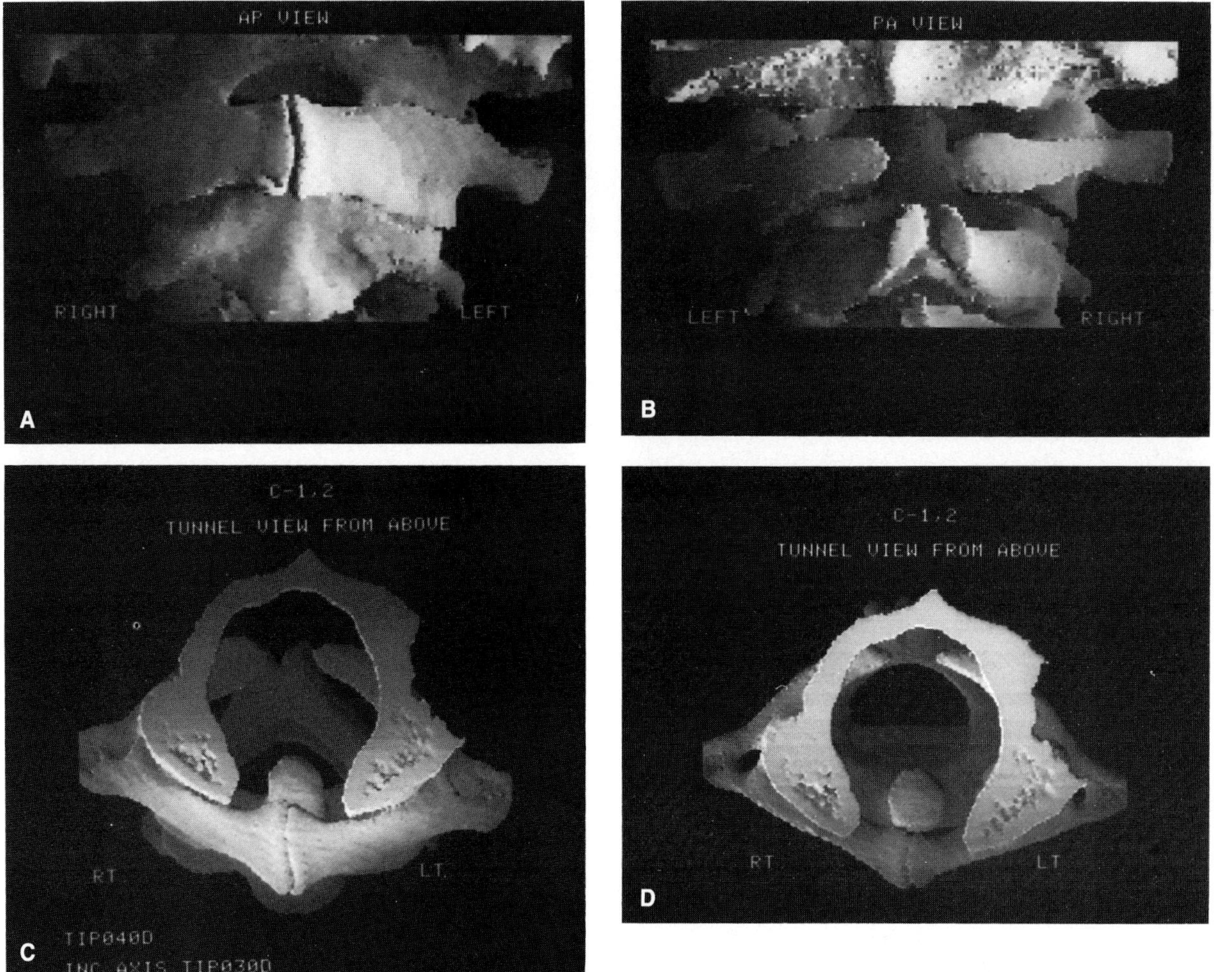

Fig. 3-54. Congenital Incomplete C1 Arch. This automobile accident victim had a C1 fracture questioned on his plain radiographs from the emergency room. (*A*) The 3-D CT A–P view shows a midline synchrondosis in the arch of C1. (*B*) The P–A view shows an incomplete posterior C1 arch and a bifid C2 posterior spinous process. (*C* and *D*) Forward rotation views were edited to show the inferior rim of the foramen magnum, the congenital anomalies of C1, the normal spinal canal size, and the anatomic alignment.

ter soft-tissue 3-D CT analysis. Semitransparent 3-D displays are being developed, which allow multiple contours to be simultaneously viewed; if the degree of transparency is adjusted and different colors are used for each contour, the physician can look through the surface of one structure to see the structure within. Stereoscopic displays are possible. Surgical procedures may be simulated by computer before the actual operation (plastic surgical reconstruction, osteotomy, and so forth). Three-dimensional anatomic models and custom designed prostheses are already being manufactured using 3-D CT data.

The medical application of 3-D displays is in its infancy. Even in this early stage of development, the potential benefits of 3-D images appear to be very important.

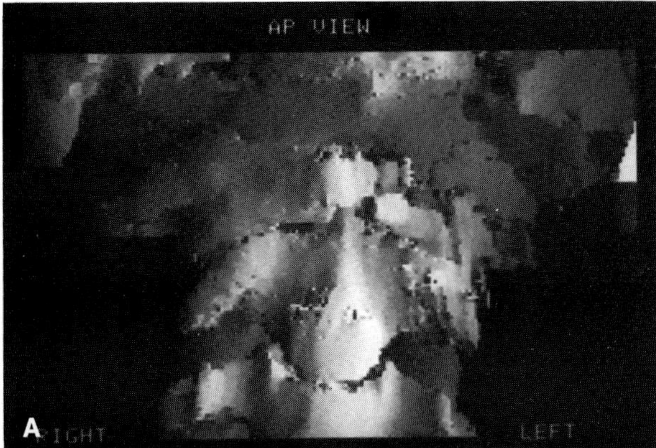

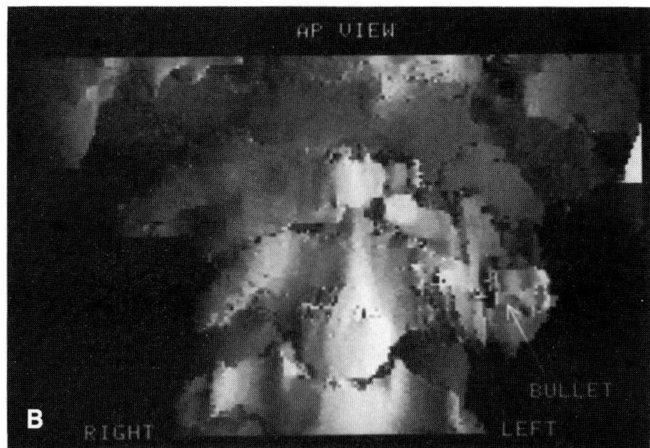

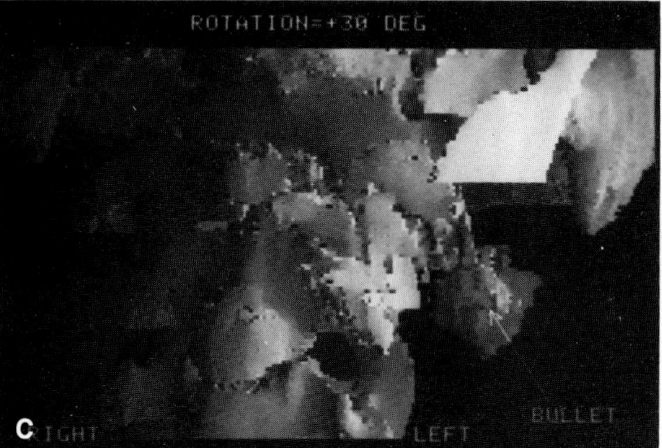

Fig. 3-55. C1–C2 Fracture secondary to gunshot wound. Three-dimensional CT images without (*A*) and with (*B* and *C*) an impacted bullet on the left at C1–C2 shows comminuted fractures of the left lateral mass and anterior arch of C1, and the left lateral mass of C2. The skull cants slightly toward the left. A 30° rotation view shows the bullet actually lies posterolateral to the spine on the left (*C*). The face has been edited out of the image to provide a clear view of C1–C2. (*B*) and (*C*) are composite images of separate bone and bullet 3-D CT images.

BIBLIOGRAPHY

Fishman EK, Drebin B, Magid D, et al: Volumetric rendering techniques: Applications for three dimensional imaging of the hip. Radiology 163:737–738, 1987

McAfee PC, Ullrich CG, Levinsohn EM, et al: Computed tomography in degenerative lumbar spinal stenosis: The value of multiplanar reconstruction. RadioGraphics 2:529–551, 1982

Pate D, Resnick D, Sartoris DJ, Andre M: 3D CT of the spine: Practical applications. Appl Radiol May:86–94, 1987

Rothman SLG, Glenn WV Jr: Multiplanar CT of the spine. Baltimore, University Park Press, 1985

Ullrich CG, Binet EF, Sanecki MG, Kieffer SA: Quantitative assessment of the lumbar spinal canal by computed tomography. Radiology 134:137–143, 1980

Ullrich CG, Kieffer SA: Computed tomographic evaluation of the lumbar spine: Quantitative aspects and sagittal-coronal reconstruction. In Post MJD (ed): Radiographic Evaluation of the Spine, Current Advances with Emphasis on Computed Tomography. New York, Masson Publishing, 1980

Zinriech SJ, Rosenbaum AE, Wang H, et al: The critical role of 3-D CT reconstruction for defining spinal disease. Acta Radiol 369:699–702, 1986

ACKNOWLEDGMENTS

I would like to acknowledge Betty Smith Hinson for preparing this manuscript and Joyce Sisk RT for photographing the illustrations for this book chapter. Without their enthusiastic effort, this chapter would not have been possible.

Magnetic Resonance Imaging of the Cervical Spine and Spinal Cord

CHRISTOPHER G. ULLRICH

Magnetic resonance imaging (MRI) is based on the physical phenomena of nuclear magnetic resonance (NMR). Physicists Edward M. Purcell of Harvard University and Felix Bloch of Stanford University independently described NMR in 1946 and received the 1952 Nobel Prize for this achievement. NMR spectroscopy has become a powerful analytic technique for studying the chemistry of molecules and their physical structure. Attempts to apply NMR techniques to medical imaging began about 1970. Working at the State University of New York Downstate Medical Center, Raymond Damadian's research team produced the first whole-body human image on July 3, 1977. Images of much smaller objects had previously been obtained by Damadian, and by other research groups including Paul Lauterbur at SUNY Stonybrook and Peter Mansfield, Waldo Hinshaw and E. Raymond Andrews at the University of Nottingham. Although crude, Damadian's image demonstrated that a powerful medical imaging device was possible. Intense commercial development followed, with the first Food and Drug Administration Market Approvals for MRI devices granted in 1984. MR technology continues to evolve rapidly.

This section briefly reviews the technical concepts related to MRI. The characteristic appearance of these images is described and specific clinical applications in the cervical spine and spinal cord are illustrated. Lastly, speculation concerning future development and medical applications of MRI is discussed.

BASIC TECHNICAL CONCEPTS OF NMR

While a detailed physics explanation of NMR is well beyond the scope of this chapter, a basic concept of the underlying physical phenomena involved in NMR is essential to understanding MRI.

Simply stated, atoms whose nuclei contain an odd number of protons and neutrons resemble a continually spinning top and behave as a small bar magnet. In nature, these atoms are randomly aligned and no magnetic forces are apparent. When an external magnetic field is applied, its force tends to align the magnetic poles of the spinning nuclei. Most of the nuclei will be in a low-energy state, in alignment with the external magnetic field. High-energy nuclei align themselves against the external magnetic field.

The spinning nuclei precess around the vector of the external magnetic field, resembling wobbling tops. Each nucleus precesses (wobbles) at its own specific frequency. This is called the Larmor or resonant frequency. It is determined by the strength of the "bar magnet" of the nucleus, and the strength of the externally applied magnetic field. If a radio wave at the exact resonant frequency is beamed at right angles to the magnetic field, some low energy nuclei will absorb energy, undergo a "spin flip," and convert to the high-energy state. This absorbed energy is emitted at the same radio frequency when the nucleus returns to the low-energy state. This characteristic absorption and release of specific radio frequencies is descriptively termed *nuclear magnetic resonance.*

The character of the high-energy nucleus can also be described by the time it takes to return to the low-energy state. The spin-lattice relaxation time, T1, is determined by the interaction between the nucleus and its environment (*lattice*). The spin-spin relaxation time, T2, describes the interaction between adjacent nuclei. Therefore, the same high-energy nucleus will emit its characteristic radio signal at different times, depending on what surrounds it. These properties (resonant frequency, T1, and T2) form the basis of NMR spectroscopy and make it a powerful technique for analyzing molecules and their environment.

MAGNETIC RESONANCE IMAGING

The terms NMRI and MRI are equivalent, but the latter term is preferred in the diagnostic radiology literature. This is due to the prevalent public phobia about anything identified as "nuclear," and to distinguish this method from nuclear medicine techniques involving radioactive isotopes.

Magnetic field strength is measured in tesla (T) units. MRI devices are broadly categorized as low field (less than 0.3 T), midfield (0.3 to 0.9 T), and high field (1.0 T or greater). MRI devices that are 1.5 T are of the highest field strength currently approved by the FDA. A superconducting magnet is most commonly used in midfield and high-field systems. These devices produce an extremely uniform magnetic field, a very desirable feature. They are costly to build and operate. Resistive magnets, used in low-field systems, are easier to maintain and operate, but they produce a less stable magnetic field. Permanent magnets, used in low- or mid-field systems, produce a very stable magnetic field, but field uniformity comparable to that of superconducting magnets is difficult to achieve. Regardless of the magnet used or magnetic field strength employed, excellent cervical spine images can be obtained if proper imaging techniques are utilized. The images illustrating this chapter were produced with either a 0.15 T resistive magnet or 1.5 T superconducting magnet systems.

The NMR spectrometer obtains its signal from the entire sample volume. In order to mathematically reconstruct an image, the MR signal must be localized within the object being imaged. This localization is usually obtained using a gradient technique. A gradient is a small secondary magnetic field that has a known variable strength. Magnetic field strength influences the exact resonant frequency. With a gradient applied, the slightly different radio frequencies detected determine where the signal arises. This, in combination with the shape and orientation of the radio frequency pulse, determines the precise location of the signal and permits mathematical image reconstruction. Most machines use 2-D Fourier transformation mathematics to calculate the MR image from the detected signal in a manner similar to x-ray computed tomography (CT).

Two time variables describe how the machine functions and determine the nature of the image obtained. The repetition time interval between radio frequency input pulses is termed *TR*. After the input pulse, the time at which the echo (emitted resonant radio frequency signal) is detected is termed *TE*. These time values are expressed in milliseconds.

At present, virtually all clinical MRI is performed using the hydrogen nuclei signal (proton imaging). Hydrogen, as a constituent of water, is the most abundant resonant nucleus in soft tissues and therefore provides the strongest signal. Other nuclei such as sodium and phosphorus may be imaged using high-field-strength systems, but the image quality is low owing to the weak signals obtained. Well-described practical clinical applications for these additional nuclei remain to be developed.

The methods for acquiring MRI data are termed *pulse sequences*. Spin echo (SE), inversion recovery (IR), and saturation recovery (SR) are some of the techniques used. Spin-echo pulse sequences, the most commonly used MRI technique, are described by TR and TE values. By varying these factors, different tissue-contrast relationships are obtained. If short TR/TE technique (*i.e.*, SE = 500/30) is used, the image is termed *T1-weighted*, because most of the detected echo signals reflect the T1-governed nuclear interactions (spin lattice). The resulting image (Fig. 3-56*A*) shows a low signal from cortical bone owing to a paucity of water molecules. The cerebrospinal fluid is hypointense, relative to muscle and spinal cord, because of its short T1 value. Fat has an increased signal relative to the spinal cord, while most lesions are either low or isointense compared with the spinal cord. These T1-weighted images tend to have the best spatial resolution, because the strongest signal is obtained with such pulse sequences.

Long TR/TE techniques (*i.e.*, SE = 2500/120) are termed *T2-weighted* images, because most of the detected signal is determined by the T2 (spin-spin) interactions of the nuclei (Fig. 3-56*B*). The emitted signal due to T1-governed events has already dissipated. The cerebrospinal fluid now demonstrates greater intensity than the spinal cord, producing the so-called pseudomyelogram effect. The bone signal remains very low compared with the spinal cord, while fat continues to show an increased signal. Pathologic processes tend to show an increased signal compared with the spinal cord, because in most cases they are associated with increased tissue water. Small lesions lying in the spinal fluid or adjacent to it can be obscured when both the spinal fluid and the lesion demonstrate an increased signal.

Images produced using long TR and short TE technique (*i.e.*, SE = 2500/30) are termed *balanced* because relatively equal contributions of T1- and T2-governed echoes are involved. In the cervical spine, this technique may allow pathologic processes to have a high signal, while the spinal fluid remains isointense or hypointense relative to the spinal cord. Lesions that may be masked on a more heavily T2-weighted image might now be apparent.

Data acquisition in MRI is usually performed with a 2-D technique in which multiple adjacent images are simultaneously obtained. A small gap is often present between these successive images. Direct axial, coronal, and sagittal image planes are produced without moving the patient, but separate data acquisitions must be performed for each image plane. It is often possible to obtain two or more TE values simultaneously as well (so-called *dual* or *multiecho* techniques). Single-image, single-echo, rapid data acquisition techniques are also being

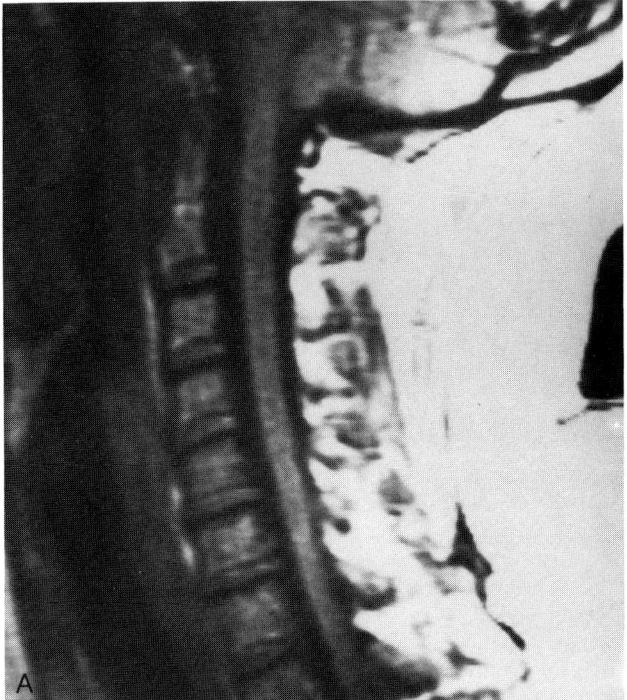

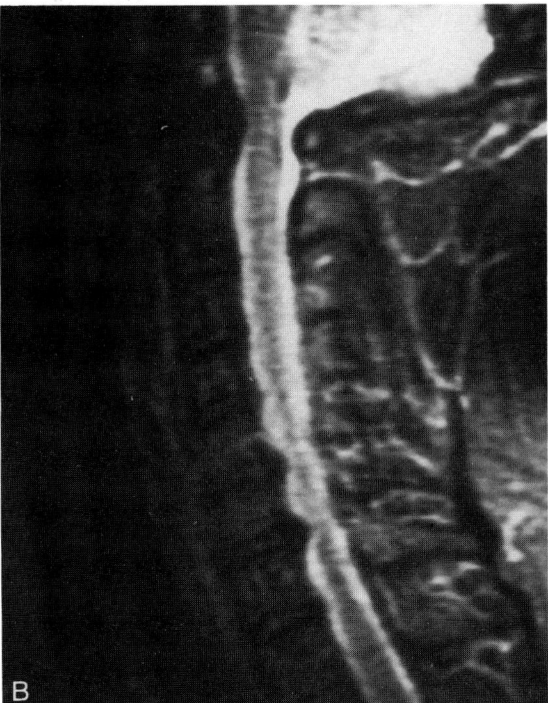

Fig. 3-56. Spin-echo technique MRI. (*A*) T1-weighted image (sagittal plane 1.5 T, SE = 600/20); (*B*) T2-weighted image (sagittal plane 1.5 T, SE = 2500/70). Making the spinal cord the reference density, cortical bone has a low signal and fat has a high signal on both T1 and T2 images. Cerebrospinal fluid (CSF) is low intensity on the T1-weighted image (*A*) and high intensity on the T2-weighted image (pseudomyelogram) (*B*). On T1-weighted images, intraaxial lesions are low or isointense compared with the spinal cord, and become high intensity compared with the spinal cord on T2-weighted images. Spinal cord lesions can be obscured by high-intensity CSF on T2-weighted images. Spondylotic anterior extradural defects are present at C5–C6 and C6–C7 in this patient.

developed. Images may be gated to cardiac or respiratory cycles to minimize physiologic motion-induced image artifacts.

Volume imaging techniques are also feasible. Once obtained, any desired image plane can be extracted from the data volume, which is a great advantage. Unfortunately, data acquisition times tend to be very long with these techniques, a factor that tends to make this approach impractical in most circumstances.

Three general types of receiver coils are employed to acquire MRI data—head, body, and surface coils (Fig. 3-57). The head coil has a field of view equivalent to that of a CT scan of the brain. Axial images are produced in a true axial plane, rather than in the angled axial plane often used for CT. The upper cervical spine down to the level of the C2–C3 interspace is usually well seen with this device. The body coil has a large field of view that is similar to a whole-body CT scan. The cervical and thoracic spine to the T8 level can usually be seen in one sagittal image with such a coil. Since the field of view is large, spinal cord image detail tends to be only fair. Nonetheless, such a coil is useful for screening purposes. The surface coil is a small device that is positioned directly over the area of interest. These coils produce the highest-resolution MR images and are very useful in cervical spine evaluations. They are often custom designed for specific anatomic examinations. The images they produce are analogous to high-resolution CT images. For the cervical spine, the surface coil is usually positioned at the back of the neck.

In summary, MRI is performed by placing the patient in an external uniform and stable magnetic

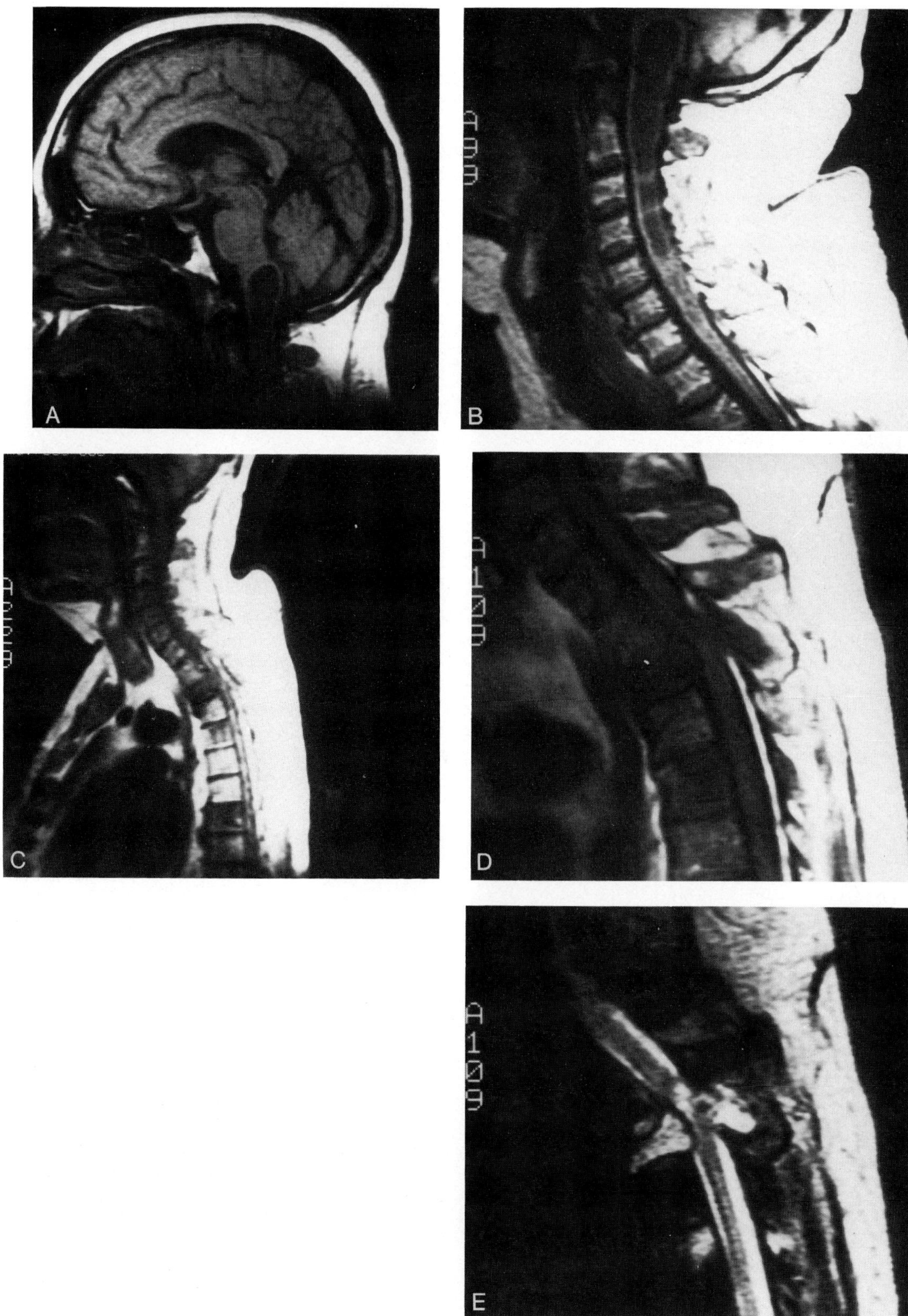
A
B
C
D
E

Fig. 3-57. Imaging coils. (*A*) Head coil (sagittal, 1.5 T, SE = 600/20): the field of view extends from the top of the head to approximately C2. The foramen magnum and upper cervical spine are well demonstrated with this coil. A cystic lesion extending from the medulla downward to the cervical spinal cord is seen. (*B*) Surface coil (sagittal, 1.5 T, SE = 600/30): the field of view extends from the foramen magnum to D2. This coil provides the best image quality of the cervical spine and is the coil of choice for most cervical spine examinations. High-quality cervical spine imaging is difficult to perform without the use of a surface coil. This lesion is a hemangioblastoma with a large cyst extending from C6 upward to the medulla. (*C*) Body coil (sagittal, 1.5 T, SE = 500/30): the field of view extends from the 4th ventricle to approximately D8. This coil is excellent for survey examinations where clinical localization is poor. The spinal cord detail is inferior to either head or surface coils, but large segments of the spinal cord can be evaluated rapidly using this coil. This patient with metastatic lung cancer shows multiple vertebral body lesions. The D2 vertebral body has collapsed. (*D*) Surface coil (sagittal, 1.5 T, SE = 500/20): the D2 vertebral body collapse and associated metastatic lung cancer with cord compression are shown in much better detail than in *C*. The D4 vertebral body shows a lesion without collapse. (*E*) Surface coil (sagittal, 1.5 T, SE = 2500/120): this is a T2-weighted image of the same area as *D*. The tumor at D2 and D4 is now white (high signal). The CSF has become white, producing a "pseudomyelogram" effect. Obvious spinal cord compression is seen.

field. A radio frequency pulse is beamed into the patient to induce the NMR phenomena. A receiver coil detects the emitted radio frequency as the nuclei revert to a low-energy state within the magnetic field. Gradients produce slight local variations in the strength of the magnetic field and permit spatial localization of the emitted resonant frequency. This detected signal is mathematically processed using 2-D Fourier transformation into the MR image. By varying TR and TE factors, spin-echo images that are T1- or T2-weighted are produced. T1 images have the best spatial resolution, while T2 images tend to accentuate pathology.

ADVANTAGES AND LIMITATIONS OF MRI

MRI involves nonionizing forms of radiation and is considered safe by current testing standards. No known deleterious effects are produced in an otherwise normal individual. The technique is noninvasive; no contrast agents are routinely employed at the present time. Its high lesion sensitivity is due to the excellent contrast resolution. By varying pulse sequences, specific tissue contrast can be enhanced and occasionally specific tissues are identified. The technique allows direct sagittal, coronal, and axial images to be obtained, and volume imaging techniques are feasible. Well known x-ray–associated imaging artifacts, such as streaks secondary to beam hardening or metal clips and dental fillings, are largely avoided.

MRI is subject to several limitations. Most of the current imaging techniques involve relatively long data acquisition time. Two-dimensional multislice spin-echo techniques can require anywhere from 3 to 15 minutes of acquisition time. Volume spin-echo imaging techniques can require 30 or more minutes of imaging time. Recently developed gradient pulse techniques (*i.e.,* GRASS by General Electric) allow rapid data acquisition (2 seconds or less per image), while retaining good image quality. Experience with these gradient pulse techniques is very limited at present.

Using spin-echo techniques, flowing blood usually produces the *flow void* effect. This results in apparent low-signal intensity in most blood vessels. This occurs when blood flow moves the high-energy nuclei in the blood stream from the image plane before the echo signal is detected. However, in very slow flowing blood vessels, or in vessels with turbulent flow, isointense or increased signals may be obtained. A similar but less severe cerebrospinal fluid flow artifact can occur (Fig. 3-58). This artifact occasionally causes diagnostic confusion on MRI cervical spine examination.

Physiologic motions, including blood vessel pulsation, cause MRI artifacts, particularly with high-field-strength systems. The vertebral arteries are especially troublesome in the cervical spine. Cardiac gating techniques can overcome the problem, but they lengthen total examination time. Swallowing also degrades cervical spine studies. If long MRI examination time is anticipated, IM atropine

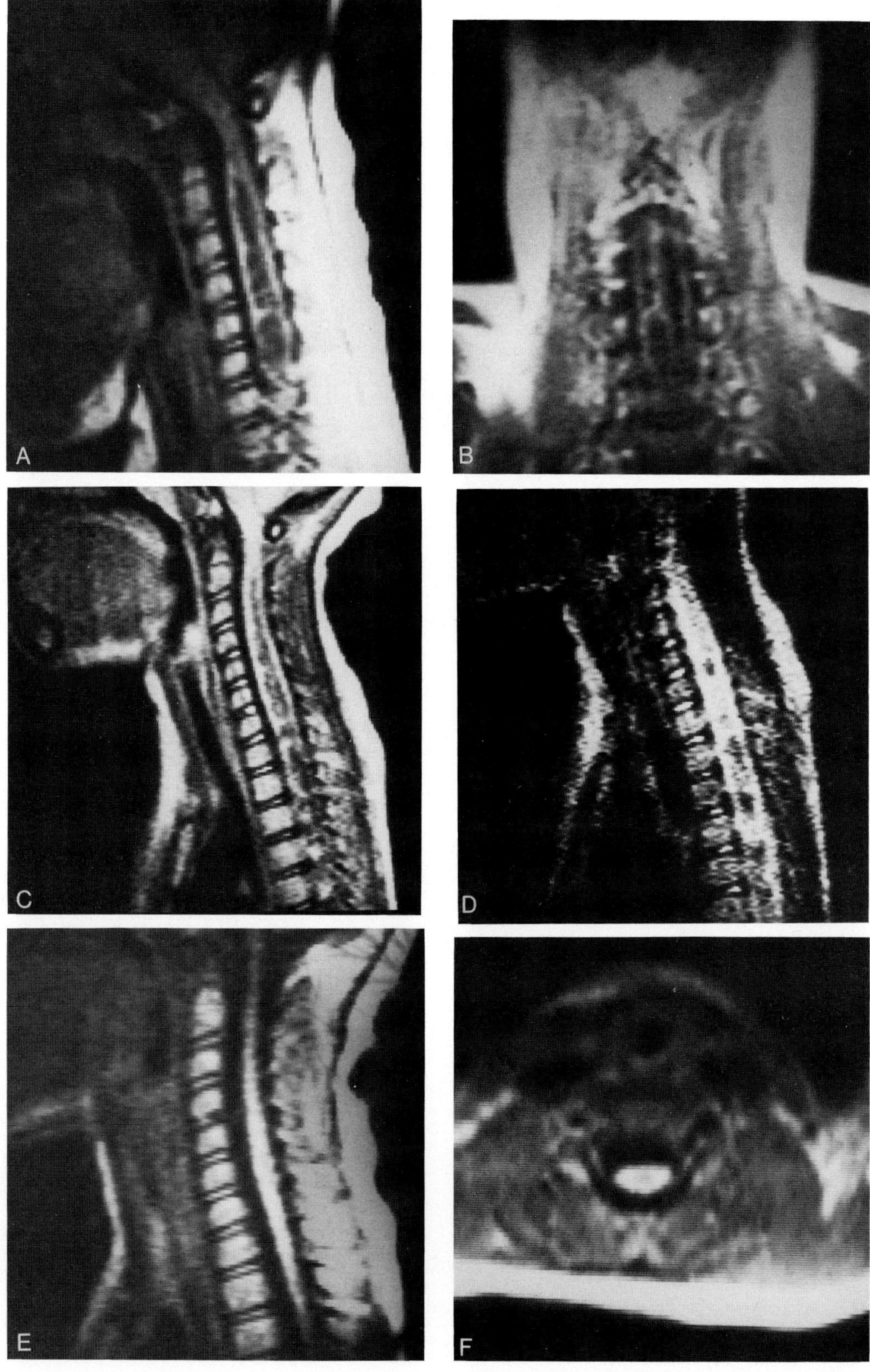
A
B
C
D
E
F

Fig. 3-58. Chiari I malformation with syringomyelia. This 7-year-old child presented with vocal cord paralysis. Sagittal (*A*) and coronal (*B*) T1-weighted MR images (SE = 500/35) show the septated syrinx (*arrow*). Very little tonsillar tissue projects into the foramen magnum. Sagittal balanced (SE = 2200/35) and heavily T2-weighted (SE = 2200/140) images (*C* and *D*) show mixed signal response within the syrinx due to variable pulsation velocities within the cyst compartments. Follow-up sagittal (*E*) and axial (*F*) T1-weighted images (SE = 500/35) show syrinx collapse 6 months after ventriculoperitoneal shunting. The patient is clinically normal at the time of follow-up examination.

reduces oral secretions, and therefore the urge to swallow. Instructing the patient to swallow between data acquisitions is also helpful.

Image artifacts associated with MRI data acquisition can cause interpretation difficulties. The *chemical shift* artifact occurs due to spatial misregistration at fat-water interfaces. The apparent margin is shifted slightly in the direction of the phase-encoding gradient. The error is most pronounced with high-field-strength MRI. Once recognized, the error is usually apparent to the trained observer.

Implanted metal, such as surgical clips and orthopedic hardware, causes local distortion of the magnetic field and therefore localized image degradation. Although the MR signal is locally disrupted, the remainder of the image is often surprisingly intact. For example, the spinal cord may be well seen in spite of Harrington rods. In addition, much of the supporting equipment and external stabilization hardware used in the treatment of severely traumatized patients cannot be safely brought into the MRI suite. This problem is most severe when high-field-strength systems are utilized.

Claustrophobic patients find the MR imager difficult to tolerate because it resembles a long narrow tube. Patient movement induces significant artifacts in most MR images. Patients with cardiac pacemakers cannot be placed within the device, owing to magnet-induced pacemaker malfunction. Cerebral aneurysm clips and embedded ferromagnetic metal fragments may cause injury if dislodged by the force of the magnetic field. Patients are routinely questioned about these factors before entering the MR suite.

Physician inexperience in performing and interpreting MRI is an additional problem that should decrease as the technique is more widely employed.

MRI examinations are not as readily available as CT. MRI is presently from 50% to over 100% more costly than comparable CT cervical spine examinations. Where MRI is not superior to CT, it is not presently cost-effective.

APPLICATIONS OF MRI IN THE CERVICAL SPINE

MRI has superior soft-tissue contrast resolution when compared with CT and conventional noninvasive x-ray techniques. Since the spinal cord is well seen without the use of intrathecal contrast agents, intraaxial spinal cord lesions are best studied using MRI. Clinical myelopathy due to an extraaxial lesion compressing the spinal cord is also well evaluated by MRI, particularly when the process is poorly localized by clinical findings. CT is often diagnostically equal to MRI if the cord compression lesion is clinically well localized. CT is superior to MRI in defining spondylotic spurs, calcifications, and bone fractures. Myelography and CT are equal or superior to MRI for the evaluation of radiculopathy secondary to small disc herniations within the neural foramen, and for small epidural and intradural metastatic lesions. CT myelography is equal to MRI in evaluation of extraaxial cord compression cases, but it is invasive. Both infections and carcinomatous meningitis are still best diagnosed by cerebrospinal fluid studies.

MRI is particularly useful in the craniocervical junction region. The commonly encountered streak artifacts due to x-ray beam hardening seen with CT are eliminated with MRI. The clear visualization of the medulla and cervical spinal cord is very helpful. The direct sagittal image plane best displays many of the important anatomic relationships in the area.

The Chiari malformation is a commonly encountered craniocervical junction lesion (Fig. 3-58). Not only is the dysplastic cerebellar tissue in the upper cervical canal reliably demonstrated, but the associated intracranial and spinal cord abnormalities are all well evaluated with MRI. Noninvasive CT evaluation is particularly limited with regard to the spinal cord findings.

Upward migration of the odontoid into the foramen magnum occurs with rheumatoid arthritis or with basilar invagination. Serious clinical effects develop if the cervicomedullary junction is compressed by the odontoid (Fig. 3-59). C1–C2 instability and its effects on the spinal cord may be studied by performing flexion and extension MRI studies. The direct sagittal MR image is particularly helpful in studying such patients.

Extraaxial foramen magnum mass lesions such as meningioma are occasionally encountered (Fig. 3-60). Meningioma usually appears as an isointense lesion to brain on T1-weighted images, but it appears hypointense if it is heavily calcified. On T2-weighted images, the lesion may be "lost" in the high-signal cerebrospinal fluid. An en plaque meningioma that does not produce much mass effect may be very difficult to demonstrate with any of the imaging techniques. CT often detects calcification in such lesions, a finding that would

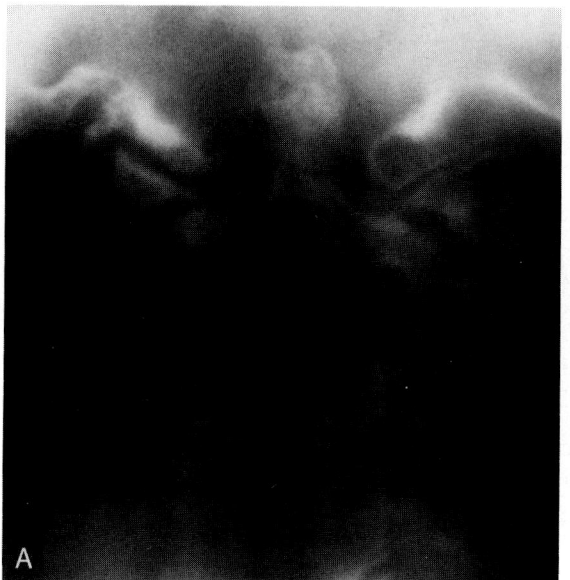

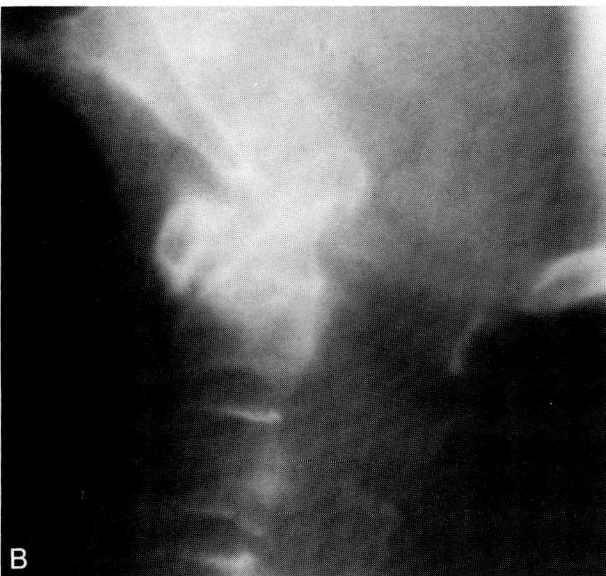

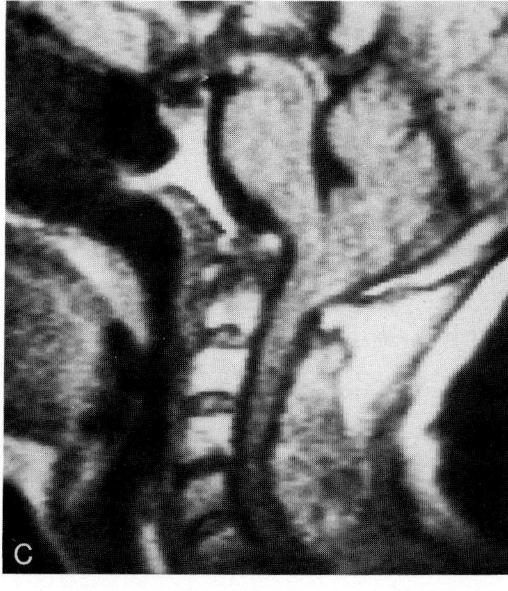

Fig. 3-59. Rheumatoid arthritis. A–P and lateral tomograms (*A* and *B*) show upward migration of an eroded odontoid process consistent with rheumatoid arthritis. Sagittal T1-weighted MRI (*C*) shows the odontoid deforming the medulla. Note that the odontoid, which is predominantly calcified, gives a very low MR signal relative to the brain.

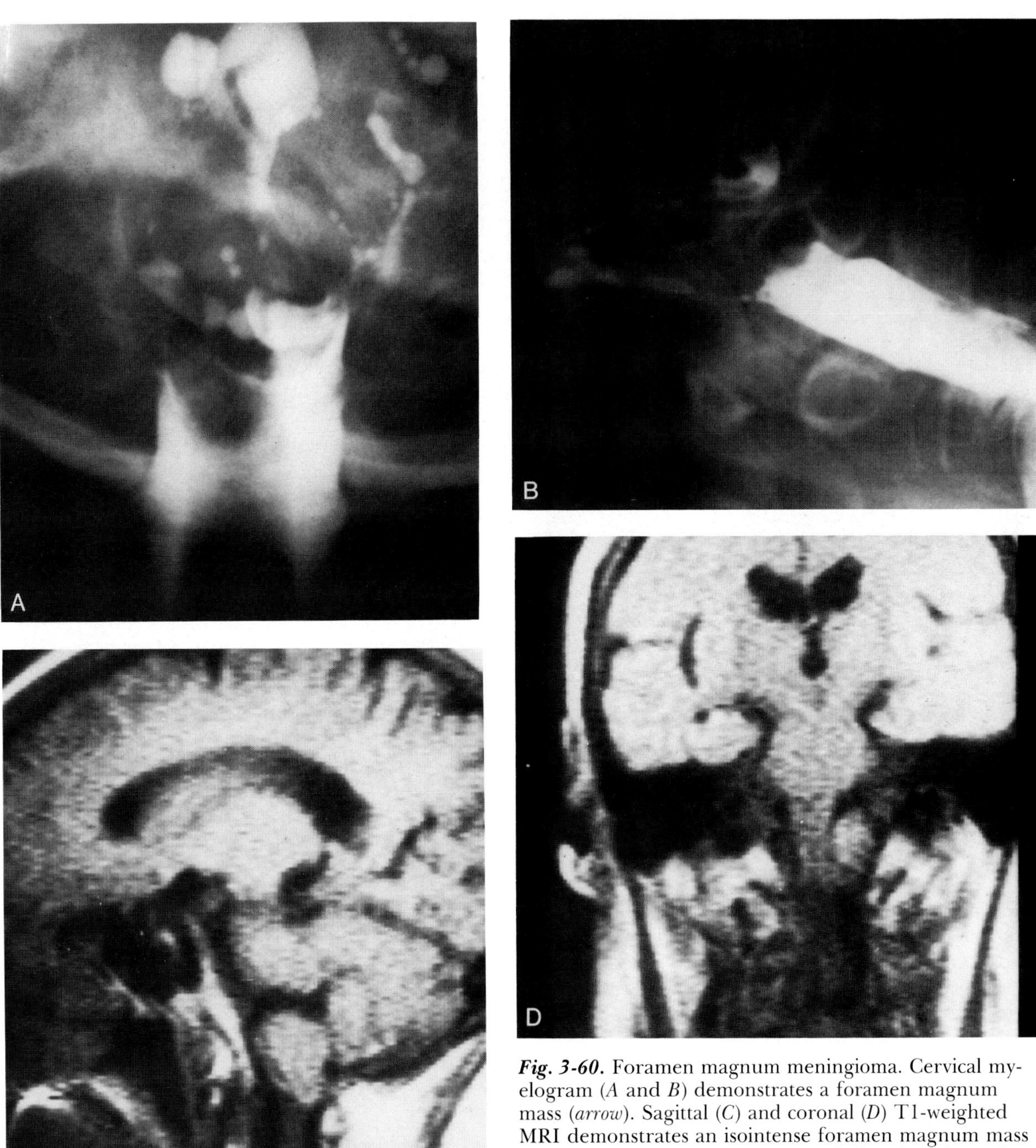

Fig. 3-60. Foramen magnum meningioma. Cervical myelogram (*A* and *B*) demonstrates a foramen magnum mass (*arrow*). Sagittal (*C*) and coronal (*D*) T1-weighted MRI demonstrates an isointense foramen magnum mass (*arrow*) compressing the cervicomedullary junction. The lesion did not show definite signal increase on T2-weighted images. A meningioma was confirmed at surgery.

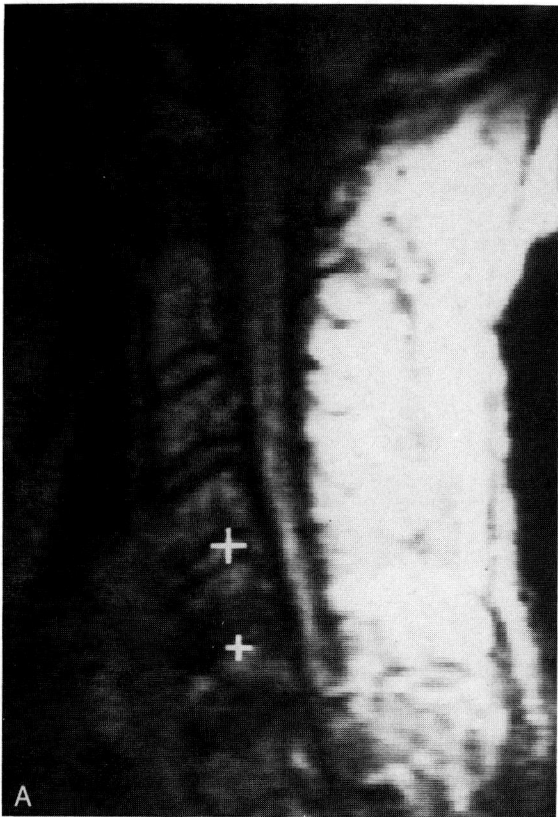

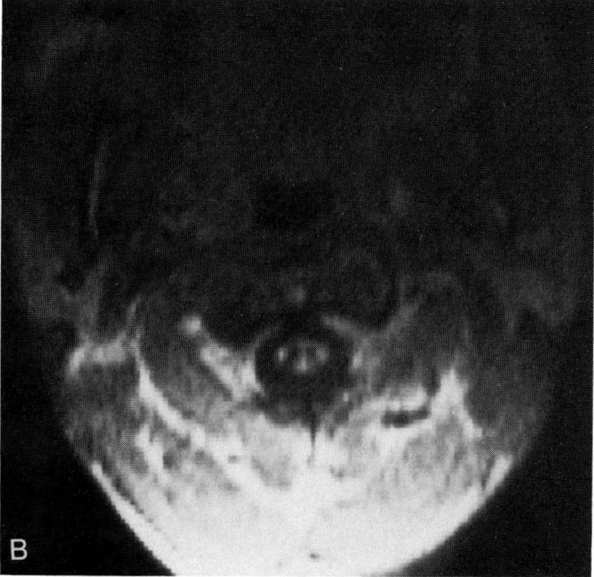

Fig. 3-61. Posttraumatic syrinx. This patient was quadriplegic following a C5 burst fracture 1 year prior to this MRI study. (*A*) Sagittal T1-weighted MRI shows what appears to be a single thin upper cervical syrinx. Residual cord compression at C5 is also noted (+). (*B*) Axial T1-weighted MRI at C2 shows two distinct syrinx cavities. Examination by MRI of the cervical spine performed only in the sagittal plane is often incomplete or inadequate.

be missed with MRI. Rarely, an exophytic tumor such as a glioma is present; MR is superior to CT for demonstrating these lesions.

Syringohydromyelia may be associated with the Chiari malformation (Fig. 3-58), spinal cord tumor, spinal cord trauma (Fig. 3-61), or a more obscure cause. If the syrinx has multiple septae, a mixed signal MRI response may be obtained owing to variable pulsation velocities in the lesion (Fig. 3-58). The resulting areas of increased MR signal should not be confused with a spinal cord tumor. The clinically unsuspected syrinx is probably more common than previously believed. MRI is superior to CT myelography for both the diagnosis and the follow-up study of syringohydromyelia. Intraoperative ultrasonography has occasionally demonstrated very small cystic spinal cord lesions that were missed by MRI or CT myelography due to inadequate spatial and contrast resolution.

Spinal cord tumor, either primary or secondary, often manifests itself as an isointense widening or distortion of the normal spinal cord contour on T1-weighted images. If fat or recent hemorrhage is present, an increased signal is seen with T1-weighted images. On T2-weighted images, a diffuse increased signal is seen within the spinal cord. It is often difficult to distinguish between the tumor and associated spinal cord edema. Unfortunately, this high-signal MRI appearance is relatively nonspecific. Acute multiple sclerosis (Fig. 3-62), infection, and cord trauma (Fig. 3-63) produce very similar MRI findings. It is important to note that the diseased spinal cord may appear normal on T1-weighted images. When an intrinsic spinal cord lesion is suspected, T2-weighted images are essential for complete examination.

Reliable MRI demonstration of the spinal cord lesions of multiple sclerosis (Fig. 3-64) has not been achieved. Clinically silent brain lesions may be identified by MRI in patients whose presenting symptoms are primarily in the spinal cord. MRI can reliably exclude compressive spinal cord lesions mimicking multiple sclerosis. Total myelography no longer needs to be performed in these patients if high-quality MRI is available.

Causes of spinal cord compression include cen-

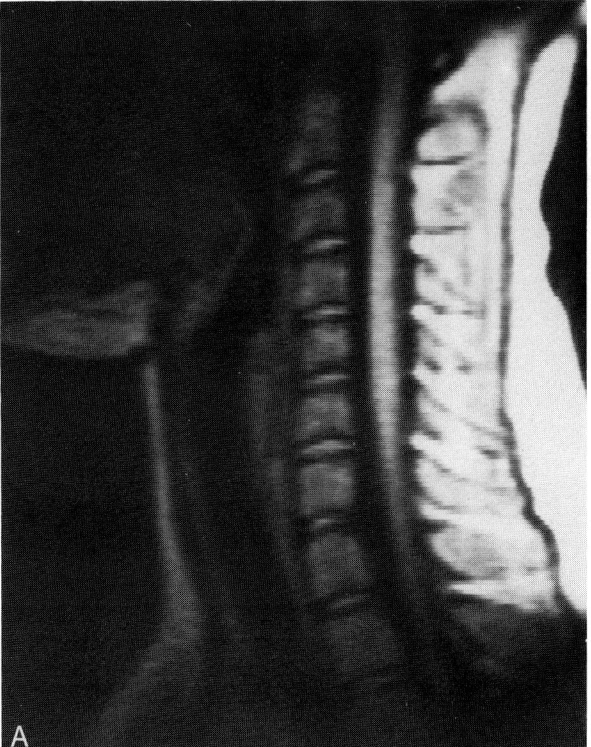

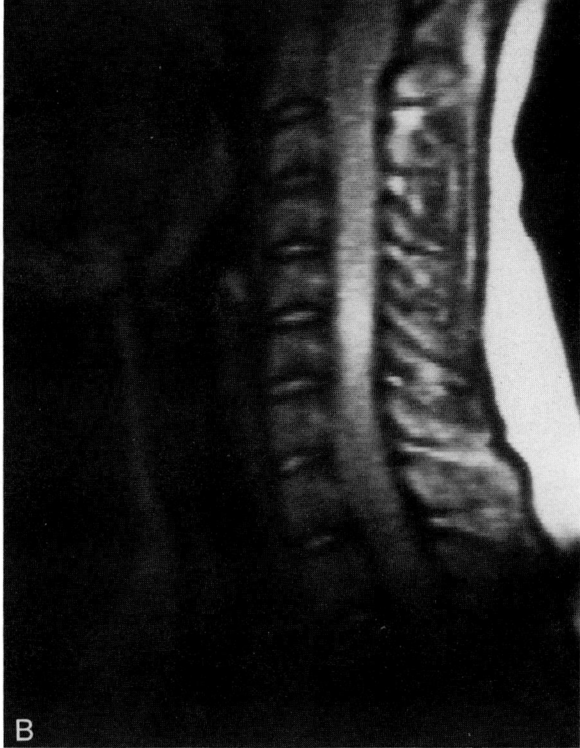

Fig. 3-62. Multiple sclerosis. This 21-year-old female presented with a rapidly progressive C5–C6 spinal cord lesion. No history of trauma or recent viral illness was obtained. Sagittal T1-weighted MRI (*A*) is normal, but a definite abnormal signal from the spinal cord at C6 (−) is seen on the T2-weighted image (*B*) (SE = 2000/70). Axial T2-weighted brain images (not shown) revealed a small periventricular white matter lesion consistent with multiple sclerosis. At present, MRI inconsistently demonstrates multiple sclerosis lesions in the spinal cord. The MR appearance of this lesion is very similar to posttraumatic myelomalacia demonstrated on Figure 3-63.

tral disc herniation (Figs. 3-65, 3-66), spondylosis (Fig. 3-67), tumor (Fig. 3-68), abscess, hematoma, and bone fragments. Spinal cord atrophy develops secondary to cord compression (Figs. 3-67 and 3-68), trauma, ischemia, or infection (Fig. 3-64). Atrophy is either focal or diffuse. Atrophy, as distinct from spinal cord compression, is irreversible. In T1-weighted MRI, the atrophic spinal cord typically appears thin in the sagittal projection and flat or triangular on axial images. A surprisingly normal appearance occurs in the coronal projection, because the dentate ligaments, which lie lateral to the spinal cord, tether the spinal cord margins. As a result, spinal cord width is relatively maintained, even though considerable spinal cord substance has been lost. This observation also explains the relatively subtle conventional myelographic findings in many cases of mild and moderate spinal cord atrophy. Hemiatrophy of the spinal cord is easily missed if only sagittal MRI is performed; obtaining axial MRI avoids this error. CT myelography is diagnostically equivalent to MRI for the evaluation of spinal cord atrophy.

Extraaxial lesions are usually best examined in both the sagittal and axial projections. If the bone or disc space is not involved, it may be very difficult to distinguish an intradural from an extradural process (Fig. 3-68) by MRI. Small intradural and epidural tumors may be "lost" with T2-weighted imaging, owing to the similar high cerebrospinal fluid and tumor signals. Thin epidural lesions can easily be overlooked if only sagittal images are obtained. Lesions large enough to produce a clinical myelopathy are difficult to miss on sagittal MRI, but complete spinal cord examination still requires axial images in many cases.

Malignant epidural tumors virtually all demonstrate increased T2 signals. Cortical bone destruc-

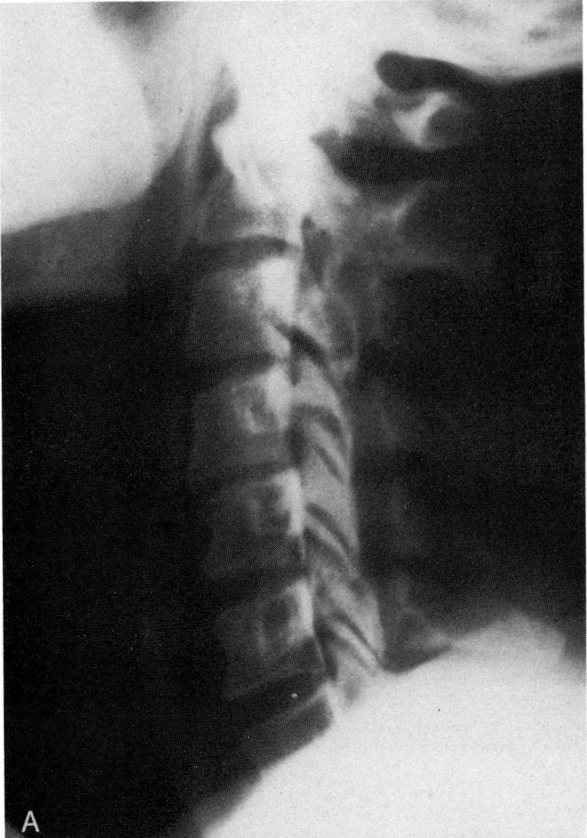

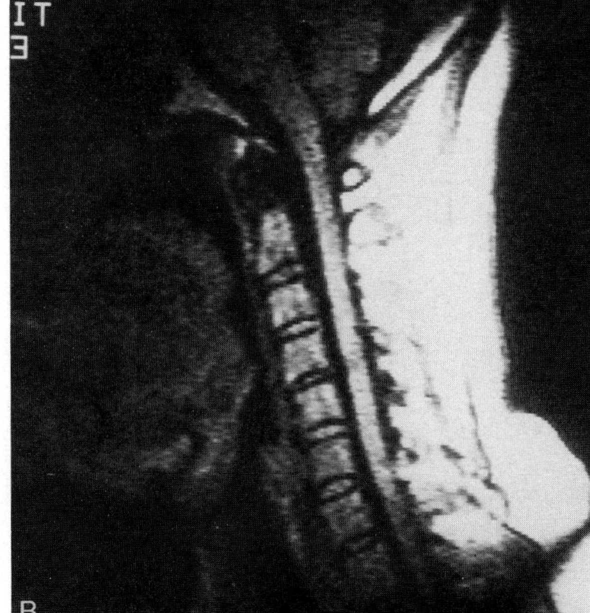

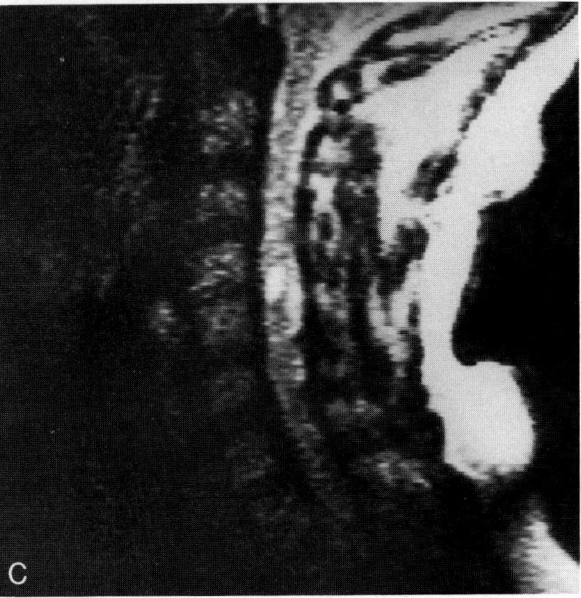

Fig. 3-63. Posttraumatic cervical myelomalacia. Six weeks prior to MRI, this 43-year-old male sustained a central spinal cord injury which had not resolved. (*A*) A lateral cervical spine radiograph shows moderate narrowing of the C4–C5 disc space. (*B*) Sagittal T1-weighted MRI shows a subtle low signal in the spinal cord at C4–C5 (*arrow*). A disc herniation or cord compression is not identified. (*C*) Sagittal T2-weighted MRI shows a definite increased signal at C4–C5 from the spinal cord. The finding is consistent with posttraumatic myelomalacia.

tion is inferred from the loss of the thin low-signal bone margin. If the bone marrow is involved, T1-weighted images show a reduced marrow signal with preservation of the disc spaces. Epidural abscess also manifests an increased T2 signal, often extends over multiple spinal segments, and may be associated with destroyed bone and disc space. Epidural non-Hodgkin's lymphoma resembles an abscess, but bone and disc spaces are spared. Clinical history is obviously very helpful in assigning an appropriate differential diagnosis in these situations.

Benign extraaxial tumors have a more variable MRI appearance. Neurofibromata and spinal cord are isodense on T1-weighted images (Fig. 3-68), but inconsistently demonstrate increased T2 signal. If a single lesion extends outward from the spinal canal through the neural foramen, a relatively confident diagnosis of neural sheath tumor (neurofibroma, schwannoma, etc.) may be made.

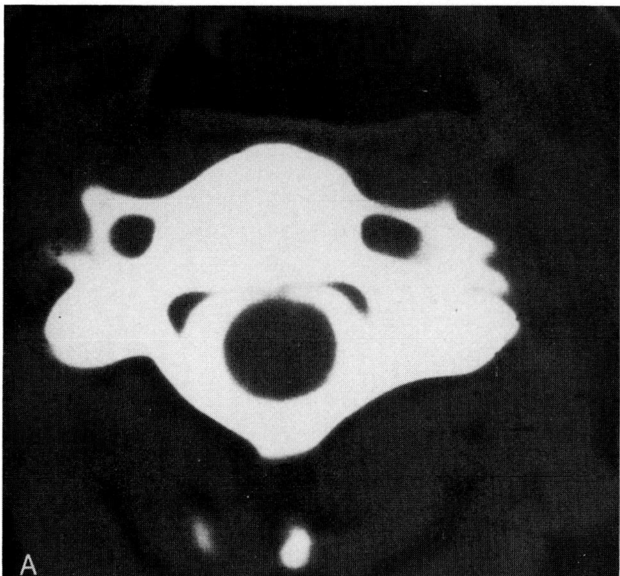

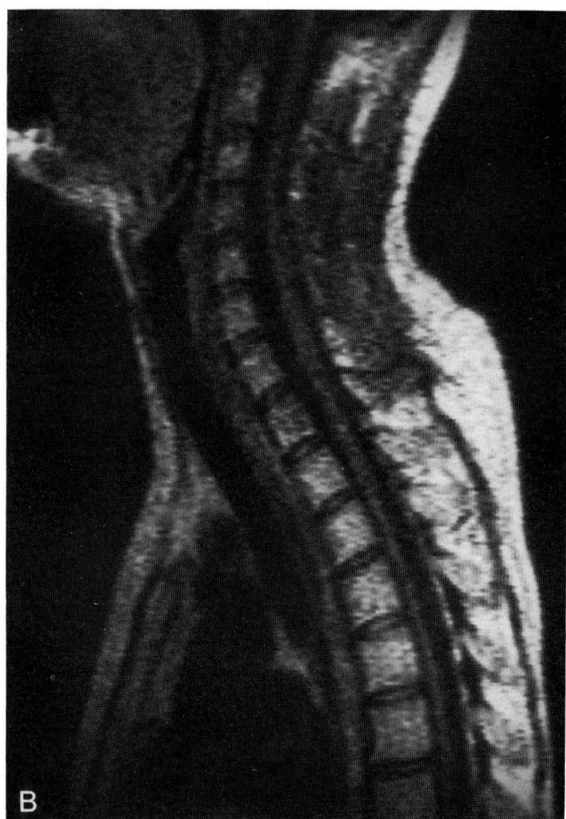

Fig. 3-64. Spinal cord atrophy secondary to presumed viral myelitis. This 25-year-old female developed a severe myelitis in May, 1984. (*A*) CT myelography demonstrates diffuse spinal cord swelling at C5. The patient survived with severe quadriparesis. (*B*) Sagittal T1-weighted MRI performed in December 1984 shows moderately severe midcervical spinal cord atrophy without evidence of a surgically treatable lesion such as a syrinx.

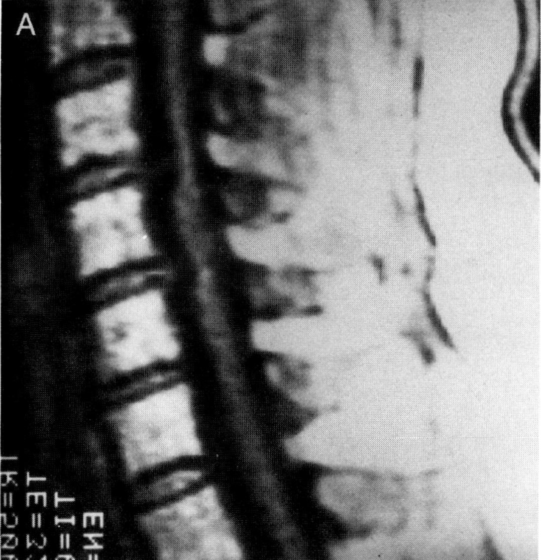

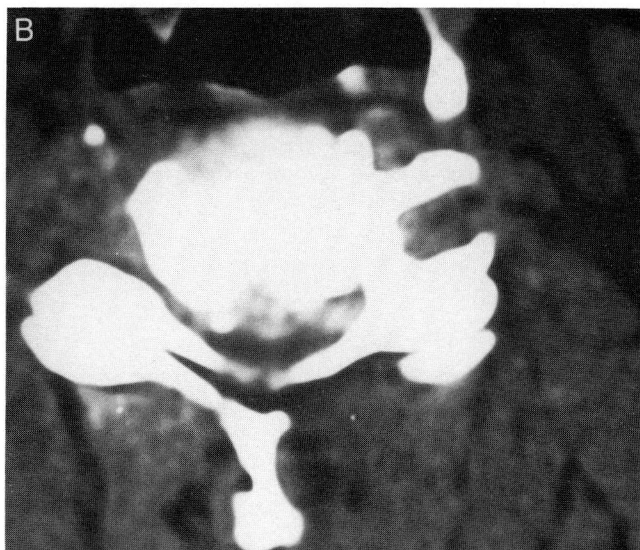

Fig. 3-65. Cervical myelopathy due to central disc herniation. This 43-year-old dentist noted progressive deterioration of his fine finger motion. Sagittal T1-weighted MRI (*A*) shows severe spinal cord compression at C4–C5 and moderate spinal cord compression at C5–C6 due to central disc herniations. Severe spinal cord compression at C4–C5 by central herniated disc is confirmed by axial CT (*B*). Two-level anterior cervical discectomy and fusion resulted in recovery of function.

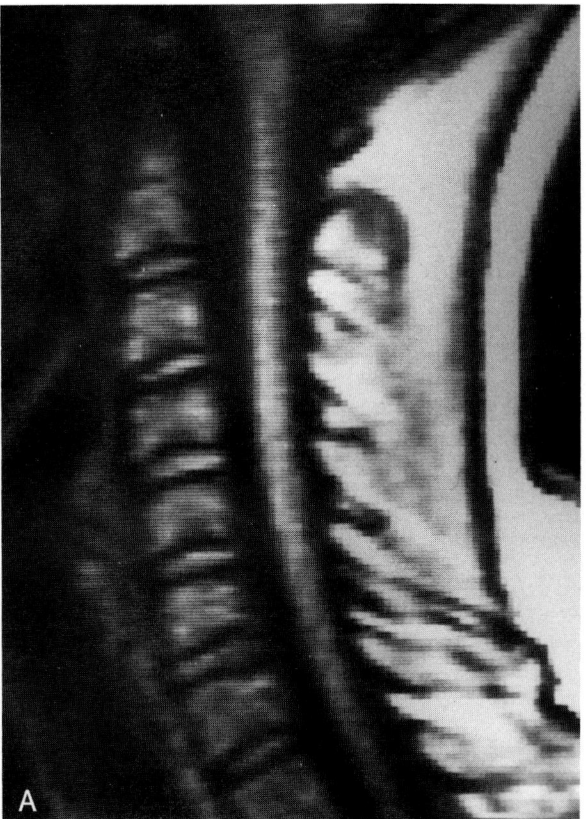

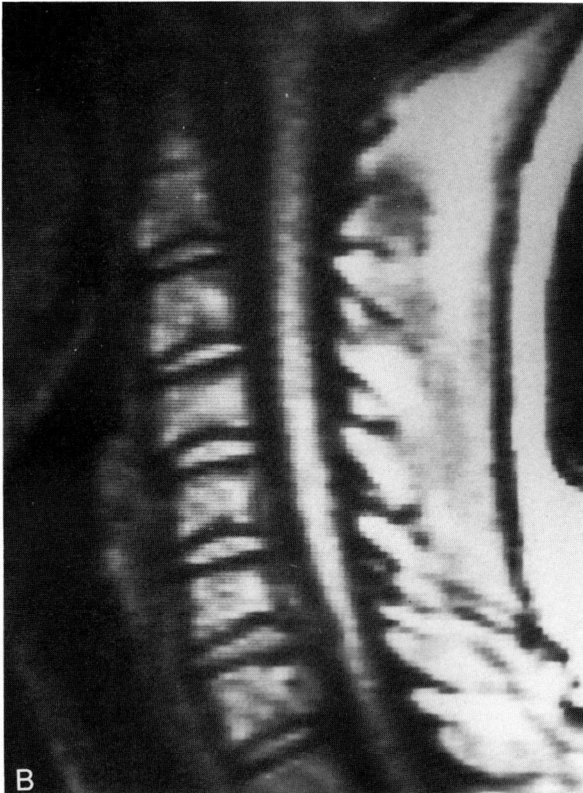

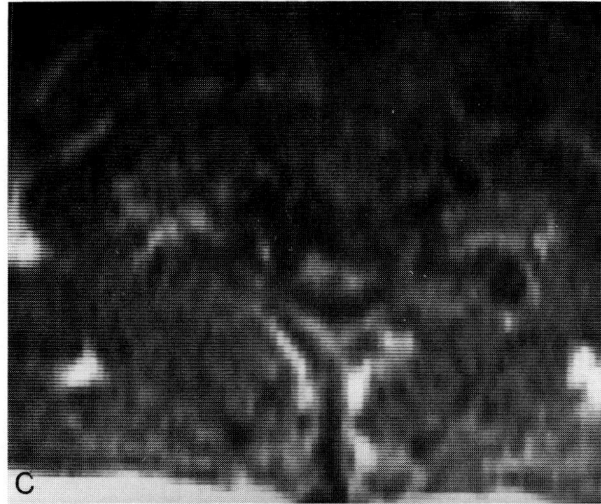

Fig. 3-66. Left cervical disc herniation. Midline sagittal MRI (*A*) appears normal, while left parasagittal MRI (*B*) shows cord deformity resulting from herniated disc at C6–C7. Axial MRI (*C*) at C6–C7 confirms left lateral disc herniation compressing the spinal cord. This image is 7.5 mm thick. Based on CT experience, MR image thickness of less than 3 mm is necessary to reliably detect very small cervical disc lesions, particularly those lesions confined to the neural foramen.

If multiple lesions are present, neurofibromatosis is the most likely diagnosis.

The youthful disc space has a low-signal anulus fibrosis and a higher signal central nucleus pulposus. A normal central nucleus pulposus signal does not exclude the diagnosis of disc herniation. With age, the nucleus pulposus becomes desiccated, and this increased central disc signal is lost. The normal central increased signal is also lost in the early stages of degenerative disc disease. Degenerative discs do not manifest an increased T2-weighted signal.

Central disc herniation is well seen with T1-weighted images (Fig. 3-65). T2-weighted images

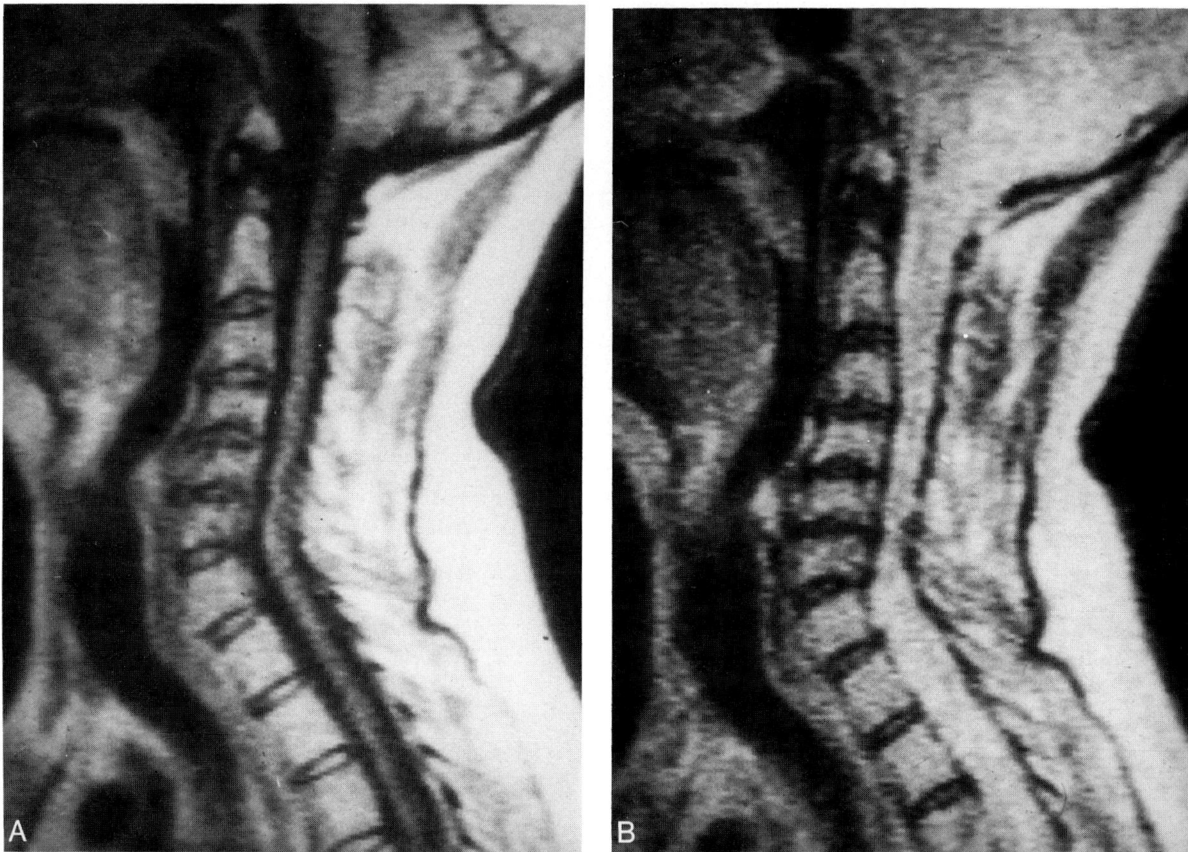

Fig. 3-67. Cervical spondylosis. (*A*) T1-weighted sagittal MRI shows narrowing of the spinal cord contour at C4–C5 and C5–C6 in an area which normally shows slight spinal cord enlargement. (*B*) T2-weighted sagittal MRI shows the "pseudomyelogram" due to increased cerebrospinal fluid and spinal cord signal. Note that the spinal cord can be faintly seen at C2 within CSF, but the spinal cord and CSF are isointense at C4–C5 and C5–C6. The spinal canal is obviously narrow from C4 to C6.

produce a "pseudomyelogram" resulting from the strong T2 signal of the cerebrospinal fluid. This outlines the margins of the thecal sac, allowing indirect assessment of bony osteophytes, calcified disc fragments, or ossification of the posterior longitudinal ligament. These calcified lesions are virtually invisible on T1-weighted MR images because of their very low MRI signal. CT directly demonstrates these calcified lesions to much better advantage.

Small lateral disc herniations residing primarily within the neural foramen are difficult to diagnose reliably by MRI techniques. Based on CT experience, an image plane (or slice) thickness of 3 mm is barely adequate for evaluating cervical radiculopathy, and slice thicknesses of 2 mm or less are more effective. The partial volume effect may obscure these very small disc herniations. Thin image plane thickness minimizes the problem. Intravenous iodine contrast opacifies the epidural veins within the neural foramen, improving CT detection of these small disc herniations by creating greater tissue contrast. Most MRI systems produce an image thickness of no less than 3 mm. Worse yet, many of these systems routinely leave 1- or 2-mm gaps between each image. These gaps are inapparent to the image interpreter. At this writing, no large comparison study is available to demonstrate conclusively that MRI is equal to CT and myelography in this group of patients. It is my

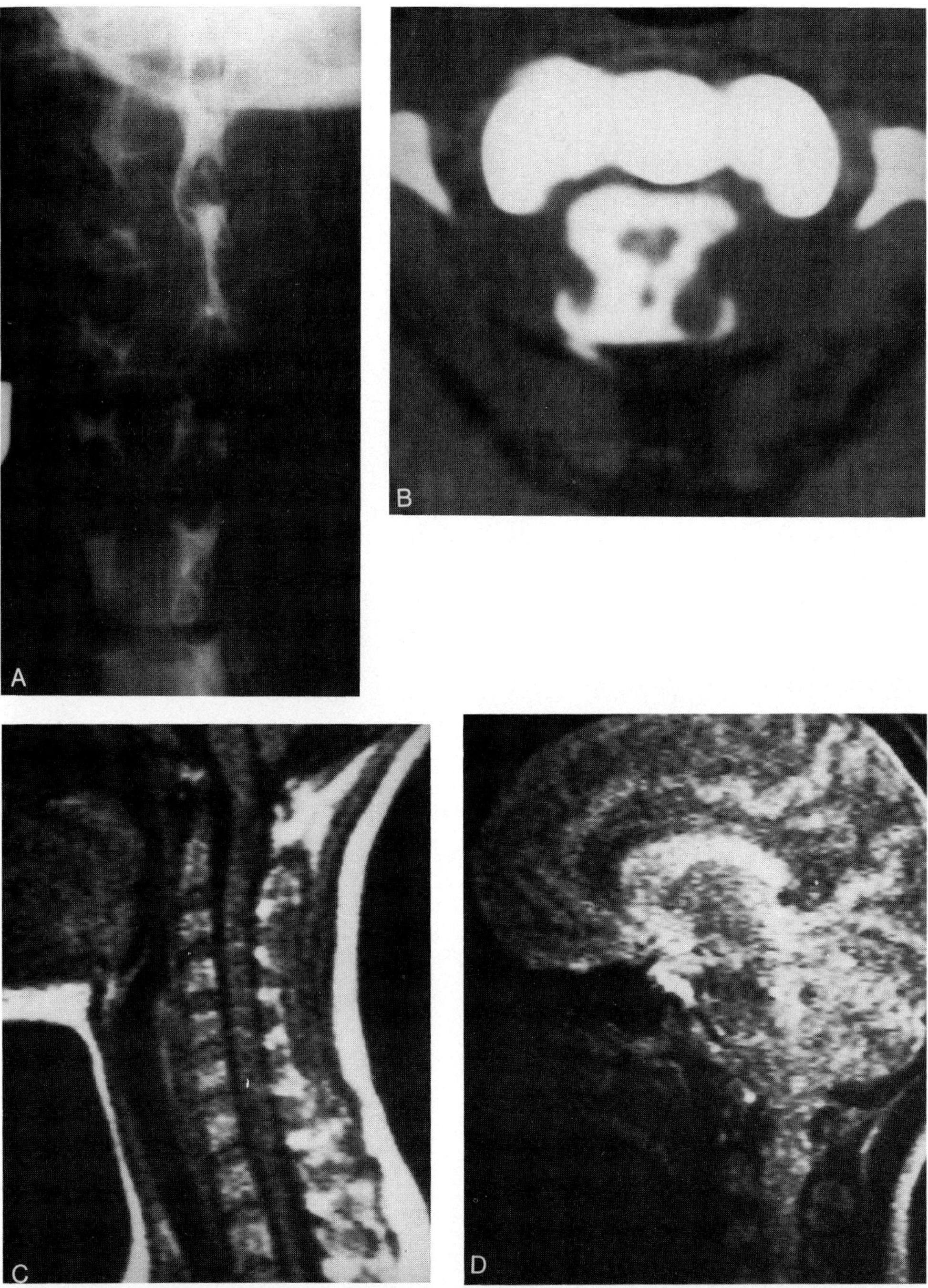

Fig. 3-68. Neurofibromatosis. This 18-year-old female presented with cervical myelopathy. (*A*) A–P myelogram reveals bilateral masses at each root level, consistent with neurofibromatosis. (*B*) Axial CT myelogram at C2 shows cord atrophy with bilateral neurofibromata. (*C*) Sagittal T1-weighted MRI shows the focal spinal cord atrophy at C2 but the individual neurofibromata are not well discriminated. The lesions are isointense with the spinal cord, and give the false impression of increased spinal cord size in the midcervical region. (*D*) T2-weighted sagittal MRI fails to definitely distinguish the tumors from the spinal cord at C1–C2.

present opinion that patients with clinically impressive radicular pain symptoms should undergo CT and/or myelography, even if the MRI examination is "negative."

Disc space infection not only causes loss of the normal nucleus pulposus signal but destroys the lucent zone representing the vertebral end-plates. An increased T2 signal emanates from the adjacent vertebral bodies, and sometimes from the disc space itself. A paravertebral inflammatory process or abscess with an increased T2 signal may also be observed.

MRI beautifully demonstrates traumatic soft-tissue injuries, but fractures are very poorly displayed because of the very low MR signal of cortical bone. Cracks in the bone are not resolved. Displaced bone is identified by its effects on the adjacent tissues, which do produce an MR signal. CT remains the most effective general imaging technique for the initial evaluation of most spinal fracture patients.

SPECULATION ON THE FUTURE

Long examination times, producing low patient "turnaround," contribute to the high cost of MRI examinations. Commercial vendors are expending considerable effort to develop rapid imaging techniques both to improve machine productivity and to minimize motion artifact problems now seen in MRI. Gradient pulse imaging techniques using very short TR/TE combinations permit single-image 2-second data acquisition with reasonably good image quality. Improved multiecho/multislice techniques allow simultaneous T1- and T2-weighted images to be obtained more quickly. Improved signal-to-noise ratio performance retains image quality while decreasing data acquisition time.

If T1 and T2 values at two different TEs are known (TR held constant), the appearance of spin-echo technique images at additional TE values can be mathematically predicted. Images may be "finely tuned" to clarify pathology (*e.g.*, tumor versus edema) without requiring repeated patient data acquisitions. No cervical spine clinical studies using this type of image manipulation have been reported.

Multislice techniques are two-dimensional (2-D) with separate data acquisitions required for each image projection desired (*i.e.*, sagittal, axial, etc.). An alternative approach is three-dimensional (3-D), or volumetric, imaging. With this technique, data are acquired simultaneously from a whole volume of interest (*i.e.*, cervical spine). Advantages of 3-D imaging include the ability to derive any desired image plane from these data, including curved or oblique images. No data gaps exist. The image plane depth (thickness) can be varied, as needed, from very thin to thick. The patient's presence is only required for the initial 3-D acquisition. Standard and additional images are all produced by processing the original 3-D data information, rather than by rescanning the patient. Disadvantages of 3-D imaging include relatively long data acquisition time. Current 3-D spine-echo techniques require 20 to 40 minutes or more, whereas gradient pulse techniques may reduce the data acquisition time to 9 to 15 minutes. A brief episode of patient motion can degrade the entire examination. 3-D imaging also requires large computer memory and data processing capacity. These requirements can add significantly to the hardware costs of an MRI system. In spite of these constraints, 3-D MRI techniques are likely to become more common for cervical spine studies in which high-resolution and multiple image planes are needed.

Inherent in 2-D multislice imaging techniques is the capability of identifying and quantifying blood or spinal fluid flow. Laminar and turbulent flow patterns can be identified, and volume and velocity values can be quantified. There may be useful applications of these techniques for clinical evaluation of syringohydromyelia and cerebrospinal fluid dynamics.

Paramagnetic contrast agents for use with MRI are also being investigated. Gadolinium-DTPA (Berlex) is the only FDA-approved agent currently available. This agent performs in a manner somewhat similar to intravenous iodine contrast for CT. In the cervical spine, paramagnetic contrast agents will be most useful in distinguishing spinal cord tumor from edema, or for identifying subtle lesions of multiple sclerosis.

New imaging coil designs, incorporating both a surface coil and a local gradient coil, are being experimentally developed. These coils, theoretically, can produce 100-μm spatial resolution. Depth of signal penetration and the field of view will be very limited. These coil designs might be referred to as "MR microscopy." They offer the possibility of studying individual nerve roots or the spinal cord in exquisite detail.

The current costs of acquisition, operation, and siting of MRI systems makes these studies very expensive. Superconducting magnets are used in most high-performance systems because of their excellent field uniformity characteristics. Costly to manufacture, their operation requires a continuous supply of expensive cryogens (*i.e.*, liquid helium and nitrogen) to cool the magnet to a temperature near absolute zero. Loss of coolant disables the system and can cause damage to the magnet itself. Elaborate magnetic shielding and/or a very large building is often required to safely contain the generated fringe magnetic field. Recently, "self-shielded" superconducting magnets (Siemens, Oxford), which promise to decrease siting expenses, have been introduced. Other design refinements may further decrease manufacture and maintenance costs.

Permanent magnets (Fonar, Field Effects) offer an alternative engineering solution. These magnets weigh up to 100 tons. Since they resemble giant bar magnets, minimal operative costs are involved and little magnetic shielding is required. Manufacture of permanent magnets to produce excellent field uniformity is considered difficult; magnetic field strengths greater than 1 tesla have not been satisfactorily achieved.

Resistive magnets are relatively easy to manufacture and maintain. Magnetic field uniformity and stability are inferior to superconducting magnets. Only low- and mid-strength magnetic fields are presently possible. Improved resistive magnet designs such as the "iron core" magnet may find a role. Hybrid resistive/permanent magnets are also being researched. These efforts may lead to both lower-cost high-field imagers and much lower-cost low- and mid-field imaging systems. These lower-cost systems could make MRI much more widely available than it is now. One hopes that the cost of MRI examinations will approach that of CT.

MR spectroscopy has been applied to test tube analysis for more than 30 years. *In vivo* MR spectroscopy offers the possibility of biochemical examination of living tissue *in situ*. Major technical problems remain to be solved before clinical spectroscopy is routinely performed. Although spectroscopy may be accomplished at 1.5 T (the highest field strength for an MR imager that is FDA approved), many researchers believe that field strengths of 3 T to 6 T will be required to adequately perform this task. Because of the high frequency of radio waves required, imaging is not easily performed at such high magnetic fields. Totally separate devices for spectroscopy may need to be built. Practical clinical applications will have to be researched and developed. It may some day be possible to assess the acutely injured cervical spinal cord by MR spectroscopy to determine the severity of injury and the prognosis. Associated MR imaging would determine the morphology of the injury.

The foregoing discussion is by no means exhaustive, but it does provide an overview of many ongoing MRI developments. MRI is now making vital contributions to cervical spine evaluation. Further technological developments will certainly expand its role in evaluating the cervical spine.

BIBLIOGRAPHY

Aubin ML, Vignaud J, Iba-Zizen MT, Stoffels O: NMR imaging of the cranio-cervical junction and cervical spine. Normal and pathological features. J Neuroradiol 11:229–37, 1984

Babcock EE, Brateman L, Weinreb JC, Horner SD, Nunnally RL: Edge artifacts in MR images: Chemical shift effect. J Comput Assist Tomogr 9:252–257, 1985

Bewermeyer H, Dreesbach HA, Hunermann B, Heiss WD: MR imaging of familial basilar impression. J Comput Assist Tomogr 8:953–56, 1984

Bradley WG, Newton TH, Crooks LE: Physical principles of nuclear magnetic resonance. In Newton TH, Potts DG (eds): Modern Neuroradiology, Vol 2. San Anselmo, Clavadel Press, 1983

Bradley WG, Jr, Waluch V, Yadley RA, Wycoff RR: Comparison of CT and MR in 400 patients with suspected disease of the brain and cervical spinal cord. Radiology, 152:695–702, 1984

Brasch RC: Methods of contrast enhancement for NMR imaging and potential applications: A subject review. Radiology 147:781–88, 1983

Bydder GM, Brown J, Niendorf HP, Young IR: Enhancement of cervical intraspinal tumors in MR imaging with intravenous gadolinium-DTPA. J Comput Assist Tomogr 9:847–51, 1985

Daniels DL, Hyde JS, Kneeland JB, Jesmanowicz A, Froncisz W, Grist TM, Pech P, Williams AL, Haughton VM: The cervical nerves and foramina: local-coil MR imaging. AJNR 7:129–33, 1986

Di Chiro G, Doppman JL, Dwyer AJ, Patronas NJ, Knop RH, Bairamian D, Vermess M, Oldfield EH: Tumors and arteriovenous malformations of the spinal cord: assessment using MR. Radiology 156:689–97, 1985

Dooms GC, Hricak H, Sollitto RA, Higgins CB: Lipomatous tumors and tumors with fatty component: MR imaging potential and comparison of MR and CT results. Radiology 157:479–83, 1985

Edelman RR, Stark DD, Saini S, Ferrucci JT Jr, Dinsmore RE, Ladd W, Brady TJ: Oblique planes of section in MR imaging. Radiology 159:807–10, 1986

Edelman RR, Wedeen VJ, Davis KR, Widder D, Hahn P, Shoukimas G, Brady TJ: Multiphasic MR imaging: a new method for direct imaging of pulsatile CSF flow. Radiology 161:779–83, 1986

Frahm J, Haase A, Matthaei D: Rapid three-dimensional NMR imaging using the FLASH technique. J Comp Assist Tomogr 10:363–68, 1986

Gawehn J, Schroth G, Thron A: The value of paraxial slices in MR-imaging of spinal cord disease. Neuroradiology 28:347–50.

Gebarski SS, Maynard FW, Gabrielsen TO, Knake JE, Latack JT, Hoff JT: Posttraumatic progressive myelopathy. Clinical and radiologic correlation employing MR imaging, delayed CT metrizamide myelography, and intraoperative sonography. Radiology 157:379–85, 1985

Goy AM, Pinto RS, Raghavendra BN, Epstein FJ, Kricheff II: Intramedullary spinal cord tumors: MR imaging, with emphasis on associated cysts. Radiology 161:381–86, 1986

Holtas SL, Kido DK, Simon JH: MR imaging of spinal lymphoma. J Comput Assist Tomogr 10:111–15, 1986

Hyman RA, Edwards JH, Vacirca SJ, Stein HL: 0.6 T MR imaging of the cervical spine: multislice and multiecho techniques. AJNR 6:229–36, 1985

Kulkarni MV, Patton JA, Price RR: Technical considerations for the use of surface coils in MRI. AJR 147:373–78, 1986

Lee BC, Deck MD, Kneeland JB, Cahill PT: MR imaging of the craniocervical junction. AJNR 6:209–13, 1985

Lee BC, Zimmerman RD, Manning JJ, Deck MD: MR imaging of syringomyelia and hydromyelia. AJR 144:1149–56, 1985

Mamourian AC, Briggs RW: Appearance of pantopaque on MR images. Radiology 158:457–60, 1986

McArdle CB, Crofford MJ, Mirfakhraee M, Amparo EG, Calhoun JS: Surface coil MR of spinal trauma: preliminary experience. AJNR 7:885–93, 1986

McArdle CB, Wright JW, Prevost WJ, Dornfest DJ, Amparo EG: MR imaging of the acutely injured patient with cervical traction. Radiology 159:273–74, 1986

Modic MT, Feiglin DH, Piraino DW, Boumphrey F, Weinstein MA, Duchesneau PM, Rehm S: Vertebral osteomyelitis: assessment using MR. Radiology 157:157–66, 1985

Modic MT, Masaryk TJ, Mulopulos GP, Bundschuh C, Han JS, Bohlman H: Cervical radiculopathy: prospective evaluation with surface coil MR imaging, CT with metrizamide, and metrizamide myelography. Radiology 161:753–59, 1986

Pavlicek W, Geisinger M, Castle L: The Effects of NMR on patients with cardiac pacemakers. Radiology 147:149–153, 1983

Quencer RM, Sheldon JJ, Post MJ, Diaz RD, Montalvo BM, Green BA, Eismont FJ: MRI of the chronically injured cervical spinal cord. AJR 147:125–32, 1986

Ramsey RG, Zacharias CE: MR imaging of the spine after radiation therapy: easily recognizable effects. AJR 144:1131–35, 1985

Reicher MA, Lufkin RB, Smith S, Flannigan B, Olsen R, Wolf R, Hertz D, Winter J, Hanafee W: Multiple-angle, variable-interval, nonorthogonal MRI. AJR 147:363–66, 1986

Rubin JM, Aisen AM, DiPietro MA: Ambiguities in MR imaging of tumoral cysts in the spinal cord. J Comput Assist Tomogr 10:395–98, 1986

Schenck JF, Foster TH, Henkes JL, Adams WJ, Hayes C, Hart HR Jr, Edelstein WA, Bottomley PA, Wehrli FW: High-field surface-coil MR imaging of localized anatomy. AJNR 6:181–86, 1985

Scotti G, Scialfa G, Colombo N, Landoni L: MR imaging of intradural extramedullary tumors of the cervical spine. J Comput Assist Tomogr 9:1037–41, 1985

Sherman JL, Citrin CM, Gangarosa RE, Bowen BJ: The MR appearance of CSF pulsations in the spinal canal. AJNR 7:879–84, 1986

Slone RM, Buck LL, Fitzsimmons JR: Varying gradient angles and offsets to optimize imaging planes in MR. Radiology 158:531–36, 1986

Smith FW: NMR—historical aspects. In Newton TH, Potts DG (eds): Modern Neuroradiology, Vol 2. San Anselmo, Clavadel Press, 1983

Spinos E, Laster DW, Moody DM, Ball MR, Witcofski RL, Kelly DL Jr: MR evaluation of Chiari I malformations at 0.15 T. AJR 144:1143–48, 1985

Sze G, Brant-Zawadzki MN, Wilson CR, Norman D, Newton TH: Pseudotumor of the craniovertebral junction associated with chronic subluxation: MR imaging studies. Radiology 161:391–94, 1986

Valk PE, Hale JD, Crooks LE, et al: MRI of blood flow: Correlation of image appearance with spin echo phase shift and signal intensity. AJR 146:931–39, 1986

Wehrli FW, MacFall JR, Glover GH, Grigsby N, Haughton V, Johanson J: The dependence of nuclear magnetic resonance (NMR) image contrast on intrinsic and pulse sequence timing parameters. Magn Reson Imaging 2:3–16, 1984

Wehrli FW, MacFall JR, Newton TH: Parameters determining the appearance of NMR images. In Newton TH, Potts DG (eds): Modern Neuroradiology. San Anselmo, Clavadel Press, 1983

Wehrli FW, Shimakawa A, Gullberg GT, MacFall JR: Time-of-Flight MR flow imaging: Selective saturation recovery with gradient refocusing (SSRGR). Radiology 160:781–85, 1986

Yenerich DO, Haughton VM: Oblique plane MR imaging of the cervical spine. J Comput Assist Tomogr 10:823–26, 1986

Scintigraphy and Selective Angiography

KEIRO ONO, KOZO OKADA, HIROSHI NAKASHIMA AND KAZUO YAMASHITA

UTILITY IN SURGERY OF THE SPINE

Since Chiewitz and Hevesy introduced phosphorus-32 (^{32}P), nuclear medical equipment and bone-seeking radiopharmaceuticals have revolutionized the diagnosis and treatment of patients with skeletal diseases.[8] Plain roentgenograms, tomograms and computed tomograms (CT) provide precise information about the morphologic changes occurring in the spine. However, occult or dynamic changes in the skeleton cannot be confirmed by such methods. Scintigraphy, particularly that using ^{99m}Tc-phosphate compounds or complexes, has proved to be the most effective method of searching for causes of dynamic change in the skeleton, such as underlying disease spread, metabolic abnormalities, and modeling or remodeling processes, and it is similarly useful for staging.[60] Scintigraphy is employed as an effective screening procedure that is supplementary to the static diagnositic methods. Its high sensitivity detects occult lesions in the spine of patients complaining of unexplainable pains. Although several kinds of radioactive tracers are used in scintigraphy, respective specificity of physical and biologic properties should be borne in mind in applying scintigraphy to skeletal diseases.

PHYSICAL AND BIOLOGIC PRINCIPLES OF SCINTIGRAPHY

In selecting or using the radioisotopes, two main properties should be noted. First, radioisotopes have different plasma concentration times, as Weber and associates reported.[64] Second, they have variable skeletal deposition, which through imaging or counting suggests the dynamics or kinematics of the skeleton.

As bone-seeking isotopes, calcium (^{47}Ca, ^{45}Ca), strontium (^{85}Sr, ^{87}Sr), fluorine (^{18}F), and technetium (^{99m}Tc) are widely utilized. Among those, ^{99m}Tc-labeled phosphate compounds are commonly used, having been first introduced by Subramanian and associates.[60] On searching for bone metabolism, calcium and strontium are useful. Fluorine is a short-lived radioisotope and has an affinity similar to calcium and strontium.[24] Currently, ^{99m}Tc-labeled methylene diphosphonate (MDP) and ethylidenehydroxy diphosphonate (EHDP) are mainstays of diagnostic bone scans. Concentrations of bone-seeking isotopes are generally evaluated in two phases: early phase and later phase.[55] The early phase involves uptake within minutes after intravenous injection of the isotope, which is purely reflected to a passive diffusion from the vascular compartment.[26] The later phase, which occurs several hours after injection, is thought to be concentrated in reactive new bone or the calcification front.[23,25,36] With respect to spine lesions, the early-phase scan rarely provides useful information. Localizing the deposition or the various factors affecting the process in the later phase continue to be investigated. In addition to increased vascularity, bone mineralization (particularly on the increased hydroxyapatite surface), immature collagen or osteoid, and enzyme systems are assumed[23,30,71] to influence late uptake. Nakashima and associates investigated ^{99m}Tc methylene diphosphonate concentration in mouse osteosarcoma.[47] They found that autoradiographs showed a concentration of the tracer in new bone laid down in response to tumor growth. Thus, the mineralization of bone matrix was considered to play a most important role in ^{99m}Tc uptake. Hypervascularity or increased blood flow, such as in Paget's disease, is accompanied by an intense uptake of tracer. However, based on the findings that an increase in vascularity by 400% leads to an increase in diphosphonate uptake of only 70%, hypervascularity cannot be highly estimated in the increased uptake of the tracer.[54] A high uptake of tracer is observed even in the normal growth plate and the adjacent areas, correlating with the accelerated bone metabolism or active bone modeling and remodeling. The metabolic bone diseases, such as Paget's disease, with an increased osteoclastic activity or hyperparathyroidism with active bone formation and resorption are also correlated with a high uptake of tracer. However, increased skeletal tracer uptake in rachitic lesions, or in osteolytic lesions in osteomalacia or bone metastases where no compensatory bone formation exists, is difficult to explain by this theory. Therefore, details on the mechanism of tracer uptake require further investigation.

Several tracers other than the bone-seeking isotopes are utilized with limited value, in infectious disease or soft-tissue tumors. Gallium-67 (^{67}Ga citrate) is one of the most intriguing radiopharmaceuticals with regard to aspects of the specific uptake mechanism. Hoffer,[34] summarizing his findings, reported the following specific mechanisms of uptake in infectious conditions:

1. Lactoferrin binding at the site of infection[66]
2. Leukocyte labeling[27]
3. Direct bacterial uptake[46]

The following are mechanisms of localization in tumor:

1. Transferrin binding[37]
2. Lactoferrin binding[33]
3. Direct tumor uptake[61]

The emphasis on the mechanism of localization in tumor is based on the similarity between the kinematics of ^{67}Ga citrate and ferric ions within the tumor, in which there are high levels of ribonucleotide reductase and an iron-dependent enzyme. Thus, the ^{67}Ga scan, since it was introduced by Edwards and Hayes, has become a useful supplement to bone scan.[21] This is because of the specific affinity of ^{67}Ga to hematopoietic tumors, various sarcomas, and infectious lesions, as compared with less specific or common high uptake of ^{99m}Tc phosphate compounds in the skeletal system. Bitran and associates reported the high uptake of ^{67}Ga citrate in the lesions of malignant schwannoma, Ewing's sarcoma, and rhabdomyosarcoma, and a low sensitivity in liposarcoma, leiomyosarcoma, malignant fibrous histiocytoma, and synovial sarcoma.[5] Based on our recent experiences, multiple myeloma, malignant lymphoma, and melanoma should be added to the tumor group with high sensitivity to ^{67}Ga citrate (see Fig. 3-74). In our clinic, suspicious tumors of the spine are usually subjected to both ^{99m}Tc and ^{67}Ga scanning on the basis of the specificity of tracers.

INDICATIONS FOR SCINTIGRAPHY

Bone scanning is highly sensitive to quantitative changes in the skeleton, but is not yet sufficiently specific to define the quality of disease or pathological condition. The greatest value of scintigraphy is probably in the evaluation of spinal tumors, particularly in the detection of bone metastases. The diseases and pathologic conditions of the spine, for which scintigraphy has proven to be of value, are as follows, according to Galasko and Weber,[26,44] and Malmud and Charkes:

1. Spine tumors
   a. Detection of bone metastases
      (i) Detection or diagnosis of symptomatic lesions
      (ii) Detection of occult lesions and extent of metastases
   b. Determining malignant or benign lesions
   c. Staging the disease, particularly in early cancer
   d. Determining appropriate plan for biopsy and therapy
   e Assessment of response to therapy
   f. Differentiation of pathologic from traumatic fractures
2. Inflammatory diseases
   a. Early diagnosis
   b. Assessment of distribution
   c. Assessment of response to therapy
3. Metabolic bone diseases
   a. Detection of extent of skeletal involvement, particularly of associated pathologic fractures
   b. Assessment of response to therapy
4. Assessment of bone graft incorporation

CLINICAL STUDIES

Normal Scintigraphy

Normal whole-body scans using ^{99m}Tc diphosphonate and ^{67}Ga citrate in a child and in two adults are shown in Figure 3-69. In ^{99m}Tc scans, a high uptake of tracer is generally localized in the epiphyseal plates and the osteochrondral junctions of the ribs in children. In adults, however, increased uptakes are in the sternum or sternoclavicular junctions, the pedicles of the dorsal vertebrae, spinous processes of the lumbar vertebrae, the acromion, and the inferior angle of the scapula. Ossicles in the ligamentum nuchae, which are found in older adults, are occasionally positive. In ^{67}Ga scans, occasional visualization of the thymus in children, and high uptake in the liver, intestine, and colon are normal. The spinal column is situated posteriorly; therefore, a posterior scan is more useful to detect or assess spinal diseases than an anterior view. In diagnosing spinal disorders, it should be remembered that high uptake of tracer in the bladder (^{99m}Tc), and liver or colon (^{67}Ga) often masks the spinal lesions (Fig. 3-69).

In general, the intensity of the radioactivity of a lesion should be evaluated in comparison to the surrounding soft tissues, normal adjacent areas, or contralateral bone. For quantitative measurements, Simon and Kirchner proposed a rating system for bone scans using ^{99m}Tc in which increased uptake by sacroiliac joints on the posterior imaging in the whole-body scans was defined as a base.[59] For ^{67}Ga scans, a similar scale was proposed based on the intensity of the liver.

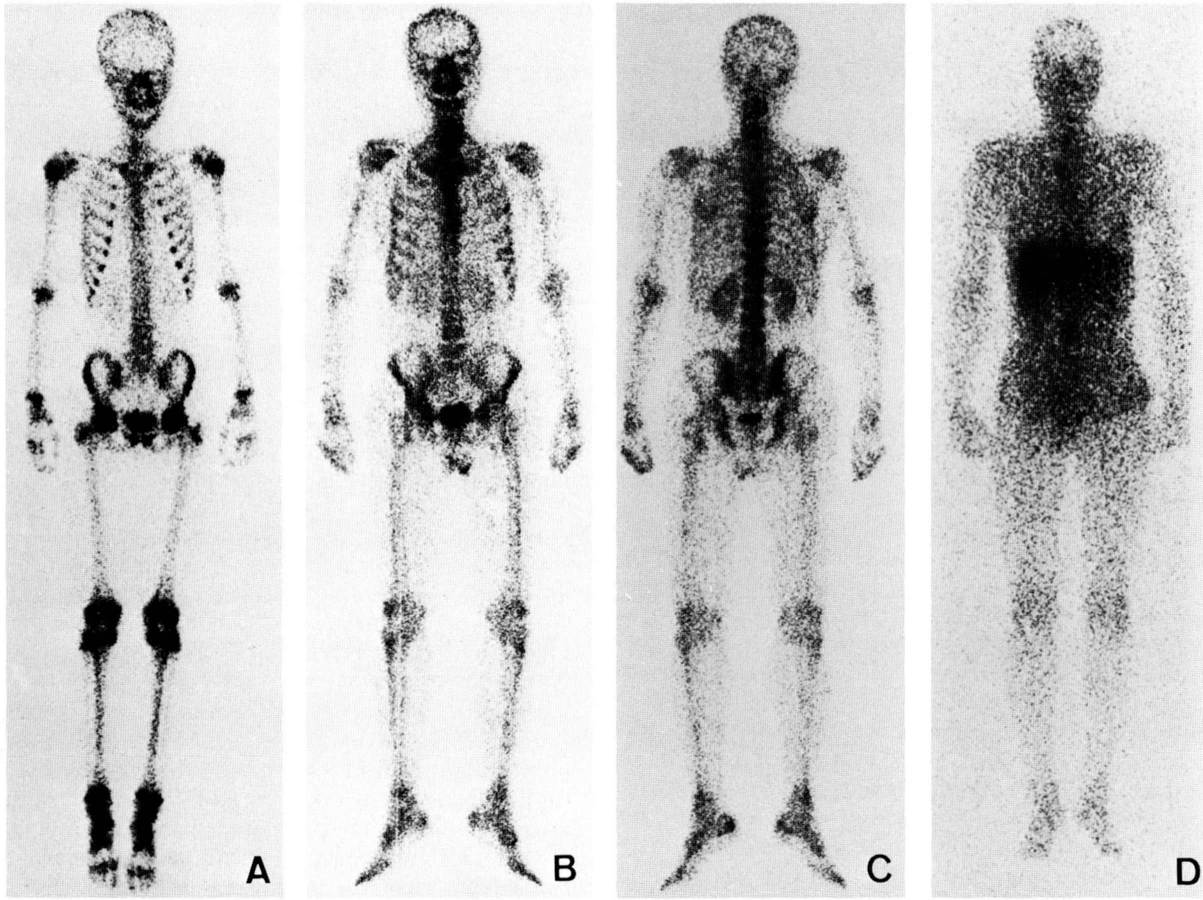

Fig. 3-69. (*A*) Normal bone scan of a 9-year-old boy, anterior view. High uptake of ^{99m}Tc-MDP is localized at the epiphyses or apophyses of the skeleton. (*B*) Normal bone scan with ^{99m}Tc-MDP of a 50-year-old man, anterior view. (*C*) Posterior view of (*B*). (*D*) Normal scintigraphy with ^{67}Ga citrate of a 32-year-old man, anterior view. High uptake of the tracer in the liver is normal.

False-Positive Images

The abnormality of bone-seeking isotopes usually results in an increased uptake, having no specific correlation to an underlying pathologic condition. Prolonged uptake at the healed fracture of the vertebra and pronounced uptake in degenerative conditions such as spondylosis or ankylosing spinal hyperostosis (Forstier's disease) are not infrequently mistaken for a positive finding (Fig. 3-70). In such patients, comparative studies including roentgenograms, CT scans, and/or bone biopsy are needed. Adams and Horton emphasized the quantitative differences between metastases and degenerative spinal diseases, in which the uptake in the metastatic lesions was greater.[2] Multiple compression fractures in the dorsolumbar spine accompanying osteoporosis and presenting hot spots of tracer are misinterpreted as metastatic lesions.

False-Negative Images

As the bone-seeking tracers have neither an exclusive nor specific affinity for pathologic conditions, there are false-negative images with invisible lesions in the spine or surrounding tissues. Galasko suggested at least four main causes: (1) characteristics of the tumors evoking no osteoblastic responses, (2) smaller deposits of tumor cells, (3) localization of the lesions situated in pubis or is-

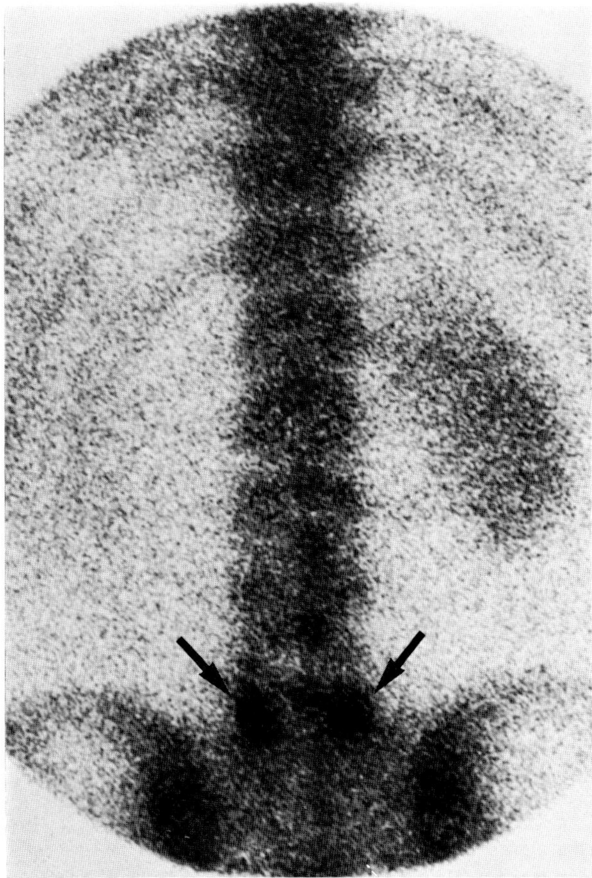

Fig. 3-70. Bone scan of a 56-year-old man, posterior view. The bilateral spotty uptake of ^{99m}Tc-MDP at the fifth lumbar vertebra (*arrows*), erroneously taken to be a metastasis, proved to be an osteoarthrotic lesion in the apophyseal joints.

chium, and (4) widespread metastatic disease presenting normal and symmetrical appearances.[26] In our series of 77 symptomatic patients with spinal metastases, 4 of 75 (5.3%) patients represented the false negatives in ^{99m}Tc scans and 14 of 36 (38.9%) in ^{67}Ga scans (Table 3-2). Spinal metastasis, which was situated mainly in the epidural space, was often not visualized, as was the case with adenocarcinoma of the lung. Widespread or advanced metastases of the spine occasionally masked the sites of lesions as Constable and Cranage described.[11] Postirradiated malignant tumors or well-controlled metastatic lesions sometimes did not show increased uptake. Other tracers presenting low lesion contrast such as ^{85}Sr, ^{87m}Sr, and ^{18}F often resulted in negative images on application to the spinal diseases, with the notable exception of metabolic bone diseases.

CHARACTERISTICS IN TUMOR, INFLAMMATION, AND MISCELLANEOUS CONDITIONS PREFERENTIALLY AFFECTING THE SPINE

Reflecting the reactive bone remodeling in the surrounding area, increased tracer uptake often extends proximal and distal to the lesions. This extension does not frequently occur in lesions of the spine. This is because increased radioactivity in the affected vertebrae does not extend beyond the adjoining discs, at least during the initial stage. When increased activity extends over multiple levels and fairly represents interposed discs between the involved levels, multiple metastases are strongly suggested (Fig. 3-71). On the other hand, increased activity extending over more than two levels without the interposed disc spaces strongly suggests inflammatory or infectious disease (Fig. 3-73). Metastatic spine tumor is most significantly detected by scintigraphy, having a coexistent high uptake, single or multiple, in remote areas of the spine. When metastases have advanced to a late stage, diffuse high uptakes of the tracer are recognized in the spine. In an anterior view, high uptakes are noted mostly in the ribs, pelvis, skull, or anterior portions of the vertebrae. With regard to spine metastasis, a posterior view is informative because of the location of the spine (Fig. 3-71*B*). A mild-to-moderate hot spot extending beyond the lateral border of the spine is a lesion of degenerative nature, and is a false positive (Fig. 3-70). Tracer usually provides a hot uptake; however, a cold area surrounded by a hot area infrequently is seen (Fig. 3-75*A*). This cold area appears on the image when a tumor (usually malignant) is aggresively invaded and no new bone formation has occurred. ^{67}Ga scan results probably coincided with the predominant area of hot spots that was shown on a ^{99m}Tc-diphosphonate bone scan (Figs. 3-71, 3-74, 3-75). Primary malignant tumor often spread into the adjoining areas, including vertebrae and surrounding soft tissues, with some variability of uptake, depending on the nature of the tumor (hot spot, or cold in a hot spot (Fig. 3-72). When a vertebra in metabolic bone disease or benign spine tumor is collapsed, it is more clearly visualized (Fig. 3-76). Among benign spine tumors, osteoid osteoma, which has either high vascularity or new bone formations, had a high uptake (Fig. 3-77). An eosinophilic granuloma, when associated with

Table 3-2. Positive Ratio of ^{99m}Tc Phosphate and ^{67}Ga Citrate in Various Diseases of the Spine

	No. of Patients	^{99m}Tc Scintigraphy	^{67}Ga Scintigraphy
Malignant spine tumor	92	85/90 (94.4%)	27/46 (58.7%)
Primary*	15	14/15 (93.3%)	5/10 (50.0%)
Metastatic†	77	71/75 (94.7%)	22/36 (61.1%)
Benign spine tumor, tumorous conditions‡	22	18/21 (85.7%)	1/ 9 (11.1%)
Spinal cord tumor	22	0/20 (0%)	1/10 (10.0%)
Inflammatory disease	26	20/23 (87.0%)	4/10 (40.0%)
Metabolic bone disease	2	2/2	

* Primary malignant spine tumor: osteosarcoma, myeloma, malignant fibrous histiocytoma, chondrosarcoma, chordoma, hemangioendothelioma, and malignant lymphoma of bone

† Sources of metastatic spine tumor: lung, stomach, breast, uterus, prostate, kidney, rectum, liver, thyroid, skin, and others.

‡ Benign spine tumor and tumorous condition: osteochondroma, giant cell tumor, chondroblastoma, hemangioma, bone cyst, osteoid osteoma, eosinophilic granuloma, osteoblastoma, and desmoplastic fibroma.

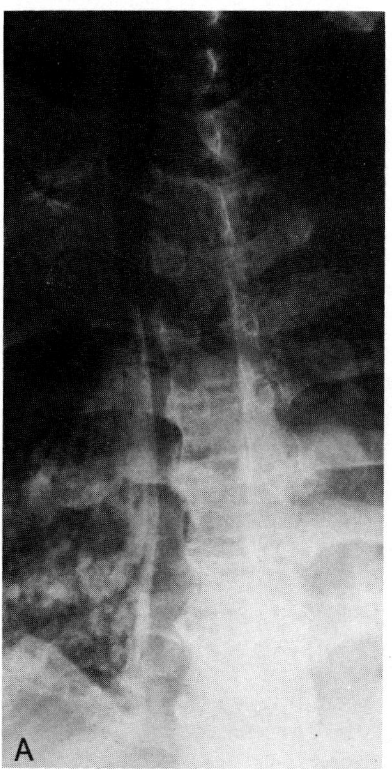

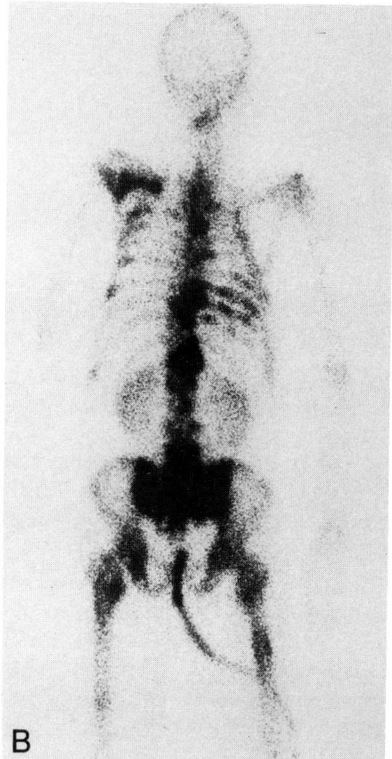

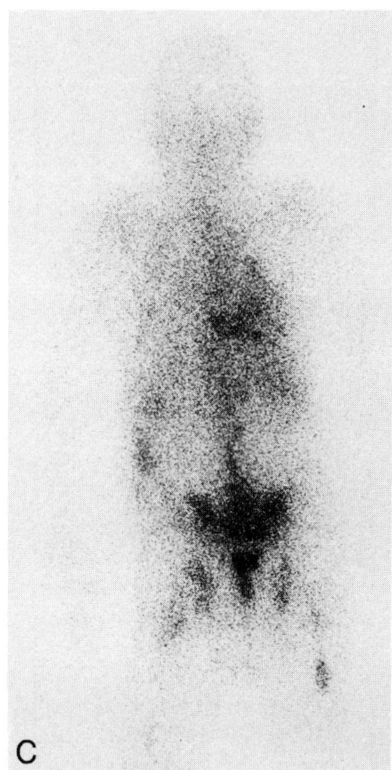

Fig. 3-71. A 60-year-old man with multiple metastases secondary to lung cancer. (*A*) A–P view of plain roentgenogram shows extensive lytic metastases of entire thorax with permanent destruction. Note the disseminated bone metastases in posterior view of bone scan using ^{99m}Tc-MDP (*B*) and ^{67}Ga citrate (*C*).

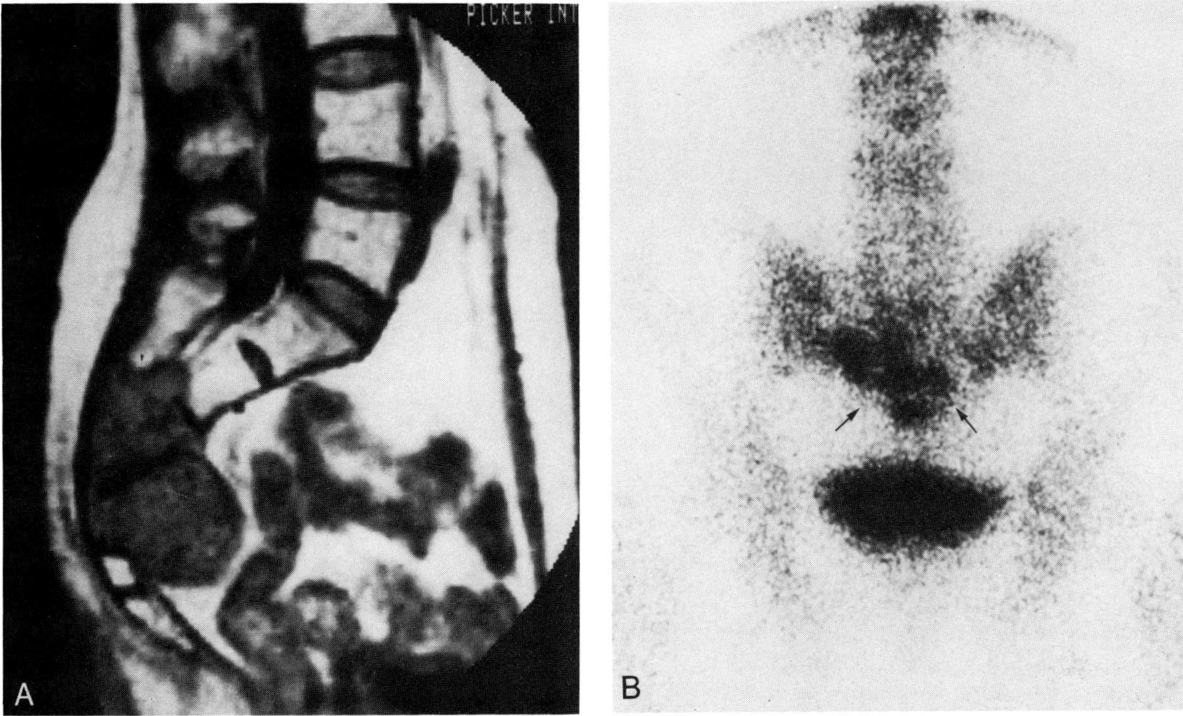

Fig. 3-72. A 53-year-old woman with chordoma. (*A*) MRI shows a tumor mass, with lytic lesion in the sacrum. (*B*) ^{99m}Tc-MDP scan shows increased uptake affecting the sacrum (*arrows*).

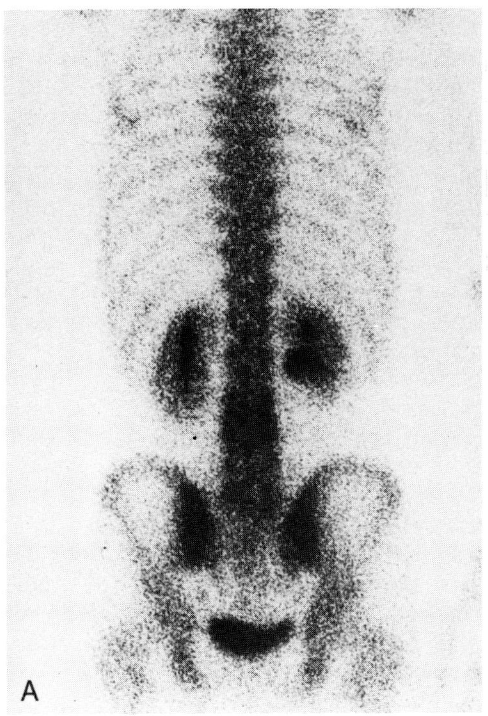

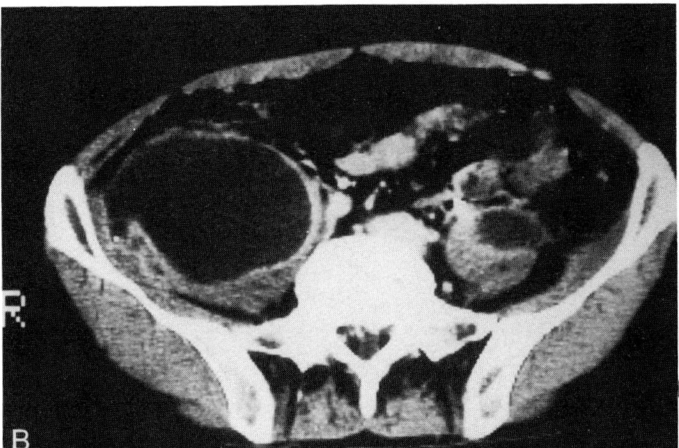

Fig. 3-73. A 37-year-old man with tuberculous spondylitis. (*A*) ^{99m}Tc-MDP scan showed an area of increased uptake affecting the third and fourth lumbar vertebrae. (*B*) Enhanced CT revealed the accompanying retroperitoneal abscesses.

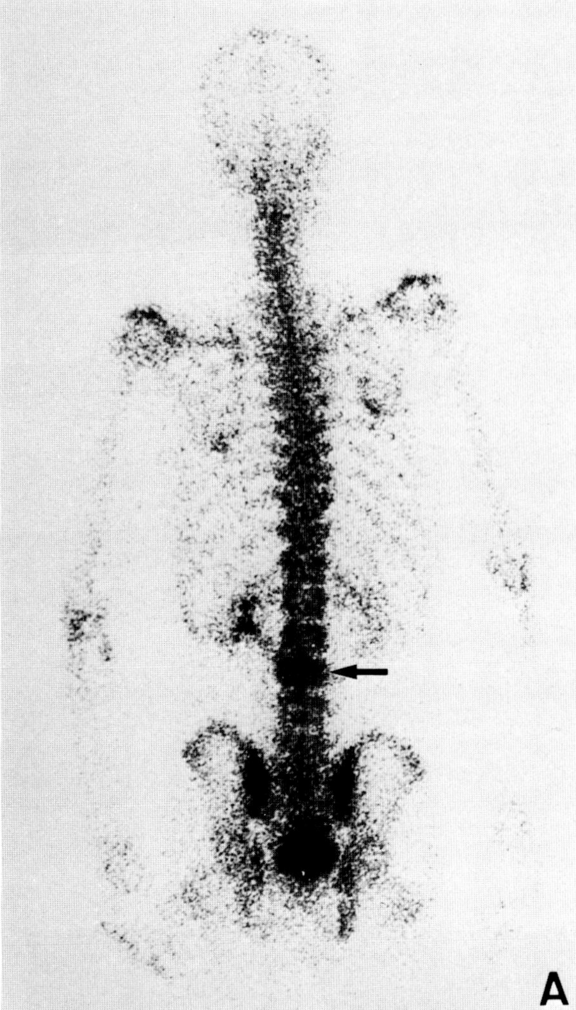

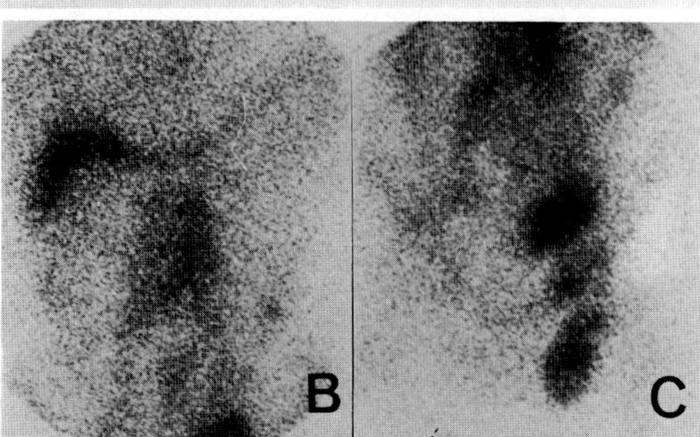

Fig. 3-74. A 38-year-old man with Hodgkin's disease and accompanying paraplegia. (*A*) In this posterior whole-body scan with ^{99m}Tc-MDP, note the increased uptake of the tracer at the third lumbar vertebra that had no remarkable roentgenographic abnormalities (*arrow*). (*B*) ^{67}Ga citrate scan focuses on the lumbar spine (*anterior view*), showing an increased uptake at the same area seen in *A*. (*C*) ^{67}Ga scan focuses on the pelvis (*anterior view*), showing intrapelvic and inguinal lymphomas.

a collapsed vertebra, also showed an unusual hot lesion.

CLINICAL EFFECTIVENESS

Scintigraphic examinations had been generally used for detection of occult lesions on roentgenograms, such as occult spine metastases.[7,9,62] However, the clinical effectiveness of scintigraphy varies among reports, depending on the nature of the lesion, stage of the disease, and the pharmaceuticals employed. In our series of 77 patients with definitely diagnosed spinal metastases, 94.7% were evident on scans using ^{99m}Tc diphosphonate and 61.1% using ^{67}Ga citrate (Table 3-2). The overall positive ratio in our series of 164 patients with spine or spinal cord lesions was 80.1% in 156 patients using ^{99m}Tc scan and 44.0% in 75 patients using ^{67}Ga citrate. The postmortem studies of patients with spine metastases of carcinoma generally revealed that a majority were evident using scintigraphy—68.8% in Clain's study and 74.7% in that of Maeyama and associates.[10,43] In another of our series of spine metastases, 201 patients with breast cancer were examined with bone scans using ^{99m}Tc-MDP for the purpose of detecting bone metastases. Among 201 patients, 57 had bone metastases. Detection by bone scintigraphy was obtained in 9 of 57 patients (15.8%) earlier than it was obtained by roentgenogram. Metastases were detected later by scintigraphy in only one patient (1.8%), whereas in 47 patients (82.5%) they were detected simultaneously. In the first group of 9 patients who were all asymptomatic, roentgenographic changes were found with an interval of 2 to 11 months (5.3 months on the average) following scintigraphic detection. Thus, even in the asymptomatic cases of spine metastases, bone scintigraphy provided a high positive ratio of detection. Moreover, the metastatic lesions in the symptomatic cases are detected with clear visualization on scintigraphy.

On the other hand, regarding the qualitative nature of lesions, especially malignancies, bone scan is not informative, as in our series there proved to be no significant differences in the positive ratio between malignant spine tumors (94.4%) and benign spine tumors (85.7%) (Table 3-2). In this regard, there was a considerably greater disparity in the positive ratio of ^{67}Ga scan to malignant and benign spine tumor, that is, 58.7% versus 11.1%. Therefore, ^{67}Ga citrate proved to be a most beneficial tracer (Fig. 3-74). In the case of a suspected malignancy, comprehensive radiologic examinations including tomograms, CT scans, and

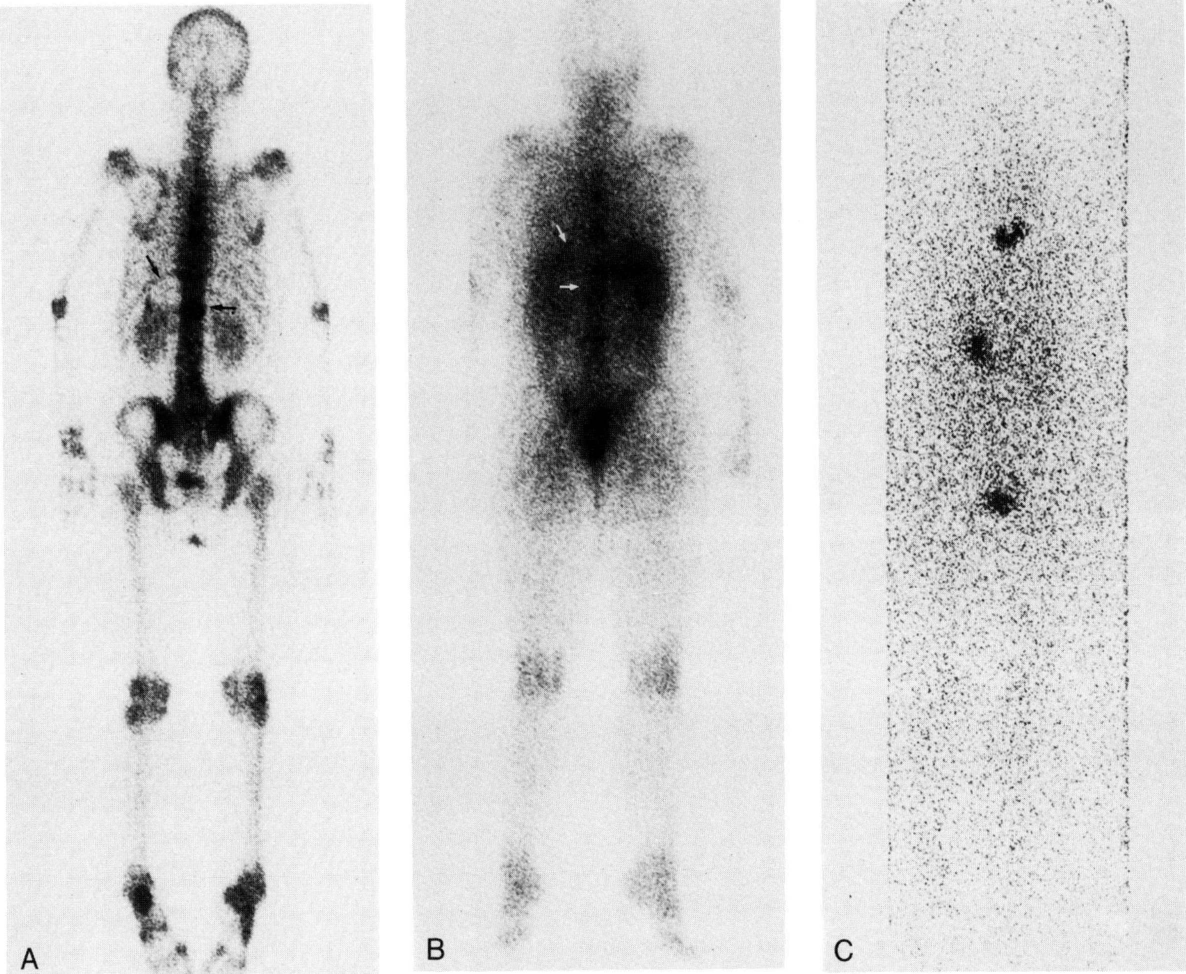

Fig. 3-75. Posterior whole-body scan in a 57-year-old woman with metastases secondary to thyroid cancer. Localization of increased uptake varied according to the tracer. (*A*) ^{99m}Tc-MDP scan shows increased uptake in the D12 vertebra and a cold area within an area of high uptake in the left eleventh rib (*black arrows*). (*B*) ^{67}Ga citrate scan showing increased uptake, which was somewhat masked, in the cold area of the left eleventh rib and the D12 vertebra (*white arrows*). (*C*)^{123} I scan shows increased uptake in the thyroid gland and the cold area of the left eleventh rib.

selective angiography should be followed for a distinct diagnosis. An evaluation of roentgenogram, bone scan, and CT scan related to their respective detection sensitivities to spine metastases was demonstrated by Onomura and associates.[49] In their study of 55 patients with definite spine metastases, the detection ratio of each exploration imaging technique was as follows: 82.1% by bone scan, 64.1% by CT scan, and 53.8% by plain roentgenogram. Even in the asymptomatic cases of spine metastases, there was a higher positive ratio of detection using bone scan. Thus, although having no specificity for the quality of diseases, bone scan is indeed a more effective modality for the detection of spine metastases. Regarding specificity to the quality of the tumor, there are few reports on the search for tumor-localizing agents to determine the accurate diagnosis of lesions as a substitute for ^{67}Ga citrate (Fig. 3-75).[21] Definite results are not established yet.

High uptake of ^{99m}Tc diphosphonate was also noted in patients with infectious spondylitis (tuberculous spondylitis, pyogenic osteomyelitis, and discitis), and noninfectious spondylitis (ankylosing

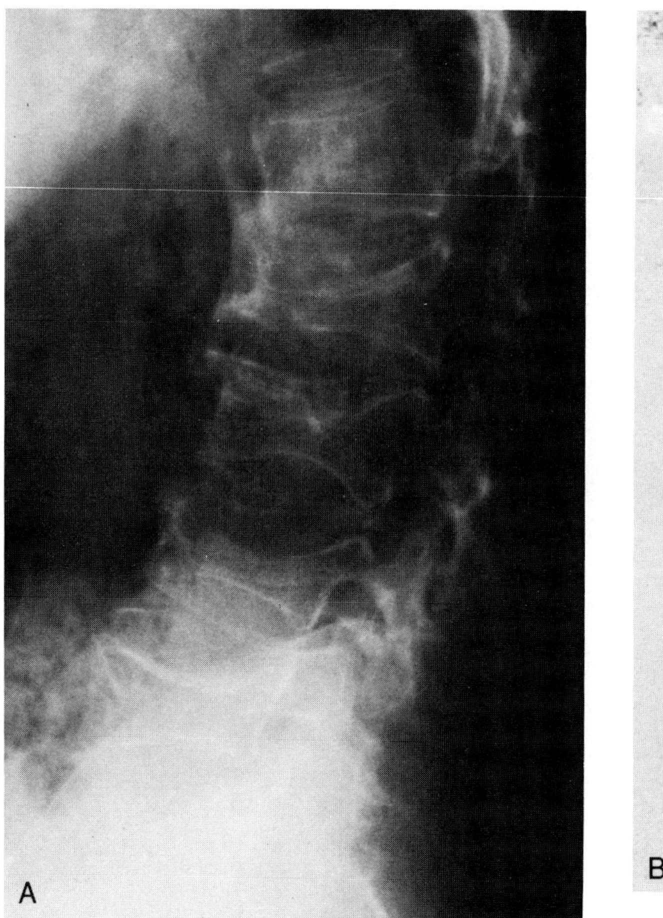

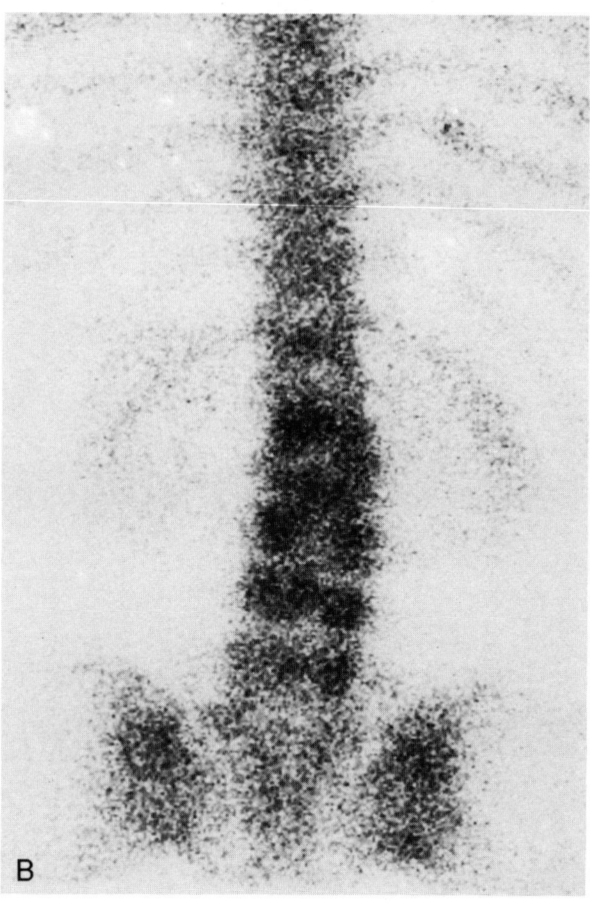

Fig. 3-76. A 46-year-old woman with a low-turnover osteomalacia, diagnosed by symptoms of low back pain, laboratory findings, and histologic evidence. (*A*) Lateral view of plain roentgenogram shows marked collapse of the lumbar vertebrae. (*B*) ^{99m}Tc-MDP scan shows the lesions by increased uptake at the same levels of the lumbar vertebrae seen in *A*.

spondylitis and erosive spondylopathy) (Fig. 3-73). The ^{67}Ga scan only showed a low uptake in such inflammatory disease. This contrasted with Hoffer's report, in which scintigraphy using inflammatory-seeking tracers (*e.g.*, ^{67}Ga-labeled leukocytes, ^{111}In oxine-labeled leukocytes and ^{99m}Tc phytate leukocytes and monocytes) is investigated.[6,33,45,56] Thus, tracers with different affinities suggesting the nature of the inflammatory disease are required.

Scintigraphic examination can be used not only for detection, but also for evaluating the extent of bone metastases to entire skeletons.[24,26] A system of staging patients with bone metastasis according to the extent of bone is essential to ascertaining the prognosis of the patient and managing the patient appropriately. There are, however, few reports available on such staging system utilized in patients suffering from advanced bone metastases. The distribution of metastatic lesions was also analyzed by bone scintigraphy in our series in 57 patients with breast cancer and skeletal metastases. They were consecutively followed (Table 3-3). A total of 933 bone lesions were detected in the positive scans, where the distribution of bone lesions was as follows: 44.3% in spine, 27.8% in ribs, 12.9% in pelvis, 5.8% in skull, 4.2% in femur, 2.4% in sternum, and 2.6% in the others. When skeletal system of metastasis was divided into the following three groups according to the distribution of bone lesions consisting of C (spine and rib), P1 (pelvis and skull), and P2 (others), a majority of the pa-

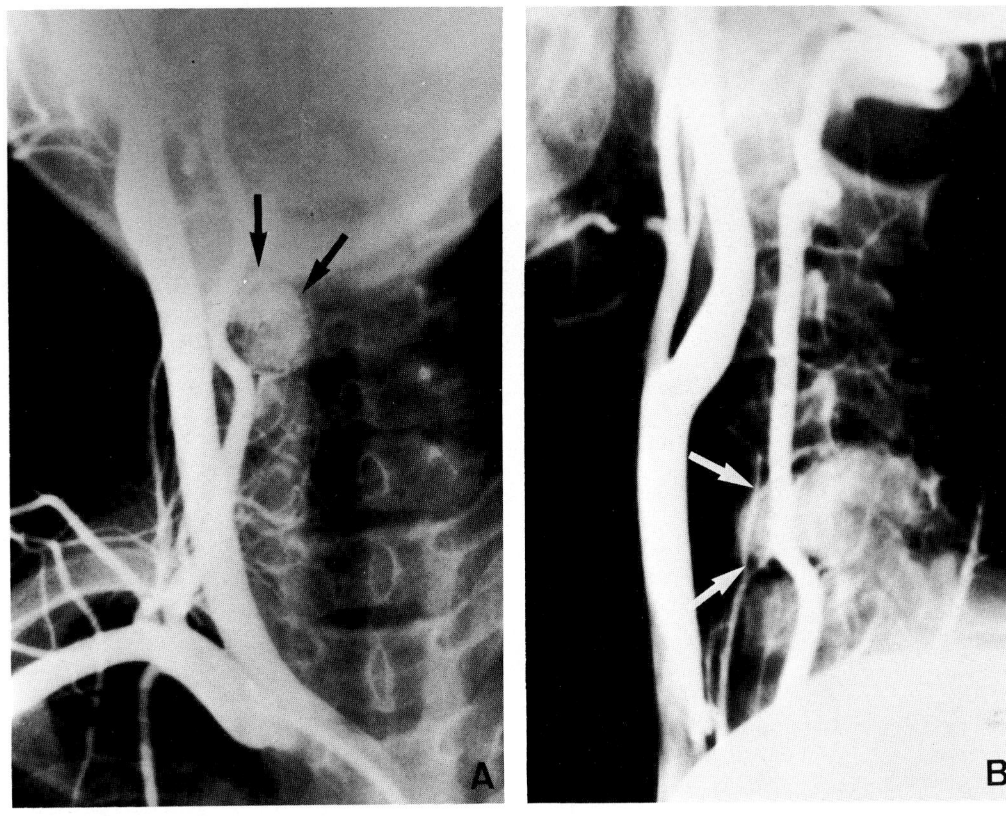

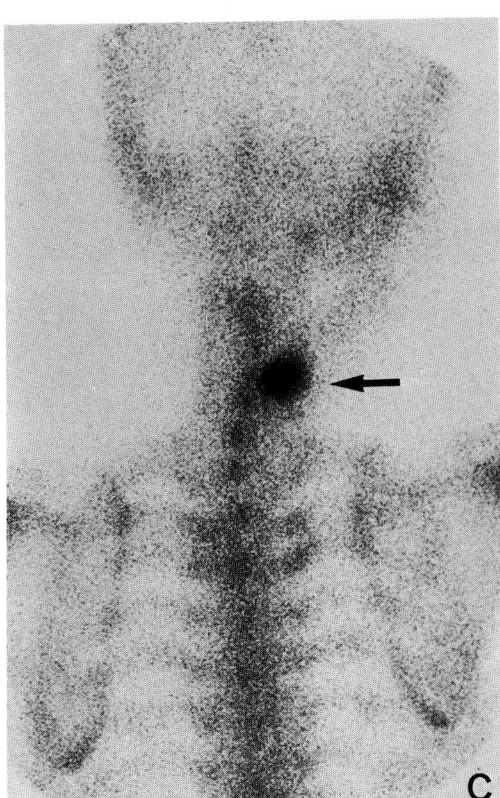

Fig. 3-77. A 12-year-old girl with osteoid osteoma at the right pedicle and body of the C5 vertebra. Selective angiography shows marked deviation of the right vertebral artery, hypervascularity, and tumor stain in the area of the vertebral and thyrocervical arteries, seen in both (*A*) the A–P view (*black arrows*) and (*B*) the lateral view (*white arrows*). (*C*) Posterior view of ^{99m}Tc-MDP shows a marked accumulation in the same area (*black arrow*).

Table 3-3. Distribution of Skeletal Metastases, Detected by Bone Scintigraphy in 148 Positive Scans in 57 Patients with Breast Cancer

SITE OF METASTASES	INCIDENCE	DISTRIBUTION OF BONE LESIONS
Spine	75.0%	44.3%*
Rib	64.9%	27.8%
Pelvis	45.3%	12.9%
Skull	25.7%	5.8%
Femur	18.2%	4.2%
Sternum	14.9%	2.4%
Humerus	4.1%	1.0%
Clavicle	4.1%	0.9%
Scapula	3.4%	0.8%

* Percentage is shown in which spine contains sacrum.

tients with bone metastases had degrees of involvement that were classifiable and of predictive value. The sequences could be classified into three patterns: C → C + P1 → C + P1 + P2, whereas the number of bone lesions also increased sequentially. Therefore, we defined a staging system according to this respective sequential distribution as follows: Stage C, Stage P1, and Stage P2. When metastases were confined to skeletal system, average survival periods for patients from the date of scintigraphy were as follows: stage C was 38.6 months, stage P1 was 18.1 months, and stage P2 was 16.3 months. There are several reports assessing the serial quantitative bone scans as an index for response to the treatment.[24,26] Regarding the prognosis or survival time of metastatic-disease patients, our staging system was significant; it correlated well with the survival periods, when skeletal metastasis was dominant.

It was of little value to apply scintigraphy to spinal cord tumor, even with hypervascularity such as occurs in hemangioblastoma, or to spinal arteriovenous malformation. A group of 22 patients with spinal cord tumor were assessed by scintigraphy; 20 were given ^{99m}Tc diphosphonate and 10 were given ^{67}Ga citrate. The bone scan showed no uptake in the lesions. These findings should be subjected to further study, including myelography and CT myelography, MRI, and selective angiography.

SELECTIVE ANGIOGRAPHY

Purpose

Since the introduction of selective angiography by DiChiro and Fisher and by Djindjian, angiography has become established in radiologic examinations of various diseases of the spine, and has facilitated vascular studies as the result of improved imaging and safety.[12,16] Nevertheless, recent advances in exploration image techniques, such as CT scanning or scintigraphy, have shown that angiography should be reappraised. These newer techniques of investigation do not replace selective angiography but rather make more efficient use of it; in fact, application of the procedure for patients with spine disorders has increased.

The objectives of selective angiography in cases of elective spine surgery are generally as follows:

1. For diagnosis of tumors (hypervascular cord tumors such as hemangioblastoma and hypervascular glioma, and hypervascular spine tumors such as primary or secondary malignant tumor, hemangioma, aneurysmal bone cyst, and osteoid osteoma)
2. For diagnosis of vascular lesions (arteriovenous malformation or hamartomatous vascular anomalies, and hypotrophic or obstructive vascular lesions of the spinal cord)
3. For prognostic assessment of paralysis by visualization of the spinal cord blood supply (posttraumatic paraplegia and tetraplegia, cervical spondylotic myelopathy, spinal cord compression by ossified posterior longitudinal ligament or ossified yellow ligament, and radiation myelopathy).
4. For prevention of spinal cord ischemia, not a rare complication during radical spine surgery, for example, in correction of advanced spine deformity or total resection of affected vertebra.
5. For treatment of hypervascular lesions, to visualize the feeder vessels (selective emboliza-

tion of main feeders to an arteriovenous malformation or other hypervascular spine lesions)

Technique and Regional Anatomy

Whereas Djindjian and associates routinely conduct the angiography examination under general anesthesia with premedication, such as a perfusion of low molecular weight dextran containing chlorpromazine 50 mg, pethidine 100 mg, promethazine 50 mg, and hydrocortisone 50 mg, we perform a percutaneous catheterization (Seldinger technique) through the femoral artery with the patient under local anesthesia whenever possible.[16,58] Young children must be given a general anesthetic or at least must be lightly sedated. Anesthesia generally masks signs and symptoms of undue cord irritation during the procedure, which would require interruption of the examination. Ioxaglate (methylglucamine iothalamate) with its greater safety is definitely preferable to other contrast dyes. Less than 8 ml in a single infusion in any one of the vessels and less than 150 ml in total are the upper limits for safety. For further detailed techniques of the procedure, see the discussions by Doppman and coworkers, Djindjian and coworkers, or Pia and Djindjian.[16,19,52]

For better imaging of a specific vascular abnormality, select a vessel that mainly feeds the lesion and avoid superimposition of vessels not specific to the area concerned. For visualization of the radiculomedullary vessels, select the proper branches of a limited number of arteries; there are considerable individual variations in the distribution or location of the main radicular arteries and the vascular sources.[18,38–40] Whereas the spinal cord has a specific long-circuit vascular system and its own hemodynamics (for safety, through the anteroposterior spinal arteries and its main feeders, the radiculomedullary vessels), the spine and its surrounding structures have a more segmental or short-circuit pattern of blood supply from the nearby major vessels. In the dorsolumbar region, for example, each vertebra receives several sets of vessels from a segmental artery. Parke described these vessels as consisting of anterior central, posterior central, prelaminar, and postlaminar branches.[50] The posterior central branch, entering the intervertebral foramen associated with the prelaminar and neural branches (the neural, meningeal, and epidural tissue), supplies the vertebral body, making an intravertebral anastomosis with the anterior central branches. Each vertebral body is supplied by four posterior central branches derived from two intervertebral levels. Therefore, at least two adjacent segmental arteries should be selected for angiography of each vertebral lesion. Pre-, para-, or retrovertebral muscles of the spine are generally supplied by either a lateral (intercostal or lumbar) or a dorsal branch of a segmental artery with rich intersegmental and intrasegmental vascular anastomoses. The cervical and sacral differ from the dorsolumbar region with regard to vascular sources but are similar to the latter with regard to segmental distribution pattern and anastomosis. Table 3-4 is a guide for the selection of an appropriate vessel for angiography. This table was based upon both Djindjian's study of the blood supply to the spinal cord and Parke's study of the nutrient arteries of the spinal column, although there are discrepancies in detail (Lazorthes *et al*, Djindjian *et al*, and Dommisse).[16,18,39,40,50]

Principal Features in Pathologic Conditions

The principal abnormalities encountered in pathologic conditions in spinal surgery are as follows.

UNUSUAL COURSE AND DISTRIBUTION OF VESSELS. Adjacent to a tumor, vessels often display a curved appearance, irrespective of the nature of the tumor. In malignant lesions, hypervascularity, abnormal distribution, and tumor vessels usually coexist.

HYPERVASCULARITY OR HYPOVASCULARITY. An increased number of vessels may be encountered, particularly in malignant tumors where the new vessels present abnormal appearances and distribution. Benign tumors often demonstrate disproportionately few vessels in relation to their large size. Postirradiation areas often exhibit true hypovascularity.

TUMOR VESSELS. Bizarre, tangled, and irregularly structured vessels may extend from a few feeders or develop into a fine network. Vessels also appear abnormal in their linear runs, sharp angles, and ramifications (Fig. 3-78). These features are well-known characteristics of tumor vessels, frequently coexisting with hypervascularity and arteriovenous shunt (Figs. 3-79 and 3-80).

VASCULAR DILATATION AND BLOOD POOLS. Dilatation of the feeder artery and blood pools within the lesion are considered to be common in malignant tumors, but, as stated by Djindjian *et al,* they are also consistently demonstrated in an angio-

Table 3-4. Guide for the Selection of the Appropriate Vessel for Angiography

LEVEL	SPINAL CORD	SPINE AND SURROUNDING TISSUES
Cervicodorsal region (C1–D2 segments)*	1. Vertebral a. → Basilar a. ↓ Anterior spinal a. Radicular a. accompanying the C3 nerve root 2. Vertebral a. or deep cervical a. →radicular a. accompanying the C6 nerve root (artery of the cervical enlargement)† 3. Costocervical trunk or 1st intercostal a. →radicular a. accompany the C8 nerve root	1. Thyreocervical trunk ascending cervical a. 2. Costocervical trunk →deep cervical a. 3. Segmental branches of vertebral a. 4. 1st intercostal a.
Mid-dorsal region (D1–D7 segments)‡	Intercostal a.; radicular a. accompanying D4 or D5 nerve root	1. Costocervical trunk 2. Intercostal a.
Dorsolumbosacral region (D8 conus terminalis)	1. Intercostal a. or lumbar a. →arteria radicularis anterior magna (Adamkiewicz) accompanying a nerve root between D9–L2 2. One or two arteries accompanying the filaments of the cauda equina Lumbar a. Iliolumbar a. Middle and lateral sacral a.	1. Intercostal a. or lumbar a. 2. Iliolumbar a. 3. Middle and lateral sacral a. superior gluteal a. or hypogastric a.

* The C1–C4 segments are unique in blood supply; they are supplied by the anterior spinal artery and generally have little or no radicular inflow. The artery is originally supplied by the suboccipital anastomotic confluence formed by the anastomosis of the vertebral, the occipital, and the ascending and deep cervical arteries. The atlantoaxial complex is supplied by the medial branch of the vertebral artery coursed from the C3 segment, the anastomotic derivatives of the carotid artery, and a number of direct branches of the vertebral artery that arches over the posterior arch of the atlas. (Lazorthes G: La vascularisation artêrielle de la moëlle. Recherches anatomiques et application à la pathologie medullaire et aortique. Neurochirurgie 4:3, 1958; Lazorthes G, Gouazé A, Djindjian R: Vascularisation et pathologie vasculaire de la moëlle épinière. Paris, Masson, 1973; Lazorthes G, Gouazé A, Zadeh JD, Santin JJ, Lazorthes Y, Burdin, P: Arterial vascularization of the spinal cord: Recent studies of the anastomotic substitution pathways. J Neurosurg 35:253, 1971; and Parke WW: Applied anatomy of the spine. In Rothman RH, Simeone FA (ed): The Spine, Vol. 19, p. 52, Philadelphia, WB Saunders, 1975)

† Lazorthes G: La vascularisation artérielle de la moëlle. Recherches anatomiques et application à la pathologie medullaire et aortique. Neurochirurgie 4:3, 1958

‡ D1, D2 segments are supplied by the extension of the anterior spinal artery of the cervical enlargement.

matous vertebra and often in an aneurysmal bone cyst in the spine (Fig. 3-81).[16]

CHANGE IN CIRCULATION TIME. Whenever arteriovenous shunts exist, often in malignant tumor and arteriovenous malformation, the circulation is rapid, as evidenced by an early venous return. These conditions often present stasis within the draining vessels.

TUMOR STAIN. An intense, relatively homogenous opacity continuing beyond the venous phase is probably one of the characteristic features of vascular lesions or malignant tumors, but is often

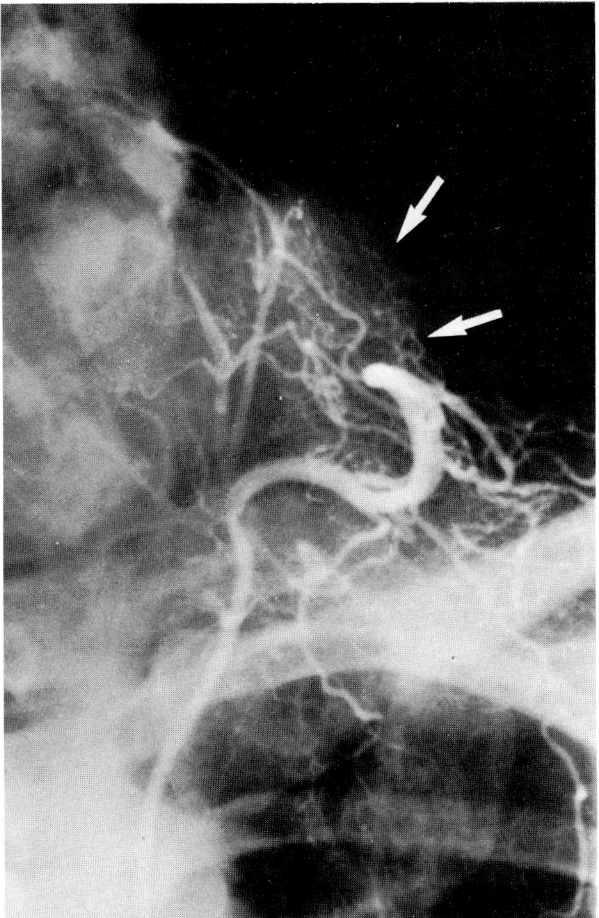

Fig. 3-78. Selective angiography of a 40-year-old woman with osteosarcoma from the C4 to C7 vertebra. Note the hypervascularity, tumor stain, and typical tumor vessels (*arrows*) suggesting malignancy, mainly in the territory of the left thyrocervical artery.

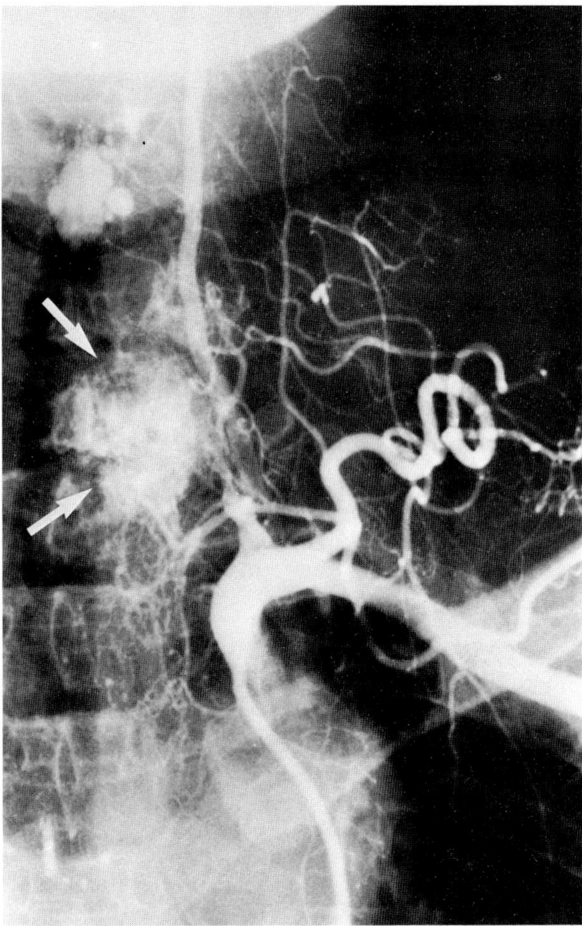

Fig. 3-79. Angiography of a 58-year-old woman with metastasis secondary to renal cancer, affecting the C7 vertebra. Note the hypervascularity, tumor stain, and tumor vessels, mainly in the territory of the thyrocervical artery.

demonstrated in vertebrae with osteoid osteoma (Figs. 3-78, 3-80, 3-81, and 3-82).*

ARTERIOVENOUS MALFORMATIONS. The best-known and most widely accepted indication for spinal cord angiography is the presence of an arteriovenous malformation. This lesion is frequently suspected because of a characteristic history, abnormalities in the cerebrospinal fluid, and the myelographic manifestations. According to morphologic characteristics, arteriovenous malformations of the spinal cord have been classified into three basic patterns by DiChiro and associates.[13] Each type is defined as follows:

Type 1 is characterized by one or two tightly coiled continuous vessels spread along a large longitudinal section of the cord (Fig. 3-83*A* and *D*).

Type 2 presents as a localized plexus or congeries of vessels into which single or multiple arterial feeders converge and from which one or several venous drainers depart. The draining veins can be

* In an attempt to discriminate the benign spine lesions (benign tumors or tumorous conditions and inflammation) from the malignancies seen in the angiography, the incidences of the foregoing vascular abnormalities were investigated respectively in 62 cases (Table 3-5). Consequently, the existence of characteristic tumor vessels and tumor stain proved to be the most specific features of the malignant nature of spine tumors, although both features were not rare in cases of giant cell tumor (Figs. 3-78, 3-79, and 3-80).

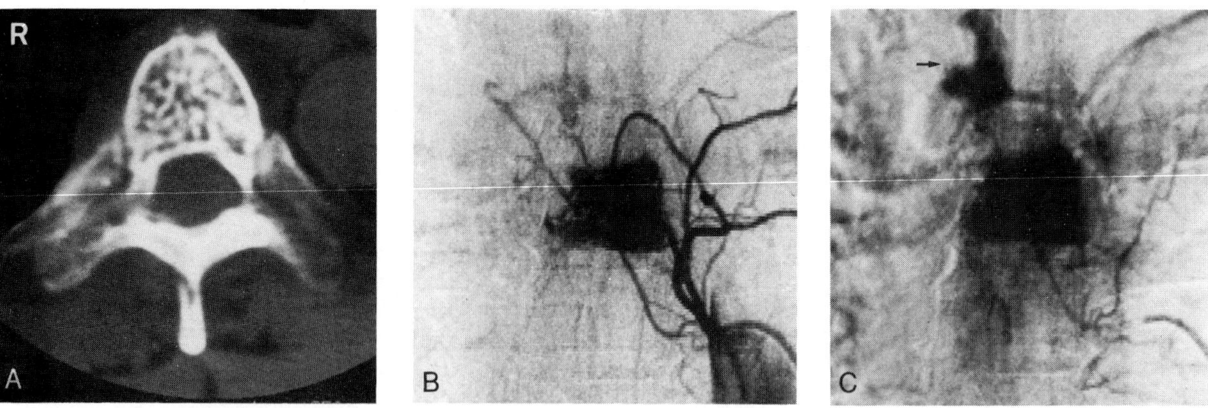

Fig. 3-80. A 59-year-old man with hemangioendothelioma in the D6 vertebra. (*A*) CT scan shows polka dot densities in the vertebral body, lytic changes of the transverse processes and ribs, and surrounding soft masses between the pleura and vertebral body. Note marked hypervascularity, tumor vessels, and tumor stain, fed mainly by the left sixth intercostal artery in the arterial phase (*B*). Further tumor stain was visualized in the adjacent proximal area in the arteriovenous phase (*arrow*).

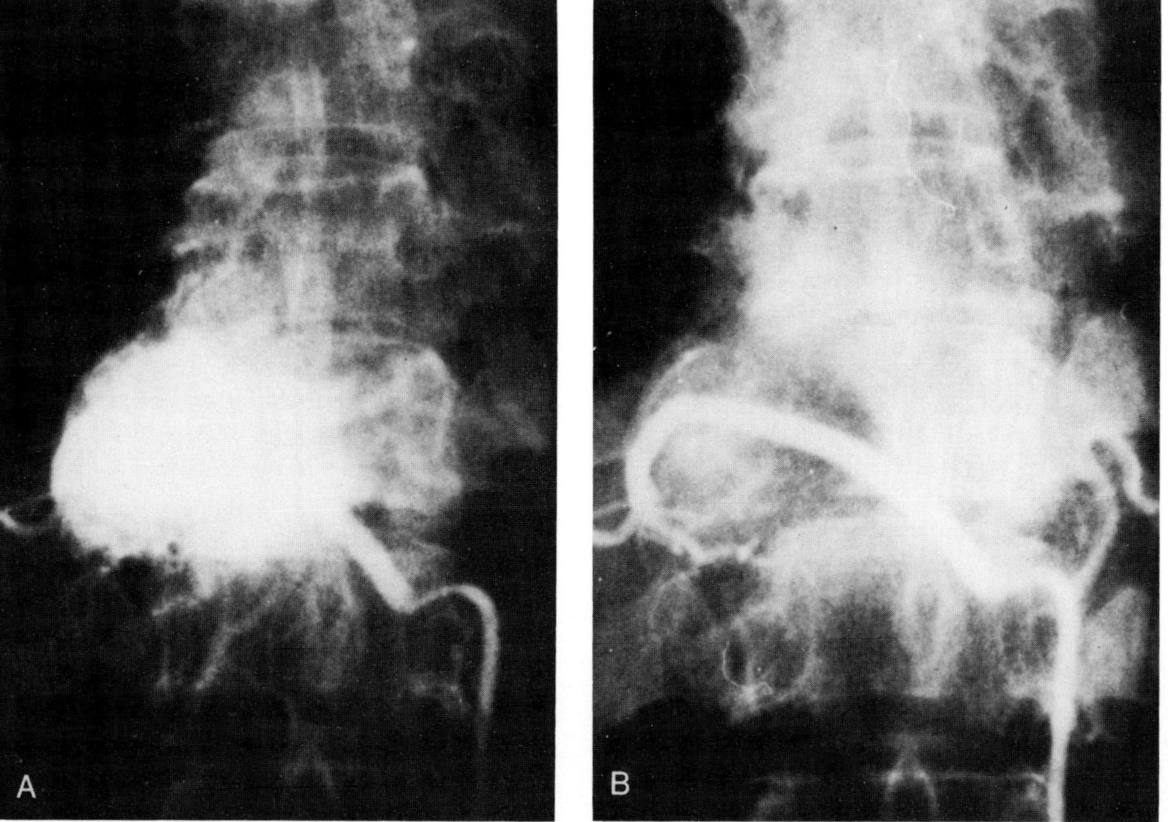

Fig. 3-81. A 53-year-old woman with metastasis secondary to thyroid cancer. (*A*) Selective angiography via the right eleventh intercostal artery shows marked dilatation of the segmental artery and hypervascularity in the lytic metastatic area of the eleventh vertebra. (*B*) Preoperative embolization was performed, using the particulates of Gelfoam. Following embolization, the vascularity was reduced.

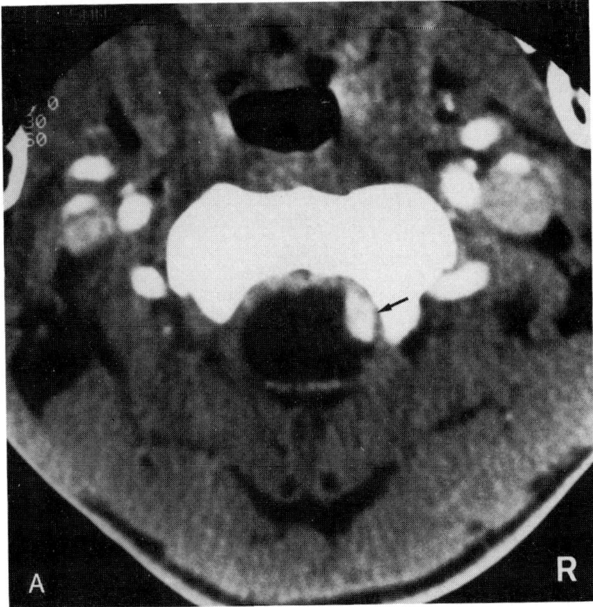

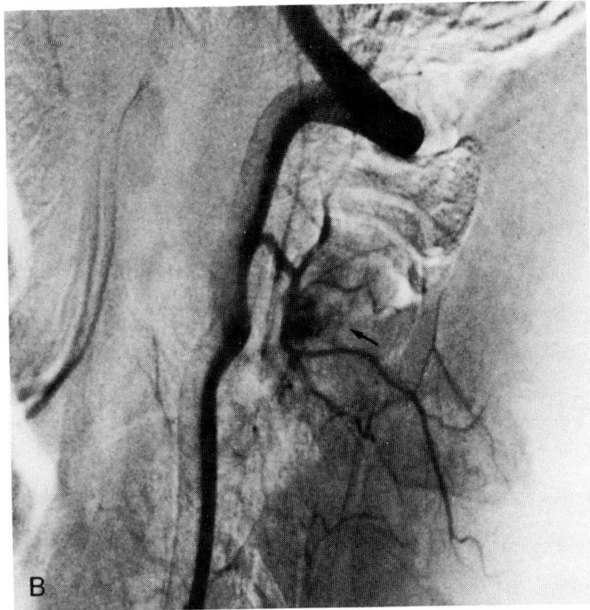

Fig. 3-82. A 29-year-old man with hemangioblastoma at the C2 and C3 level of the spinal cord. (*A*) Enhanced CT scan shows a high-intensity lesion in the spinal cord in association with syringomyelia (*arrow*). (*B*) Selective angiography via the left vertebral artery shows hypervascularity and tumor stain (*arrow*).

quite long and extend all the way to the endocranium or down to the pelvic vessels (Fig. 3-83*B*).

Type 3 is seen more frequently in children. Multiple large feeder arteries supply voluminous malformations that often appear to fill the spinal canal (Fig. 3-83*C*).

VASCULAR OBSTRUCTION. Atheromatous vascular lesions or complete obstructions are occasionally encountered in the major vessels and do not permit catheterization for radiculomedullary visualization, particularly in the elderly. The radiculomedullary vessels do not undergo atheromatous change but are frequently interrupted by various conditions, such as fracture and dislocation of the spine, tuberculous spondylitis, spondylosis, or intraspinal tumors. Based on a huge number of selective angiographies of the spine, Yonezawa and associates postulated that interruption of the radiculomedullary vessels often revealed a poor blood supply or ischemia of the spinal cord itself, and thus that selective angiography could monitor the

Table 3-5. Principal Abnormalities and Their Incidence in Selective Angiography of Spine Tumors, Tumorous Conditions, Spinal Cord Tumors, and Arteriovenous Malformations

	No. of Patients	Deviation	Hypervascularity	Tumor Vessel	Tumor Stain	Dilatation
Malignant spine tumor	27	21 (77.8%)	18 (66.7%)	25 (92.6%)	25 (92.6%)	18 (66.7%)
Primary	7	5 (71.4%)	6 (85.7%)	6 (85.7%)	6 (85.7%)	4 (57.1%)
Metastatic	20	16 (80.0%)	12 (60.0%)	19 (95.0%)	19 (95.0%)	14 (70.0%)
Benign spine tumor, tumorous condition	12	6 (50.0%)	5 (41.7%)	8 (66.7%)	8 (66.7%)	4 (33.3%)
Spinal cord tumor	6	5 (83.3%)	2 (33.3%)	2 (33.3%)	2 (33.3%)	2 (33.3%)
AV malformations	17	14/17 (81.4%)	Type1:9(64.3%)	Type2:2(14.3%)	Type3:3(21.4%)	

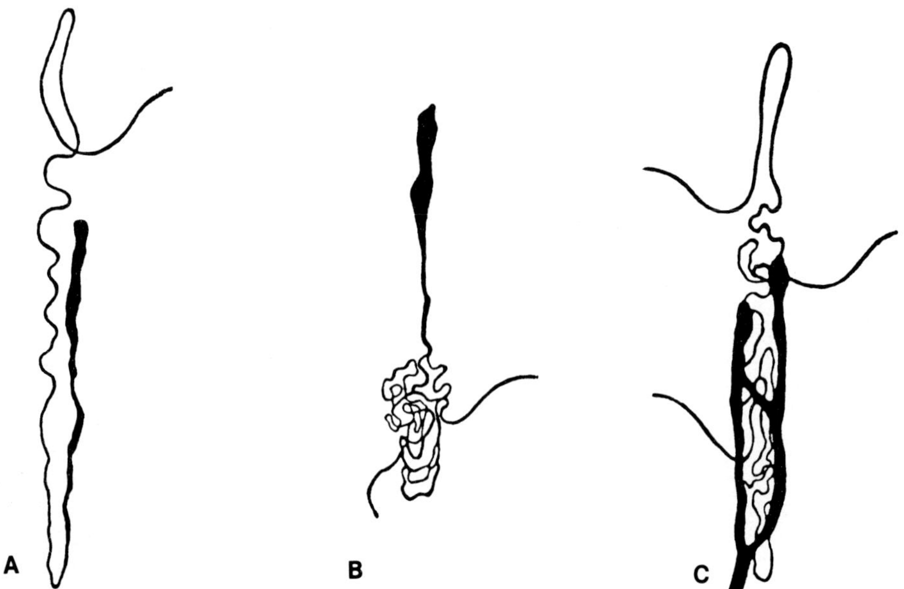

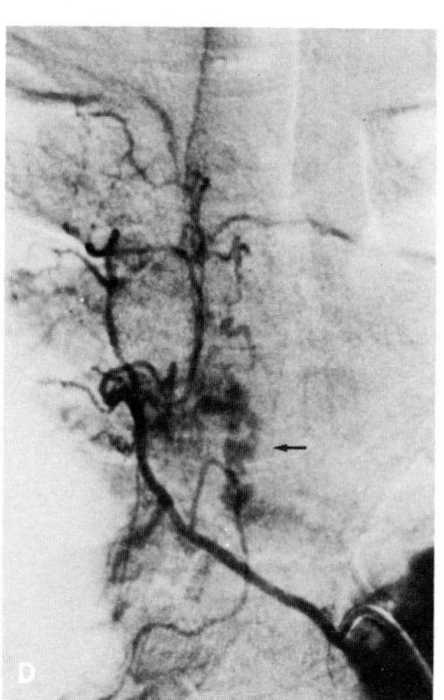

Fig. 3-83. Schematic representation (*A* to *C*) and photograph (*D*) of three types of spinal cord arteriovenous malformations. (*A*) Type 1, plain arteriovenous fistula. (*B*) Type 2, glomus. (*C*) Type 3, juvenile. (*D*) A 53-year-old woman with Type 1 arteriovenous malformation. Nidus is indicated by arrow. (Di Chiro G, Doppman JL, Ommaya AK: Radiology of spinal cord arteriovenous malformations. Prog Neurol Surg 4:329, 1971)

viability of the spinal cord under these condition.[67–70]

Clinical Effectiveness in Spine Surgery

In a puzzling case, we do not initiate the examination with selective angiography, because the findings do not provide objective data leading to a definite diagnosis, except for arteriovenous malformation or hemangioma. The examination also has inherent limitations restricting its general acceptance. But in the ever-progressing exploration of image techniques, this approach can provide pertinent information on the vascularity of the lesions. Angiography does not make biopsy superfluous but rather indicates its necessity and allows determination of the most appropriate biopsy site. We undertake the procedure to procure pertinent

Table 3-6. A Guideline to Indications for Selective Angiography in Spine Surgery

PURPOSE OF EXAMINATION	DIAGNOSTIC VALUE	PRECEDING EXAMINATIONS	
Diagnosis of inflammatory condition	Limited value, only for differentiation	Roentgenogram, bone and Ga scans	Laboratory: hematology, electrophoresis, *etc.*
Diagnosis of benign tumor of the spine	Limited value, except for hemangioma	Roentgenogram, bone and Ga scans	Cerebrospinal fluid
Diagnosis of malignant tumor of the spine	Pertinent value	Roentgenogram, bone and Ga scans	Laboratory, and search for the origin
Diagnosis of benign tumor of the spinal cord	Limited value	Roentgenogram*	Myelography, electrophysiological study
Diagnosis of vascular malformation	Pertinent value	Roentgenogram*	Cerebrospinal fluid myelography
Diagnosis of obstructive vascular lesions in the spinal cord for determination of prognosis; diagnosis of radiation myelitis	Considerable value	Past history	Cerebrospinal fluid, electrophysiological study
Diagnosis of spondylotic myelopathy	Considerable value	Roentgenogram	Cerebrospinal fluid, electrophysiological study
Diagnosis of traumatic para- or tetraplegia	Considerable value	Roentgenogram	Myelography
Diagnosis of arteriosclerosis and obstructive lesions in major and related vessels	Considerable value		Comprehensive exam of cardiovascular systems
To investigate a cause of spontaneous myelopathy (myelopathy of unknown cause)	Considerable value	Roentgenogram	Cerebrospinal fluid, electrophysiological study
To define the extent and vascularity of tumors prior to excision	Pertinent value	Roentgenogram, bone and Ga scans	Myelography
To determine the best site for biopsy	Pertinent value	Roentgenogram, bone and Ga scans	
To prevent cord or major vessel injury in spine surgery, *e.g.*, correction of kyphotic or scoliotic spine, radical excision of the affected vertebra	Pertinent value	Roentgenogram, bone and Ga scans in tumor cases	Myelography, electrophysiological study

* Roentgenography often reveals spinal canal enlargement and/or erosion of a pedicle in a certain type of hereditary teleangiectasia.

supplementary data in the later stages of investigation.

A guideline to the practice of selective angiography and its diagnostic value in various conditions is shown in Table 3-6.

The detection rates for various spine lesions in 96 patients subjected to a comprehensive exploration (x-ray examination and scintigraphy, or selective angiography) were as follows: In cases of primary malignant tumors (osteosarcoma, malignant fibrous histiocytoma, chondrosarcoma, and multiple myeloma) 75% were diagnosed prior to surgical confirmation as definitely malignant; 25% were undetermined. With metastatic tumors (lung, thyroid, breast, prostatic, stomach, hepatic, renal, rectal, and uterine cancer, malignant melanoma, and unknown origin), 86.8% were diagnosed as definitely metastatic, and 13.2% were undetermined. With benign tumors or tumorous conditions of the spine (giant cell tumor, osteochondroma, bone cyst, osteoid osteoma, eosinophilic granuloma), 83.3% were diagnosed as definitely benign, and 16.7% were undetermined.

Since surgery of the spine, particularly in cases of tumors, is apt to be accompanied by a large amount of blood loss and to require intensive follow-up care, the nature of the lesions should be anticipated in order to attain the desired results.

Nondiagnostic Purposes

As progress is made in the technical aspects of angiography, better imaging and a minimization of the risk of the procedure will be realized. This will allow more effective preoperative management and a more accurate assessment of the spinal cord blood supply before surgery.

Treatment of spinal angiomas or arteriovenous malformations by embolization was well documented by Newton and Adams, Doppman and coworkers, and Djindjian and coworkers.[17,20,48] Application of the procedure in the case of tumorous or vascular lesions of the skeletal system has been reported.[15,22,51] A few authors reported the effects of hemostasis in a procedure applied preoperatively for excision of vascular lesions of the spine.[3,15,32,41] Four types of material are available for embolization: detachable balloons, stainless steel coils, particulates (Gelfoam, polyvinyl alcohol foam-PVA), and liquid agents. We prefer particulates of Gelfoam. In our experience, arterial bleeding can be fairly well controlled in such cases if this procedure is used within 48 to 72 hours prior to surgery. No adverse effects on the spinal cord were observed when Gelfoam was used as an embolus. There were no apparent effects on the venous bleeding from the intraspinal plexus. An early recanalization or accidental embolization by a dislodged embolus are inherent drawbacks that prevent a wider application of this procedure.[32]

To lessen the iatrogenic ischemic complication of the spinal cord during scoliosis surgery, Hilal and Keim conducted preoperative and postoperative selective spinal angiography in cases of adolescent scoliosis.[31] Although the intersegmental flow in the anterior spinal artery at the apex of severe scoliosis was decreased in a few patients, correction of the curvature did result in an improved blood supply to the spinal cord. Hilal and Keim stressed the importance of careful procedures in the area of segmental arteries, particularly in anterior approaches, in scoliosis surgery. Hence, selective spinal angiography can be a useful preoperative test for identification of spinal cord vulnerability.

Complications

Spinal angiography is now routinely undertaken as one of the requirements prior to the radical excision of tumors.

Technical progress in angiography and the availability of a well-tolerated contrast medium (Conray) has reduced the number of complications. Cord-related complications, however, may occur below the midthoracic segment, and consequently may be associated with paraplegia and a poor prognosis.[1,28] There are protective blood flow currents in the spinal arteries ensuring a rapid washout, with fresh oxygenated blood rushing through the long arterial anastomotic channels from the near radicular supplies.[14] Damage to the spinal cord may occur through interference with the protective mechanism by one or more of the following:

1. Nonskillful technique and careless catheter manipulation.
2. Massive injection of the contrast media under high pressure.
3. Opacification of all the cervical and vertebral arteries on both sides for the purpose of obtaining anteroposterior, lateral, and oblique views in a single session.
4. Continuous lodging of a catheter tip into the ostium of a narrow artery.
5. Accumulation of excessive amounts of the contrast media in the upper and middle dorsal region (>150 ml of Conray). Paraplegia and transverse lesions have been reported as complications of thoracic aortography and of selective bronchial angiography.[1,63]
6. Repeated injections within 10 minutes.
7. Failure to detect the unconscious or hypotensive patient.
8. Neglecting the signals of an urgent danger, such as severe paresthesia or spontaneous leg movements following the initial injection.

Freqeunt irrigation of the catheter with heparinized saline solution is recommended for prevention of thrombosis.

DIGITAL SUBTRACTION ANGIOGRAPHY

As previously mentioned, there are a considerable number of complications following conventional angiography or selective angiography.[28] To reduce the complications following angiographic catheter techniques, physicians should know the details of vascular anatomy and be familiar with adequate techniques. Digital subtraction angiography (DSA) has recently been reappraised as a substitute for catheterization by insertion into an artery, such as in the Seldinger technique.[35,58] DSA was first reported by Robb and Steinberg in 1939 as a means by which the contrast medium is inserted through a vein.[53] When selective angiography was introduced, however, it had been out of favor for a long time, because it could provide neither the concentration nor the resolution necessary for satisfactory visualization. Recent advances in computerization and contrast agents have improved opacification in DSA. The new generation of contrast media with low osmolality are biologically inert, and they substitute for the conventional generation of ionic monomers.[4] Therefore, DSA is becoming more widely accepted, particularly in the diagnosis of the occlusive vascular diseases.

Intravenous DSA

Intravenous DSA is usually performed using a Venula needle with 16-gauge inserted into a cubital vein after administration of diazepam (10 mg) and atropine sulphate (0.5 mg). When the cubital vein is too small to insert, a 5- to 6-French angiocatheter is inserted into the femoral vein. The tip of the catheter is advanced up to the superior vena cava or inferior vena cava. Conray 60 (iothalmate meglumine), 40 to 50 ml, is injected at a rate of 12 to 15 ml per second into a cubital vein, and at a rate of 15 to 30 ml per second into a femoral vein. Following injection into a cubital vein, DSA is performed at intervals of 4 seconds in neck, 6 seconds in head or abdomen, 8 seconds in pelvis, and 10 seconds in lower limbs. Injection should not be repeated more than four times, while the dose of contrast medium should not exceed 200 ml total. The artifacts may occur with DSA, because it is a temporal subtraction system. Misregistration artifacts, which commonly result from the patient's motion, should be avoided by keeping the patient immobilized in the bed.

Although intravenous DSA is thought to be a noninvasive procedure, some complications are reported in the literature: damage to the valves of veins, transient ischemic attack, cellulitis, thrombophlebitis, and extravasation of contrast medium.[57] Intravenous DSA is indicated for occlusive vascular diseases occurring in the larger vessels, although many attempts have been made to use it elsewhere. It rarely has value in spine surgery because of either poor opacification or low arterial concentration. Although Little and associates reported satisfactory results with intravenous DSA in their original studies, Weinstein and associates and Hoffman and associates[35,42,65] reported little success in making accurate diagnoses. Gonzalez and associates also reported that intravenous DSA has value only for patients in whom intraarterial angiography is not possible.[29] Furthermore, indications for surgery should be determined by conventional angiography or selective angiography.

Intraarterial DSA

The keys to obtaining satisfactory diagnoses with intraarterial DSA are reducing registration artifacts and using a superior remasking system. A 4- to 5-French catheter is used. Following its insertion into the common femoral artery, the catheter is advanced up to the area of the purposed artery, as is done with the Seldinger technique.[58] Hypaque (diatrizoate meglumine), 40 to 50 ml dilated two to three times, is injected at a rate of 25 ml per second. Recently, Amypaque (metrizamide), an ionic dimer, has also been tried as an inert contrast medium. When selective catheterization is performed, 5 to 6 ml of diluted Renografin is injected at a rate of 3 to 4 ml per second.[4]

Intraarterial DSA is chosen instead of intravenous DSA when the total dose of contrast medium may exceed 200 ml, or in patients with renal failure. This technique requires a direct puncture of the femoral artery, in which case the advantage of noninvasiveness is lost. However, there are several advantages in intraarterial DSA: (1) A testing volume can provide satisfactory opacification; (2) diluted contrast media reduce the discomfort of burning pain for patients, resulting in fewer motion artifacts; (3) selective angiographies can be omitted in some cases; and (4) vessels superimposed on the film despite their disadvantage, permit efficient planning for future angiography.

Intravenous DSA can never surpass selective angiography in the evaluation of spinal or spinal cord diseases. Selective angiography may continue to be a mainstay as stressed by Gonzalez and associates.[29] We now advocate the use of selective angiography in combination with intraarterial DSA, especially in diseases of the spine (Fig. 3-80).

REFERENCES

1. *Abrams HL:* Radiological aspects of operable heart disease. III. The hazards of retrograde thoracic aortography: A survey. Radiology 68:812, 1957
2. *Adams FG, Horton PW:* Rectilinear bone scanning: Differentiation between metastases and degenerative spinal disease. Br J Radiol 51:281, 1978
3. *Benati A, Da Pian R, Mazza C, Maschiro A, Perini SG, Bricolo A, Ore GD:* Preoperative embolization of a vertebral haemangioma compressing the spinal cord. Neuroradiol 7:181, 1974
4. *Bettmann MA, Morris TW:* Recent advances in contrast agents. Radiol Clin North Am 24:347, 1986
5. *Bitran JD, Bekerman C, Golomb HM, Simon MA:* Scintigraphic evaluation of sarcomata in children and adults by ^{67}GA citrate. Cancer 42:1760, 1978
6. *Burleson RL, Holman BL, Tow DE:* Scintigraphic demonstration of abscesses with radioactive gallium labeled leukocytes. Surg Gynecol Obstet 141:379, 1975
7. *Charkes ND:* Radioisotope scanning of roentgenographically occult disorders of bone. In: Clinical Uses of Radionuclides: Critical Comparison with Other Techniques (CONF-711101), p 101. Oak Ridge, Atomic Energy Commission, 1972
8. *Chiewitz P, Hevesy G:* Radioactive indicators in the study of phosphorus metabolism in rats. Nature 136:754, 1935
9. *Citrin DL, Bessent RG, Greig WR:* A comparison of the sensitivity and accuracy of the ^{99m}Tc-phosphate bone scan and skeletal radiograph in the diagnosis of bone metastases. Clin Radiol 28:107, 1977
10. *Clain A:* Secondary malignant disease of bone. Br J Cancer 19:15, 1965
11. *Constable AR, Crange RW:* Recognition of the superscan in prostatic bone scintigraphy. Br J Radiol 54:122, 1981
12. *Di Chiro G, Fisher RL:* Contrast radiography of the spinal cord. Arch Neurol 11:125, 1964
13. *Di Chiro G, Doppman JL, Ommaya AK:* Radiology of spinal cord arteriovenous malformations. Prog Neurol Surg 4:329, 1971
14. *Di Chiro G, Wener L:* Angiography of the spinal cord: A review of contemporary techniques and applications. J Neurosurg 39:1, 1973
15. *Dick HM, Bigliani LU, Michelsen WJ, Johnston AD, Stinchfield FE:* Adjuvant arterial embolization in the treatment of benign primary bone tumors in children. Clin Orthop 139:133, 1979
16. *Djindjian R, Hurst M, Houdart R:* L'angiographic de la moëlle épinére. Baltimore, University Park Press, 1970
17. *Djindjian R, Cophignon J, Theron J, Merland J, Houdart R:* Embolization by superselective arteriography from the femoral route in neuroradiology: Review of 60 cases. 1. Technique indications, complications. Neuroradiol 6:20, 1973
18. *Dommisse GF:* The arteries and veins of the human spinal cord from birth. Edinburgh, Churchill Livingstone, 1975
19. *Doppman JL, Di Chiro G, Ommaya AK:* Selective arteriography of the spinal cord. St Louis, Warren H Green, 1969
20. *Doppman JL, Di Chiro G, Ommaya AK:* Percutaneous embolization of spinal cord arteriovenous malformations, J Neurosurg 34:48, 1971
21. *Edwards CL, Hayes RL:* Tumor scanning with ^{67}Ga citrate. J Nucl Med 10:103, 1969
22. *Feldman F, Casarella WJ, Dick HM, Hollander BA:* Selective intra-arterial embolization of bone tumors. A useful adjunct in the management of selected lesions. Am J Roentgenol Radium Ther Nucl Med 123:130, 1975
23. *Francis MD:* The inhibition of calcium hydroxyapatite crystal growth by polyphosphonates and polyphosphates. Calcif Tissue Res 3:151, 1969
24. *Galasko CSB, Westerman BLJ, Li J, Sellwood RA, Burn JI:* Use of the gamma camera for early detection of osseous metastases from mammary cancer. Br J Surg 55:613, 1968
25. *Galasko CSB:* The pathological basis for skeletal scintigraphy. J Bone Joint Surg 57B:353, 1975
26. *Galasko CSB, Weber DA:* Radionuclide scintigraphy in orthopaedics. Edinburgh, Churchill Livingstone, 1984
27. *Gelrud LG, Arseneau JC, Milder MS, Kramer RJ, Canellos GP, Johnston GS:* The kinetics of ^{67}gallium incorporation into inflammatory lesions: Experimental and clinical studies. J Lab Clin Med 83:489, 1974
28. *Gonzalez CF:* The nervous system. In the radiology of complications in medical practice, pp. 1. Edited by Schwarz ED. Baltimore, University Park Press, 1984
29. *Gonzalez CF, Doan HT, Han SS, Filipp GJ:* Extracranial vascular angiography. Radiol Clin North Am 24:419, 1986
30. *Guillemart A, Besnard JC, Pape A, Galy G, Fetissoff F:* Skeletal uptake of pyrophosphate labeled with technetium-95, and technetium-96m, as evaluated by autoradiography. J Nucl Med 19:895, 1978
31. *Hilal SK, Keim HA:* Selective spinal angiography in adolescent scoliosis. Radiology 102:349, 1972
32. *Hilal SK, Michelsen JW:* Therapeutic percutaneous embolization for extra-axial vascular lesions of the head, neck, and spine. J Neurosurg 43:275, 1975
33. *Hoffer PB, Miller-Catchpole R, Turner DA:*

Demonstration of lactoferrin in tumor tissue from two patients with positive gallium scans. J Nucl Med 20:424, 1979

34. *HOFFER P:* Gallium: Mechanisms. J Nucl Med 21:282, 1980
35. *HOFFMAN MG, GOMES AS, PAIS SO:* Limitations in the interpretation of intravenous carotid digital subtraction angiography. AJR 142:261, 1984
36. *JONES AG, FRANCIS MD, DAVIS MA:* Bone scanning: Radionuclidic reaction mechanisms. Semin Nucl Med 6:3, 1976
37. *LARSON SM, RASEY JS, ALLEN DR, NELSON NJ:* A transferrin mediated uptake of gallium-67 by EMT-6 sarcoma. 1. Studies in tissue culture. J Nucl Med 20:837, 1979
38. *LAZORTHES G:* La vascularisation artérielle de la moëlle. Recherches anatomiques et application à la pathologie medullaire et a la pathologie aortique. Neurochirurgie 4:3, 1958
39. *LAZORTHES G, GOUAZÉ A, ZADEH JD, SANTINI JJ, LAZORTHES V, BURDIN P:* Arterial vascularization of the spinal cord: Recent studies of the anastomotic substitution pathways. J Neurosurg 35:253, 1971
40. *LAZORTHES G, GOUAZÉ A, DJINDJIAN R:* Vascularisation et pathologie vasculaire de la moëlle épinière. Paris, Masson, 1973
41. *LEOPOINE J, MONTAUT J, PICARD L, HEPPNER H, MASINQUE M, ARNOULD G:* Embolization préalable à lexérèse d'un hémangiome du rachis dorsal. Neurochirurgie 19:173, 1973
42. *LITTLE JR, FURLAM AJ, MODIC MT:* Digital subtraction angiography in cerebrovascular disease. Stroke, 13:557, 1982
43. *MAEYAMA I, SATO S, GOTO S, ABE T, OYAMADA H, NAKANO M:* Metastatic bone tumors (in Japanese). Seikei Geka 17:949, 1966
44. *MALMUD LS, CHARKES ND:* Bone scanning: Principles, technique, and interpretation. Clin Orthop 107:112, 1975
45. *MCDOUGALL IR, BAUMERT JE, LAUTIERI RL:* Evaluation of 111 In leukocyte whole body scanning. Am J Roentgenol 133:849, 1979
46. *MENON S, WAGNER HN JR, TSAN MF:* Studies on gallium accumulation in inflammatory lesions. II. Uptake by staphylococcus aureus: Concise communication. J Nucl Med 19:44, 1978
47. *NAKASHIMA H, OCHI H, YASUI N, HAMADA H, ONO K:* Uptake and localization of ^{99m}Tc-methylene diphosphonate in mouse osteosarcoma. Eur J Nucl Med 7:531, 1982
48. *NEWTON TH, ADAMS JE:* Angiographic demonstration and nonsurgical embolization of spinal cord angioma. Radiology 91:873, 1968
49. *ONOMURA T, ISHIMURA T, ENDO K, YAMAMOTO S, KURASHIGE T, SAKATA T, SEKIMOTO I:* An evaluation of roentgenography, bone scintigraphy, and CT scan for metastatic spinal tumor (in Japanese). Rinsho Seikei Geka 15:284, 1980
50. *PARKE WW:* Applied anatomy of the spine. In Rothman RH, Simeone FA (eds): The Spine, Vol 19, p 52. Philadelphia, WB Saunders, 1975
51. *PATEL D, CROTHERS O, HARRIS WH, WALTMAN A, FAHMY N, CAREY R:* Arterial embolization for radical tumor resection. Acta Orthop Scand 48:353, 1977
52. *PIA HW, DJINDJIAN R:* Spinal angiomas. Berlin, Springer-Verlag, 1978
53. *ROBB GP, STEINBERG I:* Visualization of the heart, the pulmonary circulation and the great blood vessels in man: A practical approach. Am J Roentgenol 41:1, 1939
54. *SAGAR V, PICCONE JM, CHARKES ND, MAKLER PT JR:* Skeletal tracer uptake and blood flow in dogs. J Nucl Med 19:705, 1978
55. *SAGAR VV, PICCONE JM, CHARKES ND:* Studies of skeletal tracer kinematics. III. ^{99m}Tc(Sn) methylene-diphosphonate uptake in the canine tibia as a function of blood flow. J Nucl Med 20: 1257, 1979
56. *SCHROTH H, MÜLLER KP, BERBERICH R, OBERHAUSEN E, WILHELM H:* The application of radioactive labeled leukocytes for the proof of inflammations. Eur J Nucl Med 4:359, 1979
57. *SEEGER JF, CARMODY RF:* Digital subtraction angiography of the arteries of the head and neck. Radiol Clin North Am 23:193, 1985
58. *SELDINGER S:* Catheter replacement of the needle in percutaneous arteriography: A new technique. Acta Radiol 139:368, 1953
59. *SIMON MA, KIRCHNER PT:* Scintigraphic evaluation of primary bone tumors. J Bone Joint Surg 62A:758, 1980
60. *SUBRAMANIAN G, MCAFEE JG, BLAIR RJ, KALLFELZ FA, THOMAS FD:* Technetium-99m-methylene diphosphonate: A superior agent for skeletal imaging: Comparison with other technetium complexes. J Nucl Med 16:744, 1975
61. *THESINGH CW, DRIESSEN OMJ, DAEMS WT, FRANKEN C, PAUWELS EKJ, SCHEFFER E, VERMEIJ J, WISSE E:* Accumulation and localization of gallium-67 in various types of primary lung carcinoma. J Nucl Med 19:28, 1978
62. *TOFE AJ, FRANCIS MD, HARVEY WJ:* Correlation of neoplasms with incidence and localization of skeletal metastases: An analysis of 1355 diphosphonate bone scans. J Nucl Med 16:986, 1975
63. *VIAMONTE M JR, PARKS RE, SMOAK WM III:* Guided catheterization of the bronchial arteries. I. Technical considerations. Radiology 85:205, 1965
64. *WEBER DA, KEYES JW JR, WILSON GA, LANDMAN S:* Kinetics and imaging characteristics of Tc-99m

labelled complexes used for bone imaging. Radiology 120:615, 1976

65. *WEINSTEIN MA, MODIC MT, BUONOCORE E, MEANEY TF:* Digital subtraction angiography: Clinical experience at the Cleveland Clinic Foundation. Appl Radiol 10:53, 1981

66. *WRIGHT DG, PIZZO PA, JONES AE, GREENWALD D, DEISSEROTH AB:* Studies of ^{67}Ga uptake at sites of neutrophil exudation (abstr). Clin Res 27:360, 1979

67. *YONEZAWA M, IKATA T:* Clinical and angiographical studies of spinal artery occlusion (in Japanese). Blood Vessels 7:289, 1976

68. *YONEZAWA M, NARUSE A:* Spinal Angiography (in Japanese). Osaka, Japan Shering, 1978

69. *YONEZAWA M:* Angiographical study of cervical spondylotic myelopathy. Tokushima J Exp Med 26:115, 1979

70. *YONEZAWA M, IWASAKI K, WATANABE O, OHKUBO H, MATSUMORI S, NARUSE A, YAGI S, IKATA T:* Obstruction of vertebral artery of the cases with cervical vertebral injury (in Japanese). Cent Jap J Orthop Traumat 22:1358, 1979

71. *ZIMMER AM, ISITMAN AT, HOLMES RA:* Enzymatic inhibition of diphosphonate: A proposed mechanism of tissue uptake. J Nucl Med 16: 352, 1975

CHAPTER 4

Neurologic Evaluation

Evaluation of Patients with Cervical Spine Lesions

J. DONALD MCQUEEN AND MOE I. KHAN

HISTORICAL ASPECTS

In this history of the evaluation of patients with cervical spine lesions, there are three highlights out of many possible references. The first of these is the 5000-year-old Edwin Smith papyrus, the first surgical treatise. Central nervous system trauma was emphasized in this treatise, with 33 of 48 case presentations in this category. Six of these were cases of spinal trauma and at least four were cervical spine problems. Quadriplegia, paraplegia, and associated urinary incontinence and priapism were described for the first time, and an attempt was made to classify these injuries. Two groups of patients are noted: those with so-called sprains and those with fractures or dislocations. Treatment was based on this classification system.[8]

The next event of significance was the first experiment in neurophysiology, which was achieved by Galen who sectioned spinal cords of monkeys and other animals and provided early data on differential lesions.[27] He noted that a full cord section abolished all function below the level of the incision and that hemisection induced ipsilateral motor loss. Upper cord section resulted in quadriplegia and cessation of breathing. Diaphragmatic breathing persisted with lower cord injury but was eliminated when the phrenic nerves were cut. Thoracic breathing was suspended with compression or transection of the intercostal nerves. Galen was thus the first to differentiate the two basic types of respiratory muscle activities.

Third, the notebooks of Leonardo Da Vinci contain an interesting reference to the physiology of the spinal cord: a description of an unusual experiment on the frog. He noted: "The frog instantly dies when the spinal cord is pierced; and previous to this it lived without head, without heart or any bowels or intestine or skin; and here therefore it would seem lies the foundation of movement and life."[22] This may not have been Leonardo's greatest contribution, but it served to emphasize the importance of the segment of the central nervous system under consideration.

GENERAL CLINICAL MANIFESTATIONS

A thorough knowledge of the underlying anatomy and physiology of the nervous system is necessary for the interpretation of neurologic findings in cervical spine lesions. The neurologic examination requires accurate observation and recording in conjunction with a detailed neurologic history. The chronological evolution of the symptoms often provides a clue to the nature of the pathologic process.

Happily, many patients improve, both spontaneously and after fusions. Unfortunately, a small but definite number deteriorate—some spontaneously, some after a variety of surgical procedures, and some owing to respiratory and other complications. For this reason, neurologic examinations should be repeated.

Signs and symptoms of lesions of the cervical spine result from involvement of the spinal cord, nerve roots, or vertebrae. In addition, lower cranial nerve and medullary dysfunction may be produced by various pathologic processes at the junction of the medulla and rostral cervical cord. In eliciting the history, pay particular attention to pain, paresthesia, and numbness. The pain may be of vertebral, cord, or radicular origin. The last is of the most significance in localization and is restricted to the affected dermatome. It is usually described as sharp or lancinating, precipitated or aggravated by postural changes of the head and neck or maneuvers that increase the intraspinal pressure, such as coughing, sneezing, and straining. Pain is much more diffuse and ill defined when due to lesions within the cervical cord. It is usually experienced in areas several segments below the level of the lesion. Destructive lesions of the vertebra produce a localized deep, boring ache or pain that may well precede radiographic changes of the spine by several months. Paresthesias may occur along specific dermatomes due to radicular irritation. It is often not associated with any objective sensory loss. Accurate localization of this symptom by the patient may be helpful in localization of the lesion. Numbness is a vague but common symptom. It may indicate a host of sensory disturbances including pain, paresthesia, hypoesthesia, and hypoalgesia. When it is the result of cervical radioculopathy, the sensory disturbance usually follows the specific dermatome pattern of the root involved. However, with intramedullary cord lesions, these symptoms are likely to be more diffuse and dissociated.

The motor deficit manifested in lesions of the cervical spine can be classified as being either upper or lower motor neuron. Classically, lesions of the corticospinal tract produce upper motor neuron findings of spasiticity, hyperreflexia, hypertonicity, extensor plantar responses, reduced or absent superficial reflexes, and weakness of muscles distal to the lesion. Lesions involving the ventral horn motor neurons, ventral roots, and peripheral nerves give rise to lower motor neuron signs of hypotonicity, flaccidity, hyporeflexia or areflexia, fasciculations, fibrillations, and weakness and atrophy of the muscles involved. Sustained prominent fasciculations point to anterior horn cell disease. Fasciculations are also associated with extrinsic cord tumors; that is true only to a minor degree and probably points to pressure on the anterior cord or root (Table 4-1). A combination of both upper and lower motor neuron signs may be found, as in syringomyelia and amyotrophic lateral sclerosis.

LOCALIZATION OF LESIONS

Localization of the cervical spine lesion requires thorough familiarity not only with cross-sectional anatomy but also with details of the longitudinal axis. In general, the higher the lesion in the cervical spinal canal, the greater the loss in motor, sensory, and autonomic function. A high, complete transection of the cervical cord results in complete quadriplegia with respiratory impairment and is usually fatal. Lesions that involve multiple segments of the cervical cord and are incomplete may give rise to upper and lower motor neuron signs and long tract sensory and autonomic disturbances to a variable degree.

The neurologic assessment of patients with suspected cervical spinal pathology must be accompanied by a general physical examination. Patients suffering from acute quadriplegia due to cervical spinal injury often have head injuries in addition, but they may also have associated life-threatening abdominal and chest injuries. This subgroup of injuries should be emphasized because of the extraordinary diagnostic problems it presents. The features of traumatic shock such as from a ruptured spleen may well be overlooked because of the presence of spinal shock. Bradycardia is a common finding with spinal shock and is discussed below.

In settings other than traumatic ones, examination of the posterior neck and occipital regions may require local shaving. Cutaneous angiomas

Table 4-1. Clinical Features of Intramedullary and Extramedullary Lesions of the Cervical Spine

CLINICAL FEATURES	INTRAMEDULLARY LESIONS	EXTRAMEDULLARY LESIONS
Motor distrubances		
Spastic paresis	Late onset, lower limbs	Early onset, more marked distally
Flaccid paresis	Early onset, upper limbs	Often absent, except at segmental level
Atrophy of muscles	Often prominent, upper limbs	Uncommon but may be segmental
Fasoiculations*	Present	Present
Reflex changes		
Muscle stretch reflex	Depressed early in upper limbs, late hyperactivity in lower limbs	Early hyperactivity with possible segmental depression
Babinski sign	Late appearance	Early sign
Sensory disturbances		
Root pains	Often absent	Often presenting symptom
Local vertebral pain	Usually absent	Often present
Sensory loss	Dissociated sensory loss, maximal at level of lesion	Usually begins below level of lesion
Others		
Trophic skin changes	Often present	Rare
Bladder function	Early incontinence	Late incontinence

* See text for details.

may be present with spinal cord arteriovenous malformation, whereas the presence of café-au-lait spots, cutaneous nodules, and multiple tumors of peripheral nerves indicates von Recklinghausen's disease.[6] A short web neck suggests the Klippel-Feil anomaly. Less commonly, alteration of mobility and neck posture or abnormal curvature of the cervical spine may be present in association with a cervical spinal tumor or a herniated intervertebral disc.

Peripheral nerve and brachial plexus lesions may simulate lesions of the cervical spinal cord and nerve roots in their clinical presentations. The sensory and motor supply of each cervical nerve root differs from that of a peripheral nerve in the upper limbs. A variable number of cervical nerve roots contribute to the formation of a peripheral nerve. Consequently, several dermatome and peripheral nerve charts have been devised. Minor variation patterns are noted in the various dermatome charts as well as the peripheral nerve charts. These charts are used to differentiate peripheral from nerve root lesions. The nerve root and peripheral nerve fields are indicated in Figures 4-1 and 4-2 respectively.

Sensory symptoms following cervical root compression or irritation involve the specific dermatome distribution. There is a slight overlap so that complete anesthesia usually occurs when two or more posterior nerve roots have been interrupted. The sensory disturbance from a peripheral nerve lesion is usually better defined than that of a cervical nerve root and is often accompanied by motor deficit. While pain may be a prominent feature with irritation of a single cervical nerve root, demonstrable sensory deficit is often less conspicuous. The symptoms of peripheral nerve root lesions are not affected by coughing, straining, or head and neck movements as commonly noted with cervical nerve root compression. Brachial plexus lesions are often difficult to differentiate from those involving multiple cervical nerve roots. Upper, middle, or lower plexus lesions produce neurologic deficits related to the 5th and 6th cervical, 7th and 8th cervical, and 1st thoracic nerves respectively. Lesions of the posterior cord affect radial and axillary nerve function, whereas those of the lateral and medial cords produce a disturbance in musculocutaneous, median, and ulnar nerve function. Electrodiagnostic studies and cervical myelography are often of considerable value in differentiating these conditions.[7]

Lower motor neuron signs may be due to pathologic changes anywhere from the ventral horn cells in the gray matter of the cervical spinal cord to the distal branch of the peripheral nerve. When the lesion is located at the intervertebral foramen or within the peripheral nerve, both the sensory

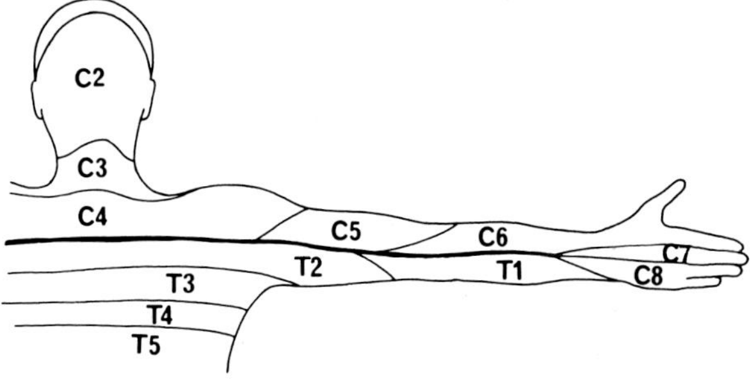

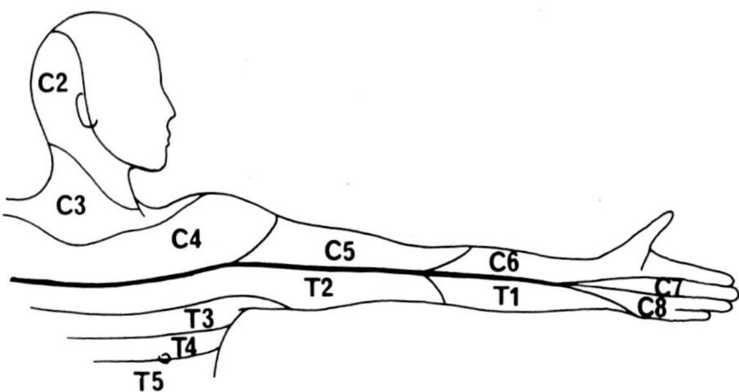

Fig. 4-1. Dermatome chart. (Modified from Haymaker W, Woodhall B: Peripheral nerve injuries, 2nd ed, p 19. Philadelphia, WB Saunders, 1953)

and motor roots are usually affected. A single ventral root lesion is more often associated with paresis of one or more muscles than complete paralysis. This is explained on the basis that more than one myotome contributes embryologically to the formation of a muscle, and each myotome is supplied by more than one ventral root.[21] Hence, complete paralysis of one or more muscles in the upper limb indicates multiple ventral root involvements or a peripheral nerve lesion, whereas paresis of a group of muscles, each of which has the same radicular innervation, suggests involvement of a single ventral root or the anterior horn cells of the appropriate segment of the cervical spinal cord. The myotomes are indicated in Fig. 4-3.

CLINICAL MANIFESTATIONS OF LESIONS AT SPECIFIC LEVELS

Lesions of the cervical spine may be located along its vertical or horizontal axis. The clinical manifestations are the result of irritation, compression, and destruction of the bony vertebra or structures within the cervical vertebral canal. Mass lesions may be located anteriorly, posteriorly, laterally, or centrally within the cervical spinal canal. Thus they may be intramedullar or extramedullar and intradural or extradural anatomically with characteristic clinical manifestations (Table 4-1). This classification of mass lesions within the cervical spinal canal correlates well pathologically and clinically, particularly when considering neoplasms.[9,14,28]

Complete Lesions

In complete lesions of the cervical cord there are many individual differences, variations within segments, and concomitant features such as local edema. It is convenient to consider segmental lesions at different levels starting from below, including T1 because of the hand involvement. The relationship between cord segments and vertebral levels is given in Fig. 4-4. Note that the spinal cord levels are higher than the vertebral levels. A simple rule to determine the segmental cord levels is to add one to the spinous process level for the cervical cord and two for the upper thoracic cord.

Complete transection at the T1 segment results in partial loss of power of interossei, lumbricals, and adductor pollicus, plus complete paralysis of the abductor pollicus brevis and all voluntary motion below save for that of the diaphragm (Fig. 4-5). Sensation is absent over the medial forearm and in all areas below it excluding the C3-C4 innervation extending below the clavicle. Horner's syndrome is present.

Complete transection at the C8 level results in clinical findings that include the above signs plus paralysis of the lumbricals and interossei with a claw hand (*main en griffe;* Fig. 4-4). Parietal weakness of the finger flexors and other hand muscles persists, but there is usually good recovery of flexion and extension at the wrist. The sensory loss extends to the hand to include the fourth and fifth fingers.

Injury at the C7 segment follows the pattern noted above with the addition of marked and abiding weakness of the finger and wrist flexors and the triceps muscle. The extensor carpi radialis longus receives innervation from C6, and accordingly extension of the wrist is present and usually predominates in wrist movement and with deviation to the radial side. The position of the hand with extended wrist and flexed fingers is often known as preacher's hand or *main du predicateur.* This retained function is all-important for later rehabilitation. Horner's syndrome may occur at this or higher levels but is usually not as well defined as

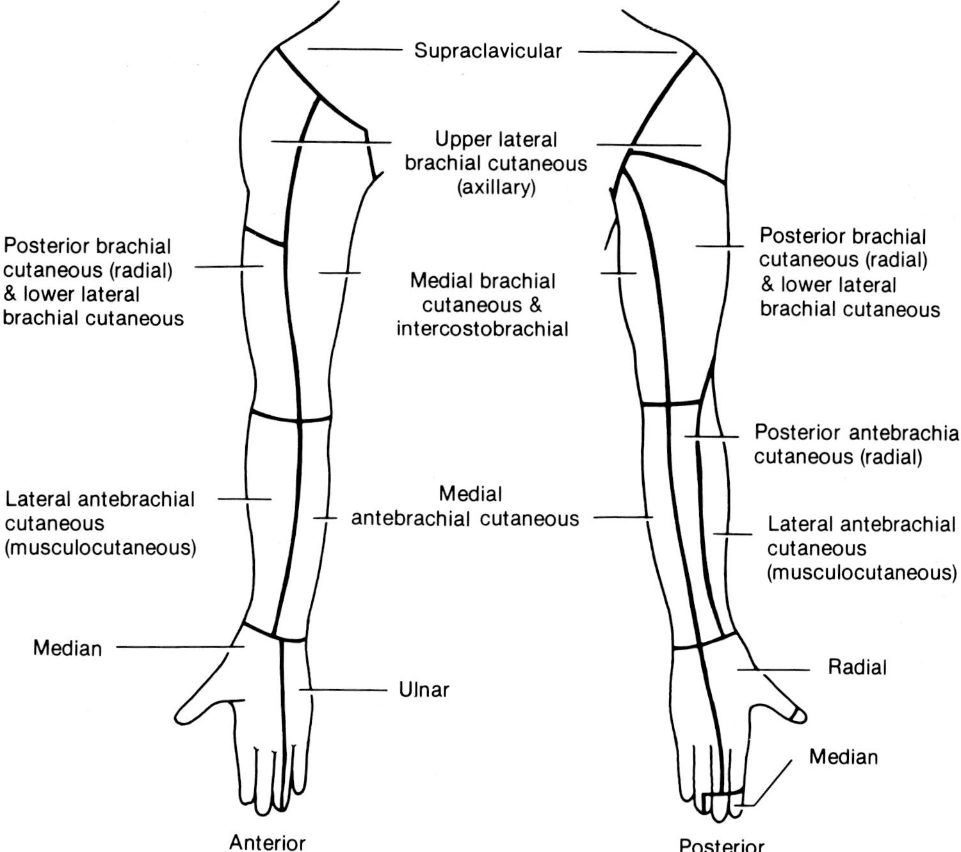

Fig. 4-2. Approximate areas of cutaneous nerve distribution to the upper limb. (From Gardner E, Gray DJ, O'Rahilly R: Anatomy, 4th ed, p 771. Philadelphia, WB Saunders, 1975)

the C8, T1, and T2 lesions, presumably because of involvement of the ciliospinal center of Budge and Waller with lower lesions.

The shift from a C7 to a C6 level lesion involves changes that are particularly marked. Triceps and extensor carpi radialis groups are more weak and may function insignificantly. Biceps, brachialis, and brachioradialis muscle power is not normal but is unopposed at the elbow to give a fairly constant flexed posture. The deltoid muscle is weakened but remains functional. The arm may be gently abducted if the patient lies in the supine position since the adductors of the shoulder are preferentially weakened. The clavicular head of the pectoralis major muscle receives innervation from C5 and hence function may be demonstrable. This is not true for the sternal head since its innervation comes solely from the lower segment. The biceps reflex is absent or diminished. The sensory loss extends to include the thumb, lateral aspects of the forearm, and the arm.

Complete transections at the C5 level result in added paralyses of the biceps, brachialis, brachioradialis, and deltoid muscles. Elevation of the shoulders is preserved, with some external rotation. The arm is otherwise flail and is areflexic. Diaphragmatic breathing is reduced initially but recovers and stabilizes with time. Anesthesia is almost complete over the arm save for a strip extending down over the shoulder and the anterior aspect of the upper arm.

Complete transections in the upper cervical segments above C5 lead to respiratory failure because of the loss of phrenic innervation from C3 through C5. Most of these patients were lost in the past. However, the current emphasis on early resusci-

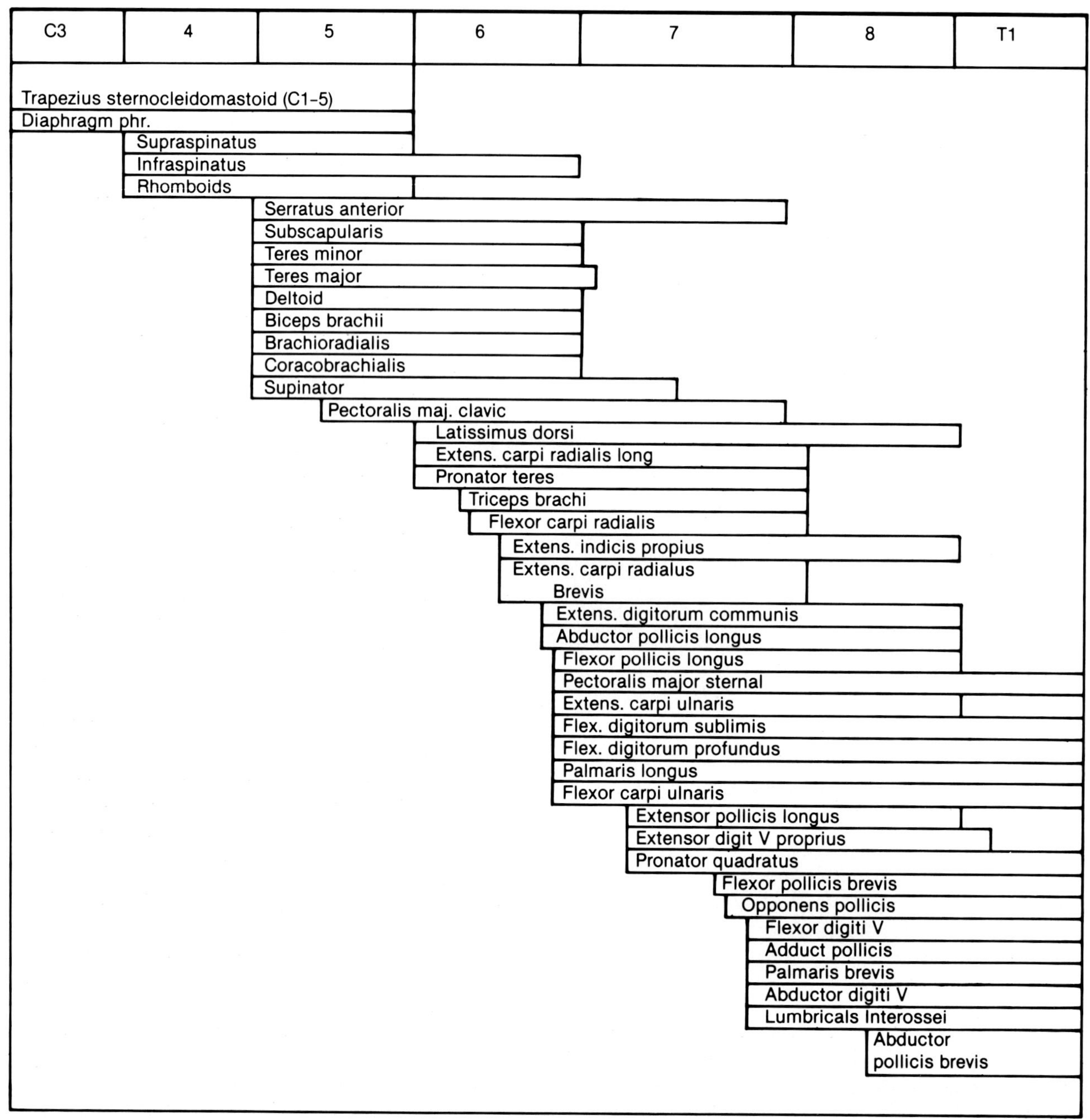

Fig. 4-3. Myotomes. (Modified from Guttmann L: Spinal Cord Injuries: Comprehensive Management and Research, pp ix, 694. Oxford, Blackwell Scientific Publications, 1973)

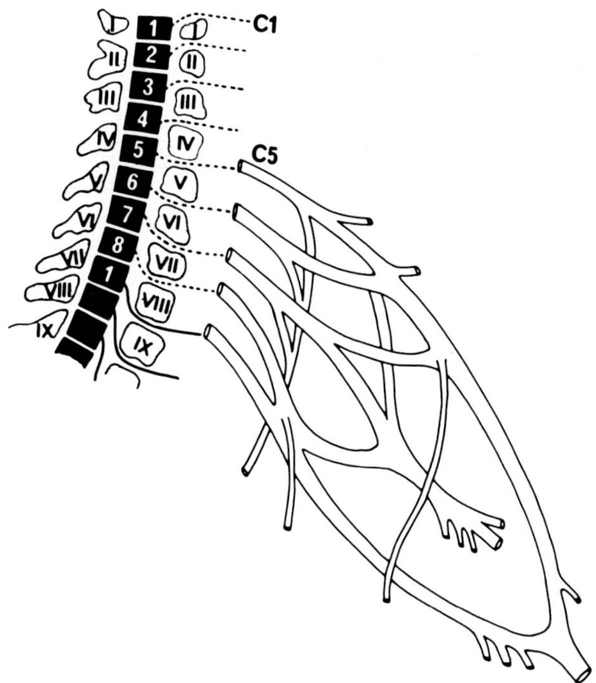

Fig. 4-4. Relationship between spinal cord segments, vertebrae, and nerve roots. (From The Neuroanatomic Basis for Clinical Neurology by TL Peele. Copyright © 1961 by McGraw-Hill Book Company. Used with the permission of McGraw-Hill Book Company.)

tation plus adequate artificial ventilation and potent antibiotic coverage results in the survival of significant numbers of quadriplegics with high-level transections. In time, some phrenic nerve function may return and may, with auxiliary respiratory muscle function, provide adequate spontaneous respiration. Phrenic nerve stimulation may also be used in other selected patients.

SHOCK, SPASTICITY, SENSORY, LOSS, AND AUTONOMIC CHANGE. There are two distinct types of shock. The term *spinal shock* was introduced by Marshall Hall, who described the neurogenic form, that is, the early areflexia and flaccidity. He first described the phenomenon in 1840 from both clinical and experimental observations.[12] His animal studies were carried out on frogs, in which reflex activity returned and increased within a few minutes. In humans, this latency extends to a few weeks (or longer with complications). In the interval, marked hypotonia is present and virtually all reflex action is absent, with the exception of the anal reflex. The presence of spinal shock indicates that, in the primate and especially the human, cord function is highly dependent on influences from above, and that the capacity for independent action is much less than in lower animals. Spasticity appears after the period of spinal shock; this has been defined by Lindsley, Schreiner, and Magoun as an exaggerated activity of extensor posture mechanisms.[19] This group and their coworkers also demonstrated the basic mechanism, which is an interruption of the descending inhibitory fibers of the corticobulbarreticular, the caudatospinal, the cerebelloreticular, and the reticulospinal pathways. Hypertonicity is found, together with hyperflexia and clonus. The latter is, in effect, an expression of repeated stretch reflexes that travel through simple monosynaptic pathways.

Reflex activity other than that found with deep tendon responses appears (or reappears) as well, and precedes the appearance of spasticity. This is of two types: one involves the sacral parasympathetics with reappearance or strengthening of the anal and bulbocavernous reflexes; the other is the primitive withdrawal response, which is quite variable but which consists primarily of flexion at the knee, and flexion and adduction at the hip. These movements are often combined with extension of the great toe and fanning of the toes, as in the Babinski response. The extension movement is actually a primitive flexion withdrawal; *dorsiflexion* may be the better term.[18] Another manifestation of the withdrawal response is the fact that the afferent discharges for the plantar responses can be elicited from wide areas on the leg and thigh. The mass reflex, or mass response, may develop later; this involves violent bilateral flexion and adduction action of the legs and abdominal contractions that are coupled with evacuations of the bladder and rectum, plus reflex sweating. Its presence points to a wide spread of activity through much of the isolated cord. The stimulus is usually excessive and is associated with an infected or full bladder on a large decubitus with sepsis. Fortunately, modern care of the paraplegic or quadriplegic is such that these problems can be largely eliminated, and consequently the mass reflex is (or should be) seen uncommonly now. Paraplegia-in-flexion was a frequent finding in the past. Its presence was felt to point to a complete lesion (as opposed to an incomplete one, as in paraplegia-in-extension). Paraplegia-in-flexion has largely disappeared, again because of better care. The flexor spasm constitutes the third phenomenon in this group. These spasms are frequently violent; they may be initiated by stimulation of intact skin or by stimu-

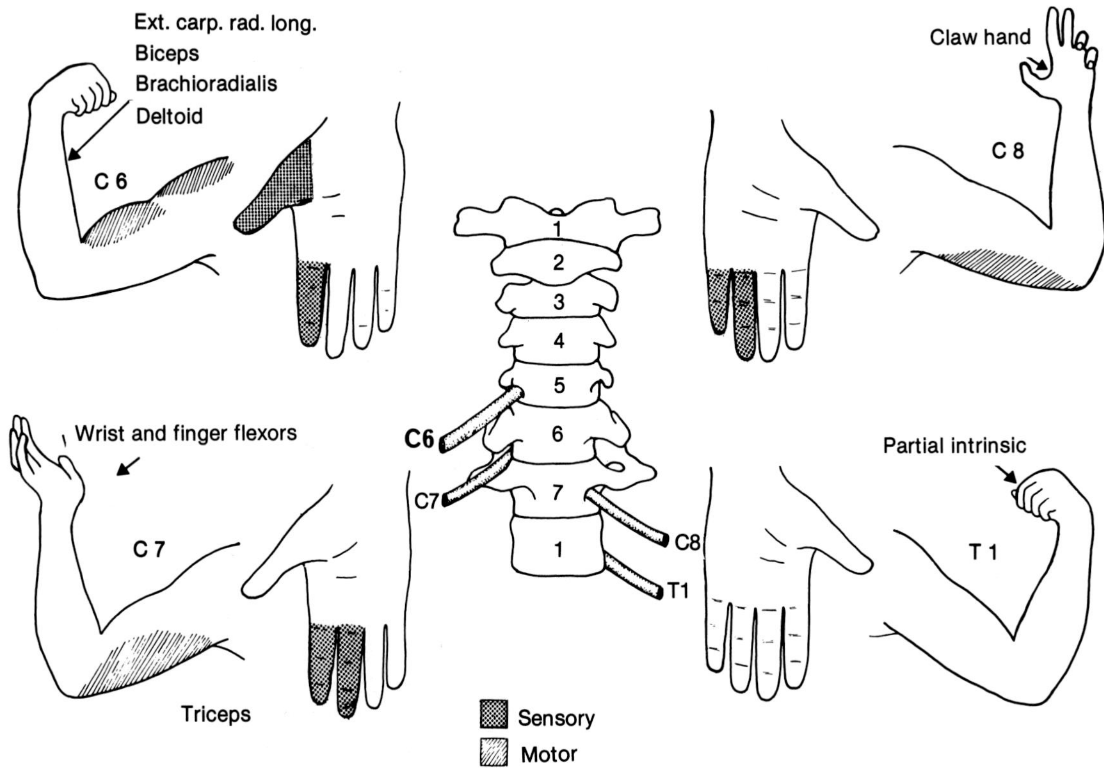

Fig. 4-5. Segmental motor and sensory changes, C6 to T1. Note: Only sensory loss is shown in the shaded hand and only muscle involvement is shown in the arm. For details, see text. (Modified from Hollinshead WH: Anatomy for Surgeons, Vol 3, The Back and Limbs, pp xii, 901, New York, Hoeben-Harper, 1958)

lation from a decubitus. These are less common than in the past but have not disappeared. Other parts of the mass reflex, such as reflex sweating, may be seen in isolation.

There is a complete loss to all sensory modalities with complete lesions. This is often associated with a zone of hyperpathia at the level of the injury. These patients are later aware of what would normally be appreciated as visceral pain. Sensations may be transmitted by way of the phrenic nerves, which contain sensory fibers although they are primarily motor. These enter the cord at the C3, C4, and C5 levels and hence are at least partly above most cervical lesions. Impulses may also travel along the autonomic nervous system. A third mechanism associated with autonomic hyperreflexia is a reflex vasoconstriction in the paralyzed area that occurs in response to visceral overdistention, which usually involves the bladder. A hypertensive crisis ensues, and the patient notes severe headache, flushing of the face, stuffiness of the nose, and a pounding heart beat.

Patients are sometimes aware of unpleasant phantom sensations in the acute phase; these often involve localized areas such as the genitals. They may be severe initially but tend to disappear during rehabilitation.

Changes in vasomotor control are very important in considering autonomic changes. Spinal shock is noted above. The second type of shock is vascular; this occurs in the acute period and is due to a sudden loss of sympathetic control. Experimental and clinical studies place the vasomotor pathways in the ventrolateral white matter.[3] Blood pressures are low for a brief period of 1 or 2 days. Many patients show only minimal changes. This hypotension is different from that found with the usual traumatic shock in that it is accompanied by a slow rather than a fast pulse. The second phase is that of postural hypotension; this persists for many weeks after the injury and can be detected by placing the patient on a tilt table. The presence of postural hypotension reflects the slow return of vasomotor tone. Careful monitoring of the blood pressure is required during tilting in this phase, because the pressures may fall precipitously and may pass the lower level for autoregulation of blood flow for the brain as well as for the spinal cord above the lesion.

Bladder involvement is prominent.[20] In the state of spinal shock, there is absence of active or reflex contraction of the detrusor muscle, and the bladder therefore distends behind the passive obstruction at the neck. If this is unchecked, urinary retention occurs with overdistention and eventually overflow incontinence. The period of bladder shock roughly parallels the period of spinal shock (1 to 6 weeks). Reflex detrusor contractions then appear under ideal circumstances; age and the quality of bladder care are important factors. These contractions may be noted prior to the reappearance of deep tendon reflexes. The mechanism is that of a simple reflex action with afferent and efferent arcs through S2, S3, and S4 paralleling the monosynaptic reflex for skeletal muscle. The end result is a full autonomatic bladder, which is now common. We find that at least 25% of men at our center are also catheter-free.* Unfortunately, this is rare for women.

Sexual malfunction is another prominent manifestation of interruption of the control of the autonomic nervous system. In the male, priapism or passive engorgement is common in the acute phase. Reflex erections return later at about the same time as reflex detrusor action. Bors gives an overall figure of 86.6% for reflex return at all spinal sites. The majority of these patients had incomplete lesions.[4] Our figure is at least 80% for complete or incomplete cervical lesions.* The frequency is clearly higher for cervical lesions as compared with low lumbar lesions with lower motor neuron involvement. Ejaculations are usually not possible with complete cervical cord transections. These require more complicated integrated reflex action through the lumbar sympathetic system. Orgastic sensations are absent with complete lesions, but alternate site for similar feelings may develop above the level of transection. Ovulation may be suppressed in the female for 1 or 2 months but is unaffected thereafter. Pregnancy and normal delivery are possible.

* A. R. Kirby, personal communication

Gastrointestinal function is also seriously impaired. Ileus and fecal retention are routine in the acute phase. Ulcerations in the upper gastrointestinal tract are uncommon but are well known. These may result from the unbalanced actions of the vagus. Bowel function returns after the period of initial spinal shock and proceeds to the establishment of an autonomatic rectum with reflex defecation, which parallels reflex bladder and reflex erection activities.

The loss of sweating is another feature of autonomic involvement. Complete cervical transections lead to a loss of sweating throughout the body since the entire sympathetic outflow is interrupted. Reflex action returns later, as noted. Pilomotor function is also affected. Heat control is a major problem and one that is particularly difficult with high lesions.[16] Late adaptations occur with the return of local vasomotor responses.

Incomplete Lesions

At attempt has been made to classify the findings with various incomplete lesions into central, hemisection, anterior, lateral, and posterior syndromes, and to add the upper cord group because of their special features.

The classical central cord syndrome is that found with syringomyelia. The cavity lies at the midline or in a paracentral position, and interrupts the decussating pain and temperature fibers to give a dissociated sensory loss. The arms, shoulders, and upper thorax are often involved in a capelike distribution. Weakness and atrophy of the small muscles of the hands are early symptoms and are due to anterior horn cell involvement. Later, muscle power in the forearm, arm, and shoulder is lost as the syrinx enlarges and fibrillations and fasciculations become widespread. The lesions progress to include the corticospinal tracts with spastic pareses, hyperreflexia, up-going plantar responses, and a neurogenic bladder, and the dorsal columns with loss of proprioception, vibration sensation, and hypoesthesia. Trophic changes are common in the hands, and a Horner's syndrome may be present due to involvement of the ciliospinal center at C8 and T1. The cavitation often extends into the thoracic area and kyposcoliosis is frequent. Many individual variations are found. Clearly, many of these findings are present with intramedullary gliomas, and the two conditions may be difficult to distinguish.

Schneider and associates described acute central cervical cord injury as a specific syndrome in

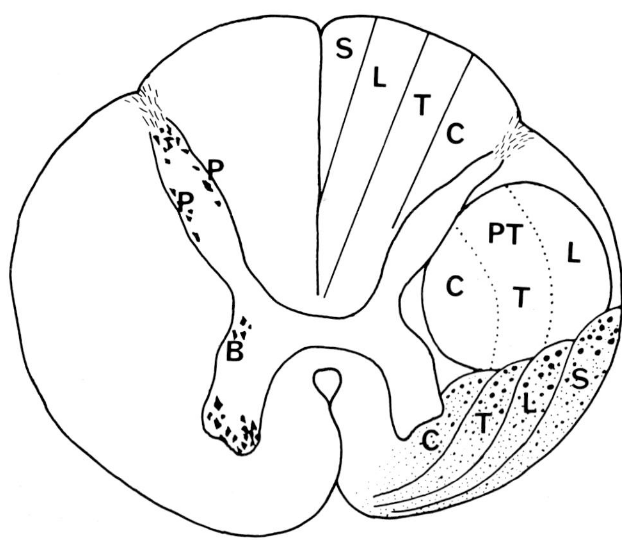

Fig. 4-6. Diagrammatic transverse section of the spinal cord to show the somatotopic lamination of the lateral spinothalmic pathway, dorsal columns, and pyramidal tract. (Walker AE: The spinalthalmic tract in man. Arch Neurol Psychiatr 43:294, 1940)

1954.[25] The cardinal feature is the presence of disproportionate weakness of the arms as compared with the legs. Variable bladder and sensory changes are also present. The lesion usually follows hyperextension of the neck, although flexion injuries were noted in some of the author's cases. Complete recovery is possible; hence, the authors felt that the lesion was edematous in nature in some instances. The classical lamination of the corticospinal tract is shown in Figure 4-6. The special involvement of the arms in this syndrome is explained by the fact that the longest fibers are on the periphery.

Hematomyelia is commonly found in the traumatic setting and is associated with varied syndromes. One of these is a persisting central syndrome, as noted above. In addition, hematomyelia is present in many of the complete lesions to the point that all or most of the cord is replaced by blood. The results of one large series suggest that 55% of patients with major cervical and thoracic spine injuries present with total sensory-motor losses.[23] Hematomyelia is present in many of the virtually complete lesions, with destruction of much of the cord.

Sacral sparing is a sign and not a syndrome. Its presence often points to an intrinsic lesion, with preservation of the outermost sensory fibers in parallel fashion to the motor sparing of the legs noted above. Unfortunately, it is not reliable as an isolated sign and may occur in other ways. It may, for example be found with external compression and also with the anterior spinal artery syndrome. The Brown-Séquard or hemisection syndrome was described in 1850 and was almost recognized by Galen. It is seen with unilateral lesions of the cord and consists of ipsilateral upper motor neuron weakness, posterior column sensory loss, and vasomotor and sudomotor changes, plus contralateral loss of pain and temperature sensibilities. These findings are present at a level one or more segments distal to the lesion. Segmental ipsilateral lower motor neuron weakness and analgesia (or hypalgesia) are found over a narrow band at the site of injury due to local damage to incoming or outgoing fibers or their cells of origin. In practice, the classical syndrome is rarely seen. Instead, a partial Brown-Séquard syndrome is commonly found with cervical cord involvements of many kinds, and consists of a simple combination of the two most prominent features of the syndrome: ipsilateral spastic weakness and contralateral analgesia and thermoanesthesia. Incomplete Brown-Séquard syndromes may also be seen as a result of lateral compression on the cord.

The posterior columns may become selectively involved following trauma, and demyelinating and degenerative processes. However, pure posterior cord syndromes are uncommon. Tabes is probably one of the best examples. This pathology consists of extensive involvement of the posterior columns due to degeneration of the incoming dorsal roots; the clinical findings are sensory ataxia plus pain and varied sensory losses. Combined lesions of the dorsal column and the corticospinal tract present as a dorsolateral syndrome and are seen more frequently. This is true for intrinsic processes such as Friedreich's ataxia and subacute combined degeneration. External compression may be exerted from a tumor. Pressure may also be applied, preferentially from the back, in a small subgroup of patients with cervical spondylosis who have unusual posterior encroachment from hypertrophy of the posterior facets and laminae. The site of involvement is shown in both the plain films and myelograms. The clinical picture is that of sensory ataxia, which is combined with corticospinal tract damage in most instances.[10]

Interestingly, a common lateral cord syndrome is found with anterior compression. In 1949, Kahn defined a lateral sclerosis syndrome which was found in association with such anterior masses as central cervical disc protrusions.[17] The clinical findings included prominent corticospinal tract involvement with only scanty sensory deficits. It was postulated that the special involvement of the corticospinal tracts resulted from local traction applied through the attachment of adjacent dentate ligaments. However, it may be true that the spasticity and weakness point to an increased intrinsic vulnerability of these tracts. One common example is the group of patients with advanced cervical spondylosis who present with marked upper motor neuron weakness in the absence of a satisfying level for pain and temperature change.

Pure anterior cord syndromes are rare, although poliomyelitis may be cited as one example. In this syndrome, the anterior horn cells are selectively damaged so that lower motor neuron signs of flaccid weakness, atrophy, and areflexia are present. Combined anterior and lateral lesions are more frequent and occur with anterior horn cell disease plus corticospinal tract involvement, as in amyotrophic lateral sclerosis, and cause both segmental lower motor neuron problems plus distal spastic weakness. The deficit after an anterolateral cordotomy is due to interruption of the spinothalamic tracts and is another example of an anterolateral syndrome. The original procedure was based on a case of Spillers in which pain and temperature sensibilities were abolished over the lower part of the body owing to the presence of bilateral tuberculomas at anterolateral sites in the spinal cord.[29]

The anterior spinal artery syndrome is much more extensive, with involvement of the anterior two thirds of the cord in the distribution of the artery. Only posterior column function is preserved, with position and vibration sensation and some touch. The syndrome commonly occurs with thrombosis or embolism but may be noted with anterior compression. Schneider reported on this clinical pattern in 13 trauma patients in terms of an acute anterior spinal cord injury.[24] Compression occurred from herniated disc fragments of dislocated bony fragments in some; destruction of the anterior portion of the cord occurred in others. Significant improvement occurred in almost half of his patients.

Foramen Magnum and Upper Cervical Spine (C1–C3) Lesions

Acute and complete spinal cord lesions above the C3 segment are almost invariably fatal unless immediate respiratory support is provided. An incomplete lesion in this region may involve the lower cranial nerves or nuclei, pyramidal decussation, sensory and motor tracts and nuclei, respiratory and autonomic centers and tracts, and upper cervical nerve roots. Not uncommonly, mass lesions may extend into the posterior fossa of the cranial cavity, producing a combination of neurologic deficits secondary to cerebellar and brain stem compression or hydrocephalus. Less commonly, compression and occlusion of the vertebral artery or anterior spinal artery may result in an infarction extending through the cervicomedullary area, simulating a concurrent upper cervical cord and brain injury.

Lesions in the upper cervical spinal cord occasionally produce a peculiar pattern of sensory deficit over the face. This is described as the Déjerine "onion-peel" pattern of sensory loss and results from involvement of the descending tract of the trigeminal nerve, which extends down as far as the C4 segment of the spinal cord.[15] The most caudal portion of this tract carries impulses from the outermost part of the face, whereas the central areas are represented at higher levels. Pain and temperature sensation become altered in a centripetal manner from the outermost part of the face as the lesion in the trigeminal tract extends upward, hence, an onion-peel pattern of sensory loss.

The sensory supply to the back of the head comes from the dorsal root of C2, which extends to about the level of the interaural line. The C1 segment is devoid of a dorsal root. Suboccipital headache is a frequent complaint of patients harboring mass lesions in the rostral cervical spinal canal and foramen magnum regions. Sensory disturbances in the form of pain, paresthesia, or numbness over the C2 dermatome may direct attention to the location of the lesion. Abnormal head and neck posture associated with active limitation of neck movements may be related to the pain. The fibers transmitting dorsal column sensibility from the lower and upper limbs are located medially and laterally, respectively, in the posterior column.[32] Hence, there may be selective impairment in dorsal column sensibility related to the portion of the column involved. The spinal accessory nerve arises from the rostral cervical cord segments and, when involved, results in impaired function of the sternocleidomastoid anpezius and trapezius muscles, which it innervates.

Various patterns of weakness and spasticity in the limbs may result when the pyramidal decussation is affected. This may range from ipsilateral monoparesis to quadriplegia. The majority of corticospinal fibers decussate in the first cervical segment or at its junction with the medulla oblongated. Although some degree of somatotropic lamination of the pyramidal decussation does exist, several patterns of decussation have been described. This partly accounts for the variation in motor disturbances even with lesions in similar location at the level of the foramen magnum. However, the lateral corticospinal tract is directly adjacent to the surface of the spinal cord in the 2nd, 3rd, and 4th cervical cord segments, whereas at lower levels it is separated from the surface by the dorsal spinocerebellar tract. In the region of the upper cervical spinal canal and foramen magnum mass lesions may first present with spastic monoparesis of the ipsilateral arm, then the ipsilateral leg, followed by the contralateral leg, and the opposite arm.[5] Less frequently, atrophy of small muscles of the hand and forearm may present, presumably on an ischemic basis.

Less commonly, paralysis of both upper limbs with relative sparing of the lower limbs may be caused by lesions involving the midline and upper portions of the pyramidal decussation. This syndrome was designated *cruciate paralysis* by Bell and may result from odontoid fractures, odontoid mass lesions (tuberculoma, chordoma), and hyperextension cervical spine injuries in the presence of basilar impression.[2] An even less common syndrome described by Wallenburg in 1901 as *hemiplegia cruciate* owing to involvement of the lateral part of the pyramidal decussation, is characterized by paralysis of the ipsilateral arm and contralateral leg.[13,33]

Serious respiratory disturbances often follow high cervical cord lesions. Irritation of the phrenic nerve may lead to hiccups, dyspnea, and coughing, whereas destruction of this nerve results in paralysis of the diaphragm. Bradycardia is less common and is attributed to interruption of fibers ascending to the cardiovascular center in the medulla oblongata. Occlusion of the vertebral arteries or thrombosis of the anterior spinal artery may cause a high cervical cord infarction, resulting in quadriplegia, impairment of various sensory modalities, bladder and bowel dysfunction, and respiratory and vasomotor disturbances.

The C1 and C2 spinal cord segments are most susceptible to injury. Direct cerebral vertex impact force may be transmitted to the C2 segment of the cord. This is well documented clinically and experimentally.[11,26] The atlantoaxial junction may be disrupted by sudden and excessive forces, whereas acute torsion of the cervical spine may damage the vertebral arteries as they exit over the C1 laminae. In addition, Turnbull and co-workers have demonstrated a paucity of radicular vessels at the upper three cervical segments that may be a significant contributory factor to this susceptibility.[31]

FALSE LOCALIZING FINDINGS

Findings with intracranial lesions may mimic those noted with cervical cord involvements. For example, the presence of a hemiparesis in association with a supratentorial mass may cause diagnostic problems (at least initially) when facial sparing is present. These problems are now resolved with the CT scanner, although not a few needless myelograms were carried out in the past. Uncertain or false localization may occur with lesions at the cervicomedullary junction, as noted above. Contralateral weakness may occur because of involvement of the corticospinal tract above the decussation. High cervical lesions may also cause such low cervical signs as weakness of the small hand muscles; this is often explained on the basis of ischemia in the lower cervical segments from interruption of blood flow down the anterior spinal artery. Changes in venous outflow may also be important. Taylor and Byrnes stress the fact that the direction of venous outflow is upward in the cervical region and so postulate that high cervical venous obstruction may have a preferential action on the lowest and most dependent cervical areas.[30] Errors may be made in matching the level of the lesion to the level of sensory loss. In practice, the lesion may be found at the indicated site or at any level above it. Finally, the absence of reliable levels of hypoalgesia with such processes as spondylosis is noted above.

REFERENCES

1. *ALEXANDER E JR, DAVID CH JR, FIELD CH:* Metastatic lesions of the vertebral column causing cord compression. Neurology 6:103, 1956

2. *BELL HS:* Paralysis of the arms from injury of the pyramidal decussation: "Cruciate paralysis." J Neurosurg 33:376, 1970
3. *BELMUSTO L, BROWN E, OWENS G:* Clinical observations on respiratory and vasomotor disturbance as related to cervical cordotomies. J Neurosurg 20:225, 1963
4. *BORS F:* Sexual function in patients with spinal cord injuries. Proceedings of Symposium on Spinal Injuries, p 62. Edinburgh, Royal College of Surgeons, 1963
5. *DAVIS L, DAVIS RA:* Principles of Neurologic Surgery. Philadelphia, WB Saunders, 1963
6. *DOPPMAN JL, WIRTH FP JR, DI CHIRO G, OMMAYA AK:* Value of cutaneous angiomas in the arteriographic localization of spinal cord arteriovenous malformations. N Engl J Med 281:1440, 1969
7. *DYCK PJ, THOMAS PK, LAMBERT EH:* Peripheral neuropathy Vol 1, pp 663–664. Philadelphia, WB Saunders, 1975
8. *ELSBERG CA:* The Edwin Smith surgical papyrus and the diagnosis and treatment of injuries to the skull and spine 5,000 years ago. Annals of Medical History 3:271, 1931
9. *ELSBERG CA:* Surgical Diseases of the Spinal Cord, Membranes and Nerve Roots: Symptoms, Diagnosis and Treatment. New York, Paul B Hoeber, 1941
10. *EPSTEIN JA, EPSTEIN BS, LAVINE LS, CANAS R, ROSENTHAL AD:* Cervical myeloradiculopathy caused by arthrotic hypertrophy of the posterior facets and laminae. J Neurosurg 49:387, 1978
11. *GOSCH HH, GOODING E, SCHNEIDER RD:* Mechanism and pathophysiology of experimentally induced cervical spinal cord injuries in adult Rhesus monkeys. Surg Forum 21:455, 1970
12. *HALL M:* Four Memoirs of the Nervous System. London, 1980
13. *HAYMAKER W:* Localization of lesions involving brain stem and emergent nerves. In Bing R (ed): A Textbook of Nervous Diseases, p 838. St Louis, CV Mosby, 1939
14. *HAYMAKER W:* Bing's Local Diagnosis in Neurological Diseases, 15th ed. St. Louis, CV Mosby, 1969
15. *HUMPHREY T:* The central relations of the trigeminal nerve. In Kahn E, Crosby E, Schneider R, Taren J (eds): Correlative Neurosurgery, 2nd ed. Springfield, IL, Charles C Thomas, 1969
16. *HUTCHINSON J:* Temperature and circulation after crushing the cervical cord. Lancet 1:713, 1975
17. *KAHN EA:* The role of the dentate ligaments in spinal cord compression and the syndrome of lateral sclerosis. J Neurosurg 4:191, 1947
18. *LANDAU WM, CLARE MH:* The plantar reflex in man with special reference to some conditions where the extensor response is unexpectedly absent. Brain 82:321, 1959
19. *LINDSLEY DB, SCHREINER LH, MAGOUN, HW:* An electromyographic study of spasticity, J Neurophysiol 12:197, 1949
20. *NATHAN P, SMITH M:* The centrifugal pathways for micturition within the spinal cord. J Neurol Neurosurg Psychiatry 21:177, 1958
21. *RANSON WS, CLARK SL:* The Anatomy of the Nervous System, 9th ed, pp 115–120. Philadelphia, WB Saunders, 1953
22. *RIESE W:* A History of Neurology, p 223. New York, MD Publications, 1959
23. *RUSSO GL, BELLARRIQUE R, LUCAS J, DUCKER TB:* Injuries of the spine and spinal cord. In Zuidema GD, Rutherford RB, Ballinger WF II (eds): The Management of Trauma, p 235. Philadelphia, WB Saunders, 1979
24. *SCHNEIDER RC:* The syndrome of acute anterior spinal cord injury. J Neurosurg 12:95, 1955
25. *SCHNEIDER RC, CHERRY G, PANTEK H:* The syndrome of acute central cervical spinal cord injury with special reference to the mechanisms involved in hyperextension injuries of the cervical spine. J Neuro 11:546, 1954
26. *SCHNEIDER RC, CROSBY EC, RUSSO RH, GOSH HH:* Traumatic spinal cord syndromes and their management. Clin Neurosurg 20:424, 1972
27. *SIEGEL RE:* Galen on psychology, psychopathology and function and diseases of the nervous system pp ix, 310. Basel, S Karger, 1X + 310, 1973
28. *SLOOF JF, KERNOHAN JW, MACCARTY CS:* Primary intramedullary tumors of the spinal cord and filum terminale. Philadelphia, WB Saunders, 1964
29. *SPILLER WG:* The location within the spinal cord of fibers for pain and temperature sensations. J Nerve Ment Dis 32:318, 1905
30. *TAYLOR AR, BYRNES DP:* Foramen magnum and high cervical cord compression. Brain 97:473, 1974
31. *TURNBULL IM, BRIEG A, HASSLER O:* Blood supply of the cervical spinal cord in man: A microangiographic cadaver study. J Neurosurg 24:951, 1966
32. *WALKER AE:* The spinothalamic tract in man. Arch Neurol Psychiatry 43:284, 1940
33. *WALLENBERG A:* Neuere fortschritte in der topischen diagnostik des pons und der oblongata. Deutsche Ztschr Nervenheilk 41:8–41, 1911

Electrodiagnostic Studies in Cervical Spine Disorders

DENNIS MAIMAN, M.D., Ph.D. AND MARTIN HOFFMAN, M.D.

In this section, electrodiagnostic studies, including the electromyogram (EMG), the nerve conduction velocity (NCV) examination, and somatosensory evoked potential (SSEP) are presented. Specific technical considerations and interpretations are not discussed, however, and the reader is referred to several excellent works for this information.[5,8,18,22,28,48] Rather, the emphasis is on reviewing the recent literature in the field. Because the nature and use of the evoked potential are not well understood, experimental work in this area is stressed.

Although a great deal of published material is available on electrodiagnostic studies, their clinical utility is imprecisely defined. Because of this, an accurate clinical paradigm cannot be developed; in a group of patients with evidence of a particular diagnosis, any one of these examinations, or some combination of them, may be valuable.

Ideally, the electrophysiologic examination represents a sensitive and quantifiable extension of the physical examination.[8,48] This kind of study can often (1) confirm abnormalities observed or suspected based on the history and/or clinical examination, (2) distinguish between overlapping pathologic conditions, which may be asymptomatic, (3) aid in the anatomic localization of a lesion (*i.e.*, peripheral nerve entrapment versus radiculopathy), and (4) allow an objective monitoring of changes in neurologic status over time.

Unfortunately, the electrodiagnostic studies are limited in their ability to assist the clinician. For example, few conventions in technique exist for the SSEP evaluation, with electrode placement and stimulus parameters varying between institutions. Nomenclature also varies, in spite of extraordinary efforts toward standardization: A guidelines committee, composed of representatives of several international scientific societies, recommended that evoked potential wave forms be named by polarity (positive or negative) and by latency (time from stimulus to peak). However, many investigators prefer and use other terminology.[8,18] The results of the electrodiagnostic evaluation may vary, depending on the skill of the examiner. For example, in the EMG much of the interpretation is done at the time of the study and depends on the observer's reliability and ability. Last, these studies provide few pathognomonic pictures for most neurologic disorders, and the results must be considered in concert with the neurologic examination and radiologic studies.

ELECTROMYOGRAPHY (EMG)

EMG is the visualization and measurement of action potentials produced by depolarization and repolarization of a muscle fiber or a group of such fibers. These actions may occur as the result of voluntary contraction or injury from a probing needle electrode, or they may be due to a disease process. With amplification, these signals can be displayed both visually and aurally. In common usage, the term electromyography includes the measurement of the nerve conduction velocity (NCV), which measures how rapidly a depolarization wave travels along a nerve segment. The two tests are complementary and have been compared to measuring how fast a man can run (NCV) versus the severity of his arthritis (EMG).[3]

Electromyography serves as both a confirmation and extension of the clinical examination. It is useful in localizing the level of a specific lesion, distinguishing between partial and complete lesions, differentiating primary muscle or nerve pathology, and evaluating malingerers.[44] Although electromyographic studies are highly sensitive, the results are nonspecific and when viewed apart from the clinical examination may be misleading.

In the context of the examination of the cervical spine, electromyographic studies are particularly helpful in differentiating lesions at the level of the root, plexus, or peripheral nerve (Fig. 4-7). They may also be helpful in evaluating localized myelopathies but have no practical role in the diagnosis of upper motor neuron diseases. The purpose of this section is to assist the nonelectromyographer in understanding some basic principles of the technique to allow proper utilization of these studies and the results obtained.

Historical Note

The first clinical use of EMG in patients was by Proebster in 1928.[37] He described spontaneous, irregular activation potentials in denervated muscles, after brachial plexus injury at birth and in longstanding poliomyelitis. With the introduction of the concentric needle electrode in 1929 by Ad-

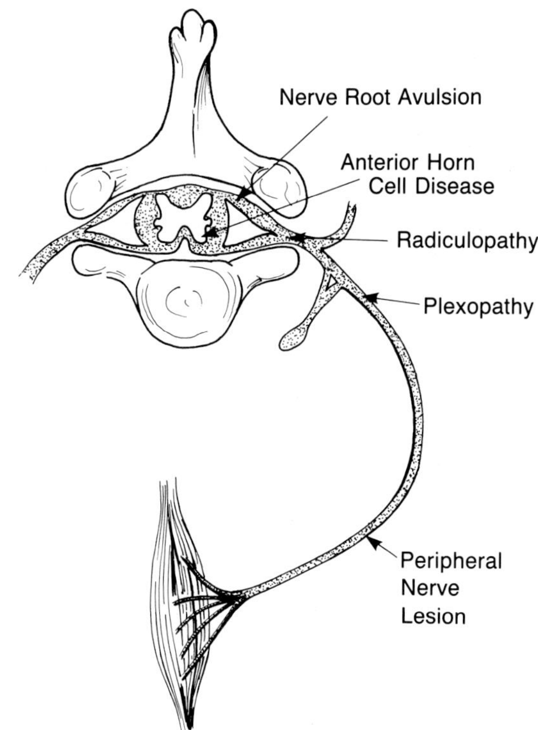

Fig. 4-7. Sites of lesions where electromyography may be helpful in differentiation of cervical spine disorders.

rian and Bronk,[1] EMG developed into a useful technique for clinical examination. Since that time, extensive experience in both health and disease, as well as refinement of instrumentation, has permitted EMG to become a practical diagnostic procedure.

Technique

The utility of EMG in the diagnosis of nerve injuries lies in its ability to detect abnormalities in the electrical activation of a muscle as a result of injury to the nerve innervating that muscle. As normal muscle function is dependent upon normal nerve supply, nerve injury is often reflected in the EMG.

The EMG examination includes four steps: the evaluation of spontaneous (resting) activity, insertional activity, activity during minimal muscle contraction, and activity during maximal muscle contraction. During these four steps, abnormal electrical activity is sought. The common EMG changes that are observed include fibrillation potentials, fasciculation potentials, positive sharp waves, and polyphasic potentials (Fig. 4-8).

Fibrillation potentials are the electrical activity resulting from the spontaneous discharge of a single muscle fiber. They result from muscle cell membrane instability produced by a variety of circumstances including inflammation, degeneration, electrolyte disturbances, trauma, and upper motor neuron disease, but they are most often seen in denervated muscle. In rare instances they may be recorded in normal muscles.

Fasciculation potentials result from the spontaneous discharge of all or part of a motor unit. The discharge may arise from any portion of the lower motor neuron, but many probably originate from the myoneural junction. They may be observed in normal persons as well as in those with a wide variety of diseases, so are considered pathologic only in association with other EMG abnormalities.

Positive sharp waves are usually seen accompanying fibrillation potentials and have similar significance. They are intercellularly recorded injury potentials, and are induced by mechanical stimuli such as tapping the muscle near the needle electrode or abruptly advancing the needle. They are considered abnormal when they persist after the electrode has stopped moving.

Polyphasic potentials are motor unit action potentials with over four phases (crossing the isoelectric line more than three times). They are the result of temporal dispersion of a muscle fiber potential and may be secondary to differences in conduction

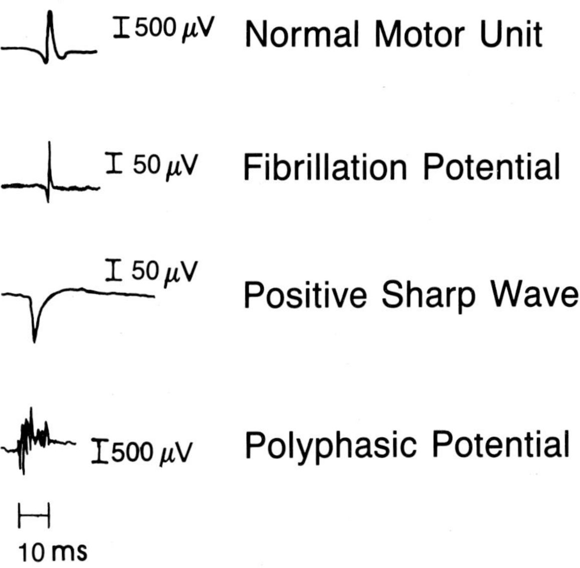

Fig. 4-8. Common action potentials in electromyography.

time along the terminal branch of a nerve or over the muscle fiber membrane. It may be normal to observe up to 5% to 15% of motor unit action potentials as polyphasic.[4] Increased polyphasic potentials are a nonspecific finding and may be present in myopathy, neuropathy, and motor neuron disease.

If abnormal potentials are observed, identification of the anatomic distribution of the affected muscles help define the site of the lesion. The extent and chronicity of the injury is determined by the pattern of abnormal electrical activity.

NERVE CONDUCTION STUDIES

Historical Note

Although von Helmholtz performed the first nerve conduction studies on humans in 1850,[47] it was Harvey and Masland in 1940 who introduced motor nerve stimulation with recording of the muscle action potential as a diagnostic tool in clinical medicine.[19] In 1948 Hodes, Larrabee, and German reported values for the motor conduction velocity in patients with peripheral nerve injuries and hysterical paralysis.[20] The first purely sensory nerve studies were not recorded until 1956 by Dawson.[14] Although determination of the NCV is still a relatively new field of interest, it is now a valuable part of the electrodiagnostic evaluation.

Technique

Traditional nerve conduction studies consist of the electrical stimulation of a nerve and recording of the evoked potential, either from the muscle (as in the study of motor nerves) or from the nerve itself (as in the study of sensory nerves). By measuring the time between stimulation and response at two stimulation sites and the distance between the stimulation sites, a conduction velocity is easily calculated (Fig. 4-9). This value represents the conduction velocity of the fastest, large myelinated group-A fibers. Although the methods are relatively simple, a number of technical factors influence the results and can lead to misinterpretation of the findings.

The goals of nerve conduction studies are to assess the number of functioning axons and the state of the myelin of the functioning axons. This is accomplished by studying the conduction velocity, amplitude of the evoked response, and duration of the evoked response (Fig. 4-10).

In sensory nerves, each axon contributes to the magnitude of the evoked response; therefore, the amplitude reflects the number of functioning axons. However, traditional motor nerve studies are limited because the amplitude of the evoked response is indicative of the number of activated muscle fibers, not the number of motor axons in the nerve. The number of axons can be diminished, yet the evoked response is normal if collateral reinnervation by the remaining axons is complete. Demyelination is observed as a decreased conduction velocity and temporal dispersion of the evoked response.

Although several peripheral nerves can be studied by stimulation at Erb's point, more proximal study is impractical because of difficulties in reaching these deep nerves for stimulation. Nerve root

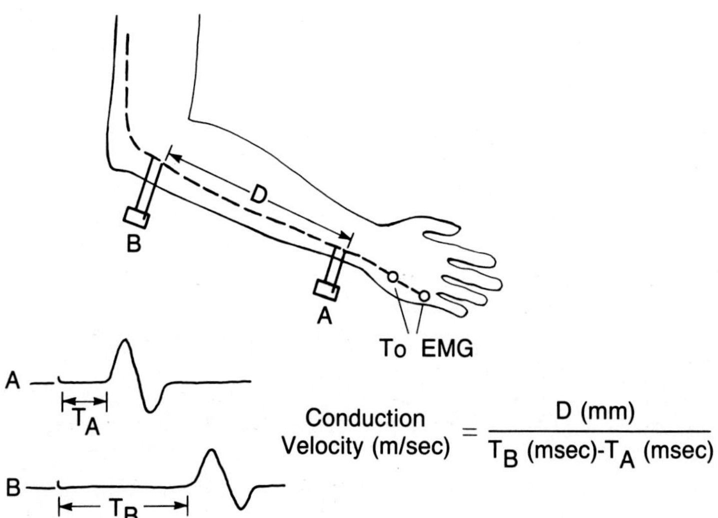

Fig. 4-9. Calculation of nerve conduction velocity. Stimulation at distal location A results in a response latency T_A, and proximal stimulation at B results in a latency of T_B. The conduction velocity of the nerve segment is the distance between proximal and distal sites divided by the difference in latencies.

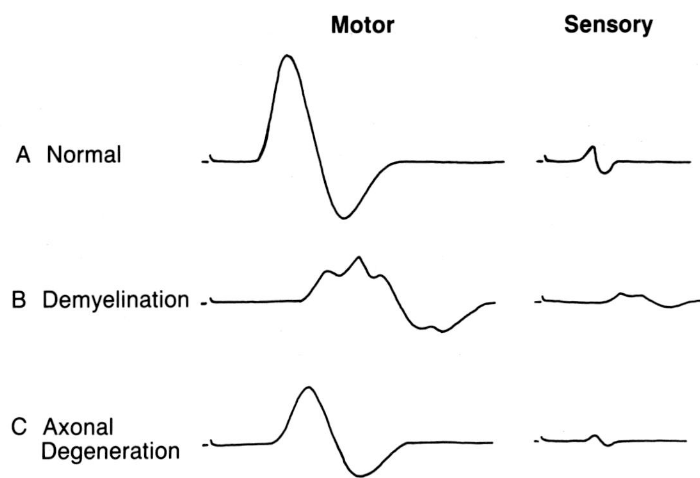

Fig. 4-10. Schematic representation of normal (*A*) and pathologic motor and sensory evoked potentials. In demyelinating processes (*B*), the action potentials show temporal dispersion, increased latency and decreased amplitude. With axonal degeneration (*C*), the latency is normal or slightly increased and the amplitude is reduced.

stimulation with needle electrodes is one technique that can be performed but is not commonly used. The F-response, another method that is sometimes used for studying the proximal segments of nerves, is a muscle action potential induced by the back firing of antidromically activated anterior horn cells. To produce an F-response, action potentials must travel antidromically through a motor nerve, where a small percentage of anterior horn cells produce an orthodromic activation potential response for the F-response. Unfortunately, this relatively easy means of studying the proximal segments of nerves has not been proven to be reliable in the diagnosis of radiculopathy.[48]

An electrodiagnostic technique for indirectly evaluating peripheral nerve segments is to record compound sensory nerve action potentials (SNAPs). This method can aid in distinguishing peripheral nerve lesions from root, spinal cord, or upper motor neuron lesions. In peripheral nerve injuries at or distal to the level of the dorsal root ganglion and involving at least some axonal degeneration, the distal-recorded SNAP is small or absent. In contrast, nerve root, spinal cord, upper motor neuron or proximal neurapraxic lesions do not abolish the distal SNAP. The recording of SNAPs has been clinically useful in distinguishing traumatic cervical root avulsions from brachial plexus injuries.[44] SNAPs persist in syringomyelia[16] and chronic cervical radiculopathies,[2] and thus are useful in distinguishing these proximal pathologic findings from other distal lesions. A decrease in SNAP amplitude also seems to be a relatively sensitive electrodiagnostic parameter for identifying thoracic outlet syndrome.[33]

A new electrodiagnostic approach is to record compound mixed nerve potentials (MNAPs), consisting of summated motor as well as sensory action potentials, to attempt to distinguish upper from lower motorneuron lesions.[7] Such MNAP recordings may prove useful in predicting outcome and in monitoring neurologic progression in cervical myelopathies.

Radiculopathy

Radiculopathy is the most common clinical disorder for which electromyography is ordered.[22,23] EMG is particularly useful, since it may show abnormalities in the absence of objective neurologic or radiologic findings.[39]

Following acute nerve root compression, there is a typical sequence of EMG abnormalities observed.[48] During the first 72 hours, the only EMG abnormalities are reflective of a conduction block in the nerve root axon. Significant involvement may result in a decrease in the number of motor unit action potentials relative to the strength of the muscle contraction. However, because of multilevel innervation of most peripheral muscles, this finding is not consistently helpful.

After approximately 72 hours, wallerian degeneration usually begins to occur. This accounts for the finding of a decreased amplitude of the motor response on peripheral nerve stimulation. Additionally, between 4 and 7 days after nerve injury, there is an increase in the number of polyphasic potentials.

The most important EMG findings in nerve root injury are first seen 7 to 10 days after the injury. These first consist of positive waves in the paraspinal muscles. Then, after 2 to 3 weeks, fibrillation potentials in the paraspinals and positive waves in the limb muscles are seen. Chronic changes following nerve root injury are less obvious. The most common abnormalities are an increased proportion of polyphasic potentials and increased insertional activity.

Evaluation of the paraspinal muscles is an important part of the EMG examination for radiculopathy. In one third of patients with lumbar radiculopathies, EMG abnormalities were found in the paraspinals only.[23] This is probably also the case for cervical radiculopathies.[32]

The literature on the use of postoperative EMG is conflicting. Some authors believe that persistent abnormal paraspinal muscle findings result from operative trauma and that they will obscure any possible findings from a new nerve injury. This may be true under some circumstances; however, useful information may still be obtained when the paraspinal findings are correlated with the clinical presentation and remainder of the EMG examination.

In summary, the EMG diagnosis of radiculopathy is based on the findings of abnormalities in muscles innervated by a specific nerve root. These abnormalities are usually first observed in the paraspinals as early as 7 days after injury and are frequently localized to the paraspinals. They consist primarily of positive waves, an increased proportion of polyphasics, and fibrillation potentials.

The Double Crush Syndrome

Patients with clinical and electromyographic evidence of peripheral nerve entrapment syndromes at the wrist or elbow frequently complain of pain in the upper arm, shoulder, or neck. These proximal symptoms are often attributed to referred pain from the distally located entrapment. However, these symptoms may be the result of a concomitant cervical radiculopathy.[46] It is postulated that the cervical lesion causes the primary damage to the nerve fiber, making it more susceptible to a superimposed distal entrapment. This has been referred to as the *double crush* syndrome.

When there is clinical suspicion of a double crush syndrome, electromyography can provide an objective analysis. EMG abnormalities compatible with a radiculopathy, and nerve conduction and EMG findings of a concomitant peripheral nerve entrapment verify the diagnosis.

Brachial Plexus Injury

Brachial plexus injuries usually result from traumatic causes such as penetrating wounds, local pressure, and traction. These injuries more often involve the roots and trunks rather than the more distal segments. For prognostic purposes, it is important to distinguish between a lesion proximal to the dorsal root ganglion (preganglionic or root avulsion) and a lesion distal to the dorsal root ganglion (postganglionic). Similarly, distinguishing the brachial plexopathy from compression of multiple cervical roots is important.

The clinical findings of Horner's sign or intact triple response suggest a preganglionic lesion, but frequently the site of lesion is difficult to determine clinically. EMG abnormalities of the paraspinal muscles indicate that the lesion involves the root or anterior horn cell. Since the dorsal root ganglion remains intact with preganglionic lesions, a root avulsion is suggested by the finding of an intact distal sensory nerve action potential in the presence of sensory loss. If the paraspinal muscles are spared and motor or sensory action potentials are low or absent, a brachial plexus lesion should be suspected. Somatosensory evoked potentials can also be helpful.

Upper Motor Neuron Lesions

Numerous studies have shown transient EMG abnormalities following spinal cord injury and cerebrovascular accidents. In patients with spinal cord injury, the EMG abnormalities are generally bilateral, diffuse, and below the level of the lesion, whereas in stroke patients the findings are confined to the hemiplegic extremities. The clinical significance of these EMG findings lies in the difficulty they may present in determining if a lower motor neuron disorder is present in addition to the upper motor neuron lesion. EMG abnormalities do not automatically mean that a lower motor neuron lesion is present. Knowledge of typical distribution and sequence of disappearance of the EMG abnormalities following upper motor neuron lesion are necessary for EMG studies to be helpful in identifying lower motor neuron disorders.

Anterior Horn Cell Disease

Disease of the anterior horn cell can result from a number of causes, including mechanical compression, vascular insult, infection, direct trauma, and genetic disorders. Amyotrophic lateral sclerosis, the most common disorder primarily affecting the motor neuron, may initially simulate a radiculopathy. Early myelopathies from cervical spondylosis, infiltrating tumors, vascular insults, infection, and syringomyelia may also occasionally present diagnostic problems. EMG can be helpful in determining the site, pattern, and extent of the disease process in addition to following the disease progression, once a diagnosis has been made.

Regardless of the cause, anterior horn cell disease or injury results in lost function of the neuron, cell inexcitability, and drop-out of individual motor units. When the process has become sufficiently extensive, clinical weakness is observed. However, reinnervation of denervated muscle fibers by nearby functioning neurons usually occurs, which may delay the onset of clinical weakness.

As a result, several typical EMG findings are observed. These usually include (1) a decreased number of motor unit action potentials recruited for the strength of the contraction, (2) fasciculation potentials, (3) positive sharp waves, (4) increased amplitude, duration, and phasicity of motor unit action potentials, (5) an alteration in the recruitment pattern of motor unit action potentials as the strength of contraction increases, and (6) essentially normal motor and sensory nerve conduction studies. As with other disorders, there are no specific EMG findings that are pathognomonic for anterior horn cell disease, but when the clinical and electromyographic findings are correlated the diagnosis can be confirmed.

In the EMG analysis for amyotrophic lateral sclerosis, the distribution of abnormal findings can be particularly helpful. Abnormal EMG findings are often present in clinically unaffected muscles. Additionally, the findings of EMG abnormalities in the tongue sometimes prevent the need for myelographic studies.

SENSORY EVOKED POTENTIALS

The SSEP, simply stated, is the response of nervous system response to an electrical stimulus. Because the response is contingent on conduction through the neurosensory pathways, it depends not only on the nature and duration of the stimulus, but also on the status of the entire nervous system between the stimulus and measured response. Therefore, it is an indirect measure of the anatomic and physiologic integrity of the system.

Caton in 1875 suggested that a peripheral stimulus could be measured as a nervous system response. Fifty years later, Berger utilized this principle in his work on electroencephalography (EEG).[26] Unfortunately, the SSEP is of low amplitude (EEG:SSEP is greater than 100:1) and is therefore buried in the EEG. It was not until 1947, when Dawson used photographic superimposition for signal averaging, that evoked potentials could be reasonably obtained.[13] Today, signal-averaging computers are used to extract the evoked potential. These responses are extracted during a specific interval following a stimulus; after several repetitions of the stimulus, the wave forms are averaged.

The response itself is a multiple-peak wave form extending over a specific period of time (Fig. 4-11 and 4-12). By convention, downward waves are positive; upward waves are negative. By international convention, as discussed earlier, the waves are further named by the peak latency: that is, the time from the stimulus to the maximum re-

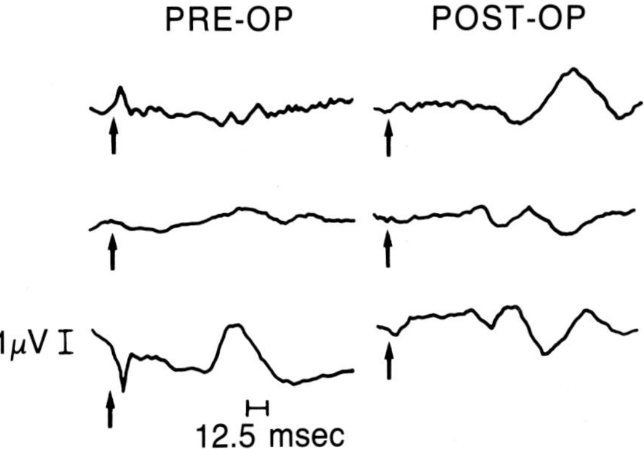

Fig. 4-11. Preoperative and postoperative SSEPs in patients with spinal cord injury.

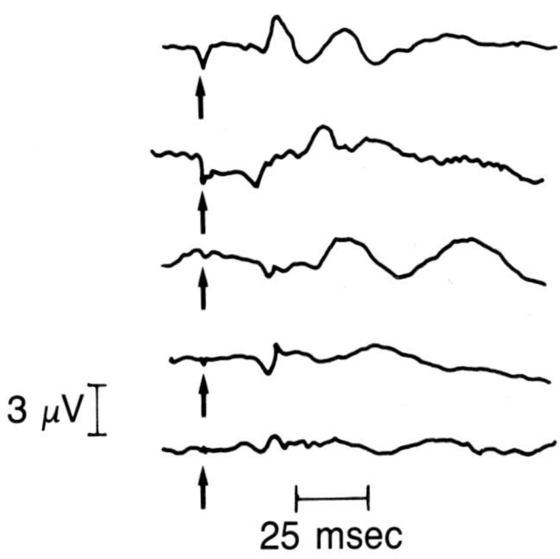

Fig. 4-12. Serial SSEPs from patient with CSM using median nerve stimulation. The second trace was obtained 3 months after the first, then at 12, 18, and 24 months. (Adapted from Cusick JF, Myklebust, JB: Temporal alterations in somatosensory evoked potentials in cervical spondylotic myelopathy. In Weidner A (ed.): Cervical Spine I, pp 131-136. Wien, Springer-Verlag, 1987

sponse.[18] Several major groups do not accept these conventions, however. Placement of electrodes, stimulus strengths, and other technical parameters can vary significantly.[8] Clinical considerations, which are complicated and fill volumes, are available.[6,8,18] Often these works also include information on standard latency and amplitude values.

Most early studies of the evoked potential concentrated on the shape and nature of the later waves in the response, or the long-latency components,[15] partly because of their greater amplitude. Unfortunately, the long-latency components tend to be inconstant and sensitive to behavioral changes.[34] In addition, interpretation of the specific peaks is difficult, since little is known of the anatomic generators.[15]

In recent years, more emphasis has been placed on the early component of the response. Isolation of these low-amplitude wave forms has become possible with improved techniques. These earlier components have been localized to some degree; it is significant that they are highly stationary.[41] In studies by Myklebust and colleagues, sleep had no effect on the first 20 to 30 msec of the brain-stem/cortical response owing to median nerve stimulation. However, later portions of the response in sleeping subjects were of both lower amplitude and delayed latency.[34]

Determination of the pathologic basis for abnormal wave forms should be approached with caution. Dorfman and coworkers have suggested that changes in latency may be of more value in the analysis of the somatosensory system than amplitude changes, particularly in the evaluation of spinal lesions.[15] Needless to say, others have disagreed, including those who suggest that latency shifts are produced by segmental demyelination (as in multiple sclerosis), while actual axonal loss (which is presumably more common) produces decreased amplitudes during conduction at normal velocities.[8] Actually, most spinal lesions include both axonal loss and demyelination; therefore, precise determination of the cause of an abnormal wave form is impossible.

Extraordinary efforts have been made to determine the anatomic generators of the SSEP. The utility of such information in clinical diagnosis is obvious; unfortunately, results to date have been disappointing.

Sances and colleagues looked at the origin of the early response (secondary to median nerve stimulation) in primates. In animals undergoing midpontine section, early responses recorded from thalamic nucleus ventromedial (VM) and the dorsal column nuclei at C1 were intact. When depth electrodes were placed into the dorsal column nuclei, the responses were synchronous with the early thalamic potential. They suggested that the generator site of the early response is between the dorsal column nuclei and the pons.[41,42]

The dorsal column conduction of the SSEP in primates was clearly established by Cusick and associates in their primate studies.[10] Segmental dorsal column resection in the thoracic spinal cord was carried out. In the immediate postoperative period, evoked potentials recorded from the spinal cord above the resection, as well as those from thalamic nucleus ventropostero lateral (VPL) and the sensory cortex, were markedly attenuated. Thalamic nucleus centromedial (CM) responses were normal several hours after the ablation; no improvement in the cortical responses was seen acutely, however, with stimulation above or below the lesion. In animals surviving 6 weeks, markedly decreased amplitudes were seen, with only minimal changes in latency. In monkeys with preservation of only the dorsal columns, responses measured in the spinal cord, thalamic nucleus VPL, and cortex were normal; CM responses were obliterated. These studies add credence to the popular conception that cortical and spinal cord responses to peripheral stimulation depend on the integrity of the dorsal columns, with little evidence for any other spinal or supraspinal effect.

Cohen and associates performed ultrasonic surgical aspiration of the spinal cord in cats, again in order to identify the pathway of the SSEP.[9] Sequential tracts were interrupted, including the dorsal and lateral columns. They found that the consistent initial positive wave, occurring at 17 to 19 msec latency after sciatic nerve stimulation, was completely obliterated following dorsal column interruption. However, some large-latency bizarre components persisted. These are presumably conducted in the spinocervical tract, a fast-conducting tract found in cats, but not primates. In unilateral dorsal column interruptions, only the ipsilateral SSEP was lost, and the contralateral response was not affected. Thus, they suggested that bilateral recording may be of benefit in measuring the asymmetry of a given lesion, both clinically and experimentally.

Most other studies attempting to define generators have based their determination on small clinical series. Such conclusions must be approached with caution, since there is a lack of rigid anatomic verification. Most investigators agree that P9 (a downward deflection 9 msec after median nerve stimulation) localizes from the distal brachial plexus.[8,50] This conclusion is based on several large series of patients with brachial plexopathies or peripheral neuropathies: preservation of P9 with loss of later peaks suggests a proximal lesion; if P9 is absent, the lesion is likely to be distal to the dorsal root ganglia. Yamada and colleagues found abnormalities at N13 and beyond in patients with mid to lower cervical lesions[50]; Chiappa and Sances and coworkers suggest a dorsal column nuclear origin of this peak.[8,41,42] Some agreement exists that N18 is thalamic in origin and that subsequent peaks originate in the parietal cortex. Again, this suggestion is based on the analysis of responses from patients with lesions in those areas.[8,50] Firm conclusions await experimental validation. In the interim, probably only the very early components can be considered accurately defined.

The Evoked Potential in Spinal Cord Injury

An early application of the SSEP was in the evaluation of spinal cord injury and prognosis for neurologic recovery. In 1963, Donaghy and Numato reported that early return of the SSEP, even with some abnormality of the wave form, was associated with good prognosis for motor recovery. This report has subsequently been verified by other investigators.[10,11,25,28,53] The high correlation between changes in the SSEP and recovery reflect the fact that, at least experimentally, spinal cord injury affects the entire cord. Most experimental studies in this area, however, have been based on the dorsal impact model, with its direct trauma to the dorsal columns.

In studies performed in cats, the above conclusion was confirmed using a tension model of spinal cord injury that prominently involves white matter. In animals with incomplete quadriplegia, some recovery of the amplitude of the cord-cord evoked potential was seen within 24 hours, with further improvement paralleling neurologic recovery. Little early recovery of the response was seen in animals suffering initially complete quadriplegia. After 4 to 5 weeks, when the latter animals had shown some nonfunctional motor recovery, some return of the primary component was evident, as well as aberrant late waves. Histologic changes seen in the white matter also closely paralleled neurologic status. Neuronal chromatolysis, axonal stretching, and demyelination/remyelination were evident in both anterior and posterior white matter, proportionate to the evoked response. Thus, the experimental validity of the use of the evoked potential extends across spinal cord injury models.

Young has identified some general patterns of evoked potential changes in clinical spinal cord injury, which may occur in combination depending on the nature of the injury.[53] The first pattern is that of an amplitude change with normal latency; in our experimental and clinical experience, improvements in amplitude tend to be associated with neurologic recovery if latencies are unaltered. An intermediate pattern includes moderate latency shifts in the early wave forms without major amplitude changes; finally, a pattern that includes long latency negative waves typically seen at 6 weeks or beyond is observed. The last pattern was found to be associated with a poor prognosis, although our experience suggests that any complex is better than no complex at all.

Perot was an early proponent of the prognostic value of the SSEP in acute spinal cord injury. In his series, presence of the response after injury suggested a favorable clinical outcome.[36] Larson measured the SSEP in 28 patients undergoing vertebral surgery for decompression of the traumatized spinal cord. Evoked potentials were typically abnormal in patients with decreased position sense, but not in those with altered pain or temperature sensation. In several patients, the SSEP improved along with the neurologic examination after surgery (Fig. 4-11). However, some patients improved clinically, although the SSEP did not change.[25] The converse was seen in a series reported by York and colleagues: Sixteen patients showed evidence or recovery of the SSEP, but no clinical improvement.[51] This may reflect that the SSEP is a more sensitive indicator of cord status than the neurologic exam.[6]

Rowed has suggested that early return of the SSEP after an incomplete injury with a reasonably normal wave form suggests a good prognosis for clinical recovery.[40] He found an excellent correlation between the initial (postinjury) SSEP and the initial neurologic grade ($p < .001$), although the correlation between the initial SSEP and discharge (to rehabilitation institute) neurologic exam was poor. He did find, however, that the more normal the initial evoked potential (in terms of latency, amplitude, and quality of the wave form), the shorter the time interval to reach a functional neurologic level in incomplete patients ($p < .01$). The SSEP tended to improve earlier than the neurologic status.

Of greater significance, perhaps, were the differences between quadriparetic patients who improved neurologically and those who did not. The primary complex (P_{30} and N_{41}) was typically found in patients showing subsequent neurologic improvement. The amplitude of this primary response was near normal in patients showing major neurologic improvement; it was (statistically) significantly lower in those without these clinical changes. Thus the initial SSEP correlated with the functional neurologic grade. The initial components which are generated within the dorsal columns were found to be the most significant; again, long-latency waves in the absence of short-latency components were often associated with a poor prognosis. Further, recovery of early-component amplitude tended to precede clinical improvement. Indeed, even in the absence of neurologic improvement, amplitude of the early components tends to improve.[53]

Others have also compared the results of the initial evoked potential examinations with ultimate clinical status. In Young's series,[53] the admission SSEP correlated better than the 6-week neurologic examination than with the admission examination. However, the follow-up SSEPs did not correlate with the follow-up exam as well as did the admission SSEP.

In a recent series by Chabot and coworkers,[6] some conclusions that seem to take a middle course (and represent a good summation of the section) were presented. The SSEP is useful in determining the extent of physiologic injury to the spinal cord and has some value in predicting the likelihood of sensory and/or motor recovery. Paralyzed patients with total absence of the response presumably have complete injuries and are unlikely to recover.[6] Our experience emphasizes the need for caution in this assumption, as we have seen several patients with clinically complete quadriplegias and absent SSEPs who showed significant neurologic improvement, with or without subsequent recovery of the SSEP.

The Evoked Potential in Cervical Radiculopathy and Myelopathy

The SSEP has been used with varying degrees of success in the evaluation of cervical root and peripheral nerve injuries. Much of the value of the technique has been previously discussed in the sections describing the nerve conduction velocity (NCV), as well as in the introduction of the SSEP. In peripheral nerve lesions, the SSEP can be used to document nerve continuity if technical problems (*i.e.*, an arm cast) do not allow examination of the nerve conduction velocity. As is true for the NCV, one can obtain SSEPs by stimulating at different sites along the nerve to determine segmental changes. In traumatic peripheral nerve lesions, return of the SSEP may be seen prior to that of the NCV; therefore, the former may be more useful in predicting regeneration.[8]

Similarly, in cervical radiculopathy the SSEP may demonstrate abnormalities of conduction earlier than the NCV. Because the NCV abnormality requires wallerian degeneration over substantial portions of the root and its peripheral nerve, significant time may pass before the electrodiagnostic study is abnormal. The SSEP, on the other hand, may be abnormal shortly after root compression. The most common finding in cervical radiculopathy is decreased amplitude of the primary component of the response using peripheral nerve stimulation. Comparison with the contralateral root may also be of value. It is important that the stimulus be applied to the main peripheral nerve supplied by that root. Unfortunately, the value of the SSEP in diagnosing cervical radiculopathy is diminished because most nerve trunks contain both motor and sensory fibers with multisegmental composition.[8]

When positive, these studies may define not only the segmental level, but also the severity of the physiologic impairment. Eisen and associates suggested that reduced amplitudes or abnormal wave forms (reflecting sensory fiber conduction blocks) are the most valuable electrodiagnostic criteria of root compression. They found the SSEP to be a highly sensitive indicator of sensory abnormality in cervical radiculopathy and suggested that an abnormal segmental SSEP in the presence of a normal NCV is diagnostic for a cervical root lesion.[16]

Because the dorsal columns are typically involved in cervical spondylotic myelopathy (CSM), the SSEP should be of value diagnostically and in monitoring patient status over time. While not practical for clinical use, the work of Kotani and colleagues[24] in CSM patients has interesting implications. After passing electrodes into the epidural space via Touhy needles, responses were measured at each cervical segment.

When the median nerve was stimulated and the response was recorded at the spinal cord (*segmental*), the normal latency of the primary component was 5 to 6 msec. When both stimulation and recording took place at spinal cord levels (*conductive*), durations and amplitudes were greater.

In patients with CSM, abnormalities of the segmental SSEPs were almost universally seen. Conductive (cord-cord) responses were abnormal, particularly when there were abnormalities of leg function; they suggested that this response emanates in part from the pyramidal tract.[24]

Cusick and Myklebust have used noninvasive

SSEP techniques to evaluate patients with cervical spondylotic myelopathy (CSM), both episodically and serially, and in association with neck motion.[12] In serial recordings, they found changes in the secondary components of the primary response (Fig. 4-12); that is, the initial peak at 16 to 20 msec (with median nerve stimulation) was unaffected until the disorder was well advanced. Over time, the latencies of later peaks increased, suggesting that a mechanical distortion of axons and resultant alterations in conductivity, represent the primary pathophysiologic basis of CSM. Of particular interest were the changes frequently seen with neck motion, especially when patients went into extension (Fig. 4-13), emphasizing that mechanical changes in the integrity of the cord can produce almost instantaneous physiologic changes. The clinical utility of these techniques appears to lie in monitoring progression of the disorder, and analyzing changes associated with neck motion as a part of the assessment of pathologic severity.

Intraoperative Evoked Potentials

In any surgical procedure on the spine, the maintenance of spinal cord integrity is of paramount importance. Measurement of the SSEP represents an ideal physiologic measure of intraoperative changes in spinal cord function if one accepts that the evoked potential is not only highly sensitive but that changes are highly specific for cord injury (an assumption that is often not correct).[26,27] For measurement of the SSEP to be useful, changes need to occur early enough that recognition can lead to modification of the procedure and to recovery.[49]

The evoked potential is also a potentially valuable measure, because it is independent of the level of consciousness and can be performed under anesthesia, although not without difficulties, as will be discussed later. Moreover, the patient serves as his own control, improving the sensitivity of the study.

Experimental studies have suggested that the SSEP is a reliable means of intraoperative monitoring. Schramm and associates reported little change in the SSEP in early compression of the spinal cord. However, once amplitude changes were seen, slight increases in compression forces resulted in more significant degrees of wave form deterioration.[43] Similar patterns have been observed by others using distraction applied to the spinal cord. Moreover, the SSEP is relatively resistant to ischemia,[11,12] indicating that conduction failure in spinal cord distortion is primarily due to (potentially reversible) mechanical factors.[11,27]

Unfortunately, there are several limitations in the use of the SSEP in spinal surgery. The response, particularly its later components, is adversely affected by anesthesia. For example, everything later than the primary response in the SSEP is eliminated by inhalational agents, particularly halothane and enflurane. Latencies may also be affected. Barbiturates and opioids, on the other hand, have a potentiating effect on the primary response.[21] The SSEP may also be temperature sensitive, with increases in conduction time associated with altered core temperatures.

Technical problems can also wreak havoc: the poor signal-to-noise ratio is degraded by the electrical artifacts of the operating room. In addition, activity in the room can be picked up as SSEP changes, owing to the high sensitivity of the technique. Electrodes can pop off, unseen, because of patient draping.

A more fundamental problem with the intraoperative use of the evoked potential is that it monitors only dorsal column integrity and therefore does not indicate direct anterior (motor) tract compromise.[20] In many instances, the entire cord in subjected to equal pathologic forces; for example, in the reduction of a dislocation of the cervical spine, the entire cord is distracted. On the other hand, in anterior surgery for a compression fracture, the anterior aspect of the spinal cord is at a

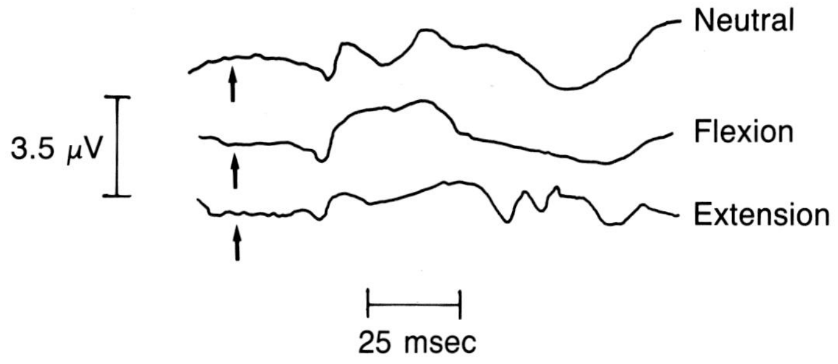

Fig. 4-13. The effects of neck motion on the SSEP in patients with CSM (median nerve stimulation). (Adapted from Cusick JF, Myklebust JB: Temporal alterations in somatosensory evoked potentials in cervical spondylotic myelopathy. In Weidner A (ed.): Cervical Spine I, pp 131-136. Wien, Springer-Verlag, 1987

greater risk of injury. Monitoring of the motor evoked potential, discussed later in this chapter, may offer aid in this area in the future. Although it is not the purpose of this review to discuss techniques, it is worth noting that a variety of stimulus/recording points have been used in intraoperative monitoring during spinal surgery. In addition to work with the SSEP using median nerve stimulation, recording with electrodes placed into the epidural space or through spinous processes is popular. In our experience, epidural techniques are particularly advantageous. First of all, the presence of electrodes both rostral and caudal to the area of interest allows for both orthodromic and antidromic stimulation.[28] The cord-cord response is extremely rapid; the primary response (probably the only one consistent enough to monitor) is very stable, and the signal-to-noise ratio is relatively low. Technical problems include the need to extend the surgical exposure for electrode placement, or conversely, the need to limit the operative field.

Clinical results to date have been mixed. In a large series, 82% of the studies carried out intraoperatively were technically satisfactory.[38] There was a false-positive rate of 6.5%, presumably due to technical problems. The false-negative rate of 3.6% is of greater concern. This latter finding may be related to progressive infarction of the cord, which would show a late effect on the dorsal column response; more likely, it may be related to a small number of surviving sensory fibers being activated by repetitive and high intensity pulses. According to Raudzens, this means that surgery was interrupted unnecessarily 62% of the time because of abnormal SSEPs, and deficits were not predicted 4.3% of the time.[38]

Clearly, the overall question of the utility of intraoperative monitoring remains to be answered. The effort is probably not as valuable in cases where the spinal cord is directly visualized, such as anterior decompression fusions of the cervical spine. In cases of scoliosis or in the closed reduction of cervical spine dislocation, the distraction effects on both motor and sensory fibers should be similar, and the value is apparent. Absolute decisions regarding surgery should not be made solely on the basis of the evoked potential, since both false positives and false negatives may occur.

MOTOR EVOKED POTENTIALS

Recently, a great deal of work has been carried out analyzing the neurophysiologic responses produced by stimulation of the motor cerebral cortex and recorded peripherally. In practice, efferent evoked potentials have been used experimentally for many years,[42] but the techniques required—and the imprecision of the results—have prevented clinical use.

Interest in the motor evoked potential (MEP) arose from the recognition that an intraoperative measure of anterior cord (motor) function is highly desirable in spinal surgery.[29] Just as for the SSEP, the methods need to be relatively noninvasive, reproducible, and sensitive.

In experimental studies of the utility of the motor evoked potential in spinal cord injury, the spinal cords of cats were subjected to varying degrees of impact injury, and both SSEPs and MEPs were obtained.[30] The investigators found the MEP (particularly that measured at the peripheral nerve) to be highly sensitive to intermediate degrees of cord injury. The SSEP was rarely affected until 200 gm/cm impacts were used, at which point marked decreases in amplitude occurred. Effects on the MEP were more gradual, however, with small decreases in amplitude first seen at 50 gm/cm impacts, becoming more pronounced at 100 to 200 gm/cm. At severe impact levels, both the MEP and SSEP were lost. In some animals, the cord response returned to some extent; both the cord and peripheral nerve responses eventually deteriorated. However, limited data on neurologic and prognostic correlates were presented.

In clinical studies by Levy and colleagues, a stimulating (anode) electrode was placed over the motor cortex, and a second stimulating electrode was placed against the hard palate to direct the current.[29] Responses were recorded at the spinal cord level (via needle electrodes onto the laminae or epidural ball electrodes) or peripherally, using EEG electrodes over motor nerves. In addition, EMG activity resulting from cortical stimulation was measured, although this was not reliable enough to be used clinically.

The first component of the wave form, a large initial positivity, has been hypothesized to be due to direct activation of large pyramidal cells; later components are due to recurrent activation through interneurons and (finally) to local and gray-matter stimulation.[29] The amplitude of the response was found to correlate in a general way with motor performance: that is, preservation of the peripheral nerve response was consistent with some degree of motor activity. If the peripheral nerve response became a slow, diffuse wave form, rather than showing sharp, discrete waves, significant motor impairment could be expected. Unfortunately, the peripheral nerve response was affected more rapidly than was the cord response; in addition, the former was sensitive to both anesthesia and metabolic alterations, making changes difficult to interpret.

Machida and colleagues recorded muscle and peripheral nerve action potentials after spinal cord stimulation.[31] While technically satisfactory tracings were obtained, the results were hard to interpret. Wave forms varied significantly between subjects, and amplitudes between sides often differed. A greater problem identified by both groups was an inability to determine when irreversible injury to the nervous system had occurred.

Several other problems have been identified that limit the MEP to investigational use. The level of currents required to produce adequate stimulation is uncomfortable, and therefore measurement of the MEP can now be performed only on anesthetized patients. In the near future, magnetic stimulation techniques may solve this problem, however. Levy and co-workers note that because the MEP tests axonal continuity, it does not distinguish between the important primary fibers as opposed to other parts of the neuronal circuit. They suggest that the use of lower motor neuron activation (*i.e.*, EMG) may enhance the reliability of MEP measurements.[29]

Others have been much more critical of the shortcomings of the technique as discussed. Young and Cracco emphasize lack of specificity: Although it has been stated that the cortical stimulation is specific for the corticospinal tract, many others would recognize that even single shocks applied to cortical gyris stimulate multiple cortical interneurons.[52] Indeed, the emphasis on the corticospinal tract may be unwise, since a great deal of motor function, even in humans, is related to multisynaptic systems. Most fibers ending in the spinal cord have arisen caudal to the cerebral cortex, including neurons arising in the basal ganglia and brain stem.

Lack of specificity in stimulation is also seen in the use of the palate or surface electrodes. In addition to cord stimulation, alpha motor neurons—particularly at the proximal segment of the lower motor neuron—are stimulated. EMG responses during cervical stimulation are not enhanced by voluntary contraction of arm muscles, which is further evidence that the actual stimulus site is distal to the ventral root.[52]

In summary, the MEP has the potential to be a valuable part of the neurophysiologic examination. However, a great deal of work remains, including improvement of the definition of the anatomic pathways being stimulated, and simplification of the techniques used. Last, studies need to be carried out to correlate changes in the MEP with neurologic phenomena, including the threshold at which neurologic abnormalities become irreversible. When this has been accomplished, the MEP will have wide clinical application.

ACKNOWLEDGMENT

This work was supported in part by Veteran's Administration Medical Research Funds.

REFERENCES

1. *Adrian ED, Bronk DW:* The discharge of impulses in motor nerve fibers. Part II. The frequency of discharge in reflex and voluntary contractions. J Physiol (Lond) 67:119–151, 1929
2. *Benecke R, Conrad B:* The distal sensory nerve action potential as a diagnostic tool for the differentiation of lesions in dorsal roots and peripheral nerves. J Neurol 223:231–239, 1980
3. *Bralliar F:* Electromyography: its use and misuse in peripheral nerve injuries. Orthop Clin NA 12:229–238, 1981
4. *Buchthal F, Rosenfalck P:* Action potential parameters in different human muscles. Acta Psychiatr Neurol Scand 30:125–131, 1955
5. *Bunch WH, Scarff TB, Trimble J:* Current concepts review: spinal cord monitoring. J Bone Joint Surg 65A:707–710, 1983
6. *Chabot R, York DH, Watts C, et al:* Somatosensory evoked potentials evaluated in normal subjects and spinal cord-injured patients. J Neurosurg 63:544–551, 1985
7. *Chassin SL, Little JW, DeLisa JA:* Compound nerve action potentials from the median and ulnar nerves. Arch Phys Med Rehab, 68:31–35, 1987
8. *Chiappa KH:* Evoked Potentials in Clinical Medicine, p 340. New York, Raven Press, 1983
9. *Cohen AR, Young W, Ransohoff J:* Intraspinal localization of the somatosensory evoked potential. Neurosurgery 9:157–162, 1981
10. *Cusick JF, Myklebust JB, Larson SJ, et al:* Spinal cord evaluation by cortical evoked responses. Arch Neurol 36:140–143, 1979
11. *Cusick JF, Myklebust J, Zyvoloski M, et al:* Effects of vertebral column distraction in the monkey. J Neurosurg 57:651–659, 1982
12. *Cusick JF, Myklebust JB:* Temporal alterations in somatosensory evoked potentials in cervical spondylotic myelopathy. In A. Weidner (ed): Cervical Spine I, pp 131–136. Wien: Springer-Verlag Publishers, 1987

13. *DAWSON GD:* A summation technique for the detection of small evoked potentials. Electroenceph Clin Neurophysiol 6:65–84, 1954
14. *DAWSON GD:* The relative excitability and conduction velocity of sensory and motor nerve fibers in man. J Physiol (Lond) 131:436–451, 1956
15. *DORFMAN LJ, PERKASH I, BOSLEY TM, ET AL:* Use of cerebral evoked potentials to evaluate spinal somatosensory function in patients with traumatic and surgical myelopathies. J Neurosurg 52:654–660, 1980
16. *EISEN A, HOIRCH M, MOLL A:* Evaluation of radiculopathies by segmental stimulation and somatosensory evoked potentials. Can J Neurol Sci 10:178–182, 1983
17. *FINCHAM RW, CAPE CA:* Sensory nerve conduction in syringomyelia. Neurology 18:200–201, 1968
18. *GUIDELINES COMMITTEE:* Guidelines for clinical evoked potential studies. J Clin Neurophysiol 3(Suppl):43–92, 1986
19. *HARVEY AM, MASLAND RL:* A method for the study of neuromuscular transmission in human subjects. Bull Johns Hopk Hosp 68:81–93, 1941
20. *HODES R, LARRABEE MG, GERMAN W:* The human electromyogram in response to nerve stimulation and the conduction velocity of motor axons. Studies on normal and on injured peripheral nerves. Arch Neurol Psychiatry 60:340–365, 1948
21. *HUME AL, DURKIN MA:* Central and spinal somatosensory conduction times during hypothermic cardiopulmonary bypass and some observations on the effects of fentanyl and isoflurane anesthesia. Electroencephalogr Clin Neurophysiol 65:46–58, 1986
22. *JOHNSON EW, STOCKLIN R, LABAN MM:* Use of electrodiagnostic examination in a university hospital. Arch Phys Med Rehab 46:573–578, 1965
23. *JOHNSON EW, MELVIN JL:* Value of electromyography in lumbar radiculopathy. Arch Phys Med Rehab 52:239–243, 1971
24. *KOTANI H, SAIKI K, YAMASAKI H, ET AL:* Evaluation of cervical cord function in cervical spondylotic myelopathy and/or radiculopathy using both segmental and conductive spinal-evoked potentials (SEP). Spine 11:185–190, 1986
25. *LARSON SJ, HOLST RA, HEMMY DC, ET AL:* The lateral extracavitary approach to traumatic lesions of the thoracic and lumbar spine. J Neurosurg 45:628–637, 1976
26. *LARSON SJ, SANCES A JR, CHRISTENSON PC:* Evoked somatosensory potentials in man. Arch Neurol 15:88–93, 1966
27. *LARSON SJ, WALSH PR, SANCES A JR, ET AL:* Evoked potentials in experimental myelopathy. Spine 5:299–302, 1980
28. *LARSON SJ, WALSH PR, ACKMANN JJ, ET AL:* Neurophysiological aids in diagnosis evaluation and prognosis. J Am Paraplegia Soc 7:66–69, 1984
29. *LEVY WJ, YORK DH, MCCAFFREY M, ET AL:* Motor evoked potentials from transcranial stimulation of the motor cortex in humans. Neurosurgery 15:287–302, 1984
30. *LEVY W, MCCAFFREY M, YORK D:* Motor evoked potential in cats with acute spinal cord injury. Neurosurgery 19:9–19, 1986
31. *MACHIDA M, WEINSTEIN SL, YAMADA T, ET AL:* Spinal cord monitoring. Electrophysiological measures of sensory and motor function during spinal surgery. Spine 10:407–413, 1985
32. *MITZ M:* Personal communication
33. *MORALES-BLANQUEZ G, DELWAIDE PJ:* The thoracic outlet syndrome: an electrophysiological study. EMG Clin Neurophysiol 22:255–263, 1982
34. *MYKLEBUST JB, SANCES A JR, CUSICK JF, ET AL:* Stationarity of the somatosensory evoked potential. Med Biol Eng Comp, 22:558–563, 1984
35. *NORTHRUP BE:* Electrophysiologic evaluation of spinal cord lesions. In Bailey RW (ed): The Cervical Spine, pp 140–146. Philadelphia, JB Lippincott Co, 1983
36. *PEROT PL JR:* The clinical use of somatosensory evoked potentials in spinal cord injury. Clin Neurosurg 20:367–381, 1973
37. *PROEBSTER R:* Uber muskelaktionsstrome am gesunden und kranken menschen. Zeit fur Orthopadische Chirurgie (Suppl 2)50:1–154, 1928
38. *RAUDZENS PA:* Sensory evoked potentials: an outline for surgical monitoring. Barrow Neurological Institute Quarterly 1:40–48, 1985
39. *REYNOLDS GG, PAVOT AP, KENRICK MM:* Electromyographic evaluation of patients with post traumatic cervical pain. Arch Phys Med Rehab, 49:170-172, 1968
40. *ROWED DW:* Value of somatosensory evoked potentials for prognosis in partial cord injuries. In Tator CH (ed): Early Management of Acute Spinal Cord Injury, pp 167–180. New York, Raven Press, 1982
41. *SANCES A JR, LARSON SJ, CUSICK JF, ET AL:* Early somatosensory evoked potentials. Electroencephalogr Clin Neurophysiol 45:505–514, 1978
42. *SANCES A JR, WEBER R, MYKLEBUST JB, ET AL:* The evoked potential: an experimental method for biomechanical analysis of brain and spinal injury. Proc 24th STAPP Car Crash Conf, pp 63–100. Society of Automotive Engineers, Warrendale, 1980
43. *SCHRAMM J, HASHIZUME K, FUKUSHIMA T, ET AL:* Experimental spinal cord injury produced by slow, graded compression. Alterations of cortical and spinal evoked potentials. J Neurosurg 50:48–57, 1979
44. *SPINNER M:* Injuries to the Major Branches of Pe-

ripheral Nerves of the Forearm, 2nd Ed, pp 57–63. Philadelphia, WB Saunders, 1978

45. *Stanwood JE, Kraft GH:* Diagnosis and management of brachial plexus injuries. Arch Phys Med Rehabil 52:52–60, 1971
46. *Upton ARM, McComas AJ:* The double crush in nerve entrapment syndromes. Lancet 2:359–362, 1973
47. *von Helmholtz H:* Messungen uber den zeitlichen verlauf der zuckung animalischer muskeln und die fortpflanzungsgeschwindigkeit der teizung in den nerven. Muller's Arch Anat Physiol, pp 276–364, 1850
48. *Weingarden HP, Mikolich LM, Johnson EW:* Radiculopathies. In Johnson W (ed): Practical Electromyography, pp 91–109. Baltimore, Williams & Wilkins, 1980
49. *Whittle IR, Johnston IH, Besser M:* Recording of spinal somatosensory evoked potentials for intraoperative spinal cord monitoring. J Neurosurg 64:601–612, 1986
50. *Yamada T, Kimura J, Wilkinson T, et al:* Short- and long-latency median somatosensory evoked potentials. Arch Neurol 40:215–220, 1983
51. *York DH, Watts C, Raffensberger M, Spagnolia T, Joyce C:* Utilization of somatosensory evoked cortical potentials in spinal cord injury. Prognostic limitations. Spine 8:832-839, 1983
52. *Young RR, Cracco RQ:* Clinical neurophysiology of conduction in central motor pathways. Ann Neurol 18:606-610, 1985
53. *Young W:* Correlation of somatosensory evoked potentials and neurological findings in spinal cord injury. In Tator CH (ed): Early Management of Acute Spinal Cord Injury, pp 153–165. New York, Raven Press, 1982

CHAPTER 5

Congenital Malformations

Congenital Malformations of the Base of the Skull: The Arnold-Chiari Malformation

RICHARD B. RAYNOR

Congenital anomalies of the base of the skull and atlantooccipital region involve both the nervous and osseous systems. Though an isolated defect may appear, various combinations involving bone and nerve are the norm. The frequent occurrence of these patterns and combinations suggests an interrelationship, if not a common cause, of their origin and development. To appreciate this, a brief review of the embryology outlining the developmental sequence and timing of the structures in this region is in order. Treatment is discussed separately with each condition but is essentially the same for all of them, because signs and symptoms are mostly due to brain stem and upper cervical cord compression.

EMBRYOLOGY

During the third week of gestation, a definitive notochord forms between the ectoderm and the endoderm. At the cephalic end of the embryo, the ectoderm immediately above the notochord begins to thicken and differentiate into neuroectoderm, which forms the neural plate. The neural plate then begins to buckle along its midline to shape the neural groove, walled in by a neural fold on either side. While this is occurring, a loose collection of intraembryonic mesenchymal cells begins to coalesce into three regions. The most medial becomes a solid mass, the paraxial mesoderm, which is just lateral to the notochord and on either side of it. The paraxial mesoderm is the anlage of the skeletal muscle, bone, and skin. By the end of the third week, this mesoderm begins to segment in a cranial to caudal direction.

During the fourth and fifth week, a total of about 42 somites is formed. There are 4 occipital, 8 cervical, 12 thoracic, 5 lumbar, 5 sacral, and 8 to 10 coccygeal pairs. Each somite differentiates into 3 parts, with the ventromedial part, called the sclerotome, destined to form the vertebral bodies. These bilateral ventromedial cells migrate to the midline and surround the notochord. Each somite eventually separates into a caudal and a cephalic portion, with the cells of the middle portion condensing to form the intervertebral disc. The caudal half of one sclerotome unites with the cranial half of its neighbor and forms the earliest manifestation of a vertebral body.[39] Only the second, third, and fourth somites do not follow this course. They eventually fuse to form the occipital bone and posterior part of the foramen magnum. The fate of the first somite is still not completely understood.

At the cranial end of the notochord, another collection of mesenchymal cells condenses to form a platelike mass between the notochord and brain stem. This basal plate unites with the occipital somites and forms the basioocciput, which completely encircles the neural tube in the region of the foramen magnum. These events are occurring at about the same time the somites are dividing and fusing to form vertebral bodies.[12]

Simultaneous with development of the cartilaginous skeleton, differentiation of the nervous system progresses. The neural plate begins to take on a tubelike appearance by the end of the third week. During the fourth week, the neural folds that form the side walls start to fuse in the midline to form a true tube. This occurs in the region of the fourth and fifth somites, the location of the atlantooccipital junctions. Fusion of the neural tube proceeds simultaneously in a cephalad and caudad direction, closing along its entire length by the end of the fourth week. Both ends of the tube remain open, however.[38] The size of the neural tube determines the diameter of the developing spinal canal.[15]

During the fifth and sixth week, further differentiation of the various parts of the brain and spinal cord occurs. Of note is the roof of the fourth ventricle, which thins out especially in the midline where the foramen of Magendie will appear and bilaterally where the paired foramina of Luschka develop. These will not actually open until about the seventh week, when they establish a direct connection between the subarachnoid space and the fourth ventricle.[38]

BASILAR IMPRESSION

Basilar impression is the most common congenital anomaly affecting the atlantooccipital region, though it may also occur as a secondary manifestation of other lesions, as discussed in later chapters. This discussion is limited to the congenital variety. Some form of the condition has been recognized from ancient times; early dynasty Egyptian carvings appear to have displayed this anomaly, as do some early Mexican sculpted figures.[26] The first formal description with a case report was by Homen in 1901.[16] A familial incidence of this malformation has been reported.

Confusion has arisen over the terms *basilar impression* and *platybasia.* Some authors have used them interchangeably, but most people consider them to be two separate conditions. Platybasia indicates an increase in the basal angle of the skull, which is determined by one line drawn along the plane of the sphenoid and another drawn along the clivus on a lateral roentgenogram of the skull.[21] Platybasia exists when this angle exceeds 145°, although there is slight variation in this figure.[34]

The confusion between the two conditions originated following a paper in 1939 by Chamberlain in which the terms were used interchangeably.[2] This same paper defined the most common method of measuring basilar impression using Chamberlain's line. A line is drawn between the posterior edge of the hard palate to the posterior lip of the foramen magnum. If the tip of the odontoid process is above this line, basilar impression exists. Other authors, though using this measurement, have considered intracranial projection of up to one third of the length of the odontoid to be normal.[36] McGregor's line, which is drawn from the upper surface of the posterior edge of the hard palate to the most caudal point of the occipital curve, is another commonly used measurement. Though platybasia and basilar expression can occur simultaneously, it is uncommonly found (Fig. 5-1).

Basilar impression is an upward movement of the base of the skull in the region of the foramen magnum and is measured by the intracranial extension of the tip of the odontoid process. In the acquired form the measurement is significant because symptoms are usually secondary to pressure effect of the odontoid, whereas in the congenital variety other anomalies are often present and it may not be possible to distinguish the primary cause of symptoms. Patients with severe cases who tend to present in childhood or early adult life do develop primary symptoms because of the upward and forward displacement of the odontoid into the cranial cavity, which results in cerebellar and brain stem signs.[23] In most patients, problems do not appear until the third to fifth decade of life.[33] The Arnold-Chiari malformation or syringomyelia is common in conjunction with basilar impression[34] and, less frequently, severe kyphoscoliosis may occur.[34]

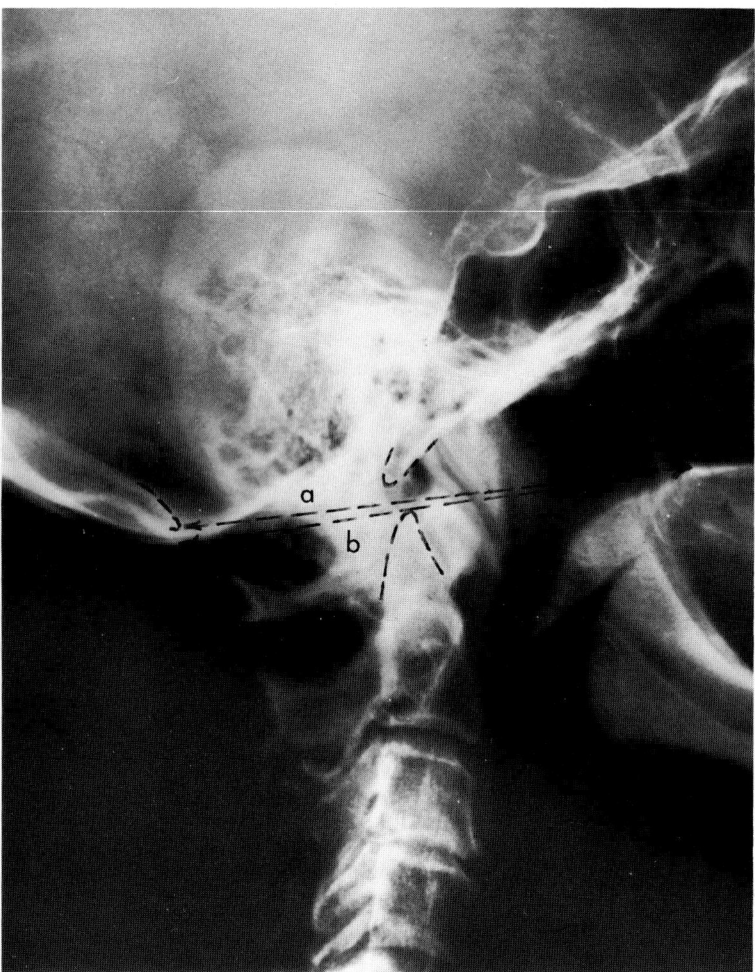

Fig. 5-1. Chamberlain's line (*a*) extends from the posterior margin of the foramen magnum to the posterior margin of the hard palate. McGregor's line (*b*) extends from the upper surface of the posterior edge of the hard palate to the most caudal point of the occipital curve. In this case they are close together, but frequently they are widely separated.

Signs and Symptoms

Clinical symptoms are due mainly to the neurologic structures involves. Long tract involvement, sometimes including all four extremities, is common and causes weakness with or without spasticity, depending on the duration of symptoms. The nature of sensory defects, which are frequent and variable, is dependent on whether they are caused by direct pressure or a central cavity from syringomyelia. Cerebellar ataxia and lower cranial nerve dysfunction can occur, causing dysarthria and dysphagia in some instances. Nystagmus is not uncommon and bizarre respiratory patterns have been reported.[33] Taylor and coworkers noted altered consciousness and periods of confusion, which were attributed to vertebral artery insufficiency.[37]

Treatment

Treatment consists of surgical decompression. In most instances this is best accomplished by laminectomy and suboccipital craniectomy, especially if an Arnold-Chiari malformation with tonsillar herniation or a syrinx is present. Less frequently in this condition, compression occurs anteriorly when the odontoid protrudes into the foramen magnum; in this case, a transoral resection of the offending bone is indicated.[27]

OCCIPITALIZATION OF THE ATLAS

Occipitalization of the atlas is one of the most common skeletal abnormalities of the upper cervical spine. It was found in 25% of a group of patients who presented with congenital malformations of the foramen magnum.[34] Fusion usually occurs anteriorly between the arch and rim of the foramen, with some segment of the posterior arch of C1 present in most instances. This fragment can frequently constrict the spinal canal, causing intermittent symptoms depending on the position of the head.[21]

Abnormal size or position of the odontoid is a significant finding and is usually present when there are neurologic signs. On occasion the odontoid may actually indent the medulla. Posterior displacement of the odontoid from the anterior foramen magnum–anterior arch complex is common, and can occur without clinical findings, depending on the size of the canal.

Other skeletal abnormalities of the upper cervical spine are frequent, especially fusion of the second and third cervical vertebrae. McRae noted this anomaly at the C2–C3 level in 17 of 25 patients with occipitalization of the atlas.[21] Other levels may be involved, but the incidence of vertebral fusion in the lower cervical spine is considerably lower than in the upper. Whether these fusions represent a true Klippel-Feil anomaly or a forme fruste is not clear because many of the patients do not have the short neck and low hair line typically seen in this condition. The Arnold-Chiari malformation and tonsillar herniation also can occur in conjunction with atlantoocipital fusion.

Signs and Symptoms

Though symptoms may not be present in many instances, the majority of patients do have them. The clinical presentation of lesions at or near the foramen magnum is notoriously confusing and may include ataxia of the extremities in various combinations along with numbness and pain in the limbs. Long tract signs with hyperflexia, Babinski response, spasticity, and weakness are frequent. Neck pain may or may not be present in conjunction with abnormal head posture. Intracranial manifestations include headache, visual disturbances, buzzing in the ears, and lower cranial nerve palsies causing dysphagia and dysarthria. Horner's syndrome has been reported, as has downbeat nystagmus.[22] Considering the wide range of symptoms, which span spinal cord, brain stem, cerebellar, and supratentorial locations, it is not surprising that a diagnosis of multiple sclerosis is frequently made before the true nature of the problems is appreciated.

Diagnostic Studies

Diagnostic studies include plain and tomographic x-ray examinations of the skull base and upper cervical spine. Positive-contrast myelography has been the definitive study for outlining the cord and brain stem along the clivus. CT scanning with intrathecal contrast provides excellent visualization of neural and osseous structures and is the preferred method of visualizing these structures in most institutions. CT simultaneously shows the actual relationship of bone, soft tissue, and brain stem–spinal cord, which is an advantage in planning treatment.

Several factors must be kept in mind, however. The cross-sectional cuts must be thin enough to satisfactorily cover the area in question and must be appropriately angled to obtain a true projection. Intracranial contrast material may cause reactions such as seizures, respiratory problems, or transient organic mental syndromes. Furthermore, this method is essentially static, since the structures visualized maintain a constant cranial-spine relationship. Though this problem can be overcome by altering the head position and repeating the study, additional x-ray exposure is necessary. Magnetic resonance imaging (MRI) has been a helpful adjunct in problem situations. The craniocervical junction can be visualized in flexed, neutral, and extended positions.

Treatment

Treatment is aimed at decompressing the affected structures.[22] When compression occurs posteriorly, upper cervical laminectomy and suboccipital craniectomy are indicated. It may be necessary to open dura in both the spinal and suboccipital region to obtain the desired space. Dura may be left open or a graft may be inserted using either artificial dural substitutes or fascia lata. When compression occurs anteriorly, the procedure of choice is a transoral approach to resect the odontoid, and possibly the rim of the foramen magnum. In this case, care must be taken not to open dura, since cerebrospinal fluid leakage and infection can result. Recently, an extraoral approach to this area has been described. It is an extension of the classical Smith Robinson technique of anterior fusion. The multiplicity of nerves and vascular structures encountered is the limiting factor in this procedure.[20]

ARNOLD-CHIARI MALFORMATION

The Arnold-Chiari malformation frequently occurs in conjunction with most of the other congenital malformations of the upper cervical spine. The pathologic entity was first described by Cleland in 1883,[4] when he noted elongation of the brain stem and extension of the fourth ventricle into the cervical canal. Chiari's first paper did not appear until 8 years later, and in it he described two lesions.[3] In the first instance, a tonsillar elongation occurs that projects into the upper cervical canal, along with some of the medial part of the inferior lobe of cerebellum. The medulla is not displaced, and hydrocephalus is not present. This is now called the Chiari Type I malformation.[1]

Chiari described a second anomaly in which the cerebellar tonsils and parts of the cerebellum were again found in the upper cervical canal. In addition, the fourth ventricle was elongated and was also in the upper cervical canal. In about half the cases a medullary kink was present, and hydrocephalus was very common. The cervical roots frequently had an upward course as they left the spinal cord. It was to this group of cases, the Chiari Type II, that two of Arnold's students attached the eponym of Arnold-Chiari malformation in 1907.[32]

The infantile presentation of the Arnold-Chiari malformation is its most severe form. Besides the defects mentioned above, hydrocephalus is almost always present. Spina bifida is a very frequent occurrence, and along with this, myelomeningocele may be found. The adult presentation usually lacks these last features and represents a less severe form of the anomaly. Many patients do not develop clinical symptoms until the third to fifth decade of life.

Other anomalies are usually found in patients who have an Arnold-Chiari malformation. Basilar impression, atlantooccipital fusion, Klippel-Feil syndrome, and spina bifida occulta are common, occurring either singly or in various combinations. The most common accompaniment of the Arnold-Chiari malformation, however, is syringomyelia or hydromyelia.[29] This association between the two lesions and several other similar conditions, especially the Dandy-Walker syndrome, was observed by Gardner in 1957.[9]

Full blown, the Dandy-Walker anomaly is usually seen in infants and children. It consists of a large posterior fossa with a dilated fourth ventricle. The lateral sinuses and tentorium are high as in the fetal position, and hydrocephalus is usually present.[6] The cause of this condition appears to be atresia of the foramina of Luschka and Magendie, resulting in their failure to open and establish communication between the central canal of the developing nervous system and the subarachnoid space. This normally occurs during the seventh week of embryonic life. The adult form of this condition is much less severe than that seen in the younger age group. In the adult, the Arnold-Chiari malformation and the Dandy-Walker syndrome may be indistinguishable in their clinical presentation. According to Gardner, these lesions are just different manifestations of the same problem. Both frequently have basilar impression, outlet obstruction of the fourth ventricle, and hydromyelia or syringomyelia.[7,9,19]

During normal development, the central canal of the nervous system gradually expands into the brain ventricles while the roof of the rhombencephalon, which covers the developing fourth ventricle, becomes thinner. Fluid pressure in the central cavity of the neural tube is dependent upon the cardiovascular system and is pulsatile in nature. Normally, these pulsations aid in development of the ventricular system. During the seventh week of embryonic life, the rhombic roof thins sufficiently for the foramen of Magendie to become patent, as do the lateral foramina of Luschka. Fluid pressure is transmitted into the potential subarachnoid space, which becomes a real space with this stimulus. Because the fluid now has a means of midline egress through the foramen of Magendie, it no longer goes into the central canal of the spinal cord, and this decreases in size.

If the foramen of Magendie fails to become patent, the fluid wave that results from normal vascular pulsations continues to be propagated into the central canal of the spinal cord, causing overdistention. The end result is syringomyelia or hydromyelia. Pressure is also exerted cranially, with hydrocephalus developing. Depending upon the resistance of the intracranial structures, the effect may be concentrated in the hind brain with marked dilatation of the fourth ventricle and posterior fossa, giving rise to the Dandy-Walker syndrome. If the hydrocephalic enlargement is concentrated in the forebrain, a posterior fossa too small to contain its neural structures will result, forcing some of the structures into the cervical canal. The Arnold-Chiari malformation then occurs.[7,9] Atresia of the openings from brain to subarachnoid space does not have to be an all-or-nothing phenomenon. The openings may be sufficient to allow significant flow of cerebrospinal fluid, and if sufficient time is allowed, equilibration of mean pressure occurs between the compartments. However, the peak of the pulse pressure wave is still directed into the central canal of the spinal cord, and this "water hammer" effect results in the development of a syrinx without hydrocephalus.[8] If fluid egress from the canal is blocked by a one-way valve effect, the cord remains distended.[11]

Though Gardner presents a reasonable mechanistic explanation for many of the events described above, there are disturbing factors that must be clarified. The size discrepancy of the posterior fossa in the Dandy-Walker and Arnold-Chiari malformations warrants further study. The frequent presence of other developmental anomalies such as atlantooccipital fusion, Klippel-Feil syndrome, and basilar impression suggests that other factors are present at the time these symptoms are developing and may influence many of them simultaneously.

Several other theories should be mentioned. According to one, traction due to caudal fixation of the cord prevents upward migration of the cervical structures and pulls the brain stem into the cervical canal. Though tethering of the cord with traction may occur in the infantile form where myelomeningocele is common, it is rare in the adult variety. Cervical segments should also be elongated by this traction, but the cervical segments are foreshortened in the Arnold-Chiari malformation.[31] Another theory considers the possibility that the nervous system overexpands in relation to the bony coverings, but this does not take into account the multiple skeletal anomalies frequently seen in conjunction with the neural defects.

Signs and Symptoms

In infants particularly and in children, the clinical presentation is dominated by the presence of hydrocephalus and frequently a myelomeningocele. These conditions tend to overshadow spinal cord compression and abnormalities at the craniocervical junction, especially since the foramen magnum tends to be large. When the Chiari II malformation is present, brain stem compression may predominate, secondary to severe tonsillar and fourth-ventricle herniation into the cervical canal. Lower cranial nerve dysfunction results in dysarthria, dysphagia, and dysphonia that can be extremely serious in the infant. Increased intracranial pressure and hydrocephalus usually occur after repair of a myelomeningocele, if they are not already present.[24] This tends to exacerbate the lower cranial nerve and brain-stem dysfunction, even causing internuclear ophthalmoplegia.[25] Altered respiratory patterns, hypotonia, or spasticity may occur, as may ataxia and nystagmus.[35]

In the adult, clinical signs and symptoms develop more slowly and tend to accentuate spinal cord dysfunction. Significant hydrocephalus is rare.[29] Many patients are initially diagnosed as having a chronic degenerative disease. A frequent early symptom is loss of pain sensation in the cervical dermatomes due to central cavitation of the spinal cord. This may be followed by atrophy and weakness of the upper extremities as the cavity extends into the anterior horn cell area and produces a central cordlike syndrome. Foramen magnum compression is common, with cerebellar ataxia, nystagmus, and lower cranial nerve dysfunction resulting.[30] Headaches occur when the normal circulation of spinal fluid is interrupted by impaction of medulla, cerebellar tonsils, and sometimes vermis into the foramen magnum and cervical canal.

The Chiari I also has the potential to cause a mild form of sleep apnea, of which the patient may be unaware but that others may observe. Laminectomy, including opening of the foramen magnum, relieves symptoms.*

Diagnostic Studies

Radiologic examination should include plain films of the cervical spine and base of the skull to check canal size and to evaluate other possible abnormalities such as basilar impression. Tomographic studies may be necessary to accurately measure the position of the dens, using either Chamberlain's or McGregor's line. The pedicles may be flattened and the cervical canal enlarged in its transverse diameter if a syrinx is present.

MRI is the easiest and most informative study available. The brain stem and spinal cord can be visualized and their relationship to the vertebrobasilar junction seen (Fig. 5-2). Syringomyelic cavities are well seen in the spinal cord. Cuts of the brain should be obtained, since enlargement of the ventricles has important therapeutic implications.

The availability of MRI is limited, however, and myelography with CT scanning is the method of choice. These provide excellent visualization and information, if appropriately performed. A problem may arise, however, if the diagnosis is unsuspected and the initial myelogram does not outline the relationship of the brain stem–spinal cord to the foramen magnum and upper cervical spine (Fig. 5-3). A CT scan performed shortly after subarachnoid instillation of contrast material outlines the cord size but may not show a syrinx cavity (Fig. 5-4). A lag of several hours usually occurs before contrast material enters the syrinx cavity, and it may be necessary to repeat the scan at 4 and even 8 hours to obtain a good study (Fig. 5-5). Sections should be done through the cervical and thoracic cord, even though clinically the problem appears to be in the cervical region (Fig. 5-6). The delayed study may show unsuspected lesions.

* Personal communication from Dr. Philip Levitt

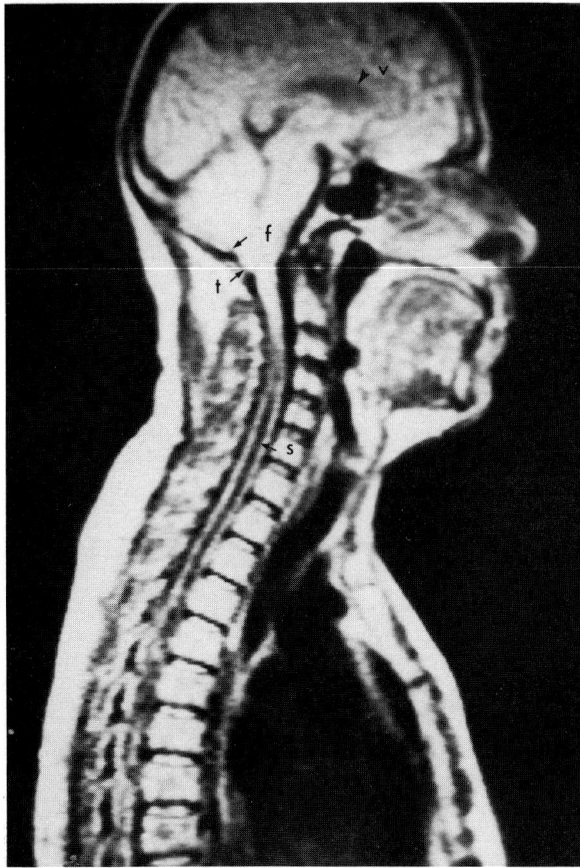

Fig. 5-2. MRI of patient with Chiari I malformation. Symptoms were mostly in the upper extremities with significant hand weakness and sensory changes. CT scan was performed shortly after instillation of subarachnoid metrizamide: (*f*) foramen magnum, (*s*) syrinx cavity in spinal cord, (*t*) cerebellar tonsil extending into cervical canal below level of C1, (*v*), normal-sized lateral ventricle.

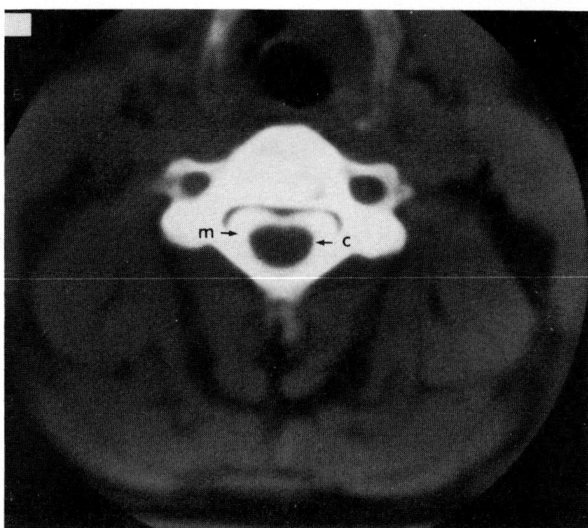

Fig. 5-4. CT scan of upper cervical cord obtained shortly after instillation of contrast. Same patient as Figures 5-2 and 5-3. (*c*) cervical cord; (*m*) metrizamide in subarachnoid space outlining spinal cord.

On occasion, the syrinx can be multiloculated with narrow channels connecting the larger chambers. Complete visualization of the cavity can be delayed under the circumstances.

Treatment

Treatment for this condition is surgical and must be adjusted to the individual problem. In children, a myelomeningocele should be properly repaired. Hydrocephalus, if it is not already present, develops in almost all cases and requires a shunting procedure.[24] When the problem is upper cervical and medullary compression due to herniation, cervical decompression is necessary. Since the fora-

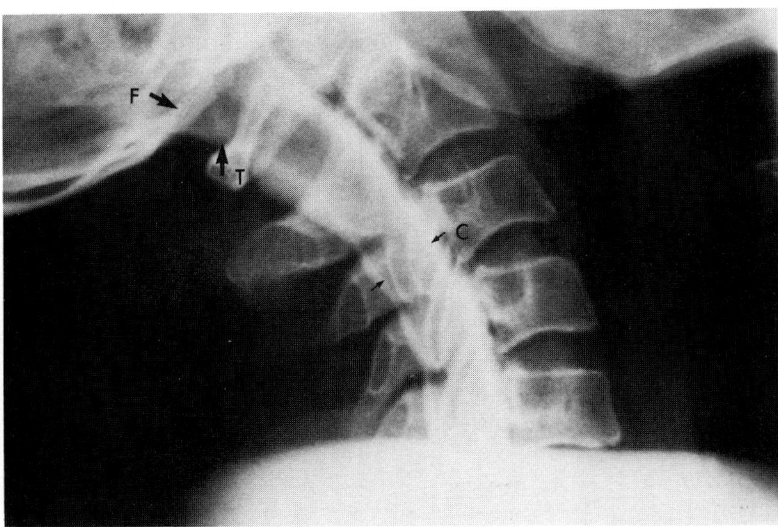

Fig. 5-3. Metrizamide myelogram outlining enlarged upper cervical cord and tonsillar herniation. This is the same patient as in Figure 5-2. (*C*) enlarged cervical cord; (*F*) foramen magnum; (*T*) outline of tonsil, which is obscured by arch of C1.

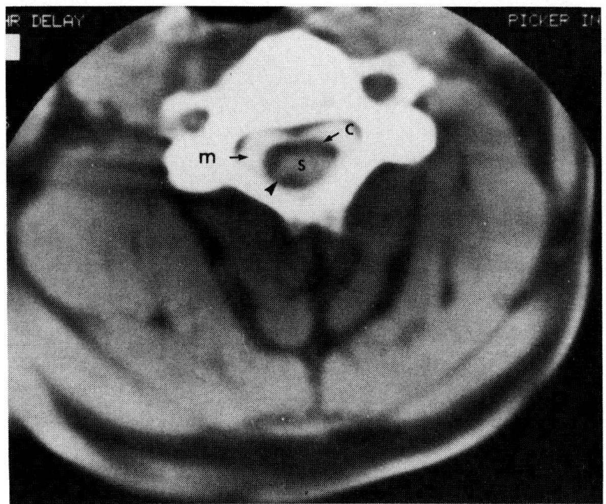

Fig. 5-5. CT scan 6 hours after instillation of contrast. Same patient as Figures 5-2 through 5-4. (*c*) cervical cord; (*m*) metrizamide in subarachnoid space outlining cord; (*s*) syringomyelic cavity, which now contains contrast. Arrowhead shows small channel connecting to larger, more distal cavity.

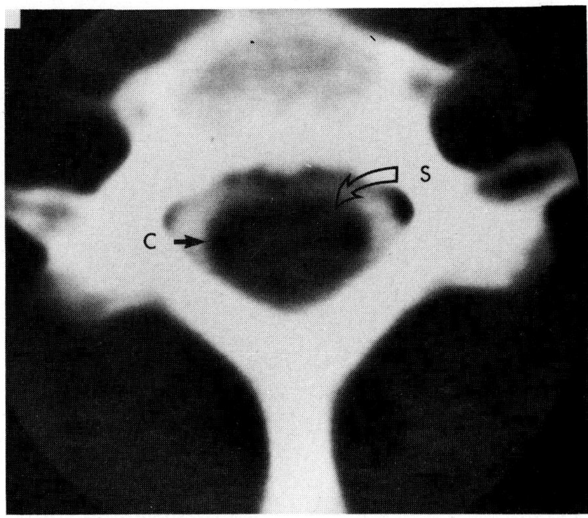

Fig. 5-6. Delayed CT scan of thoracic cord showing syrinx though myelogram did not outline an enlarged cord. Same patient as in Figures 5-2 through 5-5. (*C*) thoracic cord, (*S*) syrinx cavity containing contrast material.

men magnum is usually large in these children, it may not be necessary to open it,[13] although good radiographic studies are essential in order to make this decision. Patients in whom respiratory compromise occurs with lower cranial nerve dysfunction are quite sick and have a more severe form of the abnormality, usually the Chiari II. The maximum decompression possible is advised, including opening of the foramen magnum and laminectomy of the upper cervical segments. Unless severe adhesions are found between dura and brain stem, a dural decompression with a patch graft should be considered.

Symptoms in the adult are due to a pathologic condition at or near the foramen magnum. There are two principal causes. First is herniation of brain stem and cerebellar structures through the foramen and into the cervical canal, causing local pressure on these structures and interfering with circulation of cerebrospinal fluid. Treatment consists of laminectomy to below the level of the tonsillar herniation and opening of the foramen magnum, which, in contrast to that in children, is frequently constricted. The dura should be opened to afford adequate decompression, and here care is necessary. Large dural sinuses can be present and should be obliterated by clipping or bipolar cauterization as the dura is opened from below upward, into, and above the foramen magnum. At the level of the foramen, the dural thickening normally seen can become quite marked in these cases. Severe adhesions between the pia and arachnoid are also present in the area, and it is necessary to dissect these where possible to obtain adequate decompression. This may be tedious and difficult, and the operating microscope or some form of magnification is extremely helpful, if not essential. If the adhesions are too severe they should be left alone. A dural graft is frequently employed to make full use of the bony decompression. In some instances the dura may be left open, but muscle and fascia closure then must be done carefully in layers to prevent a spinal fluid leak.

The second main cause of symptoms is the presence of syringomyelia or hydromyelia. Gardner presents a good argument that these are probably the same condition.[8] An opening into the central cavity is frequently present around the obex. If this can be located, it should be plugged with a piece of muscle. Teflon has also been used.[28] However, some people have seen no difference in results when a foramen magnum decompression was performed alone or with a simultaneous obex plugging.[18] In those instances where an opening is not easily located, the cord is often very thin over one of the dorsal columns. This region should be opened at its thinnest point for a distance of about 1 cm to allow the cavity to decompress. Rhoton advocates leaving a silastic wick anchored to the dura to insure the patency of the opening (Fig.

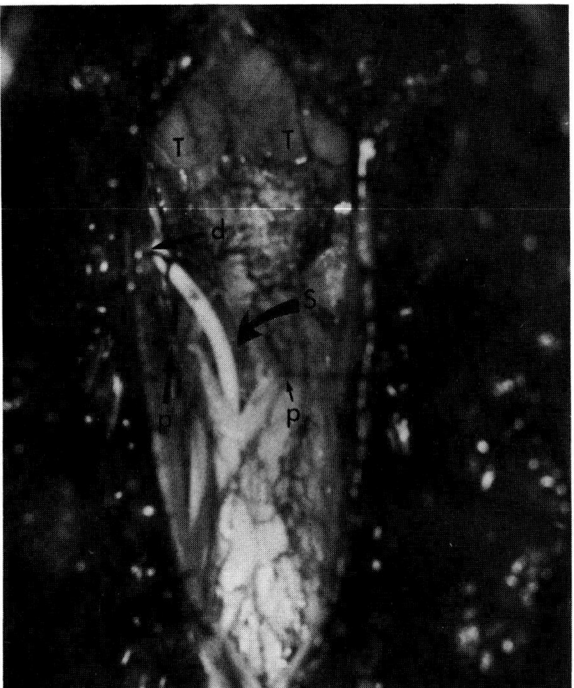

Fig. 5-7. Upper cervical cord with Arnold-Chiari malformation type I. This is the same patient as in Figures 5-2 through 6. The left dorsal column, which is about 1 mm thick, has been incised and the syrinx cavity (*s*) exposed. The distal end of the white silastic tube has been passed into the cavity. The proximal end of the tube has been sutured to the dura (*d*). Sutures have been placed in the pia (*p*) to keep the walls of the cavity open while the silastic tube is positioned. On the left (p with large arrow) the pial suture crosses a dentate ligament. The tonsils (*T*) extend below C1 which has been laminectomized, as have C2 and C3.

5-7).[29] An adequate length of tubing, usually 1 to 2 cm, is inserted into the cord cavity to prevent it from slipping out.

The results of surgical treatment are variable. About 20% of patients continue to deteriorate, especially patients presenting with a central cordlike syndrome. Most patients stabilize, but some authors have reported that up to 65% of adult patients benefit from surgery.[30] In other series, less than half the patients were helped, and no procedure was clearly superior.[17]

The outcome in children is determined by the severity of the hydrocephalus or myelomeningocele, which are usually present. The more severe these conditions, the more likely it is that the accompanying Chiari malformation is a Type II with more severe abnormalities of the nervous system. As a corollary to this, it should be noted that the younger the child when symptoms present, the more guarded is the prognosis.

The use of brain-stem auditory-evoked responses has been suggested as a means of predicting the response to surgical decompression.[14]

ACHONDROPLASIA

Neurologic manifestations of achondroplasia, especially those affecting the spine, are well known. In the adult, symptoms are caused by stenosis affecting the lower thoracic and lumbar spine. Stenosis of the lower canal is rare in the pediatric patient, however. The problem is at the opposite end of the spine, namely, a small foramen magnum.[19] Yamada *et al* have recently reported six patients with respiratory problems and quadriparesis who responded to foramen magnum decompression.[40] They point out that mortality in the first year of life is high among patients with achondroplasia, possibly because of the respiratory complications secondary to brain stem pressure, which in turn may be caused by a narrow foramen.

REFERENCES

1. *Carmel PW, Markesbery WR:* Early descriptions of the Arnold-Chiari malformation. J Neurosurg 37:543, 1972
2. *Chamberlain WE:* Basilar impression (platybasia): A bizarre developmental anomaly of the occipital bone and upper cervical spine with striking and misleading neurological manifestations. Yale J Biol Med 11:487, 1939
3. *Chiari H:* Ueber Veränderungen des Kleinhirns infolge von Hydrocephalie des Grosshirns. Deutsche Medicine Wochenschrift 17:1172, 1891
4. *Cleland J:* Contribution to the study of spina bifida, encephalocele and anencephalous. J Anat Physiol 17:257, 1883
5. *Derome P, Caron JP, Hurth M:* Indications de la voie trans-bucco-pharyngée et malformations di la charnière cranio-vertébraie. Neurochurgie 23:282, 1977
6. *Fischer EG:* Dandy-Walker syndrome: An evaluation of surgical treatment. J Neurosurg 39:615, 1973
7. *Gardner WJ:* Anatomic features common in the Arnold-Chiari and Dandy-Walker malformations suggesting a common origin. Cleve Clin Q 26:206, 1959
8. *Gardner WJ:* Hydrodynamic mechanism of syringomyelia: Its relationship to myelocele. J Neurol Neurosurg Psychiatr 28:247, 1965
9. *Gardner WJ, Abdullah AF, McCormick IJ:* The

varying expression of embryonal atresia of the fourth ventricle in adults: A-C malformation, Dandy-Walker syndrome, "arachnoid" cyst of the cerebellum, and syringomyelia. J Neurosurg 14:591, 1957

10. *Gardner WJ, Smith JL, Padget DH:* The relationship of Arnold-Chiari and Dandy-Walker malformations. J Neurosurg 36:481, 1972
11. *Hall P, Turner M, Aichinger S, Bendick P, Campbell R:* Experimental Syringomyelia: The relationship between intraventricular and intrasyrinx pressures. J Neurosurg 52:812, 1980
12. *Hamilton WJ, Mossman HW:* Human Embryology, 4th ed, pp 526–547. Baltimore, Williams & Wilkins, 1972
13. *Hoffman H, Hendrick E, Humphries E, Humphries R:* Manifestations and management of Arnold-Chiari malformations in patients with myelomeningocele. Child's Brain 1:255–59, 1975
14. *Holliday PO, Pillsbury D, Kelly DL, Dillard R:* Brain stem auditory evoked potentials in Arnold-Chiari malformation: Possible prognostic value and changes with surgical decompression. Neurosurg 16:48–53, 1985
15. *Holtzer H:* Experimental analysis of the development of the spinal column: Response of precartilage cells to size variations of the spinal cord. J Exp Zool 121:121–47, 1952
16. *Homen EA:* Zur Kenntnis der Rhachitischm-Deformationem der Schädelbasis und der basalen Schädelhyperostosen. Deutsch Zeitschrift Nirvenheilkunde 20:1–15, 1901
17. *Levy WJ, Mason L, Hahn JF:* Chiari malformation presenting in adults: A surgical experience in 127 cases. Neurosurg 12:377–90, 1983
18. *Logue V, Edwards MR:* Syringomyelia and its surgical treatment—an analysis of 75 patients. J Neurol Neurosurg Psychiatr 44:273–84, 1981
19. *Luyendÿk W, Matricale B, Thomeer R:* Basilar impression in an achondroplastic dwarf: Causative role in tetraparesis. Acta Neurochir 41:243–53, 1978
20. *McAfee P, Bohlman H, Riley L, Robinson R:* Anterior extraoral approach to the atlas and the axis. 14th Annual Meeting, Cervical Spine Research Society, Palm Beach, Dec 10, 1986
21. *McRae DL, Barnum AS:* Occipitalization of the atlas. AJR 70:23–46, 1953
22. *Menezes AH, Van Gilder JC, Graf CJ, McDonnel DE:* Craniocervical abnormalities: A comprehensive surgical approach. J Neurosurg 53:444–55, 1980
23. *Merritt HH:* A Textbook of Neurology, 3rd ed, p 424. Philadelphia, Lea & Febiger, 1964
24. *Mori K, Handa H, Okuna T, Hazama F:* Arnold-Chiari Type II malformation: A clinicopathological study with special reference to its surgical treatment. Neurochirugia 21:9–14, 1978
25. *Nishizaki T, Tamaki N, Nishida Y, Matsumoto S:* Bilateral internuclear ophthalmoplegia due to hydrocephalus: A case report. Neurosurg 17:822–25, 1985
26. *Pardis RW, Sax DS:* Familial basilar impression. Neurology 22:554–60, 1972
27. *Pasztor E, Vajda J, Piffko P, Horvath M:* Transoral surgery for basilar impression. Surg Neurol 14:473–76, 1980
28. *Peerless SJ, Durward QJ:* Management of syringomyelia: A pathophysiological approach. Clin Neurosurg 30:531–76, 1982
29. *Rhoton AL:* Microsurgery of Arnold-Chiari malformation in adults with and without hydromyelia. J Neurosurg 45:416–22, 1976
30. *Saez RJ, Onofrio BM, Yanagihara T:* Experience with Arnold-Chiari malformation. 1900–1970. J Neurosurg 45:416–22, 1976
31. *Schut L, Bruce DA:* The Arnold-Chiari malformation. Orthop Clin North Am 9:913–23, 1978
32. *Schwalbe E, Gredig M:* Ueber Eintwicklungs störungen der Kleinherns Hirrstamms und Halsmarks bei spina bifida (Arnold'sche und Chiari'sche Missbildung). Beitrage zur Patholgischen Anatomie 40:132–94, 1907
33. *Scoville WB, Sherman IJ:* Platybasia, report of 10 cases. Ann Surg 133:496–502, 1951
34. *Spillane JD, Pallis C, Jones AM:* Developmental abnormalities in the region of the foramen magnum. Brain 90:11–48, 1957
35. *Suben RL, Hamida MD, Shulman K:* Multiple cranial nerve defects associated with the Arnold-Chiari malformation. Neurology 21:673–81, 1971
36. *Taveras JM, Wood EH:* Diagnostic Neuroradiology, pp 64–66. Baltimore, Williams & Wilkins, 1964
37. *Taylor AR, Chakravorty BC:* Clinical syndromes associated with basilar impression. Arch Neurol 10:475–84, 1964
38. *Thomas JB:* Introduction to Human Embryology. Philadelphia, Lea & Febiger, 1968
39. *Truex RC, Johnson CH:* Congenital anomalies of the upper cervical spine. Orthop Clin North Am 9:891–900, 1978
40. *Yamada H, Nakamura S, Tajima M:* Neurological manifestations of pediatric achondroplasia. J Neurosurg 54:49–57, 1981

Congenital Anomalies of the Atlantoaxial Joint

ROBERT N. HENSINGER

The clinical significance of a bony anomaly in the region of the atlantoaxial joint is primarily related to its influence on the stability of this articulation. The precipitating factor may be an abnormal odontoid, atlantooccipital fusion or laxity of the transverse atlantal ligament, but the end result is narrowing of the spinal canal and impingement on the neural elements. It is important not to lose sight of this basic problem, but frequently it becomes obscured in radiologic detail, conflicting reports, and unusual clinical symptoms and signs. Atlantoaxial instability is commonly associated with other anomalies of the spine, many of which lead to scoliosis. Patients with congenital scoliosis, Down's syndrome, bone dysplasias, such as Morquio's syndrome, spondyloepiphyseal dysplasia, osteogenesis imperfecta, Larson's syndrome, and neurofibromatosis, all are capable of having significant atlantoaxial instability that may initially be unrecognized. Radiologic survey, particularly flexion–extension views of the C1–C2 articulation, should be obtained prior to a general anesthetic or preliminary spine traction in the management of their scoliosis.

PATHOMECHANICS

The articulation between C1 and C2 is the most mobile part of the vertebral column and normally has the least stability of any of the vertebral articulations. The odontoid acts as a bony buttress to prevent hyperextension, but the remainder of the normal range of motion is maintained by and solely dependent on the integrity of the surrounding ligaments and capsular structures. The articulation between the condyles of the skull and the atlas (atlantooccipital joint) normally allows only a few degrees of flexion–extension, a slight nodding motion of the head. In rotation, the atlas and head turn as a unit. The articulation between the axis and the third cervical vertebra permits some flexion–extension but is similarly restricted in rotation. Thus, the atlantoaxial joint is extremely mobile but structurally weak, and it is between two relatively fixed points, the atlantooccipital and C2–C3 joints.

Motion of the atlantoaxial articulation is usually accentuated in patients with bony anomalies of the occipitocervical junction. An excellent example is the patient with atlantooccipital fusion, who is frequently found to have compensatory hypermobility of the atlantoaxial joint. If this same patient has an associated synostosis of C2–C3, it is reasonable to expect that the additional stress on the atlantoaxial articulation may eventually lead to significant instability.[20] This assumption has clinical support, in that 60% of patients with symptomatic atlantooccipital fusion have an associated fusion of C2–C3.[14]

SYMPTOMS AND SIGNS

The symptomatic patient often presents with a puzzling clinical picture. Only a few patients present initially with a history of head or neck trauma, neck pain, torticollis, quadriparesis, or signs of high spinal cord compression. A changing intermittent pattern of symptoms is more typical than the localized pattern suggested by the roentgenograms alone.

In patients with basilar impression or atlantooccipital fusion, the clinical findings suggest that the major neurologic damage is occurring anteriorly from the odontoid. The symptoms and signs of pyramidal tract irritation, muscle weakness and wasting, ataxia, spasticity, hyperreflexia, and pathologic reflexes are common.[14] If the primary area of impingement is posterior from the rim of the foramen magnum, dural band, or the posterior ring of the atlas (typical of odontoid anomalies), there will be symptoms referable to the posterior columns with alteration of sensation for deep pressure, vibration, and proprioception. If, in addition, there is an associated cerebellar herniation, nystagmus, ataxia, and incoordination can be observed. Symptoms referable to vertebral artery compression—dizziness, seizures, mental deterioration, and syncope—may occur alone or in combination with those of spinal cord compression.[9]

RADIOLOGIC APPEARANCE OF CONGENITAL C1–C2 INSTABILITY

The atlas–dens interval (ADI) is the space seen on the lateral roentgenogram between the anterior aspect of the dens and the posterior aspect of the anterior ring of the atlas (Fig. 5-8). In children the ADI should be no greater than 4.0 mm,[11] particularly in flexion where the greatest distance can be noted. The upper limit of normal in adults is

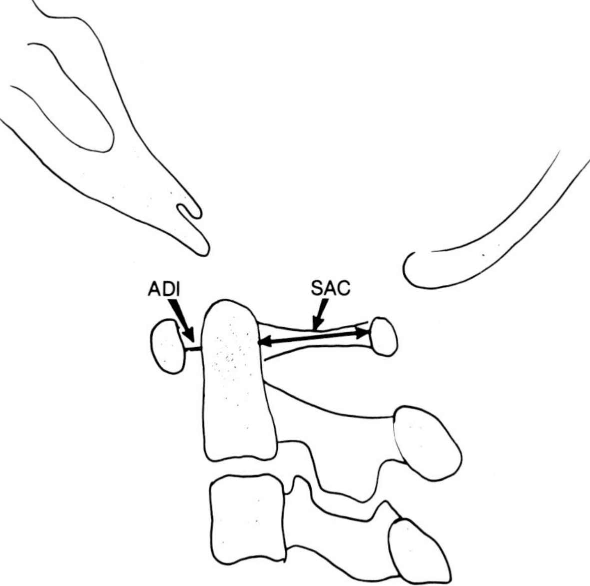

Fig. 5-8. Illustration of the atlantoaxial joint demonstrating the normal atlas–dens interval (ADI) and the normal space available for the spinal cord (SAC), the distance between the posterior aspect of the odontoid or axis, and the nearest posterior structure, usually the posterior ring of the atlas.

less than 3 mm.[10] A subtle increase in the ADI in the neutral position may indicate disruption of the transverse atlantal ligament. This is a valuable aid in the evaluation of acute injury, in which standard flexion–extension views would be potentially hazardous.[11] Fielding noted that the shift of C1–C2 does not exceed 3 mm in the adult if the transverse ligament is intact and that this ligament ruptures within the range of 5 mm.[3] The ADI is of limited value in evaluating chronic atlantoaxial instability due to congenital anomalies, rheumatoid arthritis, or Down's syndrome. In these conditions the odontoid is frequently found to be hypermobile with a widened ADI, particularly in flexion (Fig. 5-9); yet not all are symptomatic, nor do they require surgical stabilization. In this situation (Fig. 5-10), attention should be directed to the amount of space available for the spinal cord (SAC). This is accomplished by measuring the distance from the posterior aspect of the odontoid or axis to the nearest posterior structure (foramen magnum or posterior ring of the atlas). This measurement is particularly helpful when evaluating a patient with nonunion of the odontoid or os odontoideum (Fig. 5-11), as in both conditions the ADI may be normal. In flexion or extension, however, the space available for the spinal cord may be considerably reduced (Fig. 5-12).

Lateral flexion–extension stress views should be conducted voluntarily by the patient, particularly by those with neurologic deficit (Fig. 5-12). Patients with an intact or normal odontoid process are especially at risk; with anterior shift of the atlas over the axis, the spinal cord is more easily damaged by direct impingement against the odontoid process, such as in patients with atlantooccipital fusion.

In patients with multiple anomalies, abnormal bone, or dysplastic bone, adequate visualization can be obtained by using lateral tomography techniques (Fig. 5-13*B*, and *C*). Extension views should not be ignored. Many patients have been found to have significant posterior subluxation.[5,8]

Obtaining a satisfactory radiograph may be hampered by the patient's limited ability to cooperate, by fixed bony deformity, and by overlapping shadows from the mandible, occiput, and foramen magnum. A helpful guide is that the atlas moves with the occiput, and if the x-ray beam is directed 90 degrees to the lateral of the skull, a satisfactory view of the occipitocervical junction usually results. Visualization may be enhanced further with flexion–extension or tomographic views (Fig. 5-13*A*, *B*, and *C*). Carefully supervised motion studies often are necessary to establish cervical spine instability. Computed tomograms, especially those providing coronal and sagittal reconstructions, are helpful in evaluating the occipitocervical junction (Chapter 3). Careful clinical correlation is necessary, because the cross-sectional bony anatomy is not only as confusing as the sagittal anatomy but is also less familiar. Magnetic resonance imaging (MRI) may provide further information regarding the relationship of the brain stem and spinal cord to the surrounding structures (Chapter 3).

McRae[14] was the first to call attention to the relationship of neurologic symptoms and the sagittal diameter of the spinal canal (SAC). He noted that in his patients with atlantooccipital fusion, those with less than 19 mm of available space behind the odontoid or atlas were always symptomatic. However, with the availability of more clinical data, this measurement has been defined more specifically. It generally is agreed that a reduction of the lumen of the spinal canal to 13 mm or less may be associated with neurologic problems.[17] Spinal cord impingement can be either posterior from the ring of C1 or anterior from the body of C2. However, even those with an absent ring of C1 are in jeopardy, because the spinal cord can be stretched over the body of C2 in flexion or in-

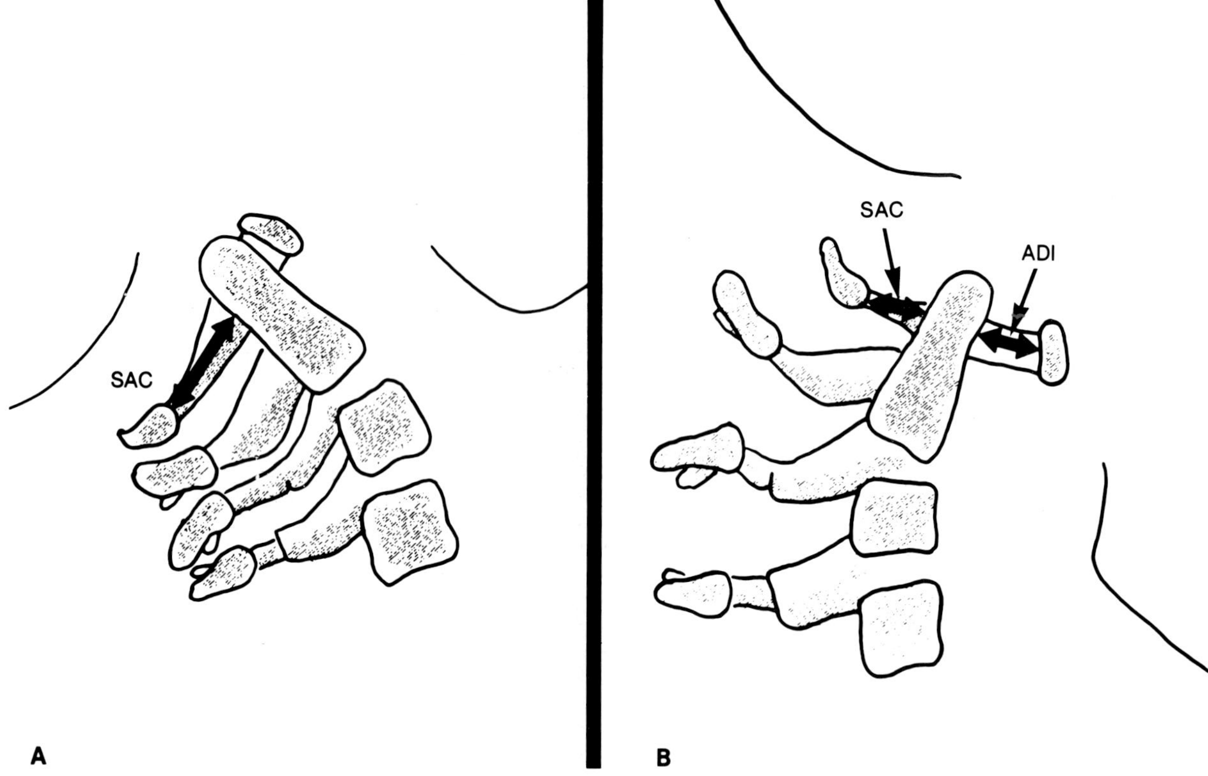

Fig. 5-9. Atlantoaxial instability with intact odontoid. (*A*) Extension. The ADI and SAC return to normal as the intact odontoid provides a bony block to subluxation in hyperextension. (*B*) Flexion. Forward sliding of the atlas with an increased ADI and decreased SAC.

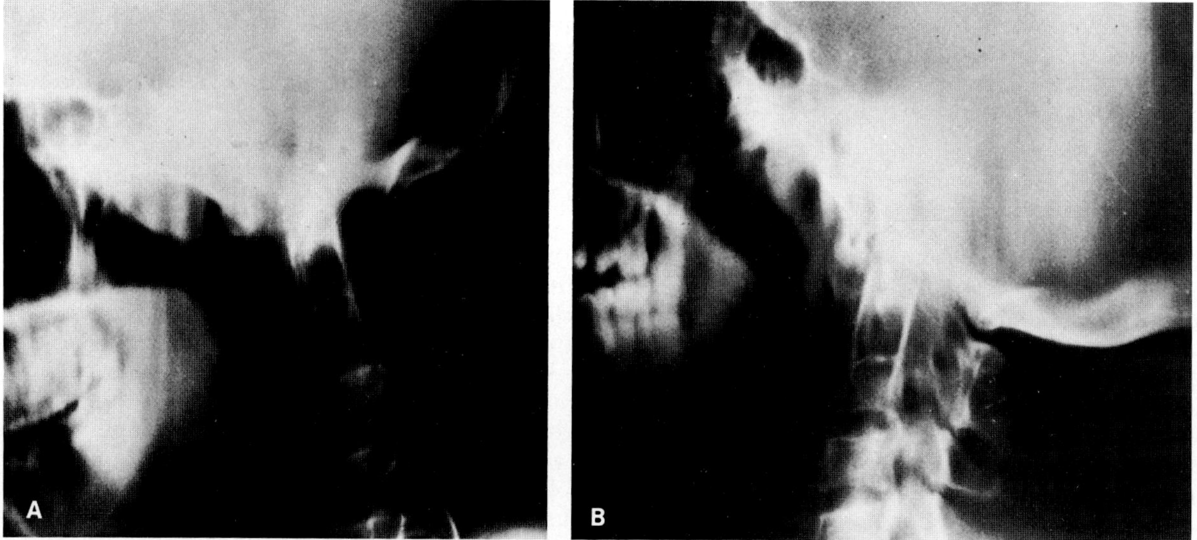

Fig. 5-10. Twenty-two-year-old patient with symptomatic atlantooccipital fusion and hypermobile odontoid. Lateral laminagraphic views in (*A*) flexion and (*B*) extension. The odontoid extends into the opening of the foramen magnum (McRae's line) and, with flexion, the odontoid moves posteriorly with impingement of the brain stem. Note the congenital C2–C3 fusion. (McRae DL: Am J Roentgenol 84:3–25, 1960)

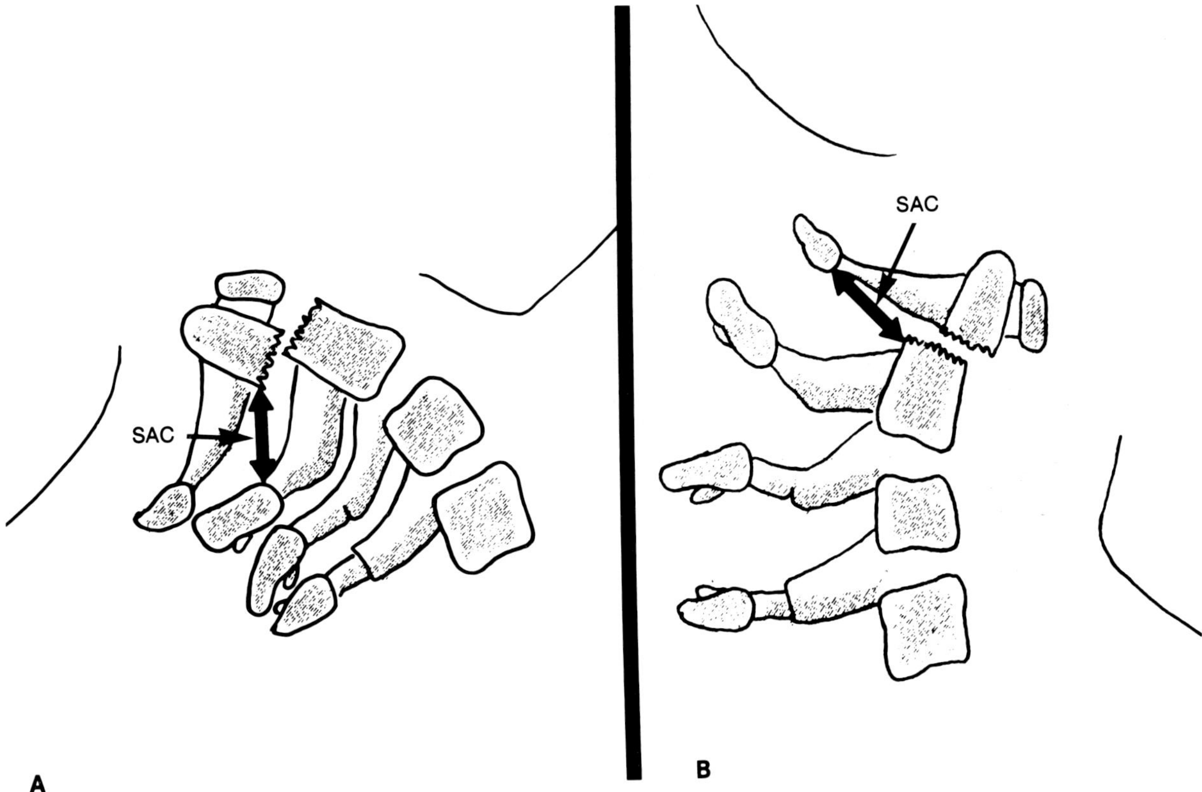

Fig. 5-11. Atlantoaxial instability with os odontoideum, absent odontoid, or traumatic nonunion. (*A*) Extension. Posterior subluxation with reduction in SAC and no change in the ADI. (*B*) Flexion. Forward sliding of the atlas with reduction of the SAC, but no change in ADI.

dented posteriorly by a fibrous band that has replaced the arch of C1. Similarly, variation in patient size and the presence or absence of soft-tissue elements affect the clinical significance of the measurement.

Steel[19] has called attention to the checkrein effect of the alar ligaments and to how they form the second line of defense after disruption of the transverse atlantal ligament (Fig. 5-14). This secondary stability plays an important role in patients with chronic atlantoaxial instability.[4] Steel's anatomic studies provide a simple rule that is helpful to physicians evaluating this area. He defined the "rule of thirds," by which the area of the vertebral canal at the first cervical vertebra can be divided into one third spinal cord, one third odontoid, and one third "space." The one third space represents a safe zone in which displacement can occur without neurologic impingement and is roughly equivalent to the transverse diameter of the odontoid (usually 1 cm).[3] In chronic atlantoaxial instability, it is of prime importance to recognize when the patient has exceeded the safe zone defined by Steel and enters the area of impending spinal cord compression. At this point the second line of defense, the alar ligaments, has failed and there is no longer a margin of safety (Fig. 5-14). In experiments, Fielding and colleagues found that after rupture of the transverse ligament, the alar ligaments are usually inadequate to prevent further displacement of C1–C2, when a force similar to that which ruptured the transverse ligament is applied.[3]

Myelographic evaluation can be of great help in defining an area of constriction. Myelography has demonstrated in some patients a ventral impingement due to a thick wad of radiolucent soft tissue posterior to the dysplastic odontoid and the body of the axis.[15] Gas or a water-soluble contrast agent (metrizamide) should be used in preference to oil contrast media.[7,12,14–16] Computerized tomography (CT) in conjunction with metrizamide myelography is particularly helpful in evaluating chil-

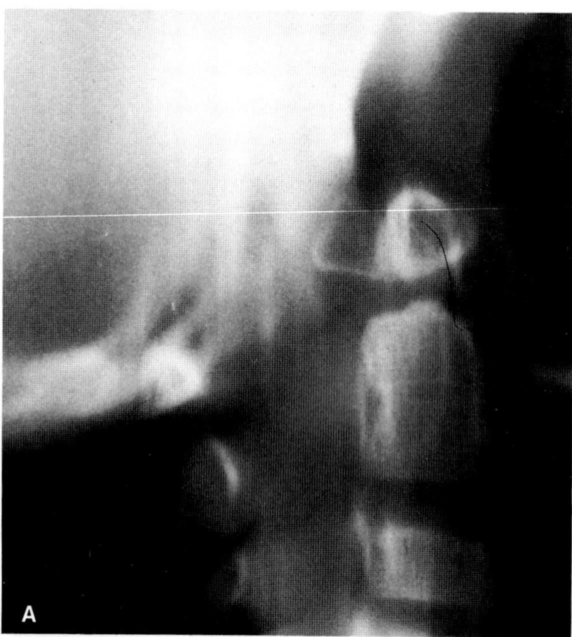

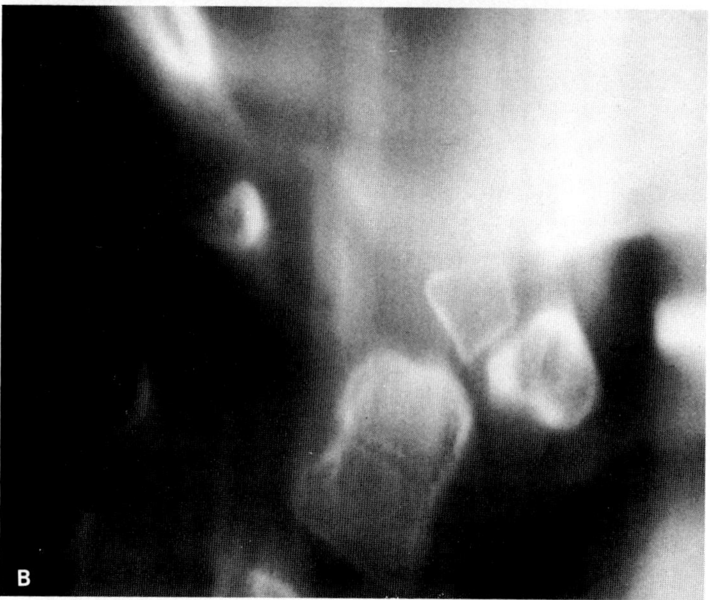

Fig. 5-12. Lateral flexion–extension roentgenograph of an os odontoideum. (*A*) Extension and (*B*) flexion. The odontoid ossicle is fixed to the anterior ring of the atlas and moves with it in flexion and extension and lateral slide. The SAC decreases with flexion and the ossicle moves into the spinal canal with extension (Fielding JW, Hensinger RN, Hawkins RJ: J Bone Joint Surg 62A:376–383, 1980)

dren with rotational deformities or compromise of the neural canal in the upper cervical spine.[7,16] Similarly, MRI is a noninvasive method of evaluating this region and enjoys an increasing application. These advances will allow a more complete and accurate examination of the brain stem, an area of considerable importance in the patient with occipitocervical anomalies.[7,16] Vertebral arteriography is helpful in evaluating patients who exhibit symptoms of transient brain stem ischemia.

CONGENITAL LAXITY OF THE TRANSVERSE ATLANTAL LIGAMENT

This is a diagnosis of exclusion suggested by the clinical occurrence of chronic atlantoaxial dislocation without a predisposing cause.[9] There is no history of trauma, congenital anomaly, infection, or systemic disorders such as rheumatoid arthritis to account for the radiologic finding. The majority of discovered patients (excluding those with

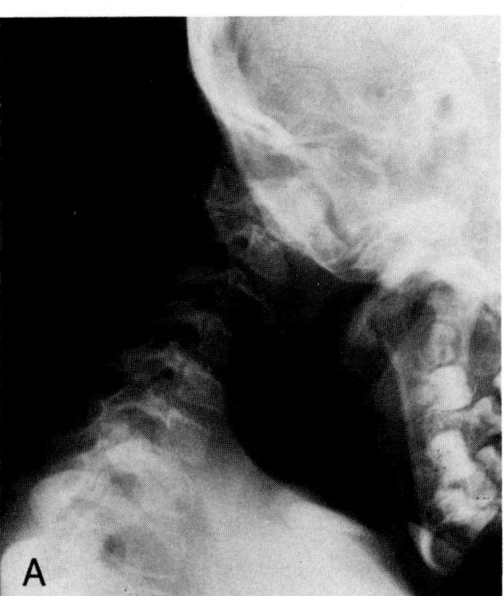

Fig. 5-13. Seven-year-old with torticollis due to a fixed bony deformity. (*A*) The overlapping shadows from the mandible, occiput, and foramen magnum prevent satisfactory radiographic study of the occipitocervical junction. (*B*) A helpful guide is that the atlas moves with the occiput, and if the x-ray beam is directed 90 degrees to the lateral of the skull, a satisfactory view usually results. (*C*) Same patient with a properly focused x-ray study, flexion–extension tomographic views, demonstrating an os odontoideum, anterior subluxation of C1 on C2 and a severely compromised SAC space available for the spinal cord.

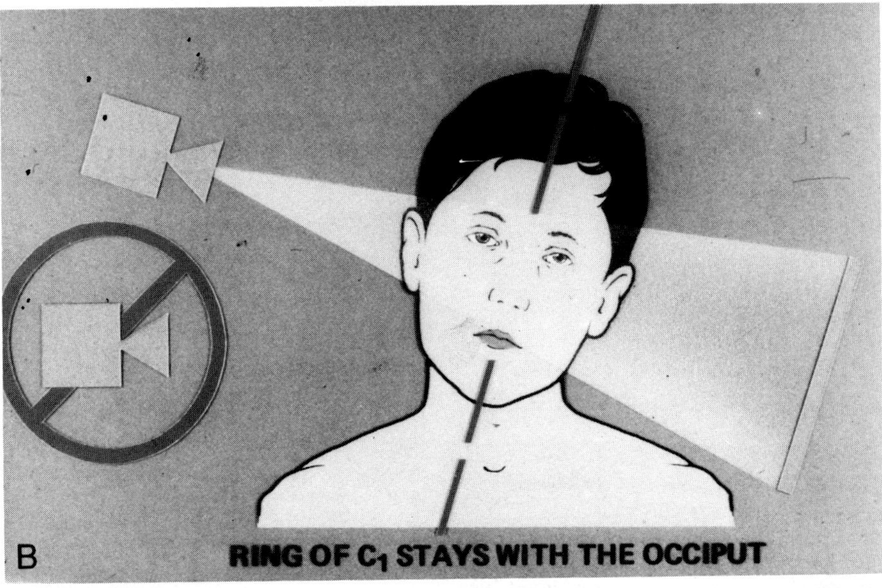

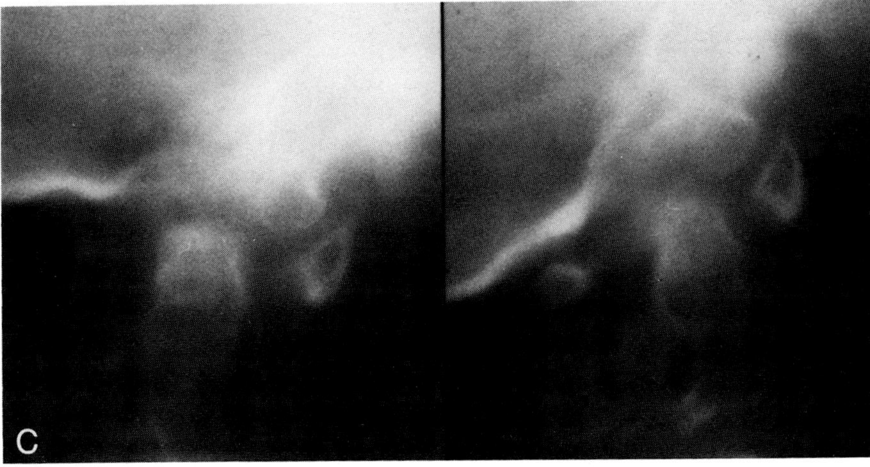

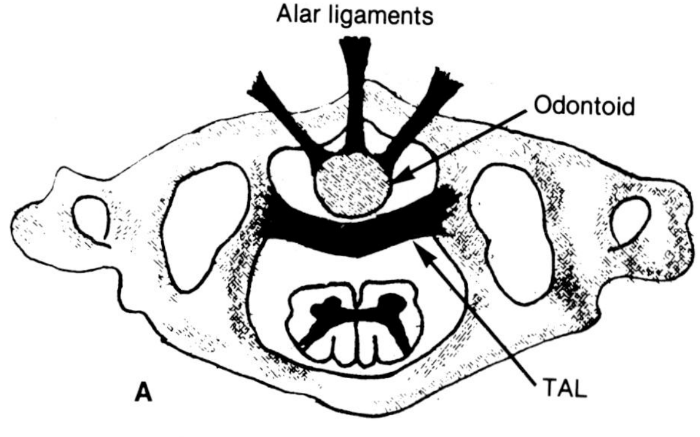

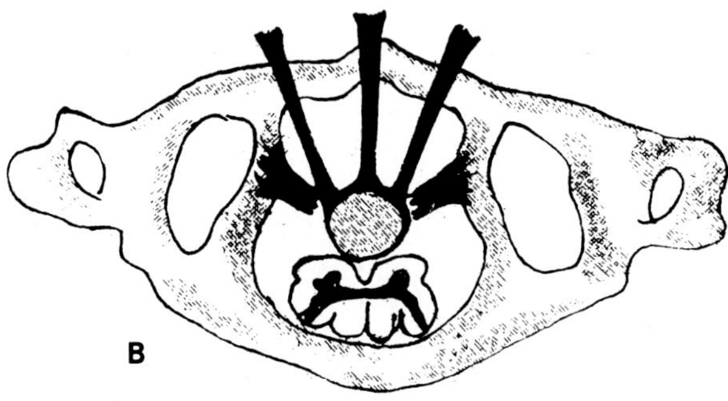

Fig. 5-14. Atlantoaxial joint as viewed from above. (*A*) Normal. (*B*) Disruption of transverse atlantal ligament (TAL); odontoid now occupies the "safe zone of Steel." The intact alar ligaments (second line of defense) prevent spinal cord compression.

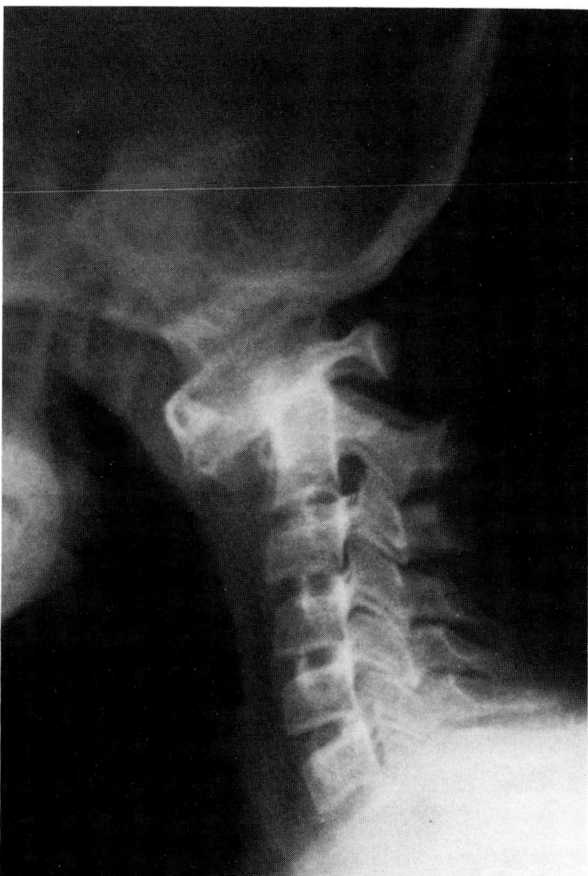

Fig. 5-15. Eleven-year-old with Down's syndrome and severe atlantoaxial instability. The patient's gait was clumsy, and physical examination revealed poor coordination of the extremities. There was no other evidence of motor-sensory impairment or pathologic reflexes. The patient had no symptoms referable to the cervical spine 2 years following surgical stabilization.

Down's syndrome) have the typical symptoms of atlantoaxial instability and require surgical stabilization.

Laxity of the transverse atlantal ligament is unusually common in patients with Down's syndrome, with a reported incidence of 20% (Fig. 5-15).[13,18] The lesion may be found in all age groups, without a preponderance at any age. Thus, the C1–C2 articulation should be evaluated in all patients with Down's syndrome prior to a general anesthetic or to participation in activities that may lead to head and neck trauma. It appears that these patients have rupture or attenuation of the transverse atlantal ligament with encroachment of the "safe zone of Steel" but are initially protected by checkrein action of the alar ligaments from spinal cord compression. In other words, many have excessive motion, but few are symptomatic, and the majority are discovered only by radiologic survey.[1,2,13] With our present knowledge, prophylactic stabilization does not seem to be indicated, but more clinical information is required.

There is general agreement that if an episode of neurologic symptoms or motion of 1 cm or greater has occurred, the patient should be stabilized by fusion of the C1–C2 articulation.[3,4] Children who are found to be unstable should be restricted from activities that might cause trauma to the head and neck.[6] Interestingly, a recent longitudinal follow-up study of Down's patients demonstrated a progressive instability in some children, rather than an acute event. In addition, several patients who were unstable became stable.[6]

REFERENCES

1. *Curtis, BH, Blank S, Fisher RL:* Atlanto-axial dislocation in Down's syndrome. JAMA 205:464–465, 1968

2. *Dzenitis, AJ:* Spontaneous atlanto-axial dislocation in mongoloid child with spinal cord compression: case report. J Neurosurg 25:458–460, 1966

3. *Fielding JW, Cochran GV, Lawsing JF III, Hohl M:* Tears of the transverse ligament of the atlas. J Bone Joint Surg 56A:1683–1691, 1974

4. *Fielding JW, Hawkins RJ, Ratzan SA:* Spine fusion for atlanto-axial instability. J Bone Joint Surg 58A:400–407, 1976

5. *Fielding JW, Hensinger RN, Hawkins RJ:* Os odontoideum. J Bone Joint Surg 62A:376–383, 1980

6. *French HG, Burke SW, Whitecloud TS, Edmunds JO:* Chronic atlanto-axial instability in Down's syndrome. Orthop Trans 9:135, 1985

7. *Geehr RB, Rothman SLG, Kier EL:* The role of computed tomography in the evaluation of upper cervical spine pathology. Comput Tomogr 2:79–97, 1978

8. *Giannestra NJ, Mayfield FH, Provencio FP, Maurer J:* Congenital absence of the odontoid process: a case report. J Bone Joint Surg 46A:839–843, 1964

9. *Greenberg AD:* Atlanto-axial dislocations. Brain, 91:655–684, 1968

10. *Hinck VC, Hopkins CE, Savara BS:* Sagittal diameter of the cervical spinal canal in children. Radiology 79:97–108, 1962

11. *Locke GR, Gardner JI, Van Epps EF:* Atlas-dens interval (ADI) in children; a survey based on 200 normal cervical spines. AJR 97:135–140, 1966

12. *Lowman RM, Finkelstein A:* Air myelography for demonstration of the cervical spinal cord. Radiology 39:700–706, 1942

13. *Martel W, Tishler JM:* Observations on the spine in mongoloidism. AJR 97:630–638, 1966

14. *McRae DL:* Bony abnormalities in the region of the foramen magnum: correlation of the anatomic and neurologic findings. Acta Radiol 40:335–354, 1953

15. *Perovic MN, Kopits SE, Thompson RC:* Radiologic evaluation of the spinal cord in congenital atlanto-axial dislocations. Radiology 109:713–716, 1973

16. *Resjo M, Harwood-Nash DC, Fitz CR:* Normal cord in infants and children examined with computed tomographic metrizamide myelography. Radiology 130:691–696, 1979

17. *Spierlings ELH, Braakman R:* Os odontoideum: analysis of 37 cases. J Bone Joint Surg 64B:422–428, 1982

18. *Spitzer R, Rabinowitch JY, Wybar KC:* A study of the abnormalities of the skull, teeth and lenses in mongolism. Can Med Assoc J 84:567–572, 1961

19. *Steel HH:* Anatomical and mechanical considerations of the atlanto-axial articulations. J Bone Joint Surg 50A:1481–1482, 1968

20. *von Torklus D, Gehle W:* The Upper Cervical Spine. New York, Grune & Stratton, 1972

Anomalies of the Atlas

ROBERT N. HENSINGER

ATLANTOOCCIPITAL FUSION (OCCIPITALIZATION; ASSIMILATION OF THE ATLAS)

This condition is characterized by partial or complete congenital fusion of the bony ring of the atlas to the base of the occiput. Atlantooccipital fusion is the most commonly recognized anomaly of the craniovertebral junction[16] and, as a consequence, has been the subject of numerous reports in the literature, including autopsy findings and detailed clinicopathologic correlations. These studies share some common findings and provide adequate information with which to plan a treatment program.

Clinical Findings

Spillane and coworkers[14] noted that none of their patients with atlantooccipital fusion had a normal appearing neck, which is in contradistinction to other bony anomalies of the craniovertebral junction. This finding is remarkably consistent,[1,8,14] and the patients are commonly found to have low hairline, torticollis, short neck, and restricted neck movements, not unlike the Klippel-Feil syndrome. Of these patients, 20% have associated congenital abnormalities including anomalies of the jaw, incomplete cleft of the nasal cartilage, cleft palate, congenital deformities of the external ear, cervical ribs, hypospadius, and anomalies of the urinary tract.[1,8,14]

Symptoms are characteristic of the conditions that lead to chronic atlantoaxial instability and may have wide variation, depending on the area of spinal cord impingement. McRae and Barnum[8] is supported by other authors[1,4,17] in his impression that the most significant finding in the symptomatic patient with atlantooccipital fusion is an odontoid process of abnormal size, position, or mobility. In this regard, he has suggested a simple rule: If the dens lies below the foramen magnum (McRae's line), the patient will probably be asymptomatic. If the dens lies in the foramen magnum or is angled posteriorly, there is likely to be crowding of the anterior neurologic elements, particularly in the region of the medulla oblongata. The clinical findings support McRae's observation that the major damage is occurring anteriorly from the odontoid, as symptoms and signs of pyramidal tract irritation, muscle weakness and wasting, ataxia, spasticity, hyperreflexia, and pathologic reflexes are commonly found in atlantooccipital fusion.[1,8] Autopsy findings consistently demonstrate that the brain stem is indented by the abnormal odontoid.[1,10] Other less common complaints include diplopia, tinnitus, earaches, dysphagia, and poor phonation, all of which are believed to be due to cranial nerve or bulbar irritation anteriorly.

Compression posteriorly by the posterior lip of the foramen magnum or a dural band is less common and results in symptoms and signs referable to the posterior columns. Thus, loss of deep pain sensation, light touch, proprioception, or vibration are less common complaints. As in basilar impression, nystagmus is a prominent finding and generally indicates herniation of the cerebellar tonsils. Headache is a frequent complaint, its pain being characterized as dull, never shooting, and it is located over the posterior two thirds of the cranium (greater occipital nerve), sometimes initiated by coughing or neck movements. Tenderness of the scalp in the same distribution may be noted.

The onset of symptoms is usually in the third or fourth decade. Symptoms usually begin insidiously and progress slowly, but sudden onset or instant death has been reported.[6] Trauma has been implicated as a precipitating factor in about one half of the patients but is usually not severe, nor does it often result in immediate onset of symptoms.[1,8,17] Local swelling from infection of the pharynx or nasopharynx has initiated symptoms.[1] Occasionally, patients present with a sudden onset of symptoms without any precipitating cause and may be wrongly suspected of having multiple sclerosis or amyotrophic lateral sclerosis.

Several explanations have been advanced to account for late onset of symptoms. Gradual laxity of the ligaments about the odontoid may occur from repeated flexion and extension of the neck, particularly if the vertebral segments below are fixed (*i.e.*, synostosis C2–C3), requiring compensatory motion of the atlantoaxial joint.[1,4,8,17] With aging, the central nervous system itself may become less tolerant of repeated blows from the odontoid, as a hearing deficit results from repeated noise injury. Symptoms are more likely due to intermittent narrowing of the spinal canal rather than to static situations to which the central nervous system has adapted.[14] Bony spurs secondary to degenerative arthritis or swelling from infection of the nasopharynx may compromise a marginally adequate space. Finally, arteriosclerotic changes in the vertebral arteries may render these vessels more susceptible to transient compression with diminished blood supply to the brain stem.

Roentgenographic Findings

Standard roentgenographic views of the craniovertebral junction can be difficult to interpret, and the condition may range from total incorporation of the atlas into the occipital bone to a bony or even fibrous band uniting one small portion of the atlas to the occiput. Rarely, complete fusion of the occiput, atlas, and odontoid has been reported.[5] Laminagrams are often necessary to demonstrate bony continuity of the anterior arch of the atlas with the occiput. Posterior fusion is not usually evident, as this portion of the ring may only be represented by a short bony fringe on the edge of the foramen magnum. Despite its innocuous radiologic appearance, this fringe is frequently directed downward and inward and can compromise the spinal canal posteriorly, and it has been found to groove the spinal cord. It is usually assumed that the assimilated atlas is fused symmetrically to the occipital opening, but several autopsy specimens have demonstrated a posterior positioning of the atlas.[8] In effect, this pushes the odontoid posteriorly, further narrowing the spinal canal and the space available for the spinal cord. CT and/or myelography[7,12] may be necessary to further delineate the degree or site of impingement.

In the young child, radiologic interpretation may be difficult, as a significant portion of the ring of C1 is unossified at birth. Ossification of the atlas begins in the paired lateral masses and progresses posteriorly into the cartilaginous neural arches. At birth there is a 5- to 9-mm radiolucent gap in the posterior neural arch. This gap is usually ossified by 4 years of age.[16] At birth, the anterior arch of the atlas is not yet ossified in 80% of children.[15] Ossification of this area is variable but usually develops from a single midline center that appears during the first year and gradually extends to the facets (lateral masses) by the third year. Ossification of the atlas is usually completed between 7 and 10 years of age.[16]

Approximately half of the patients have "relative" basilar impression due to the diminished vertical height of the ring of the atlas. This brings the tip of the odontoid closer to the opening of the foramen magnum and the medulla oblongata (Fig. 5-16). McRae[8] suggested that the position of the dens is the key to the development of neurologic problems. If the odontoid projects into the opening of the foramen magnum, the patient will probably be symptomatic, and if below, asymptomatic.

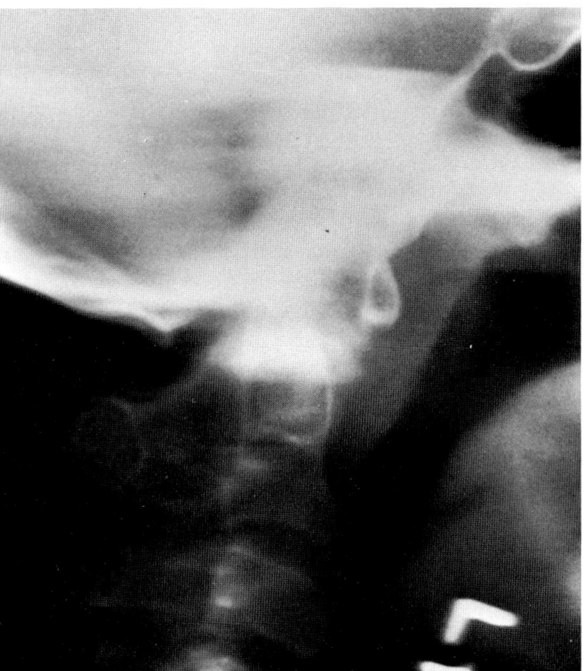

Fig. 5-16. Twenty-three-year-old male with Klippel-Feil syndrome, ataxic gait, hyperreflexia, and a history of several episodes of unconsciousness. Lateral laminographic view of the cervical spine and base of the skull demonstrates a C2–C3 fusion and fusion of the ring of C1 to the opening of the foramen magnum (occipitalization). The increased ADI suggests that the transverse atlantal ligament has failed. Patients with this pattern of fusion are at great risk. With aging, the odontoid may become hypermobile and the space available for the spinal cord posteriorly may be compromised.

The odontoid itself often has an abnormal shape and direction, frequently longer, and its angle with the base of the axis is directed more posteriorly.[8,17] McRae[8] noted that in 60% of patients with atlantooccipital fusion, the odontoid was displaced behind the anterior arch of the atlas greater than 3 mm and occasionally as much as 12 mm (see Fig. 5-16). Equally important is the width of the spinal canal between the odontoid and the posterior lip of the foramen magnum. McRae,[8,9] noted that a neurologic deficit is usually present if this distance was less than 19 mm. This measurement should be done with the neck in flexion, as this is where maximum narrowing occurs due to an abnormal dens (see Fig. 5-10).

The superior facets of the atlas are generally absorbed in the fusion, and the inferior facets, although present, are often asymmetrical. The transverse processes are usually abnormal, either missing or fused with the occiput, and the foramen for the vertebral artery may be absent.

McRae[9] was first to note the frequent occurrence of congenital fusion of C2–C3 (70%) in patients with atlantooccipital fusion. This suggests that greater demands are placed on the atlantoaxial articulation, particularly in flexion and extension when the joints above and below are fused.[1,8] Von Torklus notes that approximately 50% of patients develop the late onset of atlantoaxial instability and the resultant potential for compromise of the spinal cord.[16]

Another commonly associated abnormality is a constricting band of dura posteriorly. This has been found to groove the spinal cord and may be the primary symptom cause. The band cannot be visualized on routine roentgenograms, nor does it correlate with the presence or absence of the posterior bony fringe of the atlas. Consequently, metrizamide myelography should be an integral part of the evaluation. Alone, or in conjunction with CT (Chapter 3), this can provide excellent visualization of the lumen of the spinal canal and its contents.[7,12] A properly performed study yields valuable information regarding the presence or a dural band, cerebellar tonsillar herniation, and the size, shape, and position of the spinal cord in the spinal canal. Spillane and colleagues[14] have demonstrated that a block of the myelographic material at the foramen magnum frequently indicates cerebellar herniation. Vertebral angiography has been helpful with the demonstration of the posterior inferior cerebellar arteries looped down into the cervical canal.

Treatment

Some patients respond to nonoperative measures. Immobilization in plaster, traction, and cervical collars have been reported as helpful in management, particularly in patients who become symptomatic following minor trauma or infection.[1,11,17] An adequate trial of conservative measures is preferred, as surgical intervention represents a serious risk of morbidity and mortality to the patient.

A predominance of anterior symptoms usually stems from hypermobility of the odontoid (see Fig. 5-10) and can be controlled by posterior spine fusion, occiput to C2. Success of this procedure can be predicted if, during preliminary traction, the odontoid can be reduced and the patient's symptoms remit. Operative reduction should be avoided, as this has frequently resulted in death.[13,17] No satisfactory solution for the irreducible odontoid has been determined.

If the majority of symptoms originate from posterior spinal cord compression, then suboccipital craniectomy, excision of the posterior arch of the atlas, and removal of the dural band, if present, are suggested. Several patients have had full recovery following posterior decompression. However, many have remained unchanged, and a few have died during or shortly after this procedure.[1,11,17]

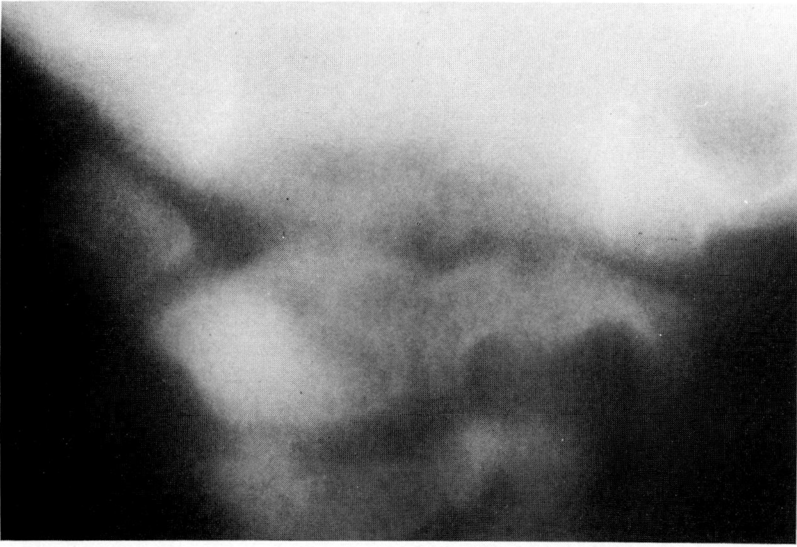

Fig. 5-17. Hemiatlas. Congenital absence of one facet of the first cervical vertebra. Clinically, the child presents with a severe and progressive torticollis. When the child is young, the neck is flexible and the torticollis can be passively corrected. However, with aging the deformity may become fixed.

Absent Facet of the Atlas

Recently Dubousset[2] described the hemiatlas, a congenital failure of formation of one facet of the first cervical vertebra (Fig. 5-17). Clinically, this can present as a severe and progressive torticollis. Interestingly, when the child is young and the neck is flexible, the torticollis can be passively corrected. However, in some aging patients, the deformity becomes increasingly severe and fixed. Roentgenographically, anteroposterior tomograms and CT scans are often necessary to document the anomaly. This can occur as an isolated anomaly, but more often is associated with other anomalies of the cervical. spine, including atlantooccipital fusion, anomalies of the odontoid, and the Klippel-Feil syndrome. To date, none have demonstrated atlantoaxial instability. Interestingly, four of the five patients who underwent arteriographic studies demonstrated an anomalous vasculature in the region on the side of the aplasia, which was frequently accompanied by neurologic problems such as the Arnold-Chiari malformation.

For those in whom the deformity is mild, or in those in whom the lower cervical deformities compensate the upper one, no treatment is necessary. In the more severely involved children, early stabilization should be considered while the upper cervical spine is still flexible, before the deformity becomes fixed. Dubousset found that if the torticollis could be corrected passively or preoperatively by a halo cast, a good result could be obtained by fusion of the occiput to the second or third cervical vertebrae.[2]

REFERENCES

1. *BHARUCHA EP, DASTUR HM:* Craniovertebral anomalies (a report of 40 cases). Brain 87:469–480, 1964
2. *DUBOUSSET J:* Torticollis in children caused by congenital anomalies of the atlas. J Bone Joint Surg 68A:178–188, 1986
3. *GRANTHAM SA, DICK HM, THOMPSON RC JR, STINCHFIELD FE:* Occipito-cervical arthrodesis: indications, technic and results. Clin Orthop 65:118–129, 1969
4. *GREENBERG AD:* Atlanto-axial dislocations. Brain 91:655–684, 1968
5. *GUENTHER SF:* Congenital anomaly of the cervical spine; fusion of the occiput, atlas and odontoid process. A case report. J Bone Joint Surg 62A:1377–1378, 1980
6. *HADLEY LA:* The Spine. Springfield, IL, Charles C Thomas, 1956
7. *GEEHR RB, ROTHMAN LG, KIER EL:* The role of computed tomography in the evaluation of the upper cervical spine pathology. Comput Tomogr 2:79–97, 1977
8. *MCRAE DL, BARNUM AS:* Occipitalization of the atlas. AJR 70:23–46, 1953
9. *MCRAE DL:* Bony abnormalities in the region of the foramen magnum: correlation of the anatomic and neurologic findings. Acta Radiol 40:335–354, 1953
10. *MCRAE DL:* The significance of abnormalities of the cervical spine. AJR 84:3–25, 1960
11. *NICHOLSON JT, SHERK HH:* Anomalies of the occipito-cervical articulation. J Bone Joint Surg 50A:295–304, 1968
12. *RESJO J, HARWOOD-NAS CD, FITZ CR, CHUANG S:* Normal cord in infants and children examined with computed tomographic metrizamide myelography. Radiology 130:691–696, 1979
13. *SINH G, PANDYA SK:* Treatment of congenital atlanto-axial dislocations. Proc Aust Assoc Neurol 5:507–514, 1968
14. *SPILLANE JD, PALLIS C, JONES AM:* Developmental abnormalities in the region of the foramen magnum. Brain 80:11–48, 1957
15. *TOMPSETT AC, DONALDSEN SW:* The anterior tubercle of the first cervical vertebra and the hyoid bone. Their occurrence in newborn infants. AJR 65:582, 1951
16. *VON TORKLUS D, GEHLE W:* The Upper Cervical Spine. New York, Grune & Stratton, 1972
17. *WADIA NH:* Myelopathy complicating congenital atlanto-axial dislocation. Brain 90:449–472, 1967

Congenital Anomalies of the Odontoid (Congenital Agenesis, Hypoplasia, and Os Odontoideum)

ROBERT N. HENSINGER

Congenital anomalies of the odontoid are uncommon[34] and are usually discovered in patients roentgenographically examined following trauma to the neck. This trauma may initiate atlantoaxial instability or precipitate symptoms in an already compromised, previously asymptomatic atlantoaxial joint.[22] Knowledge of these deformities is important, as they have great potential for neurologic sequelae, even death, from spinal cord pressure due to the abnormal atlantoaxial shift.

Three variations of odontoid anomalies have been described: aplasia (complete absence) (Fig. 5-18*A*), hypoplasia (partial absence), and the most common, os odontoideum[20,24,37,43,54] (Figs. 5-11, 5-18*B*). Aplasia is an extremely rare anomaly and is associated with complete absence of the base of the odontoid. Hypoplasia presents as a short stubby peg of odontoid projecting just above the C1–C2 facet articulation. The most common, os odontoideum, is a radiolucent oval or round ossicle with a smooth dense border of bone, separate from the axis and suggesting a congenital nonunion. The ossicle may be of variable size, located usually in the position of the normal odontoid tip (orthotopic) or near the basal occiput in the area of the foramen magnum, where it may fuse with the clivus (dystopic).[50] Separating aplasia or hypoplasia from os odontoideum is of limited importance, as they all usually lead to atlantoaxial instability, and their clinical signs, symptoms, and treatment are identical. The only distinctive features are radiographic.

The frequency of odontoid anomalies is unknown. As with many conditions that may be asymptomatic, it is probably more common than is appreciated. The majority are discovered following trauma to the head or neck, or after the spontaneous onset of symptoms sufficient to require radiologic investigation.[15] Rarely, the lesion is found as an incidental finding. Aplasia is extremely rare, and many previous reports have confused aplasia for hypoplasia. Aplasia probably has been a misnomer, since it almost never describes an associated absence of the portion of the odontoid below the articular facets of C2, which contributes to the body of the axis. Hypoplasia and os odontoideum are infrequently reported and can be considered rare.[20,24,37,43,54] With increased awareness, however, these lesions are being recognized more commonly. In a large series reported by Wollin, the average age of diagnosis was 30 years,[55] but in a series by Fielding it was 18.9 years, suggesting earlier recognition.[15] An increasing number of children are being discovered. In conditions such as Down's syndrome,[16] the Klippel-Feil syndrome, and certain skeletal dysplasias, such as Morquio's syndrome[4,28,35] and spondyloepiphyseal dysplasia,[27,52] odontoid anomalies are more common than in the general population.[7,9,26,31,46,47,50] It is interesting to note the relative infrequency of associated regional malformations with os odontoideum.[3,15,43,50] One would expect that such a fundamental congenital anomaly would be more frequently associated with other anomalies, similar to those described in the Klippel-Feil syndrome.[26]

EMBRYOLOGY AND NORMAL ANATOMY

The body of the odontoid is derived from the mesenchyme of the first cervical sclerotome and is actually the centrum of the first cervical vertebra. During development, the odontoid becomes separated from the atlas to fuse with the superior portion of the axis.[30,44,46,50,54] At birth, the odontoid is separated from the body of the axis by a wide cartilaginous band that represents the vestigial disc space and is referred to as the neurocentral synchondrosis. On the lateral radiograph it resembles an epiphyseal growth plate (Fig. 5-19*A*). It is not at the anatomic base of the dens at the level of the superior articular facets of the axis, but lies well below this level within the body of the axis (Fig. 5-19*B*). Therefore, the embryologic base of the odontoid contributes a substantial portion of the body of the axis. On the open-mouth view, the odontoid fits like a cork in a bottle, lying sandwiched between the neural arches[12] (Fig. 5-19*B*). The neurocentral synchondrosis is present in nearly all children by 3 years of age and in 50% of children by 4 years of age, and it is absent in most by 6 years of age.[6,12]

At birth, the apex or tip of the odontoid is not ossified, and roentgenographically appears as a V-shaped depression, known as the dens bicornis. A separate ossification center or ossiculum terminale usually appears at age 3 and fuses with the body of the dens by age 12.[2,5,40,50] Cattell and Filtzer[6] found an ossiculum terminale to be present in 26%

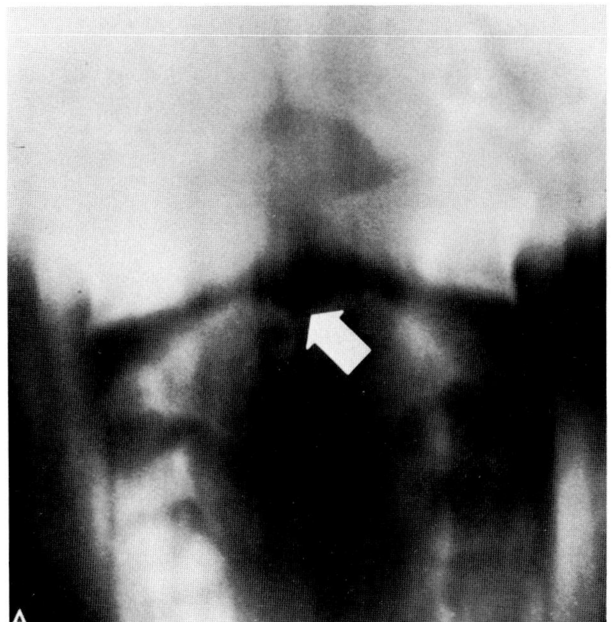

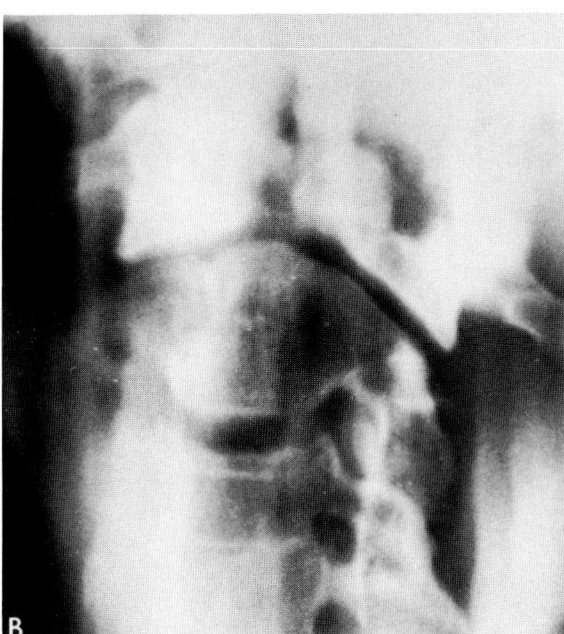

5-18. (*A*) Agenesis of the odontoid (open-mouth laminagraphic view). Note the slight depression between the superior articular facets of the axis (*arrow*). A short bony remnant in this position is termed *odontoid hypoplasia.* (*B*) Os odontoideum (open-mouth laminagraphic view). The os odontoideum is an oval or round ossicle, usually approximately half the normal size of the odontoid, with a smooth cortical border of uniform thickness. There is a jointlike articulation between the os odontoideum and the body of the axis, which appears radiologically as a wide radiolucent gap, and usually extends above the level of the superior facets.

of normal children between ages 5 and 11. It may never appear, or it may occasionally fail to fuse with the odontoid and is then called ossiculum terminale persistens. Such anomalies are rarely of clinical significance,[10,46,50] as this terminal portion is usually firmly bound to the main body of the odontoid by fibrous tissue. In the young child, the unossified portions of the odontoid may give the false impression of odontoid hypoplasia. Similarly, one may erroneously conclude that the child has C1–C2 instability as commonly the anterior arch of the atlas may slide upward and actually protrude beyond the ossified portion of the odontoid, on the lateral extension roentgenogram.[6]

The blood supply to the odontoid, delineated by Schiff and Parke (see also Chapter 1), is from two sources[42]: (1) The vertebral arteries provide both an anterior and posterior ascending artery that arise at the level of C3 and pass ventral and dorsal to the body of the axis, and the odontoid, anastomosing in an apical arcade in the region of the alar ligaments. These arteries supply small penetrating branches to the body of the axis and the odontoid. (2) Lateral to the apex of the odontoid, the anterior ascending arteries and apical arcade receive anastomotic derivatives from the carotids, by way of the base of the skull and the alar ligaments. This curious arrangement of the blood supply is due to the embryologic development and anatomic function of the odontoid. The transient neurocentral synchondrosis between the odontoid and the axis prevents the development of any significant vascular channels between the two structures. The body of the odontoid is surrounded entirely by synovial joint cavities, and its fixed position relative to the rotation of the atlas precludes vascularization by direct branches from the vertebral arteries at the C1 segmental level.

ETIOLOGY AND PATHOGENESIS

A congenital etiology of the os odontoideum has been assumed, and two theories have been advanced: (1) Failure of fusion of the apex or ossiculum terminale to the odontoid. This is unlikely as the fragment is too small and never approxi-

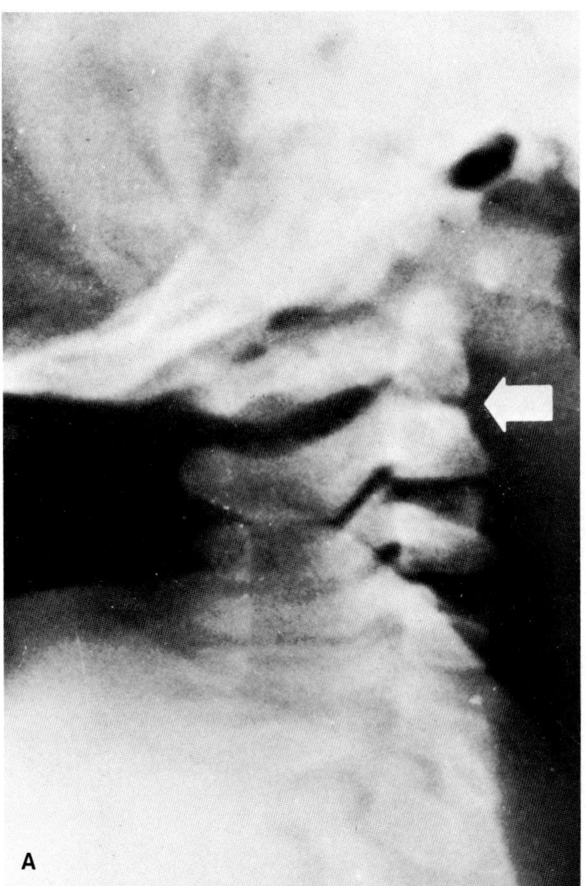

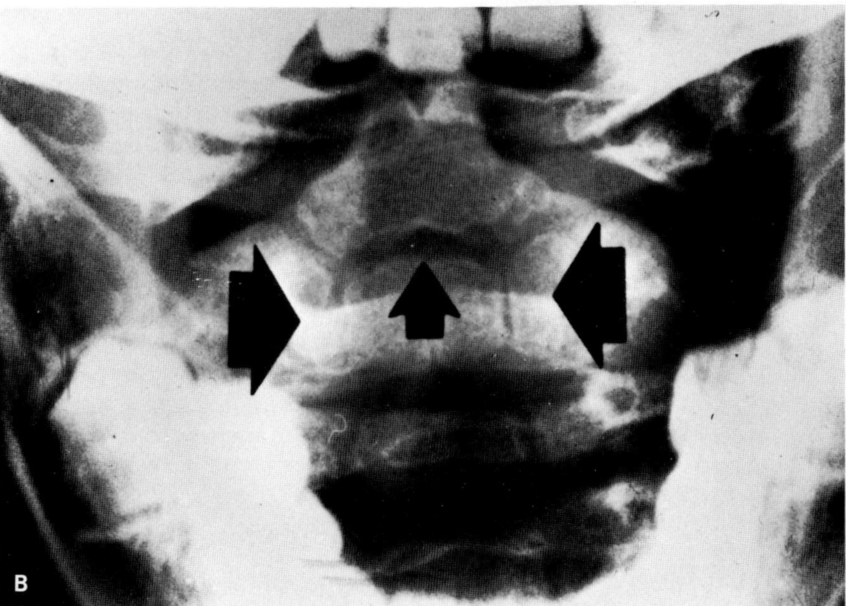

Fig. 5-19. (*A*) Six-month-old infant. The odontoid is normally formed and recognizable on routine roentgenograms at birth but separated from the body of the axis by a broad cartilaginous band (*arrow*), similar in appearance to an epiphyseal plate. It represents the vestigial disc space and is referred to as the neurocentral synchondrosis. (*B*) The neurocentral synchondrosis is not at the anatomic base of the dens, at the level of the superior articular facets of the axis. This open-mouth view demonstrates that the embryologic base of the odontoid is below the articular facets and contributes a substantial portion to the body of the axis. The odontoid appears to fit like a cork in a bottle, lying sandwiched between the neural arches. (Fielding JW, Hensinger RN, Hawkins RJ: Os odontoideum. J Bone Joint Surg 62A:376–383, 1980)

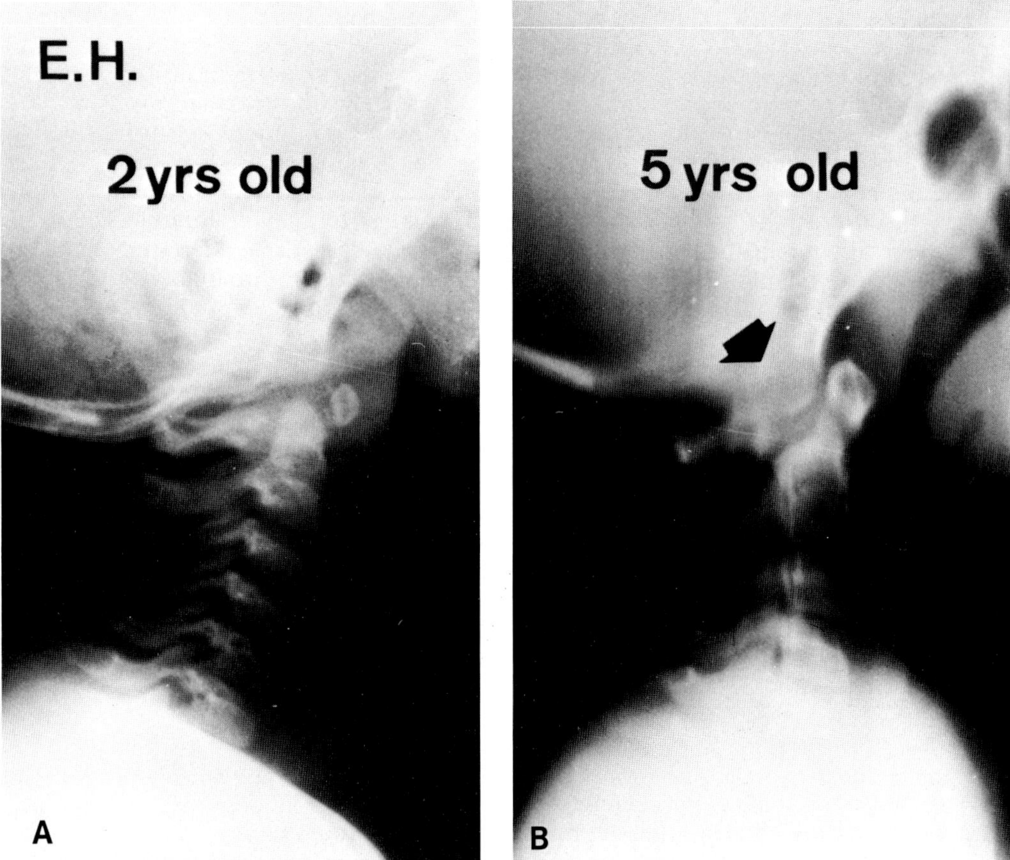

Fig. 5-20. Five-year-old boy (E.H.) who at age 2 fell from a couch. (*A*) Lateral roentenogram taken at age 2 demonstrates a normal-appearing odontoid and cervical spine. He complained of pain in the neck and occiput, and presented with torticollis. Symptoms and signs gradually resolved over 1 month. (*B*) The child was asymptomatic until age 5, when over a period of 6 months he developed increasing neck pain and stiffness without neurologic complaints or findings. Roentgenograms revealed an os odontoideum and 7 mm of flexion–extension motion. The patient subsequently underwent C1–C2 stabilization. (Fielding JW, Hensinger RN, Hawkins RJ: Os odontoideum. J Bone Joint Surg 62A:376–383, 1980)

mates the size of the os odontoideum.[46] (2) Failure of fusion of the odontoid to the axis. This too is doubtful, as one would expect a crater or depression in the body of C2, because a substantial portion of C2 is derived from the odontoid; however, this has not been reported. Rather, there is more often an associated short, stubby projection or hypoplastic odontoid remnant in the area of the odontoid base.[36,54] Hypoplasia and os odontoideum can be acquired secondary to trauma or rarely infection.[1,7,11,13,18,25,33,39,40,54] Nine cases of os odontoideum have been reported, which developed several years after trauma, where a normal odontoid was initially present (Fig. 5-20).[11,13,15,18,25,39] The majority of patients have a significant episode of trauma prior to the diagnosis of os odontoideum.[15]

Fielding and associates submit that the weight of evidence favors an unrecognized fracture in the region of the base of the odontoid as the most common cause and less often suggests a congenital origin.[15] They postulate that, following fracture of the odontoid, there may be only slight separation of the fragments, but that eventually contracture of the alar ligaments, which attach to the tip of the odontoid, exert a distraction force that pulls the odontoid fragment away from C2 and closer to their origin at the occiput (Fig. 5-21). The blood supply to the odontoid is precarious as it passes up along the sides of the odontoid and is easily traumatized, and it contributes to poor fracture healing or callus formation that might prevent retraction of the fragment. The position of the odontoid adjacent to the ring of C1 is maintained by the intact transverse atlantal ligament. The blood supply to the fragment is maintained by the proximal arterial arcade, from the carotid through the alar ligaments, and may be sufficient to maintain only a portion of the odontoid. Similarly, the blood supply to the proximal portion of the odontoid can be interrupted by excessive traction on these ligaments.[49]

CLINICAL SIGNS AND SYMPTOMS

Patients may present clinically with no symptoms, local neck symptoms, or transitory episodes of paresis following trauma, or with frank myelopathy secondary to cord compression.[48,51] Minor trauma is commonly associated with the onset of symptoms, often of sufficient degree to warrant radiologic evaluation of the cervical spine. Symptoms may be mechanical and due to local irritation of the atlantoaxial articulation, such as neck pain, torticollis, or headache. Neurologic symptoms are due to C1–C2 displacement and spinal cord compression. An important differential point from other anomalies of the occipitovertebral junction is that these patients seldom have symptoms referable to cranial nerves,[37] as the area of the spinal cord impingement is below the foramen magnum.

If the clinical manifestations are limited to neck pain and torticollis (local joint irritation) without neurologic involvement (40%),[24] the prognosis is excellent.[15,32,37,41] Similarly, patients who exhibit only transient weakness of the extremities and dysesthesia following trauma usually have complete return of function. However, patients with insidious onset and slowly progressive neurologic impairment have a greater potential for permanent deficit.[15] Damage may be mixed, with involvement of both the anterior and posterior spinal cord structures. Patients more commonly complain of weakness and ataxia than of sensory loss. However, spasticity, increased deep tendon reflexes, clonus, loss of proprioception, and sphincter disturbances in various combinations have all been described.

A small number of patients[41] may have symptoms and signs of cerebral and brain-stem ischemia, seizures, mental deterioration, syncope, vertigo, and visual disturbances.[14,17,41,43] These patients typically have a paucity of cervical cord signs and symptoms, and it is presumed that they are experiencing vertebral artery compression at, or just below, the foramen magnum.[32] Thus, the diagnosis can be quite confusing, and many patients are misdiagnosed or thought to have progressive neurologic illness. Whenever the diagnosis of Friedreich's ataxia, multiple sclerosis, or other unexplained neurologic complaints are encountered, survey of the occipitocervical junction is suggested.[38]

RADIOLOGIC FINDINGS

Agenesis or Hypoplasia of the Odontoid (see Fig. 5-18*A*)

The diagnosis of odontoid aplasia can be made at birth with standard roentgenograms. There should be a recognizable odontoid, although it is not yet fused at its base to the axis. If the odontoid is absent, a slight depression may be noted between the superior articular facets in the open-mouth view (see Fig. 5-18*A*). A short, bony remnant in this position is termed odontoid hypoplasia.

In patients with multiple anomalies, the usual roentgenographic views are not always reliable in confirming the presence or absence of an odontoid. Similarly, in patients with abnormal bone, such as Morquio's syndrome and spondyloepiphyseal dysplasia,[28,35] the odontoid may be present but dysplastic, blending with the surrounding abnormal bone, and it cannot be differentiated. In these situations, good results have been obtained by using lateral laminagraphic techniques. When the exact cut at the level of the odontoid is determined, it is repeated in flexion and extension to ascertain the stability of the atlantoaxial articulation. The extension view should not be ignored. Many patients have been found with significant posterior subluxation.[15,20] Giannestras reported a youngster who became quadriparetic from prolonged hyperextension while lying prone watching television.[20]

Os Odontoideum

In os odontoideum, there is a jointlike articulation between the odontoid and the body of the axis, which appears radiologically as a wide radiolucent gap (see Fig. 5-12). This gap may be confused with the normal neurocentral synchondrosis (see Fig. 5-19). Therefore, in children under 5 years of age, the diagnosis of os odontoideum is confirmed by demonstrating motion between the odontoid and the body of the axis. In the adult, the diagnosis of os odontoideum is suggested by observing a radiolucent defect between the dens and the body of

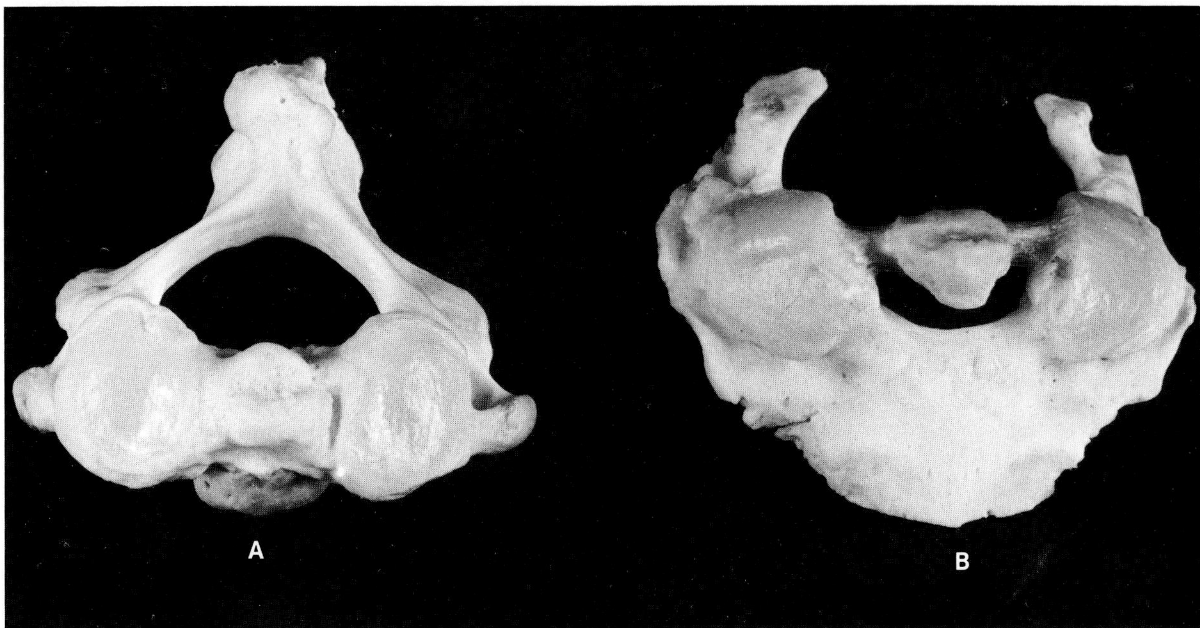

Fig. 5-21. (*A*) Anatomic specimen of an os odontoideum from a 17-year-old boy with multiple congenital anomalies, who died from renal disease. The previous bony attachment of the odontoid to the axis was rough and blunted. There was a fibrocartilaginous pseudarthrosis between the os odontoideum and C2. (*B*) The occiput and occipital events, with the os odontoideum suspended between the facets. The transverse ligament was intact, but loosened during the preparation of the specimen. The alar ligaments remain attached to the tip of the os odontoideum. They are shortened, and appear to have pulled the residual odontoid tip closer to their origin on the occiput. The os odontoideum was firmly attached by soft tissue to the occiput and ring of C1, and moved freely with these structures on C2. The foramen magnum is incomplete posteriorly. The posterior ring of C1 (not pictured) was intact. (Fielding JW, Hensinger RN, Hawkins RJ: Os odontoideum. J Bone Joint Surg 62A:376–383, 1980)

the axis. However, the radiologic appearance of the condition may be quite similar to the traumatic nonunion, and frequently the two cannot be differentiated.[33,54] In os odontoideum, the gap between the free ossicle and the axis usually extends above the level of the superior facets and is wide with a smooth edge. The ossicle is usually approximately one half the normal size of the odontoid and is rounded or oval in shape, and the cortex is of uniform thickness. In the traumatic nonunion, the gap between the fragments is characteristically narrow and irregular, and it frequently extends into the body of the axis below the level of the superior facets of the axis. The bone fragments appear to "match," and there is no marginal cortex at the level of the fracture or rounded-off appearance that is found with os odontoideum.[39] Laminagrams may be helpful in determining these subtle differences. The odontoid ossicle is fixed firmly to the anterior ring of the atlas and moves with it in flexion, extension, and lateral slide. The anterior portion of the atlas is usually hypertrophied, and the posterior portion of the ring may be hypoplastic or absent.[15,37]

Recommended roentgenographic views are the open-mouth and lateral flexion–extension. Lateral laminagrams are indicated when routine views are not satisfactory in demonstrating the anomaly. Lateral flexion–extension stress views should be conducted voluntarily by the patient, particularly those with neurologic deficit. The degree of anterior–posterior displacement of the atlas on the axis should be documented (Fig. 5-12). The os odontoideum will move with the ring of C1, and, consequently, measurements of its relationship to C1 are of little value. Measurements can be made using a line projected superiorly from the posterior border of the body of the axis to a line projected

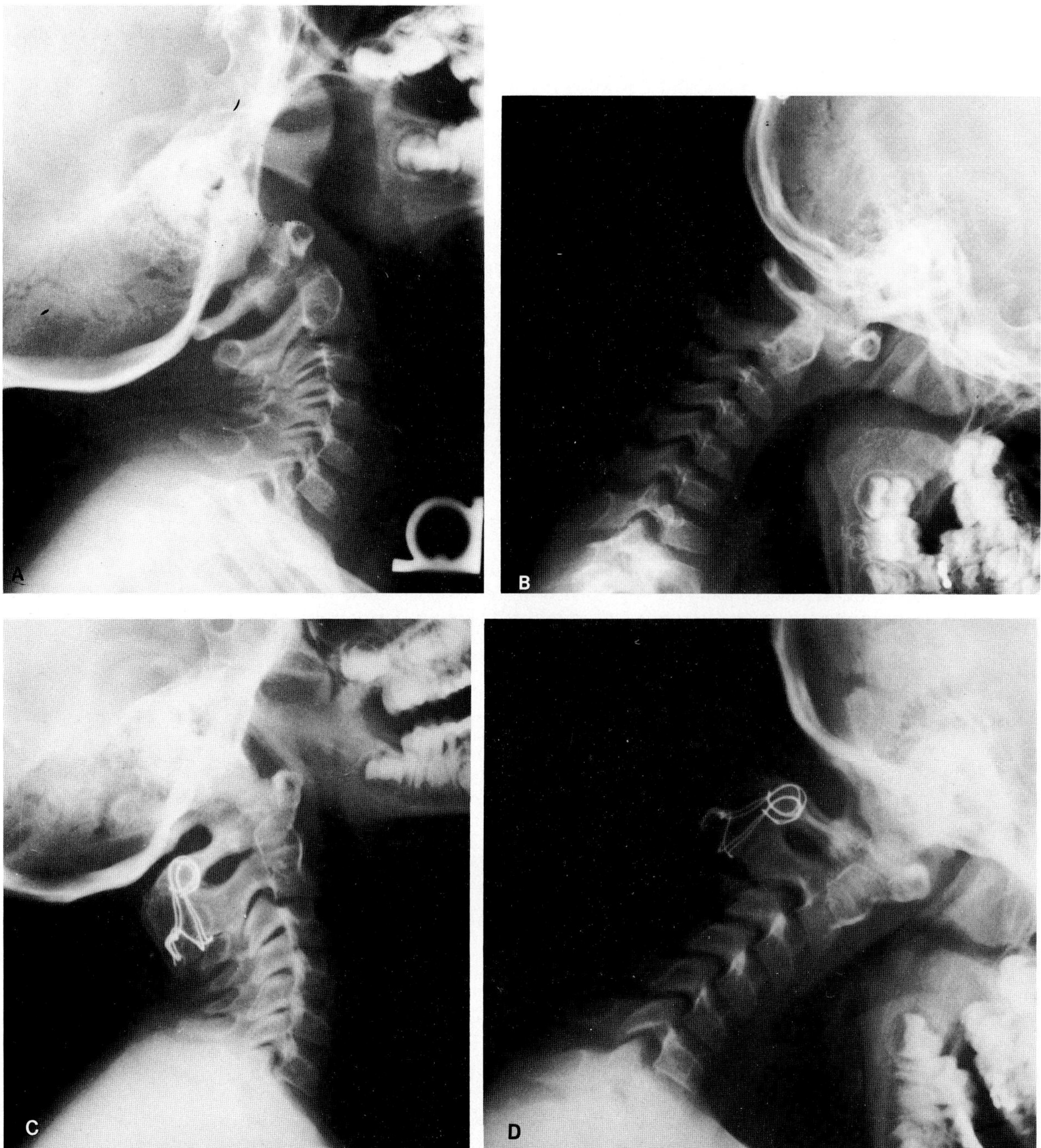

Fig. 5-22. This 6-year-old had a history of peculiar posturing and stiffness of the neck beginning at age 11 months and persisting for 5 years. Subsequent roentgenograms demonstrated (*A*) an os odontoideum and (*B*) subluxation of C1–C2 in flexion. (*C*), (*D*) Roentgenographic appearance following posterior stabilization. Reduction must be accomplished prior to surgery, and if wire stabilization is selected, care must be taken to avoid further flexion of the neck during surgery.

inferiorly from the posterior border of the anterior arch of the atlas. Measurements greater than 3 mm should be considered pathologic. The majority of symptomatic patients exhibit significant instability.[15] In a large series reported by Fielding and coworkers, the average was 10 mm, the majority being either anterior or posterior, although some were unstable in all directions.[15] Posteriorly, the lumen of the spinal canal or the space available for the spinal cord should be determined. Cineradiography may be valuable in understanding the pathomechanics of odontoid anomalies, particularly those with atlantoaxial instability.

TREATMENT

Patients with congenital anomalies of the odontoid are leading a precarious existence. The concern is that a trivial insult superimposed on an already weakened or compromised structure may be catastrophic. Patients with local symptoms or transient myelopathy can expect to recover, at least temporarily.[32,37,41] Cervical traction or plaster immobilization may be helpful in such circumstances.

Nonoperative treatment is sufficient for the patient presenting with relatively stable os odontoideum, little compromise of the SAC, and only minor mechanical symptomatology.[19,21,32,37,41] Those with significant diminution of the SAC (13 mm or less) or excessive instability (greater than 10 mm), history of myelopathy, or progressive neurologic deterioration should be considered for surgical stabilization.[15,47] The C1–C2 articulation should be reduced by simple positioning or traction prior to traction. Open reduction during surgery is discouraged, as it has proven extremely hazardous and may result in respiratory distress, apnea, or death.[19] Ideally, the patient should be maintained in the reduced position 1 to 2 weeks prior to surgery to allow recovery of neurologic function and to lessen spinal cord irritation.

The suggested method of stabilization is posterior cervical fusion of C1–C2, employing wire fixation and an iliac bone graft (Fig. 5-22).[14,15] This is not without risk, as slight flexion is often required to pass the wire beneath the posterior ring of the atlas, and the procedure can have tragic results.[37] In the patient with a marginally functioning neurologic status, it may be wiser to perform an occiput-to-C2 arthrodesis and plan to maintain immobilization in extension during the postoperative course.[37] In this regard, the halo cast is helpful. Incomplete development of the posterior ring of C1 is uncommon but occurs with increased frequency in patients with an os odontoideum.[15,29] The completeness of the C1 arch should be evaluated preoperatively, as a large gap may preclude wire fixation. If wire fixation is employed, excessive tightening of the wire should be avoided (Fig. 5-22*C,D*). The articulation is frequently unstable both in flexion and extension, and posterior dislocations due to overcorrection, may occur with disastrous results.

Patients in whom the C1–C2 dislocation cannot be reduced in preoperative traction pose a difficult problem.[8] Manipulative reduction during surgery is extremely hazardous and should be avoided.[50] Similarly, attempting to pass the wire through the narrow space under the arch of C1 is dangerous and not recommended.[47] Posterior decompression and laminectomy alone have been associated with an increased morbidity and mortality.[37] In addition, posterior decompression alone may potentiate C1–C2 instability and if performed must be accompanied by occiput-to-C2 arthrodesis.[8,16] For patients who are neurologically intact, posterior *in situ* fusion is the least hazardous procedure.[14,23] If there is anterior cord compression, an anterior decompression should be considered after adequate posterior stabilization.[22,23,53] The lateral retropharyngeal approach, as described by Whitesides and McDonald, has provided adequate anterior exposure of the C1–C2 articulation to perform decompression, reduction and stabilization.[54] This route is preferred over the transoral or mandibular and tongue-splitting approach, which are associated with an increased incidence of infection.[23,53]

REFERENCES

1. *Ahlbacks S, Collert S:* Destruction of the odontoid process due to atlanto-axial pyogenic spondylitis. Acta Radiol (Diagn) (Stockh) 10:394–400, 1970
2. *Bailey DK:* The normal cervical spine in infants and children. Radiology 59:712–719, 1952
3. *Bassett FH III, Goldner JL:* Aplasia of the odontoid process. AAOS, J Bone Joint Surg 50A:833–834, 1968
4. *Blaw ME, Langer LO:* Spinal cord compression in Morquio-Brailsford's disease. J Pediatr 74:593–600, 1969
5. *Caffey J:* Paediatric X-ray Diagnosis, 5th ed. Chicago, Yearbook Medical Publishers, 1967
6. *Cattell H, Filtzer DL:* Pseudosubluxation and other normal variations in the cervical spine in children. J Bone Joint Surg, 47A:1295–1309, 1965
7. *Curtis BH, Blank S, Fisher RL:* Atlanto-axial dislocation in Down's syndrome. JAMA, 205:464–465, 1968

8. *DYCK P:* Os odontoideum in children: neurological manifestations and surgical management. Neurosurgery 2:93–99, 1978
9. *DZENITIS AJ:* Spontaneous atlanto-axial dislocation in mongoloid child with spinal cord compression. Case report. J Neurosurg 25:458–460, 1966
10. *EVARTS CM, LONSDALE D:* Ossiculum terminale—an anomaly of the odontoid process; report of a case of atlanto-axial dislocation with cord compression. Cleve Clin Q 37:73–76, 1970
11. *FIELDING JW:* Disappearance of the central portion of the odontoid process. J Bone Joint Surg 47A:1228–1230, 1965
12. *FIELDING JW:* Selected observations on the cervical spine in the child. Curr Pract Orthop Surg, 5:31–35, 1973
13. *FIELDING JW, GRIFFIN PP:* Os odontoideum: an acquired lesion. J Bone Joint Surg 56A:187–190, 1974
14. *FIELDING JW, HAWKINS RJ, RATZAN SA:* Spine fusion for atlanto-axial instability. J Bone Joint Surg 58A:400–407, 1976
15. *FIELDING JW, HENSINGER RN, HAWKINS RJ:* Os odontoideum. J Bone Joint Surg 62A:376–383, 1980
16. *FINERMAN GA, SAKAI D, WEINGARTEN S:* Atlanto-axial dislocation with spinal cord compression in a mongoloid child. J Bone Joint Surg 58A:408–409, 1976
17. *FORD FR:* Syncope, vertigo and disturbances of vision resulting from intermittent obstruction of the vertebral arteries due to defect in the odontoid process and excessive mobility of the second cervical vertebra. Bull Johns Hopkins Hosp 91:168–173, 1952
18. *FREIBERGER RH, WILSON PD JR, NICHOLAS JA:* Acquired absence of the odontoid process. A case report. J Bone Joint Surg 47A:1231–1236, 1965
19. *GARBER JN:* Abnormalities of the atlas and axis vertebrae; congenital and traumatic. J Bone Joint Surg, 47A:1782–1791, 1964
20. *GIANNESTRAS, NJ, MAYFIELD FH, PROVENCIO FP, MAURER J:* Congenital absence of the odontoid process. A case report. J Bone Joint Surg 46A:839–843, 1964
21. *GILLMAN EL:* Congenital absence of the odontoid process of the axis; report of a case. J Bone Joint Surg, 41A:345–348, 1959
22. *GREENBERG AD:* Atlantoaxial dislocations. Brain 91:655–684, 1968
23. *GREENBERG AD, SCOVILLE WB, DAVEY LM:* Transoral decompression of atlanto-axial dislocation due to odontoid hypoplasia; report of two cases. J Neurosurg 28:266–269, 1968
24. *GWINN JL, SMITH JL:* Acquired and congenital absence of the odontoid process. AJR 88:424–431, 1962
25. *HAWKINS RJ, FIELDING JW, THOMPSON WJ:* Os odontoideum: congenital or acquired. J Bone Joint Surg 58A:413–414, 1976
26. *HENSINGER RN, LANG JR, MACEWEN GD:* The Klippel-Feil syndrome: a constellation of associated anomalies. J Bone Joint Surg 56A:1246–1253, 1974
27. *LANGER LO JR:* Spondyloepiphyseal dysplasia tarda. Hereditary chondrodysplasia with characteristic vertebral configuration in the adult. Radiology 82:833–839, 1964
28. *LIPSON SJ:* Dysplasia of the odontoid process in Morquio's syndrome causing quadriparesis. J Bone Joint Surg 59A:340–344, 1977
29. *LOGAN WW, STUARD ID:* Absent posterior arch of the atlas. AJR 118:431–434, 1973
30. *MACALISTER A:* Notes on the development and variations of the atlas. J Anat Physiol 27:519–542, 1892
31. *MARTEL W, TISHLER JM:* Observations on the spine in mongoloidism. AJR 97:630–638, 1966
32. *MCKEEVER FM:* Atlanto-axiad instability. Surg Clin North 48:1375–1390, 1968
33. *MCRAE DL:* Bony abnormalities in the region of the foramen magnum; correlation of the anatomic and neurologic findings. Acta Radiol 40:335–354, 1953
34. *MCRAE DL:* The significance of abnormalities of the cervical spine. AJR 84:3–25, 1960
35. *MELZAK J:* Spinal deformities with paraplegia in two sisters with Morquio-Brailsford syndrome. Paraplegia 6:246–258, 1969
36. *MICHAELS L, PREVOST MJ, CRANG DF:* Pathological changes in a case of os odontoideum (separate odontoid process). J Bone Joint Surg 50A:965–972, 1969
37. *MINDERHOUD JM, BRAAKMAN R, PENNING L:* Os odontoideum; clinical, radiological, and therapeutic aspects. J Neurol Sci 8:521–544, 1969
38. *NICHOLSON JS, SHERK HH:* Anomalies of the occipito-cervical articulation. J Bone Joint Surg 50A:295–304, 1968
39. *RICCIARDI JE, KAUFER H, LOUIS DS:* Acquired os odontoideum following acute ligament injury. J Bone Joint Surg 58A:410–412, 1976
40. *ROTHMAN RH, SIMEONE FA:* The spine, Vol 1. Philadelphia, WB Saunders Co, 1975
41. *ROWLAND LP, SHAPIRO JH, JACOBSON HG:* Neurological syndromes associated with congenital absence of the odontoid process. Arch Neurol Psychiatr 80:286–291, 1958
42. *SCHILLER F, NIEDA I:* Malformations of the odontoid process. Report of a case and clinical survey. Calif Med 86:394–398, 1957
43. *SHAPIRO R, YOUNGBERG AS, ROTHMAN SLG:* The differential diagnosis of traumatic lesions of the

occipito-atlanto-axial segment. Radiol Clin North Am 11:505–526, 1973

44. *SHEPARD CN:* Familial hypoplasia of the odontoid process. J Bone Joint Surg 48A:1224, 1966
45. *SHERK HH, NICHOLSON JT:* Rotatory-atlanto-axial dislocation associated with ossiculum terminale and mongolism. A case report. J Bone Joint Surg, 51A:957–964, 1969
46. *SCHIFF DCM, PARKE WW:* Arterial blood supply of the odontoid process (dens). Anat Rec 172:399–400, 1972
47. *SPIERLINGS ELH, BRAAKMAN R:* Os odontoideum: analysis of 37 cases. J Bone Joint Surg 64B:422–428, 1982
48. *SPITZER R, RABINOWITCH JY, WYBAR KC:* A study of the abnormalities of the skull, teeth and lenses in mongolism. Can Med Assoc J 84:567–572, 1961
49. *STRATFORD J:* Myelopathy caused by atlanto-axial dislocation. J Neurosurg 14:97–104, 1959
50. *TREDWELL SJ, O'BRIEN JP:* Avascular necrosis of the proximal end of the dens. A complication of halo-pelvic distraction. J Bone Joint Surg 57A:332–336, 1975
51. *VON TORKLUS D, GEHLE W:* The Upper Cervical Spine. New York, Grune & Stratton, 1972
52. *WADIA NH:* Myelopathy complicating congenital atlanto-axial dislocation (a study of 28 cases). Brain 90:449–472, 1967
53. *WEINFELD A, ROSS MW, SARASOHN SH:* Spondylo-epiphyseal dysplasia tarda: a cause of premature osteoarthritis. AJR 101:851–859, 1967
54. *WHITESIDES TR, MCDONALD AP:* Lateral retropharyngeal approach to the upper cervical spine. Orthop Clin North Am 9:1115–1127, 1978
55. *WOLLIN DG:* The os odontoideum; separate odontoid process. J Bone Joint Surg 45A:1459–1471, 1963

Klippel-Feil Syndrome

PETER D. PIZZUTILLO

HISTORICAL BACKGROUND

Variations from the norm have always captivated human interest and imagination. The examination of such variations is its own reward, and has often stimulated the search for clues leading to new developments. In 1912, Klippel and Feil expressed their belief that each variant should be reported in the hope of shedding light on the process of human evolution "towards a being more simple and more perfect." Their contribution involved a detailed clinical and anatomic description of a 46-year-old male, L. Joseph, who had a prolonged history of abdominal problems suggestive of appendicitis or ileitis, and recurrent bouts of "pleurisy" with effusions in early adulthood.[43] Monsieur Joseph presented to Doctors Klippel and Feil with pleurisy, pulmonary congestion, and nephritis on December 13, 1911, and 1 month later he expired with the additional complications of albuminuria, an enlarged heart, and tachycardia. Clinical examination revealed the apparent absence of the neck (Fig. 5-23), a low hairline, and severe limitation of neck motion; at autopsy a total of 12 vertebrae were noted in the spinal column. The upper four vertebrae displayed a bizarre morphology as an ill-defined fusion mass with rudimentary ribs upon which the occiput moved in flexion and extension.

These findings suggested to Klippel and Feil the diagnosis of congenital absence of the neck with ribs arising from the base of the skull as a "cervical thorax." The remainder of the axial skeleton revealed other anomalies, including dorsal kyphosis and dorsolumbar scoliosis. The report by Klippel and Feil represents the first detailed description of congenital fusion of the cervical vertebrae, although earlier reports suggested similar findings.

The oldest known example of congenital fusion of the cervical spine was noted in an Egyptian mummy (*circa* 500 B.C.) by Smith in a report published in 1908.[34,74] Herodotus wrote of the ancient race, the Acephala in western Libya, whose heads appeared to rest on their trunks. In the 16th century, Aldrovani explained the existence of a similar "monstrosity" by simply stating that the neck was absent. In 1743, Haller described an anencephalic fetus with five cervical vertebrae.[10,34] Three years later, Morgagni described a second anencephalic fetus with similar cervical spine changes, in addition to an elderly man with occipitoatlantal fusion and C2–C3 fusion.[34] Rokitansky, in 1850, reported C2 to C7 congenital fusion in a 70-year-old tailor. The advent of x-ray investigation allowed Sick to describe cervical spine fusions in a living 4-year-old girl with concomitant Sprengel's deformity.[34]

Feil continued his investigations with a review of the literature and found 13 related cases,[28] which he used as the basis of classification of the deformity according to the degree of involvement. Mass fusion of many cervical and upper thoracic vertebrae was classified as Type I; fusion at one or two interspaces only was classified as Type II; and cervical fusion in combination with lower thoracic or lumbar fusion was classified as Type III.

Early writings on the Klippel-Feil syndrome included observations on stillborn infants with multisystem disorders, anencephaly, iniencephaly—essentially, any change involving cervical spine morphology, such as occipitalization of the atlas, fusion of the vertebrae, hemivertebrae, and platyspondylia.[7-9,17,19,34] There is yet no clear agreement on the anatomic criteria for inclusion in this syndrome, and although occipitalization of the atlas, hemivertebrae, and basilar impression do occur more frequently in patients with this syndrome, their isolated occurrence is not generally accepted as part of the syndrome.[75] Klippel and Feil's initial patient had complete fusion of all cervical vertebrae with no identifiable atlas or axis. If such an extreme case were used as the basis for classifying patients with this syndrome, few would be found in the world literature. Because Joseph also demonstrated clinical manifestations of associated system disease (in his case, the pulmonary and renal systems were compromised), the term Klippel-Feil syndrome could have been reserved for cases of congenital fusion of the cervical spine in combination with other major system anomalies. In its current usage, however, the term Klippel-Feil syndrome refers to persons with congenital fusion of the cervical vertebrae (Fig. 5-24). Neither severity of involvement of the cervical spine nor presence of concomitant anomalies are considered necessary for inclusion in the syndrome.

CLINICAL FINDINGS

Classically, the patient with the Klippel-Feil syndrome exhibits a short neck, a low posterior hairline, and a limited range of neck motion (Fig. 5-25). This triad is usually seen in cases of massive

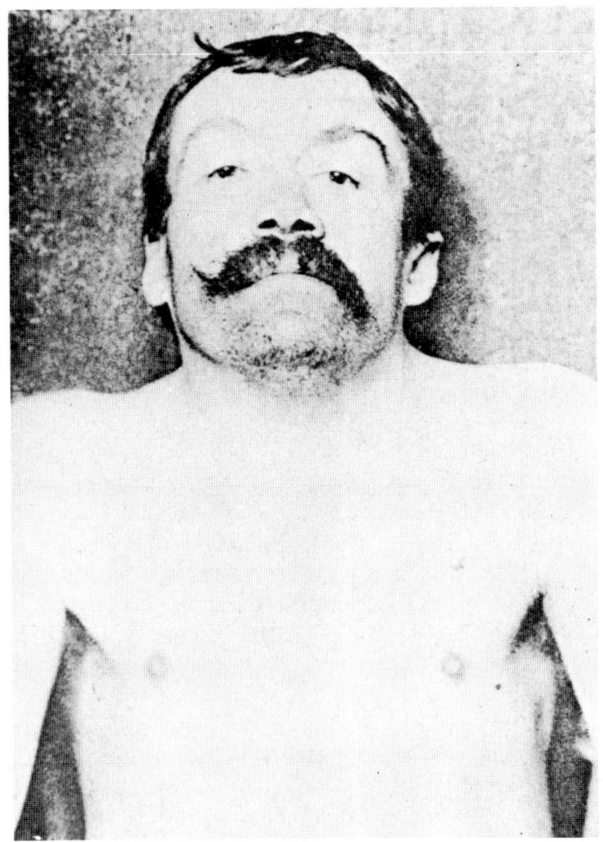

Fig. 5-23. Frontal photograph of L. Joseph.

involvement of cervical vertebrae and may create a characteristic appearance as early as birth. However, fewer than 50% of patients have all three elements of the triad; in fact, many patients with Klippel-Feil syndrome have a normal appearance.[34,37] The latter have been diagnosed through incidental radiologic findings or through family surveys of known patients with the Klippel-Feil syndrome.

A short neck and low posterior hairline are seen in patients with severe involvement. Lesser changes become quite difficult to detect because of their subjective nature, and hair styles may be altered to mask the low hairline. Other associated clinical findings such as facial asymmetry, torticollis, and webbing of the neck may facilitate detection but were seen in only 20% of patients.[30,34,37,71] It is important to differentiate torticollis that is secondary to congenital changes of the cervical spine from that due to muscular contracture. Surgical release of contracted muscles will improve head alignment, range of motion, and facial asymmetry in the latter form, but will have no beneficial results in the type associated with bony changes.

The most consistent clinical finding in Klippel-Feil syndrome is limitation of neck motion. When examining for motion, it is important to test in all planes, not merely in flexion and extension, because the atlantoaxial joint is usually normal and will preserve a fairly normal range of flexion–extension even in advanced cases. In addition, Hensinger and associates have reported patients who demonstrate full clinical flexion–extension occurring through only one open interspace (Fig. 5-26).[37] Attention must then be addressed to lateral rotation and lateral side bending for critical evaluation. Patients with fusion of the lower cervical spine or with a single-level fusion exhibit normal motion in all planes; however, with greater involvement, loss of lateral bending is frequently observed. Occasionally, patients present with no observable neck motion; this is usually associated with massive cervical spine involvement, a short neck, and torticollis. If a low posterior hairline and fixed hyperextension of the neck are present, iniencephaly (*i.e.*, an enlarged foramen magnum with absent posterior elements of the upper cervical spine) must be considered.[66] Clinical appearance may also be altered by the presence of the frequently associated Sprengel's deformity and by scoliosis.

RADIOLOGIC FINDINGS

Routine radiography, tomography, cineradiography, and the CT scan have enhanced our understanding of the congenital changes that have been included in the Klippel-Feil syndrome. The initial evaluation of these patients should include anteroposterior, anteroposterior open-mouth, and lateral flexion–extension radiographic views of the cervical spine. This series will frequently define the pattern of congenital fusion, demonstrate coexisting occipitalization of the atlas, and determine instability at the atlantoaxial joint, at interspaces above and below the fused area or at an open interspace between two congenitally fused areas.

The lateral radiograph of the very young child may appear normal until ossification develops to define the congenital changes. It is interesting to witness the obliteration of apparently normal disc spaces as ossification occurs with maturation (Fig. 5-27). Occasionally, bony union of the posterior elements is seen at an early age and heralds the existence of congenital fusion of the anterior spinal elements (Fig. 5-28).[37] When viewed on lateral radiograph, the fused vertebral bodies appear to be smaller in width than the more normal ver-

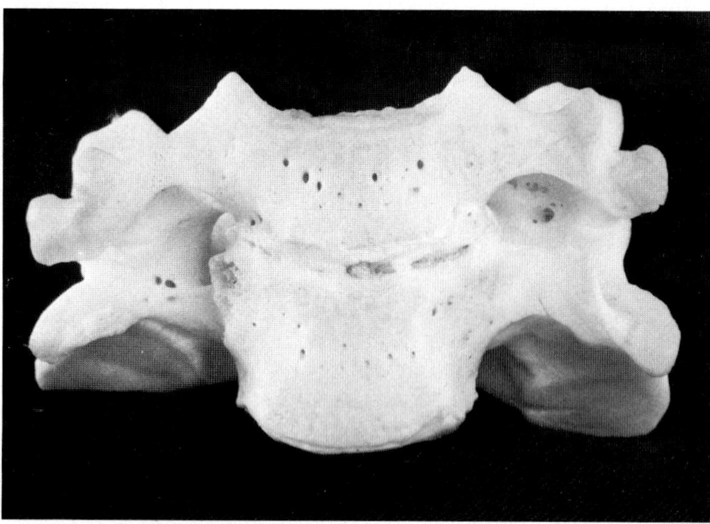

Fig. 5-24. Single-level congenital fusion of cervical vertebrae.

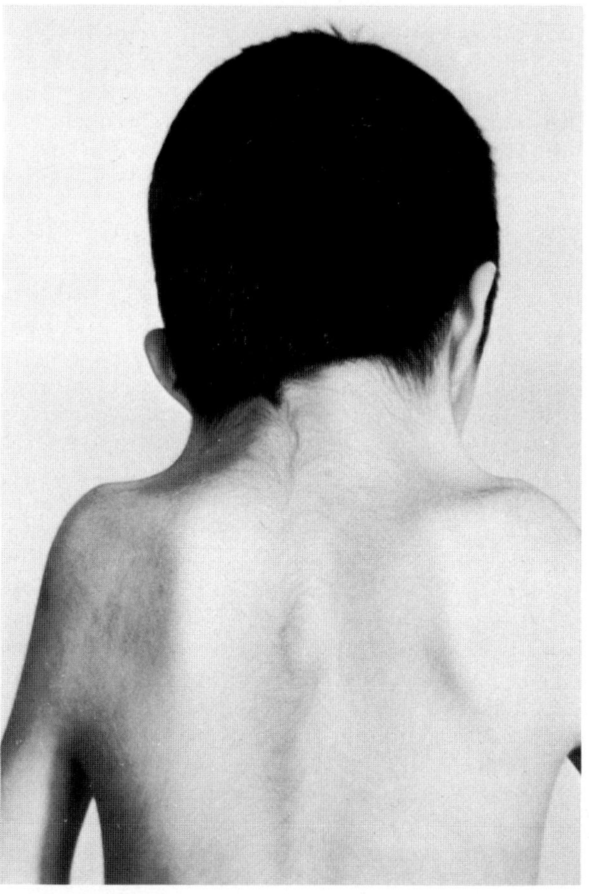

Fig. 5-25. The patient with Klippel-Feil syndrome exhibits a short neck and low posterior hairline.

tebral bodies above or below and have been described as having a "wasp-waist" appearance.[20] The spinal canal is usually normal in width; however, if the canal is enlarged, syringomyelia, hydromyelia, or Arnold-Chiari malformation must be ruled out.[21] Spina bifida occulta is frequently noted (45% of cases), whereas complete dysraphism rarely occurs.

Rudimentary disc spaces that occur at appropriate levels in the spine may be seen. In the young child, lateral flexion–extension views are helpful in diagnosing immobile areas of fusion in the partially ossified spine, whereas in the older patient these views are essential in diagnosing and in monitoring intersegmental vertebral instability (Fig. 5-29).

When multiple levels of vertebrae are fused, either alone or in combination with hemivertebrae, evaluation by routine radiography may become difficult. Rotational differences at various levels of a shortened cervical spine in conjunction with overlapping shadows from the mandible, occiput, or shoulder contribute to this difficulty (Fig. 5-30).[37] Anteroposterior and lateral flexion–extension tomography are helpful in detailing anatomic change at the occipitocervical junction and throughout the remainder of the cervical spine, and may demonstrate bony compromise of the spinal canal (Fig. 5-31). Cineradiography is a dynamic technique that allows precise positioning of the head and neck in order to evaluate axial rotation, lateral bending, and flexion–extension while avoiding the confusion of malrotation. An-

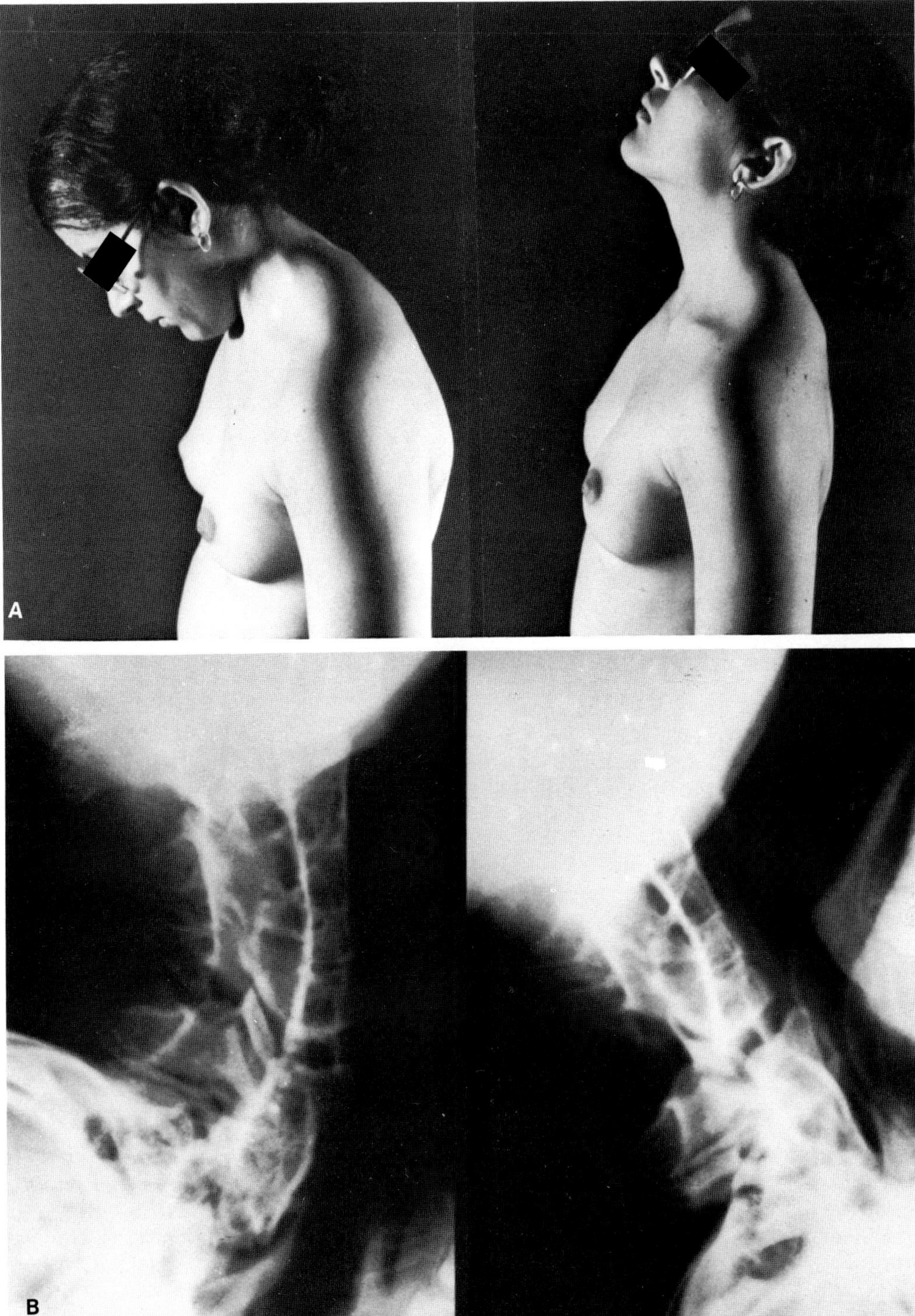

Fig. 5-26. (*A*) Clinical photographs and (*B*) lateral flexion–extension radiographs demonstrate apparent full flexion and extension through one open interspace.

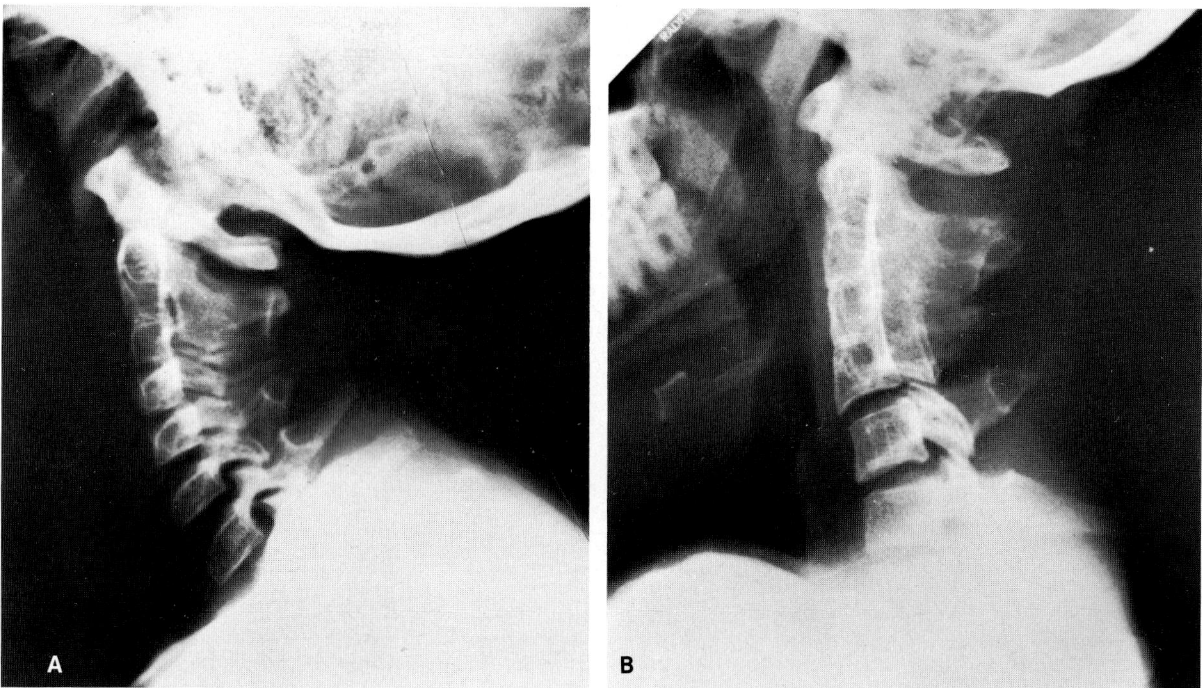

Fig. 5-27. (*A,B*) Obliteration of apparently normal disc spaces occurs with progressive ossification of the cervical spine.

terior gaping of a disc space or sudden translation of one vertebral body on another during cineradiography may indicate intersegmental instability but must be interpreted carefully in the young, because children under the age of 8 may display pseudosubluxation or sharp angulation at one interspace and yet be normal.[13] Anomalies of the brain stem, spinal cord, and bone at the occipitocervical junction, in addition to spinal stenosis, may be more critically evaluated by the use of the CT scan.

Osseous defects of the thorax, such as fused or deformed ribs, may be found when the lower cervical and upper thoracic spine are involved.[62] Anomalies of the thoracic spine noted on routine chest radiographs have served as clues to congenital changes in the cervical spine. Complete evaluation of congenital scoliosis requires a lateral radiograph of the cervical spine to rule out existing anomalies.

EMBRYOLOGY

During the first 3 weeks of life, the human blastema undergoes morphologic changes that result in the formation of a neural tube in close association with a ventrally situated notochord. The surrounding mesenchyme condenses to form a lateral column on either side of the neural tube. As development continues, the columns segment into 44 pairs of mesodermal somites that ultimately contribute to the formation of the base of the skull and to the cervical, thoracic, lumbar, sacral, and coccygeal vertebrae. While a number of the more caudal somites undergo cellular degeneration, the remaining somites differentiate into an outer dermatome, an inner myotome, and a medial sclerotome.[1] Each sclerotome develops a central cleft, the fissure of von Ebner, that divides a loose collection of cells cranially from a dense cellular area caudally. In the development of the normal spine, cells from the fissure of von Ebner migrate toward and encase the notochord to become the precursors of the intervertebral disc. The sclerotomes completely divide, and the stage of resegmentation concludes as the cranial half of one sclerotome migrates to unite with the caudal half of the adjacent sclerotome.[76]

No proven theory exists to explain the development of congenital fusion of cervical vertebrae. Similar changes have been produced in animals with teratogenic agents, but no corresponding hu-

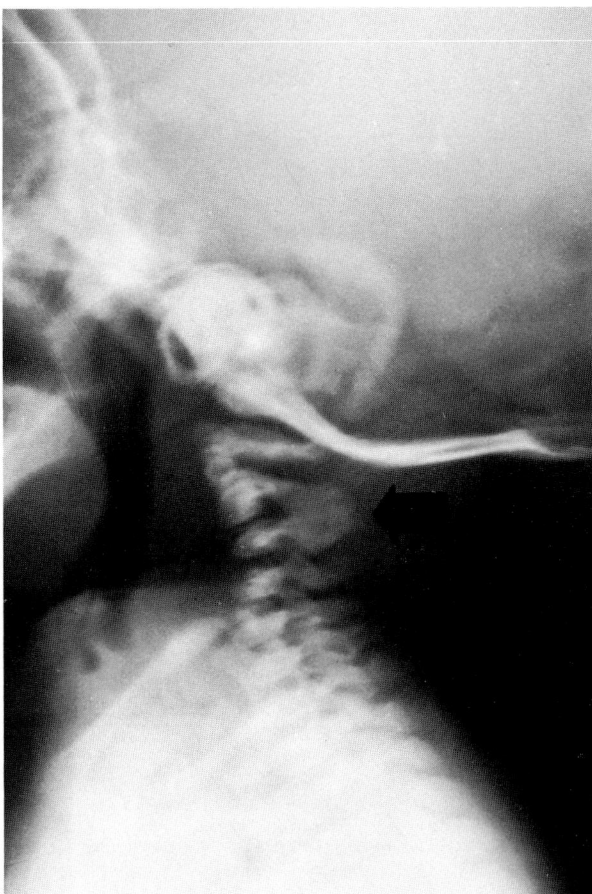

Fig. 5-28. Bony union of posterior elements of the spine may be seen at an early age and indicates congenital fusion of the anterior spinal elements.

man documentation exists. Gardner suggests that overdistention of the neural tube in the precartilaginous sclerotome stage may adversely influence notochord development and foster congenital fusion.[31] Others speculate that bilateral failure in the development of the fissure of von Ebner halts development of the spine prior to the stage of resegmentation.[76] The resultant vertebral bodies appear to be fused with primitive disc formation at appropriate levels, since normal somite segmentation had been completed. Recently, maternal alcoholism has been suggested as a significant factor in the production of the Klippel-Feil anomaly; however, supporting information is scant at present.[47,55] Although the exact nature of the insult to the embryo is not known, it seems to occur between the fourth and eighth weeks of fetal life.

A cross section of a 28- to 30-day human embryo at a lower cervical somite reveals marked proximity of the neural tube with paired dorsal aorta, pronephric ducts, upper limb buds, and developing mesonephros.[1,22] An insult at this time will not only affect the cervical spine but may also cause changes in the nearby developing organ systems that may be of serious consequence to the person's general health.

ASSOCIATED PROBLEMS

Numerous medical reports confirm that a variety of congenital problems have been associated with congenital fusion of the cervical vertebrae.[37, 54] Facial development has been involved, with cleft lip, cleft palate, high-arched palate, coloboma, ptosis of the eye, Duane's contracture of the lateral rectus muscle, lateral rectus palsy, and facial nerve palsy.[3,11,16,41,65,73] Deafness was first associated with this problem by Jalladeau in 1936, when he reported a 30% incidence of deafness in his group of 20 patients with Klippel-Feil syndrome.[39] In 1952, Wildervanck associated deafness with Klippel-Feil syndrome, abducens nerve palsy, and retraction of the eyeball (cervicooculoacoustic syndrome).[76] Several reports document conduction defects with ankylosis of the ossicles, foot-plate fixation, or absence of the external auditory canal, and other reports suggests a sensorineural deficit. There is no common anatomic lesion, and the hearing loss may be conductive, sensorineural, or mixed.[18,34,40,49,58,68,69] Evaluation of a patient with Klippel-Feil syndrome should include audiometric examination; early detection of hearing deficits in the young child may facilitate language development and eliminate the necessity of speech training at a later age.

Stapedectomy is not an uncommon surgical treatment for stapes foot-plate fixation. The stapes gusher is a serious complication of this procedure and arises from a congenital anomaly that links the subarachnoid and perilymphatic spaces. When the footplate is drilled, a sudden profuse cerebrospinal fluid flow occurs that causes immediate deafness and requires facial grafting for control. Two cases of stapes gusher occurred among 650 stapedectomies reported by Danilides and associates; one involved a patient with concomitant Klippel-Feil syndrome. Two other patients have been reported with Klippel-Feil syndrome and subarachnoid tympanic fistula, and both suffered from recurrent meningitis.[18,62] These serious complications require detailed evaluation of the Klippel-Feil patient with stapes fixation or recurrent meningitis.

Cardiovascular anomalies are associated with

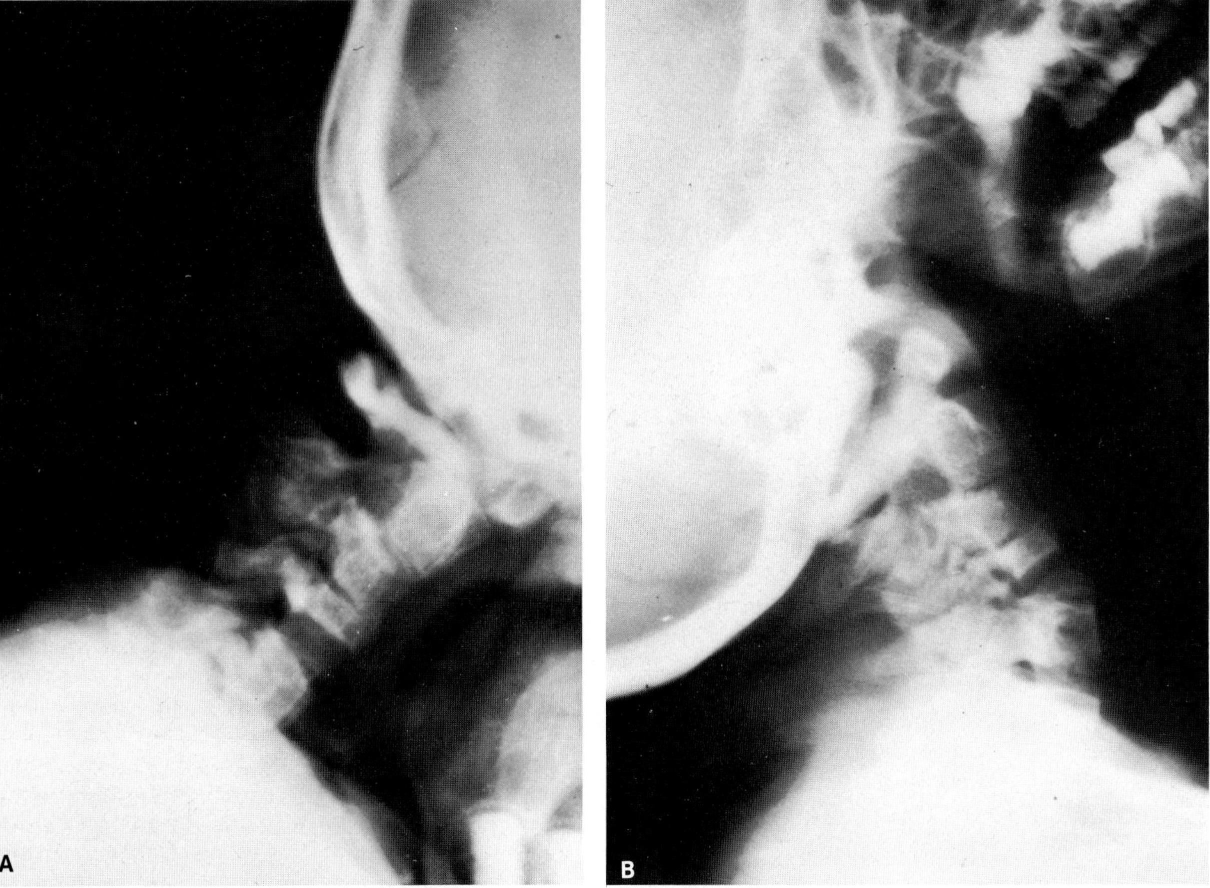

Fig. 5-29. Lateral flexion–extension radiographs are essential in diagnosing and monitoring intersegmental vertebral instability. (*A*) Flexion. (*B*) Extension.

this syndrome, with varying incidences. Gray's review of 418 patients with congenital fusion of the cervical spine noted 13 patients with cardiovascular anomalies; Nora reported five out of eight Klippel-Feil patients with cardiovascular problems.[34, 56] Ventricular septal defect, either alone or in combination with other defects, is the most frequent anomaly. Mitral insufficiency, coarctation of the aorta, right-sided aorta, patent ductus arteriosus, pulmonic stenosis, dextrocardia, atrial septal defect, truncus arteriosus, aplasia of the parietal pericardium, patent foramen ovale, single atrium, single ventricle, and bicuspid pulmonic valve have all been reported in association with the Klippel-Feil syndrome.[3,27,29,34,41,53,56]

Pulmonary complications involving failure of lobe formation, ectopic lungs, or "restrictive chest-cage" disease due to a shortened trunk, scoliosis, rib fusions, and deformed costovertebral joints have also been reported.[4,14] Furthermore, the brain stem may be involved, with intrinsic malformation, disturbance of cerebrospinal fluid dynamics, or extrinsic pressure through bony impingement or traction that may alter normal respiration.[44] These factors render the patient with Klippel-Feil syndrome more susceptible to neurologic or neurovascular injury whenever distraction forces are applied to the spine (*e.g.*, in the treatment of scoliosis) and require careful monitoring during this process.

Synkinesia, or mirror movement, is observed in the normal child, especially under the age of 5, and in 20% of patients with Klippel-Feil syndrome.[26,37] It is a disorder of motor control in which a voluntary motion of one limb is accompanied by a similar but involuntary motion of the opposite limb. The involuntary motion is usually less distinct and weaker than the voluntary motion

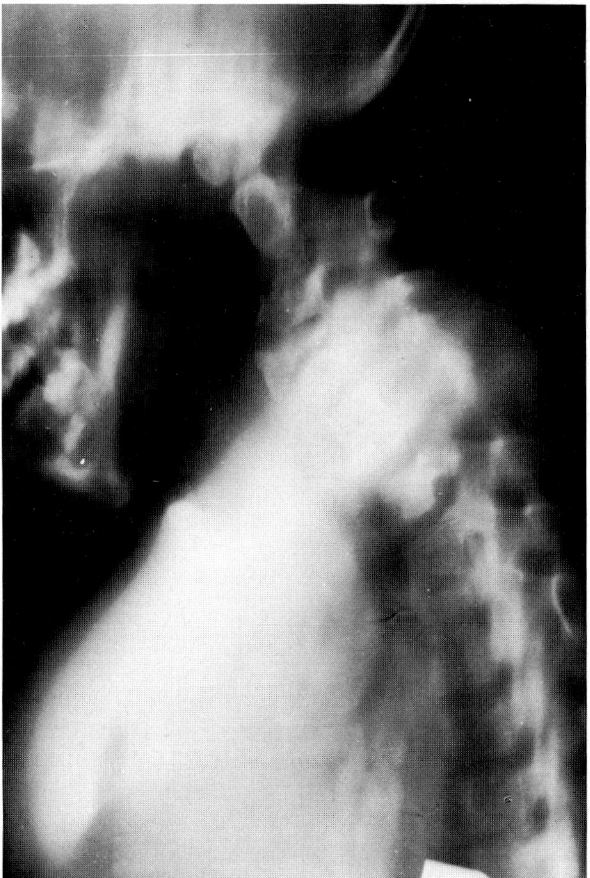

Fig. 5-30. Overlapping shadows from the mandible, occiput, or shoulder may preclude adequate evaluation of the cervical spine by routine radiography.

and has been observed in both the upper and lower extremities.[29,31] Mirror movements have been more frequently reported in the upper extremity and usually involve the hand rather than the arm. Discrete finger motions are a more sensitive indicator of synkinesia than gross pronation–supination of the forearm or flexion–extension of the elbow.

Synkinesia may be quite severe and may hamper bimanual activities, but it usually tends to become less obvious with increasing age, and is not clinically obvious beyond the second decade of life. Occupational therapy has been helpful in improving bimanual dexterity. Mirror movements have also been observed in patients with cerebral palsy, basilar impression, occipitalization of the atlas, and hemiparkinsonism, but in these conditions it tends to persist.

The association of synkinesia and the Klippel-Feil syndrome was first made by Bauman in 1932.[7] Autopsy reports of two patients with Klippel-Feil syndrome and synkinesia were published by Avery and Rentfro in 1936, and by Gunderson and Solitare in 1968.[2,36] No bony compromise of the cord was observed in either patient; however, both exhibited incomplete decussation of the pyramidal tracts in the upper cervical cord that anatomically could account for the mirror movements. Gunderson and Solitare suggest that incomplete decussation of the pyramidal tracts requires alternate and less specific extrapyramidal pathways to control motion in the upper limbs. The repetitive use of these secondary pathways may result in greater skill, which would explain the improvement seen in young children with time.[36] Electromyographic studies in patients with Klippel-Feil syndrome reveal electrical activity consistent with synkinesia even in patients in whom no clinical mirror motion is observed.[6,31,57] No physiologic mechanism for this phenomenon is yet known.

Urogenital anomalies have been observed in more than 30% of Klippel-Feil patients; the most common is unilateral absence of the kidney.[37,48,52] Other findings include absence of the hemitrigone, absence of both kidneys, absence of the ureter, hydronephrosis, ectopic kidney, horseshoe kidney, and congenital fusion of renal pelves in two distinct kidneys.[22,23,32,61,62] Genital anomalies most frequently involve female patients and include absent vagina, duplication of uterus, absent or rudimentary uterus, unilateral agenesis of the uterus, absent fallopian tube, and ovarian agenesis; male anomalies include small or undescended testes.[5,22,50,59] It is interesting that Joseph, Klippel and Feil's initial patient, died of nephritis and not of neurologic complications secondary to his massive congenital spinal involvement.

Embryologically, the urogenital system originates from the pronephric ducts that form from mesoderm in proximity to the somites destined to become the cervical spine. At 28 to 30 days of embryologic life, the pronephric ducts induce the formation of the mesonephros and ureteral buds, which will develop into the renal system. At 44 to 48 days, the pronephric ducts induce müllerian duct formation, which gives rise to the female ovaries, fallopian tubes, uterus, and vagina. An insult to the cervical somites between the fourth and eighth week of life could result in concomitant failure of resegmentation of sclerotomes and, through its effects on the pronephric ducts, either partial or total absence of the urogenital system. In one reported series, 14 of 167 female patients

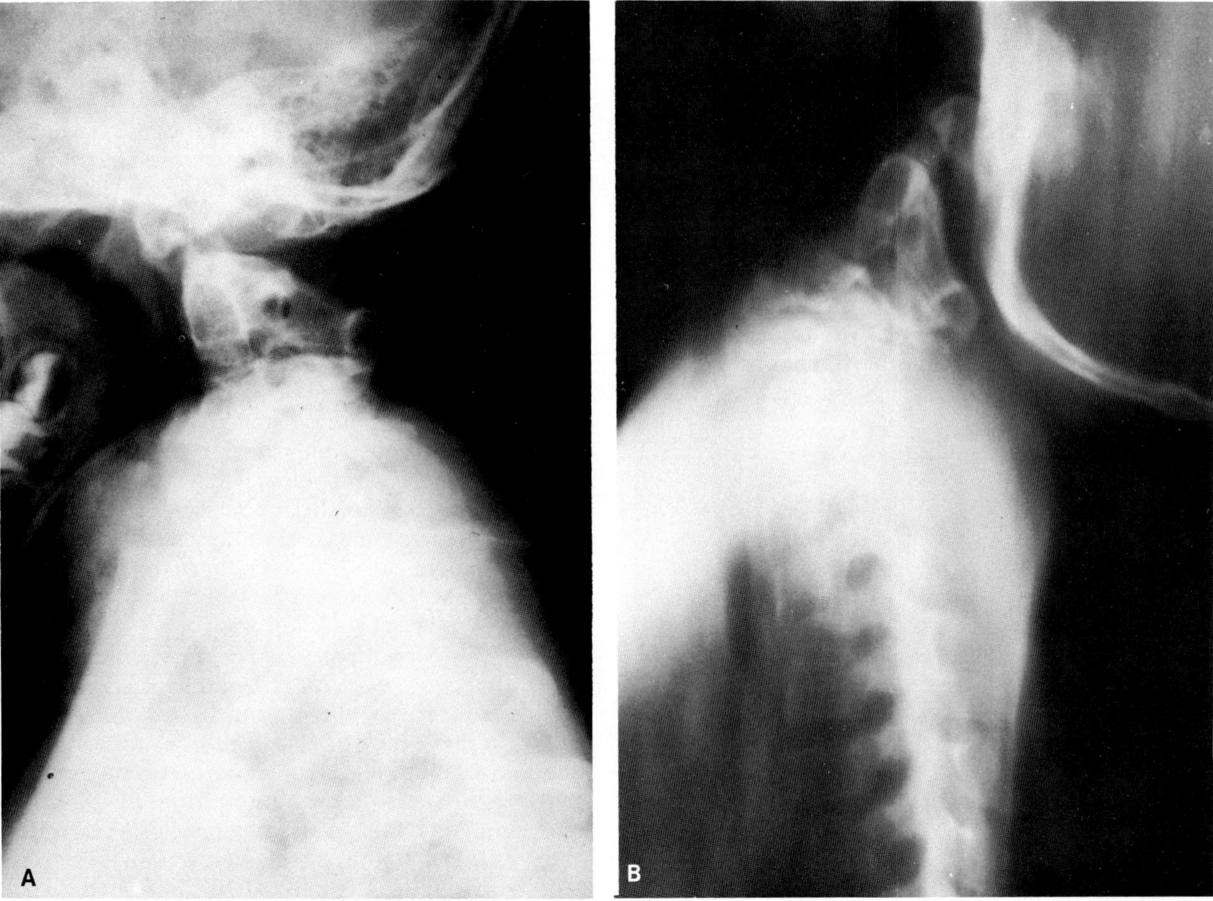

Fig. 5-31. Lateral flexion–extension tomography is helpful in detailing anatomic change at the occipitocervical junction and throughout the remainder of the cervical spine, and may demonstrate bony compromise of the spinal canal. (*A*) Flexion. (*B*) Extension.

(8%) with unilateral absence of the kidney and no cervical spine anomalies demonstrated unilateral or total absence of the uterus, while 9 of 10 females (90%) with unilateral absence of the kidneys and Klippel-Feil syndrome had no uterus.[22] The higher incidence of absent uterus and renal agenesis in patients with the Klippel-Feil syndrome emphasizes the significant risk of injury to the pronephric ducts, since both ureteral bud and müllerian duct induction require an intact pronephric duct system. Sprengel's deformity, deafness, and upper extremity anomalies were also reported in this group of patients.

Comprehensive evaluation of the patient with Klippel-Feil syndrome requires ultrasonic study of the renal system. If structural abnormality is detected, then intravenous pyelography is indicated for complete analysis. If unilateral renal agenesis is noted, then continued ultrasonic evaluation of the ovaries, fallopian tubes, and uterus should be pursued to rule out agenesis of these structures.

Abnormalities of the upper extremity occur in the form of syndactyly, hypoplasia of the thumb, absent thumb, hypoplasia of the thenar eminence, supernumerary digits, and absence of the ulna.[15,37,72] Sprengel's deformity, or congenital elevation of the scapula, has been reported in 20% of Klippel-Feil patients and may be unilateral or bilateral.[2,17,35,37,67-69] This is usually of cosmetic concern rather than a functional problem, although the range of motion of the shoulder may be significantly compromised, especially when an omovertebral bone fixes the scapula to the cervical spine. At 31 days of life, the mesodermal scapula is at the C4 level, and by 42 days it descends to a level below the first rib.[22] Again, the time of descent of the scapula coincides with the critical period in the development of the Klippel-Feil anomaly, and a single insult to the embryo at this time could reasonably be implicated in the production of both anomalies.

Scoliosis is the most commonly associated condition and has been noted in more than half of reported cases, either alone or in combination with kyphosis.[34, 37, 48, 52] Congenital changes may extend into the upper thoracic area or may exist anywhere along the thoracic and lumbar spine. Congenital scoliosis accounts for the majority of curvatures, but a second type of scoliosis, due to compensatory change in the structurally normal spine below the cervical anomaly or above and below the area of congenital scoliosis, also occurs. Focusing exclusively on the obvious congenital elements must be avoided if early changes in other areas of the spine are to be detected. Spinal orthoses may be successfully used to control truncal–pelvic alignment if curvatures are detected at an early stage. Unfortunately, many patients with this problem exhibit progressive curves that require stabilization.[37] When surgical intervention is indicated, the concern of neurologic compromise and malalignment that exists in the treatment of congenital scoliosis is compounded by the existence of anomalies and possible instability at the occipital–cervical junction and in the cervical spine.

NATURAL HISTORY

Children with congenital fusion of the cervical spine rarely develop neurologic problems or signs of instability. The lateral flexion–extension radiographs may reveal anterior gaping at an open interspace, but clinical evidence of a problem is not usually present. Occasional ill-defined pain complexes involving neck, shoulder, or chest pain may develop but are not accompanied by objective neurologic loss and usually require only symptomatic treatment. The most common age at onset of symptoms is between the second and third decades of life.[34,37] The literature reveals more than 90 cases of neurologic problems in association with the Klippel-Feil syndrome that develop as a consequence of occipitocervical anomalies, late instability, disc disease, or degenerative joint disease (Fig. 5-32). The reports include problems of cervical radiculopathy, spasticity, pain, quadriplegia, and even sudden death.[12,24,25,33,38,42,45,46,51,54,60,63-65,67,69,70,72] More than two thirds of these neurologically involved patients had single-level fusions of the upper cervical area, whereas many patients with extensive fusions of five to seven levels had no associated neurologic loss. This may relate to the excessive stress at the occipitoatlantal junction or the atlantoaxial junction in a spine with essentially normal motion, whereas the more involved spine may be protected by virtue of its marked limitation motion.

When two fused areas are separated by a single open interspace, the risk of excessive mobility and secondary degenerative changes at the open area must be considerable, even though review of the literature has yet to confirm this clinical concern. In patients with multiple short areas of fusion separated by more than one open interspace, the risks do not seem to be significant because of a more equitable distribution of stress in the cervical spine.

TREATMENT

The young patient with Klippel-Feil syndrome requires serial reevaluation with repeat lateral flexion–extension roentgenograms of the cervical spine to determine the development of instability at the occipital–cervical junction or at open intervals between fused areas. In addition, the remainder of the spine should be examined at frequent intervals during the growing phase for the development of scoliosis that may involve a congenital component or an idiopathic pattern. More immediate treatment objectives include evaluation to rule out associated system disease. A clinical evaluation of the cardiac system and electrocardiogram with chest roentgenogram are necessary to rule out congenital heart disease; ultrasound evaluation or intravenous pyelogram is required to evaluate urogenital anomalies; and audiometric evaluation should be accomplished to determine whether a hearing deficit exists. These tests should be part of the comprehensive evaluation of all patients with Klippel-Feil syndrome because of the high incidence of reported association.

In the more mature patient with Klippel-Feil syndrome, evaluation should center about the development of intersegmental instability of the cervical spine, degenerative disc disease, degenerative joint disease, and the development of radiculopathy. Pain complexes secondary to any of these problems may be relieved by conservative measures to quiet inflammatory changes; however, surgerical stabilization of degenerative and hypermobile levels may be required. The association of other axial anomalies, such as occipitalization of

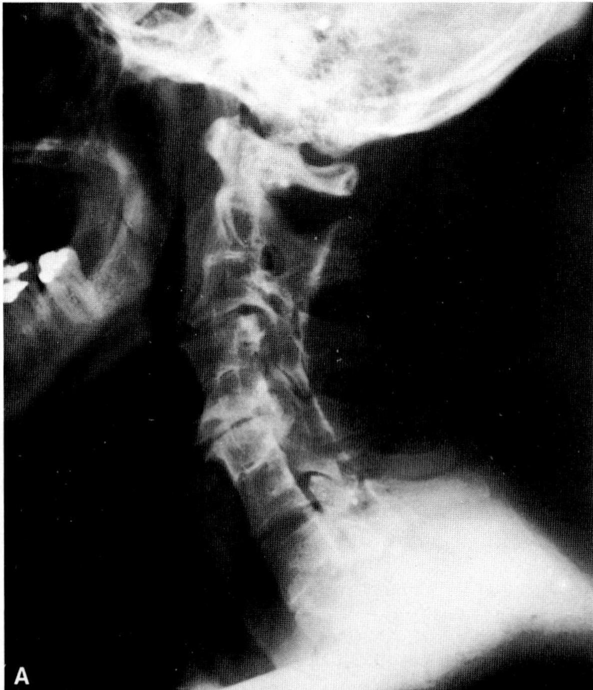

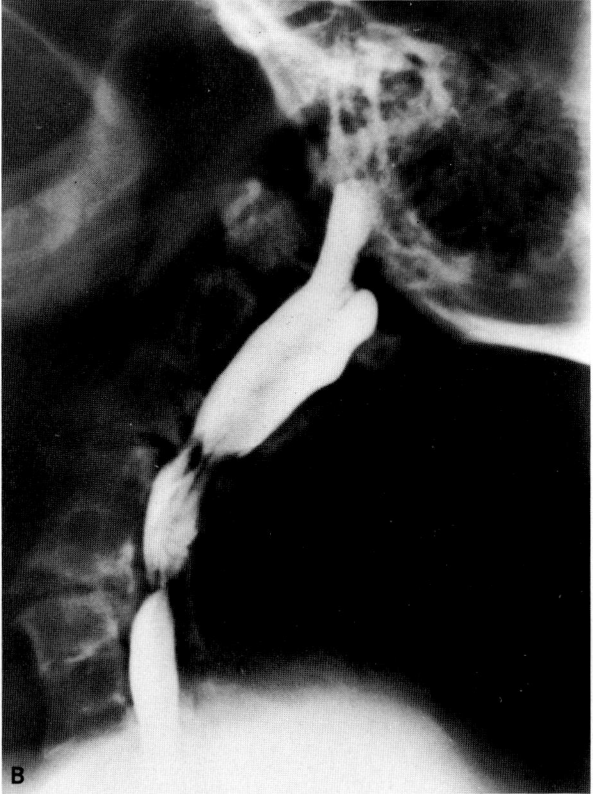

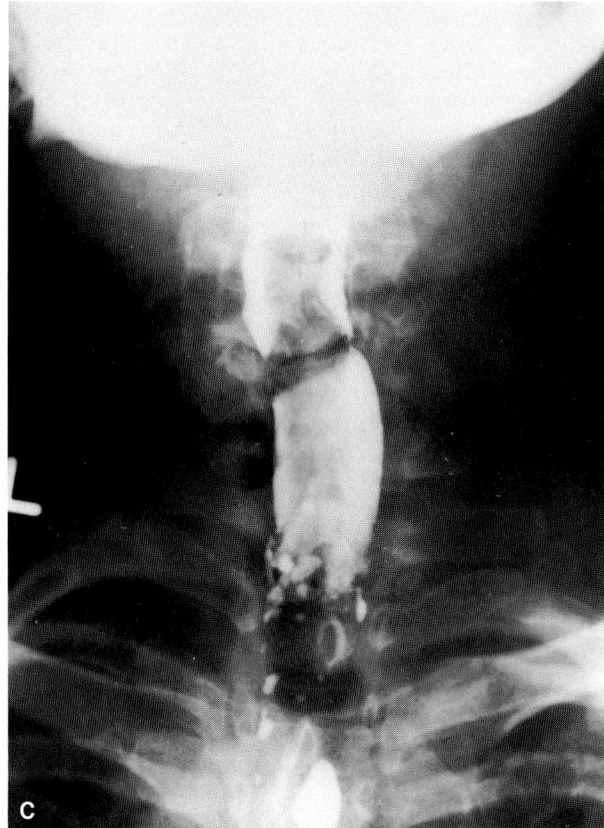

Fig. 5-32. (*A*) A lateral radiograph of the cervical spine and (*B*) a cervical myelogram of an adult patient with Kippel-Feil syndrome demonstrate degenerative disc disease, intersegmental instability, and osteophytic encroachment of the spinal canal.

the atlas and iniencephaly, should alert one to the existence of anomalies involving the brain stem and upper cervical cord.

The treatment of cosmetic problems has not been very successful because of fixed bony anomalies. Attempts to realign the cervical spine by osteotomy may result in neurologic catastrophe. Bracing of fixed torticollis has been reported but is not used extensively because of the need for long-term treatment and continued patient compliance. Bonola used resection of the upper ribs to cosmetically gain neck length; however, this was also at significant risk to the patient.[10] Surgical correction of Sprengel's deformity with resection of the omovertebral bone and realignment of the scapula may successfully improve neck cosmesis and function of the shoulder. In general, cosmetic surgery has not been commonly used in the Klippel-Feil patient because of the inherent high risks of neurologic compromise and because of the limited possible gains.

REFERENCES

1. *Arey LB:* Developmental Anatomy: A Textbook and Laboratory Manual of Embryology, 7th ed, pp 404-407. Philadelphia, WB Saunders, 1965
2. *Avery LW, Rentfro CC:* The Klippel-Feil syndrome: A pathologic report. Arch Neurol Psychol 36:1068, 1936
3. *Awan KJ:* Association of occular, cervical, and cardiac malformations. Ann Ophthamal 9:1001, 1977
4. *Baga N, Chusid EL, Miller A:* Pulmonary disability in the Klippel-Feil syndrome. Clin Orthop 67:105, 1969
5. *Baird PA, Lowry RB:* Absent vagina and the Klippel-Feil anomaly. Am J Obstet Gynecol 118:290, 1974
6. *Baird PA, Robinson CG, Buckler WSJ:* Klippel-Feil syndrome. A study of mirror movement detected by electromyography. Am J Dis Child 113:546, 1967
7. *Bauman GI:* Absence of the cervical spine. Klippel-Feil syndrome. JAMA 98:129, 1932
8. *Bertolotti M:* Le anomalie congenite del rachide cervicale. Chirurgia Degli Organi di Movimento 4:395, 1920
9. *Bertolotti M:* Gli uomini senza collo (Aplasia e fusione del rachide cervicale con spina bifida). Minerva Medica 41:481, 1950
10. *Bonola A:* Surgical treatment of the Klippel-Feil syndrome. J Bone Joint Surg 38B:440, 1956
11. *Brik M, Athayde A:* Bilateral Duane's syndrome, paroxysmal lacrimation and Klippel-Feil anomaly, Ophthalmologica 167:1, 1973
12. *Bucy PC, Ritchey H:* Klippel-Feil's syndrome associated with compression of the spinal cord by an extradural hemangiolipoma. J Neurosurg 4:476, 1947
13. *Cattell HS, Filtzer DL:* Pseudosubluxation and other normal variations in the cervical spine in children. J Bone Joint Surg 47A:1295, 1965
14. *Chaurasia BD, Singh MP:* Ectopic lungs in a human fetus with Klippel-Feil syndrome. Anat Anz 142:205, 1977
15. *Chemke J, Nisani R, Fischel RE:* Absent ulna in the Klippel-Feil syndrome: An unusual associated malformation. Clin Genet 17:167, 1980
16. *Cooper JC:* Klippel-Feil syndrome: A rare case of cervico-fascial deformity. Br Dent J 140:264, 1976
17. *Critchley M:* Sprengel's deformity with paraplegia. Br J Surg 14:243, 1926-1927
18. *Danilides J, Maganaris T, Dimitriadis A, Iliades T, Manolidis L:* Stapes gusher and Klippel-Feil syndrome. Laryngoscope 88:1178, 1978
19. *Dikshit SK, Agarwal SP, Gupta RC, Singh RS:* Klippel-Feil syndrome. Indian J Pediatr 36:245, 1969
20. *Dolan KD:* Developmental abnormalities of the cervical spine below the axis. Radiol Clin North Am 15:167, 1977
21. *Dolan KD:* Expanding lesions of the cervical canal. Radiol Clin North Am 15:203, 1977
22. *Duncan PA:* Embryologic pathogenesis of renal agenesis associated with cervical vertebral anomalies (Klippel-Feil phenotype). Birth Defects 8:91, 1977
23. *Duncan PA, Shapiro LR, Stangel JJ, Klein RM, Addonizio JC:* The Mircs Association: Müllerian duct aplasia, renal aplasia, and cervico-thoracic somite dysplasia. J Pediatr 95:399, 1979
24. *DuToit F:* A case of congenital elevation of the scapula (Sprengel's deformity) with defect of the cervical spine associated with syringomyelia. Brain 54:421, 1931
25. *Epstein JA, Carras R, Epstein BS, Levine LS:* Myelopathy and cervical spondylosis with vertebral subluxation and hyperlordosis. J Neurosurg 32:421, 1970
26. *Erskine CA:* An analysis of the Klippel-Feil syndrome. Arch Pathol 41:269, 1946
27. *Falk RH, MacKinnon J:* Klippel-Feil syndrome associated with aortic coarctation. Br Heart J 38:1220, 1976
28. *Feil A:* L'absence et la diminution des vertebres cervicales (etude clinique et pathogenique): Le syndrome de reduction numerique cervicale. Theses de Paris, 1919
29. *Ford FR:* Diseases of the Nervous System in Infancy, Childhood and Adolescence, 5th ed, pp 167–170. Springfield, IL, Charles C Thomas, 1966
30. *Frawley JM:* Congenital webbing. Am J Dis Child 29:799, 1925
31. *Gardner WJ:* Klippel-Feil syndrome, iniencephalus, anencephalus, hind-brain hernia, and mirror movements. Overdistention of the neural tube. Child's Brain 5:361, 1979
32. *Gehring GG, Shenasky JH:* Crossed fusion of renal pelves and Klippel-Feil syndrome. J Urol 116:103, 1976
33. *Giannini V, Paterno M:* Sindromi neurologiche associate o complicanti il morbo di Klippel-Feil. G Psichiat Neuropat 88:955, 1960
34. *Gray SW, Romaine CB, Skandalakis JE:* Congenital fusion of the cervical vertebrae. Surg Gynecol Obstet 118:373, 1964
35. *Gunderson CH, Greenspan RH, Glaser GH, Lubs HA:* Klippel-Feil syndrome: Genetic and clin-

ical reevaluation of cervical fusion. Medicine 46:491, 1967

36. *Gunderson CH, Solitare BH:* Mirror movements in patients with the Klippel-Feil syndrome: Neuropathic observations. Arch Neurol 18:675, 1968
37. *Hensinger RN, Lang JR, MacEwen GD:* Klippel-Feil syndrome: A constellation of associated anomalies. J Bone Joint Surg 56A:1246, 1974
38. *Illingsworth RS:* Attacks of unconsciousness in association with a fused cervical vertebrae. Arch Dis Child 31:8, 1956
39. *Jalladeau J:* Malformations congenitales associees au syndrome de Klippel-Feil. Theses de Paris, 1936
40. *Jarvis JF, Sellars SL:* Klippel-Feil deformity associated with congenital, conductive deafness. J Laryngol Otol 88:285, 1979
41. *Kauffman RL, McAllister WH, Ho C, Hartmann AF:* Familial studies in congenital heart disease. Birth Defects 8(5):82, 1973
42. *Kirkham TH:* Cervico-oculo acusticus syndrome with pseudopapilloedema. Arch Dis Child 44:504, 1969
43. *Klippel M, Feil A:* Un cas d'absence des vertebres cervicales avec cage thoracique remontant jusqu'a base du craine. Nouv Icon Salpetriere 25:223, 1912
44. *Krieger AJ, Rosomoff HL, Kuperman AS, Zingeresser LJ:* Occult respiratory dysfunction in a craniovertebral anomaly. J Neurosurg 31:15, 1969
45. *Lee ZK, Weiss AB:* Isolated congenital cervical lock vertebrae below the axis with neurological symptoms. Spine 6:118, 1981
46. *List CF:* Neurologic syndromes accompanying developmental anomalies of occipital bone, atlas and axis. Arch Neurol Psychiatr 45:577, 1941
47. *Lowry RB:* The Klippel-Feil anomalad as part of the fetal alcohol syndrome. Teratology 16:53, 1977
48. *MacEwen GD, Winter RB, Hardy JH:* Evaluation of kidney anomalies in congenital scoliosis. J Bone Joint Surg 54A:1451, 1972
49. *McLay K, Maran AGD:* Deafness and the Klippel-Feil syndrome. J Laryngol 83:175, 1969
50. *Mecklenburg RS, Krueger PM:* Extensive genitourinary anomalies associated with Klippel-Feil syndrome. Am J Dis Child 128:92, 1974
51. *Michie I, Clark M:* Neurological syndromes associated with cervical and craniocervical anomalies. Arch Neurol 18:241, 1968
52. *Moore WB, Matthews TJ, Rabinowitz R:* Genitourinary anomalies associated with Klippel-Feil syndrome. J Bone Joint Surg 57A:355, 1975
53. *Morrison SG, Perry LW, Scott LP:* Congenital brevicollis (Klippel-Feil syndrome) and cardiovascular anomalies. Am J Dis Child 115:614, 1968
54. *Mosberg WH Jr:* Klippel-Feil syndrome: Etiology and treatment of neurologic signs. J Nerv Ment Dis 117:479, 1953
55. *Neidengard L, Carter TE:* Klippel-Feil malformation complex in fetal alcohol syndrome. Am J Dis Child 132:929, 1978
56. *Nora JJ, Cohen M, Maxwell GM:* Klippel-Feil syndrome with congenital heart disease. Am J Dis Child 102:858, 1961
57. *Notermans SLH, Go KG, Boonstra S:* EMG studies of associated movements in a patient with Klippel-Feil syndrome. Psychiatr Neurol Neurochir 73:257, 1970
58. *Palant DI, Carter BL:* Klippel-Feil syndrome and deafness. Am J Dis Child 123:218, 1972
59. *Park IJ, Jones HW Jr:* A new syndrome in two unrelated females: Klippel-Feil deformity, conductive deafness and absent vagina. Birth Defects 311, 1971
60. *Peters JJ:* Two cases of Klippel-Feil syndrome associated with severe mental subnormality. Radiography 28:316, 1962
61. *Ramsey J, Bliznak J:* Klippel-Feil syndrome with renal agenesis and other anomalies. AJR 113:460, 1971
62. *Richards SH, Gibbin, KP:* Recurrent meningitis due to congenital fistula of stapedial foot plate. J Laryngol 91:1063, 1977
63. *Rinvik R:* A case of the Klippel-Feil syndrome. Acta Paediatr Iatr 31:417, 1944
64. *Sava GM, Gohn DF, Rothner AD:* Anterior decompression for progressive brainstem compression in the Klippel-Feil syndrome. Cleve Clin Q 45:325, 1978-1979
65. *Sherk HH, Dawoud S:* Congenital os odontoideum with Klippel-Feil anomaly and fatal atlantoaxial instability: Report of a case. Spine 6:42, 1981
66. *Sherk HH, Nicholson JT;* Cervico-oculo-acusticus syndrome. J Bone Joint Surg 54A:1776, 1972
67. *Sherk HH, Shut L, Chung S:* Iniencephalic deformity of the cervical spine with Klippel-Feil anomalies and cogenital evaluation of the scapula. J Bone Joint Surg 56A:1254, 1974
68. *Shoul MI, Ritvo MP:* Clinical and roentgenologic manifestations of the Klippel-Feil syndrome (congenital fusion of the cervical vertebrae, brevicollis): Report of eight additional cases and review of the literature. AJR 68:369, 1952
69. *Smith GE:* Significance of fusion of the atlas to the occipital bone and manifestations of occipital vertebrae. Br Med J 2:594, 1908
70. *Southwell RD, Reynolds AF, Badger VM, Sherman FC:* Klippel-Feil syndrome with cervical cord compression resulting from cervical subluxation in association with an omovertebral bone. Spine 5:480, 1980
71. *Stark EW, Borton TE:* Hearing loss in the Klippel-Feil syndrome. Am J Dis Child 123:233, 1972

72. *STRAKX TE, BARAN E:* Traumatic quadriplegia associated with Klippel-Feil syndrome: Discussion and case reports. Arch Phys Med Rehabil 56:363, 1975

73. *THOMSON J:* A case of the Klippel-Feil syndrome. Arch Dis Child 12:127, 1937

74. *TURNER EL, SHOULDERS HS, SCOTT LD:* Klippel-Feil syndrome with unusual clinical manifestations. Am J Roentgenol Rad Therapy 40:43, 1938

75. *VON TORKLUS D, GEHLE W:* The Upper Cervical Spine, pp 38–43. New York, Grune & Stratton, 1972

76. *WILDERVANCK LS:* Klippel-Feil syndrome associated with abducens paralysis, bulbar retraction, and deaf-mutism: Case. Ned Tijdschr Geneeskd 96:2752, 1952

BIBLIOGRAPHY

Albright JA, Brand RA: The Scientific Basis of Orthopaedics, pp 51-58, New York, Appleton-Century-Crofts, 1979

Brown MW, Templeton AW, Hodges FJ III: The incidence of acquired and congenital fusion in the cervical spine. AJR 92:1255, 1964

Eisemann ML, Sharma GK: Wildervanck syndrome: Cervico-occulo-acoustic dysplasia. Otolaryngol Head Neck Surg 87:892, 1979

Forney WR, Robinson SJ, Pascoe DJ: Congenital heart disease, deafness, and skeletal malformations: A new syndrome? J Pediatr 68:14, 1966

Gupta M, Singh RN: The Klippel-Feil syndrome: A case report. Indian Pediatr 15:437, 1978

Juberg RC, Gershanik JJ: Cervical vertebral fusion (Klippel-Feil) syndrome with consanguineous parents. J Med Genet 13:246, 1976

Singh SP, Rock EH, Shulman A: Klippel-Feil syndrome with unexplained apparent conductive hearing loss: A case report. Laryngoscope 79:113, 1969

Zook EG, Salmon JH: Anomalies of the cervical spine in the cleft-palate patient: An operative danger. Plast Reconstr Surg 60:96, 1977

Risk Factors in Congenital Stenosis of the Cervical Spinal Canal

JOSEPH S. TORG

The purpose of this section is to define as a distinct clinical entity the phenomenon of cervical spinal stenosis with cord neurapraxia and transient quadriplegia.

Characteristically, the clinical picture involves an athlete who sustains an acute transient neurologic episode of cervical cord origin with sensory changes. The episode may be associated with motor paresis involving either both arms or both legs, or all four extremities following forced hyperextension, hyperflexion, or axial loading of the cervical spine.

Sensory changes include burning pain, numbness, tingling, or loss of sensation, while motor changes consist of weakness or complete paralysis. The episodes are transient; complete recovery usually occurs in 10 to 15 minutes, although in some cases gradual resolution does not occur for 36 to 48 hours. Except for burning paresthesia, neck pain is not present at the time of the injury. Motor function returns completely, along with full, pain-free cervical motion. Routine roentgenograms of the cervical spine show no evidence of fracture or dislocation.

On the basis of a retrospective review of 32 patients in whom an acute transient neurologic episode resulted from forced hyperextension, hyperflexion, or axial loading of the cervical spine, the following four questions have been answered:[26]

1. What factor or factors explain the neurologic picture, in the face of both benign roentgenograms and subsequent clinical course?
2. What was the incidence of cervical spinal cord neurapraxia during a collegiate football season?
3. Is the individual who experiences an episode of cervical spinal cord neurapraxia predisposed to permanent neurologic injury?
4. Are activity restrictions indicated for those who present this clinical picture?

The study group consisted of 32 athletes, nine of whom were either patients of or had been seen in consultation by the author. Records for the remaining 23 patients were obtained from the National Football Head and Neck Injury Registry.[25] The patients were all males, 15 to 32 years of age (mean age, 20 years). A group of 29 were injured while playing football, one while playing ice hockey and one while playing basketball. One was a professional boxer. Of the 29 patients who played football, four were professional, 16 were college, and nine were high school players. All had reported experiencing one or more episodes of cervical spinal cord neurapraxia. Clinical records and radiographic reports were reviewed in all cases. Clinical material was reviewed for information pertaining to a previous history of cervical spine injury; delineation of mechanism of injury; extent of either motor or sensory involvement, or both; duration of neurologic signs and symptoms; presence and character of pain; roentgenographic evaluation; range of cervical spine motion; treatment; recovery pattern; subsequent activity restriction; and history of recurrence of cervical spinal cord neurapraxia.

Lateral cervical spine roentgenograms available for 24 patients were reviewed for congenital anomalies, instability, disc disease, and spinal stenosis. Measurements to determine spinal stenosis were made at the level of C3 through C6 on the lateral view of the cervical spine. The presence of spinal stenosis was determined by two methods. The first was the standard method in which the sagittal spinal canal diameter is determined from the midpoint of the posterior aspect of the vertebral body to the nearest point of the corresponding spinolaminar line.[2,12,15,19,27,29] The second was devised by Pavlov and is called the ratio method.[26] The ratio method compares the sagittal spinal cord diameter measured, as described, to the anteroposterior width of the vertebral body measurement through the midpoint (Fig. 5-33). Lateral cervical spine roentgenograms of 49 males of similar age but without neurologic complaints were used as a control group, and measurements for spinal stenosis were performed at the C3 through C6 level by both the standard and ratio methods.

In an attempt to establish whether or not individuals experiencing one or more episodes of transient cervical spinal cord neurapraxia were predisposed to permanent neurologic injury, a mail and telephone survey was conducted of all known patients with permanent quadriplegia listed with the National Football Head and Neck Injury Registry[25] to ascertain whether or not they had experienced prodromal neurologic symptoms. Also, the Registry listings were cross checked with all of the subjects in the study group to determine

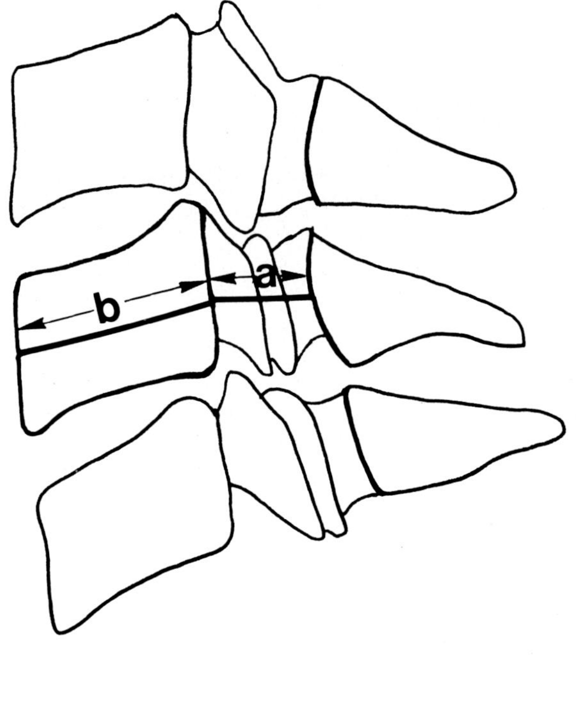

$$\text{ratio} = \frac{a}{b}$$

Fig. 5-33. The spinal canal – to – vertebral body ratio is the distance from the midpoint of the posterior aspect of the vertebral body to the nearest point on the corresponding spinolaminar line (*A*) divided by the A–P width of the vertebral body (*B*). (Torg JS, Pavlov H, Genuario SE, et al: Neurapraxia of the cervical spinal cord with transient quadriplegia. J Bone Joint Surg 68A:1354–1370, 1986)

whether any of them had subsequently sustained any permanent neurologic injury.

In order to ascertain the nature and incidence of cervical spinal cord neurapraxia during the 1984 football season, a mail survey of 503 schools participating in National Collegiate Athletic Association football (Divisions I to III) was conducted.

Evaluation of the medical records, including radiographic reports in all 32 patients and lateral cervical spine roentgenograms, which were available for review in 24 of the patients, revealed that the 32 individuals in this group who sustained cervical spinal cord neurapraxia could be subdivided into the following four subgroups; none of these patients had "normal" cervical spines.

DEVELOPMENTAL STENOSIS

Seventeen of the subjects had roentgenographic evidence of developmental stenosis of the spinal canal (Fig. 5-34). In this group the mechanism of injury was hyperflexion in five patients, hyperextension in eight patients, and axial loading in four patients. All 17 had experienced sensory manifestations; 11 had experienced paralysis, three weakness in four extremities, one weakness in both lower extremities, and two no motor involvement.

LIGAMENTOUS INSTABILITY

Four patients had roentgenographic evidence of ligamentous instability: one between C1 and C2 (Fig. 5-35), one between C2 and C3, and two between C5 and C6 (Fig. 5-36). In three patients the initial insult was reported to result from axial loading of the spine. One case followed a hyperextension injury. However, in one younger patient with instability between C5 and C6, the symptoms followed a hyperflexion injury. Two of the patients in this group had paralysis of all four extremities, while two had no motor impairment. All four had sensory manifestations, one having upper extremity paresthesias and the remainder having involvement in all four extremities.

INTERVERTEBRAL DISC DISEASE

Intervertebral disc disease was demonstrated in six patients, one having a myelogram (Fig. 5-37) and another a magnetic resonance imaging scan compatible with an acute disc herniation (see Fig. 5-44) while the remaining four had chronic changes manifested by intervertebral disc-space narrowing and posterior osteophyte formation (Fig. 5-38). Both subjects with acute disc herniation had a stenotic canal at the involved level. Axial loading of the spine was the mechanism identified in two patients, hyperflexion in one, and hyperextension in the remaining three. Five of the six subjects had motor paralysis, one had weakness in four extremities, and five had sensory manifestations in all four extremities, while one had bilateral upper extremity sensory manifestations only.

CONGENITAL CERVICAL ANOMALIES

There were five patients with congenital cervical anomalies. Two patients had failure of segmentation involving C2 and C3 (Fig. 5-39), one involving C3 and C4 (Fig. 5-40), and one involving C2, C3, and C4 (Fig. 5-41). The fifth patient had marked

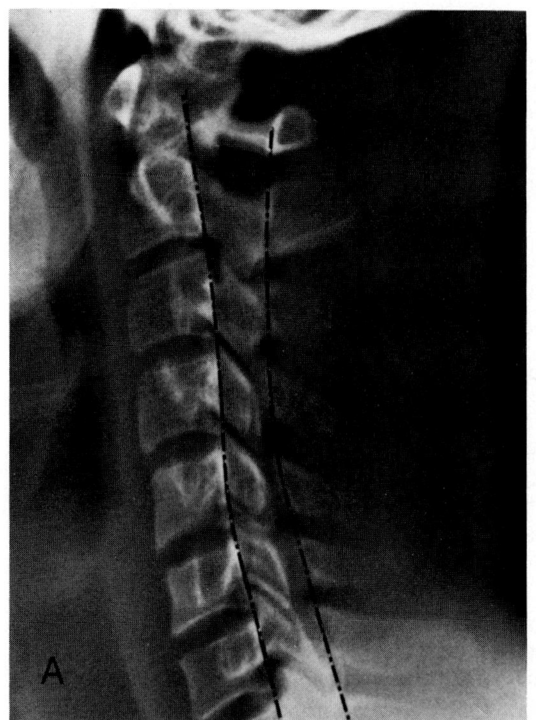

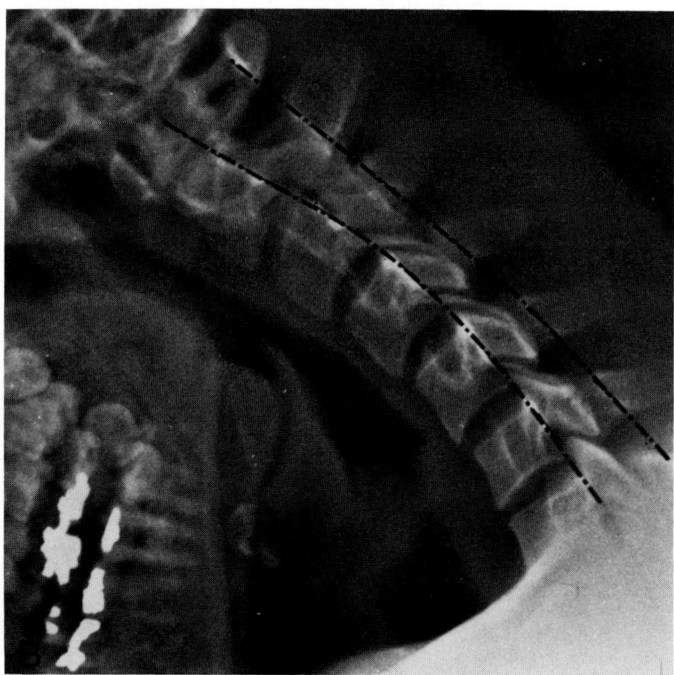

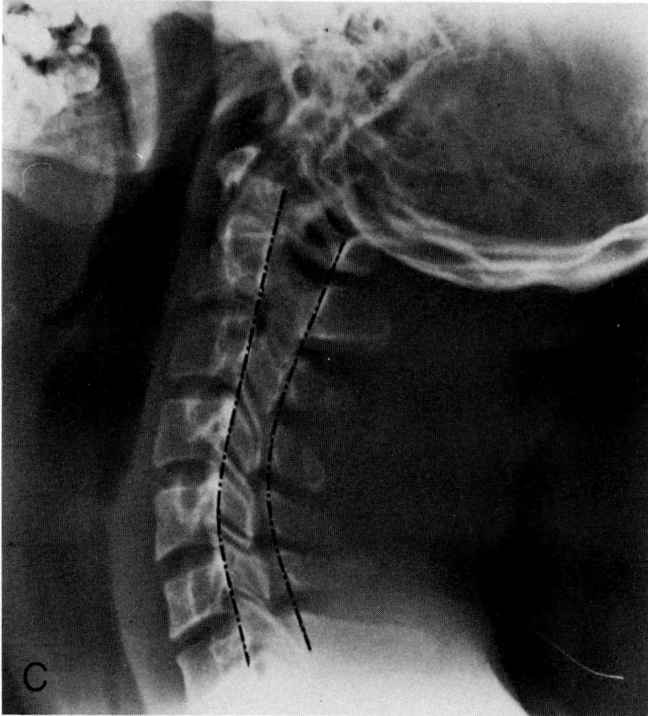

Fig. 5-34. The anterior and posterior aspect of the spinal canal are demarcated. There is marked narrowing of the sagittal diameter at the level of C3 and C4 on the (*A*) neutral, (*B*) flexion, and (*C*) extension views. (Torg JS, Pavlov H, Genuario SE, et al: Neurapraxia of the cervical spinal cord with transient quadriplegia. J Bone Joint Surg 68A:1354–1370, 1986)

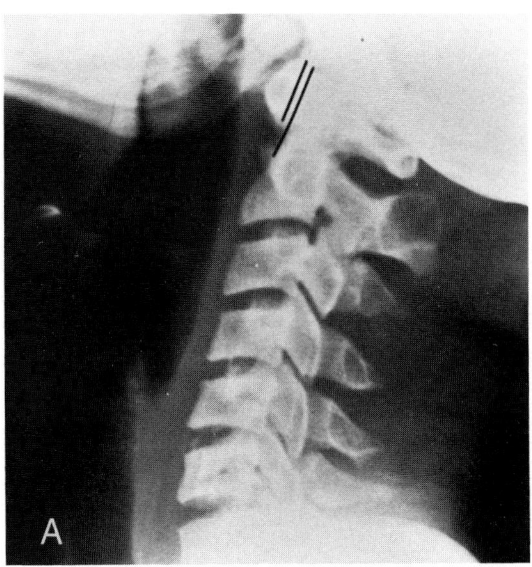

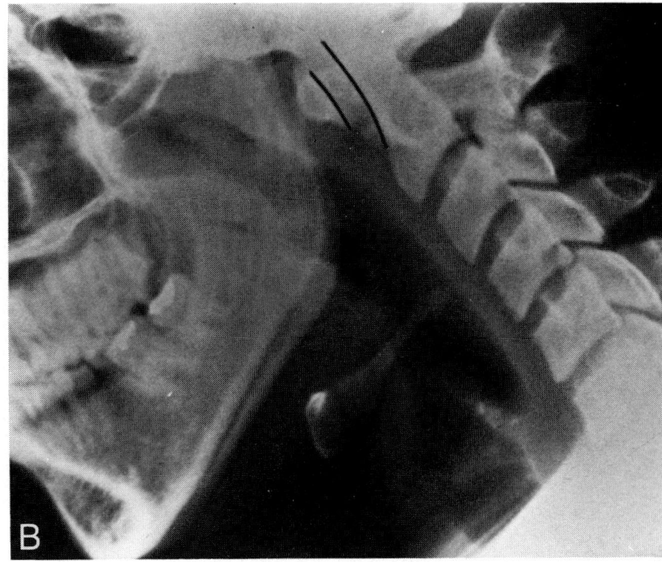

Fig. 5-35. Atlantoaxial subluxation. (*A*) In neutral position, the ADI (atlantodens interval) measures within the normal limits of 2.5 mm between the posterior aspect of the anterior arch of C1 and the anterior aspect of the odontoid. (*B*) In flexion, the ADI increases beyond the normal limits indicating an atlantoaxial subluxation. (Torg JS, Pavlov H, Genuario SE, et al: Neurapraxia of the cervical spinal cord with transient quadriplegia. J Bone Joint Surg 68A:1354–1370, 1986)

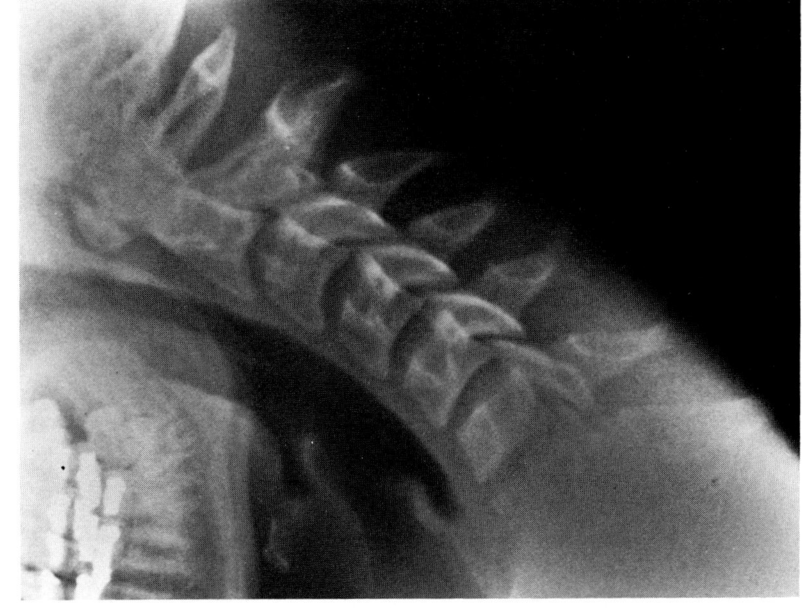

Fig. 5-36. Lateral view of the cervical spine in flexion demonstrates instability and laxity of the posterior ligamentous complex at C5–C6. Laxity is identified by a "fanning" or increase in the intraspinous distance, loss of parallelism between the facet joints on the lateral view (the inferior aspects of the apophyseal joints diverge, as opposed to being parallel), widening of the posterior aspect of the intervertebral disc space and narrowing the anterior intervertebral disc space at this level. There is no evidence of anterior subluxation. (Torg JS, Pavlov H, Genuario SE, et al: Neuropraxia of the cervical spinal cord with transient quadriplegia. J Bone Joint Surg 68A:1354–1370, 1986)

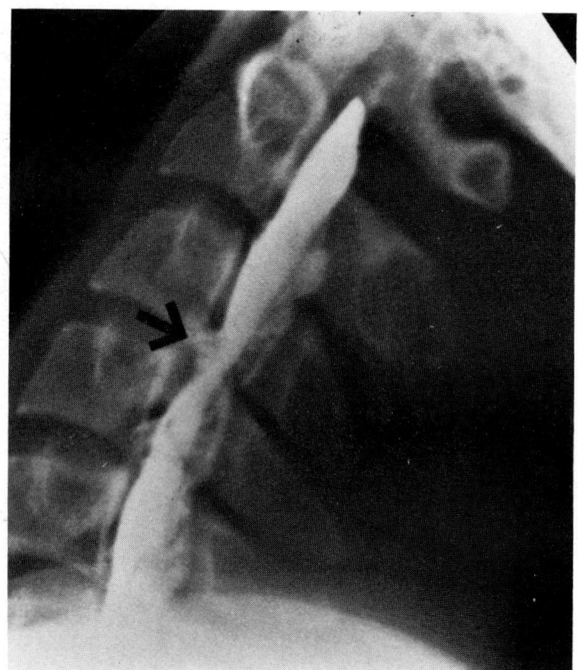

Fig. 5-37. Lateral view obtained during myelography demonstrates an anterior extradural defect at the C3–C4 intervertebral disc space consistent with a herniated nucleus pulposus. (Torg JS, Pavlov H, Genuario SE, et al: Neurapraxia of the cervical spinal cord with transient quadriplegia. J Bone Joint Surg 68A:1354–1370, 1986)

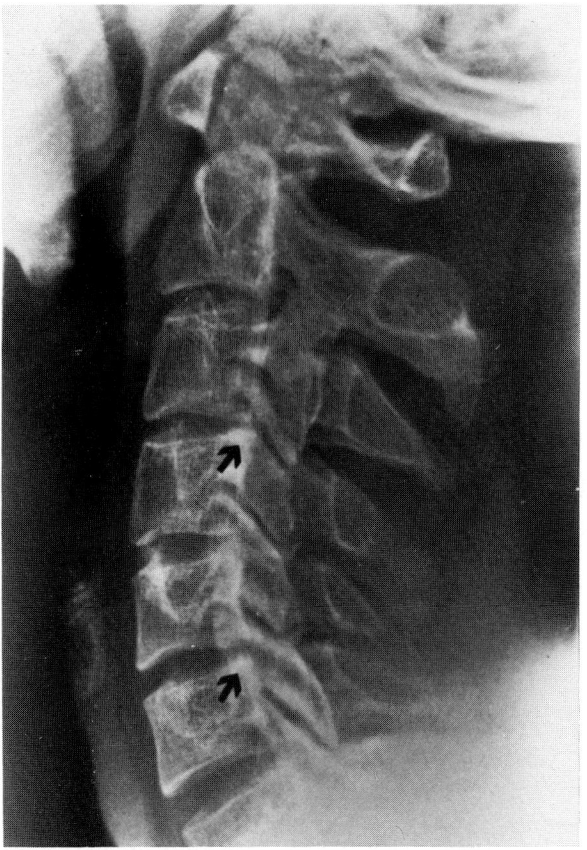

Fig. 5-38. There are small hypertrophic spurs and sclerosis in the posterior corner of C4 and C6. The intervertebral disc spaces are narrowed at these locations, and the spurs extend beyond the posterior border of the vertebral bodies, decreasing the sagittal diameter of the spinal canal. (Torg JS, Pavlov H, Genuario SE, et al: Neurapraxia of the cervical spinal cord with transient quadriplegia. J Bone Joint Surg 68A:1354–1370, 1986)

proliferative changes of the anterior aspect of C4, C5, and C6 characteristic of diffuse idiopathic skeletal hyperostosis (Fig. 5-42).[21] Hyperextension was the precipitating mechanism in all five cases. Sensory manifestations consisted of burning pain, numbness, and paresthesias, which were limited to the upper extremity in four patients and were present in all four extremities in one patient. One patient had weakness in the upper extremities, and one had paralysis of all four extremities. Three patients had no motor involvement.

For statistical purposes, the controls and the 24 individuals in the patient group in which lateral views of the cervical spine were available for review were divided into the following subgroups:

Group A—Controls, N = 49
Group B—Developmental spinal stenosis, N = 12
Group C—Instability, disc disease, congenital anomalies, N = 12
Group D—Entire patient group, N = 24

The sagittal spinal canal diameter (Table 5-1) and the spinal canal: vertebral ratio (Table 5-2) was statistically analyzed at the level of C3 through C6. The Mann-Whitney test was used to compare each subgroup with the controls and the entire patient group with the controls. There was statistically significant spinal stenosis in both subgroups B and C and in the entire patient group D, as compared with the control Group A, by both the standard and the ratio methods at all levels.

In a telephone survey of 223 known patients with quadriplegia listed with the National Football Head and Neck Injury Registry, 117 individuals were contacted personally. None of these patients recalled any episodes of transient motor paresis

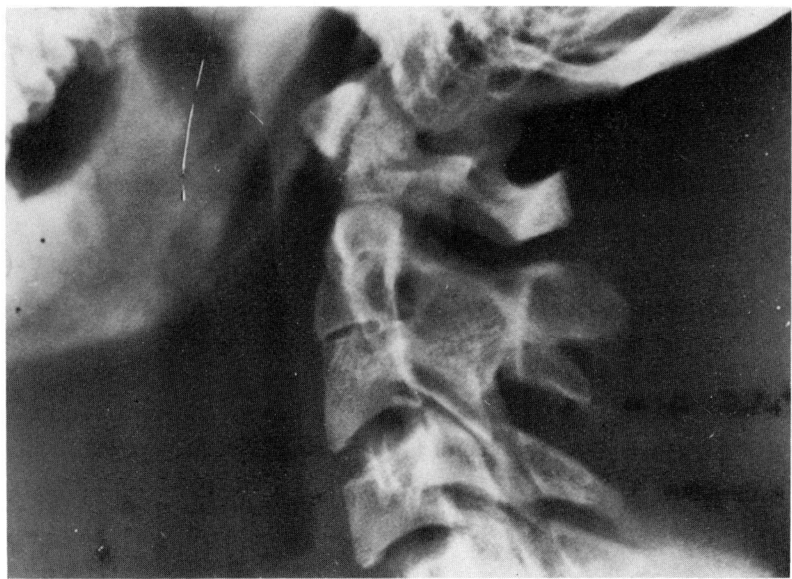

Fig. 5-39. Lateral view of the upper cervical spine demonstrates a congenital fusion between the apophyseal joints at C2 and C3 and a partial interbody fusion between C2 and C3, especially posteriorly. The intervertebral disc space is markedly reduced and obliterated in the posterior aspect. (Torg JS, Pavlov H, Genuario SE, et al: Neurapraxia of the cervical spinal cord with transient quadriplegia. J Bone Joint Surg 68A:1354–1370, 1986)

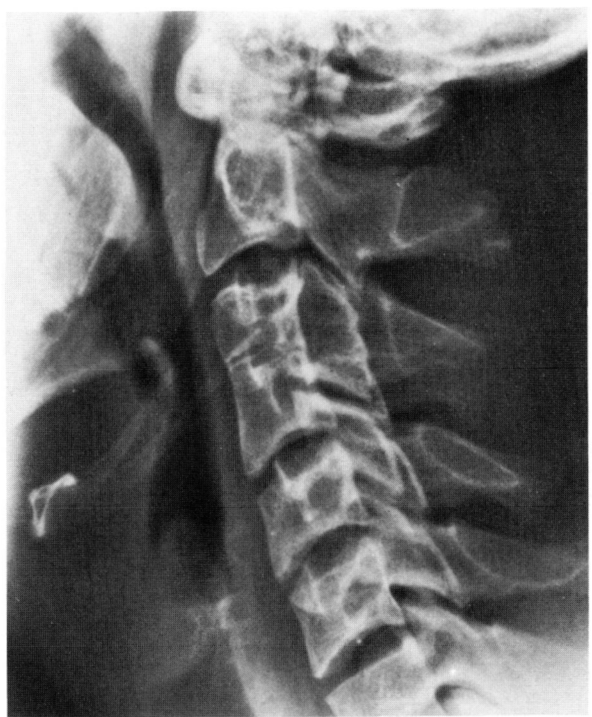

Fig. 5-40. Congenital anterior interbody fusion between C3 and C4 is shown with almost complete obliteration of the intervertebral disc space and with apophyseal joint fusion. (Torg JS, Pavlov H, Genuario SE, et al: Neurapraxia of the cervical spinal cord with transient quadriplegia. J Bone Joint Surg 68A:1354–1370, 1986)

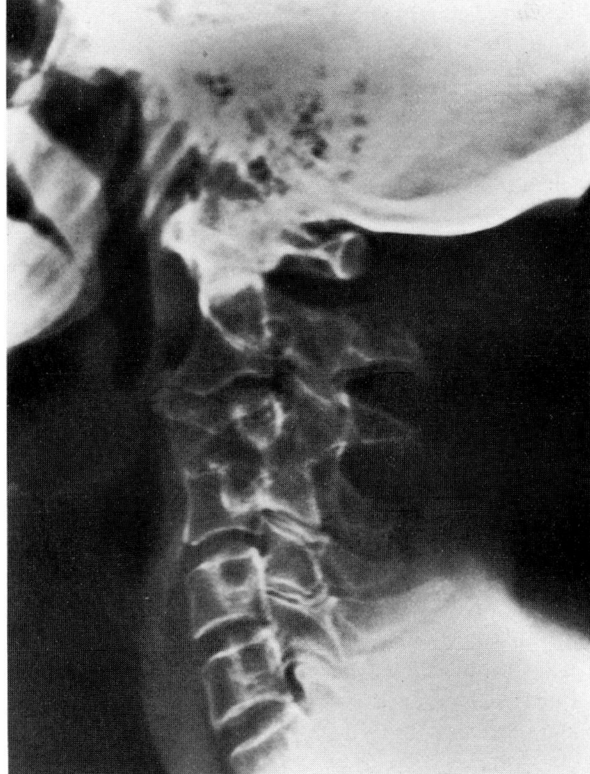

Fig. 5-41. Malformations involving C2, C3, and C4, including congenital fusions at these levels. (Torg JS, Pavlov H, Genuario SE, et al: Neurapraxia of the cervical spinal cord with transient quadriplegia. J Bone Joint Surg 68A:1354–1370, 1986)

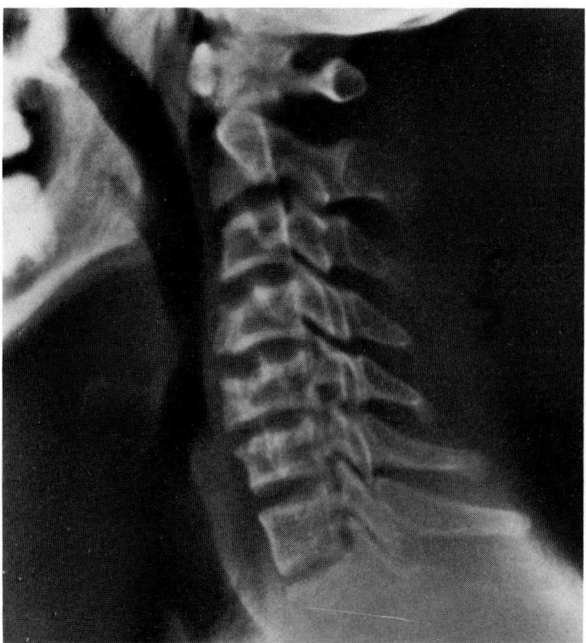

Fig. 5-42. Lateral roentgenogram demonstrates anterior proliferation changes involving C4, C5, and C6, with decreased A–P diameter of the spinal canal of these levels. (Torg JS, Pavlov H, Genuario SE, et al: Neurapraxia of the cervical spinal cord with transient quadriplegia. J Bone Joint Surg 68A:1354–1370, 1986)

prior to their permanent lesion. When asked about any sensory episodes, 115 said they had had none, one was equivocal but described unilateral numbness lasting for 1 minute, and one was positive with numbness and tingling involving all four extremities and lasting for 1 minute.

In an attempt to determine the nature and incidence of cervical spinal cord neurapraxia during the 1984 collegiate football season, a mail survey was conducted of the 503 National Collegiate Athletic Association schools participating in football. Of these, 344 schools (68%) responded, representing 39,377 football players. Two distinct groups were identified: Group I (N = 5) had experienced transient quadriplegia with paresthesia, while Group II (N = 24) had experienced transient paresthesia in either the upper or the lower extremities, or both.

Group I, which had experienced both transitory paresis and paresthesia, described classic examples of cervical spinal cord neurapraxia. Numbness was reported as lasting from 1 minute to 12 hours. Tingling in all four extremities persisted anywhere from 30 minutes to several weeks. Paralysis in this group ranged from 1 minute to 24 hours, with five subjects reporting quadriparesis. The incidence rate for Group I was 5 in 39,377 or 1.3 per 10,000 participants.

Group II reported only sensory involvement. Numbness and tingling was reported as lasting from 30 seconds to 48 hours. The sensory symptoms were confined to the upper extremities in the majority of patients, and only seven subjects reported paresthesia in all four extremities. The incidence rate for Group II was 24 in 39,377 or 6.0 per 10,000 participants.

An attempt was made to establish recurrence patterns in the 32 patients we studied. Of the 17 individuals with developmental cervical stenosis, nine did not attempt to return to their activity after the one episode. Three did return to football, had a second episode, and withdrew from the activity. One patient returned to football and, despite a second episode, continued to play without further problems at 3 years follow-up. Three individuals returned to football without any problems at 2 years follow-up. A professional boxer, who had a cervical laminectomy following two episodes of transient quadriplegia, continues to box and has had no further problems at 5 years follow-up.

Of the five patients with congenital fusion of the upper cervical spine, four withdrew from football after the one episode. One has continued to play collegiate ice hockey without a problem at 3 years follow-up.

Of the four individuals with cervical instability, two withdrew from football. One of the younger patients with ligamentous instability between C5 and C6 had three episodes of whole-body numbness precipitated by cervical spine hyperflexion while wrestling. He stopped wrestling and is asymptomatic at 2 years follow-up. One college player with instability between C5 and C6 was allowed to return to football with the use of a neck roll, and by keeping his head up while tackling. He has had no further problem at 1 year followup.

Three of the six patients with degenerative disc disease withdrew from football following the initial episode. A professional football player discontinued his activity after one recurrence and was lost to follow-up. Two patients with acute intervertebral disc herniation, one basketball player, and one football player underwent anterior discectomy and interbody fusion. Both are without recurrence; however, neither returned to his sport.

There is sparse documentation in the literature of the syndrome that we have described as cervical spinal cord neurapraxia. Grant and Puffer reported a case of quadriparesis that occurred in an 18-year-old football player with developmental

Table 5-1. Stastical Analysis of Sagittal Spinal Canal Diameter

LEVEL	GROUP	MEAN (MM)	SD	RANGE (MM)	N
C3	A: Controls	19.24	.188	13.7–23.5	49
	B: Stenosis	14.38*	.221	9.5–17.0	12
	C: Inst., HNP, Cong. Fus.	17.45§	.285	13.5–23.5	12
	D: Combined	15.92	.297	9.50–23.50	24
C4	A: Controls	18.56	.195	14.3–23.5	49
	B: Stenosis	14.17*	.221	9.0–17.0	12
	C: Inst., HNP, Cong. Fus.	16.67‡	.183	13.5–19.5	12
	D: Combined	15.42	.241	9.00–19.50	24
C5	A: Controls	18.71	.183	14.7–23.5	49
	B: Stenosis	13.50*	.218	8.5–17.0	12
	C: Inst., HNP, Cong. Fus.	16.25†	.187	13.0–19.0	12
	D: Combined	14.87*	.247	8.50–19.00	24
C6	A: Controls	19.03	.193	15.0–23.5	48
	B: Stenosis	14.13*	.206	10.0–17.0	12
	C: Inst., HNP, Cong. Fus.	15.59*	.219	12.0–18.5	11
	D: Combined	14.83*	.221	10.00–18.50	23

* $p < .0001$
† $p < .001$
‡ $p < .01$
§ $p < .05$
Inst. = Instability

Table 5-2. Statistical Analysis of Spinal Canal: Vertebral Body Ratio

LEVEL	GROUP	MEAN	SD	RANGE	N
C3	A: Controls	1.008	.118	.69–1.27	49
	B: Stenosis	.652	.143	.33–.81	12
	C: Inst., HNP, Cong. Fus.	.807*	.156	.591.18	12
	D: Combined	.730*	.166	.330–1.180	24
C4	A: Controls	.973	.110	.76–1.19	49
	B: Stenosis	.648*	.134	.32–.81	12
	C: Inst., HNP, Cong. Fus.	.764*	.061	.64–.86	12
	D: Combined	.707*	.118	.320–.860	24
C5	A: Controls	.975	.091	.80–1.17	49
	B: Stenosis	.637*	.116	.31–.770	12
	C: Inst., HNP, Cong. Fus.	.734*	.087	.57–.90	12
	D: Combined	.685*	.112	.310–.900	24
C6	A: Controls	.978	.104	.80–1.23	48
	B: Stenosis	.648*	.098	.36–.75	12
	C: Inst., HNP, Cong. Fus.	.686*	.090	.55–.85	11
	D: Combined	.665*	.094	.360–.850	23

* $p < .0001$
† $p < .001$
‡ $p < .01$
§ $p < .05$

cervical stenosis.[11] Stratford published an account of a professional football player who had a minimal transient neurologic deficit following a hyperextension injury to his cervical spine.[23] Funk and associates presented two cases of temporary quadriplegia occurring in football players.[10] One, who had suffered two episodes of generalized numbness and paralysis that lasted only a few seconds following hyperextension of his neck had reportedly normal roentgenograms, myelogram, and neurologic examination. The second, a professional player, was temporarily rendered quadriplegic following neck hyperflexion. Although cervical roentgenograms were negative for fracture, flexion views showed a definite forward shift of the first on the second cervical vertebra.

Payne and Spillane reported the association between developmental stenosis of the spinal canal and the development of myelopathy.[19] They recognized that a decrease in the sagittal diameter is further accentuated by encroachment of osteophytes, degenerative disc disease, or vertebral subluxation.

Moiel and coworkers subsequently reported on the significance of the congenitally narrow cervical canal in the absence of degenerative osteoarthritic changes.[15] They reported the case of an 18-year-old male involved in an automobile accident who developed a central cord syndrome caused by a hyperextension injury. This was associated with a congenitally narrow cervical spinal canal, which measured 13 mm at levels C4 through C6. Congenital stenosis associated with quadriplegia following trauma was reported by Countee and Vijayanathan and was found to occur primarily in black males with a cervical canal diameter of 14 mm or less.[7]

Narrowing of the sagittal diameter of the cervical spine may occur secondary to either a diffuse developmental condition or an acquired stenosis predicted on spondylolytic changes. Several investigators have observed that symptoms may be associated with both types of stenosis.[2,3,6,7,9,13,15,16,19,28,29]

Kessler has observed that the most critical radiographic measurement for cord compression in the cervical region is the sagittal diameter of the spinal canal.[14] He noted that values below 14 mm are uncommon and fall below standard deviations in any cervical segment.

Variations in the landmarks and methods used for determining the sagittal distance as well as different target distances used for obtaining the roentgenograms have resulted in inconsistencies in the "normal" values. The most commonly employed method for determining the sagittal canal diameter is to measure the distance between the middle of the posterior surface of the vertebral body to the nearest point of the spinolaminar line.[2,12,19,27,29] Using this technique, Boijsen reported that the average sagittal diameter of the spinal canal from the fourth to the sixth cervical vertebrae in 200 healthy subjects was 18.5 millimeters (14.2 to 23 mm). The target distance used was five feet. Wolf, Payne and Spillane, Moiel and other investigators,[3,13] reported an average diameter of 17 mm (± 5 mm) between C2 and C7, using a target distance of 6 feet. Countee reported that the normal average of the sagittal diameter of the cervical spinal canal averages 18.3 to 18.5 mm at the level of C3, and 17.8 mm between C4 and C7 using a target distance of 6 feet.[7] Narrowing of 14 mm or less at any cervical segment falls below two standard deviations from normal.[7] Epstein reported that the normal sagittal diameter for the midcervical canal from the floor to the spinal lamina line is normal if it is over 15 mm, and values less than 13 mm are significant, although he does not indicate exactly to what point on the spinolaminar line the measurement was taken.[8,9] Hinck evaluated the sagittal diameter of the cervical spine in children of ages 3 to 18 years and found the mean sagittal diameter at the level of the C3 to be 17.3 ± 1.4 (14.3 to 20.3 mm), at C4 to be 17.1 ± 1.3 (14.2 to 20 mm), and at C5 to be 16.7 ± 1.2 (13.9 to 19.4 mm), at a target distance of 5 feet.[14]

Wilkinson and associates measured the sagittal diameter of the cervical spinal canal by two methods.[28] The first method, the preexisting sagittal diameter, is similar to that described above and is the distance from the midposterior body of each vertebra to the midpoint (as opposed to the nearest point) of the corresponding lamina. The second is the absolute anteroposterior diameter, and it is the distance from the posterior aspect of the spondylotic spur to the closest point on the spinolaminar line at the particular interspace. The measurements were performed on four clinical subgroups: a group of patients with neck and arm pain but without neurologic symptoms, one group with radicular pain, one group with myelopathic symptoms, and a group with mixed symptoms. The preexisting sagittal diameter and absolute anteroposterior diameter values for patients in these groups were largest in those patients without radicular pain and smallest in the patients with mixed symptoms. Specifically, the average preexisting sagittal diameter range of values in these two groups were 17.1 to 14.3 mm for C3, 16.3 to 13.2 mm for C4, and 16.4 to 12.4 mm for C5. The average absolute anteroposterior diameter values were 15.5 to 12.5 mm between C3 and C4, 15.7 to 13.1 mm between C4 and C5, and 14.8 to 12.6 mm between C5 and C6, using a target distance of 6 feet.

Penning, emulating the work of Buetti-Bauml, measured the sagittal diameter of the cervical spinal canal as it is affected by flexion and extension.[5,20] These investigators measured the sagittal diameter of the spinal canal from the inferior portion of the superior vertebral body to the closest portion of the spinolaminar line of the inferior vertebrae. Penning called this the "pincers mechanism" (Fig. 5-43), in which the cord is pinched

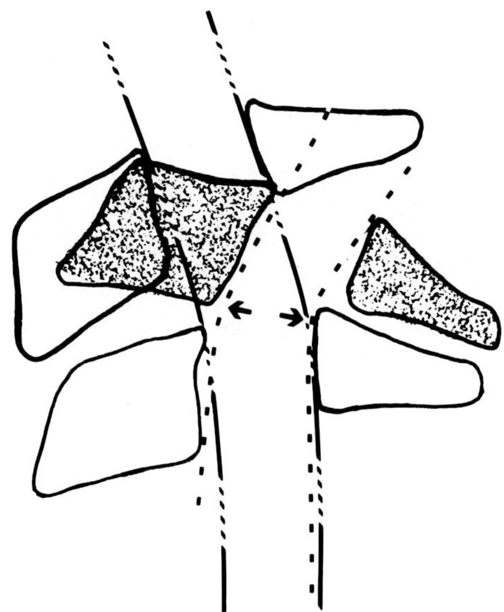

Fig. 5-43. The pincers mechanism as described by Penning occurs between the posterior inferior aspect of the vertebral body and the anterior superior aspect of the spinolaminar line of the subjacent vertebra. (Torg JS, Pavlov H, Genuario SE, et al: Neurapraxia of the cervical spinal cord with transient quadriplegia. J Bone Joint Surg 68A:1354–1370, 1986)

between the two opposing body processes. The degree of pinching of the spinal cord is dependent on the sagittal diameter of the spinal canal and the degree of extension. The degree of cord compression is compounded by the presence of spondylotic degenerative spurs. He noted that if the sagittal diameter is less than 11 mm in extension, there is a strong suspicion of spinal cord compression.

Symptomatic patients with spondylotic spurs generally have a cervical spine sagittal diameter smaller than the lower limits of normal.[16,18,19] Nugent reported preexisting sagittal diameter measurements of 14.7 mm in patients with spondylosis and absolute anteroposterior diameter measurements from the osteophyte spur to the spinolaminar line of 10.9 mm.[16] Payne reported sagittal diameter in symptomatic patients with spondylotic spurs to be 14 mm.

Patients with cervical spinal stenosis, either developmental or secondary to spondylosis and degenerative diseases, are especially at risk during hyperextension.[20] It has been noted that patients with hyperextension injuries have cervical sagittal diameters of less than average size.[1,16,17] Spinal cord compression during hyperextension has been reported by several investigators to result from the inward indentation of the ligamentum flavum, and Taylor has reported that infolding of the laminar ligaments during hyperextension can narrow the canal by 30% of its width.[8,9,18,19,20,21,23,28] In addition to the ligamentum flavum, hyperextension also causes the posterior longitudinal ligament and ligamentum flavum to thicken secondary to relaxation, the dural diameter to decrease in size, and the spinal cord diameter to increase in size as described by Breig.

The method most commonly referred to for determining the sagittal spinal diameter in the literature is the standard method. The ratio method for determining the sagittal spinal canal diameter devised by Torg and Pavlov[26] compares the standard measurement of the canal with the anteroposterior width of the vertebral body at the midpoint of the corresponding vertebral body. The actual millimeter measurement of the sagittal diameter as determined by the conventional method is misleading both as reported in the literature and in actual practice, owing to variations in the target distances used in obtaining the roentgenogram and the landmarks used for obtaining the measurement. Using the standard method, the actual millimeter measurements of the canals in our patients were occasionally within the "acceptable normal" range. Using the ratio method, the ratios were abnormal and indicated stenosis in all the patients. The ratio method compensates for variations in x-ray technique because the sagittal diameters of both the canal and vertebral body are affected similarly by magnification factors. The ratio method is independent of technique variations, and the results were statistically significant. Using the ratio method of determining the canal dimension, a spinal canal–to–vertebral body ratio of less than 0.80 is indicative of significant cervical spinal stenosis.

Evaluations of the lateral roentgenograms available for review in 24 of the 32 patients with cervical spinal cord neurapraxia reported here have revealed, when compared with a series of 49 controls, statistically significant decreases in the anteroposterior diameter of the spinal canal between C3 and C6 (Fig. 5-44). Because of the aforementioned variation in radiographic technique and differences in target distances, we believe that the ratio of the anteroposterior diameter of the spinal canal to the anteroposterior diameter of the vertebral body is the more reliable method of determining cervical spinal stenosis. Using this method, it has been demonstrated in all 23 patients that the ratio was less than 0.80 for those with developmental spinal stenosis, congenital fusions, post-

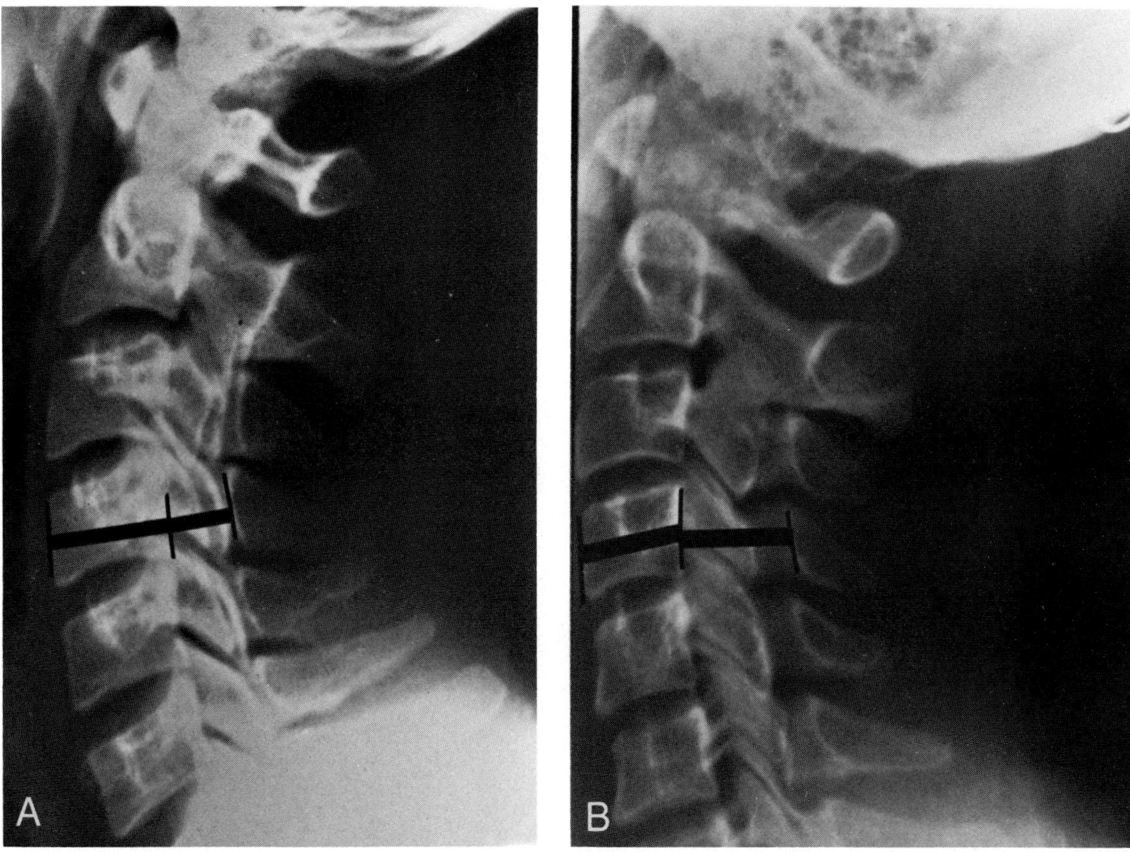

Fig. 5-44. Comparison between the spinal canal – to – vertebral body ratio of the stenotic (*A*) versus the control (*B*) patient is demonstrated on lateral views of the cervical spine. The spinal canal – to – vertebral body ratio is approximately 1:2 (.50) in the stenotic (*A*) patient compared with 1:1 (1.00) in the control (*B*) patient. (Torg JS, Pavlov H, Genuario SE, et al: Neurapraxia of the cervical spinal cord with transient quadriplegia. J Bone Joint Surg 68A:1354–1370, 1986)

traumatic instability, and acute and chronic degenerative changes, and that these were significantly different from the ratios in the control group (Fig. 5-44*A*). Specifically, the mean ratios for the control group from C3 through C6 were 0.98 or greater (Fig. 5-44*B*).

On the basis of these observations, we conclude that the factor identified that explains the described neurologic picture of cervical spinal cord neurapraxia is diminution of the anteroposterior diameter of the spinal canal, either as an isolated observation or associated with intervertebral disc herniation, degenerative changes, posttraumatic instability, or congenital anomalies. In instances of developmental cervical stenosis, forced hyperflexion, or hyperextension of the cervical spine, a further decrease in the caliber of an already stenotic canal occurs as explained by the pincer mechanism of Penning (Fig. 5-43). In patients with stenosis associated with osteophytes or a herniated disc, direct pressure can occur, again with the spine forced in the extremes of flexion or extension. This phenomenon of mechanical compression of the cervical cord with flexion is vividly demonstrated by a magnetic resonance imaging scan of one of our patients with an acute herniated pulposus at C3–C5 (Fig. 5-45). We further postulate that with an abrupt but brief decrease in the anteroposterior diameter of the spinal canal, the cervical spinal cord is mechanically compressed, causing transient interruption of either its motor or sensory function, or both, distal to the lesion. The neurologic aberration that results is transient and completely reversible.

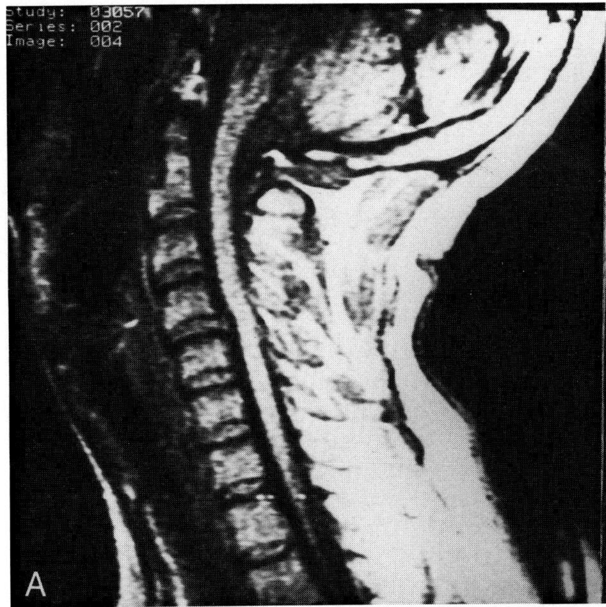

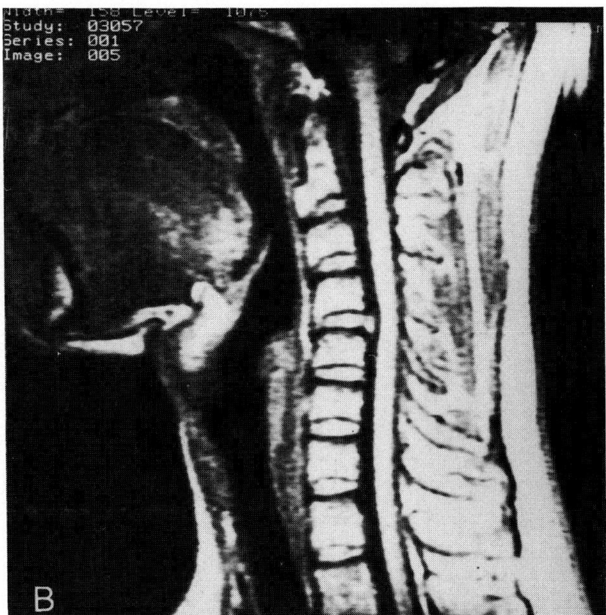

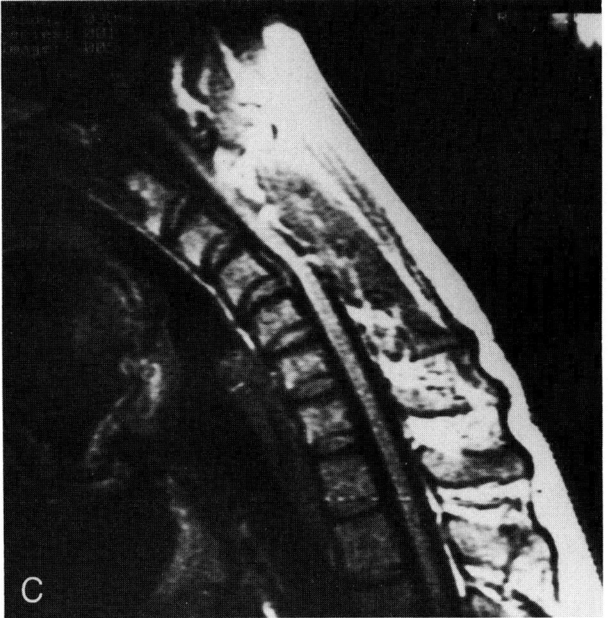

Fig. 5-45. (*A*) Magnetic resonance image of the midsagittal cervical spine of a 29-year-old recreational basketball player who experienced paresthesias and weakness in all four extremities following forced hyperflexion injury to his neck. In the neutral position, a herniated nucleus pulposus is observed to protrude posteriorly at the C4–C5 level. Note that the vertebral body – to – spinal canal ratio at the C4 level was 0.789, and at the C5 level was 0.750. On the basis of our data, these ratios indicate developmental spinal stenosis. (*B*) Magnetic resonance image of the same patient with mild flexion of the neck and cervical spine demonstrates the disc herniation with displacement of the posterior longitudinal ligament and compression of the cord with a decrease in its A–P diameter at the C4–C5 level. (*C*) Magnetic resonance image of this patient with a greater degree of neck flexion demonstrates further decrease in the A–P diameter of the cord due to compression or tenting over the herniated nucleus palposus. (*A, B,* and *C,* Torg JS, Pavlov H, Genuario SE, et al: Neurapraxia of the cervical spinal cord with transient quadriplegia. J Bone Joint Surg, 68A:1354–1370, 1986)

A review of the literature has revealed few reported cases of transient quadriplegia occurring in the athlete. Attempts to establish the occurrence rates indicate that the problem is more prevalent than expected. Specifically, in the population of 39,377 exposed participants, the reported incidence rate for transient paresthesia in all four extremities was 6 per 10,000, while the incidence rate reported for paresthesia associated with transient quadriplegia was 1.3 per 10,000 in the one football season surveyed. From these data we conclude that the prevalence of this problem is relatively high and that an awareness of the etiology, manifestations, and appropriate management principles is warranted.

Characteristically, following an episode of the

cervical spinal cord neurapraxia with or without transient quadriplegia, the first question raised concerns the advisability for activity restrictions. In an attempt to address this problem, we have interviewed 117 young athletes who sustained cervical spine injuries associated with complete permanent quadriplegia while playing football between the years 1971 and 1984. None of these patients recalled a prodomal experience of transient motor paresis. Conversely, none of the patients in this series who had experienced transient neurologic episodes subsequently sustained an injury that resulted in permanent neurologic injury. On the basis of these data, we conclude that the young patient who has had an episode of cervical spinal cord neurapraxia with or without transient quadriplegia is not predisposed to permanent neurologic injury because of it.

With regard to activity restrictions, no definite reoccurrence patterns have been identified to establish firm principles in this area. However, we believe that athletes who have this syndrome associated with demonstrable cervical spine instability or acute or chronic degenerative changes should not be allowed further participation in contact sports. Athletes with developmental spinal stenosis or spinal stenosis associated with congenital abnormalities should be treated on an individual basis. As indicated, of the six youngsters with obvious cervical stenosis who returned to football, three had a second episode and withdrew from the activity, and three returned without any problems at 2 years follow-up. Our data clearly indicate that those with developmental spinal stenosis are not predisposed to more severe injuries with associated permanent neurologic sequellae. However, in view of the apprehensions and demands placed on the responsible medical personnel, it appears that the most reasonable course of action is to exclude the individual from further participation.

REFERENCES

1. *Alexander E, Davis CH, Field CH:* Hyperextension injuries of the cervical spine. Arch Neurol Psychiatr 79:146–157, 1958
2. *Boijsen E:* Cervical spinal canal in intraspinal expansive processes. Acta Radiol 42:101–115, 1954
3. *Brain L Wilkinson M (eds):* Cervical Spondylolysis and Other Disorders of the Cervical Spine, 1st ed. Philadelphia, WB Saunders, 1967
4. *Breig A:* Biomechanics of the Central Nervous System. Stockholm, Almqvist and Wiksell, 1961
5. *Buetti- Bauml C:* Funktionelle Rontgendiagnostik der Halswirbelsaule. Stuttgart, Thieme, 1954
6. *Burrows EH:* The sagittal diameter of the spinal canal in cervical spondylolysis. Clin Radiol 17:77–86, 1963
7. *Countee RW, Vijayanathan T:* Congenital stenosis of the cervical spine: diagnosis and management. J Nat Med Assoc 71:257–264, 1979
8. *Epstein JA, Carras R, Epstein VS, Lavine LS:* Myelopathy in cervical spondylolysis with vertebral subluxation and hyperlordosis. J Neurol Surg 32:421, 1970
9. *Epstein VA, Epstein JA, Jones MD:* Cervical Spinal Stenosis. Radiol Clin North Am 15:215–281, 1977
10. *Funk FJ, Wells E:* Injuries of the cervical spine in football. Clin Orthop Rel Res 109:50–58, 1975
11. *Grant T, Puffer J:* Cervical stenosis: A developmental anomaly with quadriparesis during football. AM J Sports Med 4:219–221, 1976
12. *Hinck VC, Hopkins CE, Savara BS:* Sagittal diameter of the cervical spinal canal in children. Radiology 79:97–108, 1962
13. *Hinck VC, Sachdev NS:* Developmental stenosis of the cervical spinal canal. Brain 89:27–36, 1966
14. *Kessler JT:* Congenital narrowing of the cervical spinal canal. J Neurol Neurosurg Psychiatr 38:1218–1224, 1975
15. *Moiel RH, Raso E, Waltz TA:* Central cord syndrome resulting from congenital narrowing of the cervical canal. J Trauma 10:502–510, 1970
16. *Nugent GR:* Clinico-Pathologic Correlations in Cervical Spondylolysis. Neurology, 9:273–281, 1959
17. *Pallis C, Jones AM, Spillane JD:* Cervical spondylolysis: incidence and implications. Brain 77:274, 1954
18. *Payne EE:* The cervical spine and spondylolysis. Neurochirurgia 1:178–196, 1959
19. *Payne EE, Spillane JD:* The cervical spine: an anatomico-pathological study of 70 specimens (using special technique) with particular reference to problems of cervical spondylolysis. Brain 80:571–596, 1957
20. *Penning L:* Some aspects of plain radiography of the cervical spine in chronic myelopathy. Neurology 12:513–519, 1962
21. *Resnick D, Niwayama G:* Diffuse idiopathic skeletal hyperostosis (DISH) or ankylosing hyperostosis of Forestier and Rotes-Querol. In Resnick D, Niwayama G (eds): Diagnosis of Bone and Joint Disorders with Emphasis on Articular Abnormalities. pp 1416–1452. Philadelphia, WB Saunders, 1981
22. *Stoltmann HF, Blackward W:* The role of the ligamentum flavum in the pathogenesis of mye-

lopathy in cervical spondylolysis. Brain 87:45, 1974

23. *STRATFORD J:* Congenital Cervical Stenosis: A factor in myelopathy. Acta Neurochir 41(1–3):101–106, 1978
24. *TAYLOR AR:* The mechanism of injury to spinal cord in the neck without damage to the vertebral column. J Bone Joint Surg 33B:543–546, 1951
25. *TORG JS, VEGSO JJ, SENNETT B, DAS M:* The national football head and neck injury registry, 14-year report on cervical quadriplegia, 1971 through 1984. JAMA 254:3439–3443, 1985
26. *TORG JS, PAVLOV H, GENUARIO SE, ET AL:* Neurapraxia of the cervical spinal cord with transient quadriplegia. J Bone Joint Surg, 68A:1354–1370, 1986
27. *WELLS CE, SPILLANE JD, BLIGH AS:* The cervical spinal canal in syringomyelia. Brain 82:23–40, 1959
28. *WILKINSON HA, LEMAY ML, FERRIS EJ:* Roentgenographic correlation in cervical spondylolysis. AJR 105:370–374, 1969
29. *WOLF BS, KHILNANI M, MALIS L:* Sagittal diameter of the bony cervical canal and its significance in cervical spondylolysis. J Mount Sinai Hosp 23:283–292, 1956

CHAPTER 6

Fractures and Dislocations

Recognition of Injuries to the Lower Cervical Spine

BEN L. ALLEN, JR.

Closed, indirect injuries to the lower cervical spine produce patterns of anatomic damage that differ from those seen in other regions of the vertebral column. To illustrate, while the most common serious musculoskeletal pathologic condition in thoracolumbar fractures is retropulsion of vertebral bone into the neural canal, this problem is uncommon in the cervical spine, where *translation through a motion segment* is the most frequent severe pathologic finding. Since ligament failure must occur to permit motion segment translation, the main challenge to the treating physician is *accurate identification of the ligamentous component of the injury* to a cervical motion segment. An associated neurologic injury is of paramount importance as far as the functional outlook for the patient is concerned, but at this time reduction and immoblization of the musculoskeletal lesion is the main treatment for the injured spinal cord or nerve root.[3]

Although sophisticated techniques for imaging the cervical vertebrae and spinal cord are available, the initial judgments about cervical pathology are usually based on history, physical examination, and plain lateral x-ray views of the cervical spine. The history suggests the possibility of neck injury, the initial physical examination establishes the presence or absence of neurologic injury, and the lateral x-ray is the initial diagnostic study. For that reason, this section emphasizes findings on the initial lateral x-ray film. Knowledge of the common patterns of cervical fractures and dislocations facilitates prompt, appropriate decisions about the need for more elaborate assessment and about specific management of the patient.

A classification of cervical fractures and dislocations is helpful because it organizes the injuries into an easily remembered format and provides a means for analyzing the tissue failure in a specific injury. Several years ago, we published a classification that we developed to meet these goals in our clinical service; for the most part it is not original, but rather a restructuring of the voluminous material on the subject.[1] Since that work, there have been additional conceptual advances and increased documentation of the natural history of specific lesions.

Conceptualizing the spine as consisting of three elements or columns is as helpful in the cervical as in the thoracolumbar spine, and it will be developed as it applies to our classification of cervical injuries.[2] By definition, the vertebral arches and their supporting ligaments constitute the posterior element or column. The posterior half or so of the intervertebral disc, including the posterior longitudinal ligament and the vertebral centra, constitutes the middle element or column. The anterior half or so of the intervertebral disc, including the anterior longitudinal ligament and vertebral centra, are the anterior elements or column. Labeling the ligaments in each of these elements as posterior, middle, or anterior ligamentous complex, respectively, is a useful shorthand.

The identification of bone failure as the significant injury may be erroneous. Since bone is readily seen radiographically and other tissues are not, the tendency to emphasize its significance is understandable. However, bone failure *per se* is rarely of great significance, except as a marker for the actual or expected ligament failure. The best way, in my experience, to control this bias is to consider all cervical spine injuries to affect a motion segment. Thus, when a fracture is seen on the plain lateral x-ray, the two vertebrae constituting the injured motion segment need to be recognized.

The use of adjectives descriptive of the altered shape of the damaged vertebral centrum to categorize fractures may also lead to errors in diagnosis. Terms such as "wedge fracture," "burst fracture," or "teardrop fracture" can apply to a variety of lesions with differing degrees of ligamentous injury and differing prognoses, and should probably not be used.

A recent study by the orthopedic group concerned with spinal injuries at Rancho Los Amigos Hospital, based on the classification described here, reported new data on the healing of various lesions when they are reduced and treated in a halo device.[4] Where possible, their findings will be integrated into this discussion. This should not be construed, necessarily, as an endorsement of treating specific lesions in a halo, but rather as an opportunity to understand the range of outcomes that may be expected with such conservative management.

Indirect fractures and dislocations at the lower cervical spine can be divided into groups that are characterized by graduated or sequential increments of similar tissue failure—an injury spectrum or phylogeny. When this is done, six groups are delineated: three occur very commonly, one is of intermittent frequency, and two happen much less often. The three common groups, named for the presumed dominant mode of loading and the presumed posture of the neck at the time of injury, are compressive flexion, distractive flexion, and compressive extension. Vertical compression is the intermediate group. Distractive extension and lateral flexion are the less common groups (see Figure 6-1).

Within each group, the risk of neurologic injury rises with the increasingly severe damage to the cervical motion segment, but the relationship is not always evident and direct. For example, total quadriplegia may occur with no apparent injury or with trivial injury to the cervical spine, and, conversely, severe displacement of a cervical motion segment sometimes occurs without significant neural injury. One cannot conclude that a normal neurologic examination rules out a dangerous spine injury or vice versa. Thus, the importance of adequate protection of the cervical spine during the initial assessment phase of management is self-evident.

COMPRESSIVE FLEXION

The compressive flexion phylogeny (CF), shown in Figure 6-2, is characterized in the early stages (S) by compressive failure of the anterior elements of the uppermost vertebra in the injured cervical motion segment. In the advanced lesion, there is ligamentous failure through the middle and posterior elements with posterior translation of the fractured vertebra posterior with respect to the lowermost intact vertebra in the motion segment (see Fig. 6-2*E*). The neural canal narrows as the inferior vertebral margin of the upper vertebra approaches the lamina of the lower vertebra.

When an A–P x-ray is obtained, in addition to the initial lateral, one may see a vertical fracture of the centrum, which is more common as one moves up the phylogeny. When this fracture occurs, fracture of the lamina, usually not evident on plain film, is consistently present on computerized tomographic (CT) views. Occasionally, a displaced bilaminar fracture is evident on plain films and, also occasionally, an axial splitting fracture of the spinous process may occur. Sometimes the middle element fails by a fracture of the posterior inferior portion of the centrum, rather than by rupture of the middle ligamentous complex (see Fig. 6-8*B*). The anterior vertebral segment of the fractured vertebral centrum is occasionally rectangular,

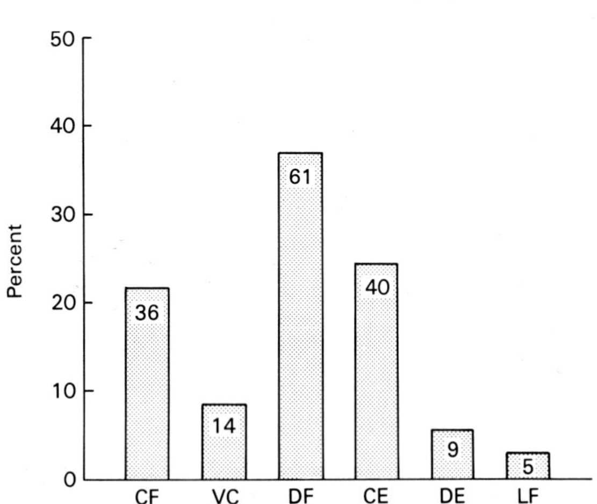

Fig. 6-1. The distribution of lesions according to groups is shown as a percentage of total cases in our original study, in which case identification was keyed to radiographic abnormality. Frequency keyed to presence of a serious neurologic deficit, as in the Rancho series, differed in that CF, DF, and VC, in that order, were the most common lesions.

rather than triangular; this does not seem to affect the pattern of subsequent ligamentous failure of the middle and posterior elements.

These injuries have a strong predilection for the midcervical spine, with a peak incidence at C4–C5 and C5–C6.

CF Stages 1 and 2 are risk-free for pathologic displacement, and any immobilization is for treatment of an associated neural injury or associated pain. With Stages 3 and 4, pathologic angulation through the injured motion segment is possible. Because there is postural stability in extension, conservative management with a device that maintains an extended cervical posture is usually effective. The Stage 5 lesion is often grossly unstable, may require heavier-than-usual weight for maintenance of reduction when treated in traction, and may show a strong propensity to redisplacement when early mobilization is attempted without traction treatment of a duration sufficient for stabilization to occur. These guidelines apply to management of the spinal lesion and may sometimes need modification for neurologic considerations (Fig. 6-2).

With progression up the phylogeny, there is an increasing trend for the lesions to heal by bony ankylosis of the motion segment: in the Rancho series, the rate of spontaneous interbody fusion was over 90% for CF 4 and 5 lesions.

As shown in Figure 6-3, there is an increasing probability of serious concurrent neurologic injury as one progresses from the milder to the more severe stages of the compressive flexion phylogeny.

VERTICAL COMPRESSION

The vertical compression phylogeny (VC), shown in Figure 6-4, is characterized by compressive failure of both the anterior and middle elements of a particular vertebra. This family of injuries is the only one in which the bony failure overrides the ligamentous component of the particular lesion in clinical significance. In the early stages, the vertebral centrum is compressed so that there is a loss of height, as measured along both the anterior and the posterior margins of the vertebral centrum. The extent of compressive injury progresses from involvement of the bone supporting one vertebral end-plate to the bone at both end-plates. Although the typical initial compressive failure results in an increased concavity of either the superior or inferior chondral plate, sometimes there is variation, with a wedgelike contour and loss of height in both the anterior and middle elements. In the advanced lesion the cancellous bone of the centrum bulges in a peripheral direction, including posteriorly into the neural canal. Often the advanced lesion occurs with no evidence of ligament injury. At other times, there is ligament failure through the anterior, middle, and posterior ligamentous complex with gross displacement. In our experience, the translation that occurs is between the fractured vertebra and the subjacent one, but the number of cases available for study is too small to make a definitive judgment. Rarely, lateral tomography or computerized axial tomography may be required to discern an advanced VC lesion with ligament failure from the CFS5.

The paramount distinction of severe VC lesions from the CFS5 is that the neural canal is narrowed by retropulsed vertebral bone, which narrows the neural canal as it approaches the lamina of the fractured vertebra. Thus, the VCS3 is an exception to our generalization that translation is usually the important displacement in a cervical spine injury.

VC lesions tend to occur low in the cervical spine with a peak incidence at C6–C7 and C7–T1. Vertebral arch fractures are commonly associted, and increase in frequency, with movement up the phylogeny.

When there is no ligamentous involvement (gen-

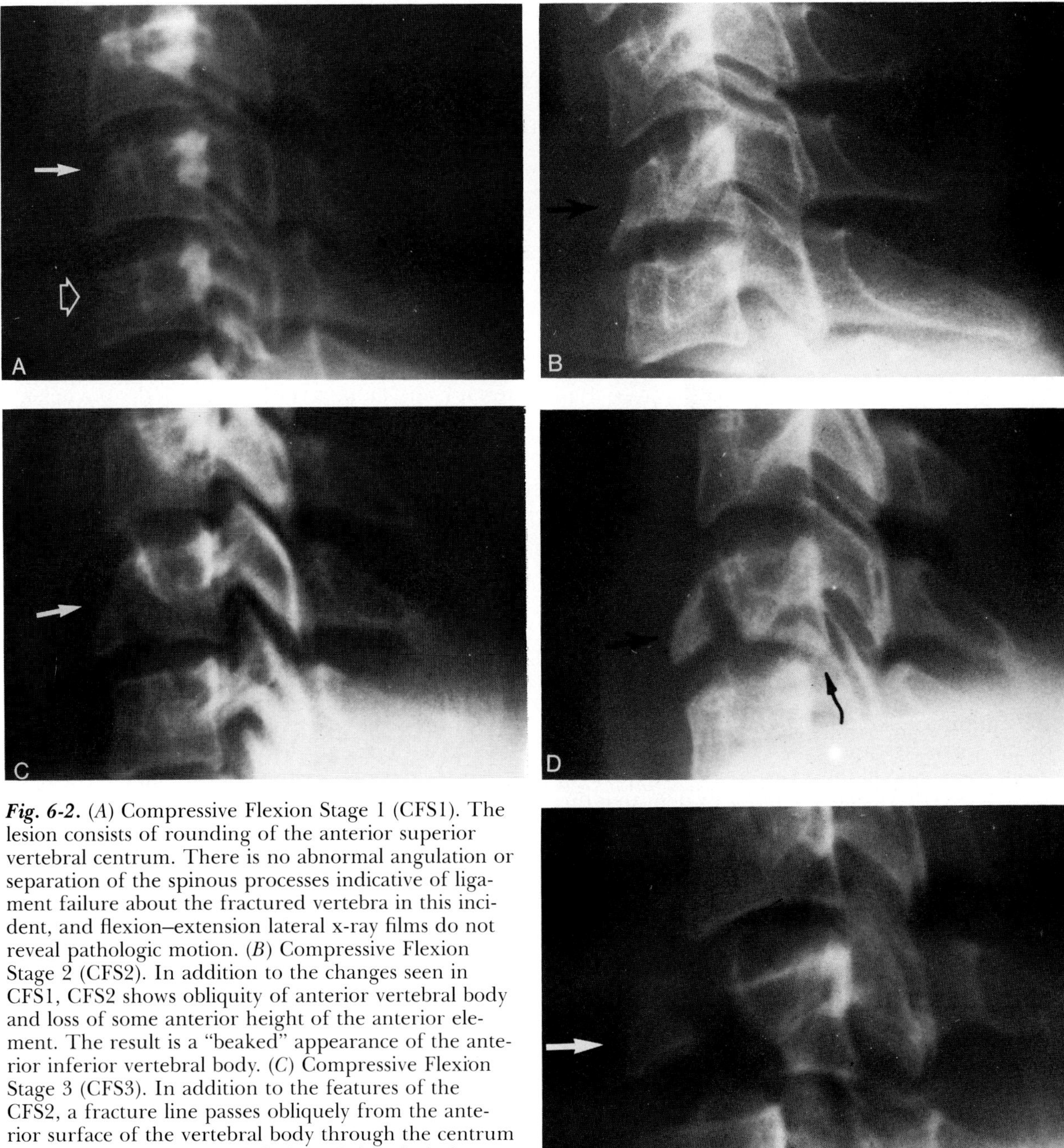

Fig. 6-2. (*A*) Compressive Flexion Stage 1 (CFS1). The lesion consists of rounding of the anterior superior vertebral centrum. There is no abnormal angulation or separation of the spinous processes indicative of ligament failure about the fractured vertebra in this incident, and flexion–extension lateral x-ray films do not reveal pathologic motion. (*B*) Compressive Flexion Stage 2 (CFS2). In addition to the changes seen in CFS1, CFS2 shows obliquity of anterior vertebral body and loss of some anterior height of the anterior element. The result is a "beaked" appearance of the anterior inferior vertebral body. (*C*) Compressive Flexion Stage 3 (CFS3). In addition to the features of the CFS2, a fracture line passes obliquely from the anterior surface of the vertebral body through the centrum and extends through the inferior subchondral plate. (*D*) Compressive Flexion Stage 4 (CFS4). In addition to the deformation of the anterior elements and the fracture of the "beak," the CFS4 demonstrates mild, less-than-3-mm translation of the inferior posterior vertebral margin into the neural canal at the involved motion segment. This indicates beginning failure through the middle and posterior ligamentous complexes. Observe that there is no evidence for additional bone deformation advancing from CFS3 to CFS4. (*E*) Compressive Flexion Stage 5 (CFS5). The lesion has the features of the bony injuries seen in the CFS3, but now there is ligamentous failure through the middle and posterior elements with posterior translation through the motion segment.

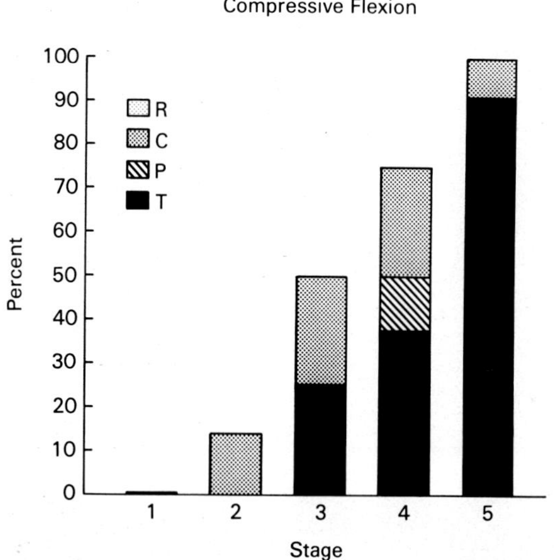

Fig. 6-3. The incidence of neurologic abnormality as a function of the particular stage of the CF phylogeny is shown as a percentage. For this and subsequent graphs, labels are as follows: (*R*) radioculopathy; (*C*) central cord syndrome; (*P*) partial cord injury; and (*T*) total cord lesion. The open space above each bar represents patients with no neurologic abnormality.

erally there is none), the lesions in this phylogeny present a low risk for translational deformity. The retropulsed bone in the VCS3 lesions may or may not reduce with traction, and it is evident that this lesion cannot be reduced by realignment of the cervical spine. Early corpectomy may sometimes be required for neural decompression.

The VC lesions, as CF lesions, have a high probability of healing by spontaneous anterior interbody fusion, if they are treated conservatively; the rate was approximately 80% with the VCS3 in the Rancho series.

As seen in Figure 6-5, the risk of neurologic injury is related to the severity of the cervical spine injury.

DISTRACTIVE FLEXION

The distractive flexion phylogeny (DF), shown in Figure 6-6, is characterized in the early stages by failure of the posterior ligamentous complex, in intermediate stages by failure of the posterior ligamentous complex and partial failure of the middle and anterior ligamentous complex, and in the advanced lesion by failure of all three ligamentous complexes with variable sparing of the anterior longitudinal ligament, which may be either stripped from the vertebral surface or ruptured.

A sometimes confusing characteristic of this family of lesions is that, often in the early stages, there is compressive failure of the anterior elements of the lowermost vertebra in the injured motion segment. This pattern of compressive injury can resemble the initial stages of the CF phylogeny, if one focuses solely on the bony abnormality. The distinguishing feature is the early presence of ligamentous injury, the pathologic displacement occurring between the fractured vertebra and its superior vertebra, rather than its inferior vertebra as in CF, and, progressing up the phylogeny, anterior translation, rather than posterior translation. As one moves up the phylogeny, displacement becomes progressively more severe, from pathologic angulation with minimal translation in the early stages, to unilateral and then bilateral interlocked facets, and finally to complete displacement through the injured motion segment. Bilateral laminar fractures are commonly associated, being present in about 40% of advanced lesions. With anterior translation through the motion segment, the neural canal may be narrowed as the posterior superior centrum of the lower vertebra is approached by the lamina of the superior vertebra.

Distractive flexion lesions tend to be more widely distributed through the lower cervical spine than the previous phylogenies and commonly occur from the C3–C4 motion segment through the C7–T1 motion segment. However as one moves up the phylogeny, there is a distinct tendency for the injury to be localized at a lower level in the cervical spine.

All distractive flexion lesions should be considered at risk for displacement and should be managed accordingly. One should keep in mind that only the minimum severity of ligamentous failure can be inferred from the abnormal bony relationships on the initial film. Special studies may be required to delineate the full extent of the problem. Following reduction, good postural stability in extension may be present for DFSI, S2, and S3; however, Stage 4 lesions are often grossly unstable.

In the Rancho experience, roughly 50% of the DFS1 and DFS3 lesions stabilized, by White's criteria, with treatment in a halo. Most of the DFS2 lesions (unilateral interlocked facet) stabilized with conservative management. All of their DFS4 lesions healed by intervertebral ankylosis, but there were only three. Thus, it is evident that the DF

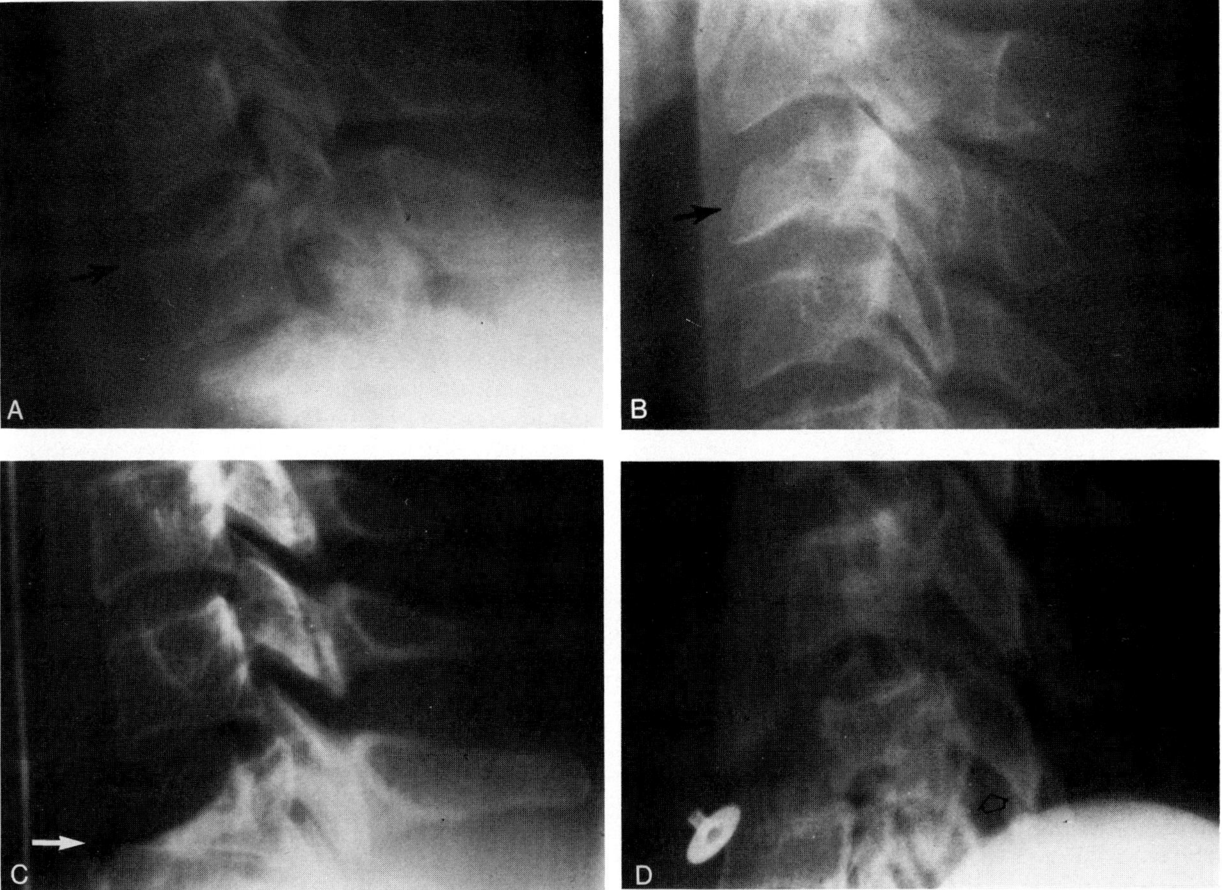

Fig. 6-4. (*A*) Vertical Compression Stage 1 (VCS1). The lesion consists of a fracture of either a superior or an inferior end-plate, usually with a "cupping" deformity. Occasionally a wedge shape may result. There is no evidence of ligamentous failure. (*B*) Vertical Compression Stage 2 (VCS2). Both vertebral end-plates are involved in the VCS2 lesion. Fracture lines through the centrum may occur, but displacement is minimal. (*C*) Vertical Compression Stage 3 (VCS3). A progression of vertebral body damage is seen as in VCS2. The centrum has fragmented, and its residual pieces have displaced peripherally in multiple directions. The posterior portion of the centrum bulges into the neural canal. VCS3 lesions in which the vertebral arch is intact may have acute kyphotic angulation at the injury level. (*D*) In the VCS3 with ligamentous failure, narrowing of the neural canal by two mechanisms occurs. Bone retropulsed from the vertebral centrum approaches the lamina at the injury level, and additionally there is posterior translation through the motion segment.

injuries present a higher risk of failure to heal with conservative management than do other groups, but the probability of achieving stability with nonoperative management is higher than generally reported in the literature.

As was true for the preceding phylogenies, and as shown in Figure 6-7, the risk of neurologic injury increases with the increasing severity of the musculoskeletal lesion. Note the more common occurrence of radiculopathy in this phylogeny than in the previous ones.

ASSOCIATED COMPRESSION FLEXION AND DISTRACTIVE FLEXION LESIONS

Distractive flexion and compressive flexion injuries to contiguous motion segments, as shown in Figure 6-8, occur commonly. The distractive flexion lesion

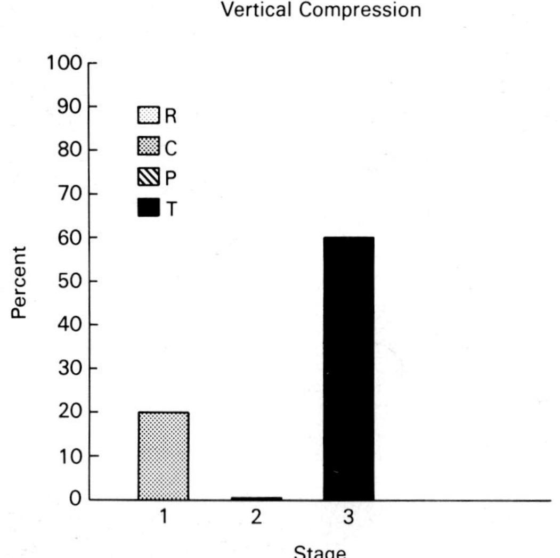

Fig. 6-5.

is consistently located above the compressive flexion lesion. Some mild degrees of compressive failure of the anterior elements commonly occur with distractive flexion injuries, and we generally do not consider there to be a double lesion when the bony failure resembles that seen in CFS1 or CFS2. But with bony failure equivalent to or greater than that seen in CFS3, we classify the patient as having a double lesion. Awareness of this common association may sometime facilitate treatment decisions.

COMPRESSIVE EXTENSION

The compressive extension phylogeny, shown in Figure 6-9, is characterized in the early stages by fracture of the vertebral arch that may assume one of several patterns. Unilateral vertebral arch fractures either involve the articular process, which may be compressed, fractured in a linear manner, or undergo a combination, or involve an ipsilateral fracture of a pedicle and lamina, making possible the so-called transverse-facet appearance. In our experience, the CES1 unilateral vertebral arch fracture is the most common single type and stage encountered in the cervical spine and, because of its frequency, deserves special comment. The injury is often not evident on the initial lateral film. Oblique views may or may not show some degree of rotary listhesis at the involved motion segment, evidenced by displacement through the ipsilateral uncovertebral joint. Nonstandard x-ray views, such as 20-degree oblique views and pillar views, may be necessary to establish the diagnosis. With rotary listhesis, the lesion may resemble the DFS2 on cursory assessment.

The remaining lesions in the CE phylogeny are relatively uncommon and are less clearly sequential than those in other phylogenies. One progresses from a unilateral vertebral arch fracture, to multiple contiguous bilaminar fractures, to a bilateral articular process fracture. For patients with bilateral articular process fractures the logical sequence would be as follows: a stage without vertebral translation, one with partial vertebral body width translation, and another with full vertebral body width translation. In our original survey, we found examples of the latter translation only. Subsequently, other clinicians have shared examples of the first two with us; therefore, they are more than hypothetical. We postulated them as Stage 3 and Stage 4 in the original work. When translation occurs in CE injuries, there is tension shear failure through the middle and anterior elements, with subsequent anterior translation through the involved motion segment.

The advanced stage in this phylogeny is confusing because of its complex radiographic appearance. Displacement involves partial failure through the posterior ligamentous complex above the motion segment, with translation of the superior vertebra. For example, consider that vertebra B has sustained a bilateral articular process fracture resulting in displacement of that vertebra forward on vertebra C, which is subjacent to it. A large fraction of the vertebral arch of B, the entire spinous process, the entire lamina, and portions of both articular processes, all are left behind with the vertebral arch of C. For this to occur, there has been a failure through the posterior ligamentous complex between vertebra A, which is superior to B, and the vertebral arch of B (see Figure 6-9*E*).

CE lesions occur throughout the cervical spine, most being concentrated at C6–C7.

The CE lesions are not at significant risk of displacement until failure of the posterior, middle, and anterior ligamentous complexes occurs. The rotary listhesis commonly seen in the CES1 appears to make no difference in outcome, with respect either to pain or to the sometimes-associated radiculopathy. Since the articular process is damaged in this injury mechanism, an attempt to reduce the rotary listhesis is generally futile because there is no point of bony or postural stability to be gained. As might be expected from the extent of bony injury, the CES5 in our experience and in the literature has healed by bony union when reduced and maintained in traction.

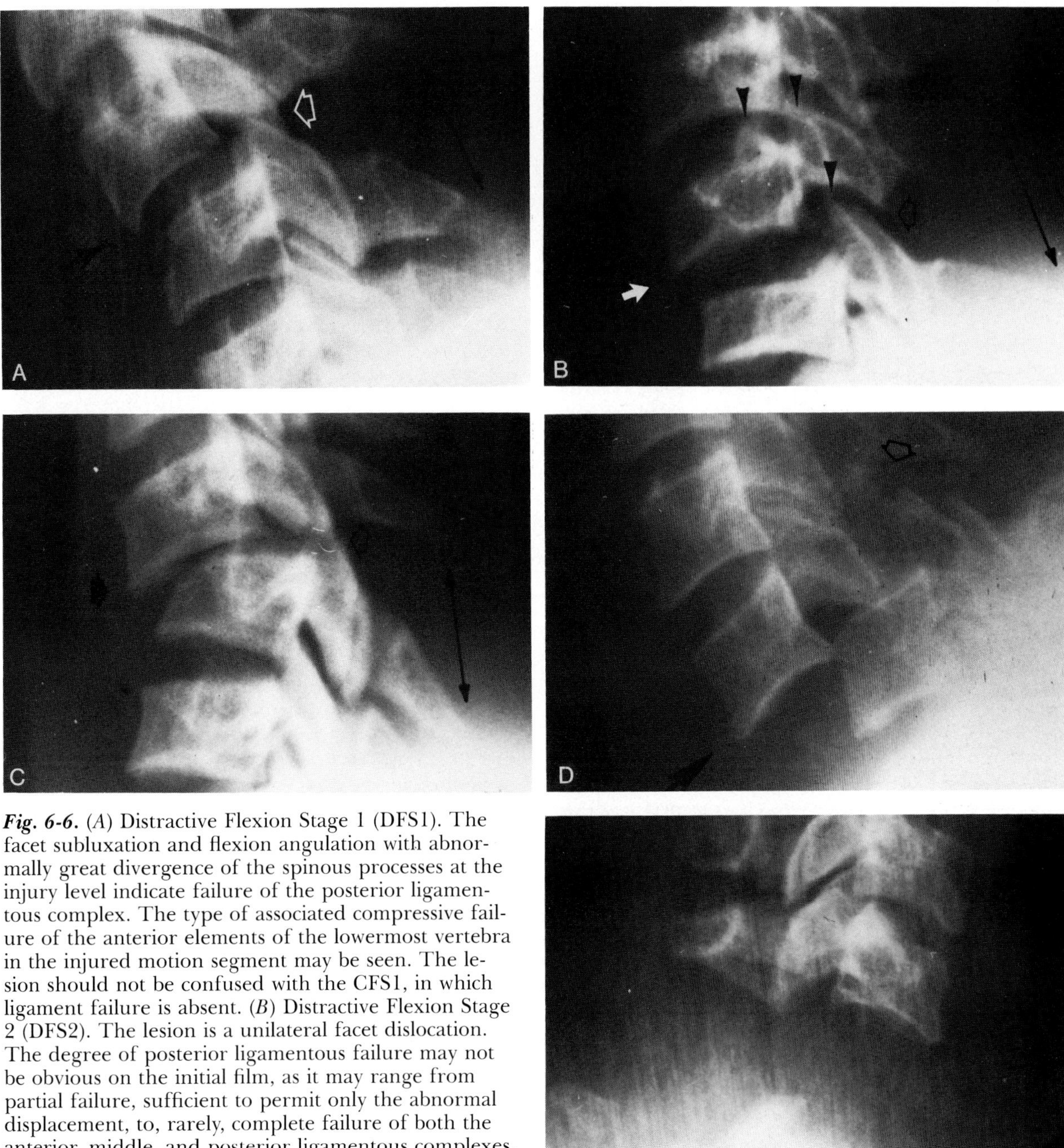

Fig. 6-6. (*A*) Distractive Flexion Stage 1 (DFS1). The facet subluxation and flexion angulation with abnormally great divergence of the spinous processes at the injury level indicate failure of the posterior ligamentous complex. The type of associated compressive failure of the anterior elements of the lowermost vertebra in the injured motion segment may be seen. The lesion should not be confused with the CFS1, in which ligament failure is absent. (*B*) Distractive Flexion Stage 2 (DFS2). The lesion is a unilateral facet dislocation. The degree of posterior ligamentous failure may not be obvious on the initial film, as it may range from partial failure, sufficient to permit only the abnormal displacement, to, rarely, complete failure of both the anterior, middle, and posterior ligamentous complexes. Oblique views of 45 degrees provide the most obvious display of the pathologic displacement. (*C*) Distractive Flexion Stage 3 (DFS3). Here is bilateral facet dislocation with approximately 50% vertebral body width translation anteriorly. The posterior surfaces of the superior vertebral articular processes lie either snugly against the anterior surfaces of the interior articular processes or in a "perched" position. Blunting of the anterior superior margin of the inferior vertebra to a rounded contour may or may not be present. (*D*) Distractive Flexion Stage 4 (DFS4). In the DFS4 there is full vertebral body width translation through the injured motion segment. (*E*) When the DFS4 lesion occurs in a patient with impaired consciousness and reduced muscle tone, the appearance of a "floating vertebra," with application of light traction, may be present.

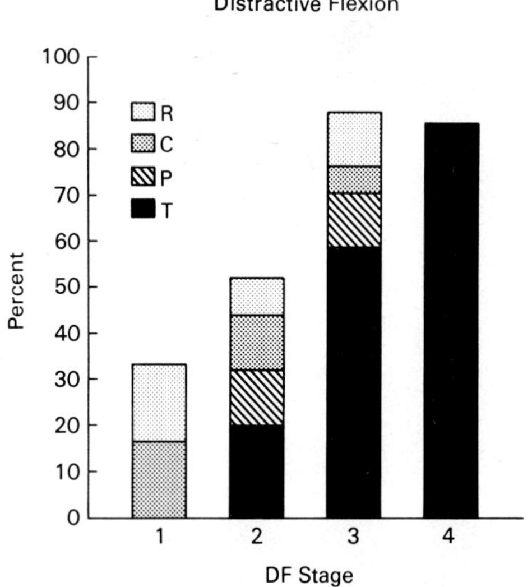

Fig. 6-7.

As shown in Figure 6-10, there are two surprises in this phylogeny. One is the high, unexpected incidence of total cord injury with multiple contiguous bilamina fractures, and the other is the absence of the total cord lesion in the severely displaced CES5 lesions.

DISTRACTIVE EXTENSION

The distractive extension phylogeny (DE), shown in Figure 6-11, is characterized by progressive anterior-to-posterior failure of the ligaments, which support a cervical motion segment. With complete ligamentous failure, the upper vertebra in the injured motion segment displaces posteriorly, and it may pinch the cord between its posterior inferior margin and the vertebral arch of the vertebra below it, as described by Taylor and Blackwood. A frequent clue to the distractive extension injury is an avulsion fracture at the site of attachment of the anterior portion of the annulus. Even when displaced, these lesions tend to reduce when the head is placed at a neutral position, and detection of them on a lateral view may be challenging. This phylogeny differs from others in that an older age group tends to be afflicted. Falls onto the face are a common mechanism of injury.

The amount of accumulated case material is too small to make a definitive comment about distribution, but distractive extension appears to occur at all levels in the lower cervical spine, with a peak incidence of the C5–C6 level. Presently, data are insufficient to suggest a reasonable probability of healing, by bony union and conservative management, for this group (Figure 6-12).

LATERAL FLEXION

The lateral flexion phylogeny (LF), shown in Figure 6-13, consists of injuries sufficiently rare that only tentative staging can be suggested at this time. At all stages, asymmetric compression of a vertebral centrum is seen on the A–P view. The initial lateral view shows evidence of a compressive injury to the vertebral centrum, but the asymmetrical nature may not be appreciated until the A–P view is

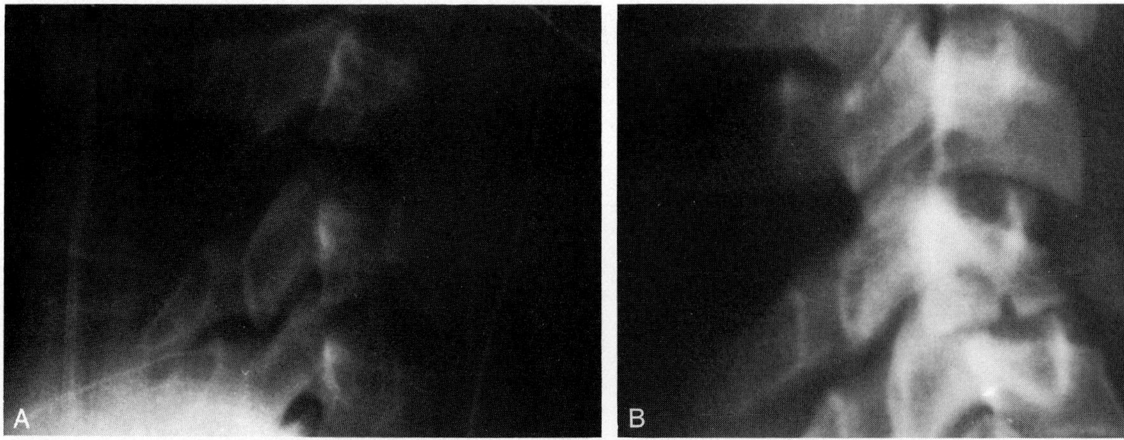

Fig. 6-8. (*A*) Here the DFS4 is the more severe lesion. The CFS3 involves the next most caudal motion segment. (*B*) Here is a DFS1 one motion segment above a CFS4. Note the brittle fracture of the middle bony element in the CF lesion—a rare pattern of bony and ligamentous failure combined.

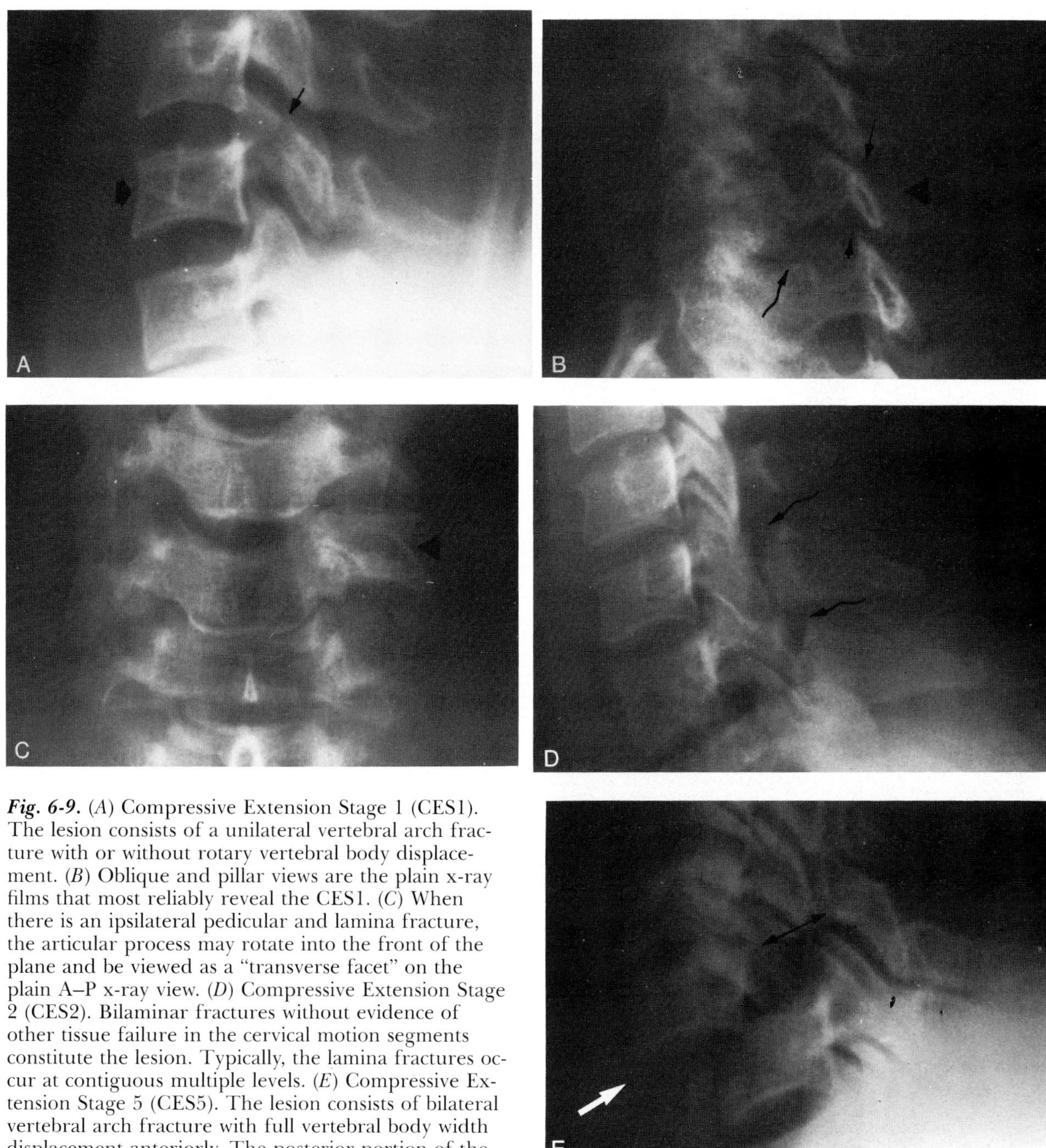

Fig. 6-9. (*A*) Compressive Extension Stage 1 (CES1). The lesion consists of a unilateral vertebral arch fracture with or without rotary vertebral body displacement. (*B*) Oblique and pillar views are the plain x-ray films that most reliably reveal the CES1. (*C*) When there is an ipsilateral pedicular and lamina fracture, the articular process may rotate into the front of the plane and be viewed as a "transverse facet" on the plain A–P x-ray view. (*D*) Compressive Extension Stage 2 (CES2). Bilaminar fractures without evidence of other tissue failure in the cervical motion segments constitute the lesion. Typically, the lamina fractures occur at contiguous multiple levels. (*E*) Compressive Extension Stage 5 (CES5). The lesion consists of bilateral vertebral arch fracture with full vertebral body width displacement anteriorly. The posterior portion of the vertebral arch of the fractured vertebra does not displace, while the anterior portion of the arch remains with the centrum. Ligamentous failure occurs at two different levels as explained in the text.

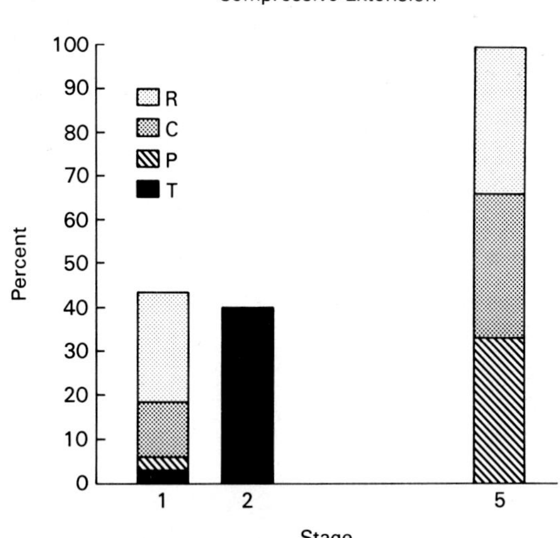

Fig. 6-10.

Fig. 6-12.

obtained. Consistently, the vertebral arch is fractured on the side ipsilateral to the compression of the centrum. In the early stages, vertebral arch fragments are not grossly displaced, whereas in the later stage gross displacement is obvious. Another type of displacement that may occur in advanced lesions is ligamentous failure lateral to the midline, such that there is separation between the vertebral arches on the side away from the vertebral compression.

The lesions tend to involve the lower cervical spine. Insufficient data are present to make a statement about the probability of healing by bony union.

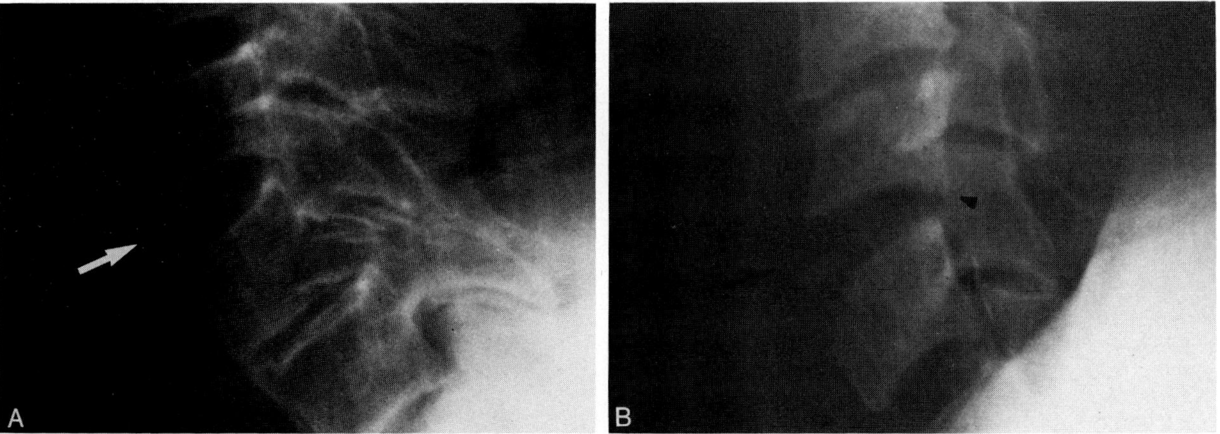

Fig. 6-11. (*A*) Distractive Extension Stage 1 (DES1). The lesion consists of either failure of the anterior ligamentous complex or a transverse nondeforming fracture of the centrum. There may or may not be an avulsion fracture of an adjacent anterior vertebral body margin. The radiographic tip to the injury is usually abnormal widening of the disc space. The DES1 involves no posterior displacement. (*B*) Distractive Extension Stage 2 (DES2). In this lesion there is evidence of failure of all three ligamentous complexes through the involved motion segment with displacement of the upper vertebral body posteriorly into the neural canal. Because displacement of this type tends to spontaneously reduce when the head posture is neutral or in flexion, radiographic evidence of the instability may be subtle.

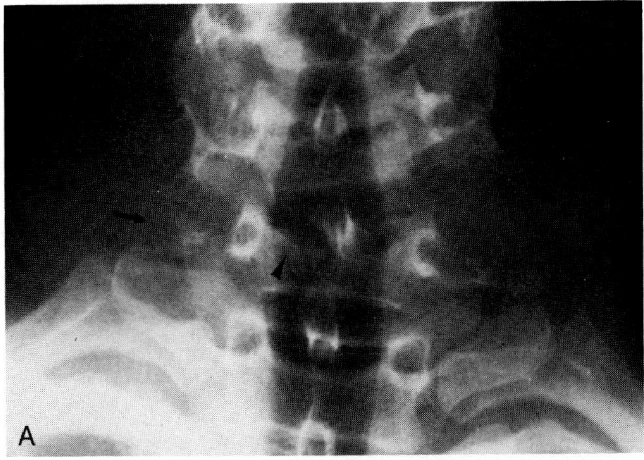

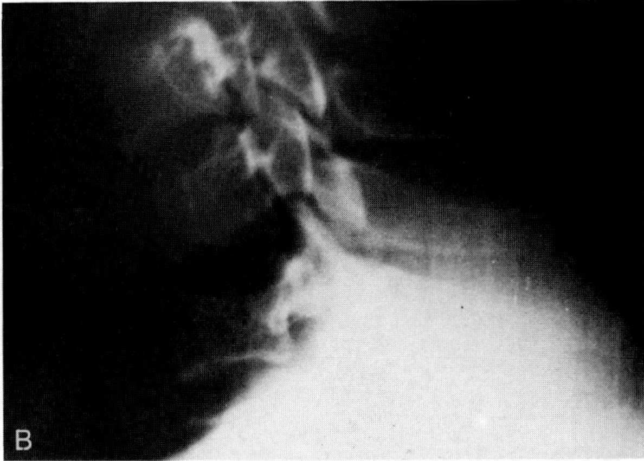

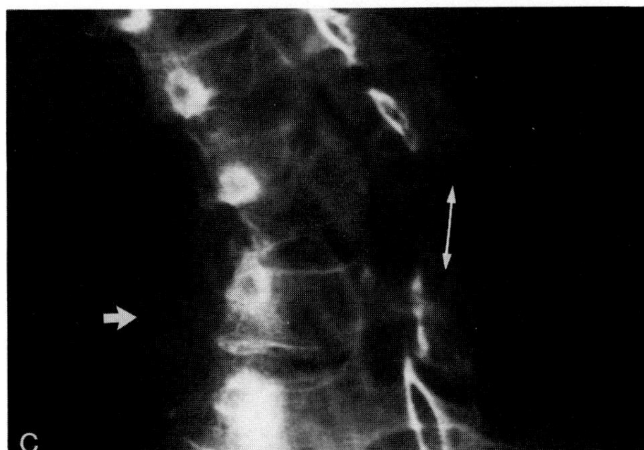

Fig. 6-13. (*A*) Lateral Flexion Stage 1 (LFS1). This lesion consists of asymmetrical compression fracture of the centrum plus vertebral arch fracture on the ipsilateral side, without displacement of the arch on the A–P view. Special views or tomography may be needed to reveal the vertebral arch fracture. (*B*) The asymmetrical compression is evident on the A–P view. (*C*) Lateral Flexion Stage 2 (LFS2). In this lesion, there are lateral asymmetrical compression of the centrum and either ipsilateral vertebral arch fracture with displacement seen on the A–P view or ligamentous failure of a contralateral side with separation of the articular processes.

Lateral flexion injuries historically have a high associated incidence of brachial plexus injury and have a higher-than-expected incidence of total cord injury in the advanced stages (Fig. 6-14).

MULTIPLE LESIONS

Double and multiple lesions sometimes occur, and generally they are easily understood, if one applies the discussed motion segment analysis to each single lesion. Compressive flexion, vertical compression, and compressive extension are the groups in which we have seen multiple lesions all in the same phylogeny.

The important association of distractive flexion and compressive flexion has already been discussed. Additional combinations of lesser frequency include a compressive flexion lesion plus a vertical compression lesion, distractive flexion plus compressive extension, and uncommonly, various

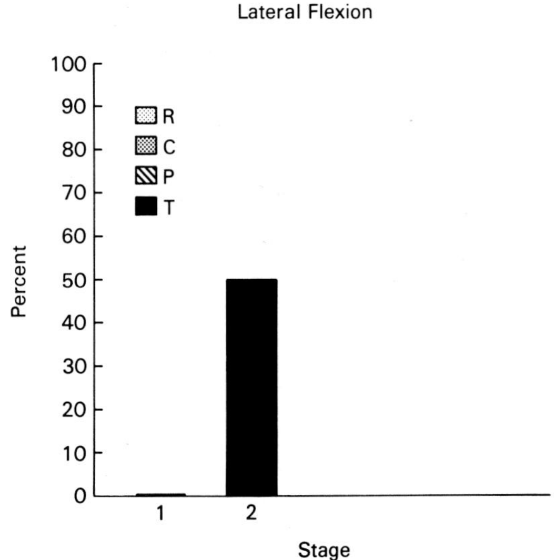

Fig. 6-14.

of the phylogenies with an upper cervical spine lesion. Herniated nucleus pulposus occasionally occurs but so infrequently that no meaningful correlations can be made.

When combined, distractive flexion lesions consistently involve the motion segment above an associated compressive flexion injury. In combination compressive flexion–vertical compression lesions, the compressive flexion consistently involves the motion segment above the vertical compression lesion.

SUMMARY

Diagnosis and formulatoin of treatment strategies for lower cervical spine injuries is facilitated by the following:

Thinking of motion segment as the injury site.
Analyzing by the three-element or column concept.
Identifying the phylogeny to which a particular injury belongs.
Forgetting "wedge," "burst," and "teardrop," as descriptive terms.
Rationally specifying the treatment strategy at the particular tissue injury.

REFERENCES

1. *ALLEN BL JR, FERGUSON RL, LEHMANN TR, O'BRIEN RP:* A mechanistic classification of closed, indirect fractures and dislocations of the lower cervical spine. Spine 7:1–27, 1982
2. *DENIS F:* Spinal instability as defined by the three-column concept in acute spinal trauma. Clin Orthop Rel Res 189:65–76, 1984
3. *DUCKER TB, BELLIGARRIGUE R, SALCMAN M, WALLECK C:* Timing of operative care in cervical spinal cord injury. Spine 9:525–531, 1984
4. *WATERS RL, ADKINS RH, NELSON R, GARLAND D:* Cervical spinal cord trauma: Evaluation and non-operative treatment with Halo-vest immobilization. Cont Orthop 14:35–45, 1987

Cranial Traction and the Halo Orthosis

JOSEPH S. BARR, JR., MARTIN H. KRAG, AND DONALD S. PIERCE

Devices that produce longitudinal traction along the cervical spine may be used to reduce deformity or to provide a degree of stabilization. Significant amounts of traction may be necessary to reduce subluxations, dislocations, or fractures of the cervical spine. There are three basic methods of applying cervical traction: the head halter, tongs, or the halo ring. Head-halter traction is easy to apply and noninvasive, but it is mainly useful to relieve muscle spasm. Neither the skin over the mandible and occiput nor the temporomandibular joints themselves tolerate a significant amount of traction for more than a brief period of time. Tongs allow relatively large amounts of traction to be placed on the cranium, and thereby to the cervical spine, and are useful for the reduction of dislocations and fractures. Tongs do not provide rigid immobilization and confine a patient to bed or a turning frame. The halo ring can be used for skeletal traction and reduction and then combined with a vest orthosis to allow the patient to be ambulatory.

DEVELOPMENT OF TONGS

The first use of tongs for cranioskeletal traction in the management of cervical spine trauma was reported by Crutchfield[5] in 1933. His original patient had a mandibular fracture that precluded the use of head-halter traction. Crutchfield modified a device that had been used for femoral traction. His tongs are placed into surgically created burr holes in the parietal region above the widest diameter of the cranium (Fig. 6-15). The position of Crutchfield tongs placed near the vertex allowed the patient to be turned in bed, but also resulted in a significant danger of the tongs pulling out of the skull. Even though the tips of the tongs are blunted, repeated tightening to prevent pull-out may cause penetration through the inner table of the skull.[10] In spite of this, Crutchfield tongs remained in widespread use up through the early 1970s.

At about the time of Crutchfield's report, in Toronto, McKenzie[12] wrote about using modified ice tongs, which had a depth stop ⅛ inch from the tong points and a mechanism for locking the points into position. These points had to be driven into place with a mallet. In 1938, Barton[2] and Blackburn[3] independently described devices that they had each developed (Fig. 6-15). Barton's tongs were similar to McKenzie's but were somewhat safer, as the points were drilled into place. Blackburn's tongs required burr holes in the parietal region for placement. This device was somewhat unwieldy and made it difficult to turn the patient. Hoen[11] described a method using wire loops through a pair of burr holes on each side of the skull to apply traction. Technically, this was more difficult, and the wires tended to pull out of the outer table of the skull. Several investigators described hooks passed under the zygoma bilaterally as a method of achieving cranial traction. Vincke[14] in 1948 developed another variation of cranial tongs, which were placed in parietal burr holes using an eccentric cutter (Fig. 6-15).

The most commonly used tongs today are those developed by Gardner[9] in 1973 and known as the Gardner-Wells tongs (Fig. 6-16). These have a one-piece bow with threaded pins on either side. One of the pins is spring loaded with an indicator that shows the amount of compressive force (30 pounds) exerted by the pin. These pins are easily placed while the patient is under local anesthesia in the emergency room. The points can be inserted below the greater diameter of the skull. They tilt upward to avoid the danger of pins being pulled out. The width of the device makes it impossible to turn the patient on his or her side. The pins of these tongs are sharp and, if over-tightened, can protrude through the inner table of the skull.[8] Gardner-Wells are the most commonly used type of tongs for patients with cervical spine injuries, mainly because of the ease of application.

TRACTION TECHNIQUES

Tong Application

Gardner-Wells tongs are readily applied under local anesthesia. Pin sites should be below the equator of the skull and just anterior to the ears. The skin is prepared and infiltrated with local anesthesia down to the galea. The pins are tightened by hand until the indicator on the spring-loaded pin protrudes 1 mm. At 24 hours following application, the spring-loaded pins should be retightened until the indicator is flush with the flat surface of the pin. Thereafter, they should not be retightened. Halo ring application is described later in this chapter (Fig. 6-17).

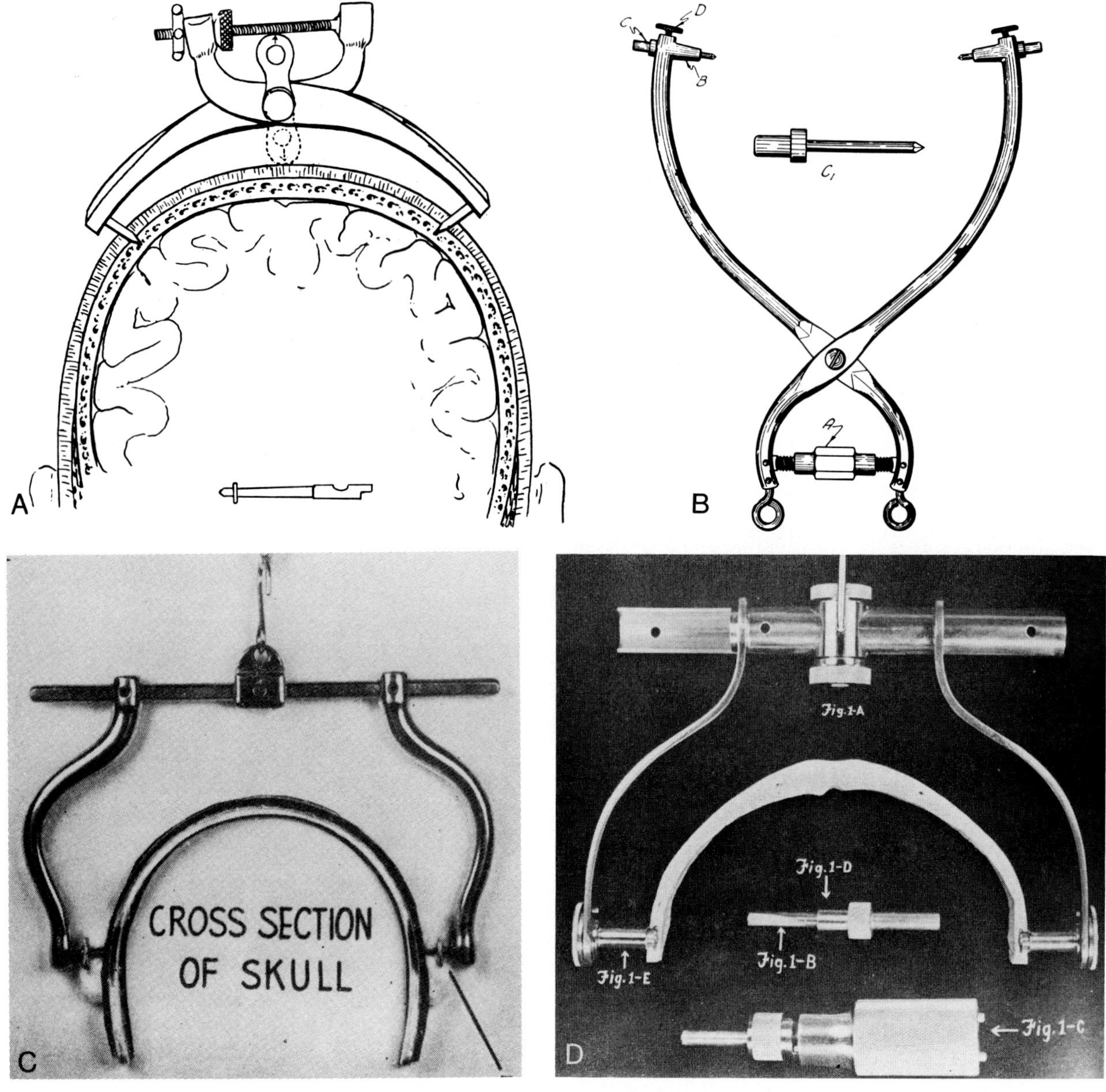

Fig. 6-15. Examples of tongs. (*A*) Crutchfield, (*B*) Barton, (*C*) Blackburn, (*D*) Vincke.

Manual Traction

This method of manipulation to reduce facet dislocations has been recommended by Evans[7] and Burke and Berryman.[4] They describe traction under general anesthesia, with lateral flexion and rotation to reduce a facet dislocation. The procedure is repeated in the opposite direction for a bilateral dislocation, followed by extension of the spine to lock the reduced facets. The safety of this procedure has been questioned by other authors,[6] and has never found wide acceptance in the United States.

Tong and Halo Traction

Muscular relaxation must be achieved to reduce facet dislocations. Active contraction of the cervical musculature in the adult may easily overcome up to 50 pounds of traction.[1] An injured cervical spine

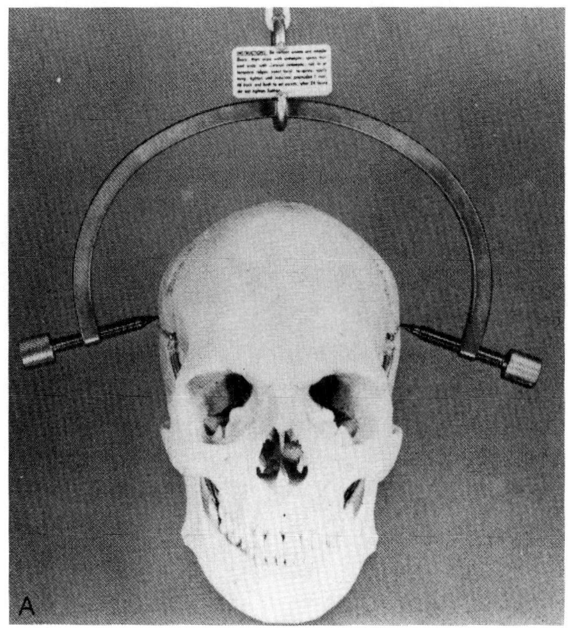

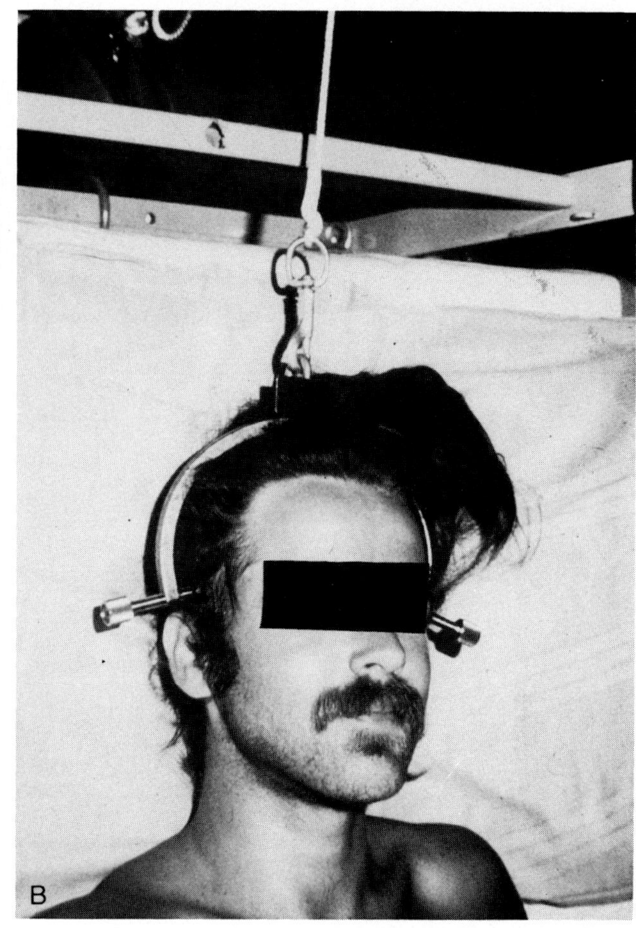

Fig. 6-16. Gardner-Wells tongs. (*A*) Instructions for use are printed on the tongs. The points are directed upward to decrease the risk of pulling out. One pin is spring loaded to indicate 30 pounds of pressure. (*B*) Patient in traction with Gardner-Wells tongs. The pins are placed just above the ears and below the equator of the skull.

may not safely sustain the same loads, and careful x-ray monitoring is necessary to avoid overdistraction. It is the generally accepted practice to add weight in 5-pound increments every 10 to 15 minutes until reduction is achieved, or to a maximum of 70 to 80 pounds.[13,15] This procedure is best carried out in the radiology department with fluoroscopic control or frequent lateral x-ray studies. Once reduction is achieved, the spine is extended and weight decreased to 5 pounds. If at first a halo was used, the vest is then applied to maintain the reduction. Occasional facet dislocations are irreducible with traction, and open reduction is necessary.

THE HALO ORTHOSIS

The halo device was first described for use in the immobilization of the cervical spine by Perry and Nickel[26] in 1959. Initially, they used it with a cast for patients with severe poliomyelitis who had suffered paralysis of the cervical musculature. Fusion of the entire cervical spine in these patients was necessary for stability and needed rigid immobili-

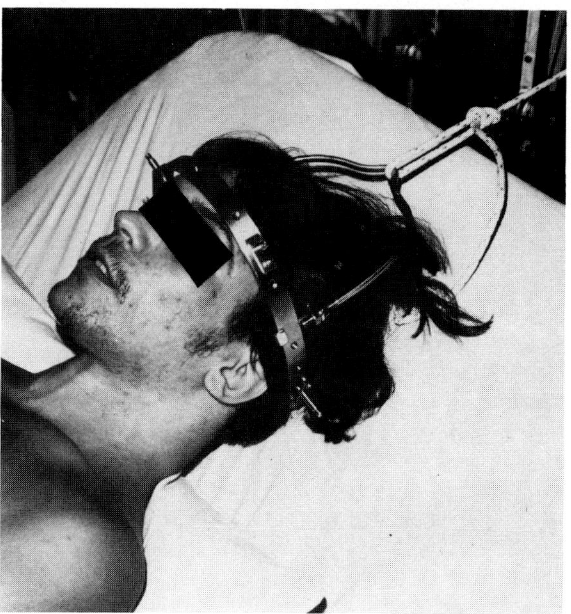

Fig. 6-17. Patient in traction with a halo ring. A "U"-shaped bail adapts the ring for traction.

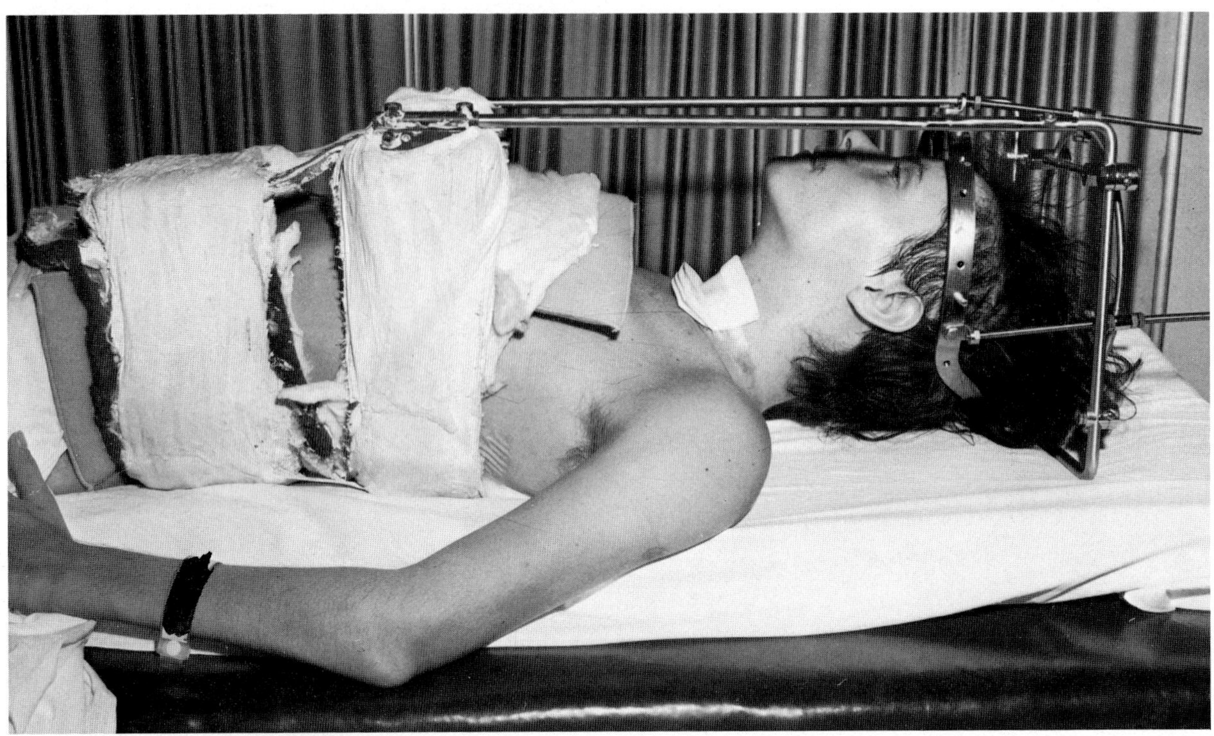

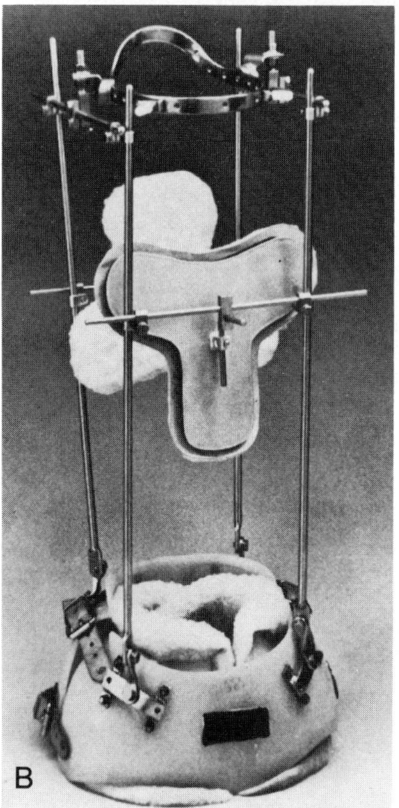

Fig. 6-18. Developmental halo configurations. (*A*) Halo cast on a quadriplegic patient. The cast was difficult to apply, bulky, and caused frequent pressure sores. The shoulder straps were removed in this instance to allow for anterior cervical fusion. (*B*) The halo and pelvic girdle. Adjustable pads were used for the thoracic spine and sternum.

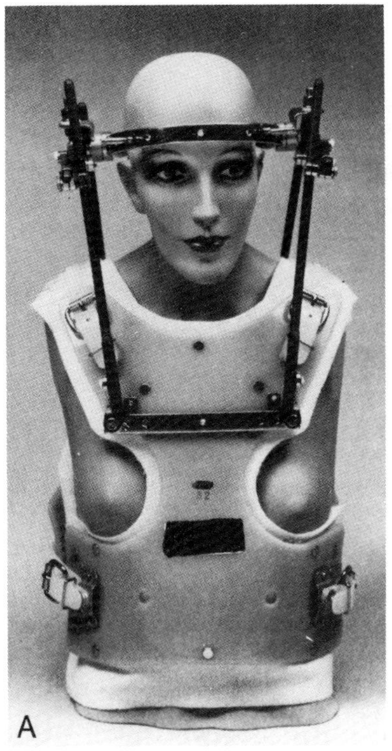

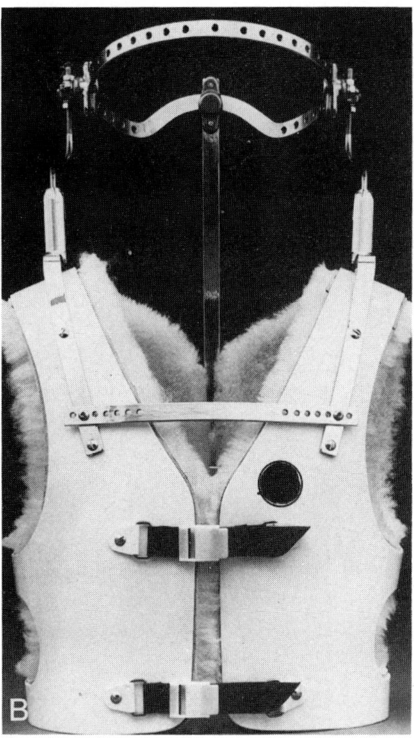

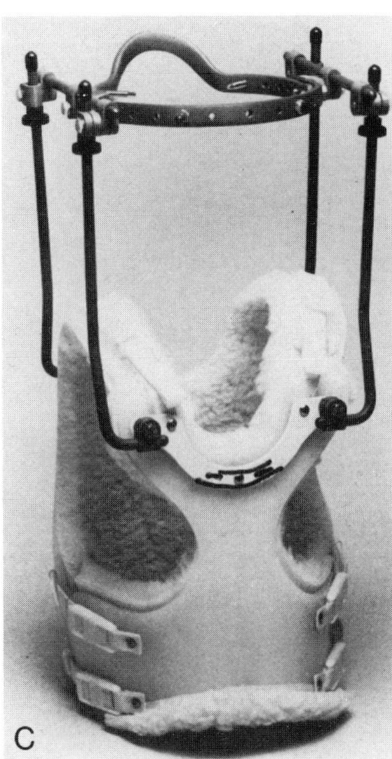

Fig. 6-19. These representative halo vest designs are currently available and in use.

zation while the fusion was healing. The halo ring was adapted from a device that had been used in maxillofacial surgery to stabilize facial fractures. Since the middle 1960s, the halo has been in common use for virtually any type of cervical spine condition that causes instability, including fractures, dislocations, tumors, infectious disease, rheumatoid arthritis, instability following laminectomy, and other rare conditions including massive osteolysis.[16,17,24,25,27]

The halo device has undergone an evolution over the past 3 decades. Originally, the framework was embedded in a body cast (Fig. 6-18). This was difficult to apply to a paralyzed patient with an unstable cervical spine injury, and the body cast over insensate skin caused many pressure sores. A removable plastic pelvic girdle was then developed that could be used with anterior and posterior uprights to attach to the halo ring. Anterior and posterior pads were used for the sternum and thorax; the spine and trunk could sag and move some within this device, causing distraction forces across the cervical spine. This device never gained much popularity.

In the early 1970s, a two-piece removable thoracic orthosis was designed that could be attached to the halo ring with uprights (Fig. 6-19). Different styles of halo vests are now available from a number of manufacturers. The halo vest was a marked improvement over the previous devices, and it reduced sagging of the spine by providing thoracic contact closer to the cervical spine. It allowed the patient to sit more easily and, if neurologically intact, to be ambulatory. Inspection of the skin and skin care were markedly facilitated by the halo vest.

Biomechanical studies done on patients wearing halo vests have shown that as little as 4% or as much as 30% of cervical spine motion can still occur as the patient moves between the supine and sitting positions.[20,21,23,29] Although the halo vest is the most effective orthosis for cervical spine immobilization, instances of loss of fracture reduction within the halo vest have been reported.[30] Recently, a new type of vest has been designed in an effort to improve the fit on the thorax, thereby decreasing motion between the vest and thorax. Preliminary results with this vest (Fig. 6-20) show

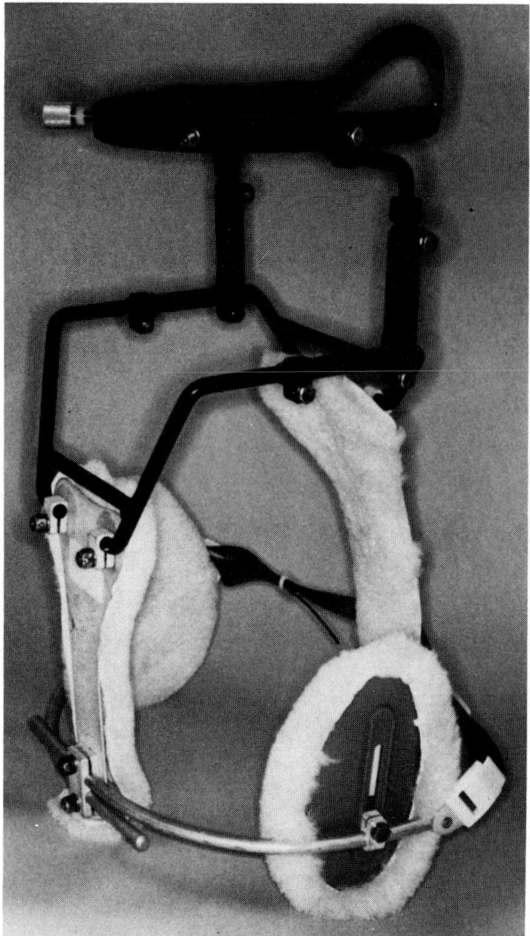

Fig. 6-20. New adjustable vest design which allows pressure to be borne over the sternum, interscapular region, and lateral rib cage. Improved fixation to the thorax is achieved.

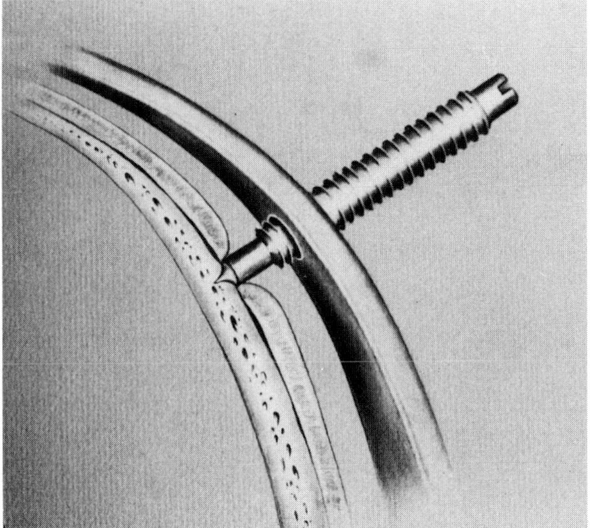

Fig. 6-21. Detail of the halo pin to show the sharp point and broad shoulder, which minimize penetration beyond the outer table of the skull.

reduction of undesirable forces on the cervical spine and halo, together with good acceptance of this device by patients.[22]

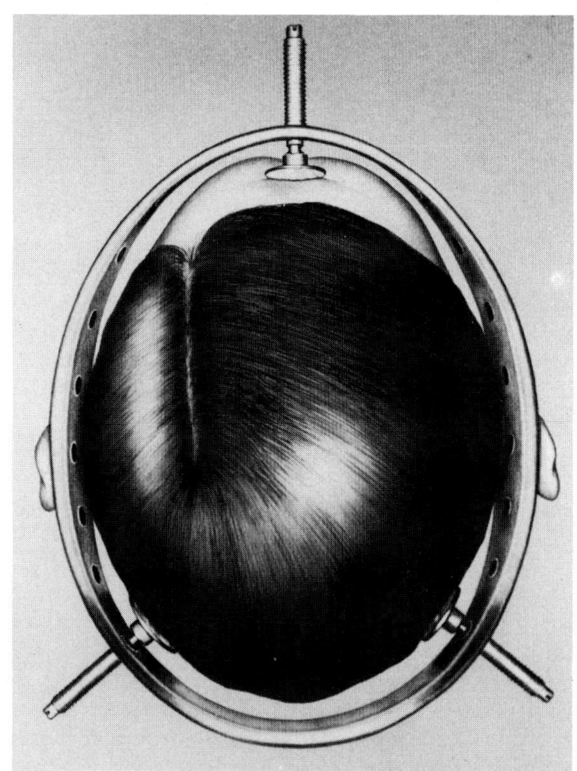

Fig. 6-22. Halo ring centered with pins and base plates. There should be at least 1 cm of clearance between the skin and the ring everywhere.

Application

The halo ring is usually applied under local anesthesia. The more unstable the spine, the more important it is to allow the patient to splint his own spine with his musculature while the halo orthosis is being applied. The halo ring is supplied in a number of sizes, one of which fits virtually anyone, including young children. The circumference of the skull is measured and compared with the manufacturer's chart to ascertain the proper halo ring size. The halo and pins are sterilized before application. The pins themselves have a sharp point but rapidly widen to a broad shoulder; this design allows the point of the pin to penetrate the outer table of the skull while avoiding penetration to the inner table or of the skull entirely (Fig. 6-21). The patient's neck may be supported during the application by a collar or an assistant. Several manufacturers make a device that supports the patient's occiput while the ring is applied. The appropriate-sized ring is carefully positioned approximately 1 cm above the eyebrows and 1 cm above the tip of the ears, and it is held in place with pins and base plates, two posteriorly and one in the midline between the eyes (Fig. 6-22). This centers the ring on the patient's skull. There should be at least 1 cm of clearance between the skin and the ring in all areas.

It is extremely important that the pin be positioned just below the greater circumference of the patient's skull, so that any pressure on the ring will not cause it to slip off. There are a number of predrilled and threaded holes in the ring, and generally two pins are positioned anterolaterally at the lateral aspect of the supraorbital ridge. Two other pins are positioned on either side posterolaterally. Osteologic study of the skull has been performed,[18] and it confirms that anterolateral placement of the anterior pins avoids the thinner areas over the frontal sinus and in the temporal fossae. Pins in the temporal area may also damage the temporalis muscle and cause pain during chewing. Anteriorly, the supraorbital nerve should be avoided; it can be located by palpating its foramen. Generally, the anterior pins are placed just lateral to that region (Fig. 6-23). The skin beneath the appropriate holes is prepared with antiseptic solution. Long hair should be tied up in a ribbon on the top of the patient's head to get it out of the way. Some hair can be clipped or shaved around the ears as necessary. After the antiseptic is applied, local anesthetic *without* epinephrine is introduced into the skin directly beneath the hole (Fig. 6-24). The needle can be placed through the appropriate hole down into the skin, a wheal of anesthetic is raised, and then the needle proceeds through the soft-tissue layers to the skull itself. Three or four cc of local anesthesia is generally adequate at each of the four pin sites. Epinephrine is *not* used because it, together with the pressure of the pin, might cause a skin slough. The person applying the ring wears sterile gloves and inserts the sterile pins into the four appropriate holes. The pins are then tightened down slowly, with care being taken to tighten opposite pins together (left anterior and right posterior, or right anterior and left posterior) until they begin to seat themselves on the skull. It is critical to keep the ring well centered on the skull while this is being done. Once the pins are finger tight on the skull, the base plates and positioning pins can be removed. Again, at this point, it is essential that the halo is no more than 1 cm above the eyebrows and ears. A torque screwdriver is then used to tighten the pins. It is useful to have two such screwdrivers available so that opposite pins can be tightened at the same time. The pins are tightened gradually, increasing about 1 inch pound of torque at a time until all four pins are at 6 inch pounds of torque. At this point, the halo ring should be stable on the skull.

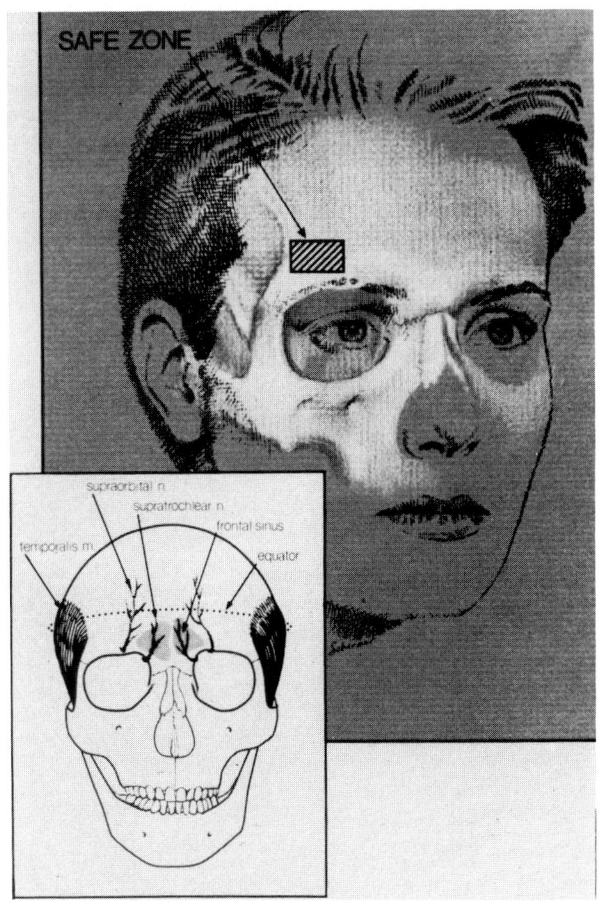

Fig. 6-23. The safe area for anterior pin placement is over the lateral eyebrow, avoiding the nerves and frontal sinus medially, and the thin temporal bone and temporalis muscle laterally. (Garfin SR, et al: Complications in the use of the halo fixation device. J Bone Joint Surg 68A:320–325, 1986)

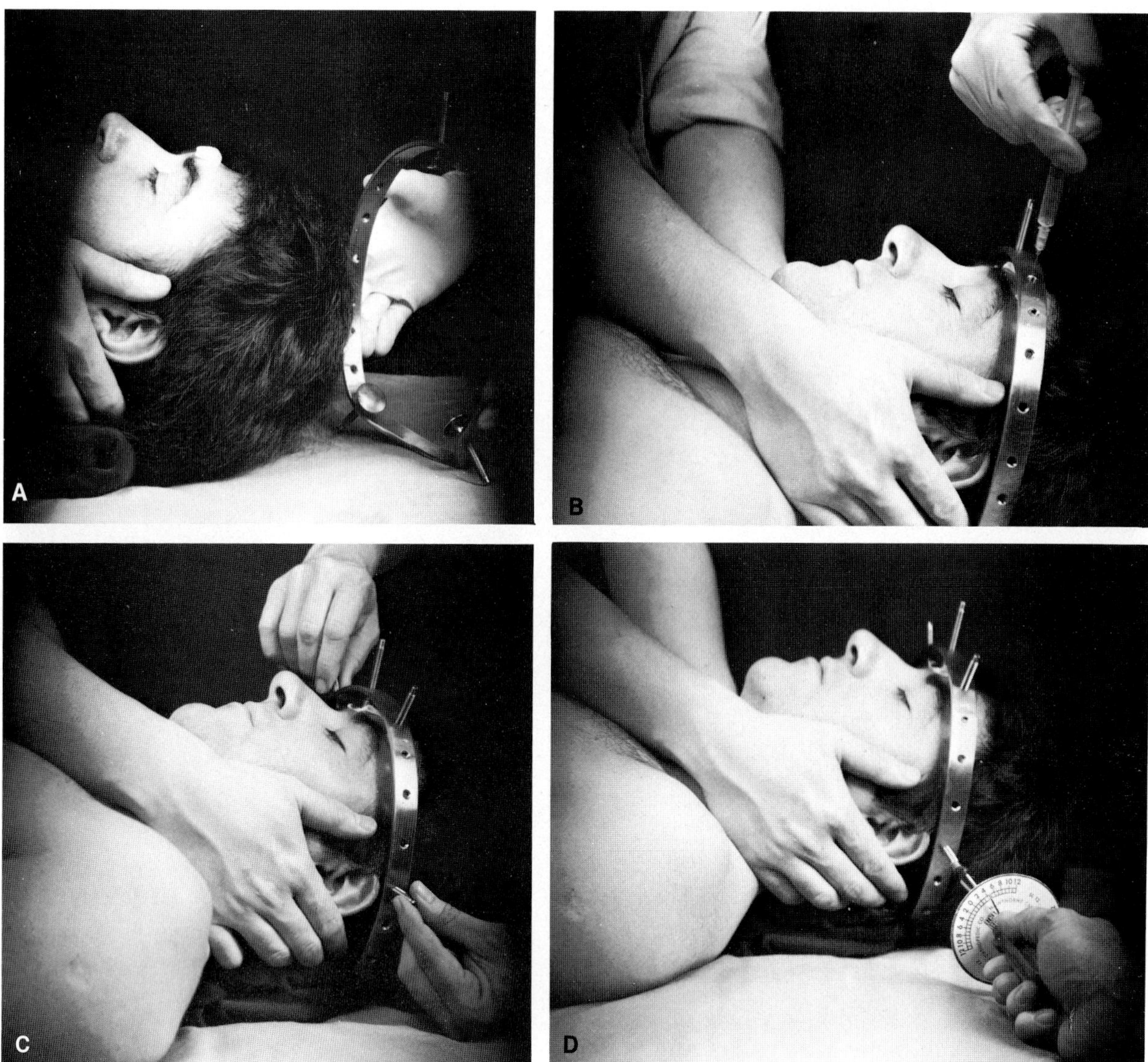

Fig. 6-24. (*A*) The patient's head is supported by an assistant while the appropriate-sized sterile halo ring is slipped over the skull. Three base plates and positioning pins are already on the halo. A piece of adhesive tape between the eyebrows helps to secure the position of the anterior base plate. (*B*) Injection of local anesthetic after the skin has been prepped. Two holes just lateral to the eyebrows and two holes at or behind the ears are chosen. The halo is positioned low over the eyebrows and ears and maintained there by the assistant and by the base plates and positioning pins. (*C*) Halo pins are finger tightened until they penetrate the skin and make contact with the outer table of the skull. Opposite pins are tightened simultaneously. (*D*) A torque screw driver is used to gradually tighten the pins to 6 inch pounds of torque. (*E*) The posterior half of the vest with the attached uprights has been slid underneath the patient. The head is still supported by an assistant. (*F*) Completed assembly of the vest and uprights. The halo is now secured by two threaded uprights. (*G*) Completed assembly of the halo apparatus with the third point of fixation to prevent flexion or extension of the halo.

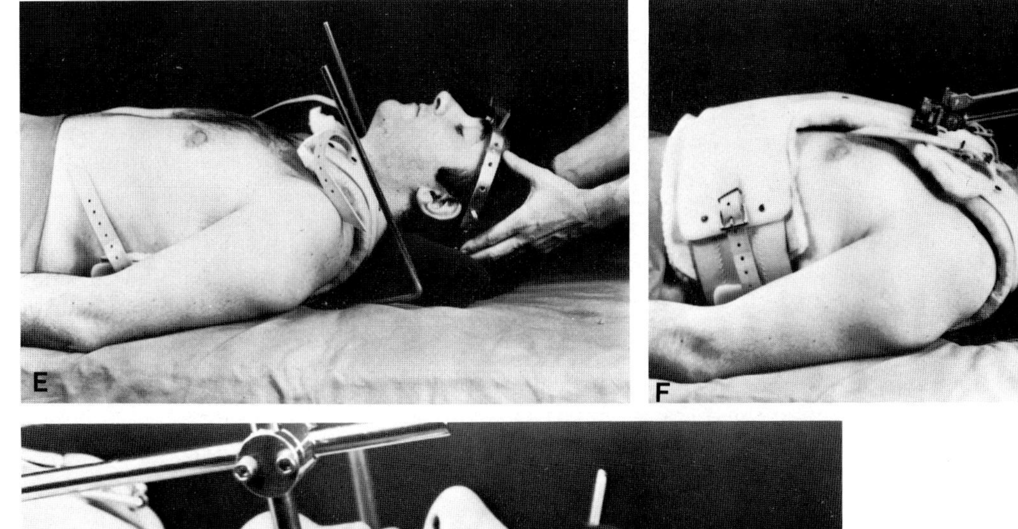

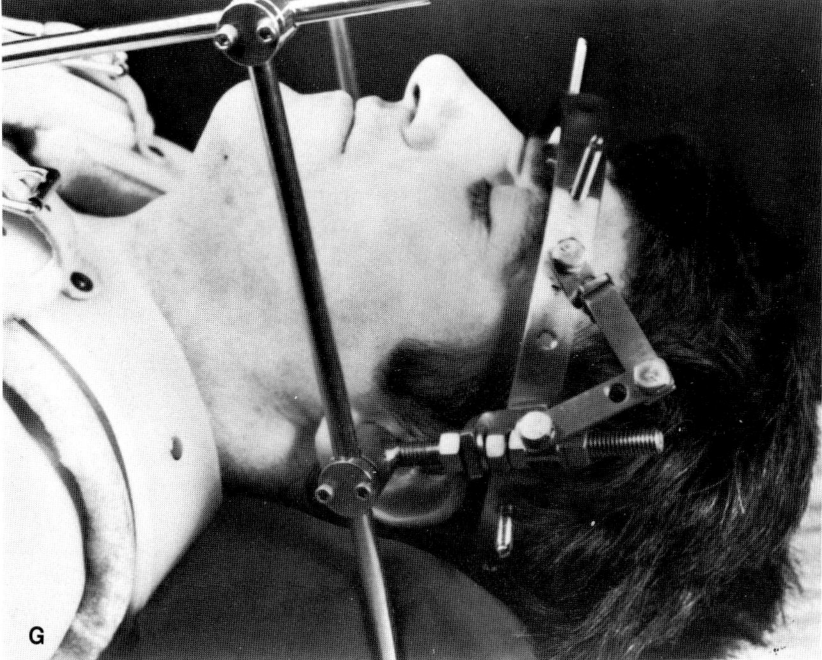

Fig. 6-24, *Cont'd*

If the procedure is performed slowly, and if some time is allowed for the local anesthetic to take effect, the patient should not suffer undue pain. It is important to reassure the patient that the main feeling will be pressure, as during dental work under local anesthetic. Some intravenous analgesic or medications similar to diazepam can be used, if necessary, but in most instances it is not needed.

Once the ring has been secured, the thoracic vest is applied. Vests are available in a number of different sizes, according to the circumference of the chest at the level of the xiphoid. The newer vest design (Fig. 6-20) has one size, which is adjustable and fits most adults. The posterior half of the vest can be slipped underneath, by rolling the patient from side to side or by several people lifting the patient, keeping the neck stable. The anterior part of the vest is then positioned, and the two halves are fastened together. The uprights are assembled to the halo ring. The total time of application should be 1 hour or less with experienced personnel.

Each manufacturer has a different hardware configuration. In general, provision is made for tilting of the ring to provide flexion or extension of the skull and to position the threaded upright anteriorly or posteriorly along the horizontal rod, providing flexion or extension of the cervical spine. Some halo vests can be detached either anteriorly or posteriorly, allowing for removal of one half of the jacket to allow for anterior or posterior surgery (Fig. 6-25).

Ambulatory patients can walk in the halo orthosis immediately and generally need 2 to 3 days to achieve a sense of balance. Patients who are bedridden or paralyzed should be turned every 2 hours; this can be done in a regular bed or on a frame. The quadriplegic patient can be elevated to a sitting position and transferred into a wheelchair very rapidly after the halo orthosis is applied. This enables the rehabilitation program to begin sooner than it would for the patient confined to a bed or a frame and tongs for 6 to 8 weeks or more.

Patient acceptance of this device is uniformly good once the rationale for its use and the alternative of extended bed rest are explained to the patient and family. Occasionally, an elderly patient with the device has a sensory deprivation type of syndrome, and in a rare patient removal of the device has been necessary because the patient was unable to tolerate it.

Care of the Patient in the Halo Orthosis

Following application of the halo orthosis, the halo pins should be checked in about 48 hours and retorqued to 6 inch pounds of torque. Subsequently, the pins should be checked weekly or every 2 weeks and kept finger tight. The pins should not be tightened continually with a torque screwdriver; that can cause penetration of the skull resulting in meningitis or brain abscess. Skin care under the vest can be given by a nurse or member of the patient's family. The buckles on the vest can be loosened slightly to allow for skin washing, application of alcohol, and so forth. Clothing can be modified to slip under the vest or fit over the vest and around the uprights. The vest itself is generally lined with a sheepskin or Kodel material. If the patient has to wear the device for months and the lining becomes soiled, half of the vest can be removed at a time to change the lining. Halo pin care must be performed daily. It is important to remove any crusts that form around the pin sites. Antiseptic ointment can be applied with a cotton applicator following crust removal. Generally, as long as the halo pins are tight, they remain sterile and no problem with infection will occur. A loose pin is prone to get infected. If this occurs, it is possible to place another pin in an adjacent hole under sterile precautions, tighten it down, and then remove the infected pin. Antibiotics are often necessary to help clear up the pin infection.

Adaptability

As previously mentioned, the halo orthosis can be used with virtually any type of cervical spine problem where stability needs to be maintained. It is generally possible to position the uprights so that roentgenograms can be taken without difficulty. At times, polytomography is necessary to accurately evaluate the cervical spine. The halo ring and upright components are now being manufactured in graphite and other nonmetallic materials to allow for the use of computed axial tomography, and magnetic resonance imaging.

Myelography can be carried out, if desired, through a C1–C2 cervical puncture, or through a lumbar route. Use of the halo ring to reduce a fracture-dislocation or jumped facets has already been described. Following reduction, the vest can be applied, and the ring attached to the vest. In addition, the ring and uprights can be manipulated to position the neck to maintain a reduction, once it is achieved. The ring itself can be tilted to flex or extend the cranium and the upper cervical spine. Flexion or extension of the lower cervical spine is best achieved by moving the ring and head anteriorly or posteriorly along the horizontal pieces of the assembly. It is important to obtain lateral x-rays with the patient supine and sitting to ensure that stability is maintained in various positions.[23]

The anterior part of the vest is often cut out for breast comfort in the female or for external cardiac massage, if necessary. Intubation of the patient for surgery or for respiratory depression can usually be performed without removing the vest or changing its configuration. Occasionally, it is necessary to use a fiberoptic laryngoscope, particularly in rheumatoid patients or patients with ankylosing spondylitis. The vest can be removed completely for surgery, if desired, and the ring can be secured through the Mayfield head rest. Alternatively, as already shown (Fig. 6-25), it is possible to remove one-half of the vest and keep the patient stabilized in the other half during surgery.

Complications

Several different types of complications have been reported with use of the halo vest.[19] Loosening or infection of halo pins has been reported in 20% or more of patients. Proper pin application and after-care can somewhat reduce this complication rate. Patients must be seen frequently to avoid loosening of the pins, and loose pins that cannot be successfully tightened, or infected pins, must be replaced promptly. Pressure areas can occur under the vest, particularly in quadriplegic patients. Careful skin care is necessary to avoid prob-

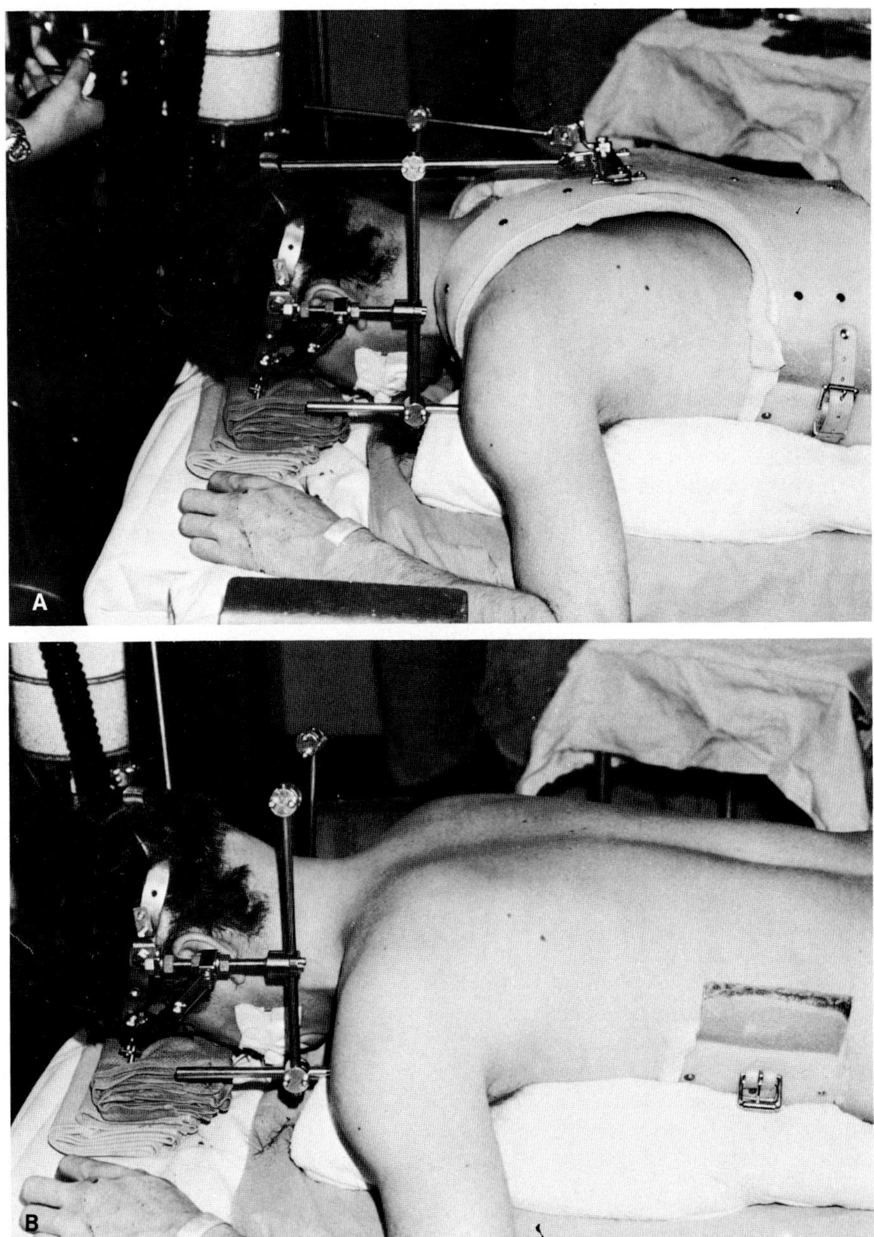

Fig. 6-25. Posterior cervical fusion using the halo vest. (*A*) The patient has been intubated and turned prone on the operating table. The uprights and connecting horizontal bar have been applied so that either the anterior or posterior half of the halo vest could be removed for surgery, as required. (*B*) The posterior half of the vest has been removed, exposing the cervical spine. The horizontal bars can be lowered out of the way, one at a time, and then resecured to maintain rigid stability of the cervical spine during the fusion procedure. The posterior half of the vest is replaced at the end of surgery and the halo apparatus reassembled.

lems. Occasional injuries to the supraorbital or suprathrochlear nerves have been reported in patients with the anterior pins placed too medially.

The most severe complication related to halo pins has been penetration of the entire skull resulting in meningitis or brain abscess. This complication must be avoided by not overtightening the pins. Occasionally, a patient has unsightly scars following removal of the pins. Severe scarring is uncommon and surgical revision of the scars is rarely necessary. Some patients complain of pin discomfort while wearing the halo. Pins must be carefully inspected to make sure they are tight and not infected. Discomfort is more common if pins are placed in the temporal fossa.

Aside from brain abscess or meningitis, the most severe complications seen with the halo orthosis are those involving loss of reduction or loss of position of the cervical spine fracture or dislocation.[30] As previously discussed, it is recognized that some change in position of the spine can occur as the patient changes position. Thus, it may be impossible to completely immobilize a very unstable cervical spine.[28]

Conclusion

Biomechanically, the halo orthosis is the most effective device available for immobilization of the cervical spine. However, it is not infallible, and complications involving the pins and vest do occur. Proper attention to application of the halo vest and detail in its care can avert many of these complications, but it must be recognized that an occasional patient will have a change in position of the cervical spine or loss in reduction while in a halo orthosis. This type of patient must be surgically stabilized to achieve the maximal result.

Advances in design of the vest and superstructure promise to improve the fixation of the vest to the thorax and thus its overall stabilizing capabilities.

REFERENCES

1. *BARD G, JONES MD:* Cineradiographic recording of traction of the spine. Arch Phys Mech 45:403–406, 1964
2. *BARTON LG:* Reduction of fracture dislocations of the cervical vertebra by skeletal traction. Surg Gyn Obstet 67:94–96, 1938
3. *BLACKBURN JD:* A new skull traction appliance. South Surg 7:16–18, 1938
4. *BURKE DC, BERRYMAN D:* The place of manipulation in the management of flexion–rotation dislocations of the cervical spine. J Bone Joint Surg 53(B):165–182, 1971
5. *CRUTCHFIELD WG:* Skeletal traction for dislocation of cervical spine: report of a case. South Surg 2:156–159, 1933
6. *DURBIN FC:* Fractures-dislocations of the cervical spine. J Bone Joint Surg 39(B):23–38, 1957
7. *EVANS DK:* Reduction of cervical dislocations. J Bone Joint Surg 43(B):552–555, 1961
8. *FELDMAN RA, KHAYYAT GF:* Perforation of the skull by a Gardner-Wells Tong. J Neurosurg 44:119–120, 1976
9. *GARDNER WJ:* The principle of spring-loaded points for cervical traction. J Neurosurg 39:543–544, 1973
10. *GRUNDY DJ:* Skull traction and its complications. Injury 15:173–177, 1983
11. *HOEN TI:* A method of cervical traction for treatment of fracture dislocations of the cervical spine. Arch Neurol Psychiatr 36:158–161, 1936
12. *MCKENZIE KG:* Fracture, dislocation, and fracture-dislocation of the spine. Canad Med Assoc J 32:263–269, 1935
13. *NORRELL H:* Treatment of unstable spinal fractures and dislocations. Clin Neurosurg 25:193–208, 1978
14. *VINCKE TH:* A skull traction apparatus. J Bone Joint Surg 30(A):522–524, 1948
15. *YASHON D, ET AL:* Rapid closed reduction of cervical fracture dislocation. Surg Neurol 4:513–514, 1975
16. *DANZIG LA, ET AL:* The treatment of cervical spine metastasis from the prostrate with a halo cast. Spine 5:395–398, 1980
17. *FREEMAN GE:* Correction of severe deformity of the cervical spine and ankylosing spondylitis with a halo device. J Bone Joint Surg 43(A):547–552, 1961
18. *GARFIN SR, ET AL:* Osteology of the skull as it affects halo pin placement. Spine 10:696–698, 1985
19. *GARFIN SR, ET AL:* Complications in the use of the halo fixation device. J Bone Joint Surg 68(A):320–325, 1986
20. *JOHNSON RM, ET AL:* Cervical orthoses: A study comparing their effectiveness in restricting cervical motion in normal subjects. J Bone Joint Surg 59(A):332–339, 1977
21. *JOHNSON RM, ET AL:* Cervical orthoses. A guide to their selection and use. Clin Orthop 154:34–45, 1981
22. *KRAG MH, ET AL:* A new halo-vest: Initial clinical experience in comparison to a "standard" halo-vest. Proc Cerv Spine Res Soc, 1986
23. *KOCH RA, NICKEL VL:* The halo vest. An evaluation of motion and forces across the neck. Spine 3:103–107, 1978
24. *KOSTUIK JP:* Indications for the use of the halo immobilization. Clin Orthop 154:46–50, 1981
25. *NICKEL VL, ET AL:* The Halo: A spinal skeletal trac-

tion fixation device. J Bone Joint Surg 50(A):1400–1409, 1968

26. *Perry J, Nickel VL:* Total cervical-spine fusion for neck paralysis. J Bone Joint Surg 41(A):37–59, 1959
27. *Schweigel JF:* Halo-thoracic brace: Management of odontoid fractures. Spine 4:192–194, 1979
28. *Stauffer ES:* The halo external fixator. (editorial). J Bone Joint Surg 68(A):319, 1986
29. *Walker PS, et al:* Forces in the halo-vest apparatus. Spine 9:773–777, 1984
30. *Whitehill R, et al:* Failure of immobilization of the cervical spine by the halo vest. J Bone Joint Surg 68(A):326–332, 1986

Fractures and Dislocations at the Base of the Skull and Upper Cervical Spine

DONALD S. PIERCE AND JOSEPH S. BARR, JR.

The anatomy of the area at the base of the skull, which includes the first three cervical vertebrae, is unique as compared with the remainder of the vertebrae in the cervical area. The shapes of the first two cervical vertebrae are completely different from those of the remaining five, and the degrees of motion that take place at this area, together with the fact that the area directly supports the skull and is intimately associated with the foramen magnum, render injuries to this area particularly serious and also particularly difficult to treat.[15]

SKULL, C1, AND C2 DISLOCATIONS

Functionally, nodding occurs in large part as a result of the skull moving on the supporting lateral masses of the first cervical vertebra. Rotation does not normally take place at this point. When rotation is forced between the skull and C1, a rare but serious condition occurs: the articular processes of the skull dislocate, either one forward and one posteriorly on the supporting lateral masses of C1 or directly posteriorly or anteriorly (Fig. 6-26).[1,2] This dislocation, if the patient survives, may go undetected despite a bizarre angulation of the skull unless tomograms of the area are taken. Such a dislocation may also be associated with a rotary subluxation or dislocation in the opposite direction, of C1 on C2. This dual dislocation may be compatible with life. However, in this situation as well, the dislocation of the skull on C1 may be missed in plain x-ray films because the standard A–P film used for discerning whether or not C1 is dislocated on C2 rarely, if ever, shows the dislocation of the skull on C1.

The occiput may be dislocated directly posteriorly with both condyles of the skull sliding off the supporting lateral masses of C1, the tip of the odontoid having been avulsed by the alar ligaments.[4] Eismont and Bohlman reported such a case, in which severe neurologic deficit persisted.[4] Anterior dislocation of the condyles of the skull on the lateral masses of C1 has also been reported by Gabrielsen and Maxwell; in this case, the diagnosis was not made until tong traction had been instituted.[6] Neurologic deficit was much less, but the normal distance from odontoid to basion was markedly decreased. There was permanent loss of flexion because of contact between the basion and the tip of the odontoid process.

JEFFERSON'S FRACTURE

Unique to the first cervical vertebra, the Jefferson's fracture is a bursting of the ring of C1 as a result of axial loading directly downward on the ring of C1, causing multiple fractures of the ring and usually a spreading of the fragment.[8,9] An A–P film generally shows widening of the distance between the odontoid and the lateral masses of C1, and the lateral film frequently shows cracks in or frank disruption of the ring posteriorly.[13] However, if there is little or no displacement of the fragments, it is sometimes difficult to make a diagnosis with certainty; it is also sometimes difficult to discern the number of breaks through the ring, particularly if one of the breaks occurs directly in the midline where tomography is less accurate than it is more laterally. Heretofore, fractures in the anterior center of the ring went undetected because they fell in the plane of the lateral roentgenogram or tomogram where it was impossible to see them. The advent of the CT scan made diagnosis of Jefferson's fracture and follow-up of the healing process easier and more accurate.

If the lateral masses are spread more than 6.9 mm the transverse ligament is torn (Figs. 6-27 and 6.28).[12] It is noted, however, that congenital abnormalities in the arch of C1 with midline posterior and anterior defects can cause spreading of the lateral masses of C1 in the absence of a Jefferson's fracture.[3] In this situation, an exaggerated Water's view will show the congenital abnormality. The posterior defect is rarely, if ever, midline.[7]

ODONTOID FRAGMENT IN THE FORAMEN MAGNUM

One additional condition that may present itself at the base of the skull and C1 is the fracture of the odontoid in which a fragment of the odontoid migrates upward into the foramen magnum, with danger of compression of the high cervical cord and the base of the brain. It is impossible to remove a fragment of a fractured odontoid from the area of the foramen magnum through a posterior approach. Although the area of the base of the skull does not lend itself easily to surgery from an anterior approach, this is possible, at high risk, by splitting the mandible and the tongue and oper-

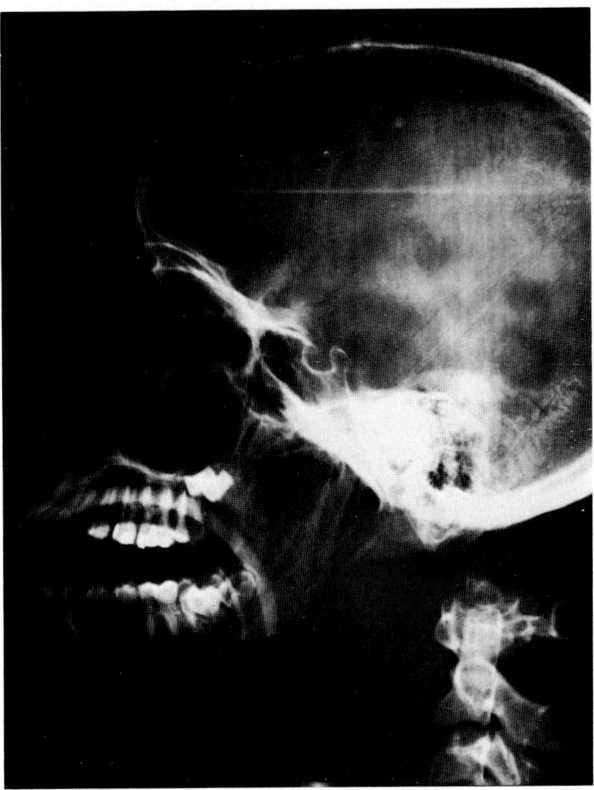

Fig. 6-26. Lateral view of a fatal decapitation injury.

ating through the oropharynx. This transpharyngeal approach is fraught with technical difficulty, and there is a danger of infection from the mouth and oropharynx. Therefore, it may be preferable to treat the condition from a posterior approach by foramen magnum decompression and posterior fusion.

COMBINATION JEFFERSON'S FRACTURE AND FRACTURE OF THE ODONTOID

A combination of Jefferson's fracture and fracture of the odontoid is a rarely seen entity that is presumably due to direct axial loading of the cervical spine through the skull coupled with a secondary posterior force, presumably from hyperextension of the skull on the anterior portion of C1. This may even take the form of an odontoid fracture with a split directly in the middle of the anterior segment of C1, as in Case 2. Such a fracture of the odontoid yields marked instability, and therefore there is danger of damage to the cord. However, because the odontoid fragment is being carried with the already fractured ring of C1, this fracture may be compatible with life and may produce no neurologic damage unless there is gross motion of the skull on the cervical spine. If any severe neurologic damage were present, the injury would be lethal. Possible damage to the vertebral arteries is

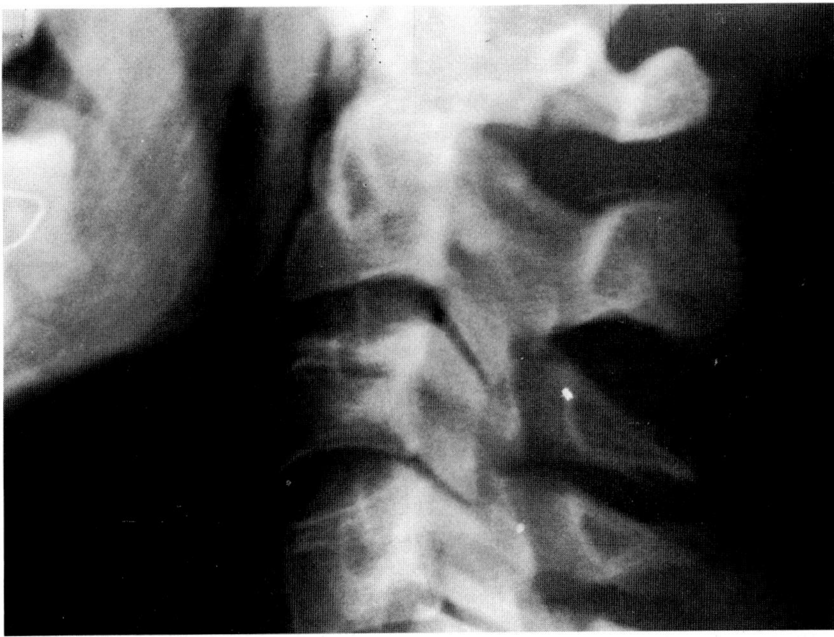

Fig. 6-27. Lateral roentgenogram angling upward to show fractures in the posterior ring of C1.

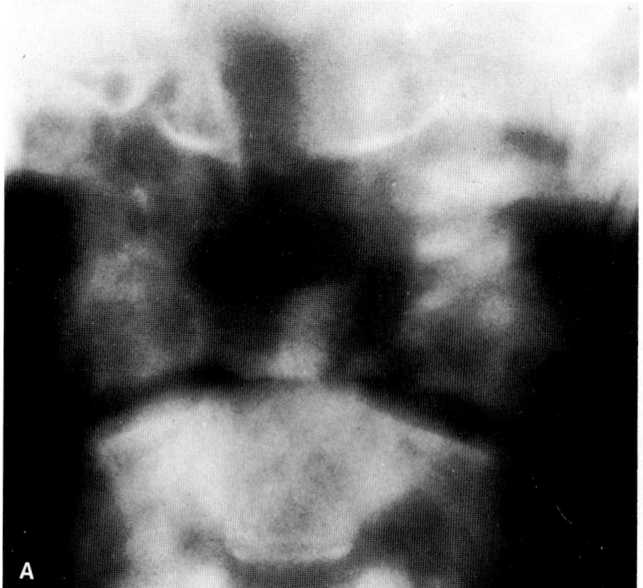

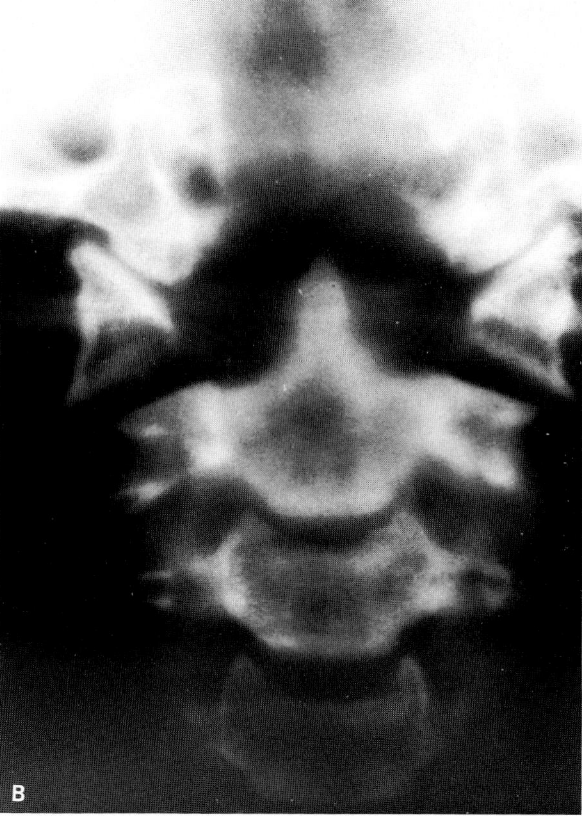

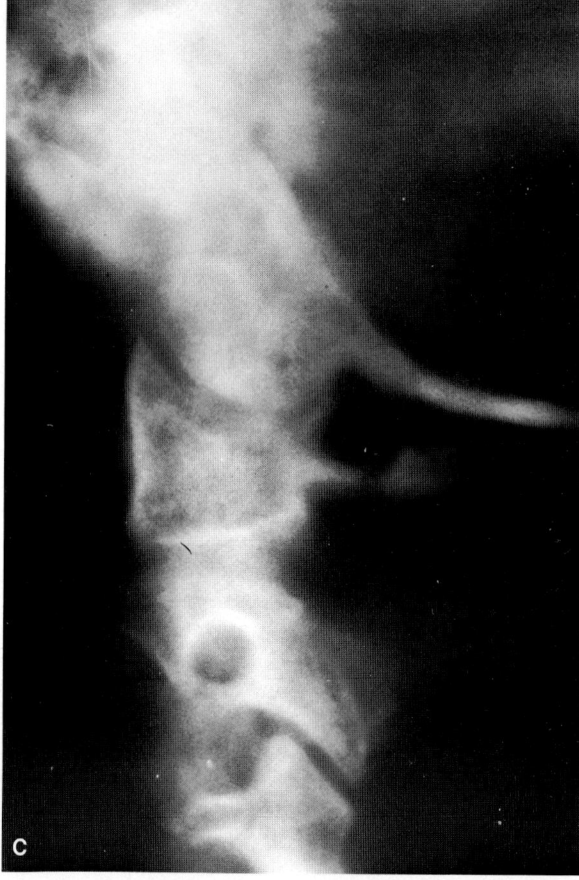

Fig. 6-28. (*A*) A–P view showing separation of lateral masses and C1, and fracture of the odontoid at the base. (*B* and *C*) At 6 weeks after the injury, tomograms show displacement of lateral masses of C1. (*C*) The lateral view shows healing fractures in the arch of C1 posteriorly. At 6 months postinjury, an A–P view (*D*) and a lateral view (*E*) of the healed Jefferson's fracture show permanent lateral displacement of the lateral masses of C1.

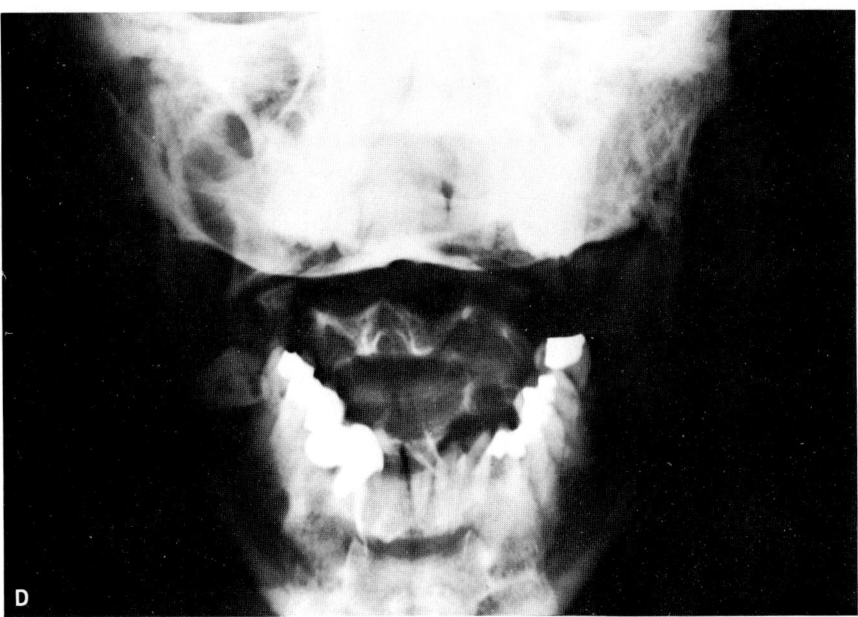

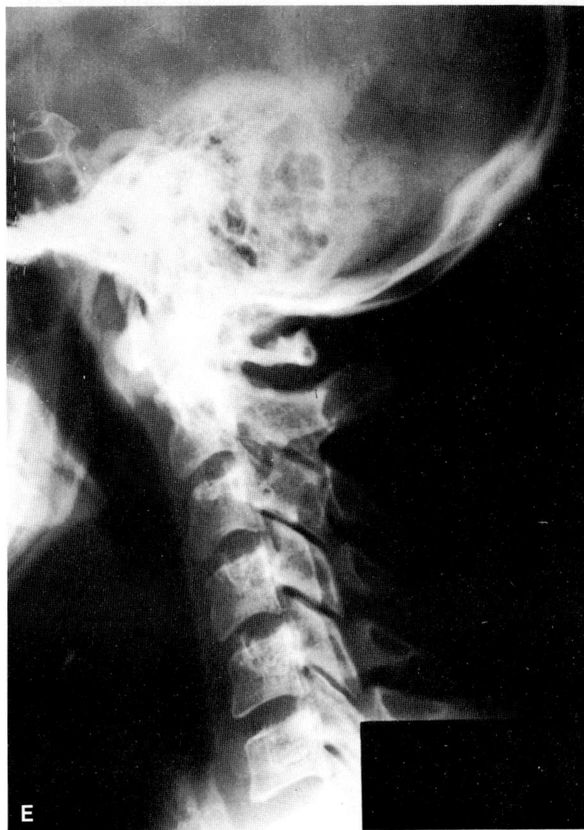

usually avoided because of the comminution of the ring of C1, which averts pressure on the vessels.

VERTEBROBASILAR INJURIES

The vertebral arteries are vulnerable to injury in the foramina of the lower cervical vertebra at the junction between C1 and C2, and as they pass over the arch of C1 through the atlantooccipital membrane. Intimal disruption may lead to acute, complete thrombotic occlusion, subintimal hematoma, dissection of the artery, or pseudoaneurysm formation. Obviously, atlantooccipital dislocation usually causes total disruption of the vertebral basilar system and death. However, there are more than 20 cases in the literature of less severe injuries to the vertebral basilar system produced by mechanisms such as chiropractic manipulations, yoga exercises, overhead work, and cervical traction. The mechanism of injury seems to be cervical hyperextension accompanied by excessive rotation. Severely diminished flow in one vertebral artery may well lead to occlusion of the posterior inferior cerebellar artery on that side, resulting in a lateral medullary infarction, Wallenberg's syndrome. This syndrome is characterized by the ipsilateral loss of cranial nerves V, IX, X, and XI, cerebellar ataxia, Horner's syndrome, and contralateral loss of pain and temperature sensation.

With increasing severity of injury, vascular involvement can ascend to the basilar, superior cerebellar, and posterior cerebral arteries. Sudden death, quadriplegia, or the "locked-in" syndrome (quadriplegia with loss of lower cranial nerves, allowing eye blinking only) can ensue. These symptoms following injury or cervical manipulation should alert one to the possibility of vascular injury, and immediate cerebral arteriography for accurate diagnosis is indicated. Arteriography also helps to assess the collateral circulation. Following arteriography, treatment consists of immediate anticoagulation with heparin to prevent further extension of thrombosis and administration of oxygen to maintain cerebral oxygenation.[11]

TREATMENT

Use of the Halo Brace

In the treatment of virtually all of Jefferson's fractures, the rare dislocation of the skull on C1 with or without dislocation of C1 on C2, and migration of an odontoid fragment into the foramen magnum requiring posterior decompression, we strongly recommend the use of the halo brace to stabilize the spine. It can be used as definitive treatment when surgery is not indicated. It can also be used during a surgical procedure and afterward during the healing process to allow the patient the freedom of ambulation. The studies of Johnson and associates have shown the use of the halo device to be the only method of stabilization that gives absolute stability to the cervical spine.[10] In the delicate area at the base of the skull, such absolute immobilization is a prerequisite for any surgical approach.

Treatment of Jefferson's Fracture

In general, Jefferson's fractures are best treated with the halo brace. The device affords adequate immobilization for undisplaced Jefferson's fractures so that they may heal without any surgical intervention. Healing is generally adequate within 3 to 6 months, and fusion is rarely if ever necessary. In a rare situation where a Jefferson's fracture fails to heal, fusion from the occiput to C2 will afford adequate stabilization of the spine in this area; in our opinion, this surgical procedure should be done only with immobilization of the patient in the halo brace, with maintenance of stabilization until adequate healing is seen on roentgenogram.

Odontoid Fragments in the Foramen Magnum

If there is migration of a fragment of the odontoid into the foramen magnum threatening the high cervical cord and basilar structures of the brain, the patient should be immobilized in a halo brace with the brace applied in such a way that it allows the posterior half to be removed for surgical procedure. Surgery should then be undertaken in the company of a qualified neurosurgeon, who will carry out the foramen magnum decompression by removal of adequate bone from the base of the skull posteriorly to allow adequate room for the upper cervical cord and the vertebral arteries. The orthopedic portion of the procedure is then carried out by fusion from the upper base of the skull posteriorly to C2—if needed, even to C3—to get adequate fixation for the graft below. The technique for this procedure will be described subsequently.

Skull, C1, and C2 Dislocations

In a case in which there is evidence of dislocation of the skull on C1, with or without subluxation of C1 on C2, set up the halo brace as described for the previous situation. After induction of anesthesia with nasotracheal intubation, turn the patient face down and remove the posterior half of the halo, leaving the halo supported by the anterior upright bars. Through a midline approach, expose the spine and base of the skull; dissect the arch of C1 free over 1 cm in the midline posteriorly; and, with great care, pass a looped #20 wire under the arch, protecting the cord carefully in the midline posteriorly and holding the arch with Kelley clamps. Grasp the wire loop so that the arch of C1 cannot sublux forward, and grasp the arch itself with Kocher clamps, while an assistant, beneath the drapes, applies traction through the vertical traction bars to take pressure off the ring of C1; then manipulate the ring into position underneath the skull on top of C2. Conduct a trial movement with traction off to be certain that the reduction has been achieved. Release of traction on the halo from underneath the drapes will then hold the reduction, and a second assistant should continue to exert gentle posterior traction after the trial of reduction to be certain that no slippage occurs until the wiring of the graft has been carried out.

One cannot emphasize strongly enough the importance of not dissecting too far laterally when dissecting under the arch of C1 in passing the loop of wire beneath it; this may lead to damage or severe hemorrhage from one or both of the vertebral arteries as they come together from their lateral position to a more central position, from which they pass to the brain through the circle of Willis.

Case 1. A 21-year-old female was seen 3 months after an automobile accident, a head-on collision without a seatbelt; she was thrown forward, striking the right side of her head over the right eyebrow on the roof of the car at the border of the windshield. She had immediate onset of pain in her neck. She could not move her head to the right without moving her entire neck below the base of the skull to the right. She was initially diagnosed as having muscle spasm and a stiff neck; she held her neck rigidly to the left at the base of the skull, correcting by bending the remainder of the cervical spine to the right. Plain roentgenograms showed no abnormality of the lower cervical spine, but they did show what was thought initially to be a rotary subluxation of C1 and C2 (Fig. 6-29*A, B, C,* and *D*). Tomograms were taken that showed, in addition, a dislocation of the skull on C1 as well as a rotary subluxation of the skull on C1 on C2. The patient was advised of the gravity of the situation and the necessity for operative correction and fusion. She was placed in a halo vest without specific attempt to change the alignment of the cervical spine. After having become used to the vest for a short period, she was taken to the operating room; under general anesthesia with a nasotracheal intubation, the posterior half of the halo was removed and, through a midline incision, the arch of C1 was exposed and grasped with two Kelley clamps. It was clear at the time that the midpoint of the posterior arch of C1 was far to the left of the midpoint of the skull and also far to the left of the midpoint of the spinous process of C2. At this point, an assistant beneath the drapes placed traction on the halo itself by increasing the length of the vertical traction bar between the halo and the horizontal supporting bar from the halo jacket. This loosened the pressure of the skull on C1. With two Kocher clamps and a wire loop passed between the arch of C1 in the midline and the spinal cord to prevent forward luxation, the arch of C1 was rotated to the right. Initially, it appeared that reduction had been achieved. However, as the hold on the Kocher clamps was relaxed, the arch of C1, held back by the wire grasped by a second assistant, rotated again to the left and retained its former position. Further traction was put on and, under careful observation, the Kocher clamps were reapplied, and once again the arch of C1 was rotated to the right. At this point, an audible pop was heard and the arch of C1 snapped into place beneath the skull, with the midpoint directly beneath the midpoint of the skull and in alignment with the spinous process of C2. At this point traction was decreased until no traction existed, and the arch of C1 could not be moved with the Kocher clamps. Fusion in the manner described in the text was then carried out (Fig. 6-29).

Combined Jefferson's Fracture and Fracture of the Odontoid

Jefferson's fracture combined with odontoid fracture is not amenable to surgical fusion, even if one wished to do an immediate fusion to stabilize the odontoid. Obviously, the fusing to the fractured posterior arch of C1, even if it were possible, would afford no stabilization of the fragment of the odontoid on its base. Therefore, treatment with the halo jacket or halo cast is the treatment of choice initially, with alignment of the odontoid fracture as well as possible, and watchful waiting until the ring of C1 is healed. If at that time the odontoid fracture has gone on to delayed or nonunion, posterior C1–C2 fusion may be carried out with the protection of the halo brace, stabilization being maintained in the halo brace for as long as desired or until healing takes place in the odontoid fracture. This will be up to the discretion of the surgeon. The length of time will depend greatly on the degree of stability achieved by the surgeon at the time of fusion.

Case 2. A 31-year-old white male carpenter fell from the roof of the house on which he was working, directly on the top of his head. He was taken to a local hospital with a towel wrapped around his neck because he felt severe pain. Roentgenograms showed a Jefferson's fracture and a fracture at the base of the odontoid (Fig. 6-30*A*). He was immobilized in a cervical brace and sent to the Massachusetts General Hospital where, after reading the roentgenograms, a halo jacket was applied and reduction of the odontoid fracture achieved without distraction of the Jefferson's fracture. Tomograms were then taken to determine whether or not there were any further fractures, and at this time a suspicion of a fracture at the center of the ring of C1 anteriorly was entertained. A CT scan of the upper cervical spine was then obtained by placing a cervical collar on the patient, disconnecting the halo from the halo jacket, and removing the jacket with the patient set up to go into the scanner. The patient was then moved carefully into the scanner, the CT scan was obtained, the patient was returned to the halo jacket, and the collar was removed. The CT scan showed the midline fracture (Fig. 6-30*B*). Three months later the same procedure was repeated (Fig. 6-30*C*). The fractures of the arch of C1 were seen to be healing, but the odontoid fracture was not healing. Stability

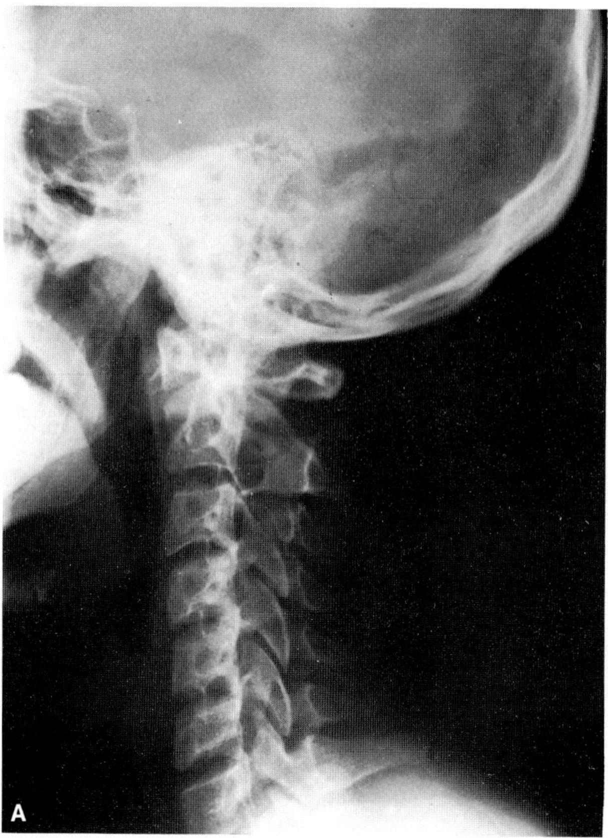

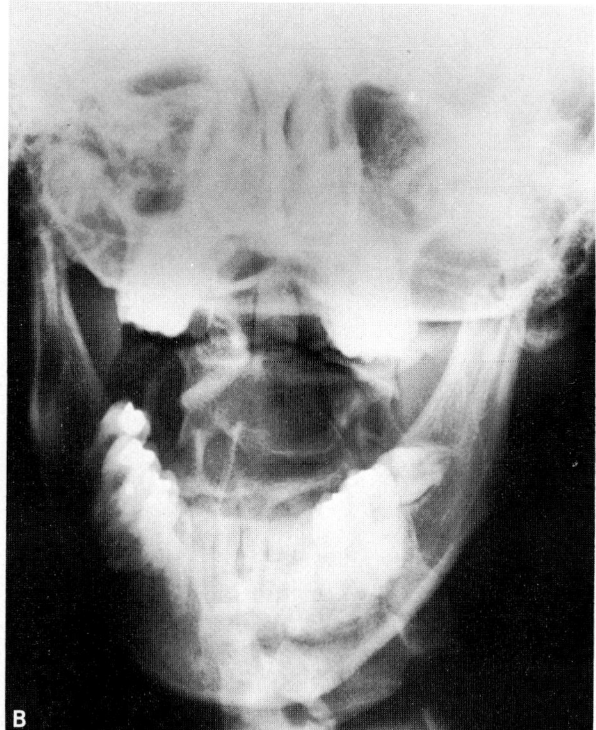

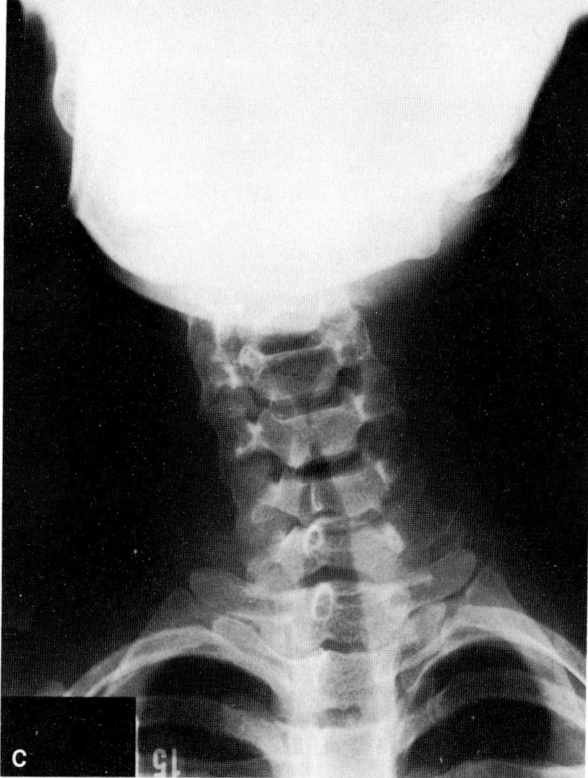

Fig. 6-29. (*A*) A preoperative lateral view of C1–C2 showing dislocation of the skull of C1 on C2. (*B*) A preoperative A–P odontoid view showing rotary dislocation of C1 on C2 with the base of skull obscured owing to angulation asymmetry. (*C*) A preoperative A–P view of the cervical spine showing marked angulation of the skull with abnormality at C1–C2. (*D*) A preoperative view showing the location of the skull on C1 and C1 on C2. (*E*) The 1-year postoperative view showing successful reduction and occipital fusion to C1–C2.

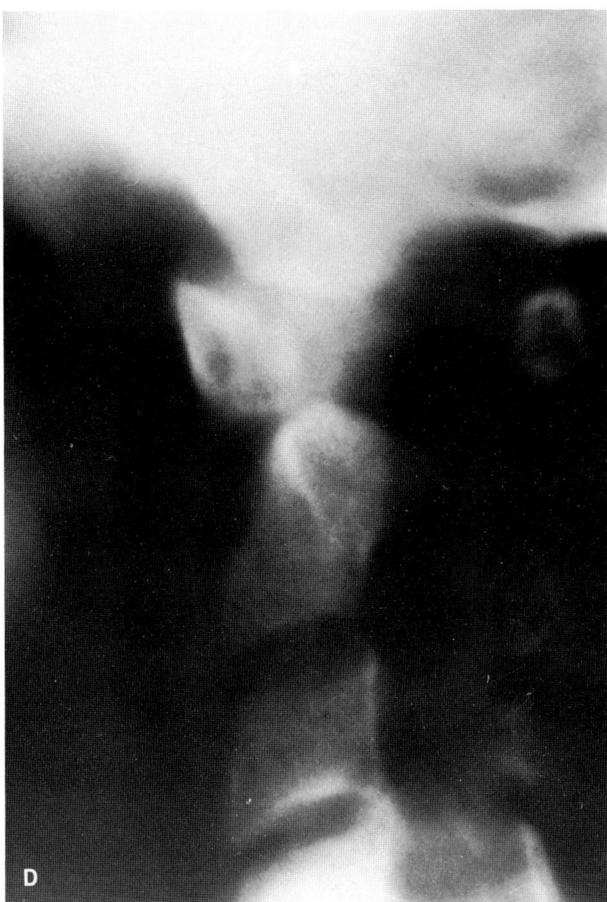

was deemed good enough to carry out a posterior fusion of C1 to C2; this was carried out in the halo brace, which was subsequently removed 6 weeks later. The patient had no neurologic deficit.

Technique of Occiput–Cervical Fusion

In the past, fusion to the occiput has been deemed difficult to achieve. We have developed a technique for securing grafts to the skull at the inion, the point at the center of the base of the skull in which the bone is extremely thick. This point still exists after quite a major decompression of the foramen magnum in most cases. It is usually thick enough so that it is possible to use the Hall air drill with a small bur to make two trenches in the sides of the inion and then to drill at an angle into the base of the inion itself. It is then possible, making one or more such drill holes on each side, to pass #20-gauge wires through the inion without having to go through the skull into the epidural space. One or two wires are thus passed through the inion, which gives extremely strong fixation for the grafts.

Next, a corticocancellus graft of adequate length is taken from the posterior iliac crest in the standard manner as a single piece. It is split on the diagonal to give two triangular segments, and these are then shaped to fit exactly the contour of the base of the skull, fitting into the two troughs made with the Hall drill beside the inion. They are also shaped to fit down onto the arch of C1 and

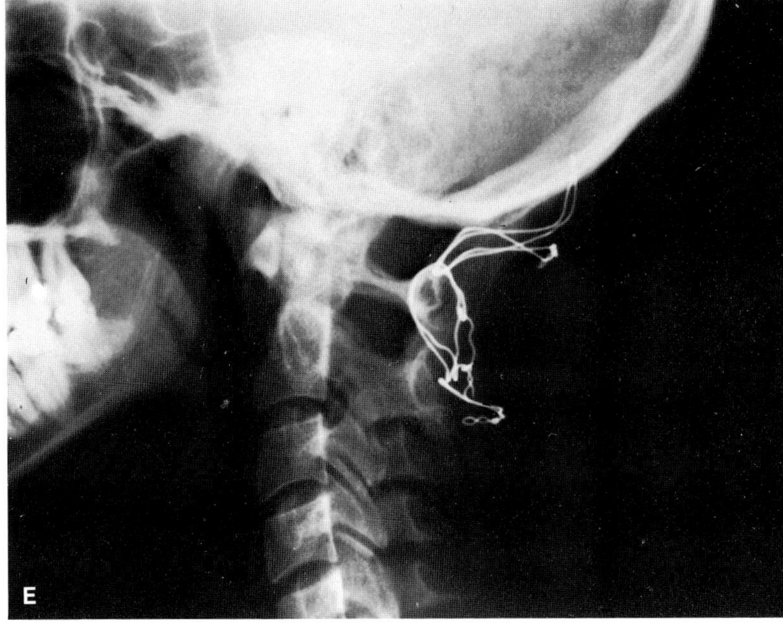

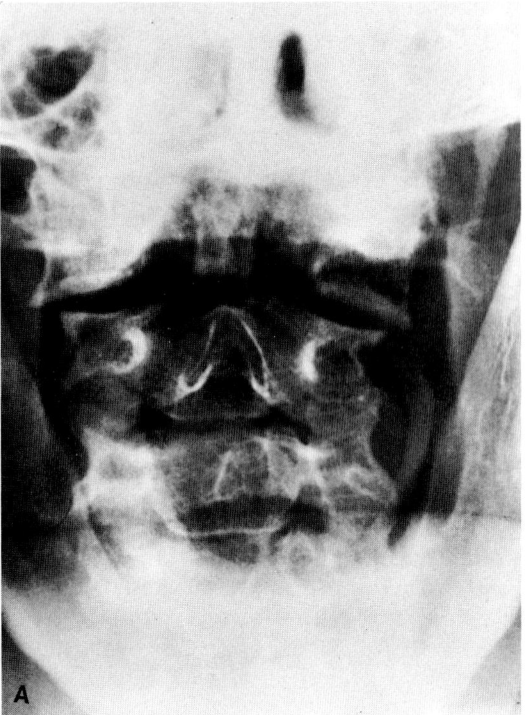

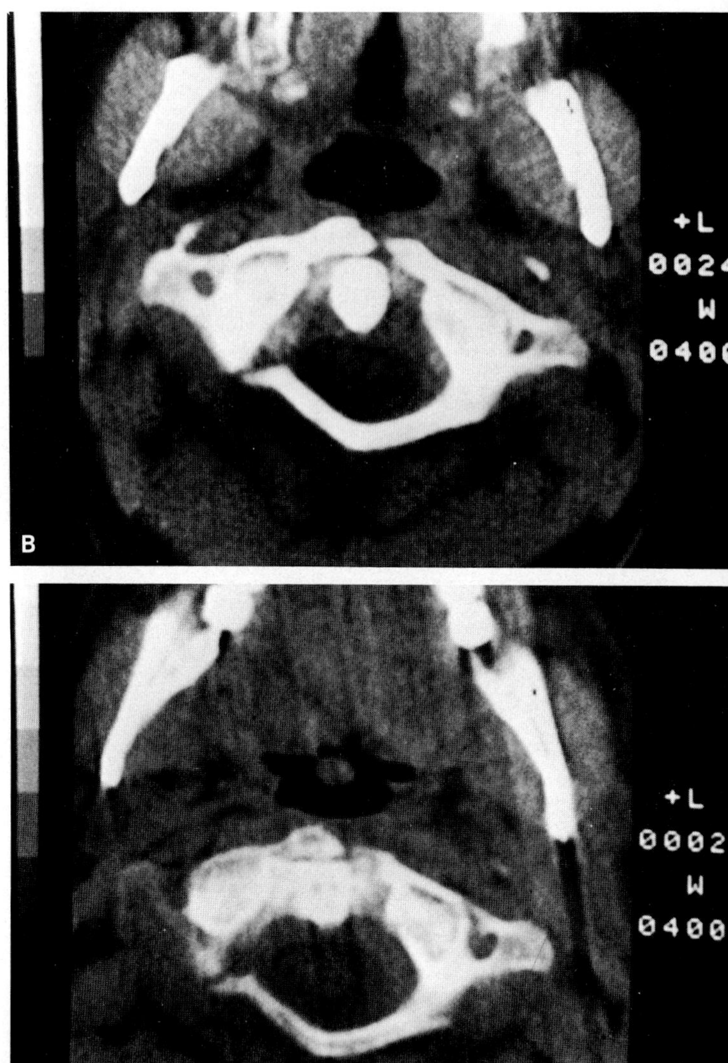

Fig. 6-30. (*A*) Open-mouth view at the time of injury showing widening of the lateral masses of C1 and a fracture at the base of the odontoid (see text). (*B*) A CT scan showing anterior fracture of C1 and left posterior arch fracture of C1. (*C*) CT scan 3 months later, showing healed fracture of anterior and left posterior portions of C1 (see text).

the laminae of C2 and, if necessary, to be continued to C3. This makes the graft roughly the shape of an isosceles triangle with the long side pointing posteriorly toward where the incision will be closed. One of the two shorter sides will rest slightly curved against the skull; the other will rest against the arch of C1 and the laminae of C2 and, if necessary, C3.

The wire loop that has been passed beneath the arch of C1 is secured around the two grafts, and the two free ends of the loop are passed from opposite sides through a drill hole or a hole made with a Towel clip in the base of the spinous process of C2. After being crossed over the graft, one end is passed up through the loop and the ends are twisted and tightened to hold the graft on the arch of C1 and to C2–C3. If desired, the free ends, may be passed through a hole in the end of the graft for even better fixation. The wire or wires passed through the inion are then passed through a drill hole in the upper end of each graft and at the upper points of the triangle as they rest against the skull. It is twisted tight and cut off. This gives an extremely stable fusion at the time of surgery and also provides a posterior bar from C2 or C3 to the skull, which pulls a reduced C1 against the

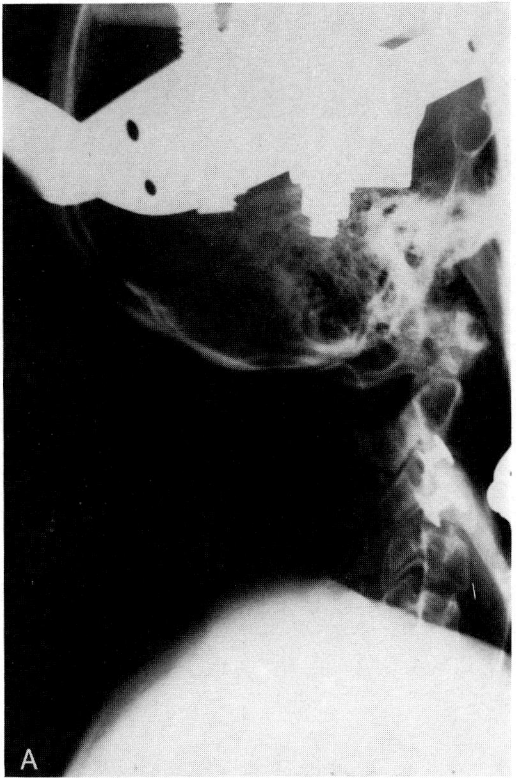

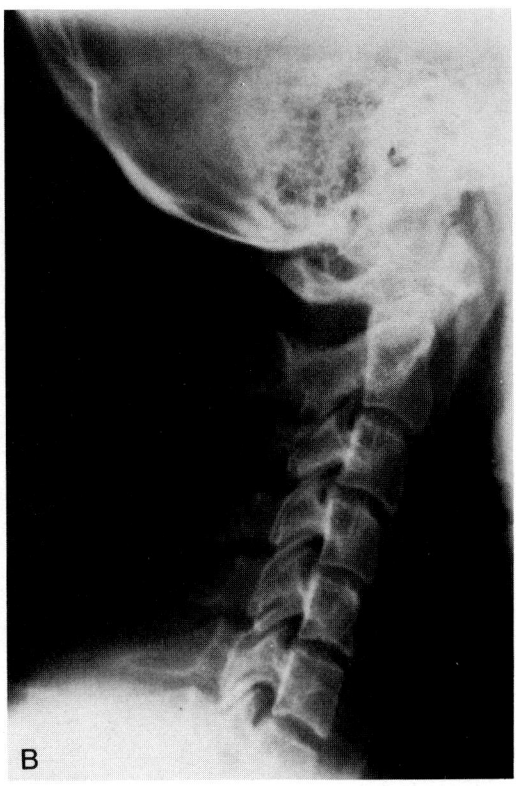

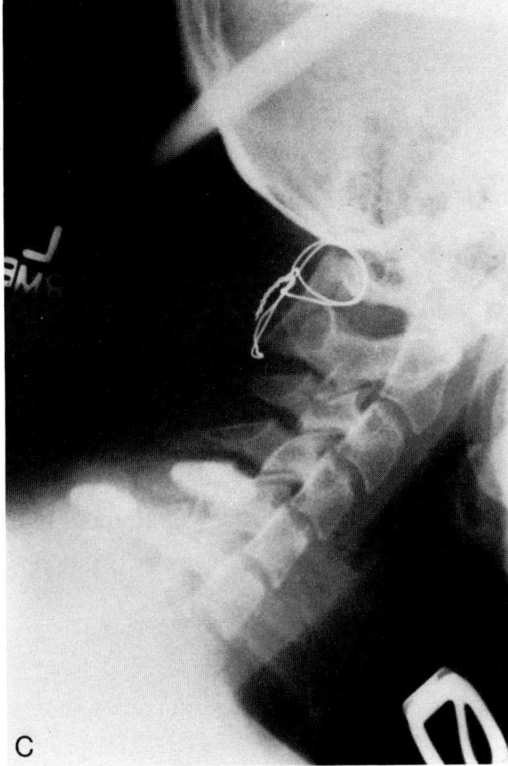

Fig. 6-31. (*A*) Lateral roentgenogram showing os odontoideum with displacement. (*B*) Lateral roentgenogram in flexion showing increased anterior subluxation. (*C*) Lateral roentgenogram postoperatively showing C1–C2 fusion.

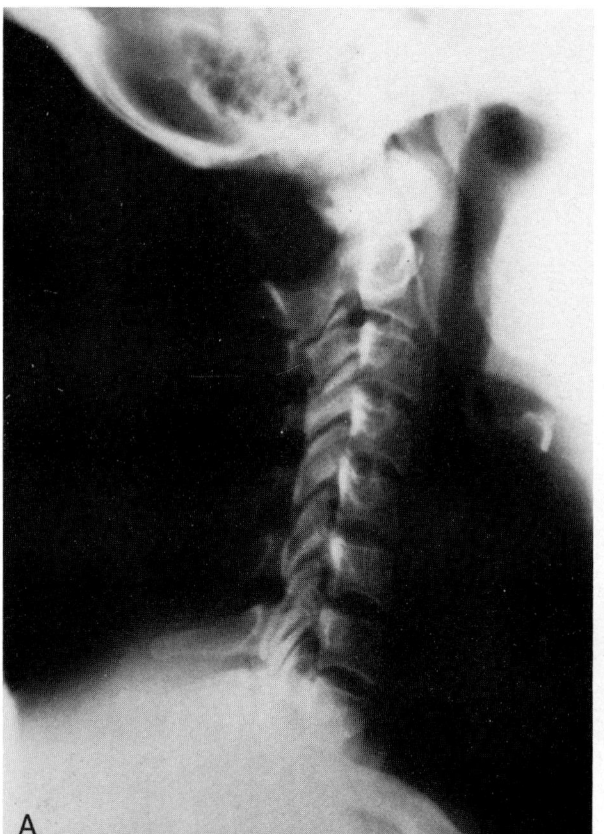

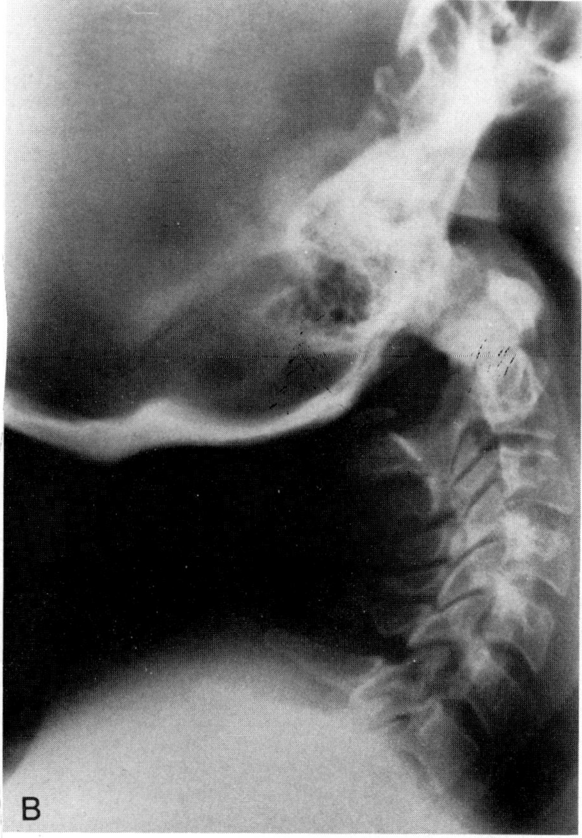

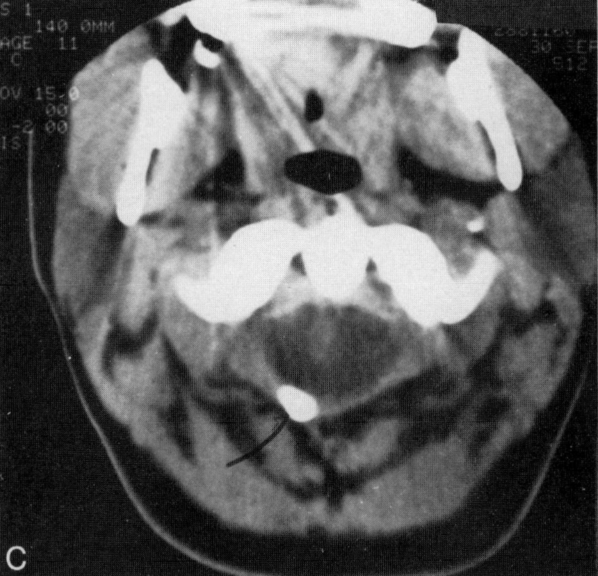

Fig. 6-32. (*A*) Lateral roentgenogram showing absent C1 posterior arch with retained spinous process. (*B*) Lateral roentgenogram showing no displacement in extension. (*C*) CT showing absence of C1 arch with ossified spinous process.

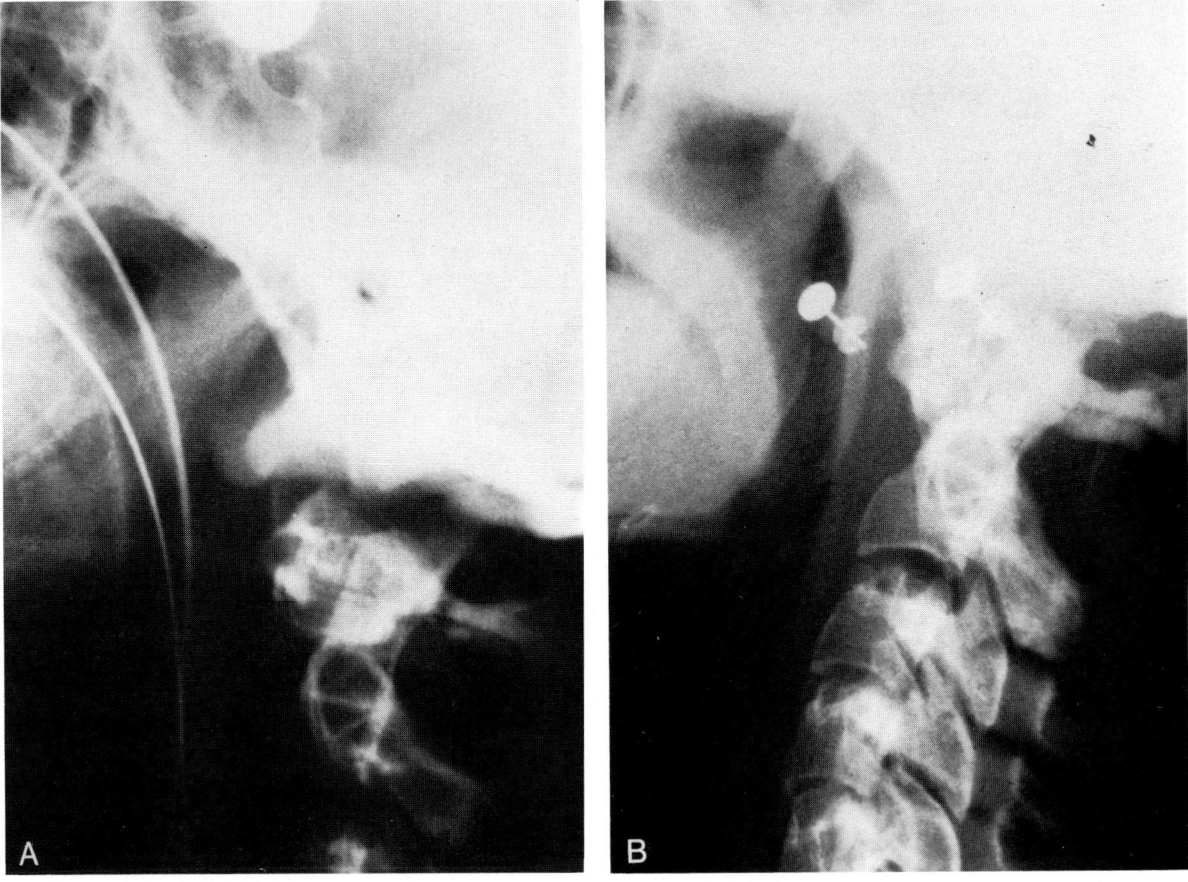

Fig. 6-33. (*A*) Lateral roentgenogram of upper cervical spine showing distraction of occiput and atlas in traction after injury. (*B*) Lateral roentgenogram of upper cervical spine after release of traction. Normal anatomic alignment has been restored.

skull and holds it in proper alignment during the healing process. This technique may be used for any situation in which the bone in the area is adequately firm and in which it is desired to fuse from the skull to C2 across C1. This technique may also be required in certain situations in which congenital anomalies render the arch of C1 either aplastic and applied closely underneath the occiput, where it is too far forward to safely pass a wire beneath it to secure a graft, or absent entirely so that there is nothing under which to pass a wire.

Case 1. This is a twenty-year-old male who was involved in a motor vehicle accident. Subsequent to the accident there were no neurologic (Fig. 6-31 *A*, *B*, and *C*) deficits. The patient had intractable pain at the base of the skull and was discovered to have an os odontoideum with marked displacement. Bending films showed displacement believed to be dangerous in a young man who stated that his intention was to continue extremely active contact sports. A spinal fusion posteriorly was deemed adequate; however, the patient had to be warned that, because of the hypoplastic arch of C1 applied to the base of the skull, it might be impossible to pass a wire beneath it, and fusion to the base of the skull might have to be carried out.

Case 2. This is a patient involved in a motor vehicle accident who felt severe pain at the base of the skull that resolved after a short period of time. X-rays show complete absence of the arch of C1, except for a tiny ossicle of bone representing the posterior process. Although no surgical intervention was indicated here, in a patient of this type, were surgery indicated, fusion of C2 to the occiput would be necessary (Fig. 6-32 *A*, *B*, and *C*).

It goes without saying that fractures and dislocations at the base of the skull and upper cervical spine require extremely careful evaluation. Sometimes injuries to other parts of the cervical spine receive attention, and less frequent injuries at the base of the skull are missed. In other situations such injuries are not appreciated, and wrong or inadequate treatment is administered.

Such is the case of an 18-year-old female struck by a car. She was brought to the emergency room quadriparetic (Fig. 6-33 *A* and *B*). The injury at the base of the skull was not initially recognized. Traction with tongs was mistakenly applied, causing distraction of the occiput and atlas and resulting in immediate pentaplegia (respirator-dependent quadriplegia). Bony union occurred after 4 months; however, the patient had no neurologic recovery and remained respirator dependent. Such tragic complications may usually be avoided by careful evaluation by polytomography and/or CT scanning before traction is applied.

Postoperatively, the halo brace is maintained for at least 6 weeks or until roentgenograms show evidence of bony healing. The patient may be ambulatory if there is no paralysis or other injury, and he can go home during this period. If for any reason, as in rheumatoid arthritis, a posterior fusion has failed, the technique of Whitesides may be used: using a modified Henry's postauricular approach to the vertebral artery, drill a hole through the lateral mass of C1 and C2, roughening the articular surface between the two and passing a lag screw through on each side to hold C1 and C2 together. This is a very difficult procedure technically; obviously, in less than experienced hands it is very dangerous. However, when a posterior fusion has failed, it is probably preferable to attempt a fusion by this method than through a transpharyngeal approach.

Surgery to the area of the skull, C1, and C2 is less common than surgery in other areas of the cervical spine and offers an especially challenging technical problem in the field of spinal surgery.

REFERENCES

1. *Alker GJ, Oh YS, Leslie EV, et al:* Postmortem radiology of head and neck injuries in fatal traffic accidents. Radiology 114:611, 1975
2. *Bucholz RW, Burkead WZ:* J Bone Joint Surg 61A:248, 1979
3. *Budin E, Sondheimer F:* Lateral spread of the atlas without fracture. Radiology 87:1095, 1966
4. *Eismont FJ, Bohlman HH:* Posterior atlantooccipital dislocation with fractures of the atlas and odontoid process. J Bone Joint Surg 60A:397, 1978
5. *Evarts CM:* Traumatic occipito-atlantal dislocation. J Bone Joint Surg 52A:1653, 1970
6. *Gabrielsen TO, Maxwell JA:* Traumatic atlanto-occipital dislocation. AJR 97:624, 1966
7. *Garber JN:* Abnormalities of the atlas and axis vertebrae: Congenital and traumatic. J Bone Joint Surg 46A:1782, 1964
8. *Hinchey JJ, Bicker WH:* Fracture of the atlas. Ann Surg 121:826, 1945
9. *Jefferson G:* Fracture of the atlas vertebra. Br J Surg 7:407, 1920
10. *Johnson R, et al:* Cervical orthoses: A study comparing their effectiveness in restricting cervical motion in normal subjects. J Bone Joint Surg 59A:332, 1977
11. *Lipson SJ:* Fractures of the atlas associated with fractures of the odontoid process and transverse ligament ruptures. J Bone Joint Surg 59A:940, 1977
12. *Schellhas KP, Latchaw RE, Wendling LR, Gold LHA:* Vertebrobasilar injuries following cervical manipulation. JAMA 244:1450, 1980
13. *Sherk HH, Nicholson JT:* Fractures of the atlas. J Bone Joint Surg 52A:1017, 1970
14. *Spence KF Jr., Decker S, Sell K:* Bursting atlantal fracture associated with rupture of the transverse ligament. J Bone Joint Surg 52A:543, 1970
15. *White A, Panjabi MM:* The clinical biomechanics of the occipitoatlantoaxial complex. Orthop Clin North Am 9:867, 1978

Fractures of the Odontoid Process of the Axis

LEWIS D. ANDERSON AND CHARLES R. CLARK

Fractures of the odontoid process of the axis (dens) have caused confusion and controversy throughout this century. There has been little agreement as to the best method of treatment, the prognosis, or the incidence of nonunion, which has been reported to be as high as 62.8% and as low as 4.8%.[2,46] Controversy has centered on treatment of fractures occurring at the junction of the dens and the vertebral body.[12]

The early history of this injury is somewhat obscure. In their article in 1956 on fractures of the odontoid process, Blockey and Purser stated that they could not identify the first description of this fracture.[6] They did note that, at the beginning of this century, odontoid fractures were thought to occur in association with fractures of the atlas. Corner, in 1907, reported in six patients fractures of the odontoid and the atlas had caused death.[14] Jefferson reported on thirteen patients with fractures of both the atlas and the odontoid.[30]

Osgood and Lund, in 1928, reviewed the literature related to fractures of the odontoid.[38] Up to that time, they found a total of only 55 reported cases of fractures of the odontoid process. They stated that most preceding authors had considered these to be rare injuries, with a high percentage accompanied by neurologic involvement and death. They reported an instability rate of 50%. Osgood and Lund suspected that the high mortality rate was related to the fact that many of the reported cases were based on autopsy material. They also discussed late neurologic involvement and found that, in ten of their reported cases, paralysis was not initially present but that it subsequently caused death after a second minor injury. They wrote that the general impression at the time of their article was that union of odontoid fractures was rare. At the time of their review, only three surgically treated patients were known to them. Two of these had previously been reported in 1910 by Mixter and Osgood.[35]

More recent articles have reported fractures of the odontoid in increasing numbers. Sherk, in 1978, found more than 500 such injuries reported in the literature.[53] Thus, over 90% of the total fractures of the odontoid in the literature have been reported in the last 50 years. It appears that the reasons for this are threefold. First, the actual number has risen because of the increase in population. Second, there is much greater susceptibility to injury in high-speed motor vehicle accidents in recent years. In the older literature, most fractures of the odontoid were caused by major falls and blows to the head. In more recent articles, motor vehicle accidents are by far the most common cause.[7,12,16,17] Third, prior to the report of Osgood and Lund, many of the cases reported were from autopsy material.[38] Radiologic techniques were not nearly so well developed as they are today. There can be little doubt that high-quality radiographs and tomograms have greatly aided the modern diagnosis of odontoid fractures.

As mentioned earlier, the treatment controversy centers on fractures at the junction of the dens and vertebral body. Because there are strong advocates of both surgical[3,8,15,21,54] and nonsurgical[2,10,13,17,40,58] management of this injury and[2] because clinical studies support both types of treatment, the surgeon is justified in selecting either form of management.[12] However, most studies have involved relatively small numbers of patients. The Cervical Spine Research Society recently reported a large multicenter study addressing the issue of the appropriate initial management of fractures of the dens.[12] This is the largest reported series of this fracture of which we are aware.

CLASSIFICATION

Several classifications of these fractures have been proposed. Schatzker and associates, in 1972, classified odontoid fractures as "high" and "low," depending on whether the fracture was above or below the accessory ligament.[46] However, in their 37 patients with an overall rate of nonunion of 63% they could find no correlation between union and the level of the fracture. They did find a higher incidence of nonunion if the fracture was displaced. In undisplaced fractures the nonunion rate was 42%. In fractures with anterior displacement the nonunion rate was 63% and in those with posterior displacement it was 93%.

In 1974, Anderson and D'Alonzo reported a series of 60 patients with fractures of the odontoid process treated at the Campbell Clinic and City of Memphis Hospital from 1964 through 1972.[3] Forty-nine of these patients were followed for a minimum of 6 months.

After reviewing the roentgenograms of each of

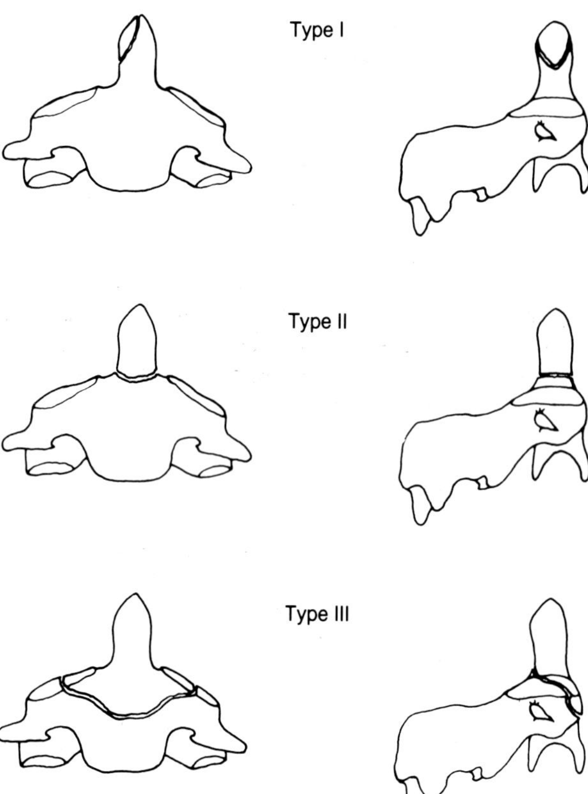

Fig. 6-34. Three types of odontoid fractures as seen in the anteroposterior and lateral planes. Type I is an oblique fracture through the upper part of the odontoid process itself. Type II is a fracture at the junction of the odontoid process with the vertebral body of the second cervical vertebra. Type III is really a fracture through the body of the atlas. (Anderson LD, D'Alonzo RT: Fractures of the odontoid process of the axis. J Bone Joint Surg 56A:1664, 1974)

these patients carefully, they found that there appeared to be three distinct types of fractures as determined by the anatomic location of the fracture line (Fig. 6-34). Type I fractures have an oblique fracture line through the upper part of the odontoid process and probably represent an avulsion fracture where the alar ligament attaches. Type II is a fracture occurring at the junction of the odontoid process and the body of the axis. Type III is a fracture that extends down into the cancellous bone of the body of the axis and in reality is a fracture of the body of C2. Type I fractures, which are rare, are stable injuries that have a good prognosis and require only minor treatment. Type II fractures, the most common type, tend to be unstable and have a high rate of nonunion when treated by conservative methods. The apical paired alar and accessory ligaments all attach to the proximal enlargement in this fracture and explain its potential instability. Type III fractures have a large cancellous surface, are more stable, and have a good prognosis for union with conservative treatment. The authors were not able to find a correlation between displacement and the end result. Anatomic and vascular considerations have been offered as explanations of why a Type II fracture may not unite (the vessels may be injured) and why a Type III injury tends to heal very well (the blood supply to the dens is not damaged).[54] Because of its clinical applicability and anatomic significance, the classification of Anderson and D'Alonzo was selected for the Cervical Spine Research Society multicenter study. In addition, most recent articles on odontoid fractures have adopted this classification.[7,12,15–17,22,33,41,42,45,48,54,58,59]

ANATOMY

Development

The second cervical vertebra is complex from both developmental and anatomic standpoints. Four ossification centers are present at birth. These include the two neural arches, the body, and the odontoid process. As Fielding has aptly described it, the odontoid, as seen in the anteroposterior projection, fits between the two neural arches and the superior articular facets of the axis like a cork in a bottle. The base of the odontoid is well below the superior articular facets of the axis.[22] (Fig. 6-35) At birth, the odontoid is joined to the body and neural arches by a cartilaginous plate. The older literature referred to this as an epiphyseal plate, but studies by Ewald have shown that this is not true.[6,18] Histologic study shows that cartilage does exist here, but not in the pattern typical of the epiphyseal line; it is more truly a synchondrosis. There are also paired synchondroses between the neural arches and the body of C2. The configuration of the paired vertical synchondroses between the odontoid and the neural arches and the body and the neural arches with the transverse synchondrosis between the odontoid and the body have the configuration of the letter H.[5,22]

It should be noted that the transverse synchondrosis of the odontoid is well below the junction of the odontoid and the body in the adult. Thus a Type II fracture is well above the level of the old synchondrosis.[22]

The odontoid fuses with the body of the axis between the age of 3 and 6 years. The synchon-

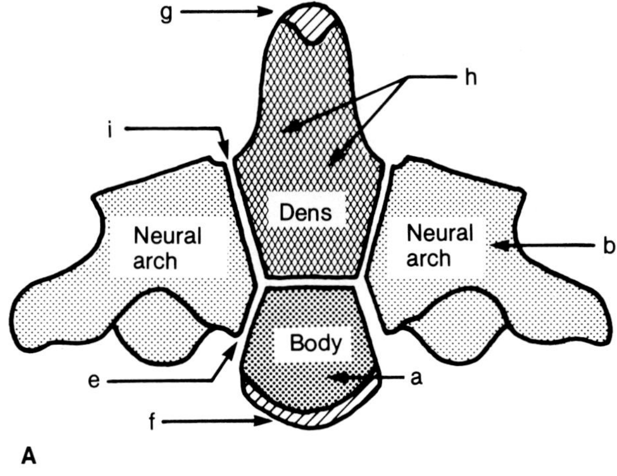

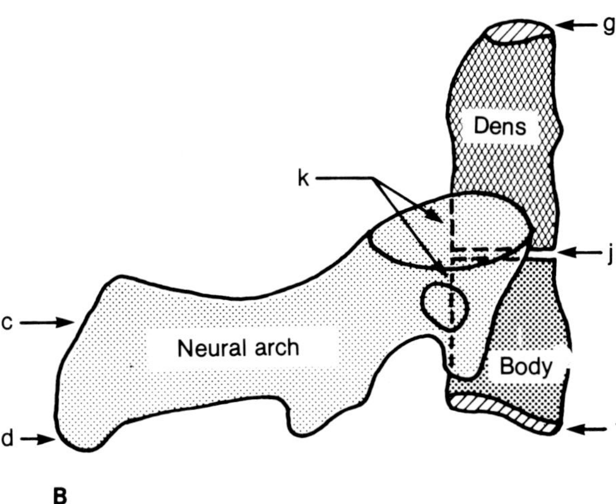

Fig. 6-35. Diagrams of the second cervical vertebra (axis or epistropheus). (*A*) Anterior view. (*B*) Lateral view. (*a*) In the body, one center (occasionally two) appears by the fifth fetal month. (*b*) Neural arches appear bilaterally by the seventh fetal month. (*c*) Neural arches fuse posteriorly by the second or third year. (*d*) Bifid tip of the spinous process (occasionally a secondary center is present in each tip). (*e*) Neurocentral synchondrosis fuses at 3 to 6 years. (*f*) Inferior epiphyseal ring appears at puberty and fuses at about 25 years. (*g*) "Summit" ossification center for the odontoid appears at 3 to 6 years and fuses with the odontoid by 12 years. (*h*) In the odontoid (dens), two separate centers appear by the fifth fetal month and fuse with each other by the seventh fetal month. (*i*) The synchondrosis between the odontoid and the neural arch fuses at 3 to 6 years. (*j*) The synchondrosis between the odontoid and the neural arch fuses at 3 to 6 years. (*k*) The posterior surface of the body and the odontoid. (Bailey DK: The normal cervical spine in infants and children. Radiology 59:713–719, 1952)

drosis between the neural arches and the body joint occurs at about the same time. By the age of 7, all synchondroses of the axis should be united. At times a residual remnant of the transverse synchondrosis may persist at least until the age of 11.[22]

In utero, the odontoid process develops with separate right and left ossification centers. These are present by the fifth fetal month and usually fuse in the midline by the seventh month. Occasionally, a vertical line between the right and left ossification centers persists at birth and should not be confused with a fracture.[22]

The most superior part of the odontoid is unossified at birth and has the shape of a V. This is known as the summit ossification center and begins to ossify at about 3 years of age.[5] It normally fuses within the remainder of the odontoid by age 12. Beyond this age, its presence as a separate ossification center is known as ossiculum terminali, but it is thought to have no clinical significance.[22]

Blood Supply

In the past it has been thought that perhaps the blood supply to the odontoid process was poor and that this might contribute to the high incidence of nonunion. More recently, the blood supply of the odontoid process has been well described by Schatzker and colleagues, Althoff and Goldie, and Schiff and Parke.[1,47,49] These authors found that just the opposite was true. Althoff and Goldie state that the odontoid process is, in fact, the center of a dense arterial network (Fig. 6-36).

Paired anterior and posterior ascending arteries from the vertebral arteries reach the base of the odontoid via the accessory ligaments and run cephalad at the periphery to reach the tip of the process. There they anastomose freely with each other and with transverse superior and inferior arteries that apparently come from the internal carotid arteries to form the apical arcade. Other arteries contributing to this arcade include branches from the ascending pharyngeal arteries that join the arcade after passing through the occipital condyle.

Schatzker and associates also describe the central arteries of the odontoid that enter the anterior surface of the body of the axis and proceed in a cephalad direction to its tip.[46] They also describe small vessels entering the superior portion of the odontoid via the apical and alar ligaments.

Thus, the odontoid has been shown to have an excellent blood supply. With the many anastomoses, it seems unlikely that injury to some of the blood vessels at the time of fracture is a significant cause of nonunion.

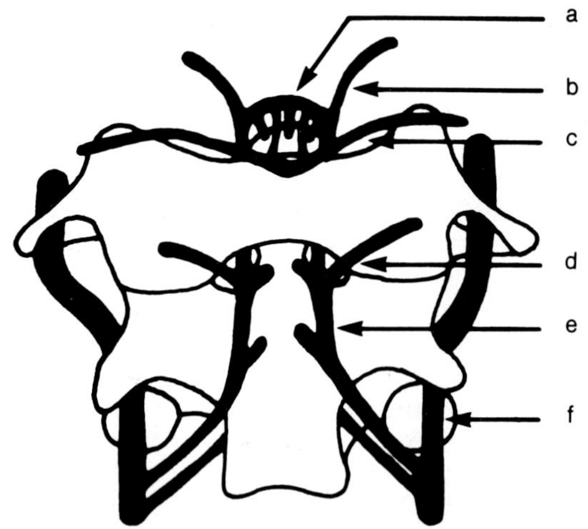

Fig. 6-36. Anterior aspect of the atlas and axis with arteries. (*a*) Apical arcade. (*b*) Posterior horizontal artery. (*c*) Superior anterior horizontal artery. (*d*) Inferior anterior horizontal artery. (*e*) Anterior ascending artery. (*f*) Vertebral artery. (Althoff B, Goldie IF: The Arterial Supply of the Odontoid Process of the Axis. Acta Orthop Scand 48:626, 1977)

In experimental studies, Schatzker and coworkers found that the anatomy and blood supply of the canine odontoid were very similar to those of the human.[47] They created osteotomies of the canine odontoid, both above and below the insertion of the accessory ligaments. The animals were sacrificed at 8 weeks, and microangiographic studies showed an extensive vascular network in the proximal fragment. These studies tend to confirm what one would expect from our knowledge of the rich blood supply of the odontoid process in humans.

Ligaments

The odontoid process, along with its accompanying ligamentous structures, is the primary stabilizer of the atlantoaxial articulation. The apophyseal joints lie in the transverse plane and contribute little to stability. The odontoid is held snugly against the posterior aspect of the atlas by the strong transverse ligament, which arises from the lateral masses of the atlas and lies posterior to the odontoid (Fig. 6-37). The paired accessory ligaments arise posterior to and in conjunction with the transverse ligaments and insert into the lateral aspect of the odontoid joint above the base. The alar ligaments are paired and run caudad from their origin on the occipital condyles to insert on the superior and lateral aspect of the odontoid. The unpaired apical ligament arises from the anterior aspect of the foramen magnum and inserts centrally at the tip of the odontoid process.[46] Note that in a Type II fracture the proximal dens fragment remains attached to the apical, alar, and accessory ligaments.[45]

INCIDENCE

The exact overall incidence of fractures of the odontoid is not known. In many fatal cases, especially those due to traffic accidents, autopsies and roentgenographic examination of the upper cervical spine are not carried out.

The incidence for those patients surviving the

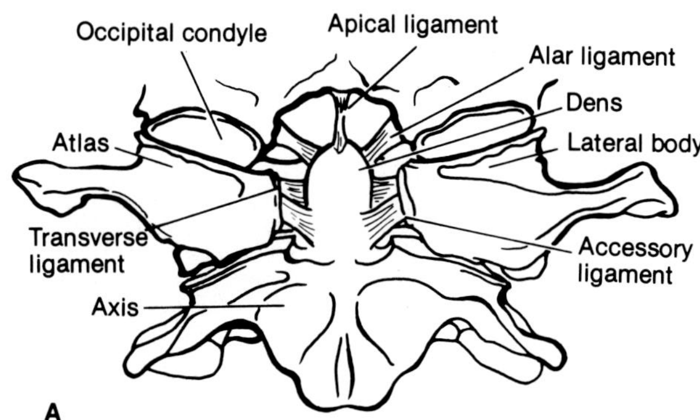

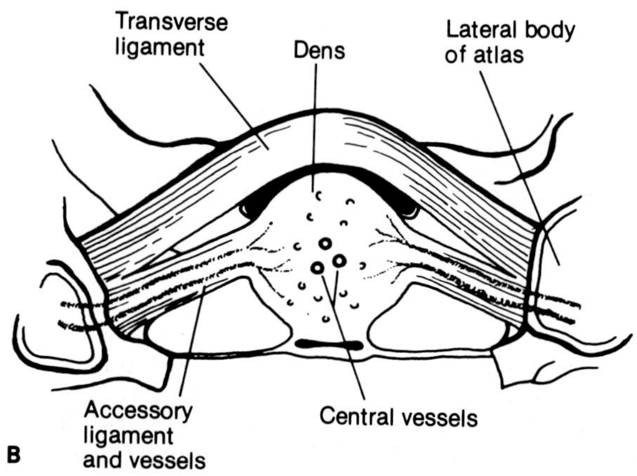

Fig. 6-37. (*A*) Coronal section of a human dens with the anterior arch of the atlas removed to illustrate the anatomic relationships and ligamentous attachments of the dens. (*B*) Transverse section through a human dens at the level of the transverse ligament to illustrate the origin and insertion of the accessory ligaments and vessels. (Schatzker J, Rorabeck CH, Waddell JP: Fractures of the dens [odontoid process]: An analysis of thirty-seven cases. J Bone Joint Surg 53B:392–393, 1971)

initial injury and reaching the hospital is better understood. Amyes and Anderson found 53 odontoid fractures in a total of 393 patients with cervical spine fractures and dislocations seen at the Los Angeles County Hospital between 1939 and 1954 (13%).[2] In the recent literature, Sherk as well as Husby and Sorensen have reported a similar incidence of 10% to 15% of all cervical spine fractures and dislocations in adults to be fractures of the odontoid.[29,53,58]

In children under the age of 7 years, all fractures of the cervical spine are rare. However, of children in this age group, odontoid fractures constitute 75% of all cervical spine fractures and dislocations.[52] Sherk and associates found a total of only 15 patients from birth to 7 years of age who had been treated at the Philadelphia Children's Hospital for cervical spine fractures. Of these, 11 involved fractures of the odontoid process. In a review of the literature prior to 1978, these authors found only 24 additional odontoid fractures in young children averaging 4 years of age, for whom enough information was given to be useful.[52]

MECHANISM AND CAUSE OF INJURY

In the older literature, most fractures of the odontoid were caused by severe falls or blows to the head from heavy objects. These two causes accounted for 80% of the 56 cases reviewed by Osgood and Lund in 1928.[38]

By the 1950s, with more widespread use of the automobile and increased speed of the vehicles, the cause of most odontoid fractures had changed. In 1955 Amyes and Anderson described 63 patients with odontoid fractures. Thirty-six (57%) were the result of motor vehicle accidents.[2] Most of the major series of odontoid fractures reported since then state that at least 50% of these fractures are traffic related.[7,12,16] Anderson and D'Alonzo found 71%, and Husby and Sorensen 81%, of the odontoid fractures in their series to be caused by motor vehicle accidents.[3,29] Clark and White reported 70% of Type II and 72% of Type III fractures resulted from such accidents.[12] The mechanism of injury varies according to age. Most fractures in patients under age 40 result from traffic accidents, and most in patients over age 60 result from falls.[41]

While many fractures of the odontoid process in children are also caused by traffic accidents, a significant number in children under 7 years of age result from less severe trauma. Seimon reported two young children with odontoid fractures that were caused by minor falls of 61 and 91 cm.[51]

In their extensive review of the literature, Blockey and Purser concluded that violence to the head that throws it into extreme flexion, extension, or rotation may fracture the odontoid process.[6] After the fracture has taken place, the relationship of C1 to C2 is no longer stable and the atlas can subluxate, carrying the odontoid with it. If the force that caused the fracture is flexion, the subluxation is anterior, and if the force is extension the subluxation is posterior. Blockey and Purser thought that rotational injuries almost never occurred alone and that the direction of displacement in these injuries depends on whether rotation was combined with flexion or extension. They noted that the mandible lies inferior to the C1–C2 articulation. Fractures of the mandible are thus flexion injuries and associated with anterior displacement of the odontoid.

The exact mechanism whereby flexion, extension, and rotation injuries fracture the odontoid is undoubtedly very complex. Several authors have found it difficult, if not impossible, to reproduce this fracture in cadaver material. In addition to the direction of the force, the various ligaments must play a major role. It seems logical that in flexion injuries the strong transverse ligament is forced against the posterior odontoid process and fractures it from the body with anterior displacement. Conversely, with extension injuries the posterior aspect of the ring of the atlas is forced against the anterior odontoid causing fracture and posterior displacement. While these explanations are probably partially true and conceptually helpful, they are undoubtedly greatly oversimplified.

In most series of odontoid fractures, anterior displacement of the odontoid is more common than posterior displacement, and in some series the ratio of anterior-to-posterior displacement is as high as six or seven to one.[4,6,29,39,46] Clark and White reported 61% of Type II and 89% of Type III fractures were anteriorly displaced.[12] Thus, it appears that flexion is a much more common cause of odontoid fractures than is extension.

CLINICAL FINDINGS

According to several authors, the average age of patients with fractures of the odontoid is the early to middle forties, although the distribution by decade is fairly even.[3,39,46] Males outnumber females in most series by a ratio of three to one, presumably because they are subject to more violent trauma.[4,39,46]

Fractures of the dens are frequently missed because the patient is unconscious or intoxicated, or has associated trauma to the head.[3,4,27,29,34,39,54] A high index of suspicion is necessary, as the clinical symptoms are frequently nonspecific. This point must be emphasized in educating emergency-ward personnel. The patient usually complains of poorly localized pain in the posterior part of the neck and has paravertebral muscle spasm, tenderness, and limited range of motion of the neck. Neurologic loss may range from high tetraplegia (with respiratory center involvement) to occipital neuralgia due to irritation of the greater occipital nerve. In addition, motor and sensory weakness involving a portion of an upper limb due to injury to one or more cervical nerve roots may also be present.[54]

The complaint of occipital and suboccipital pain is nearly always made by patients who are alert. Most patients are unable or unwilling to go from the supine to the sitting position without supporting their heads with their hands.

Paradis and Janes, and Husby and Sorensen report that over 50% of patients with odontoid fractures have significant associated injuries.[29,39] The most common of these are cerebral concussion, scalp laceration, fracture of the mandible, and extremity fractures.[3,4] Additional cervical spine fractures are not unusual, and a careful search for these should be carried out.

The true frequency of neurologic deficit is not known for patients who die before reaching the hospital. Of the patients admitted to hospitals with odontoid fractures, neurologic findings vary greatly in degree of involvement and include mild upper extremity weakness, hyperreflexic lower extremities, decreased occipital sensation, paraparesis and Brown-Séquard syndrome.[3] Fortunately, most of these early neurologic findings clear with treatment.[3,4] Late neurologic involvement is discussed in a later section on treatment.

RADIOGRAPHIC FINDINGS

Fracture is confirmed by radiographic studies, but as moving the head and neck during the evaluation is potentially dangerous, the initial diagnosis may be difficult. Since the head cannot be moved for examination or radiographs, gentle traction should be maintained on the head with the spine in the neutral position, while anteroposterior, open-mouth, and lateral radiographs are made.[12] Most fractures of the cervical spine will be demonstrated during the examination, especially if displacement has occurred. Subsequent examination includes the standard anteroposterior examination, oblique views, and the open-mouth odontoid view. The latter examination may be impossible in patients with fractures of the mandible and in unconscious patients.

If standard roentgenographic examinations do not demonstrate the odontoid clearly, then anteroposterior and lateral tomography should be carried out. The value of excellent tomographic studies cannot be overemphasized. In a recent study at our institution, we found that eight patients with cervical spine fractures had significant delays in diagnosis and treatment, owing to inadequate plain roentgenographic examination or improper interpretation. Tomographic examinations led to the correct diagnosis in all eight patients.[4] Significantly, all had head injuries involving the atlantoaxial region. Two of the eight patients incurred greater than 2-year delays each in the diagnosis of odontoid fractures, even though several series of plain roentgenograms were made during this time. Diagnosis of this fracture on plain films is often difficult. We have been surprised at the number of fractures demonstrated by tomography that were not apparent with standard roentgenograms.

Fractures of C1 appear to be the most commonly associated fracture.[41] Recognition of associated injuries is important because of their impact on treatment.

MORTALITY

Just as the true incidence of odontoid fractures is not known, neither is the true mortality rate. As discussed previously, the problem lies with the odontoid fractures causing immediate death that are never diagnosed. In the older literature, death occurred in well over 50% and many of the cases were from autopsy material.[37] In the more recent series describing patients who did reach the hospital, the mortality rate, including those dying of associated injuries, appears to be between 3.3% and 8%.[2–4,23,29,37,39]

OS ODONTOIDEUM

Os odontoideum is a round or oval ossicle with a smooth border located either in the position of the normal odontoid process or more proximally near the base of the occipital bone. A wide radiolucent zone separates the os odontoideum from the base of the remaining odontoid process, which usually projects like a peg or a mound above the articular facets of the axis.

In the past, os odontoideum was thought to be a developmental anomaly. Wollin described nine cases in 1963, and although he considered it a developmental lesion, he noted that it was difficult to explain on that basis.[60] The vestigial cartilaginous disc between the odontoid process and the body of C2 lies well below the articular facets of the axis. Failure of the disc to fuse would not explain the location of the os odontoideum and the projection of the residual base of the odontoid above the articular facets.

More recently in 1980, Fielding, Hensinger, and Hawkins reported the largest series of os odontoideum in the literature, consisting of 35 patients from three major centers.[23] Those authors believe that os odontoideum results from trauma and is not developmental. Eleven patients had lesions attributable to injuries incurred before they were 4 years old. Nine of these patients had documented roentgenographic evidence of a normal odontoid process prior to the development of os odontoideum. The authors contend that the following series of events takes place: First the odontoid process is traumatically disrupted at its base. Next, a contracture of the alar ligaments distracts the proximal fragment upward. The blood supply to the upper portion of the odontoid is maintained by the proximal arterial arcade from the carotids. However, the amount of blood supply may not be sufficient to nourish the entire odontoid, if the other vessels are interrupted. This phenomenon, along with motion, would explain resorption of bone at the lower portion of the odontoid.

A strong case is now made that os odontoideum is the result of trauma. Ricciardi and associates described os odontoideum developing in a 15-month-old infant who sustained an acute ligament injury of the transverse and accessory ligaments.[43] No fracture of the odontoid was seen. Serial roentgenograms revealed gradual resorption of the caudal portion of the odontoid. The authors postulate disruption of the blood supply by the ligament injury with subsequent avascular necrosis and resorption of the base of the odontoid.

TREATMENT

Odontoid Fractures in Children

Blockey and Purser, in their article of 1956, appeared to be the first to recognize that odontoid fractures in children under 7 years of age are different from and have a better prognosis than odontoid fractures in adults.[6] All five fractures in these young children united with conservative treatment. They pointed out that the fracture in a young child occurs at the cartilaginous plate where the odontoid process joins the body (Fig. 6-38). This is well below the articular facets, and the authors thought that the injury was in fact an epiphyseal separation. All five patients had anterior displacement of the odontoid.

Ewald, in 1971, reported a 16-month-old female with an odontoid fracture successfully treated in a halo. He noted that postmortem studies of young children reported in the literature, as well as those in his own institution, showed that the junction of the odontoid process with the body of the axis was cartilaginous but that it was no evidence of a true epiphyseal plate.[18] He concluded that the odontoid process must be considered a primary ossicle and not an epiphysis.

Griffiths, in 1972, reported four young children with odontoid fractures.[25] All united with relatively short periods of immobilization. Seimon reported two young children with odontoid fractures incurred in minor falls, such as from a cot.[51] Both complained of pain when brought to the sitting or returned to the supine position, unless the head was supported. He considered this a valuable diagnostic finding. His patients were treated in traction followed by a collar, and both fractures united.

Sherk in 1978, reviewed the literature and found 24 fractures of the odontoid process in children under 7 years of age for whom enough information was available to be useful.[52] All fractures took place through the cartilaginous plate, and, of those documented, displacement was always anterior. One of the 24 patients was treated by primary fusion. Of the remaining 23, one diagnosed but untreated patient developed a nonunion. One additional patient retrodisplaced in a Minerva and underwent C1–C2 fusion. Fractures of the remaining 22 conservatively treated patients united.

The author added 11 cases of fractures of the odontoid in children under 7 years of age. All were at the cartilaginous plate and all displaced anteriorly. These patients were reduced in traction or by the split-mattress technique followed by casts or braces for 6 to 16 weeks. All united uneventfully. Sherk concluded that almost all children under 7 years of age with this injury have done well.

Based on the results reported by the various authors above, it appears obvious that odontoid fractures in children under age 7 are different.

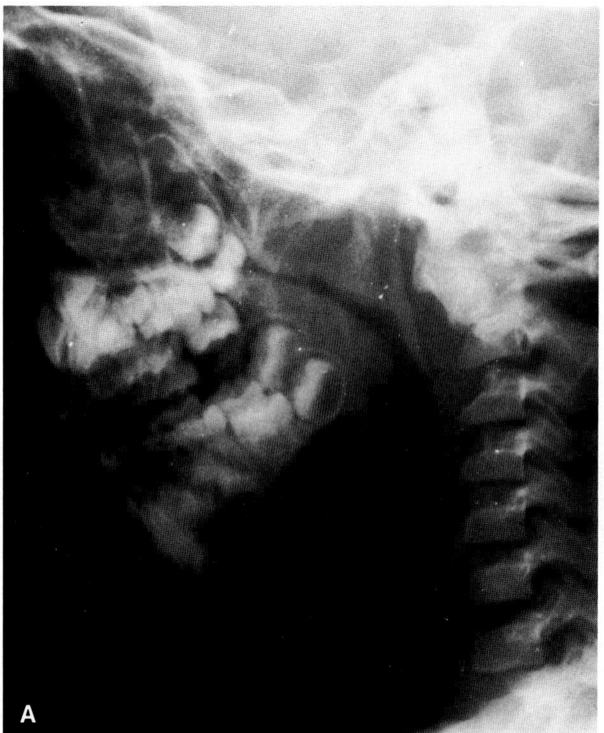

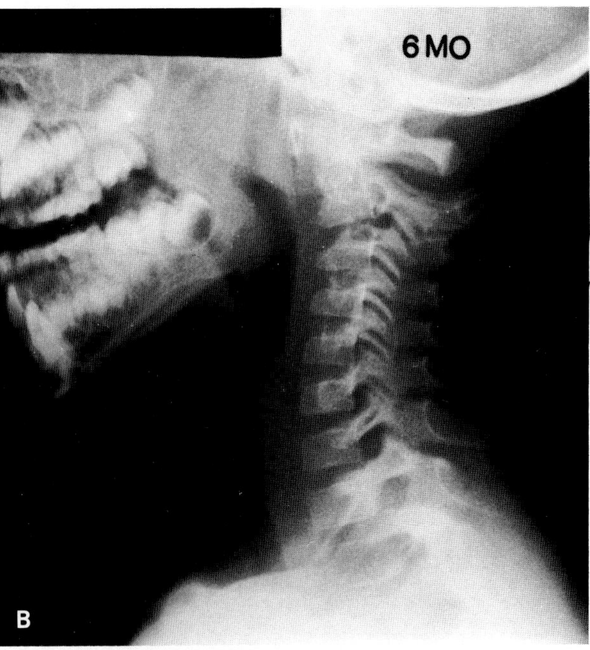

Fig. 6-38. A Type II odontoid fracture with anterior displacement in a 5-year-old child. (*A*) Lateral roentgenogram. This may represent a traumatic epiphyseal separation rather than a true fracture. (*B*) Six months after treatment in traction followed by a Minerva jacket, the fracture has united and stability has been restored. (Anderson LD, D'Alonzo RT: Fractures of the odontoid process of the axis. J Bone Joint Surg 56A:1669, 1974)

Almost all heal, if they are reduced in traction or by the split-mattress technique, followed by 2 to 3 months in a Minerva or halo cast.

Odontoid Fractures in Adults

As noted earlier in this section, the percentage of patients with fractures of the odontoid that develop nonunion varies greatly from one reported series to another.

In 1956, Blockey and Purser reviewed 35 adult patients in whom the outcome was known.[6] Nonunion resulted in 63%. However, 16 of these patients received no initial treatment. They could find no correlation between the degree of displacement and the direction of displacement with union of the fracture. They did think that older patients were more likely to develop nonunion.

Amyes and Anderson reported 63 cases of odontoid fractures in 1956.[2] All were treated conservatively in tong or halter traction for approximately 1 month, followed by a collar or a cast. Only three failed to unite, for a nonunion rate of 5%. This series represents, by far, the highest reported success rate for union. In their discussion, they note that it was often difficult "to be certain that the fracture was firmly healed" and that "sometimes the fracture line remained visible but dislocation had not occurred when the patient was last seen." It appears that at least some of the patients had fibrous rather than bony union.

Schatzker reviewed 37 patients with odontoid fractures in 1971.[46] Twenty-two of their patients were treated conservatively with 4 to 6 weeks in traction followed by a similar period in casts or braces. Fourteen of the 22 so treated failed to unite (64%). The authors classified the fractures as high or low, depending on whether the fracture was above or below the accessory ligaments, but could find no correlation of union. Unlike Blockey and Purser, they thought nonunion was more likely to develop in displaced fractures, especially if the displacement is posterior. They agreed with Blockey and Purser that nonunion was more likely in patients over 60 years of age. Fifteen of their patients were treated by primary fusion. Thirteen fusions were successful. The authors concluded that a 64% failure of union with conservative treatment is unacceptable and that most patients with odontoid fractures should have atlantoaxial fusion after a preliminary period in traction of 1 to 2 weeks to allow edema to subside.

In 1972, Roberts and Wickstrom reviewed 50 patients treated for odontoid fractures at Charity Hospital in New Orleans.[44] Forty were treated conservatively, with union developing in 32, and nonunion in 8. The overall nonunion rate was 20% with nonunion present in 30% of displaced fractures and 17% of those that were undisplaced. The authors thought that odontoid fractures should be treated in traction followed by a Minerva cast for 20 weeks. If union is not present by that time, fusion is indicated.

Paradis and Janes from the Mayo Clinic reported 17 acute fractures of the odontoid in 1973. They considered all to be of the Schatzker "low" type. Thirteen were treated conservatively, most with 4 weeks of traction in tongs followed by braces. There were only two nonunions (15%). They thought that prolonged mobilization of at least 4.5 months contributed to their success.

In 1974, Anderson and D'Alonzo reported 49 fractures of the odontoid process and devised a new classification of these fractures that has been described previously in this section.[3]

Type I fractures are rare, and the authors found only two in their series, both of which healed with minimal treatment (Fig. 6-39). Such fractures are stable, as they are above the transverse ligament. Even if nonunion develops, they should cause no problem. Type II fractures, the most common, numbered 32 in this series. Fourteen were undisplaced, and 18 were displaced. All 14 undisplaced fractures and eight of the displaced fractures were treated in traction followed by bracing. Nonunion developed in 36%. No difference in nonunion rates was found between the displaced and undisplaced fractures. Ten of the displaced Type II fractures were treated by primary fusion. There were 15 Type III fractures; one was treated by primary fusion, and fourteen were treated in traction or bracing, or both. Thirteen united promptly. The one nonunion (7%) developed in a patient who received no treatment until 5 weeks after injury.

Anderson and D'Alonzo concluded that Type I fractures are rare and require only symptomatic treatment. Type II fractures, undisplaced or displaced, are prone to nonunion (36%), and primary fusion should be considered (Fig. 6-40). Type III fractures have a broad cancellous surface and the rate of union with conservative treatment is high (93%) (Fig. 6-41). Husby and Sorensen in 1974, reported 32 patients with odontoid fractures from Denmark. They classified their fractures into high and low groups. These descriptions are very similar to Anderson's and D'Alonzo's Type II and Type III. There were nine high fractures, and eight were treated with primary fusion. All eight united with solid fusions. Twenty-one patients with low fractures were treated conservatively with only three nonunions (14%). These authors advise primary fusion in all high fractures and in unstable low fractures.

Apuzzo and colleagues, in 1978, reported 45 patients treated at the Los Angeles County Hospital between 1969 and 1974.[4] Three patients were treated by primary fusion, and there were two early deaths. Forty patients were treated conservatively with a nonunion rate of 33%. Minerva cast was the most common treatment, with nonunion in 5 of 22. Five were treated in halo, with three nonunions. The remaining thirteen were treated with various conservative measures. The authors found that nonunion was higher in displaced fractures and higher in patients over 40 years of age. They recommend conservative treatment for all undisplaced fractures and primary C1–C2 fusion for all fractures displaced more than 4 mm. They thought that patients over 40 years of age with displaced fractures are probably best handled by operative treatment. Pierce and Barr, in 1979, reported their experience with the halo cast or vest for various cervical spine problems, including 20 patients with fractures of the odontoid process.[42] They found the halo a versatile device, although they state that Type II odontoid fractures often did not heal, even with halo immobilization, and fusion is indicated in a halo vest. No figures were supplied.

On the other hand Sweigil, in the same year and same journal, reported odontoid fractures treated in halo vests with union in 21.[57] He thought the halo brace an excellent tool in the treatment of odontoid fractures. Many of the fractures in his series resulted from relatively minor trauma.

In 1979, Donovan also reported a series of 54 patients with odontoid fractures.[15] There were 33 Type II fractures and 21 Type III fractures. Of

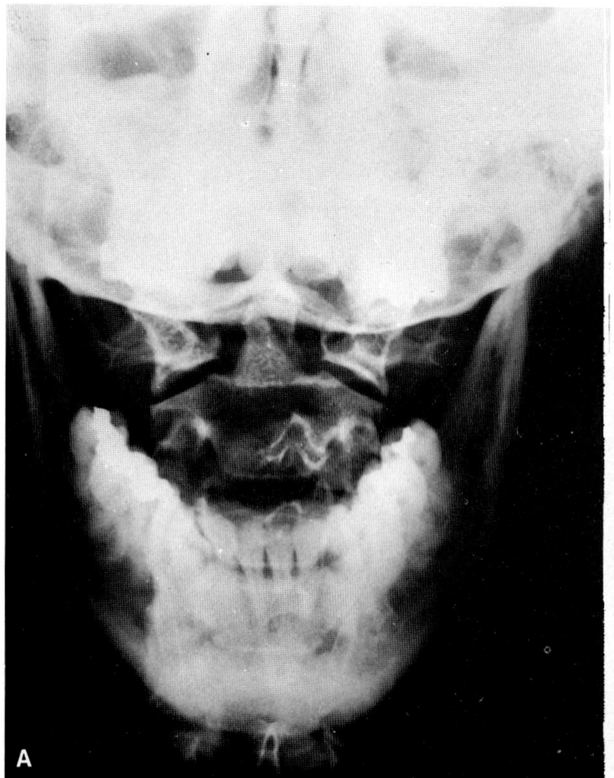

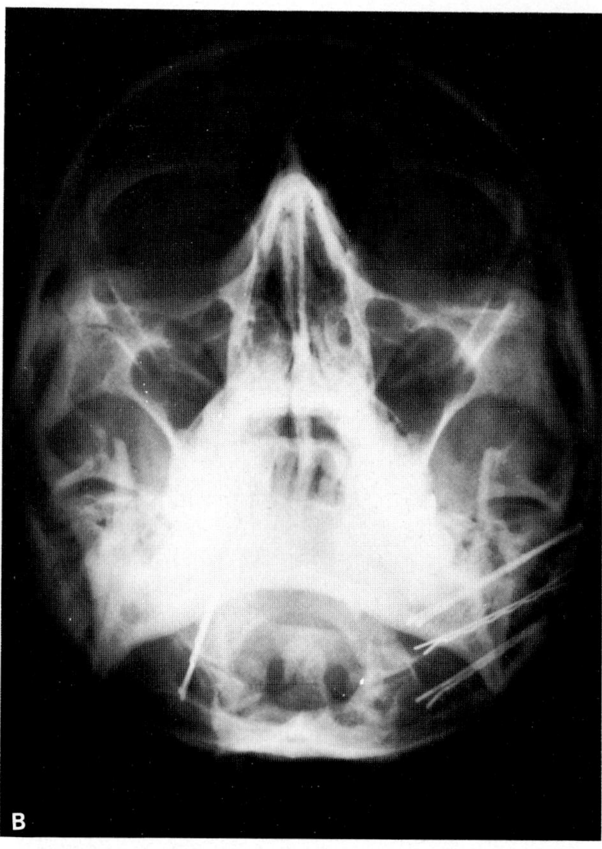

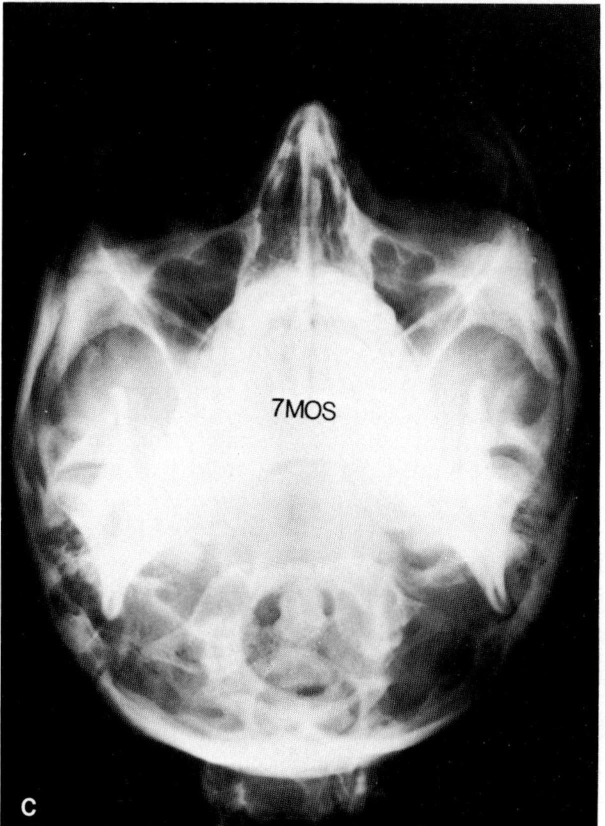

Fig. 6-39. A Type I fracture of the odontoid process located high in the odontoid process. (*A*) The open-mouth odontoid view. (*B*) Water's view. The odontoid is located at the center of the foramen magnum in this view. (*C*) The fracture healed by 7 months with conservative treatment. (Anderson LD, D'Alonzo RT: Fractures of the odontoid process of the axis. J Bone Joint Surg 56A:1665, 1974)

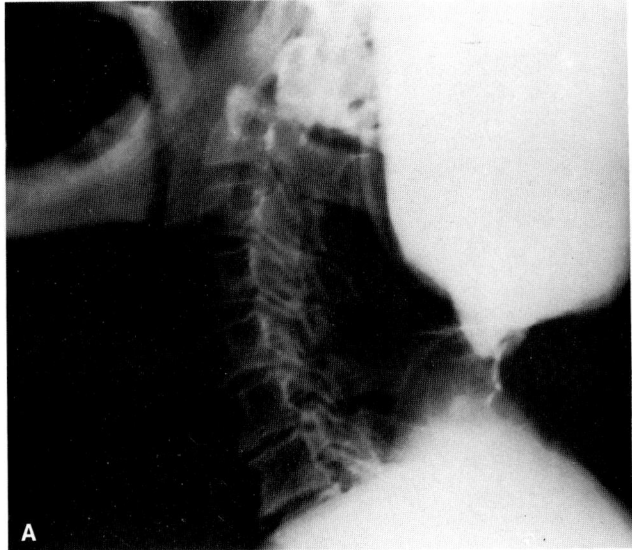

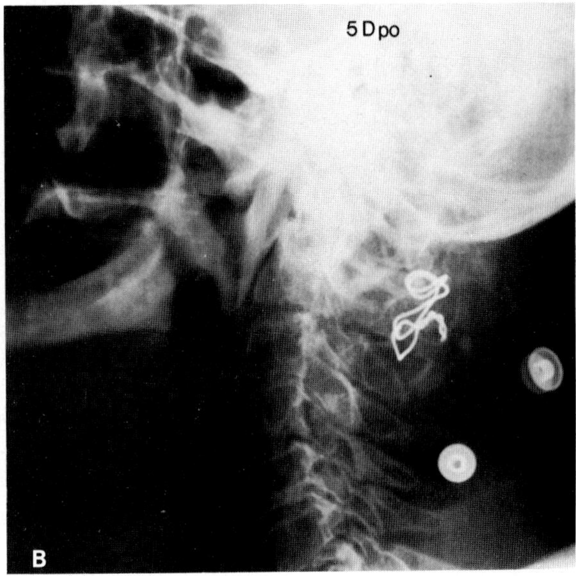

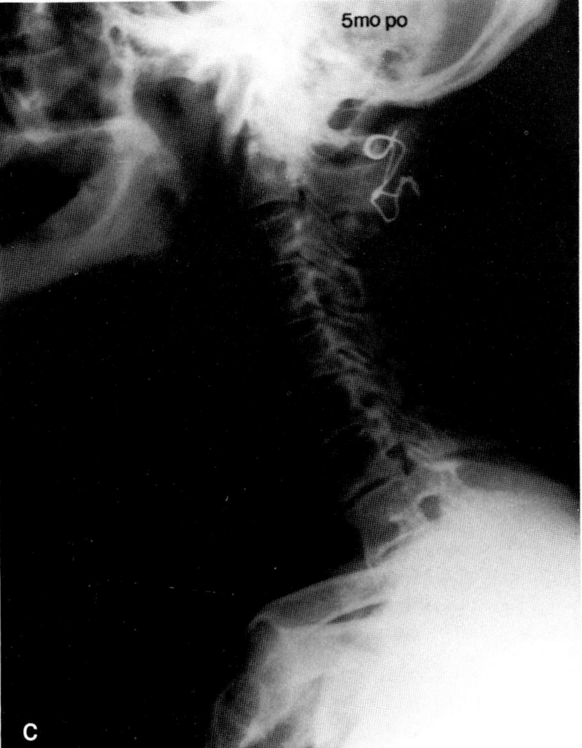

Fig. 6-40. A Type II odontoid fracture. (*A*) Lateral roentgenogram. Note the marked posterior displacement of the odontoid process in relation to the body of C2. (*B*) Five days after reduction of the fracture with skeletal traction, posterior wiring of C1 to C2, and fusion with autogenous iliac bone grafts. Reduction prior to fusion is very important in preventing delayed long-tract signs; they may develop even with a successful fusion if correct alignment is not restored. (*C*) At 5 months, the fusion appears solid and the fracture of the odontoid has united in good position. (Anderson LD, D'Alonzo RT: Fractures of the odontoid process of the axis. J Bone Joint Surg 56A:1667, 1974)

the total, 28 were treated with halo jackets and 26 by various other methods. Of those treated with halos, 75% united. On the other hand, only 27% treated by other methods healed. No correlation was found between age and the extent of displacement, and the final result. Donovan stated that as would be expected, Type III fractures showed better results than Type II, but he provided no specific figures. He concluded that results for Type II fractures were so uniformly poor that primary fusion seems justified. He thought that surgery should be delayed until the acute symptoms and edema had subsided.

Southwick concluded that it now appears that neither the halo brace nor any other form of external fixation represented adequate treatment for Type II fractures.[56] He also thought that fusion procedures could be associated with significant morbidity and mortality unless performed in a meticulous fashion by experienced surgeons.

Posterior fusion is the primary procedure in this country. The Japanese and Europeans have had extensive experience with anterior procedures. The anterior stabilization described by Bohler has the theoretical advantage of preserving motion at the atlantoaxial articulations.[7]

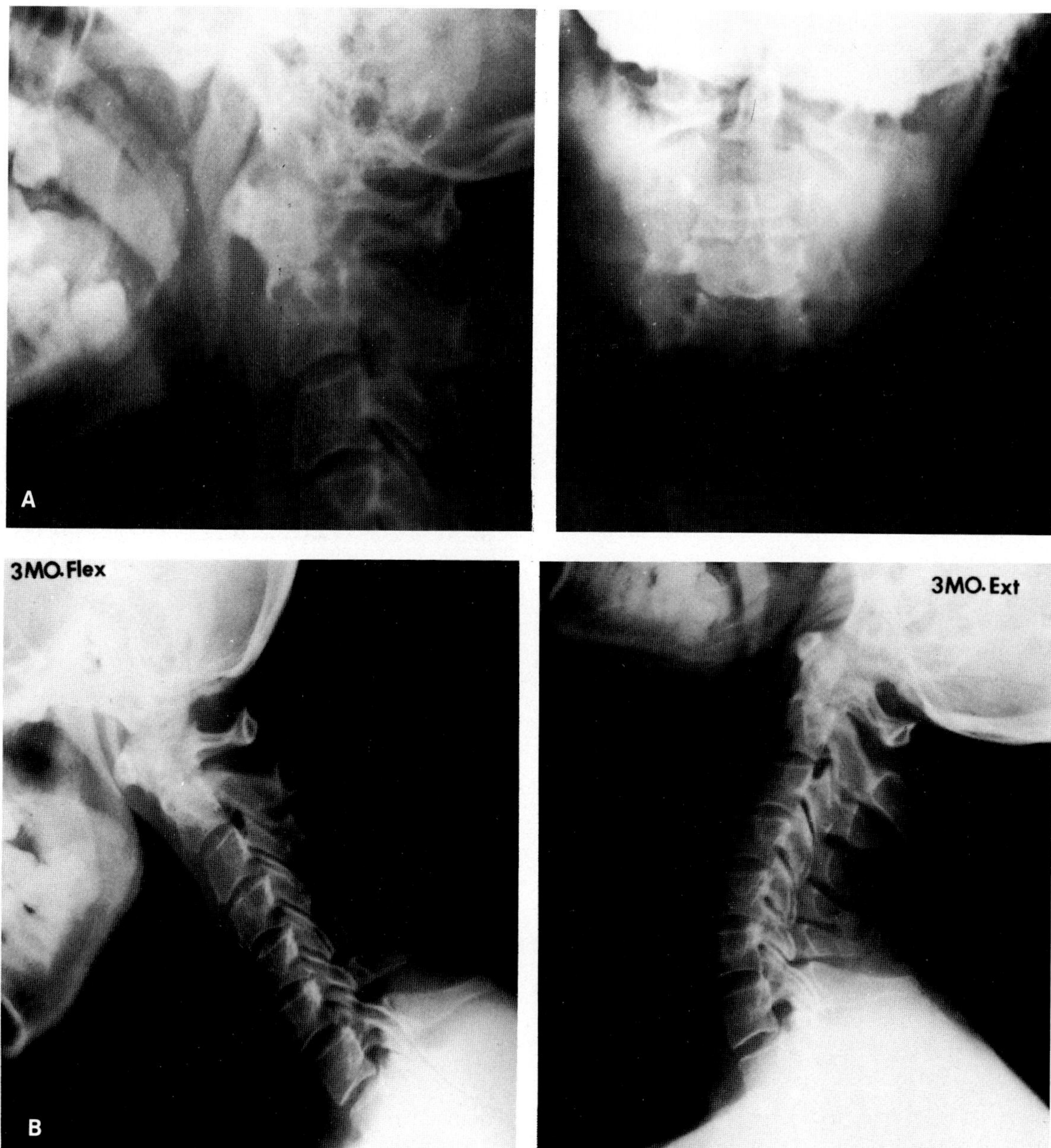

Fig. 6-41. A Type III odontoid fracture. (*A*) Lateral roentgenogram and open-mouth odontoid view. The odontoid process is displaced 5 mm anteriorly in relationship to the body of the second cervical vertebra. It was reduced almost completely with 2.6 kg of skeletal traction. (*B*) Lateral roentgenograms, inflexion and extension, after 3 months of treatment in traction followed by bracing. The fracture has united in good position and is stable. (Anderson LD, D'Alonzo RT: Fractures of the odontoid process of the axis. J Bone Joint Surg 56A:1668, 1974)

Clark and White reported 96 Type II and 48 Type III injuries in the Cervical Spine Research Society study.[12] The management of Type II fractures was particularly troublesome, as 32% of such fractures failed to unite. Although Type III injuries have been considered to be quite innocuous, they found that 13% failed to unite and 15% went on to malunion. Thus, both injuries must be carefully managed. Stability was obtained with the halo device in almost 70% of Type II fractures; however, stability was achieved in 96% of patients treated with a posterior cervical fusion.

Displacement appeared to be a significant factor affecting the outcome of the treatment of Type II fractures. Fractures with 5 mm or more of either anterior or posterior displacement had a 26% rate of nonunion and a 13% rate of malunion. Twenty-nine percent of the Type II fractures with 10 degrees of angulation resulted in nonunion. Type II fractures that were either significantly angulated or displaced, or both, had a statistically significant ($p < 0.05$) increase in nonunion or malunion, regardless of treatment. In many of the patients in this series, the fracture had not been treated immediately after injury because the diagnosis had been missed. All of these patients had symptomatic instability.[12]

The authors concluded that patients with a Type II injury who have either significant displacement or angulation, or both, should be considered for surgical stabilization. Posterior fusion was the mode of surgical management preferred by most surgeons in this series.

Clark and White further concluded that Type III fractures are not benign, despite the fact that they occur through the vertebral body. They found a significant rate of malunion in patients who were treated with an orthosis alone. They stated that the halo device appears to be the safest and most reliable form of therapy for Type III injuries, although surgery may be required for particularly unstable fractures.[12]

LATE MYELOPATHY

So-called late myelopathy associated with odontoid fractures is due to a nonunion of the fracture and the resultant instability of the antlantoaxial joint. Subsequent trauma, which may be only minor in nature, may cause pressure on the cord causing anything from minor neurologic symptoms to quadriplegia and death. In their review of 55 odontoid fractures in 1928, Osgood and Lund report at least 10 and probably 17 patients with such injuries.[38] Schwartz and Wigton reported two cases of late myelopathy that occurred at 5 years and 18 years after the original fracture.[50] Anderson and D'Alonzo found in the literature over 50 cases of delayed myelopathy, with wide variation in the degree of involvement, including spastic hemiparesis, urinary and fecal incontinence, Brown-Séquard syndrome, monoparesis, quadriplegia, and occipital neuraliga.[3] They added one case of their own with onset of symptoms 19 years after the initial injury (Fig. 6-42). Paradis and Janes found that in a group of 29 patients referred to them with nonunion 4 months to 15 years after injury, 76% had neurologic findings.[39]

There appears to be almost unanimous agreement that anything less than solid bony union is an unacceptable result, in patients with odontoid fractures treated by conservative methods. If nonunion or fibrous union develops, then posterior wiring and fusion is almost always indicated to prevent late myelopathy and possibly death.

DISCUSSION

After reviewing the older and more recent literature, a number of points seem clear. The true overall incidence of odontoid fractures is not known, but of patients surviving to reach the hospital odontoid fractures constitute between 10% and 15% of all cervical spine fractures, which are reported with increasing frequency in adults. Over 50% are due to motor vehicle accidents, with major falls and blows to the head accounting for most of the rest. In young children trauma is often less severe. The pathomechanics involve either flexion or extension forces, and in some fractures, rotation. Flexion injuries are more common and are associated with anterior displacement. Extension injuries are less common and are associated with posterior displacement.

Clinical findings include pain in the neck and occipital region. Most patients are unable to move from the supine to the sitting position without supporting their heads with their hands. Neurologic findings, varying greatly in degree, are found in approximately 15% to 25% of cases. Associated injuries are frequent, and the most common are cerebral concussions, scalp lacerations, fractures of the mandible, and extremity fractures.

Most authors believe that cervical spine films should be obtained routinely in unconscious patients to rule out odontoid and other cervical spine injuries. The mortality rate for patients with odon-

Fig. 6-42. (*A*) An undisplaced Type II odontoid fracture in a 17-year-old boy. He was treated in traction followed by bracing. A nonunion of the odontoid developed. (*B*) An open-mouth odontoid view shows the obvious nonunion 19 years after injury. (*C*) Lateral roentgenograms made in flexion and extension 19 years after injury. The odontoid reduces in extension and displaces anteriorly 3 mm in flexion. (*D*) Lateral roentgenograms made in flexion and extension 4 months after posterior wiring and fusion. The fusion mass appears solid between C1 and C2, and the odontoid process is stable. (Anderson LD, D'Alonzo RT: Fractures of the odontoid process of the axis. J Bone Joint Surg 56A:1670–1671, 1974)

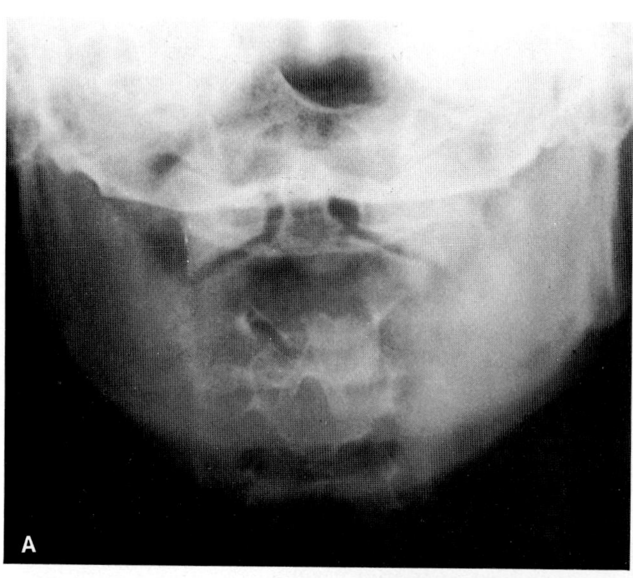

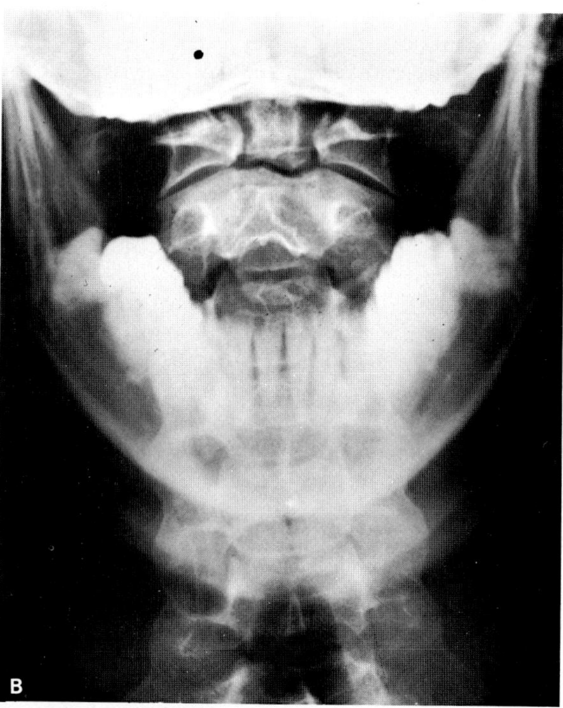

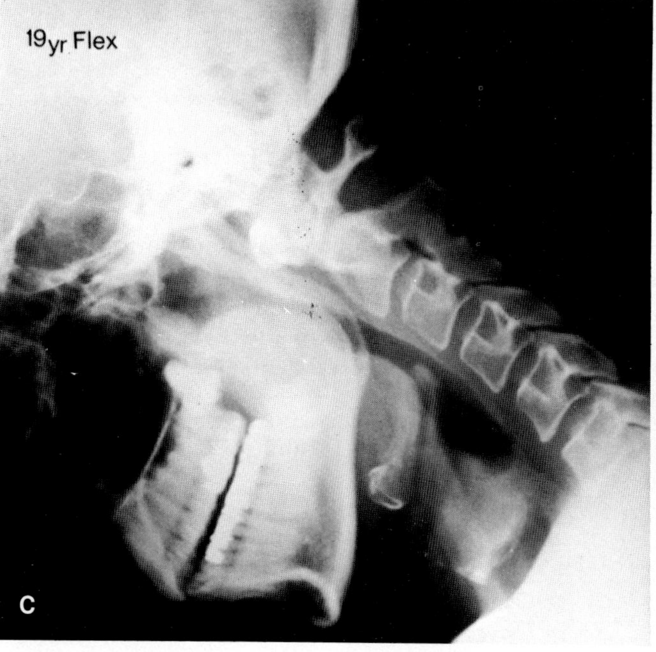

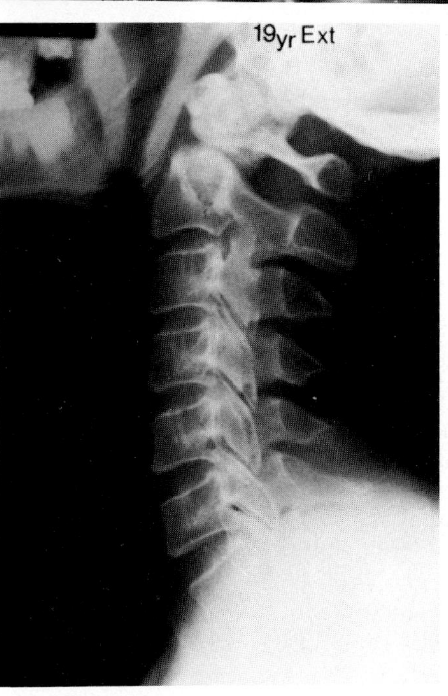

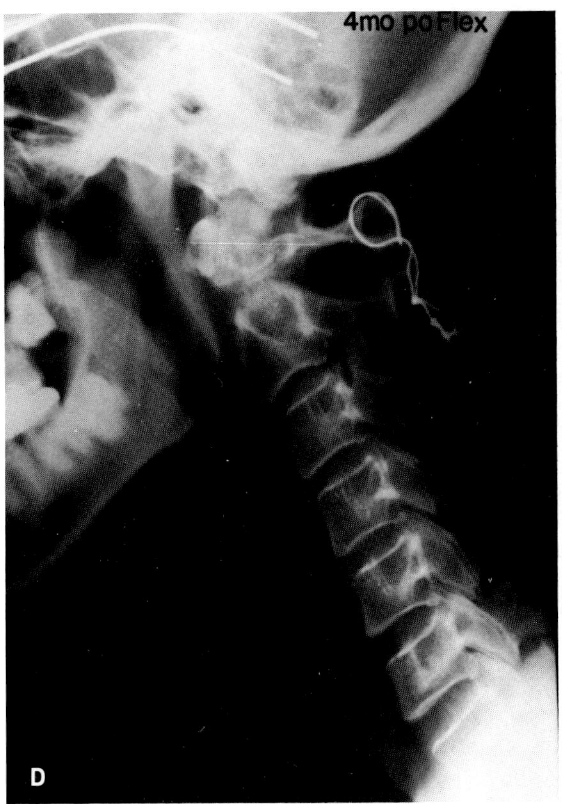

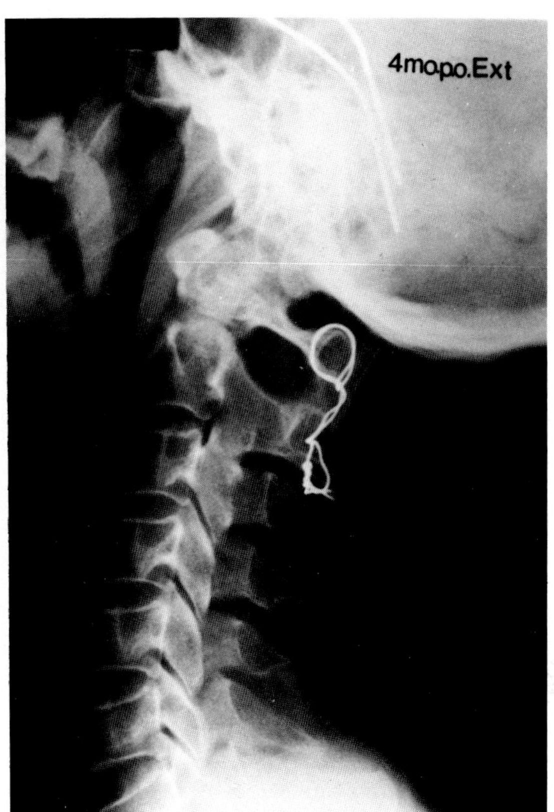

toid fractures who reach the hospital is now much lower than the more than 50% reported in the older literature. More recent series report a mortality rate between 3.3% and 8%, including those dying of associated injuries.

Fractures of the odontoid may be difficult to demonstrate on standard roentgenograms. If there is any question, tomography should be used. The value of tomographic studies cannot be overemphasized, especially in the upper cervical spine.

Excellent general agreement seems to exist about the several items related to odontoid fractures discussed above. There is also excellent agreement about the treatment and prognosis in children under 7 years of age. Almost all heal and progress well if they receive adequate reduction and external immobilization. The os odontoideum increasingly appears to be a traumatic rather than a developmental defect and perhaps results from an injury of the blood supply to the base of the odontoid at a level above the articular facets, with subsequent avascular necrosis and resorption of the base of the odontoid.

The area of greatest controversy is the treatment and prognosis of odontoid fractures in adults. Nonunion has been variously reported to be as low as 4.8% and as high as 64%. Other authors have reported results in between these extremes.

When we described a new classification for odontoid fractures in 1974 (Anderson and D'Alonzo) we hoped that we had shed some light on the controversy surrounding the prognosis of the individual types.[3] In our series the nonunion rate for Type III fractures was only 7%, but the nonunion rate for Type II fractures treated conservatively was 36%. We concluded that patients with Type III fractures progressed well with conservative management but thought that primary fusion of Type II fractures appeared to be justified in many of these patients.

Other authors since then have reached similar conclusions. Husby and Sorensen used the classification of high and low types of odontoid fractures, but their description suggests that these fractures are identical to Type II and Type III.[29] They advised primary fusion of the atlas and axis for the high fractures and conservative treatment for low fractures. Of 21 low fractures treated conservatively, only three, or 14%, were nonunions.

Apuzzo and colleagues apparently did not find

the classification of Type I, II, and III helpful and stated, in fact, that 7 of 13 Type III fractures ultimately came to fusion.[4] These authors found an overall nonunion rate of 33% in fractures treated conservatively but only 16% nonunion in undisplaced fractures. The rate of nonunion in displaced fractures treated conservatively was 60%. They concluded that undisplaced fractures could be managed by bracing, the exact type being unimportant. Primary fusion was recommended if displacement is over 4 mm. Interestingly, three of their five patients treated with halo immobilization developed nonunion. They thought that patients over 40 years of age had a poorer prognosis and recommended fusion.

Pierce and Barr stated that Type II fractures treated by halo immobilization often did not heal and thought that fusion was indicated.[42] Donovan found that Type III fractures showed better results than Type II. His experience with Type II fractures was so poor, even with halo fixation, that he recommended primary fusion for this group.[15] He did not think the degree of displacement correlated with the end result, and he thought that methods of closed treatment other than the halo had proven unacceptable.

On the other hand, Sweigil reported union in 21 of 22 patients treated in halo braces. He gave no classification of the fractures, but most of his cases appear to have been caused by less violent trauma than those in most other series.

Clark and White reported a significant rate of both nonunion and malunion after initial treatment. Thirty-two percent of the Type II lesions and 13% of the Type III fractures did not unite after initial management in the Cervical Spine Research Society series. The halo device was successful in managing 68% of Type II injuries, whereas posterior cervical fusion was successful in 96%. The complications, however, may be more significant with surgery. Clark and White concluded that patients with a Type II injury who have either significant displacement or angulation, or both, should be considered for surgical stabilization. They further stated that Type III fractures are not benign. The halo device appears to be the safest and most reliable form of therapy for Type III injuries, although surgery may be required for particularly unstable fractures.[12]

Thus, although some authors still disagree about the prognosis in fractures of the odontoid, most now appear to favor conservative treatment for Type III fractures. Many consider patients with Type II fractures, especially if the fracture is displaced, to be candidates for primary atlantoaxial fusion. Even halo vest immobilization has yielded poor results for Type II fractures.

ATLANTOAXIAL FUSION

If one accepts the premise that primary surgical treatment is indicated in certain selected odontoid fractures, what then is the treatment of choice? Almost all authorities now believe that posterior wiring and fusion of C1 to C2 or C3 is the appropriate operation. Inclusion of the occiput is unnecessary, except in unusual circumstances such as congenital absence of the posterior arch of the atlas or congenital fusion of the atlas to the occiput. If the occiput is included, the failure rate is increased approximately twofold over that for atlantoaxial fusion alone.[44] Also, McGraw points out that, according to Fielding, including the occiput results in an additional loss in flexion–extension of 30%.[32]

In the past, fracture of the ring of the atlas associated with a fracture of the odontoid was thought to be an additional indication for inclusion of the occiput in the fusion. It is commonly known that almost all fractures of the atlas heal well. Lipson has pointed out that with this combination of injuries, halo immobilization is recommended until fracture of the atlas has healed. Then atlantoaxial arthrodesis can be performed.[31]

Sherk and Snyder in 1979 found in a review of the literature that at least 386 posterior upper cervical spine fusions had been reported.[54] They found that C1–C2 fusions had a failure rate of approximately 10% and occipitocervical fusions had a failure rate of about 20%. The complications they found included nonunion, infection, and spinal cord and brain-stem infarction.

Fried, in 1973, reported less than satisfactory results in ten patients in whom posterior wiring and intraarticular facet fusions had been done by several different surgeons.[24] The wire size varied from 18 to 24 gauge. One death resulted from the operation, and in eight patients redisplacement of the fracture occurred. He concluded that C1–C2 fusion should be reserved for patients in whom conservative measures had failed.

On the other hand, most recent articles about odontoid fractures and other causes of atlantoaxial instability conclude that posterior wiring and fusion is an effective method associated with low morbidity and mortality in experienced hands.[3,4,9,12,20,26,29,32,39,46] Table 6-1 shows the number of patients undergoing atlantoaxial fusion in several reported series and the number and percent of successful fusions.

Table 6-1. Atlantoaxial Fusion in Several Recently Reported Series

AUTHOR	YEAR	NO. FUSIONS	NO. UNITED	SUCCESS (%)
Schatzker et al	1971	15	13	87
Paradis and Janes	1973	29	23	79
McGraw and Rusch	1973	15	14	93
Anderson and D'Alonzo	1974	18	16	89
Husby and Sorensen	1974	9	9	100
Fielding et al	1976	46	45	98
Brooks and Jenkins	1978	14	13	93
Griswold et al*	1978	30	29	97
Apuzzo et al	1978	13	13	100
Clark and White	1985	54	52	96
Total		243	227	932

* Patients with Brooks-type fusion.

As far as can be determined, no deaths in the series in Table 6-1 were directly attributable to the operation. One patient in the Cervical Spine Research Society series died 6 weeks after surgery from a myocardial infarction.[12] The techniques used in the different series varied somewhat, but all had in common the use of corticocancellous bone grafts that were wired securely to the posterior elements of the atlas and the axis. The series reported by Brooks and Jenkins[9] and by Griswold and colleagues[26] used wedge-shaped bone grafts wired to the posterior arches of the atlas and lamina of the axis. The other series employed modifications of the Gallie fusion.

The use of preoperative and intraoperative traction with skeletal tongs or a halo ring is most important for safety during the operative procedure, if there is instability. We use traction routinely. The patient is anesthetized and intubated in the supine position on a Stryker frame with traction in place. The patient is then turned to the prone position for the operation. An alternative is to perform an intubation with the patient awake and supine and to position him prone on a Wilson frame before the induction of anesthesia. A neurologic examination and lateral radiographs are also obtained before anesthesia is induced.[11] Some orthopedists have preferred to carry out the surgery with a halo vest applied preoperatively. We agree with Murphy, Wu, and Southwick that it is preferable to operate on a Stryker frame or Wilson frame with traction.[11,36,54] The use of a halo tends to restrict exposure and makes the operation more difficult. It must be emphasized that, for posterior atlantoaxial fusion to be effective and safe, the surgeon must be experienced and the surgery must be meticulous. Exposure must be done carefully to avoid damage to the cord and vertebral arteries. Sharp dissection should be used in exposing the posterior elements of C1 and C2, and rough stripping with a periosteal elevator must be avoided. Hemostasis must be as complete as possible. The exact method of wiring the bone grafts varies. The techniques recommended by Fielding and colleagues, McGraw and Rusch, Husby and Sorensen, Brooks and Jenkins, and Griswold and associates have all proved successful, and the reader is referred to these articles for details. They all provide good fixation of C1 to C2 and secure fixation of the bone graft to the vertebra. For grafting, it is important to use autogenous iliac bone. That from bone banks has less chance of success. The wound must be adequately drained. We often use two penrose drains, exiting at the superior and inferior margins of the wound. Closed-suction type drains should be monitored, because they can become clogged. If this clogging goes unnoticed for several hours, the resulting hematoma can be disastrous. Finally, postoperative external immobilization must be adequate and continued until amalgamation of the bone grafts has occurred, usually for about 4 months. Some surgeons prefer to use a halo, which is certainly excellent fixation. However, a good brace that immobilizes the occiput and chin and extends well down over the anterior and posterior chest is usually adequate and is more comfortable.

CONCLUSIONS

The following conclusions can be drawn concerning fractures of the odontoid process of the axis:

1. Fractures of the odontoid process of the axis have been reported with increasing frequency in recent years.
2. Fracture of the odontoid process as well as other cervical spine fractures should be ruled out in patients admitted with cerebral concussion.
3. Tomography is of great help in the diagnosis of fractures of the odontoid process. It is also helpful in differentiating Type II and Type III injuries and in determining the best treatment.
4. Fractures of the odontoid in children under 7 years of age are different. Almost all do well with satisfactory conservative treatment, and primary surgical treatment is rarely indicated.
5. The classification of odontoid fractures into Type I, Type II, and Type III has helped in determining prognosis and treatment. The degree of displacement and angulation are also important.
6. Type I fractures are rare. They are stable injuries and require only symptomatic treatment for good results.
7. Type II fractures are the most common. They tend to be unstable and have a high incidence of nonunion if treated conservatively, even with a halo vest. This is particularly evident when there is either significant displacement or angulation of the fracture.
8. Type III fractures tend to be more stable, have a large cancellous surface, and usually unite in a high percentage of cases with good conservative measures. A halo vest is the most secure form of immobilization for this fracture. If a less rigid orthosis is used, the fracture should be frequently monitored to avoid the possibility of malunion.
9. In fractures of the odontoid treated conservatively that progress to nonunion, late myelopathy is a real danger. Almost all patients in this category should undergo posterior atlantoaxial fusion.
10. Many of these fractures may be missed initially. A high index of suspicion is essential to recognize the diagnosis and initiate appropriate treatment.

REFERENCES

1. *Althoff B, Goldie IF:* The arterial supply of the odontoid process of the axis. Acta Orthop Scand 48:622–629, 1977
2. *Amyes EW, Anderson FM:* Fracture of the odontoid process. Arch Surg 72:377–393, 1956
3. *Anderson LD, D'Alonzo RT:* Fractures of the odontoid process of the axis. J Bone Joint Surg 56A:1663–1674, 1974
4. *Apuzzo Michael LJ, et al:* Acute fractures of the odontoid process. J Neurosurg 48:85–91, 1978
5. *Bailey DK:* The normal cervical spine in infants and children. Radiology 59:712, 1952
6. *Blockey NJ, Purser DW:* Fractures of the odontoid process of the axis. J Bone Joint Surg 38B:794–816, 1956
7. *Bohler J:* Anterior stabilization for acute fractures and non-unions of the dens. J Bone Joint Surg 64:18–28, 1982
8. *Bohlman HH:* Acute fractures and dislocations of the cervical spine. An analysis of three hundred hospitalized patients and review of the literature. J Bone Joint Surg 61A:1119–1142, 1979
9. *Brooks AL, Jenkins EB:* Bone Joint Surg 60A:279–284, 1978
10. *Chan DPK, Morwessel RM, Leung KYK:* Treatment of odontoid fractures with halo cast immobilization. Orthop Trans 5:118–119, 1981
11. *Clark CR, Ranawat CS:* Posterior cervical (C1–C2) fusion for atlantoaxial subluxation in rheumatoid arthritis. Strat Orthop Surg 4:1–16, 1985
12. *Clark CR, White AA:* Fractures of the dens: A multicenter study. J Bone Joint Surg 67:1340–1348, 1985
13. *Cooper PR, Maravilla KR, Sklar FH, Moody SF, Clark WK:* Hal immobilization of cervical spine fractures. Indications and results. J Neurosurg 50:603–610, 1979
14. *Corner EM:* Rotary dislocation of the atlas. Ann Surg 45:9, 1907
15. *Donovan MM:* Efficacy of rigid fixation of fractures of the odontoid process and retrospective analysis of fifty-four cases. Orthop Trans 3:309, 1979
16. *Dunn ME, Seljeskog EL:* Experience in the management of odontoid process injuries: An analysis of 128 cases. Neurosurgery 18:306–310, 1986
17. *Ekong CEU, Schwartz ML, Tator CH, Rowed DW, Edmonds VE:* Odontoid fracture: Management with early mobilization using the halo device. Neurosurgery 9:631–637, 1981
18. *Ewald FC:* Fracture of the odontoid process in a seventeen-month-old infant treated with a halo. J Bone Joint Surg 53A:1636–1640, 1971
19. *Fielding JW:* Normal and selected abnormal motion of the cervical spine from the second cervical vertebra to the seventh cervical vertebra based on cineroentgenography. J Bone Joint Surg 46A:1779–1781, 1964
20. *Fielding JW, Hawkins RJ, Ratzan SA:* Spine fu-

sion for atlantoaxial instability. J Bone Joint Surg 58A:400–406, 1976

21. *Fielding JW, Cochran GVB, Lawsing JF III, Hohl M:* Tears of the transverse ligament of the atlas. A clinical and biomechanical study. J Bone Joint Surg 56A:1683–1691, 1974
22. *Fielding JW, Hawkins RJ:* Roentgenographic diagnosis of the injured neck. AAOS: Instructional course lectures. 25:149–169, 1976
23. *Fielding JW, Hensinger RN, Hawkins RJ:* Os Odontoideum. J Bone Joint Surg 62A:376–382, 1980
24. *Fried LC:* Atlanto-axial fracture—dislocations. J Bone Joint Surg 55B:490–495, 1973
25. *Griffiths SC:* Fracture of odontoid process in children. Pediatr Surg 7:680–683, 1972
26. *Griswold DM, et al:* Atlanto-axial fusion for instability. J Bone Joint Surg 60A:285–292, 1978
27. *Hadley LA:* Atlanto-occipital fusion, ossiculum terminale and occipital vertebra as related to basilar impression with neurological symptoms. AJR 59:511–524, 1948
28. *Hawkins RJ, Fielding JW, Thompson WJ:* Os odontoideum: Congenital or acquired. J Bone Joint Surg 58A:413–414, 1976
29. *Husby J, Sorensen KH:* Fracture of the odontoid process of the axis. Acta Orthop Scand 45:182–192, 1974
30. *Jefferson G:* Fracture of the atlas vertebra. Br J Surg 7:407–422, 1919–20
31. *Lipson SJ:* Fractures of the atlas associated with fractures of the odontoid process and transverse ligament ruptures. J Bone Joint Surg 59A:940–942, 1977
32. *McGraw RW, Rusch RM:* Atlanto-axial arthrodesis. J Bone Joint Surg 55B:482–488, 1973
33. *Maiman DJ, Larson SJ:* Management of odontoid fractures. Neurosurgery 11:471–476, 1982
34. *Marar BC, Tay CK:* Fracture of the odontoid process. Aust NZ J Surg 46:231–236, 1976
35. *Mixter SJ, Osgood RB:* Traumatic lesions of the atlas and axis. Ann Surg 51:193–207, 1910
36. *Murphy MJ, Wu JC, Southwick WO:* Complications of halo fixation. Orthop Trans 3:126, 1979
37. *Nachemson A:* Fracture of the odontoid process of the axis. A clinical study based on 26 cases. Acta Orthop Scand 29:185–217, 1960
38. *Osgood RB, Lund CC:* Fractures of the odontoid process. N Engl J Med 198:61–72, 1928
39. *Paradis GR, Janes JM:* Posttraumatic atlantoaxial instability: The fate of the odontoid process fracture in 46 cases. J Trauma 13:359–366, 1973
40. *Pepin J, Bourne R, Hawkins R:* Odontoid fractures of the axis with special reference to the elderly patient. Orthop Trans 5:119, 1981
41. *Pepin JW, Bourne RB, Hawkins RJ:* Odontoid fractures, with special reference to the elderly patient. Clin Orthop Rel Res 193:178–183, 1985
42. *Pierce DS, Barr JS:* Use of halo and cervical spine problems. Orthop Trans 3:125, 1979
43. *Ricciardi JE, Kaufer H, Louis DS:* Acquired os odontoideum following acute ligament injury. J Bone Joint Surg 58A:410–412, 1976
44. *Roberts A, Wickstrom J:* Prognosis of odontoid fractures. J Bone Joint Surg 54A, 1972
45. *Ryan MD, Taylor TKF:* Odontoid fractures: A rational approach to treatment. J Bone Joint Surg 64:416–421, 1982
46. *Schatzker J, Rorabeck CH, Waddell JP:* Fractures of the dens (odontoid process): An analysis of thirty-seven cases. J Bone Joint Surg 53B:392–404, 1971
47. *Schatzker J, Rorabeck CH, Waddell JP:* Nonunion of the odontoid process—an experimental investigation. Clin Orthop Rel Res 108:127–137, 1975
48. *Schiess RJ, DeSaussure RL, Robertson JT:* Choice of treatment of odontoid fractures. J Neurosurg 57:496–499, 1982
49. *Schiff DCM, Parke WW:* The arterial supply of the odontoid process. J Bone Joint Surg 55A:1450–1456, 1973
50. *Schwarz GA, Wigton RS:* Fracture-dislocation in the region of the atlas and axis, with consideration of delayed neurologic manifestations and some roentgenographic features. Radiology 28:601–607, 1937
51. *Seimon LP:* Fracture of the odontoid process in young children. J Bone Joint Surg 59A:943–947, 1977
52. *Sherk HH:* Fractures of the odontoid process in young children. J Bone Joint Surg 60A:921–923, 1978
53. *Sherk HH:* Fractures of the atlas and odontoid process. Orthop Clin North Am 9:973–983, 1978
54. *Sherk HH, Snyder BJ:* An exceptional case analysis of upper posterior neck fusion. Orthop Trans 3:125, 1979
55. *Smith BL, Anderson LD, Harris EC:* The treatment of comminuted fracture of the distal radius with pins and plaster. Contemp Ortho 3:629–635, 1981
56. *Southwick WO:* Management of fractures of the dens (odontoid process). J Bone Joint Surg 62A:482–486, 1980
57. *Sweigil JF:* Halo thoracic brace in the management of odontoid fractures. Orthop Trans 3:126, 1979
58. *Wang GJ, Mabie KN, Whitehill R, Stamp WG:* The nonsurgical management of odontoid fractures in adults. Spine 9:229–230, 1984
59. *Wisoff HS:* Fracture of the dens in the aged. Surg Neurol 22:547–555, 1984
60. *Wollin DG:* The os odontoideum. J Bone Joint Surg 45A:1459–1471, 1963

Traumatic Spondylolisthesis of the Axis (Hangman's Fracture)

STEVEN R. GARFIN AND RICHARD H. ROTHMAN

There is no man so good, who, were he to
submit all his thoughts and actions to the
laws, would not deserve hanging ten times in
his life.

M. DeMontaigne, 1580

The fracture through the pedicle of the second cervical vertebra, separating the posterior neural arch from the body of the axis, has been a lesion of significant medical and legal concern for the last century. This fracture pattern, more precisely and scientifically termed *traumatic spondylolisthesis of the axis,* was believed by many anatomists and physicians in the late 19th and early 20th centuries to be the "ideal lesion" produced by judicial hanging and the condition hangmen should strive to achieve.[16,17,23,26] Recently, interest in this topic has been rekindled, owing to the observation of the similarities between the historical description of fractures created by the hangman's noose and certain fractures created in high-speed motor vehicle collisions. Although this chapter is primarily concerned with the more scientific aspects of the pathogenesis, diagnosis, and management of the pars interarticularis fracture of the second cervical vertebra, certainly the historical aspects and early descriptions of this fracture cannot be ignored. The chilling and often macabre nature of hangings is frequently what stimulates the interest in this fracture. Because of the morbid fascination aroused by this topic, and owing to academic interests, we briefly discuss the history of hanging and its relationship to the fracture pattern and etiology as more commonly seen today.

HISTORICAL ASPECTS

Behold a wicked, hardened Wretch,
Whose Neck in Justice must be stretched,
Upon the fatal Gallows tree,
And not a soul to pity me,
Not one will my Just Fate bewail,
I must be hurried from the Gaol,
It is for Wilful Murder I,
A Fatal Death am doomed to die

The Sorrowful Lamentation and Last
Farewell of John Price, 1718

Capital punishment for crimes against the state has been recorded since early times. The first record of hanging, however, can be traced to Deuteronomy:21 of the Old Testament, in which it was noted in the description of an early transgression: "His body shall not remain all night upon the tree, but thou shalt in any wise bury him that day; for he that is hanged is a cursed of God." Hanging was introduced to Western civilization (England) by the Angles, Jutes, and Saxons between the 5th and 10th centuries.[13,20] Before that time, the English boiled criminals but apparently found the process inconvenient and time-consuming. Hanging was selected as a more expeditious mode of public execution.

As first employed, hanging was only one of many steps of a criminal's punishment.[4] Before the actual hanging, the condemned person was drawn through the streets of town; he was then hanged by the neck and let down alive so that his body could be quartered, thereby prolonging his suffering and agony.

As the art of hanging advanced, the actual methods required to achieve the final execution were not codified. Pronouncements from the judge's bench historically condemned the victims to be "hung by the neck until dead," with no reference to the exact mechanism used to effect this end. As old prints and woodcuts depict, during this period the knot was generally placed suboccipitally and the victim was slowly asphyxiated. One can find evidence of people who were allowed to hang for over an hour until death became plainly manifested.[21]

Centuries later, in an effort to increase efficiency, the victim was turned off a ladder with a subsequent fall of several feet. Alternatively, the noose was placed about his neck while he was standing in the cart that was to carry him to his place of execution. After arriving at the designated location, the cart was withdrawn and the victim was left to hang freely from the gallows. Even in this case, however, death often remained a slow and uncertain event. Additional efforts were often required on the part of the executioner. Some applied manual traction on the feet, whereas other vigorous hangmen, in certain difficult situations, scurried to the shoulders of the victim to add their own weight to help complete the task.[21] Occasionally, a victim was prematurely released from the gallows, and resuscitation has been recorded. In fact, cases of recovery after hanging became so well known in early England that it became common practice for the friends of the hanged to carry the body immediately to a sympathetic surgeon who would try to revive the person.[21]

The long drop, apparently first employed by Newgate Gaol in London in 1784, became more common toward the end of the 18th century. When correctly performed, the long drop achieved a more rapid and humane death. Its indiscriminate employment, however, led to occasional unpleasant consequences.[1] In Ireland in 1865, the hanging of two criminals using a 15-foot drop completely decapitated one and caused near decapitation of the other.[17] During this time, however, the long drop was not the universal mode of execution. A notable exception was the hanging of the famed cadaver "supplier" Burke of the Burke-Hare partnership. In 1829, Burke was allowed a drop of only inches; as might be expected, death ensued slowly from strangulation.

These errors in judgment and lack of scientific precision aroused the ire of many physicians in England and the United States.[1] Mathematical tables and scientific testing of hanging techniques were developed. In 1866 Reverend S. Houghton devised a mathematical table relating body weight of the victim to the length of the drop.[11] Later, an English judiciary committee met and decided that a force of 1260 foot-pounds was the force necessary to rapidly fracture the cervical spine and presumably the spinal cord, and to cause death. An equation was developed by which the height of the drop was determined to be equal to 1260 foot-pounds divided by the weight of the victim in pounds. This became the official guideline for the British Commonwealth, although it was not rigidly followed. This same committee (Lord Aberdare's Capital Sentences Committee) also received a recommendation that submental knots be employed, because this technique would most surely lead to cervical fractures and instant death. The recommendation was acknowledged by Lord Aberdare and his committee but was not adopted as law.

In 1913, Frederick Wood-Jones first recognized and described two distinct types of lesions resulting from judicial hanging.[26] These findings were based on the study of two series of specimens preserved in the Royal College of Surgeons Museum. The first series was collected from the skulls of Nubians, presumably hanged during the Roman period, whose bodies were discovered along the Nile River in Egypt. Wood-Jones found that many of the Nubian skulls had fractures of the base of the skull along the basilar suture lines. All of the cervical vertebrae were found to be intact. He also examined the skull of Dr. Pritchard, an infamous British poisoner, who was hanged by a subaurally placed knot. Wood-Jones pointed out that Dr. Pritchard's skull had a basilar skull fracture similar to that of the Nubian skulls he had examined. He hypothesized that the Nubians, therefore, must also have been hanged using subaural knots.

In the second series of specimens, donated by Captain C. F. Fraser, superintendent of the Rangoon Central Gaol, all the skulls were intact and all of the cervical vertebrae showed an identical lesion, a fracture-dislocation of the axis (Fig. 6-43). It was known that this second set of skulls was from hangings using a submental knot. From these observations, Wood-Jones concluded that "the submental knot should supercede the subaural knot in [the] English judicial hangings." Similarly, J. Marshall concluded one of his articles in the British Medical Journal by noting that "overwhelming evidence as to the deadliness of the submental knot has accumulated, the adoption of which would simplify matters."[16] Marshall, convinced of the merits of this method, went to the extreme of inventing a collar to maintain the knot in a submental position during hanging.

PATHOANATOMY

To fully understand and appreciate the mechanism of injury, we must turn our attention first to the functional and applied anatomy of the axis. The second cervical vertebra is a transitional unit between the cervicocranium above and the more typical cervical vertebrae below. The phrase *cervicocranium,* as adopted by Schneider and associates, applies to the base of the skull, the atlas, the odontoid process, and the body of the axis.[23] (Fig. 6-44). The weakest link in this system is the pars interarticularis of C2, a narrow isthmus that is located between the superior and inferior facets. The superior facets are biconcave structures situated nearly in the horizontal plane and slightly deviated laterally. The large inferior facets, posterior and caudal to the pars interarticularis, are similar to the cervical facets below them and are angled obliquely with the articular surfaces directed anteriorly. The pars interarticularis is primarily a narrow tube of cortical bone with limited cancellous material, connecting the facets.[24] Im-

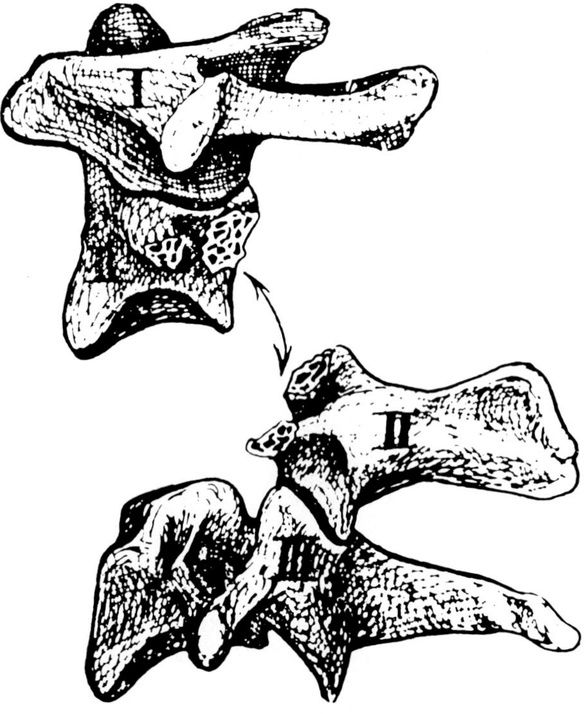

Fig. 6-43. The "ideal lesion" produced by hanging. (Wood-Jones F: The ideal lesion produced by judicial hanging. Lancet 1:53, 1913)

mediately lateral to the isthmus, and extending from it, is the foramen transversarium, which houses the vertebral artery in its course to the brain (Fig. 6-45).

According to Wood-Jones,, the ideal judicial hanging should produce an injury to the cervical spine in which the

> posterior arch of the axis is snapped clean off and remains fixed to the third vertebra, while the atlas, the odontoid process and the anterior arch of the axis remain fixed to the skull. This lesion is produced by a violent jerk which throws the man's head suddenly backwards and snaps his axis vertebra. Death in this series of cases was uniformly instantaneous, for the spinal cord was cleanly severed by the fracture of the neck. In every instance the knot was placed "a little to the left of the chin"—*i.e.,* was a submental knot [see Fig. 6-43].[26]

The modern counterpart of this hangman's fracture is termed traumatic spondylolisthesis of the axis.[2,3,7,9,10,23,25] The injury is usually sustained in a motor vehicle collision during rapid deceleration (Fig. 6-46). The victim is thrown forward in the car with this head striking the windshield; this usually occurs during either a head-on collision with

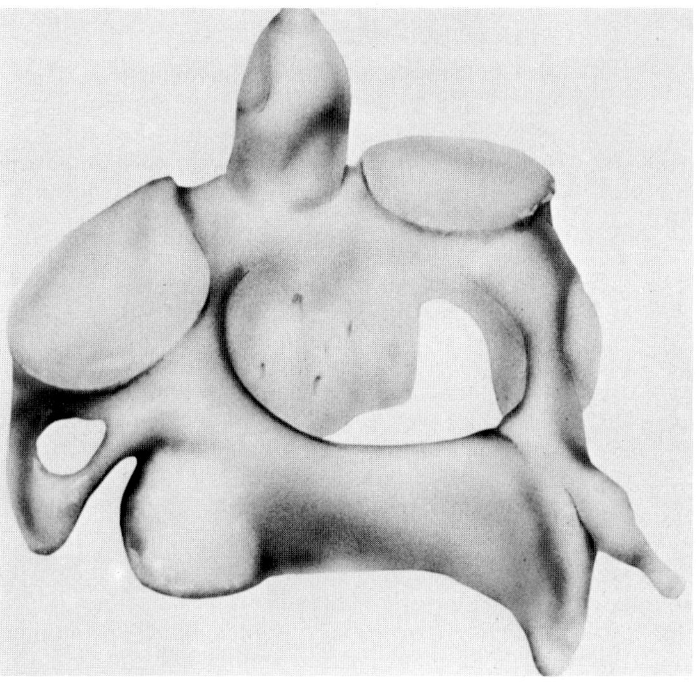

Fig. 6-44. Second cervical vertebra (axis). This oblique view shows the superiorly projecting odontoid process and the pars interarticularis and foramen transversarium separating the superior and inferior facets.

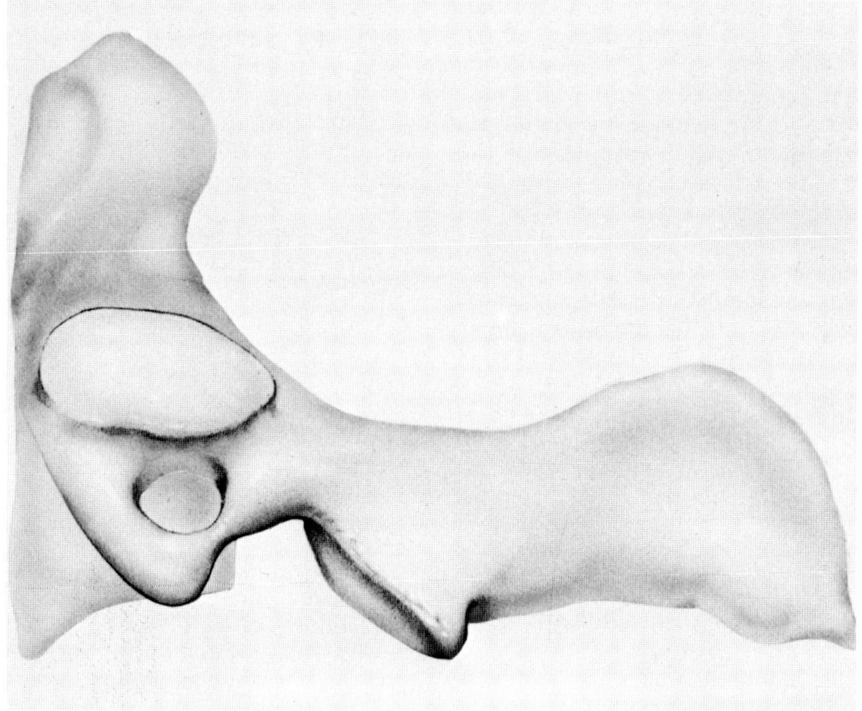

Fig. 6-45. The narrow pars interarticularis separating the superior facet from the more posteriorly positioned inferior facet. The direction of the facets is more horizontal than on other vertebrae.

another vehicle or a collision with a fixed object. At the moment of impact, the cervical spine is subjected to two vectors of force: The first of these is axial loading, and the second is extension. In effect, a disruption of the cervicocranium from the lower cervical spine occurs. Analysis of the force mechanisms involved indicates that the cervicocranium moves as one unit as axial loading and extension are applied, while the posterior arch of the axis and the lower cervical vertebrae move and act together as a counterforce.

Sequential analysis of the pathologic anatomy of this lesion is helpful in understanding not only the variety of patterns seen in clinical practice, but also

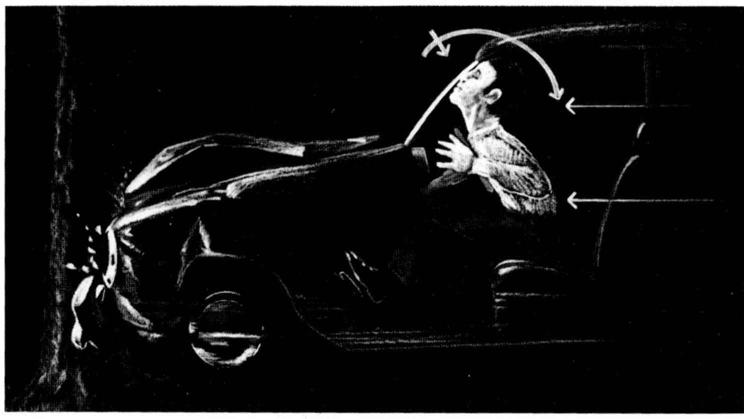

Fig. 6-46. Mechanism of injury in most front-end automobile collisions leading to hangman's fractures. Forces to the neck are applied in both axial loading and extension. After the initial impact, there may be a rebound flexion of the cervicocranium.

the treatment we will recommend. Although Holdsworth originally described the mechanism of extension injuries, which does in fact fit the primary pattern seen in the hangman's fracture very well, Cornish later specifically related the extension mechanism to traumatic spondylolisthesis of the axis.[3,12] Schneider and associates, focusing on this topic, established the extension mechanism of injury in motor vehicle accidents as a major factor in these fractures. Later, however, Effendi and associates as well as Levine and Edwards suggested that the axial load/extension mechanism of injury was not the sole cause of all hangman's fractures.[6,14]

Almost all authors[2,3,6–10,12,14,18,19,23–25] agree that most injuries are caused, at least initially, by axial load and extension. As the axial load and extension forces are applied to the cervicocranium, failure of the neural arch will occur with a bilateral fracture (Fig. 6-47). As shown by CT scans, the fractures are usually bilateral, but rarely symmetrical.[6,24] Most likely this is related to some degree of cervicocranial rotation at the time of impact. At this stage, little displacement occurs and no instability is present. As continued loading occurs and the cervicocranium is forced into further extension, disruption of the anterior longitudinal ligament and perhaps disc and posterior longitudinal ligament may take place (Fig. 6-48). Although rupture frequently occurs through the substance of the anterior longitudinal ligament, avulsion with a small accompanying bone chip off the anterior superior margin of C3 or, less often, the anteroinferior margin of C2 may develop. Continuation of these forces leads to disruption of the disc and avulsion of the disc itself from either the superior plate of C3 or the inferior plate of C2. At this point, true instability is present between the cervicocranium and the cervical spine below. As the forces subside, if the ligaments are completely disrupted anteriorly, and the posterior longitudinal ligament fails or is stretched, posterior subluxation of the body of C2 on C3 and anterior widening of the C2–C3 disc space may occur and can be observed on lateral radiographs (Fig. 6-49).

As proposed by Schneider and others, because of the failure of anterior and posterior longitudinal ligaments, as well as the intervening C2–C3 disc space, a multiplane instability between the cervicocranium and cervical spine below could develop (Fig. 6-50). It was believed that subluxation could occur anteriorly, as well as posteriorly, because of the complete disruption of the soft tissues of the anterior vertical column combined with the

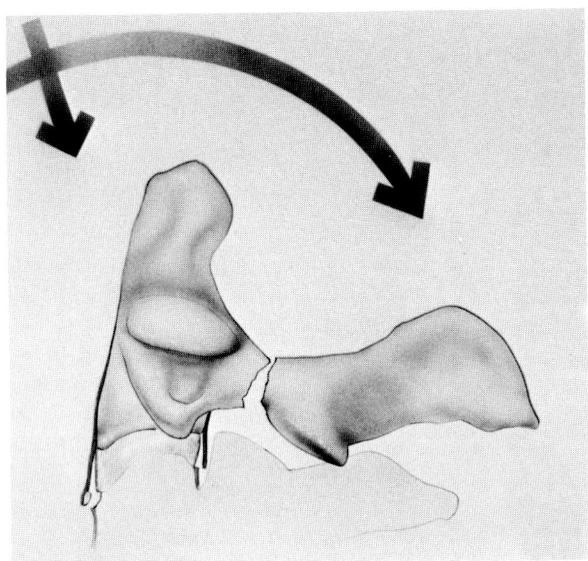

Fig. 6-48. Continued loading may cause disruption of the anterior longitudinal ligament. This allows further displacement of the fracture, particularly posteriorly. Small avulsion of anterosuperior body of C3 may also occur, as shown here.

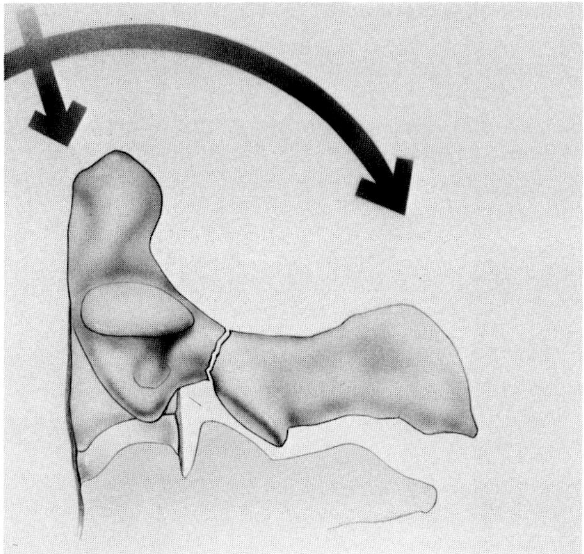

Fig. 6-47. Nondisplaced fracture occurring through the pars interarticularis of C2. This is caused by axial loading and extension, as depicted by the arrows.

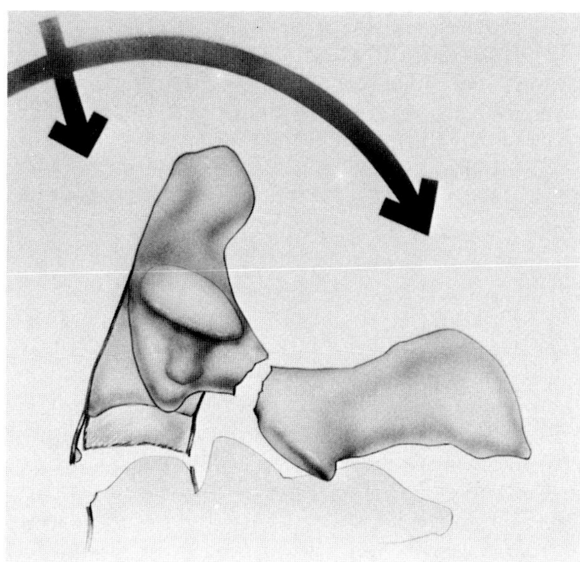

Fig. 6-49. Disc disruption may occur with sufficient extension force. This frequently increases the displacement of the pars fracture and may lead to early instability.

fractures through the pars interarticularis posteriorly (Fig. 6-51). However, subsequent descriptions attempted to clarify the various C2–C3 configurations seen on lateral radiographs by suggesting that more than one type of force coupling may be involved.[5,6,14,22,24] Rather than always assuming complete disruption of the anterior and posterior longitudinal ligaments and disc space, allowing either anterior or posterior subluxation depending on gravitational forces on the cervicocranium, it is perhaps more appropriate to relate the findings of anterior subluxation of C2 on C3 to a reflex flexion force that occurs after the hyperextension and axial load.[6,14]

Pathoanatomically, following the axial and extension forces, a fracture occurs through the pars interarticularis of C2. As the motor vehicle deceleration, and therefore the body deceleration, continues, the cervicocranium is frequently, by reflex, thrown forward (in a manner similar to mechanisms described in whiplash injuries).[15] This flexion force can lead to disruption of the posterior longitudinal ligament, disruption of the C2–C3 disc space (as described for the extension forces), and stripping of the anterior longitudinal ligament off the C3 body.[5,6,14,24] This leads to anterior subluxation of C2 on C3 and, depending on the degree of disc space disruption, can also result in a residual angulatory deformity of the body of C2 in relation to C3 (Fig. 6-51).

Rarely, a pure flexion mechanism may create a similar appearance. However, in the case of pure flexion, bilateral C2–C3 facet dislocations most likely occur before the fracture through the pars interarticularis develops. Lateral radiographs demonstrate the C2–C3 facet dislocation, which in

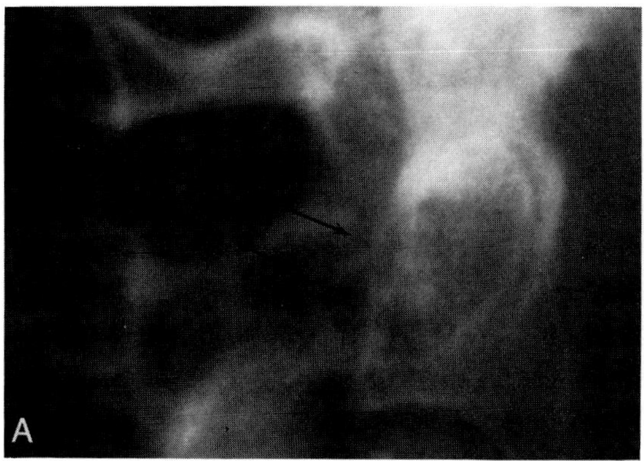

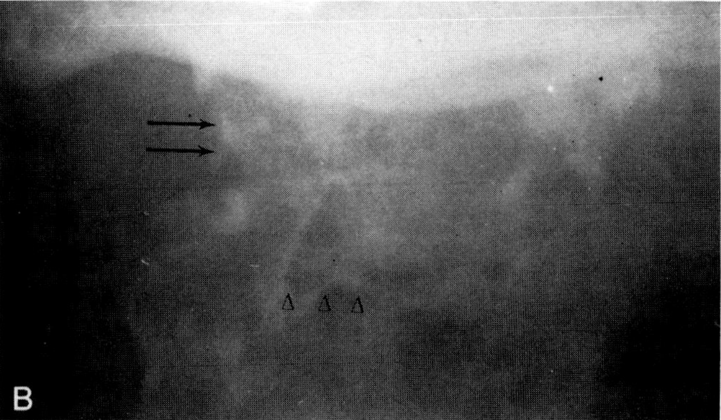

Fig. 6-50. (*A*) 67-year-old male with traumatic spondylolisthesis of the axis. The subluxation of C2 on C3 can be seen, and the fracture through the pars is identified by the arrow. (*B*) The degree of instability can be seen in this A–P projection. The body (*closed arrow*) of C2 remains with the cervicocranium and is deviated laterally compared with the spinous process of C2 (*open arrows*), which remains with C3 and the remaining caudal portions of the cervical spine. In this example, owing to the multiplane instability demonstrated, the anterior and posterior longitudinal ligaments and the C2–C3 disc space, presumably were completely disrupted.

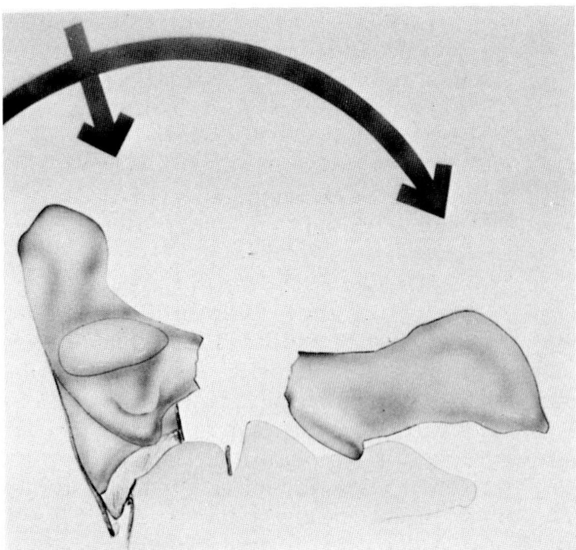

Fig. 6-51. Following the extension and axial loads, rebound flexion occurs, which may injure the posterior longitudinal ligament and lead to anterior subluxation of C2 on C3. Although disruption of the anterior longitudinal ligament is depicted, it does not always occur. Instead, it may be stripped off of C3, allowing the spondylolisthesis to occur.

this instance occurs before or without any extension force.

CLASSIFICATIONS

An understanding of the mechanism of injury is useful for developing sound treatment regimens. Additionally, classifications can be utilized to predict results or guide the treatment. A number of classifications have been proposed,[6–8,14] although not all are useful in directing patient management. Based on our understanding of the pathomechanics of the injury and for establishing a treatment regimen, the classifications of Effendi and colleagues[6] and the modified system proposed by Levine and Edwards,[14] appear to be the most useful.

Type I injuries are considered stable by both Effendi and Levine (Fig. 6-47). These are fractures through the pars interarticularis with less than 1 to 2 mm displacement at the fracture site. They are caused by axial loading and extension forces.

Type II injuries[6] demonstrate the isthmus fracture due to extension and axial loading forces and have some degree of displacement (Figs. 6-48 and 6-49). Although this can occur in extension (5% of Effendi's series), it usually is related to a rebound flexion and is associated with disruption of the posterior longitudinal ligament and C2–C3 disc structure, leading to slight angulation and anterolisthesis (Fig. 6-51).

Levine and Edwards have added a Type IIA, which consists of less displacement but more angulation than is seen in the Type II injury. They feel that the force vector leading to this injury is related primarily to flexion, since the degree of displacement and angulation increases when traction is applied, in contrast to the Type II injuries, which reduce in light traction.

Type III injuries (both Levine and Effendi) are most likely pure flexion injuries. The C2–C3 facet capsules are disrupted and a dislocation occurs. This is followed by a fracture through the pars interarticularis when a compression load is added after the facets dislocate.

SYMPTOMS AND SIGNS

The symptoms produced by this fracture are not highly specific. As with any significant neck injury, there is diffuse pain throughout the cervical spine associated with stiffness and trauma. The patient often feels marked apprehension and fear with a sense of subjective instability. Pain radiating along the course of the greater occipital nerve (C2)—so-called occipital neuralgia—is frequent.

Physical findings associated with this lesion are often nonspecific. Marked guarding of neck motion by the patient is usual. Inspection of the scalp and face usually reveals the stigmata typical of direct trauma at the point of contact between the skull and the windshield of the vehicle. Facial and skull fractures are not unusual and should be carefully looked for. These injuries are fairly direct evidence of the extension and axial compression nature of the fracture, and one can often reconstruct a fairly precise mechanism to describe the vector forces by analyzing these traumatic signs. Neurologic examination of these patients frequently reveals a paucity of dramatic findings.

ASSOCIATED FINDINGS

It is a common failing to focus on one lesion and miss occult fractures at another level. With this in mind, it should be noted that as significant force is applied to these predominant extension and compression injuries, particularly in the axial direction, associated fractures frequently occur in

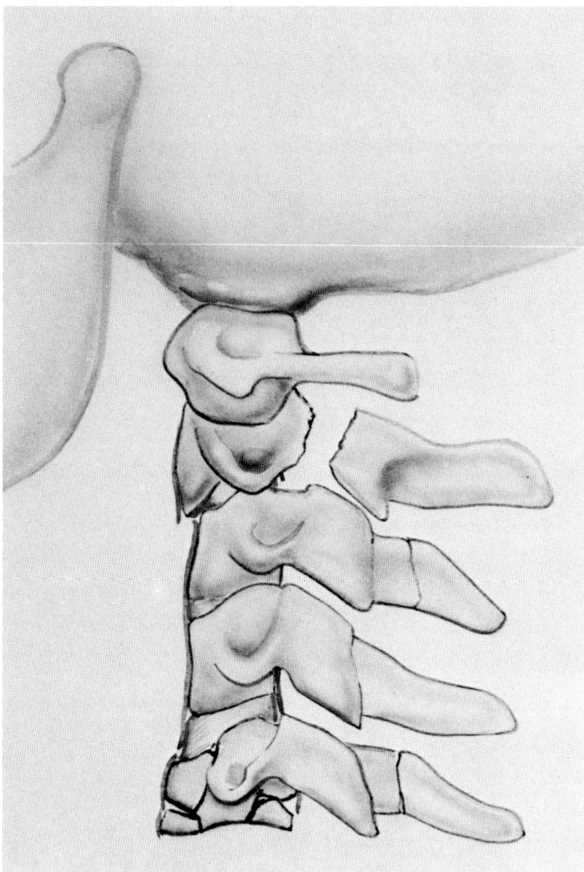

Fig. 6-52. The widened spinal canal at the level of the C2 fracture is shown. Fractures of the spinous processes of C3 and C5, as well as of the body of C5, could be missed with cursory evaluation.

the lower cervical spine (Fig. 6-52). Most frequently, these are burst injuries of the body of a vertebra in the midcervical area or fractures of spinous processes. One must be particularly alert for these additional fractures, especially when confronted with marginal radiographic views that are obtained during the patient's initial evaluation.

In this injury, there is relative sparing of the spinal cord and nervous system because of the capacious nature of the bony canal in the upper cervical spine. Additionally, as anterolisthesis develops, the spinal canal widens at the C2 level (Fig. 6-52). Catastrophic spinal cord injuries occur during actual hangings, as opposed to motor-vehicle-induced injuries, because in the former, following the fracture (which occurs because of extension), a distraction force leads to the spinal cord damage. Fortunately, except in the Levine and Edwards IIA classification, most of the injuries seen at this level today are not related to distraction.

Common associated lesions include head injuries; facial lacerations, abrasions, and fractures; cervical and/or thoracic spine injuries; tracheal ruptures; and thoracic cage (rib, lung, sternum) injuries. As mentioned, presumably because of the lack of a distraction mode combined with the widened canal that occurs with anterior spondylolisthesis, neurologic deficits are few and usually temporary. When permanent neurologic deficits do occur, they are often associated with Type III injuries. Also, on occasion, motor vehicle accident victims using a diagonal lap/sash seat belt can be partially thrown from a car, with the diagonal component of the restraint catching the neck, acting to cause a distraction–extension force. This is more closely analogous to the classic hangman's injury and has more serious impact because of the attendant cord damage. Fortunately, this is also a rare event.

TREATMENT

To determine the correct treatment, the stability and type of the fracture must be determined. Flexion and extension lateral films, as well as routine cervical spine roentgenograms, can significantly help in this determination. The unstable fracture reveals marked displacement on the initial films (A–P and lateral projections) or excessive motion on lateral flexion–extension roentgenograms.

If the fracture is believed to be stable (Type I), a cervicothoracic orthosis and early ambulation will suffice until fracture healing is complete. Prolonged recumbency and hospitalization are neither necessary nor helpful. In unreliable patients, a halo device affixed to a thoracic vest may be useful.

For the unstable fracture, prompt reduction of the subluxation is indicated (Fig. 6-53). This is usually accomplished by placing the patient in traction with the head and neck in mild extension. Occasionally, closed manipulative reduction under general anesthesia, aided by fluoroscopic visual control, is necessary. Once the fracture is aligned, a halo vest can be applied and ambulation initiated; this can often be accomplished within 24 hours of the injury. The early ambulation and rehabilitation are important in reducing the morbidity from the injury and the sequelae of prolonged immobilization and bed rest. The halo vest should be maintained for 8 to 12 weeks, and then a cervicothoracic brace should be applied until healing

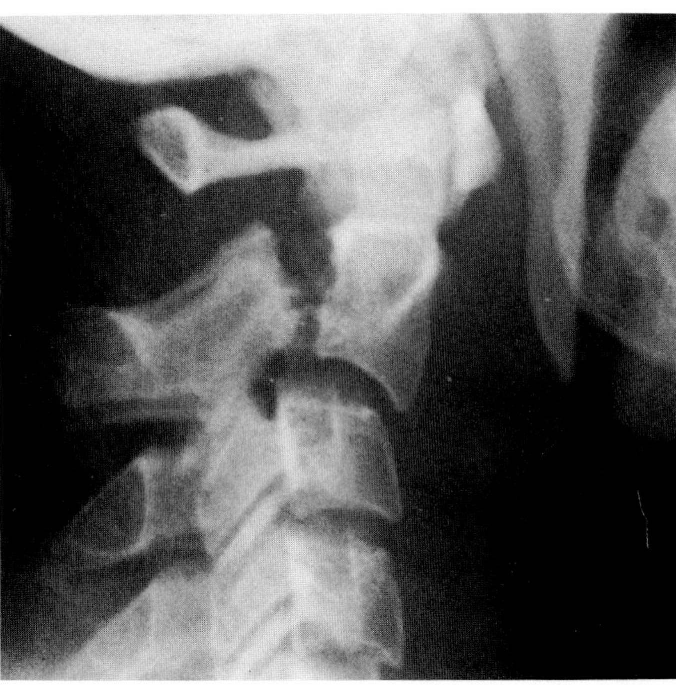

Fig. 6-53. Patient with traumatic spondylolisthesis of the axis. Wide displacement at the fracture site and anterior subluxation of C2 on C3 are evident. The patient was treated in a halo vest with his neck extended to reduce the fracture, which healed uneventfully.

is unquestionably demonstrated, usually by 3 to 4 months from the date of injury.

The traction used can be at the discretion of the surgeon, and various approaches have been tried. A simple halter is sufficient in the minimally displaced fracture where only short-term traction is indicated and the patient is cooperative. When formal skull traction is desired, Gardner-Wells tongs can be applied in the emergency room under local anesthesia. These tongs are spring loaded and require no drilling, and in our experience they have rarely been pulled loose. If a halo is used, then halo traction is most sensible and efficient, because it is easily converted to the halo vest once reduction is accomplished.

Healing follows one of two patterns; either the fracture itself unites, or spontaneous anterior fusion occurs between the bodies of C2 and C3 (Fig. 6-54). Anatomic reduction is not necessary for healing, and a modest amount of residual displacement, in and of itself, is not an indication for surgical intervention. The prognosis has been good in regard to both fracture healing and recovery from any neurologic deficits that may develop.

Surgery to stabilize or reduce this injury is seldom necessary. Our only indications for surgical intervention are (1) late pain, presumably due to disruption of the C2–C3 disc, (2) objective demonstration of late instability, and (3) a Type III injury with dislocated facets. In this context, late instability would be defined as grossly observable motion on lateral flexion–extension roentgenograms performed after 3 months of adequate immobilization. If a Type III injury is determined, a posterior approach to reduce the C2–C3 facets should be performed and a posterior C2–C3 fusion undertaken. This, however, will not stabilize the axis fracture through the pars interarticularis. Therefore, after reducing the C2–C3 facets and fusing that level, external immobilization (a halo) should be used to allow healing across the pars interarticularis and/or the C2–C3 disc space (as one would treat a pure Type II injury).

If surgery is undertaken for indications (1) and (2) above (late nonunion or instability), an anterior interbody fusion at the C2–C3 interspace is generally recommended. The anterior route obviates including C1 in the fusion, which would be necessary because of the fracture and resultant instability of the posterior element of C2, if the posterior approach were selected. Occasionally, if a persistent spinal cord deficit is noted and can be explained by a residual C2–C3 deformity, a C3 anterior vertebrectomy can be performed to free the anterior margin of the spinal cord at the time of the anterior fusion (Fig. 6-55).

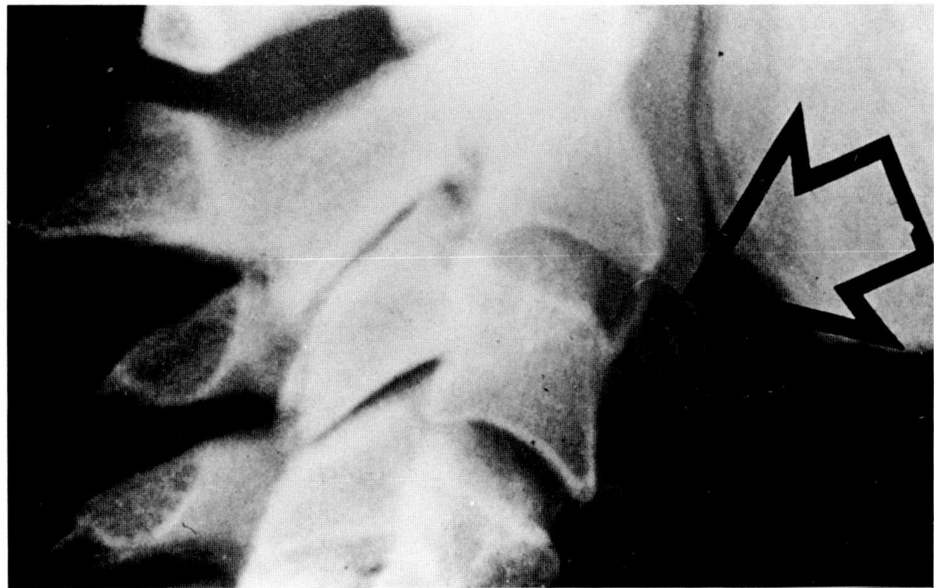

Fig. 6-54. Healed hangman's fracture. The arrow indicates calcification of the anterior longitudinal ligament.

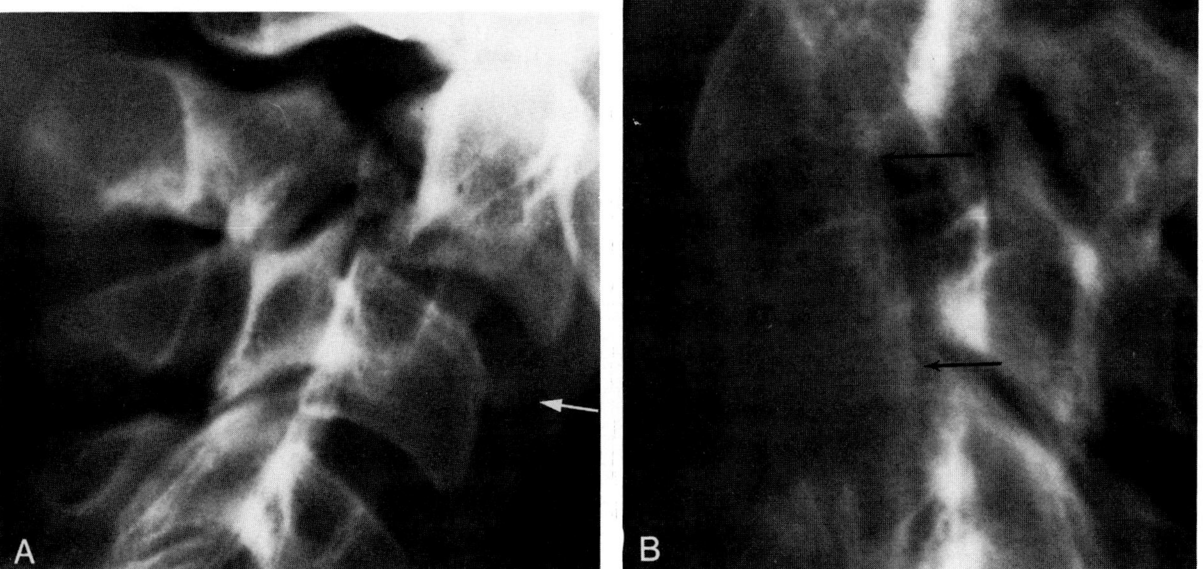

Fig. 6-55. (*A*) A 28-year-old male sustained this C2 fracture and had a spinal cord injury presumably related to this injury. He was treated in a halo for 4 months. His compliance was poor. He developed late pain and instability. Callus can be seen anteriorly at the C2–C3 disc space. This did not completely bridge the disc space to create a solid union. (*B*) Because of pain, demonstrated instability on flexion–extension films, and a persistent spinal cord injury, the patient underwent C3 anterior vertebrectomy and cord decompression followed by C2–C4 strut graft fusion. This radiograph demonstrates healing anteriorly and perhaps posteriorly.

CONCLUSIONS

Most patients who sustain a traumatic spondylolisthesis of the second cervical vertebra obtain the injury through an extension-axial loading mechanism. In some individuals, a subsequent flexion component will create an anterior spondylolisthesis due to disruption of the posterior longitudinal ligaments and disc space, with the anterior longitudinal ligament remaining intact, although being stretched or stripped off the body of C3. Primary flexion injuries undoubtedly occur (Type III and perhaps IIA), but they are rare. It is also uncommon to have any significant neurologic sequelae associated with these injuries, especially in long-term follow-up. For the great majority, nonoperative treatment suffices and leads to an excellent prognosis for fracture healing, neurologic status, and return to full function. We conclude by returning again to British history and poetry:

'Tis sweet to dance to violins,
When love and life are fair,
But 'tis not sweet with nimble feet
To dance upon the air

From the Ballad of Reading Gaol
Oscar Wilde, 1898

REFERENCES

1. *ANNOTATION:* Judicial hanging. Lancet 1:629, 1913
2. *BOHLMAN HH:* Acute fractures and dislocations of the cervical spine. J Bone Joint Surg 61A:1119, 1979
3. *CORNISH DL:* Traumatic spondylolisthesis of the axis. J Bone Joint Surg 50B:31, 1968
4. *DUFF C:* A New Handbook on Hanging. London, A Melrose Ltd, 1954
5. *DUSSAULT RG, EFFENDI B, ROY D, CORNISH B, LAURIN CA:* Locked facets with fracture of the neural arch of the axis. Spine 8:365, 1983
6. *EFFENDI B, ROY D, CORNISH B, DUSSAULT RG, LAURIN CA:* Fractures of the ring of the axis. J Bone Joint Surg 63B:319, 1981
7. *FRANCIS WR, FIELDING JW:* Traumatic spondylolisthesis of the axis. Orthop Clin North Am 9:1011, 1978
8. *FRANCIS WR, FIELDING JW, HAWKINS RJ, PEPIN J, HENSINGER R:* Traumatic Spondylolisthesis of the Axis. J Bone Joint Surg 63B:313, 1981
9. *GARVER JN:* Abnormalities of the atlas and axis vertebrae: Congenital and traumatic. J Bone Joint Surg 46A:1782, 1964
10. *GROGONO DJS:* Injuries of the atlas and axis. J Bone Joint Surg 36B:397, 1954
11. *HAMMOND DN:* On the proper method of executing the sentence of death by hanging. Med Rec NY 22:426, 1882
12. *HOLDSWORTH F:* Fractures, dislocations and fracture-dislocations of the spine. J Bone Joint Surg 52A:1534, 1970
13. *LAURENCE J:* A History of Capital Punishment. Port Washington, Kennikat Press, 1932
14. *LEVINE AM, EDWARDS CC:* The management of traumatic spondylolisthesis of the axis. J Bone Joint Surg 67A:217, 1985
15. *MACNAB I:* Acceleration extension injuries of the cervical spine. In Rothman RH, Simeone FA (eds): The Spine, 2nd ed, pp 647–660. Philadelphia, WB Saunders Co, 1982
16. *MARSHALL JD:* Letter to the Editor: The executioner surgeon. Br Med J 2:1340, 1913
17. *MARSHALL JD:* Letter to the Editor. Lancet 1:194, 1913
18. *NORTON WL:* Fractures and dislocations of the cervical spine. J Bone Joint Surg 44A:115, 1962
19. *PEPIN JW, HAWKINS RJ:* Traumatic spondylolisthesis of the axis: Hangman's fracture. Clin Orthop 157:133, 1979
20. *POTTER JD:* The Art of Hanging. New York, AS Barnes, 1965
21. *ROBERTSON WGA:* Recovery after judicial hanging. Br Med J 1:121, 1935
22. *RODA JM, CASTRO A, BLAZQUEZ MG:* Hangman's fracture with complete dislocation of C-2 on C-3. J Neurosurg 60:633, 1984
23. *SCHNEIDER RC, LIVINGSTON KE, CAVE AJE, HAMILTON G:* Hangman's fracture of the cervical spine. J Neurosurg 22:121, 1965
24. *SHERK HH, HOWARD T:* Clinical and pathologic correlations in traumatic spondylolisthesis of the axis. Clin Orthop 174:22, 1983
25. *WILLIAMS TG:* Hangman's fracture. J Bone Joint Surg 57B:82, 1975
26. *WOOD-JONES F:* The ideal lesion produced by judicial hanging. Lancet 1:53, 1913

Fractures and Dislocations of the Lower Cervical Spine

HENRY H. BOHLMAN AND ENRIQUE BOADA

Traumatic injuries of the cervical spine are among the commonest causes of severe disability and death following trauma. Often these injuries are not diagnosed in the emergency room situation, and only in recent years has the treatment become more standardized.[4,6] Approximately one third of the injuries are due to a motor vehicle accident, one third to a fall, and the remaining one third to some type of athletic injury or wound inflicted by a missile or falling object.[7] If a lower cervical fracture results in quadriplegia, the patient may become significantly dependent on others for most of the basic physiologic needs and life's activities.

The incidence of cervical spine injuries peaks during adolescence, young adulthood, and again during the sixth and seventh decades. Because of the nature of accidents resulting in cervical spine injuries, the majority involve young healthy persons: those who are very active, those who engage in physically dangerous activities, and occasionally those who exhibit sociopathic personality traits resulting in alcoholic intoxication. People in their sixth and seventh decade make up the second largest group of cervical spinal injury patients. Cervical spondylosis and a preexisting narrow spinal canal are highly associated with the injury in this age group; for this reason, lesser forces may result in severe spine and spinal cord injury.

The Edwin Smith surgical papyrus of Egypt, which dates from 5000 years ago, describes spinal cord injury as an "ailment not to be treated." This somewhat pessimistic attitude has persisted over the years, including in more recent times. With the institution of trauma and spinal cord injury centers in this country, great steps have been taken toward improving emergency care, medical and surgical treatment, and rehabilitation of the person sustaining a spine and spinal cord injury. There has been a renewed interest in research to define the electrical, pathophysiologic, biochemical, and mechanical events that occur with the acute spine and spinal cord injury.[9,10,11,12] Major treatment advances were the application of anterior and anterolateral operative approaches to the spine and improved internal fixation used with surgery.[2,8,13,15] There has been a more precise definition of instability. Various internal fixation devices of the spine have been analyzed for their effectiveness in surgically treating spine injuries. Recent investigations have reclassified spine and spinal cord injuries so that clinical analysis and various treatment modalities may be more accurately assessed.

In addition, there has been further clarification on an experimental basis of acute and chronic spinal cord compression, the effect of initial stabilization, and various treatment modalities. Studies of the experimental, as well as human, spine and spinal cord injury pathology further clarified the problem and added to our basic core of knowledge to be used in deciding the treatment of these injuries.

The management program for cervical spine injuries that is outlined in this section is based on Bohlman's review of 300 such patients and his experience as chief of the 60-bed Acute Spinal Cord Injury Service at the Cleveland Veterans Administration Medical Center since 1974, where Boada has had the opportunity to share in this experience for 4 years. Our therapeutic goals in the treatment of cervical spine and associated spinal cord injuries are to preserve life; to maintain neurologic function and avoid further damage by immediate transportation of the patient to a spinal injury center; to accomplish immediate reduction and stabilization by external or internal means; to restore as much function of the spinal cord and nerve roots as possible; and finally, to have the patient reach the best quality of life possible through adequate rehabilitation, once the above goals have been attained.

PATHOLOGY

The pathology of fractures and dislocations of the lower cervical spine may be divided into the major areas of soft tissue, osteoarticular, and central nervous system areas. In addition, one should consider the experimental work on spine and spinal cord pathology and its relationship to the clinical setting.

In 1967 and 1968 at the Baltimore City Morgue, Davis, Bohlman, and associates[22] studied the head and neck pathology of 50 persons who died as the result of craniospinal injuries. This study was carried out with initial roentgenograms of the cervical spine in various positions, including distraction, accomplished by hanging the cadaver in a head-halter traction device. Following roentgenograms, the vertebral arteries were injected with a dye solution of micropaque and gelatin to outline the vascular supply and the disruption around the cervical spine. Further roentgenograms were taken in flexion, extension, and distraction, and finally the entire cervical spine and cord was removed *in toto,* including the foramen and magnum. The spine was sagittally sectioned, and the cord was removed and examined grossly as well as microscopically with histologic sections. In addition, the brain was removed from each to determine the association of head and neck pathology.

Soft-Tissue Injuries

The soft-tissue pathology involved the muscle groups surrounding the cervical spine, which were not usually torn unless the injury was quite severe, that is, with complete osseous separation or dislocation at a single level. Hemorrhage did occur into the muscle substance and commonly into the retroesophageal space, where as much as 700 mm of blood was encountered, which would certainly be enough to cause respiratory distress in the clinical situation. The origin of the hemorrhage was not the major vertebral arteries, but rather the small radicular arteries branching from the vertebrals at the osseous foramina. The major vessel systems were resistant to damage, and the vertebral artery was torn in only two cases: one of a severe dislocation and another that thrombosed with a unilateral facet dislocation (Fig. 6-56*A* through *F*). The anterior spinal artery was thrombosed in one of the 50 cases. Ligament injuries occurred in combinations rather than as an isolated tear of the anterior or posterior longitudinal ligament, indicating that multiple forces were involved in these severe injuries, rather than a single flexion or extension force. The transverse ligament was torn in only one case of the 50 autopsies performed. Disc injuries were the most commonly encountered pathologic entity (Fig. 6-57 *A, B, C,* and *D*). Disc disruption at one or more levels occurred in 38% of the cases, unrelated to previously existing osteoarthritis, and only one disc extrusion was found in a patient with central cord quadriparesis (Fig. 6-56*B*).

Osseous Injuries

The osseous pathology occurred most often (in two thirds of the cases) at high levels between the occiput and C3, as one might expect in this fatal injury study. Vertebral body fractures so common in the clinical practice were uncommon here, occurring in only seven cases. The skull was fractured in over half of the cases, with bilateral basilar fractures extending through the petrus ridges being the most common type (Fig. 6-58).

Central Nervous System Injury

There was a high association between brain pathology and neck injuries. Brain contusions and edema occurred together in half of the cases. Contusions in these cases were caused by shearing forces within the brain substance secondary to deceleration forces. Only one subdural hemorrhage was identified in the brain, but subarachnoid hemorrhage was seen in over half the cases. The major lesions of the spinal cord were contusions or lacerations associated with petechial hemorrhages within the cord substance (22 cases), usually at the upper cervical levels. Small epidural hemorrhages were noted in only two cases; they extended over multiple levels but did not cause any significant compression of the spinal cord. On gross inspection of the spinal cords at autopsy, the petechial hemorrhages were at the level of the osseous and ligamentous disruption. There were two cases of central cord necrosis.

These pathologic findings demonstrated a very high association of head and neck pathology. One would have to believe that any force applied to the head would be transmitted to the neck, so this was not a surprising finding. Brain lesions were associated with spinal cord lesions in 61% of the cases, with osseous and ligament injuries to the cervical spine in 47% of the cases, and with both skull fractures and cervical spine lesions in 37% of the cases. On the other hand, spinal cord lesions were associated with brain lesions in 63% of the cases, with osseous and ligament injury to the cervical spine also in 63% of the cases, and with both skull fractures and cervical spine lesions in 37%. It became evident from the study that the head and neck should be considered as a unit, and in the clinical setting, one should always obtain cervical spine roentgenograms if there is any evidence of head injury, or vice versa.

Experimental Pathology

The pathophysiology of cervical spine and cord injuries has been studied experimentally, clinically, and at autopsy in humans. It is difficult to accurately correlate the degree of spinal cord pathology with clinical evaluation of neurologic deficit. In addition, there is not an easy correlation of findings at autopsy in spinal cord injury patients with the clinical situation. Bohlman has reviewed

300 cervical spine injuries, of which the autopsy findings in 48 cases indicated that only three patients had total cord disruption, and many of these patients with clinical evidence of total cord lesions had incomplete contusions or parenchymal hemorrhages. On the other hand, some patients with anterior cord syndromes had normal spinal cords microscopically without evidence of gross cord disruption. The latter finding would support the concept that ischemia is the basis for the anterior cord syndrome (Fig. 6-59). Of these 48 autopsy studies, four patients with unilateral facet dislocations demonstrated impairment of major radicular feeder vessels to the spinal cord and were associated with central cord necrosis, which would lend support to the case for early reduction of spinal fractures. Bohlman has demonstrated in the animal model of chronic anterior cord compression, as well as in the anterior weight drop contusion model, that central necrosis of the gray matter is the most common pathologic finding. Therefore, the formerly described anterior and central cord syndromes may represent varying degrees of the same pathologic process, that is, contusion of the cord initially, followed by microvascular oligemia, edema, and subsequent necrosis of the cervical spinal cord. Again, it seems appropriate that immediate reduction of fractures and dislocations with skeletal traction and removal of offending anterior compressive pathology, which may interfere with normal recovery of the spinal cord, would be beneficial to prevent further pathologic processes within the spinal cord substance.

In the past, laminectomy has been proposed as an operative procedure for the treatment of spinal cord injuries, with the indication being the mere possibility of an epidural hemorrhage occurring with the fracture. Massive epidural hemorrhage, however, is extremely rare with trauma, occurring only in four of the eight patients with ankylosing spondylitis in Bohlman's review series of 300 patients; it did not occur to any extent in Davis and Bohlman's series of 50 fatal craniospinal injuries. Compressive pathology of the spinal cord in cervical spine injuries is almost always anterior, with reference to the spinal cord, and, as a logical sequence, the approach for any decompressive operative procedure should be in that direction.

In conjunction with fractures and dislocations of the lower cervical spine, a significant portion of these patients sustaining such injuries have, in addition, injuries to the spinal cord. The question then arises of what effect compression of the spinal cord by bone or disc fragments has on recovery of that injury. Bohlman and associates have demonstrated experimentally that incomplete spinal cord injuries have the potential to recover to varying degrees, depending upon the amount of initial cord contusion, as well as mechanical factors producing compression of neural tissue. If, with the original fracture of the cervical spine, the spinal cord is incompletely damaged or contused, this indicates that varying amounts of functional cord tissue remain. It then follows that mechanical factors subjecting this remaining viable cord tissue to anterior compression may prevent optimal recovery of spinal cord function. Compressive elements may physiologically block spinal cord function and recovery for extended periods of time without totally destroying the neural tissue itself (Fig. 6-60). The spinal cord will remain ischemic and deformed as long as compression is present, so that in most instances there will be a clinical and neurologic recovery that reaches a plateau, but no further recovery of spinal cord function will occur unless the compressive element is removed. Therefore, anterior decompression of the spinal cord may aid in recovery of the spinal cord function. The important problems are as follows: How severely may the spinal cord be contused and how long may it be compressed anteriorly and still recover significant neurologic function? Bohlman and associates developed an experimental model of incomplete spinal cord injury by individually producing compression (by pressure transducer) and contusion (by weight drop) in animals through the anterior cervical spinal approach at the C5–C6 level. Approximately 800 g cm of energy were required to produce a consistent incomplete quadriparesis of marked severity in the beagle hound. This is considerably greater than the 400 g cm of energy required to produce an incomplete paraplegic from the standard thoracodorsal technique. The animal model of incomplete spinal cord injury secondary to compression was produced in dogs by inserting a pressure transducer through the fifth and sixth cervical interspace by the anterior approach (Fig. 6-61). Approximately 15 pounds per square inch of pressure applied externally through a remote spring-loaded reservoir produced immediate and incomplete paralysis, which was then maintained by chronic compression for 3 to 8 weeks until no further neurologic recovery occurred. In these animals the cord was then decompressed by removing the pressure transducer, and late recovery of paralysis was studied. It was demonstrated in this study that recovery from chronic paralysis could occur, even though the de-

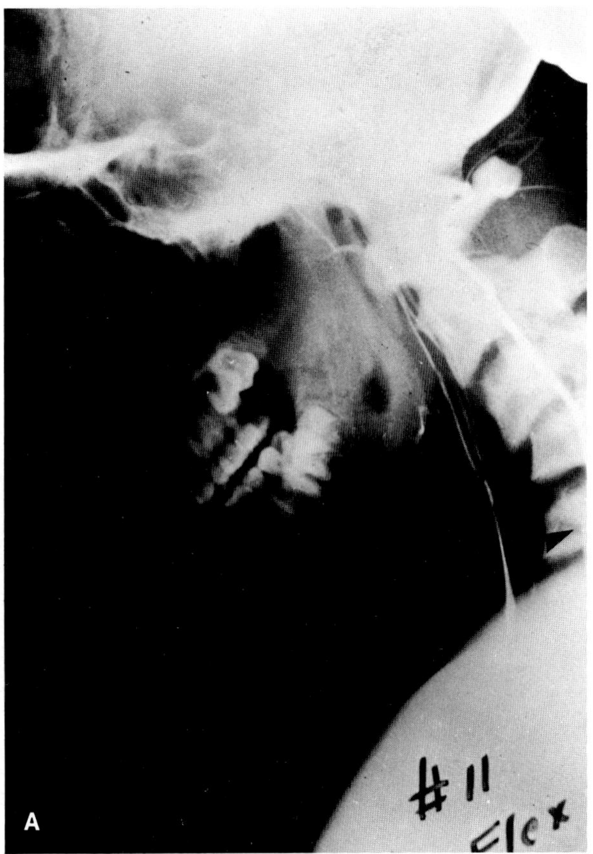

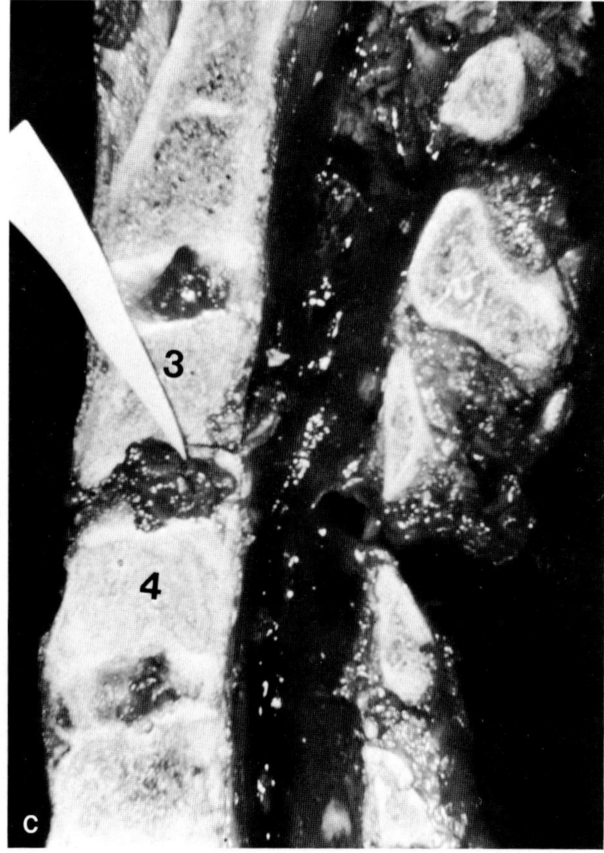

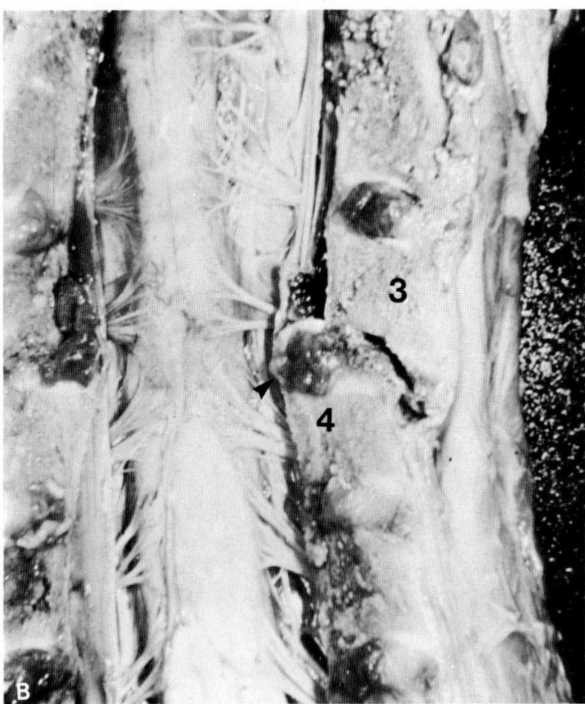

Fig. 6-56. (*A*) Lateral roentgenogram of a 16-year-old boy who sustained a fracture-dislocation of C3 on C4 diving into an ocean wave. Clinical examination revealed a central cord quadriparesis. Following the patient's death, which occurred 13 days after the injury from respiratory complications, the lateral roentgenogram was taken and a vertebral arteriogram was performed. One vertebral artery filled and the other was occluded at the C5 level (*arrow*). (*B*) Photograph of a midsagittal section of the cervical spine of the patient shown in *A*. Note the retropulsed disc at the third and fourth interspace protruding into the spinal canal and the contused spinal cord at that level. The patient also had a unilateral facet dislocation that could not be reduced in skeletal traction prior to his death. (*C*) The patient's retropulsed disc has been manually placed back into its proper position between the third and fourth cervical vertebrae, and the unilateral facet dislocation could only be reduced following replacement of the disc fragment into its original position. The spinal canal is now is normal alignment. The originally herniated disc in this patient could have easily been retrieved from the anterior approach, and possibly the patient would have obtained significant recovery of neurologic function if the osseous displacement and disc protrusion had been corrected.

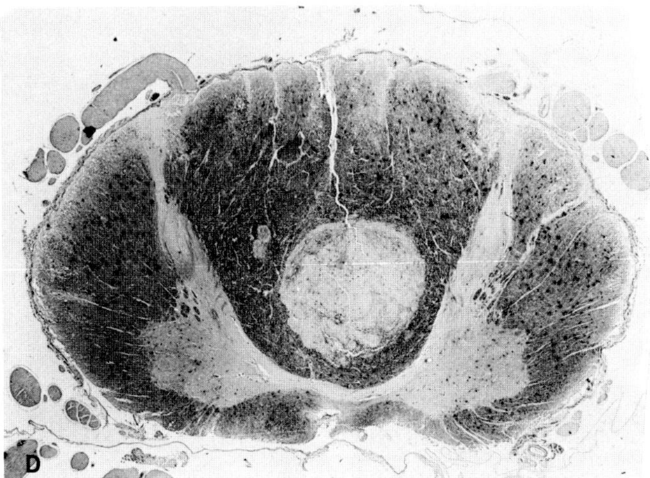

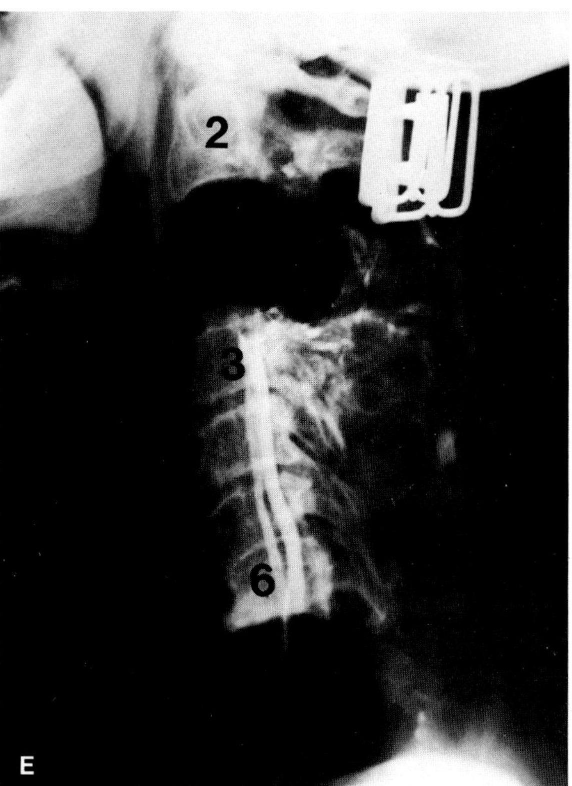

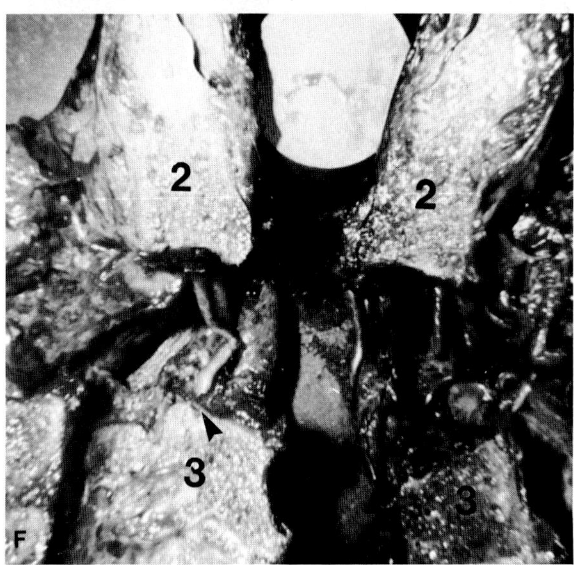

Fig. 6-56. (*Continued*) (*D*) Cross section of the spinal cord revealing central necrosis in the gray matter (myelin stain, original magnification 6.5×). (*E*) Postmortem lateral roentgenogram of a patient sustaining a severe spine injury with total disruption of the second on third and sixth on seventh interspaces. The postmortem arteriogram shows rupture of the vertebral arteries at C2, a very rare occurrence. (*F*) Autopsy specimen sectioned sagittally, demonstrating an osteoarthritic atlantoaxial joint and separation of C2 on C3, as well as disruption of the vertebral artery (*arrow*). (Davis D, Bohlman H, Walker AE, Fisher R, Robinson R: The pathological findings in fatal craniospinal injuries. J. Neurosurg 34:603, 1971)

compression was performed late after chronic paralysis had been well established and plateaued. Also, most of the dogs studied developed central cord syndromes with forepaw paralysis greater than hindpaw paralysis, regardless of which model was used to injure the spinal cord. The spinal cords of the dogs were subjected to gross and histologic examination, which revealed varying degrees of central gray matter damage as the most common finding. This would lend support to the theory that most damage occurs in the central gray matter and that central and anterior cord syndromes are various degrees of the same pathologic process. Also, in the animal studies as well as in human autopsy recoveries, a number of the spinal cords appeared normal histologically after the animals or human had been significantly quadriparetic for varying periods of time. Again, this leads one to believe that ischemia, or decreased vascular supply to the spinal cord, plays a role in subsequent paralysis and later recovery. As in other studies, the cortical evoked potentials used to study these animal models of spinal cord injury paralleled the degree of spinal cord damage as well as the degree of recovery in both animal models. A most important point to be made from this study is that late recovery of spinal cord function can occur if me-

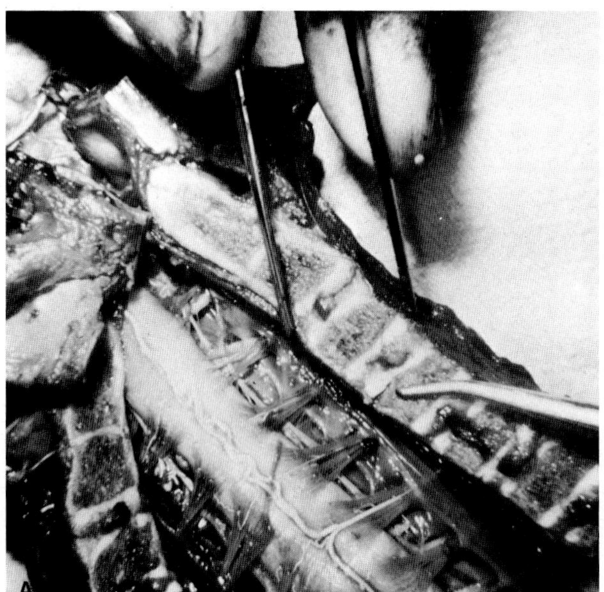

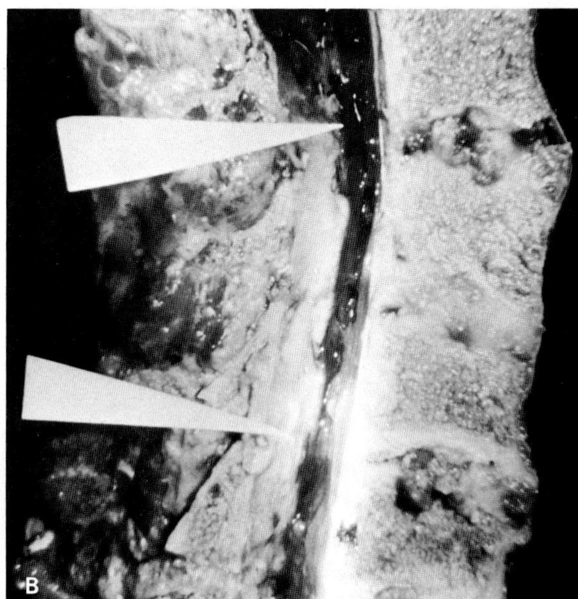

Fig. 6-57. (*A*) Photograph of a midsagittal section of the cervical spine in a 4-year-old child sustaining a fatal injury in a vehicular accident. Note the separation of the cartilaginous disc from the bony end-plate of the superior margin of C3 at the end of the probe. Younger children in this study showed separation of the cartilaginous from the osseous end-plates, whereas older people manifested their injuries by total disruption of the disc. In addition, note the anterior spinal artery filled with a solution of barium and gelatin and a very large radicular feeder vessel coming in along a nerve root on the right side of the photograph. These radicular vessels may be occluded or injured with unilateral facet dislocation and produce ischemia and necrosis of the spinal cord. (*B*) Photograph of an adult male who sustained a fatal head injury with associated disruption of his disc spaces, as pointed out by the arrows. The picture is a lateral view of the midsagittal section of the cervical spine. Note the hemorrhagic, distorted discs at two levels without protrusion of disc material into the spinal canal. It was not possible to demonstrate disc disruptions roentgenographically in this study, even with traction views of the cervical spine.

chanical impediments, such as protruding disc and bone fragments, are removed from the spinal canal by the anterior approach.

Pathologic Basis for Treatment

In the clinical setting, the same theoretic basis for treatment appears to apply in human spinal cord injury patients. Bohlman and colleagues have carried out late anterior decompressions of 172 spinal cord injuries with 2- to 12-year follow-up on the cases operated upon between 1973 and 1984. Of the 111 anterior decompressions of cervical spinal cord injuries, 57 were incompletely injured patients and 54 were complete quadriplegics without any sparing of motor function below the level of the fracture. For the most part, these patients had plateaued in their neurologic recovery prior to surgical intervention. Decompressions were carried out, at an average of 13 months following injury, although some patients have had decompressions later with measurable recovery of motor and sensory function (Fig. 6-62). Anterior decompression of a completely quadriplegic patient may be indicated in those with unreduced dislocations or major axial loading fractures of the vertebral body with significant bony protrusion against the spinal cord and nerve roots. If bone fragments are compressing remaining functioning nerve roots coming from the higher level of noninjured spinal cord, then we believe that root recovery may occur and aid in nerve root recovery and, therefore, arm function. Long-term follow-up on the 111 patients with cervical lesions having late anterior decompression revealed greater than half demonstrated nerve root or arm function recovery to a measurable degree. Of the 57 incomplete spinal

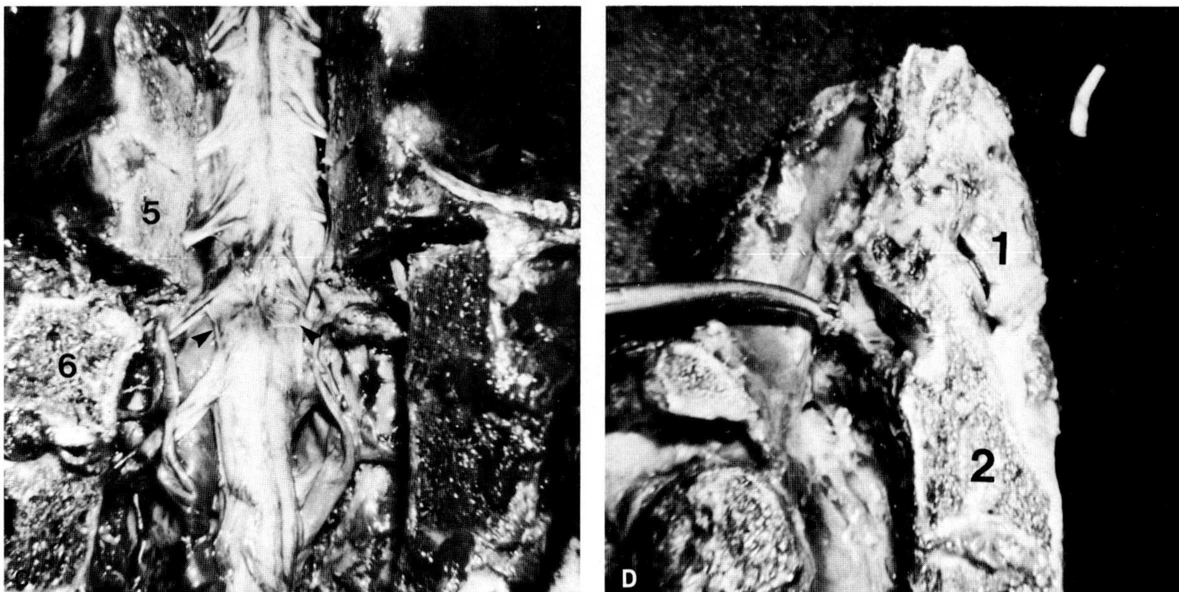

Fig. 6-57. (*Continued*) (*C*) Photograph of a midsagittal section of the cervical spine in an adult male, who sustained a fatal head and neck injury in a vehicular accident. Note the complete separation of the vertebral bodies at C5 and C6 levels, with severe contusion of the spinal cord (*arrows*). There has been total disruption of the anterior as well as posterior longitudinal ligaments and disruption of the disc. Traction views in this instance showed wide separation of the interspace because the ligamentous structures had been completely damaged, a very unstable situation from a clinical standpoint. (*D*) Saggital section of an autopsy specimen demonstrating a complete tear of the transverse ligament of the atlas (probe) secondary to trauma. This is a very rare phenomenon, occurring in only 3% of cervical spine injuries. (*C*, Davis D, Bohlman H, Walker AE, Fisher R, Robinson RA: The pathological findings in fatal craniospinal injuries. J Neurosurg 34:603, 1971)

cord injury patients only 6 could ambulate preoperatively; approximately 60% had significant or measurable motor recovery in the lower extremities, and of this group 36 patients became functional walkers with minimal or no aid. In principle, therefore, it appears necessary to evaluate spine and spinal cord injury patients for acute as well as chronic cord compression, which can be alleviated by anterior decompression and fusion.

The type of treatment called for in osseous and ligament injuries of the lower cervical spine depends upon the degree of pathologic damage that has occurred with the original injury. An axial loading compression fracture of a lower cervical vertebral body may be treated with a rigid brace or halo apparatus and will heal uneventfully; however, severe compression fractures of the vertebrae may produce osseous fragment protrusion into the spinal canal, and this necessitates skeletal traction for reduction, and possibly anterior arthrodesis. The most common severe cervical spine injury involving the posterior elements is a subluxation or dislocation in which the posterior ligament complex is completely torn. This may, in addition, be associated with anterior disc or ligament disruption. As pointed out by Bohlman, late instability is more common than frequently realized because ligamentous structures do not reconstitute normally, even with prolonged rigid external fixation. Unless spontaneous fusion occurs anteriorly with a reduced dislocation, chronic instability can commonly occur. A significant problem can arise in the case of the patient who presents with posterior instability and an incomplete spinal cord injury with evident compressive pathology against the anterior cervical cord. In this instance, we believe that the patient's dislocation or fracture should be reduced and attempted alignment carried out by skeletal traction. This should be followed by a posterior arthrodesis and wiring for stabilization, and then a staged anterior decompression and arthrodesis to relieve the spinal cord compression. The

(Text continues on p. 367)

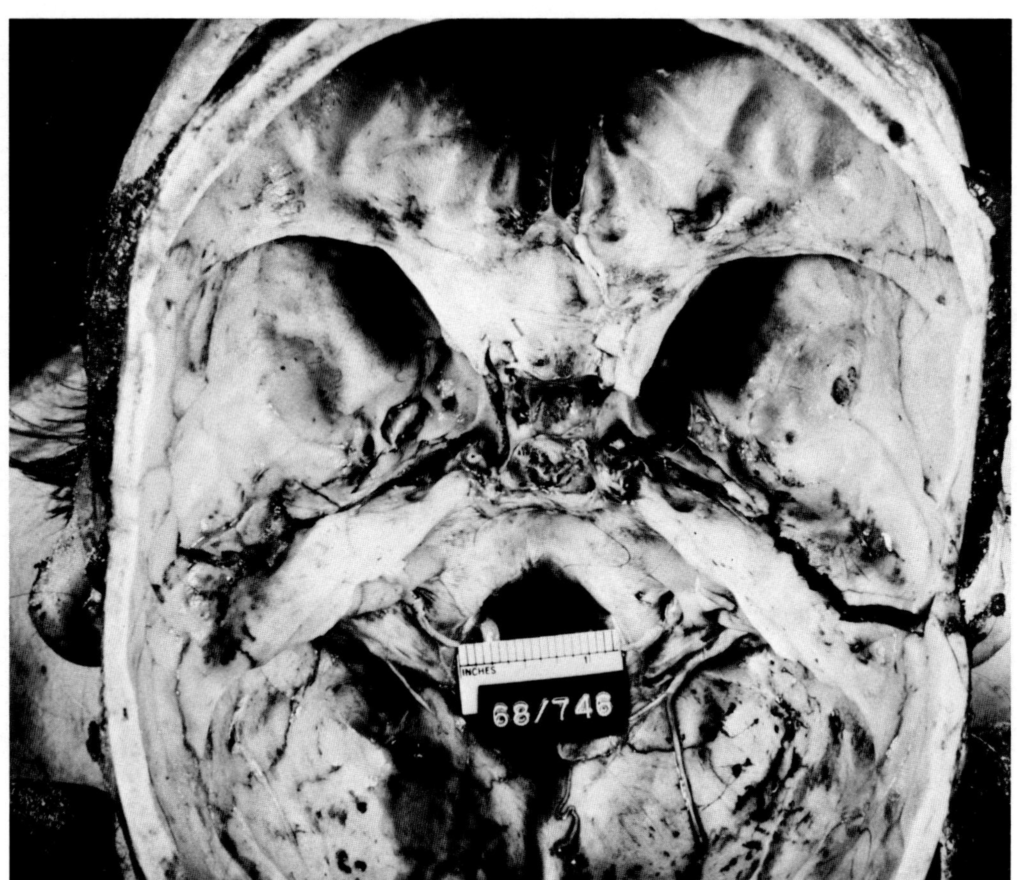

Fig. 6-58. The most common type of skull fracture in this pathology study was basilar through the petrous ridges and the clivus and extended up into the skull convexities. (Bohlman HH: Pathology and current treatment concepts of cervical spine injuries. In the American Academy of Orthopaedic Surgeons: Instructional Course Lectures, Vol XXI, pp 108–115. St. Louis, CV Mosby, 1972)

Fig. 6-59. (*A*) Lateral roentgenogram of a 53-year-old man who had a central cord quadriparesis at C3 after he fell while intoxicated. A preoperative myelogram shows protrusion of disc material between C3 and C4 (*arrows*). (*B*) Postoperative lateral roentgenogram of the patient after anterior cervical discectomy and fusion at C3 and C4. Surgery was performed 10 days after injury and there was rapid recovery of function, but the patient died of a pulmonary embolus 10 months following injury. (*C*) This histologic section of the spinal cord is at the level of C3 and C4, and shows little more than peripheral vacuolation (hemotoxylin and eosin, original magnification × 10). This patient represents the feasibility of significant recovery of neurologic function when there has been little damage to the spinal cord with the original injury. With anterior decompression, significant recovery of spinal cord function can occur. (Bohlman HH: Acute fractures and dislocations of the cervical spine: An analysis of 300 hospitalized patients and review of the literature. J Bone Joint Surg 61A:1119–1142, 1979)

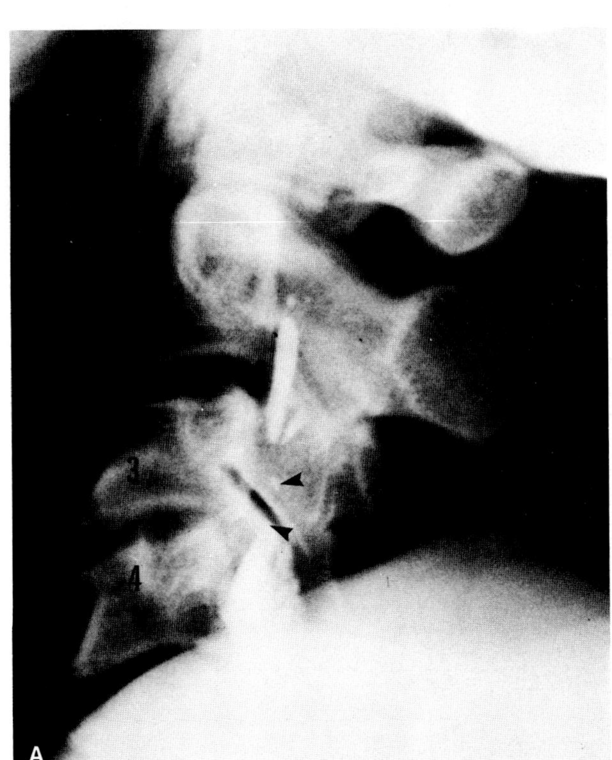
3
4
A

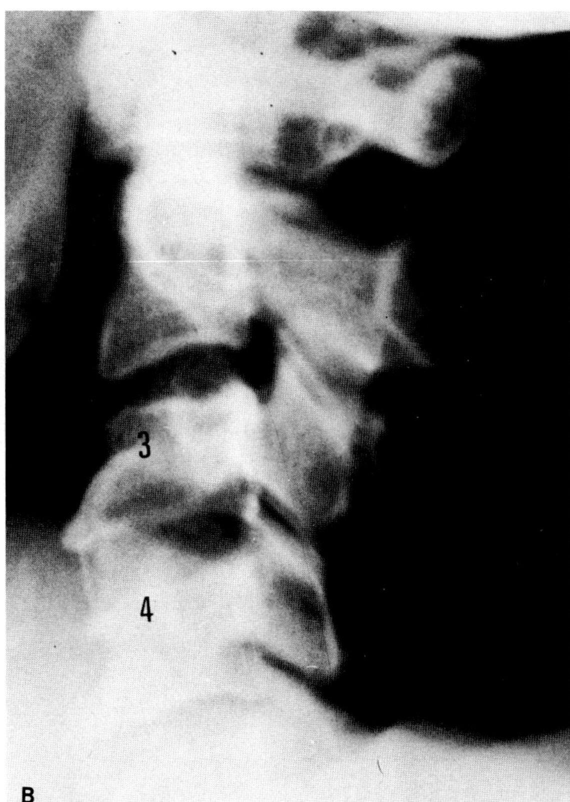
3
4
B

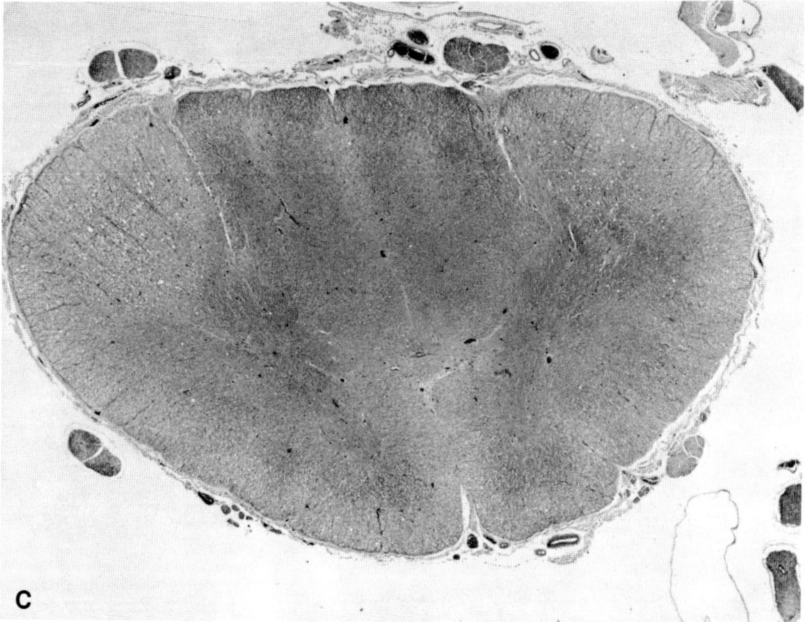
C

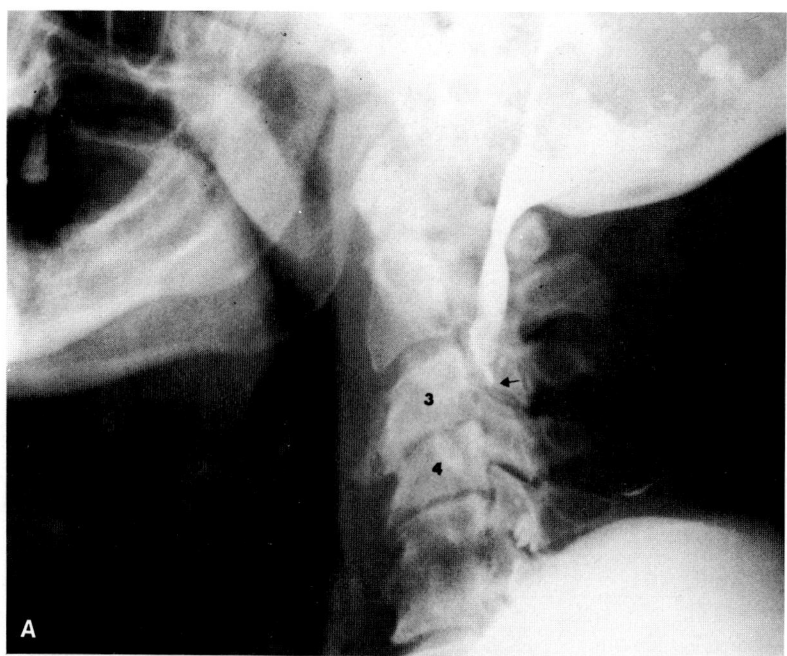

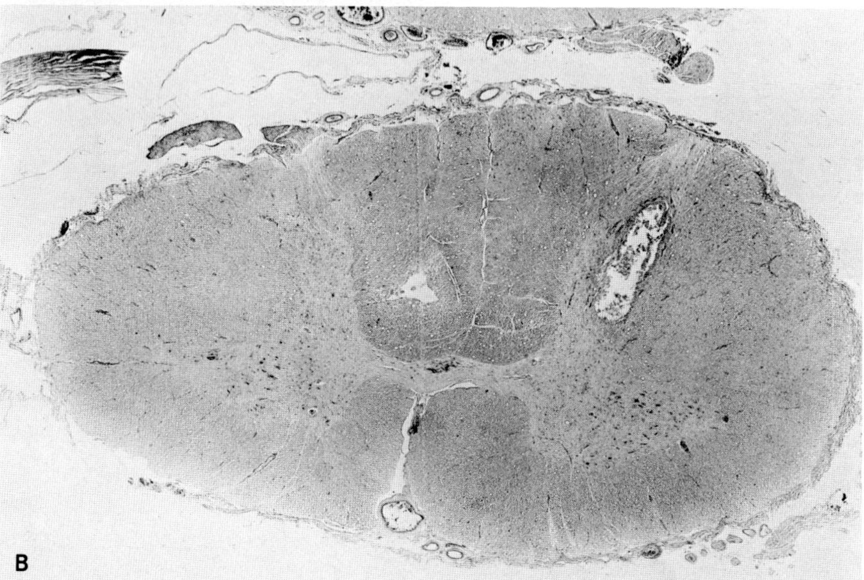

Fig. 6-60. (*A*) As a result of a fall down the stairs while intoxicated, this 65-year-old man had an occipital scalp laceration and mild central cord quadriparesis at the C4 level, but diagnosis was delayed for 2 weeks. Myelogram revealed a narrow spinal canal, a herniated disc, and a block at the C3–C4 level. Laminectomy with opening of the dura was performed 2 weeks after injury without recovery of function. The patient died of respiratory distress and pneumonia 20 days postoperatively. (*B*) Cross section of the spinal cord at the C4 level showing necrosis of the central white matter and dorsal horn, as well as focal hemorrhages and congestion in the anterior horns, but there was relatively good maintenance of cord tissue for potential recovery (hematoxylin and eosin stain, original magnification × 12.5).

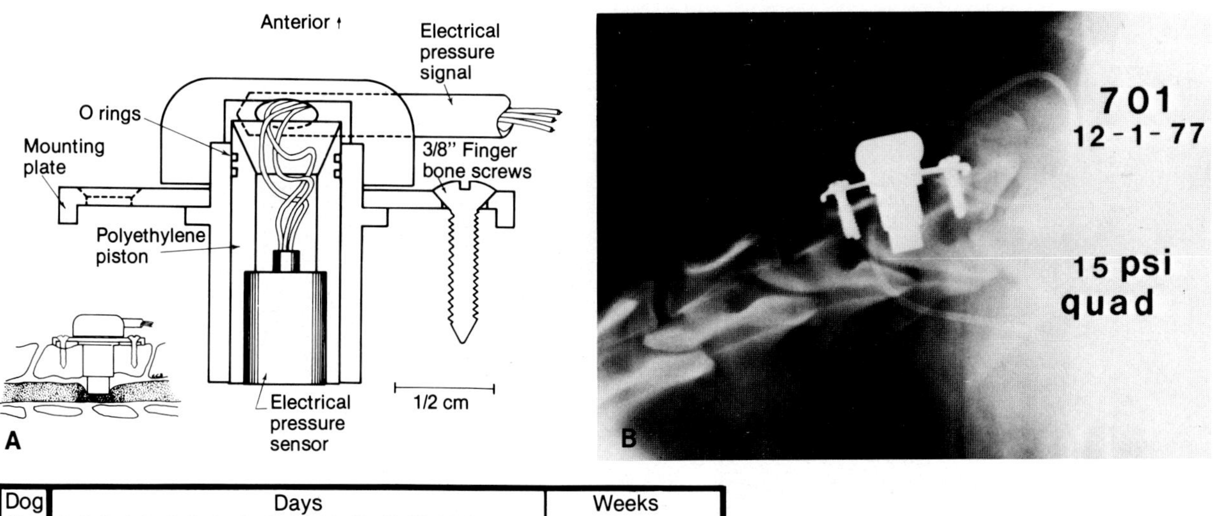

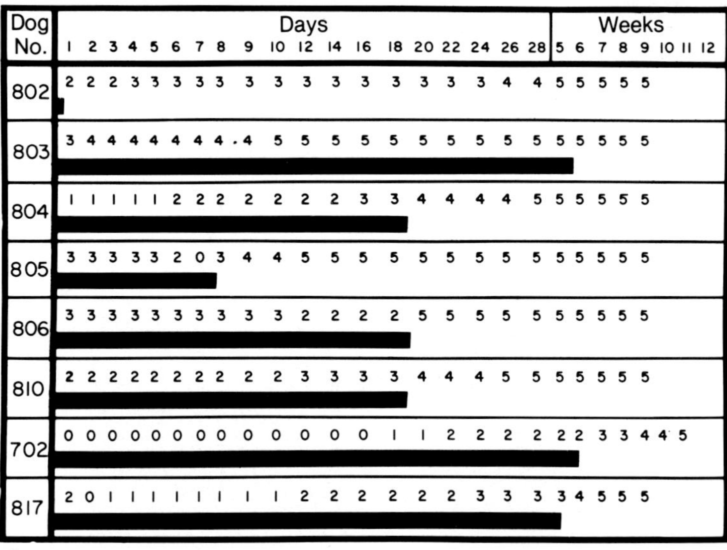

Fig. 6-61. (*A*) A newer design of the pressure transducer with a solid polyethylene piston and an incorporated electrical pressure sensor to measure pressure directly applied to the spinal cord. The transducer piston is remotely controlled and monitored, after insertion into the anterior cervical spine at the C5–C6 interspace (*inset*). (*B*) Lateral roentgenogram of a pressure transducer inserted with 15 lb/sp is applied externally, producing quadriparesis. The plunger extended into one third of the canal diameter. The transducer is at the interspace between C5 and C6. (*C*) Neurologic recovery grades during a 12-week period following initial spinal cord compression. Recovery is graded by a revision of the Tarlov classification: Grade 0 = complete quadriplegia with no extremity motion; Grade 1 = minor joint movements; Grade 2 = major joint motion; Grade 3 = animal can stand; Grade 4 = animal can walk; Grade 5 = animal can walk up a 20° inclined plane. The bar graft indicates duration of compression. Most of the animals did not recover neurologic function until anterior decompression was carried out by removing the pressure transducer. (Bohlman HH, Bahniuk E, Raskulinecz G, Field G: Mechanical factors affecting recovery from incomplete spinal cord injury: A preliminary report. Johns Hopkins Med J 145:115–125, 1979)

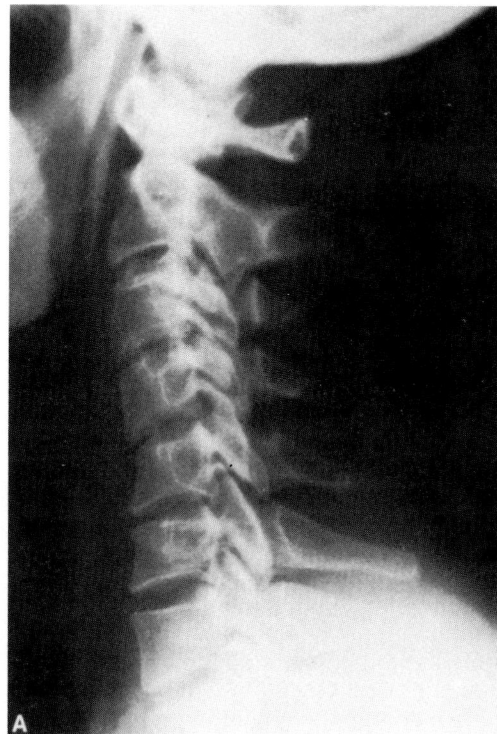

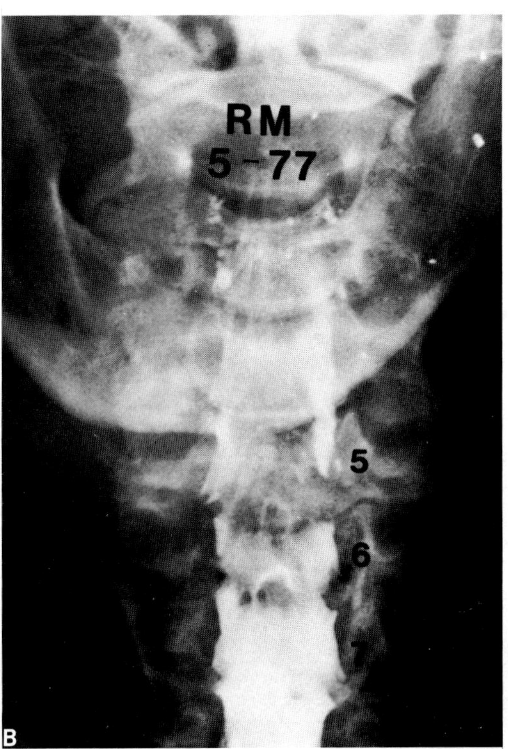

Fig. 6-62. (*A*) Lateral roentgenogram of a patient sustaining an incomplete spinal cord injury with an anterior cord syndrome following a vehicular accident. Lateral roentgenogram reveals no fractures or dislocations, but slight narrowing at the C5–C6 disc space. (*B*) A–P view of the myelogram revealing disc protrusions and obstruction of the dye column at C5–C6 and C6–C7, 5 months following injury when the patient was not recovering neurologic function. (*C*) Lateral roentgenogram of the patient following anterior discectomy and fusion at the C5–C6 and C6–C7 levels, which resulted in significant recovery of motor function and ultimately ambulatory status, even though the patient's surgery was performed 5 months after the original injury. This patient demonstrates the feasibility of carrying out late anterior decompression on incomplete spinal cord injury patients when neurologic recovery has plateaued and when further recovery can occur if anterior decompression is performed. (*B*, Bohlman HH: Indications for late anterior decompression and fusion for cervical spinal cord injuries. In Tator CH (ed): Early Management of Acute Cervical Spinal Cord Injury, pp 373–391. New York, Raven Press, 1982)

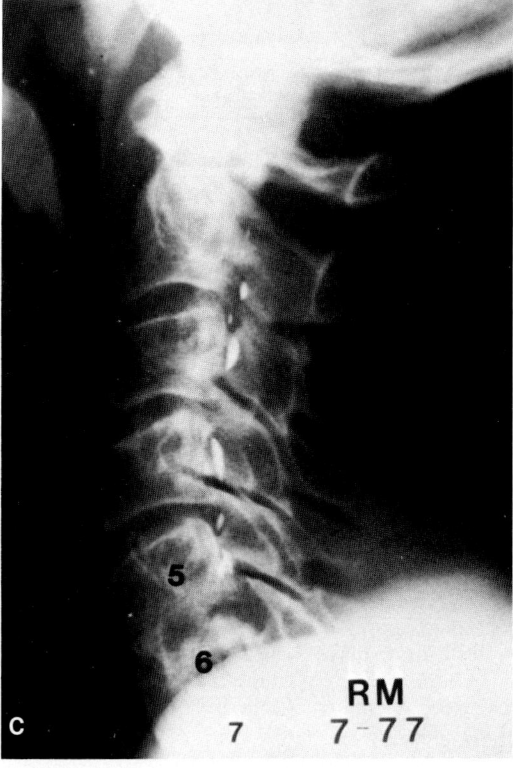

above basic principles have evolved from a study of the basic pathology of the soft tissue as well as osteoarticular structures. In addition, the central nervous system must be considered in those patients who have associated spinal cord and osseous injuries. Both experimental and clinical pathologic studies of cervical spine and spinal cord injuries lend support to the following principles of patient evaluation and treatment.

PATIENT EVALUATION

General Assessment

The general assessment of a patient with cervical spine and spinal cord injury begins with a recognition of the problem at the scene of the accident, or no later than in the emergency room. In Bohlman's review of 300 cervical spine injuries, 100 were initially missed in the emergency rooms of various hospitals. Delay in diagnosis ranged from 1 day to over 1 year, and the common causes for lack of recognition of cervical spine injuries were head injuries, acute alcoholic intoxication, and multiple injuries. Specifically, these injuries were frequently missed in patients who were in coma or had a decreased level of consciousness because roentgenograms of the cervical spine were not taken. Patients with severe scalp and head lacerations may bleed profusely as evidence of head trauma, but may distract the examiner from evaluation of the spine. The acute intoxicated patient who had fallen down the stairs, striking the head and fracturing the spine, may not complain of neck pain. Patients with polytrauma in shock may not complain of neck pain. A smaller number of traumatic injuries to the cervical spine may develop Brown-Séquard syndrome. They appear to have a hemiparesis which mimics a cerebral vascular accident and, therefore, may be admitted to an inappropriate service in the hospital or sent out of the emergency room. As we previously mentioned, there is a high correlation of head and neck injuries, and one must suspect a cervical spine injury with any evidence of head injury, and *vice versa.* The causes of delay in diagnosis (singly or in combination) in Bohlman's 300 cervical spine review group included brain injury in 25 patients, head injury with loss of consciousness in 33, alcoholic intoxication in 14, and associated fractures or multiple injuries in 33.

History

A detailed history of the mechanism of injury should be taken from the patient if he is conscious, or from relatives or others witnessing the injury. Scalp lacerations on patients will offer some clue as to the site of force applied to the head and, therefore, to the neck. It is most important to obtain a history of whether there was any initial paralysis following the spinal injury, which may have recovered by the time the patient arrives in the emergency room. That is, there are some patients who have spinal cord concussions, specifically those with a narrow cervical spinal canal, who may later arrive in the emergency room without any neural deficit whatsoever. The severity of the injury is then not appreciated. In addition, many patients who had mild motor weakness and relative sensory sparing after the injury may be mistaken as hysterical when a real spinal cord injury has occurred. A general physical examination must be performed on all patients with spinal trauma, especially the polytrauma patient with other organ systems involved and the patient with injuries in the extremities. In the emergency room it is very easy to gently palpate the posterior spinous processes in the cervical region and elicit a pain reaction from a patient with severe spinal trauma. If the patient is unconscious, this, of course, is not possible. Once any suspicion of cervical spine injury arises, the patient should be immobilized with sandbags with at least a head halter traction applied until appropriate roentgenograms can be taken.

Roentgenographic Evaluation

Visualization of the lower cervical spine can be obtained by A–P, lateral, and oblique films, which may be taken with the patient in the supine position, with the superimposed shoulder pulled down by the physician in charge to obtain a good lateral view. However, fractures of the lateral mass of the lower cervical spine and articular facets may be difficult to visualize on routine roentgenograms. In that case, laminography and computed tomography may be helpful in defining greater details of the cervical fractures, especially bone protrusion into the spinal canal. Finally, we believe that cervical myelography in the acute situation, with or without CT scanning, is extremely important to evaluate the osseous and disc fragments protruding against the spinal cord. More recently, magnetic resonance imaging has been used to define extrinsic and intrinsic cord lesions.

Neurologic Assessment

In neurologic assessment of the patient with lower cervical spine injury, initial gross motor examination can be done in the field by testing levels of cord function. This is performed by asking the patient to move the arms, then the hands, followed by legs and toes; the paramedic or emergency transportation team should elicit this information and document it at the scene of the accident. All patients with suspected cervical spine injuries, whether comatose or alert, should be stabilized with a spine board and a cervical collar. Anal sphincter tone, as well as intercostal and diaphragmatic breathing, can be documented in the field at the scene of the accident. The common neurologic syndromes that occur in lower cervical spine injuries are isolated nerve root paralysis, anterior cord syndrome, central cord syndrome, Brown-Séquard syndrome, and complete cord syndrome, or quadriplegia. Once the patient is identified as having a significant spinal cord or nerve root injury in association with a lower cervical spine fracture, skeletal traction should be immediately applied to the skull to support the head and neck in appropriate alignment. A more detailed neurologic assessment is discussed in Chapter 3.

Incidence of Osseous Lesions

In Bohlman's review of 300 cervical spine injuries, including eight patients with ankylosing spondylitis, there were 229 patients with spinal lesions between the third and seventh cervical vertebrae, 62 without neural deficit and 167 with neural deficit. The 62 patients with no paralysis had a total of 127 fractures or subluxations between the third and seventh cervical vertebrae that occurred alone or in combination at one level in each patient. Fifty-three patients had a subluxation (either unilateral or bilateral) or a fracture of one or more articular processes. Thirty-four patients had a crushed vertebral body with or without displacement of fragments; 19, a fracture of a lamina; 1, a pedicle fracture; 16, a fracture of a spinous process; and 4, one or more fractured transverse processes. Of the 167 patients with neural deficits, there were 250 fractures, subluxations, or dislocations that occurred singly or in combination at one level between the third and seventh cervical vertebrae. These spine lesions included 105 fractures, subluxations, or dislocations of one or both articular processes, 85 fractures of a vertebral body, 5 fractures of pedicles, 21 fractures of one or more spinous processes, and 34 fractures of a lamina. Excluding the comatose patients and those with spondylitis and neural deficit, there were 29 patients with nerve root lesions, 55 with a complete cord lesion, and 71 with an incomplete cord lesion. Lower cervical fractures and neural deficits were associated predominantly with a displaced fracture of an articular process, vertebral body, or pedicle; the degree of osseous displacement was related to the severity of the neural deficit. None of the 105 patients with a lesion of an articular process and nerve root involvement had bilateral displacement, whereas 46% of the incomplete and 70% of the complete cord lesions were associated with bilateral subluxation or dislocations. There were 85 patients with fracture of a vertebral body and paralysis; 73 with a lesion of the cord had significant protrusion of the vertebral fracture into the spinal canal. Therefore, as one might expect, the degree of osseous displacement is significantly related to the degree of neurologic deficit.

CLASSIFICATION AND SPECIFIC OSSEOUS LESIONS

Fractures and dislocations of the lower cervical spine may be classified as those involving the posterior elements, those involving the anterior elements, those involving the lateral elements, and those involving a combination of these. The following list is a basic classification of fractures and dislocations between the third cervical and first thoracic vertebrae.

Lower Cervical Spine Fractures and Dislocations (C3 through T1)

A. Posterior elements
   1 Unilateral facet dislocations
   2 Bilateral facet dislocations
   3 Bilateral perched facets
   4 Fractured facets
   5 Spinous process fractures
   6 Laminae fractures
B. Anterior elements
   1 Compression fracture of vertebral body without displacement
   2 Compression fracture of vertebral body with displacement
   3 Avulsion fracture
   4 Fracture through disc space (spondylitic)
C. Lateral elements: Lateral mass fracture, pedicle fracture

The lateral roentgenogram of the lower cervical spine should be sufficient to initiate the diagnosis of fracture or dislocation. On this film one of three major types of vertebral body displacement is usually evident: (1) slight (1- to 3-mm) posterior subluxation of the upper vertebra on the lower; (2) moderate (3- to 5-mm) anterior subluxation of the

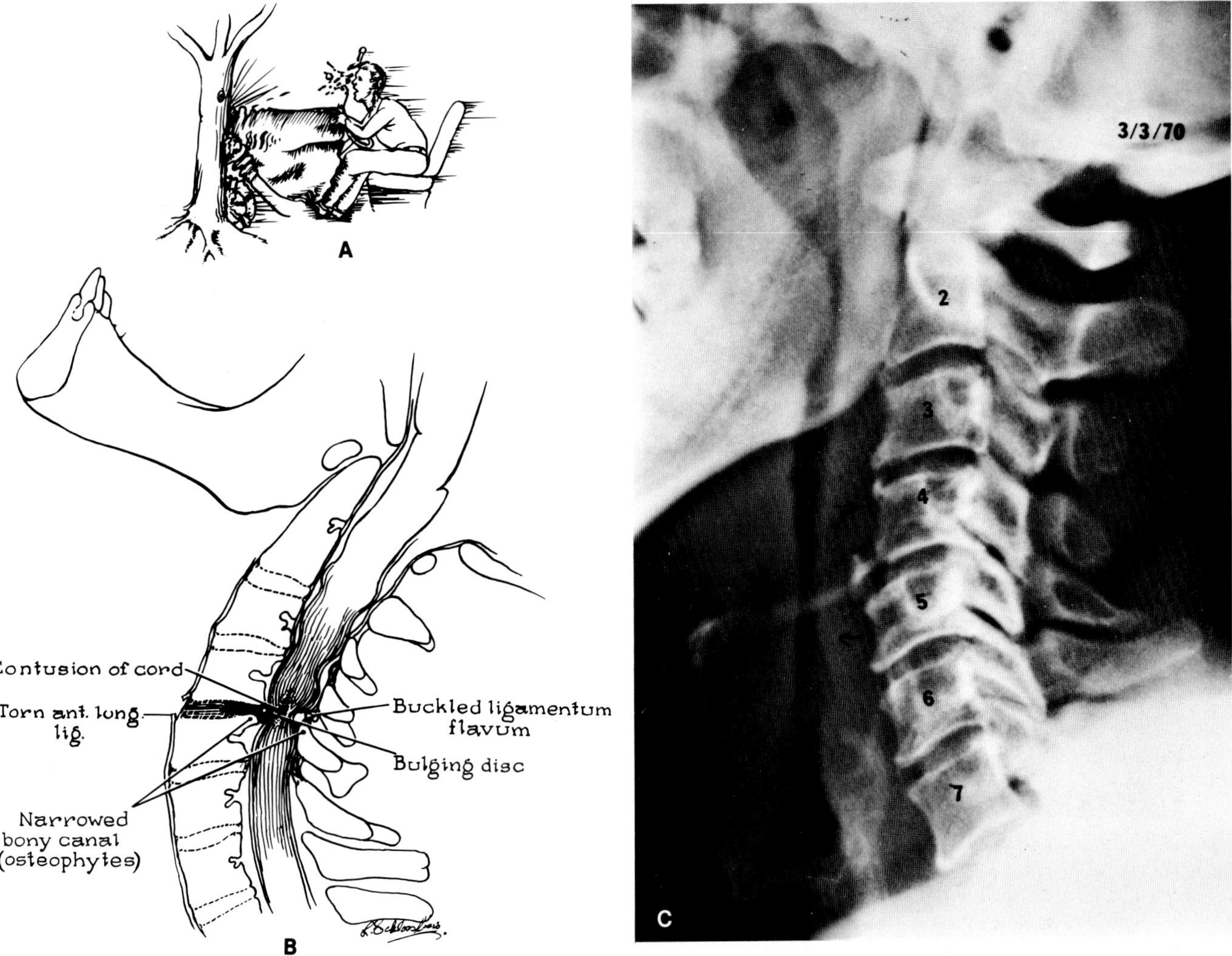

Fig. 6-63. (*A*) Frontal head injury producing hyperextension with cervical spondylosis. (*B*) Note the ligamentum flavum buckles inwardly against the posterior spinal cord while the bulging disc compresses the cord anteriorly. The combined forces contuse the cord. The disc is also disrupted. (*C*) Lateral cervical spine roentgenogram in a totally quadriplegic patient at the C5 level. Note the slight posterior subluxation of C4 on C5. Avulsion fracture of the anterior, inferior body of C4 indicates a hyperextension injury. This corresponds to the diagram. (Bohlman HH: The neck. In D'Ambrosia R (ed): Musculoskeletal Disorders, 2nd ed, pp 183–219. Philadelphia, JB Lippincott, 1985)

upper vertebra on the lower one; or (3) maximal anterior dislocation (5 mm or greater). In the patient with slight posterior subluxation, this usually occurs with extension injuries and is associated commonly with cervical spondylosis in which there is a fracture through the ossified disc space (Fig. 6-63). This may be very subtle, and one must be aware of this extension injury and measure the posterior aspects of the vertebral bodies to see if the posterior subluxation exists. Moderate anterior subluxation visualized on the lateral roentgenogram usually indicates some disruption of the posterior elements, which may be either a unilateral facet dislocation, a unilateral facet fracture, or bilaterally perched facets (Fig. 6-64). These entities may be associated with incomplete quadriparesis or nerve root compression. Maximal anterior dislocation indicates complete bilaterally dislocated

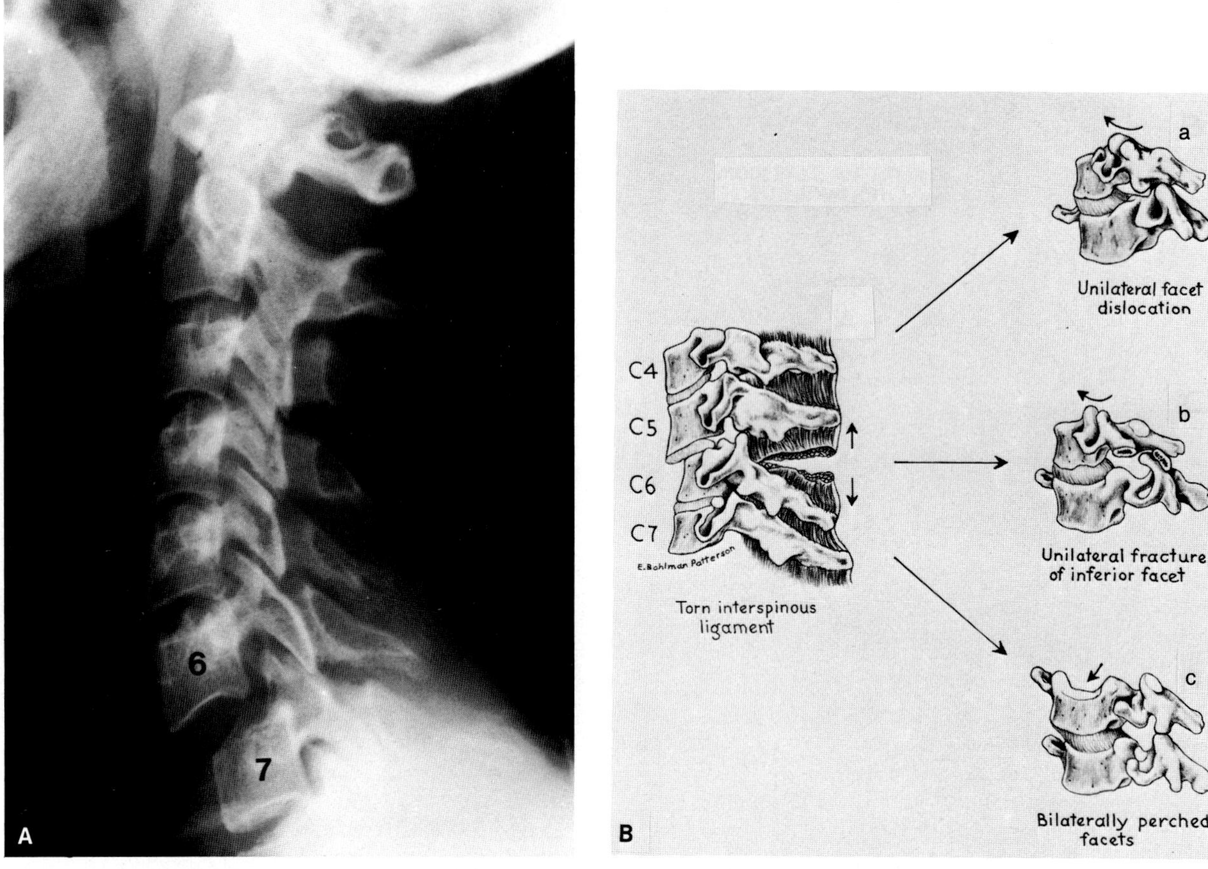

Fig. 6-64. (*A*) Lateral roentgenogram of a patient sustaining moderate anterior subluxation of C6 on C7. Note the vertebral displacement is approximately one third of the width of the vertebral body. In this situation, oblique roentgenograms must be obtained to determine the specific pathology involving the posterior elements. (*B*) Various types of fractures and dislocations (*a, b, c*) of the articular processes that may cause moderate anterior subluxation. (*A*, Bohlman HH, Ducker TB, Lucas JT: Spine and Spinal Cord Injuries. In Rothman RN, Simeone FA (eds): The Spine, 2nd ed, pp 661–756. Philadelphia, WB Saunders, 1982; *B*, Bohlman HH: Acute fractures and dislocations of the cervical spine. J Bone Joint Surg 61A:1119–1142, 1979)

osteoarticular facets; it is usually associated with complete quadriplegia and is quite evident (Fig. 6-65). It is important to identify what pathologic entity has occurred, specifically in the posterior elements, to plan the appropriate treatment method following roentgenographic evaluation.

Fractures of the Posterior Elements

A unilateral facet dislocation usually results from flexion and rotation forces applied to the neck, causing tearing of the facet joint capsule and posterior ligament complex. These fractures may be considered "stable," but they also may compress nerve roots, creating an isolated upper extremity muscle paralysis, or produce an asymmetrical spinal cord compression with resultant Brown-Séquard syndrome. The A–P roentgenogram should reveal that the spinous processes above the dislocation are displaced laterally from the midline, and the lateral view should indicate moderate anterior subluxation of the upper vertebral body on the lower one. Oblique views will confirm the exact diagnosis of the pathology occurring in the posterior elements.

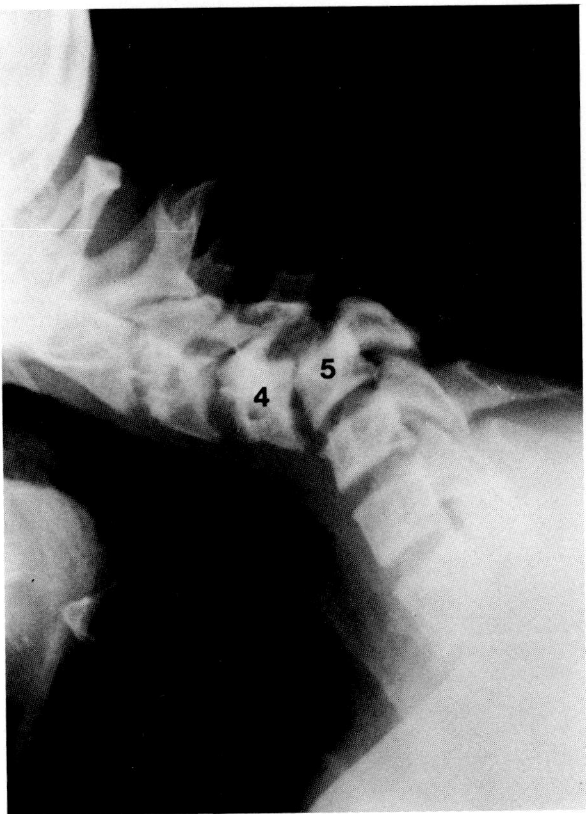

Fig. 6-65. Lateral roentgenogram of an anterior dislocation of C4 on C5 with bilateral dislocation of the articular processes in a quadriplegic patient. (Bohlman HH: Acute fractures and dislocations of the cervical spine: An analysis of 300 hospitalized patients and review of the literature. J Bone Joint Surg 61A:1119–1142, 1979)

Bilateral osteoarticular facet dislocations are a result of flexion forces and are usually associated with severe neurologic deficit or complete quadriplegia secondary to spinal cord damage. The facet capsules, as well as the posterior ligament complex, are torn and the intervertebral disc is disrupted. The only remaining element is the anterior longitudinal ligament, and the lateral roentgenogram will reveal marked displacement of the upper vertebral body by at least half its width on the lower vertebral body. Oblique views will demonstrate the completely dislocated facets. Bilaterally perched osteoarticular facets (tip-to-tip) occur as the result of a pure flexion force where the posterior ligament complex tears (Fig. 6-66). There is frequently no associated neurologic deficit except for possibly an isolated root paralysis. Lateral roentgenograms may reveal spreading of the interspinous space and an angular anterior subluxation of the upper vertebral body on the lower one involved. Oblique views will confirm the tip-to-tip position of the laminar cortices and facets. Under normal circumstances, on the oblique views the laminar cortices overlap like shingles on a roof; however, if they intersect at one level the osteoarticular facets are considered perched.

Fractured facets may occur as an isolated entity, secondary to flexion and rotation forces applied to the cervical spine (Fig. 6-67). The fractured facet may compress the nerve root in the foramina from the posterior aspect and produce single muscle paralysis. Lateral roentgenograms reveal slight forward subluxation of the vertebral bodies involved, and oblique views must be obtained to confirm the facet fracture that is causing the pathologic process.

Fractures of the spinous processes may result from strenuous muscle exertion that avulses the bone, such as the so-called clay shoveler's fracture involving the seventh cervical vertebra. These are usually not difficult to identify on lateral roentgenogram.

Fractures of the laminae are commonly missed on routine roentgenograms because the 30-degree angle that is required to identify this portion of the vertebra is difficult to obtain in the acute injury situation. Ordinarily, however, fractures of the laminae do not compress the spinal cord, heal uneventfully, and therefore are not a major treatment concern.

Fractures of the Anterior Elements

Fractures of the anterior portions of the vertebral body between the third cervical and first thoracic vertebrae are caused by axial loading as well as flexion forces. The vertebral body may be mildly compressed or severely fractured, similar to a burst fracture of the lower spinal vertebrae in which there is posterior displacement of osseous material into the spinal canal (Fig. 6-68).

Obviously, the latter more severe fractures are associated with nerve root and spinal cord compression. Tomography or computed tomography may be necessary to identify the degree of bony intrusion into the spinal canal. Axial loading and flexion injuries may produce very mild osseous injuries and yet extrude a large disc fragment into the spinal canal (Fig. 6-69). This becomes of great significance when spinal cord compression is present, especially in an incomplete cord injury. It therefore behooves the treating physician to iden-

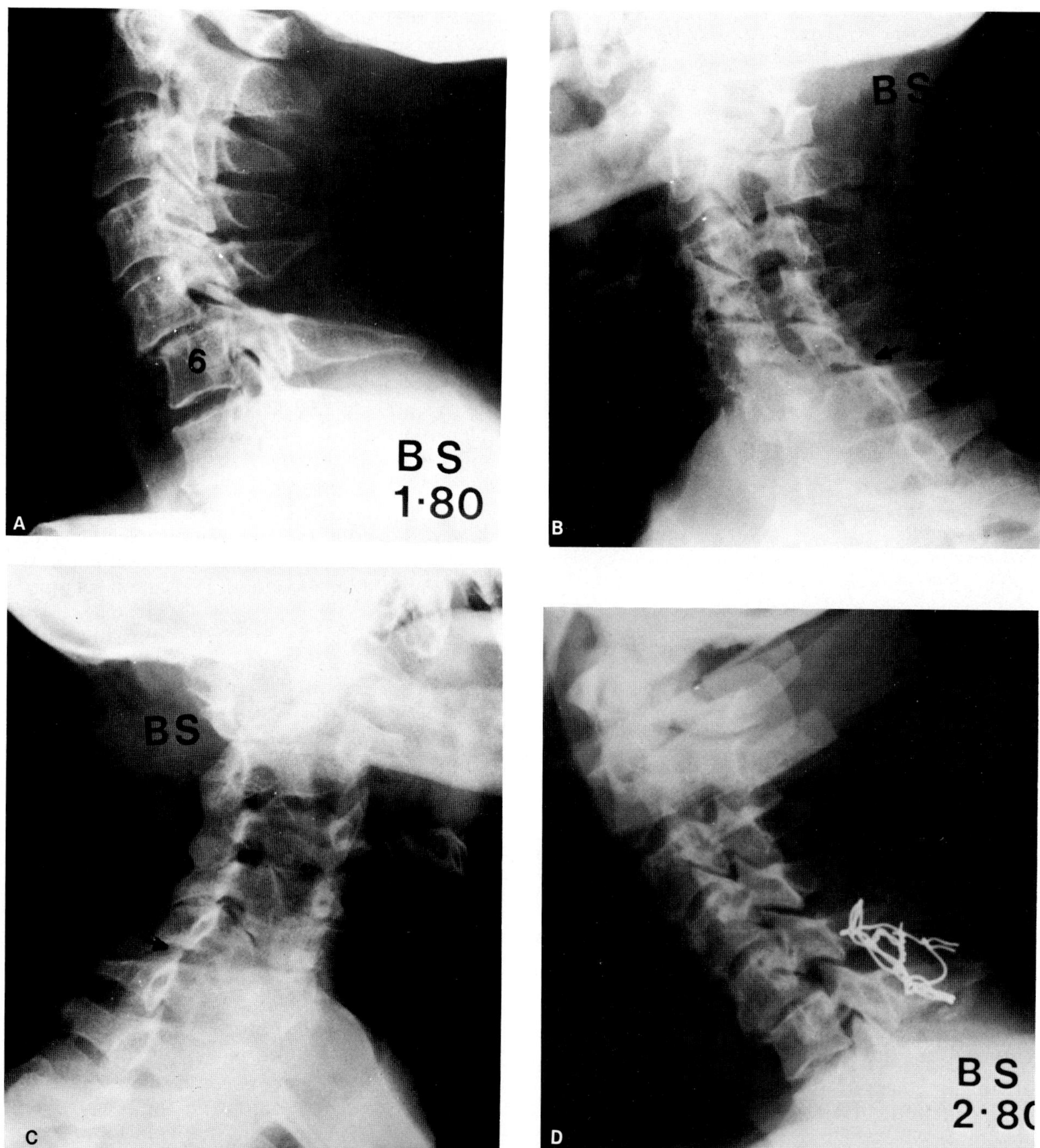

Fig. 6-66. (*A*) Lateral roentgenogram of a patient sustaining a subluxation of C5 on C6 with tearing of the posterior interspinous ligaments, manifested by spreading of the spinous processes. (*B*) Oblique roentgenogram showing perched facets at the C5–C6 level. (*C*) Oblique roentgenogram showing perched facets on the right side at the C5–C6 level. (*D*) Reduction was carried out in skeletal traction and a posterior arthrodesis was performed, using the triple-wire technique and corticocancellous iliac grafts.

tify herniated discs, although these are less common as a cause of neural compression. We know from pathologic studies previously mentioned that herniated discs and bone fragments lie anterior to the posterior longitudinal ligament and do not exist as free fragments in the spinal canal. This is extremely important when considering the anterior operative approach to decompression and stabilization.

The extension injuries previously mentioned frequently occur in patients over the age of 50 and are highly associated with cervical spondylosis, and a congenitally narrow spinal canal.[24] One may only see an avulsion fracture of the anterior vertebral body with reverse subluxation and little bony damage; however, the degenerate intervertebral disc and the longitudinal ligaments are completely disrupted, an unstable situation that should be recognized. This type of injury can actually be associated with complete quadriplegia and severe spinal cord damage.

Fractures of the Lateral Elements

Lateral flexion forces produce fractures of the lateral masses and pedicles, which are extremely uncommon in the lower cervical spine and much more common at the level of the first and second cervical vertebrae (Fig. 6-70).

Fractures with Ankylosing Spondylitis

Fractures of the lower cervical spine may occur in patients with ankylosing spondylitis. Frequently, these occur with very minor trauma or a fall, and are overlooked in the emergency room situation. In Bohlman's review series of 300 cervical spine injuries, eight patients sustained fractures of the cervical spine with ankylosing spondylitis, and seven had associated neural deficit. Massive epidural hemorrhage occurred in four of these eight patients; this was not recognized in any of the other 292 patients in the review series (Fig. 6-71). These fractures occur from any force applied to the cervical spine, but usually through the ossified intervertebral disc and more commonly at the lower cervical levels.

TREATMENT

There are five major goals to consider in the treatment of fractures and dislocations of the lower cervical spine: (1) immobilization; (2) medical stabilization; (3) spinal alignment; (4) operative decompression if there is proved cord compression; and (5) spinal stabilization. All of these goals must be carefully thought out and rationally approached based on the pathology involved in each individual injury. These steps are all important in the overall treatment of cervical spine injuries and may significantly influence the final outcome of stability and neurologic recovery.

Immobilization

As previously mentioned, immobilization is carried out as soon as the cervical spine injury is recognized, because continuous movement of an injured spinal cord may accentuate the pathologic processes that are already under way within the spinal cord. The spinal cord is a soft-tissue structure that is easily damaged by mobile fractured vertebrae, which may be compressing the cord. The principles that have been used for years in treatment of the injured extremity also apply to fractures of the spine. Ancillary medical personnel and emergency medical crews should be taught initial immobilization with a spine board and soft collar. In Bohlman's 300 cervical spine review series, a number of patients developed increasing neural deficit secondary to unintentional movement of the injured cervical spine.

Medical Stabilization

The same principles that apply to the multiply injured patient apply to the cervical spine injury patient: establishment of an airway and maintenance of circulatory status and, therefore, spinal cord perfusion. A damaged cervical cord may be extremely susceptible to loss of blood supply and oxygen, as are the organ systems. Nasotracheal intubation should be carried out if necessary to maintain the airway and, therefore, total body oxygenation. Poor perfusion pressure does not necessarily influence the complete transverse cord lesion; however, in the patient with incomplete cord lesion, there may be significant compromise of the blood flow, which is detrimental to the overall recovery rate. This is especially true in the older patient with a central cord syndrome and already existing edema of the spinal cord, who may be in hypovolemic shock. Patients with associated chest injuries should have ventilatory support to maintain adequate perfusion. This is especially true in patients who have sustained a cervical spine injury diving into a body of water and who have thereby inhaled water into the pulmonary system, which creates edema and loss of perfusion in the lungs.

Spinal Alignment

Once the patient has been stabilized medically by the team of critical care specialists, the next consideration is spinal alignment. Vertebral disloca-

(Text continues on p. 377)

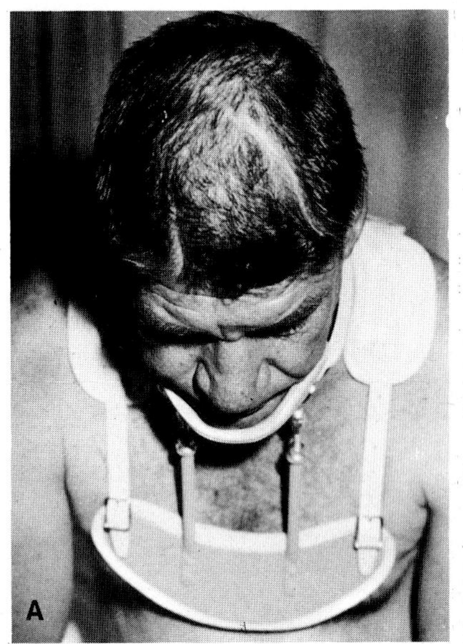
A

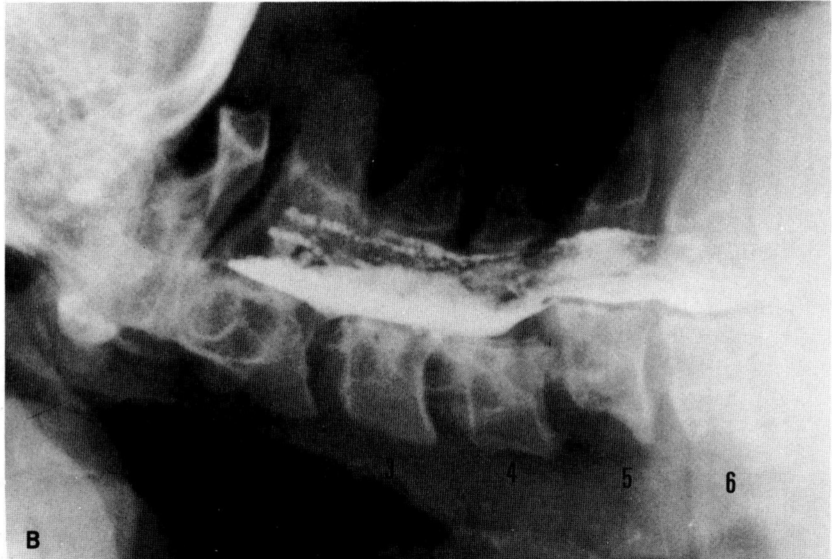
B
4
5
6

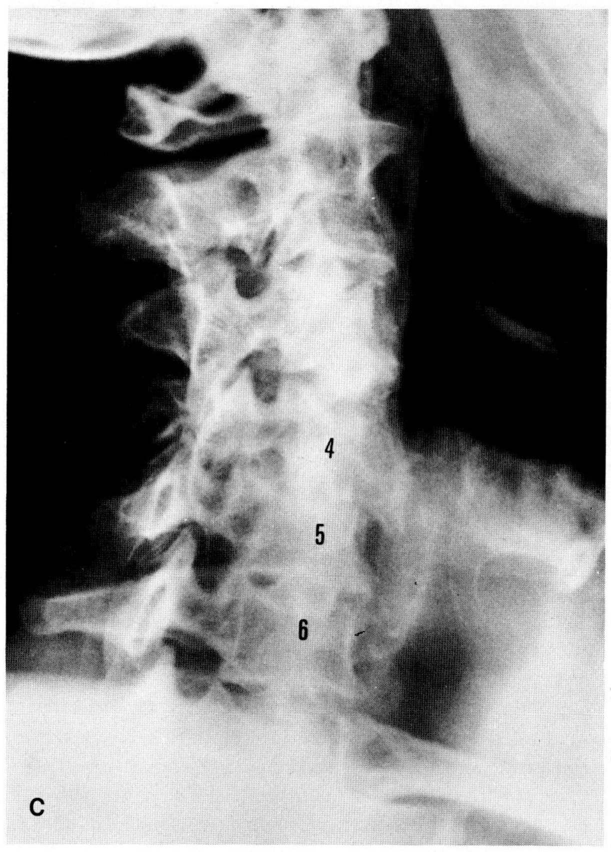
4
5
6
C

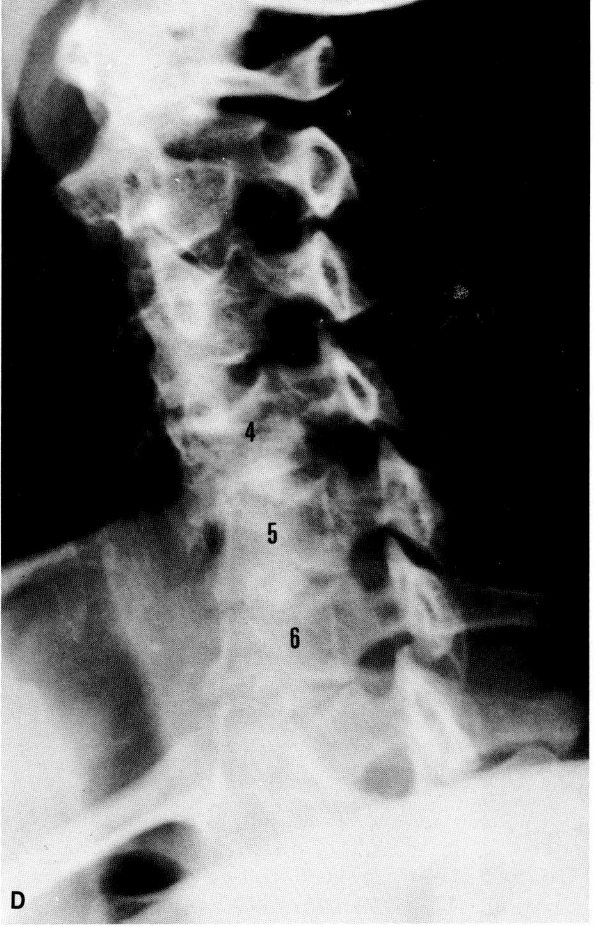
4
5
6
D

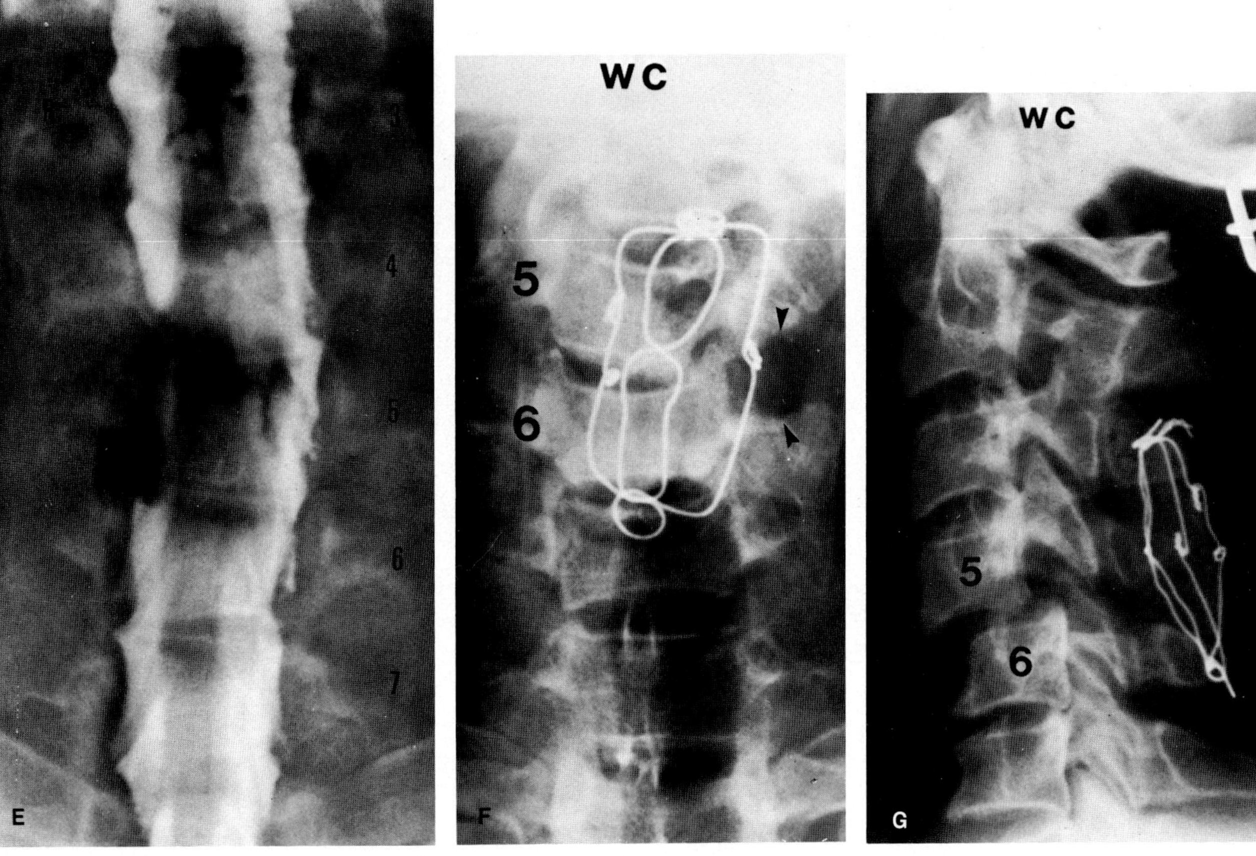

Fig. 6-67. (*A*) Photograph of a patient who sustained severe scalp lacerations in a vehicular accident 6 weeks previously while intoxicated. At that time he dislocated C4 on C5, which was unrecognized. He did not complain of pain. (*B*) Lateral view of a cervical myelogram showing the patient's displacement of C4 on C5 6 weeks following injury. He had no signs of cord compression; however, he did have a right fifth root palsy manifest by deltoid and biceps weakness. (*C*) Right oblique roentgenogram demonstrating a dislocated and fractured C4 facet, occluding the C4–C5 foramina. The latter pathology caused compression of the right fifth nerve root. (*D*) Left oblique roentgenogram of a patient demonstrating perched facets at the C4–C5 level, but on this side the foramen is still open. (*E*) A–P cervical myelogram demonstrating a significant extradural filling defect at the C4–C5 level on the right, indicating severe fifth nerve root compression. (*F*) A–P roentgenogram of postoperative foraminotomy (*arrow*) and posterior arthrodesis. Note the triple-wire technique. The first wire is placed through and around the spinous processes of the involved vertebra, locking the unstable vertebra in place; then additional wires are placed through the separate iliac bone grafts on either side, through and around the spinous processes, holding the bone grafts against the vertebrae involved. (*G*) Lateral roentgenogram showing postoperative arthrodesis with double wiring and iliac bone graft. (*A*, *B*, and *C*, Bohlman HH: The neck. In D'Ambrosia RD (ed): Musculoskeletal Disorders, 2nd ed, pp 183–219. Philadelphia, JB Lippincott, 1985; and *E*, *F*, and *G*, Bohlman HH, Ducker TB, Lucas JT: Spine and spinal cord injuries. In Rothman RN, Simeone FA (eds): The Spine, 2nd ed, pp 661–756. Philadelphia, WB Saunders, 1982)

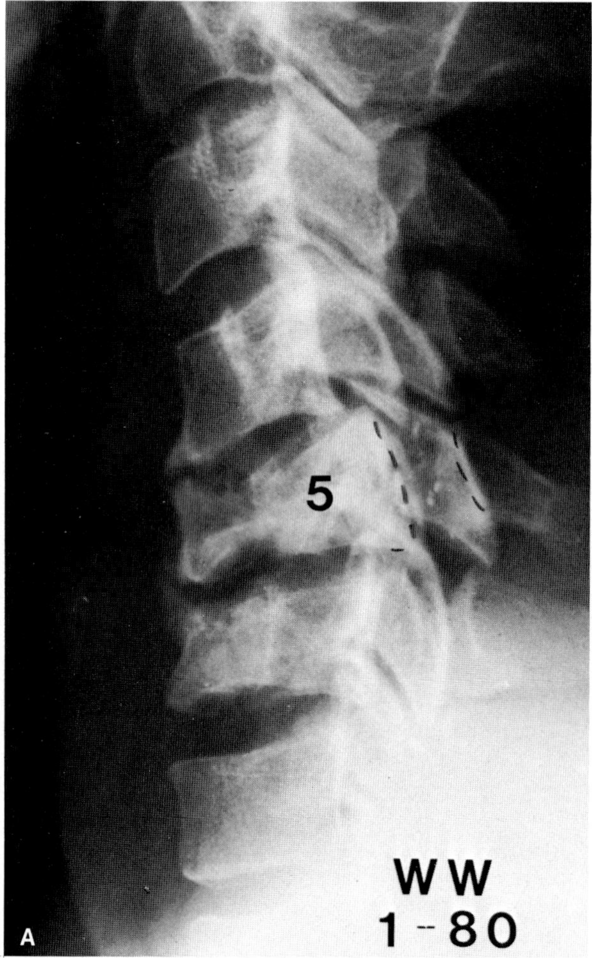

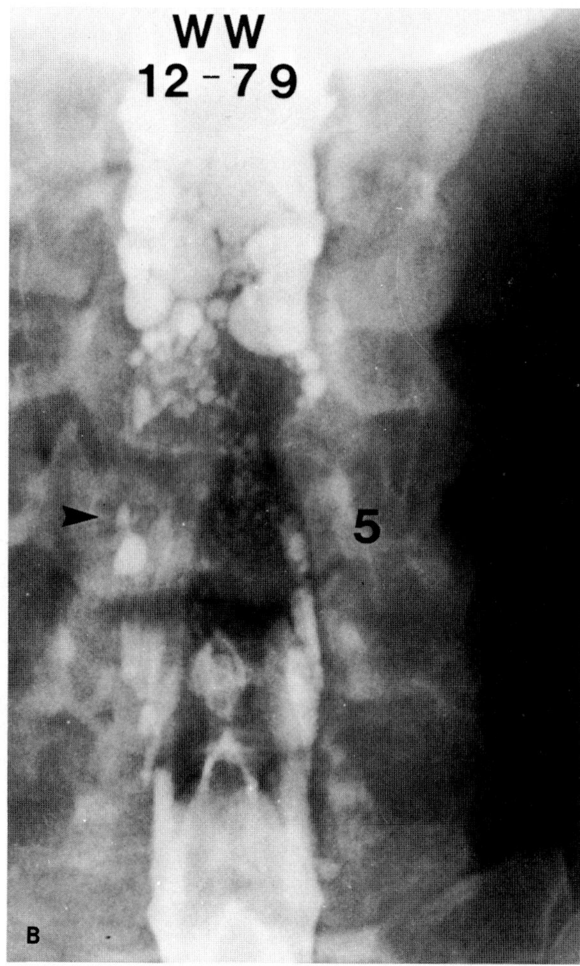

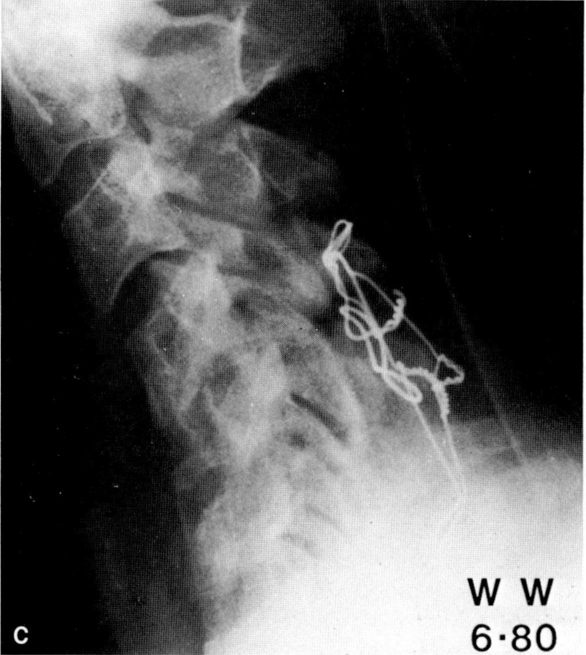

Fig. 6-68. (*A*) Lateral roentgenogram of a patient sustaining a compression fracture of C5 with retropulsed bone fragments and an anterior cord quadriparesis. The posterior ligament complex is torn, as manifested by spread of the spinous processes of C4 and C5. (*B*) A–P view of the cervical myelogram, demonstrating lack of filling of the dye column from the C4 through C6 levels. (*C*) Final roentgenogram 5 months following posterior wiring and iliac fusion. Decompression and stability have now been established and neurologic recovery occurred. (Bohlman HH: Indications for late anterior decompression and fusion for cervical spinal cord injuries. In Tator CH (ed): Early Management of Acute Cervical Spinal Cord Injuries, pp 373–391. New York, Raven Press, 1982)

tions or fractures that produce compression of the neural tissue must be realigned to prevent further damage to the spinal cord by loss of its blood supply and progressive edema. Restoring spinal alignment is the first stage of decompression of the spinal cord and nerve roots, and is usually accomplished with skeletal traction. Reduction of a fractured or dislocated cervical spine is probably much more important in the final outcome of the patient than any drug that can be administered or any operative procedure.

Decompression of the Spinal Canal

Once spinal alignment has been obtained as best possible with skeletal traction, decompressing the spinal canal or neural elements can be considered for those patients who have sustained spinal cord injuries. After spinal alignment, diagnostic procedures such as myelography can be carried out, with CT and MRI to determine if there is further neural compression. It is our belief, and it is also well documented in the literature that continued neural compression prevents optimal recovery of spinal cord function. However, one should prove absolute neural compression before considering any decompressive operation. As previously mentioned, most neural compression is anterior to the spinal cord and should be approached in that direction.

Spinal Stabilization

Following medical stabilization and spinal alignment, spinal stabilization must be considered if there has been significant vertebral displacement. Late instability secondary to ligament tearing is the major problem, as documented by Bohlman in his 300 cervical review series. Torn posterior ligaments secondary to fractures and dislocations do not reconstitute normally; therefore, consideration should be given to surgical stabilization in this situation. This is especially true when considering associated injury to the spinal cord or nerve roots; one must establish spinal stability and maintain it until osseous healing occurs.

In the patients who have sustained lower cervical spine subluxations with major osseous displacement, the ligamentous structures are torn, with a potential problem of instability. Following reduction by skeletal traction, one must then decide whether the existing potential instability is great enough to warrant operative stabilization. If this is not the case, one should proceed with a rigid orthosis for a period of 8 to 12 weeks. If the condition meets White's criteria of instability, we generally proceed with posterior surgical stabilization, because in patients with cervical subluxations the posterior ligament complex is torn and the pathology should be approached from the posterior aspect. The most severe subluxation that occurs in the lower cervical spine is that of the bilaterally perched facets where there is significant angulation of the vertebral bodies and tearing of the posterior ligaments. These patients, even if held by a rigid external fixation such as a halo device, in many instances will develop late instability with pain, with or without increasing neurologic deficit. (Fig. 6-72). If this type of instability is present, we prefer a posterior arthrodesis, using iliac bone and a triple wire technique to immediately stabilize the spine.

The cervical dislocations indicate a more severe and complete disruption of the ligament structures posteriorly as well as anteriorly, so that the facet joints are no longer in continuity. Initial treatment is, of course, skeletal traction. It is extremely difficult to reduce a unilateral facet dislocation by skeletal traction, even if the dislocation is stable, and this type of injury may frequently be associated with nerve root paralysis or incomplete spinal cord injury. Therefore, it is our preference to carry out an open reduction and posterior fusion with iliac bone rather than attempt a closed reduction with more than 40 pounds of weight applied to the cervical spine. We are not in favor of manipulative reduction as mastered by the British as an alternative to open reduction, because this is a less controlled method of obtaining the final result and does not necessarily ensure ultimate stability. Partial removal of the superior articular process of the inferior vertebra may be necessary to obtain reduction at the time of surgery, or a foraminotomy may be required to ensure adequate decompression of the nerve root, especially in the case of the fractured facet.

Bilateral osteoarticular facet dislocations are extremely unstable and usually accompanied by a profound neurologic deficit. As in the above fractures, closed reduction is initially attempted by skeletal traction and may be successful, since there is major ligament complex tearing both anteriorly and posteriorly. However, if closed reduction is not successful, we prefer a posterior open reduction followed by fusion. Although there is an option to treat patients having dislocations without surgery with rigid immobilization following reduction, not all of these patients spontaneously arthrodese the vertebra anteriorly; therefore, 3 months of time may be wasted and arthrodesis may still be neces-

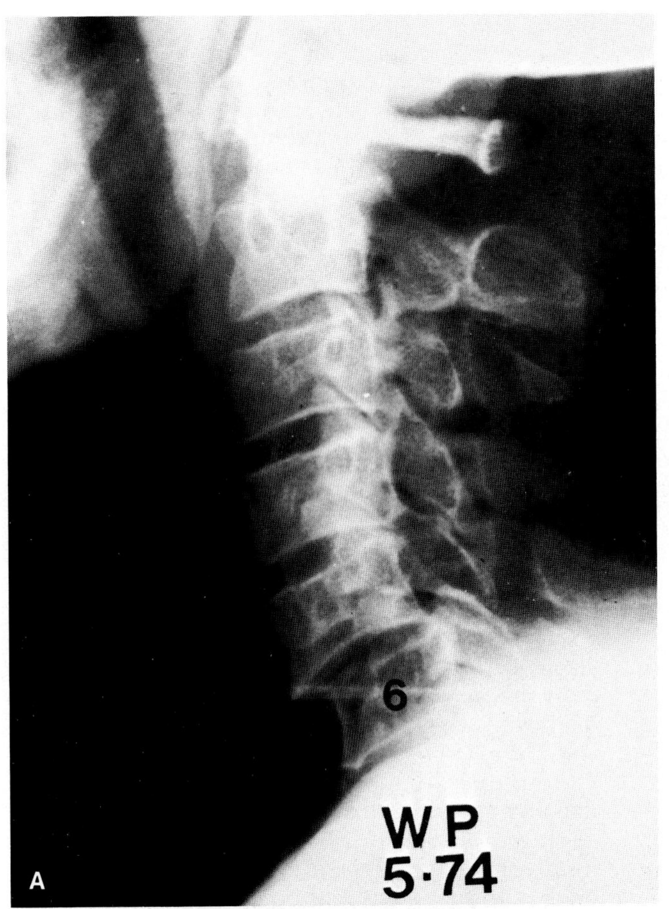
6
WP
5·74
A

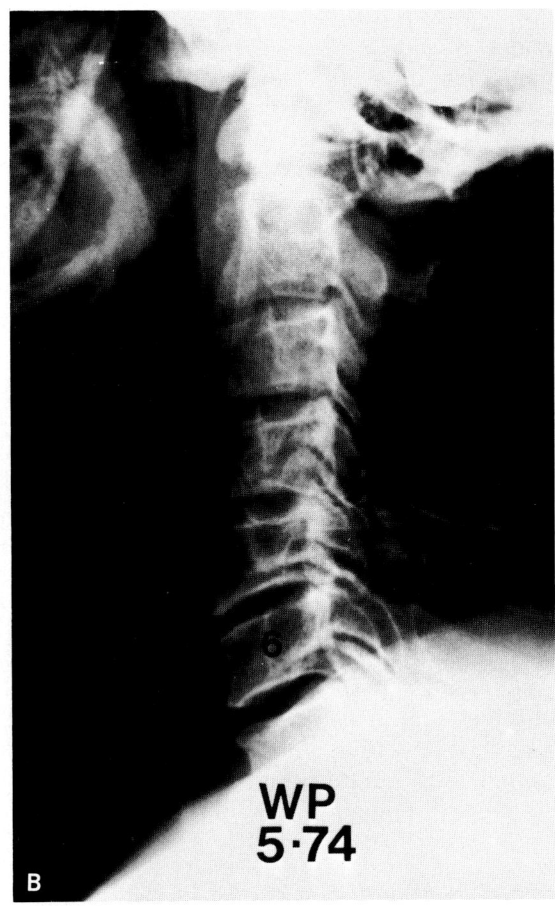
6
WP
5·74
B

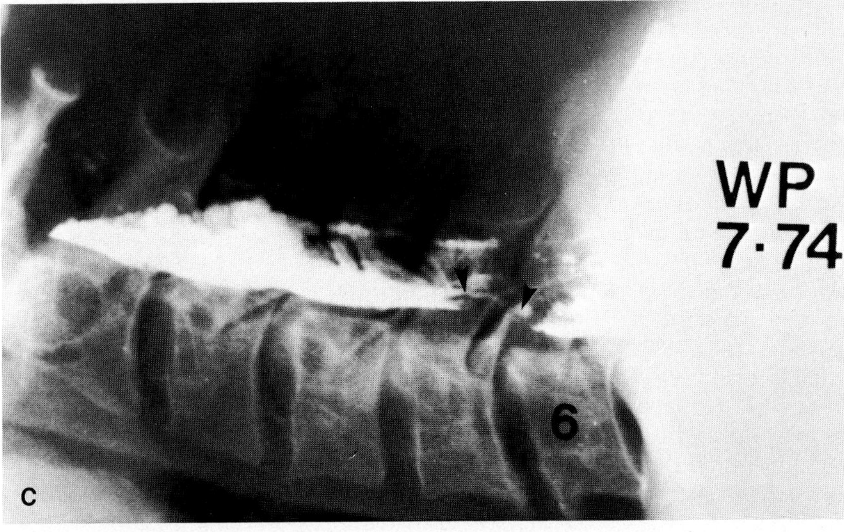
WP
7·74
6
C

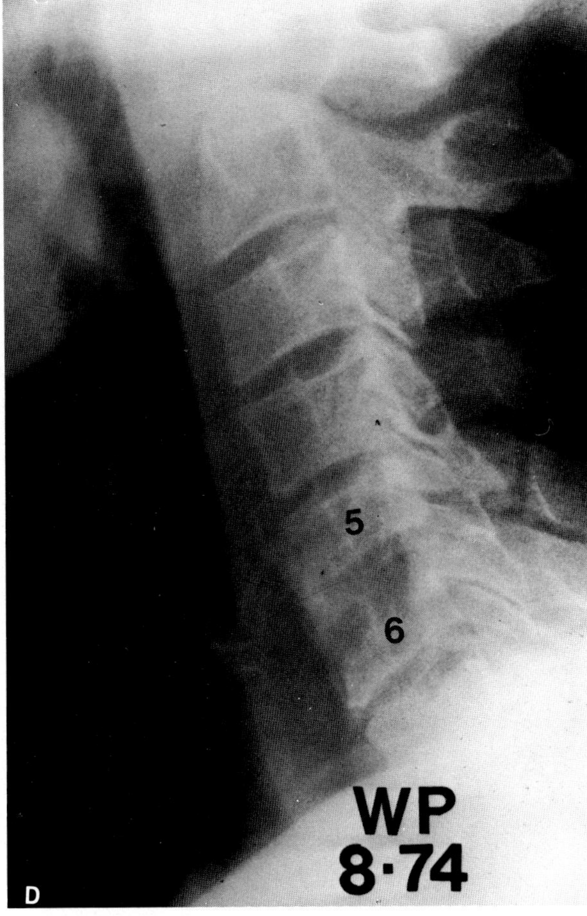

Fig. 6-69. (*A*) Lateral roentgenogram of a patient sustaining a fracture-dislocation of C5 on C6 with moderate anterior subluxation. He had an anterior cord quadriparesis. (*B*) Reduction was carried out by skeletal traction, although the pätient did not improve neurologically over the ensuing 8 weeks. (*C*) Lateral view of a cervical myelogram demonstrating a large herniated nucleus pulposus between the fifth and sixth cervical levels (*arrows*). (*D*) Postoperative lateral roentgenogram of the patient showing anterior discectomy and arthrodesis has been carried out at the C5–C6 space. Postoperatively, the patient recovered significant neurologic function.

sary, further delaying rehabilitation of the patient. In the patient with complete quadriplegia, we frequently carry out posterior operative stabilizations under local infiltration anesthesia, which is very easy for the patient to tolerate, especially in the case of high cervical cord injuries at or above the fifth cervical level.

Isolated fractures of the lateral and posterior vertebral elements without associated dislocation or neurologic deficit are usually stable injuries and will heal with immobilization in a rigid orthosis.

Treatment of Cervical Compression Fractures

Mild compression or axial loading fractures of the cervical spine without paralysis can be treated adequately with a rigid orthosis for 8 to 12 weeks until healing has occurred, as visualized by roentgenogram. However, the more severe compression fracture of the lower cervical spine may be quite unstable, especially the burst fracture; if this fracture is associated with bone fragments posteriorly protruding into the spinal canal, skeletal traction should be immediately instituted and closed reduction attempted, as described. Following skeletal traction, if bone protrusion into the spinal canal remains or if the fracture is so severe that potential kyphosis may result, then surgical intervention using the anterior approach may be indicated. It is not infrequent that severe axial-loading fractures treated with a rigid orthosis may develop progressive kyphosis after the brace is removed. In our experience, it is uncommon for the compression fracture to totally arthrodese to the vertebral body above and below, thus creating complete stability. It is, therefore, our preference to treat burst fractures with retropulsion of bone into the spinal canal with early anterior corpectomy, or vertebrectomy and iliac fusion. In patients who have sustained incomplete cord syndromes with bone or

(Text continues on p. 384)

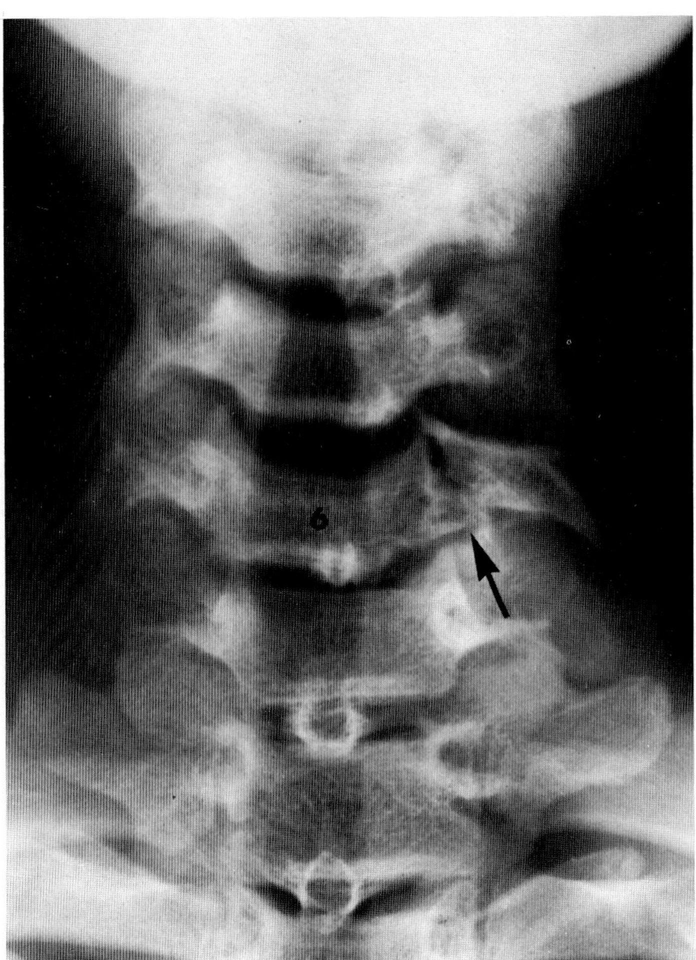

Fig. 6-70. A–P roentgenogram demonstrating a lateral mass fracture of C6 (*arrow*). (Bohlman HH: The neck. In D'Ambrosia R (ed): Musculoskeletal Disorders, 2nd ed, pp 183–219. Philadelphia, JB Lippincott, 1985)

Fig. 6-71. A 60-year-old man with ankylosing spondylitis fell and sustained a fracture of C7 without neural involvement. His facial lacerations were sutured on the day of injury and he was discharged. One week after injury he returned with progressive quadriparesis. Laminectomy revealed a massive epidural hemorrhage (*arrows*), which was confirmed at autopsy 18 days later. (Bohlman HH: Acute fractures and dislocations of the cervical spine: An analysis of 300 hospitalized patients and review of the literature. J Bone Joint Surg 61A:1119–1142, 1979)

Fig. 6-72. (*A*) A lateral roentgenogram shows redislocation of C5 on C6 following treatment in a Minerva jacket for 4 months. No paralysis had occurred. Note the completely torn posterior ligament complex, manifested by widened interspinous space and perched facets at C5–C6. (*B*) The patient later had an anterior and posterior stabilization with correction of the deformity.

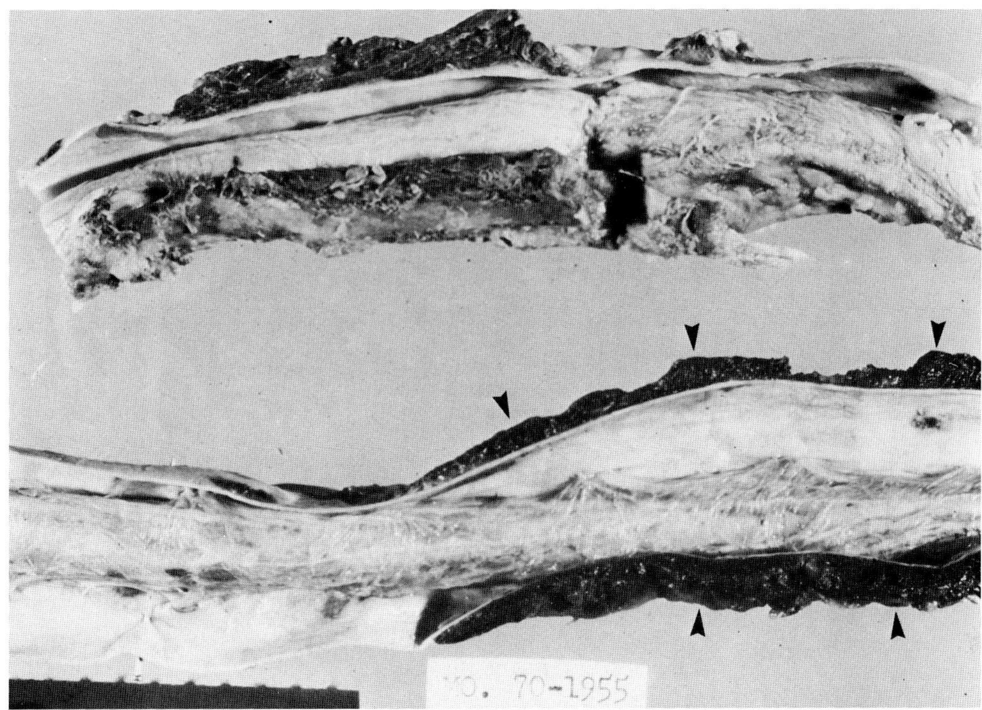

Fig. 6-71.

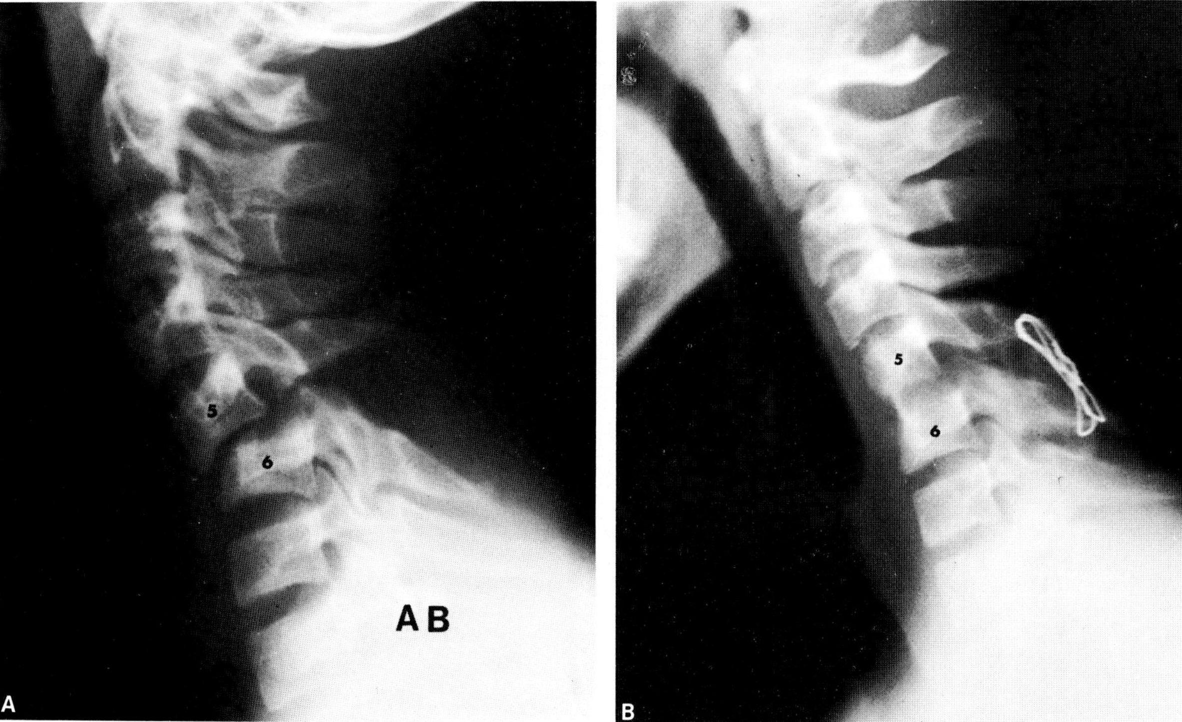

Fig. 6-72.

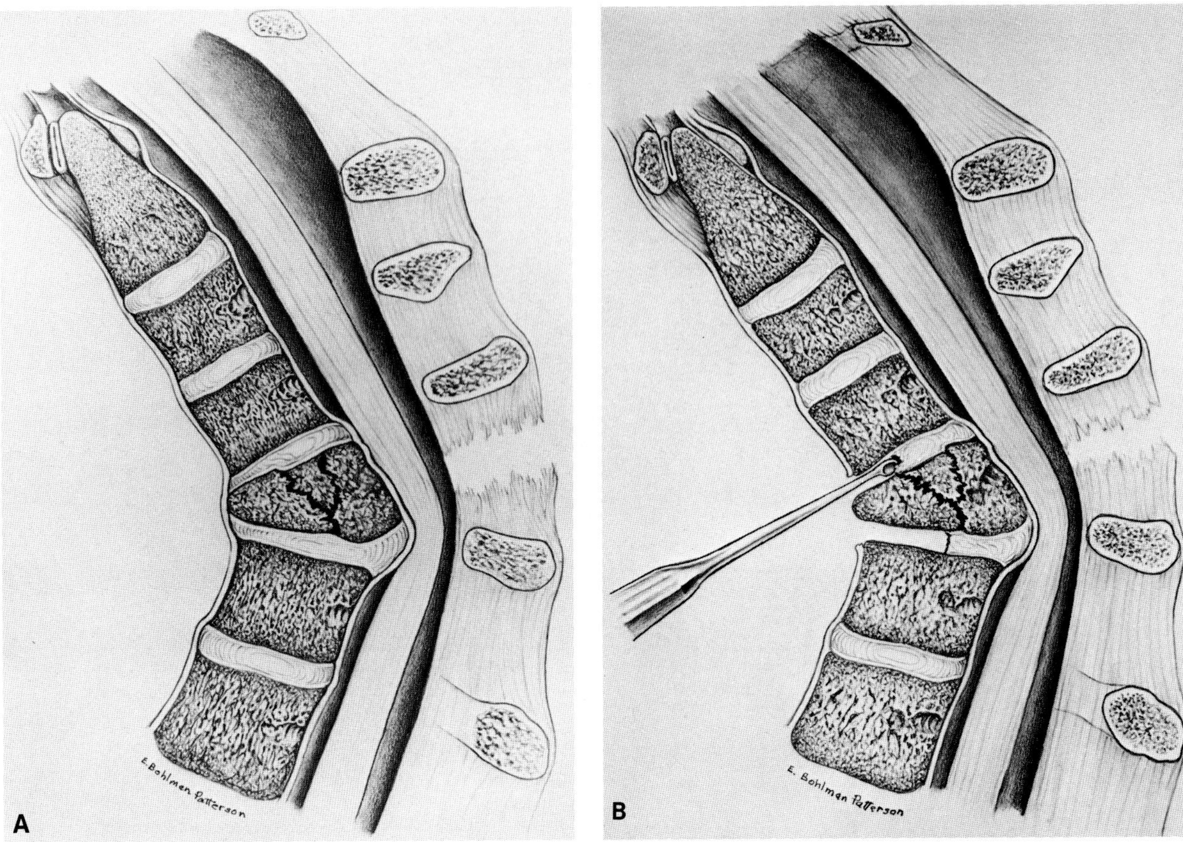

Fig. 6-73. (*A*) Artist's drawing of a lateral view of a compression fracture of the C5 vertebra, showing typical compression fracture with protrusion of disc material and bone fragment and a kyphotic deformity causing compression of the anterior aspect of the spinal cord. (*B*) Lateral view of the cervical spine showing initial removal of disc material on either side of the crushed vertebral body, which is used as a guide to identify the extent of the crushed bone superiorly and inferiorly, as well as posteriorly. (*C*) Following initial disc removal on either side of the crushed vertebral body, hand rongeurs were used to remove the first portion of the crushed vertebral body. (*D*) The portion of the remaining crushed vertebral body is then removed with a power bur. All of the disc is removed back to the posterior longitudinal ligament to identify the extent of bony protrusion. (*E*) The remaining posterior vertebral cortex is removed using a curette to peel the bone from the longitudinal ligament. (*F, left*) Anterior view of the cervical spine showing the extent of vertebral body resection to the posterior longitudinal ligament, sparing the lateral cortices to protect the vertebral arteries. The posterior longitudinal ligament is not violated and no instruments enter the spinal canal. (*F, right*) A full-thickness iliac crest graft is inserted to replace the resected vertebra. The cortical surface of the crest is placed posteriorly. This procedure corrects the kyphotic deformity and relieves the spinal cord compression. (*A* and *F*, Bohlman HH: Acute fractures and dislocations of the cervical spine. J Bone Joint Surg 61A:1119–1142, 1979; *B* and *C*, Bohlman HH, Ducker TB, Lucas JT: Spine and spinal cord injuries. In Rothman RN, Simeone FA (ed): The Spine, 2nd ed, pp 661–756. Philadelphia, WB Saunders, 1982; *D* and *E*, Bohlman HH, Eismont FJ: Surgical techniques of anterior decompression and fusion for spinal cord injuries. Clin Orthop 154:57–67, 1981)

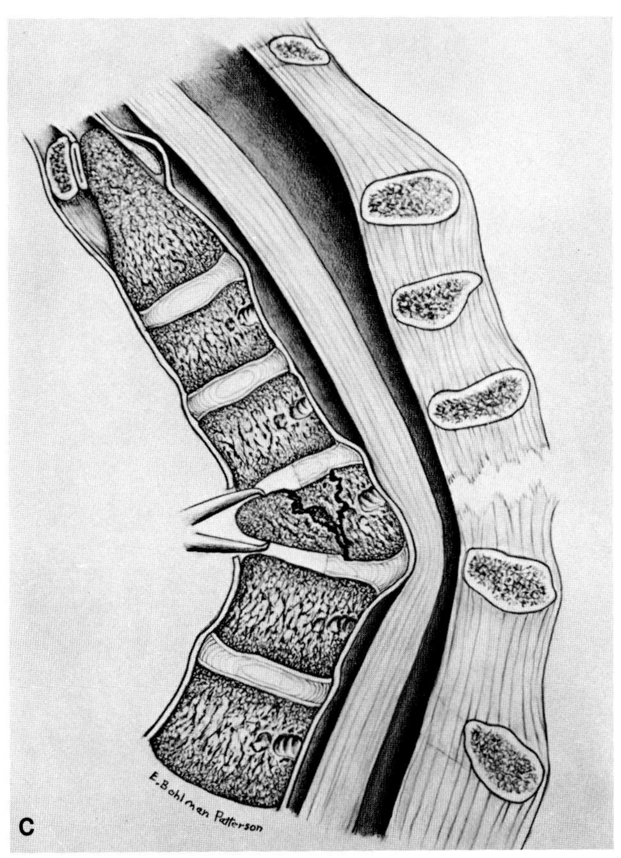
E. Bohlman Patterson
C

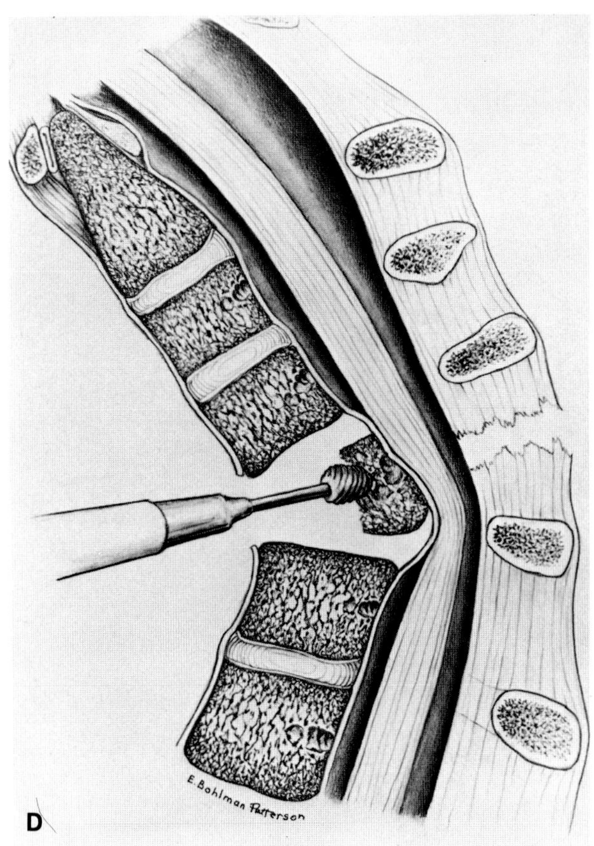
E. Bohlman Patterson
D

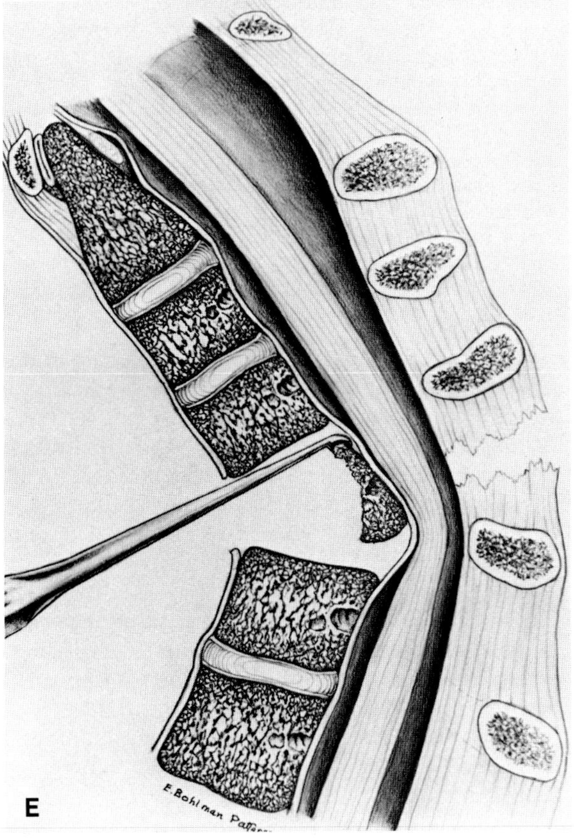
E. Bohlman Patterson
E

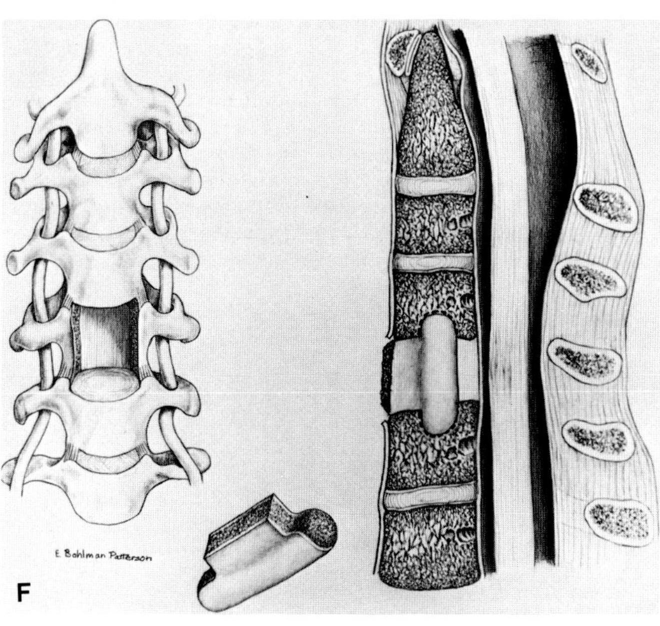
E. Bohlman Patterson
F

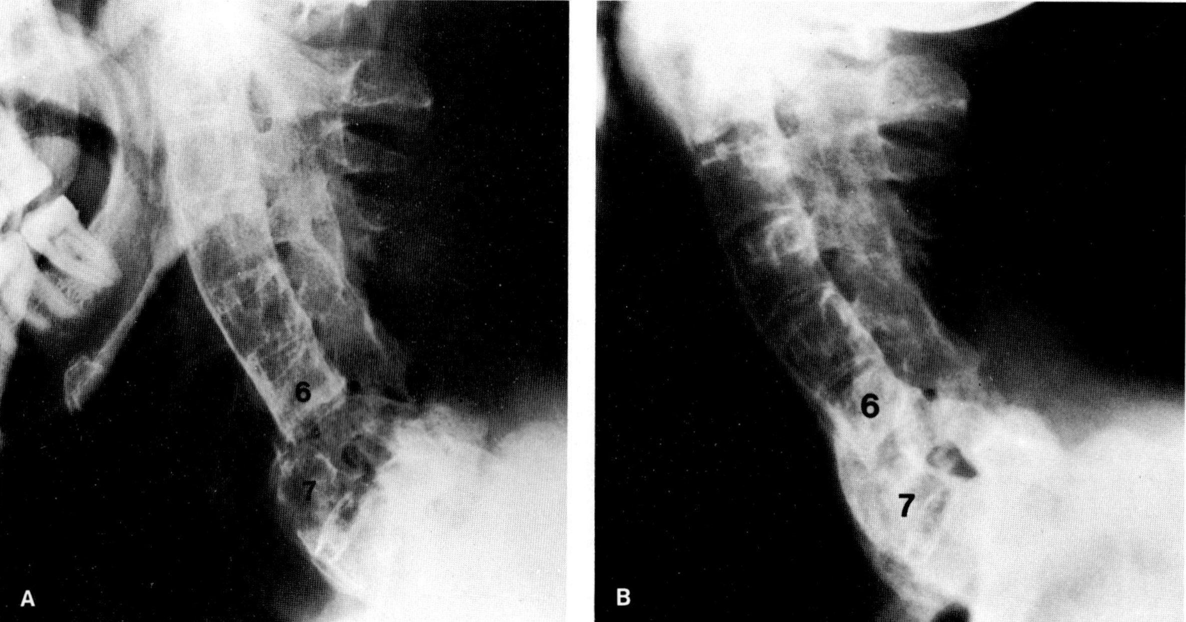

Fig. 6-74. A patient with ankylosing spondylitis sustained a fracture through the C6–C7 ossified disc space. The patient was seen in the emergency room for a chin laceration after an automobile accident and was discharged. He returned 48 hours later with quadriparesis. Myelogram revealed total block at T1 and a laminectomy was performed, extracting a large epidural hematoma. The spine was judged "stable" at operation and the skeletal tongs were removed. Four weeks later the patient became worse neurologically; a roentgenogram (*A*) was taken, revealing a posterior displacement of C6 on C7. The patient was placed back in skeletal tong traction and improved immediately. (*B*) This lateral roentgenogram demonstrates callus formation at 2 months following injury. The patient recovered to ambulatory status with a stable spine. Operative stabilization and fusion is not necessary in a patient with ankylosing spondylitis. (Bohlman HH: Complications of treatment of fractures and dislocations of the cervical spine. In Epps C (ed): Complications in Orthopaedic Surgery, 2nd ed, pp 897–918. Philadelphia, JB Lippincott, 1985)

disc fragments retropulsed into the spinal canal, anterior decompression and fusion is indicated if skeletal traction has failed to completely reduce the fragments. We carry out a cervical myelogram following attempts at closed reduction, and if bone or disc fragments still compress the anterior cervical cord, we proceed with the anterior decompressive operation and iliac fusion (Fig. 6-73). The timing of such an operative treatment of the spinal cord compression is still somewhat controversial; however, we believe that continued compression of the spinal cord in incomplete spinal cord injuries is detrimental to neurologic recovery.

Occasionally, a patient will present with an incomplete spinal cord injury who, in addition, has a severe compression fracture anteriorly as well as a flexion injury tearing the posterior ligament complex. In this instance, there is instability both anteriorly and posteriorly, as well as neural compression, which should be corrected. Even though general alignment of the vertebral bodies can be restored with skeletal traction, it is unlikely that the bone fragments protruding into the spinal canal will be pulled back into place; in addition, as mentioned, the ligament structures posteriorly do not reconstitute normally. In this instance we proceed with a posterior wiring and arthrodesis, followed by a staged anterior decompression and fusion with iliac bone. Immediate ambulation in a rigid orthosis is then possible, and the damaged spinal cord has the greatest chance for recovery of neural function.

Treatment of Fractures in Patients with Ankylosing Spondylitis

Patients with ankylosing spondylitis who sustain fractures through the lower cervical spine heal uneventfully with rigid immobilization. The above principles apply in this situation, that is, immediate reduction of the dislocation and maintenance in skeletal traction for 3 to 6 weeks, followed by application of a rigid orthosis (Fig. 6-74). Occasionally, patients with ankylosing spondylitis and preexisting flexion deformities of the spine will sustain a fracture, and skeletal traction straightens the spine and produces an increased neural deficit. The spine must, therefore, be immobilized in skeletal traction in a vertical position with the patient in a semisitting position in bed. If a patient with ankylosing spondylitis develops an ascending paralysis and it is proved by meylography or CT scanning that a massive epidural hemorrhage has occurred, this may be an indication for a posterior laminectomy and arthrodesis. However, this is very rare and probably will not occur as long as the patient is quickly immobilized and stabilized with external fixation.

The Use of Cervical Orthoses

Brief mention should be made about the types of cervical orthoses that may be used in the treatment of lower cervical spine fractures. In patients with major injuries of the cervical spine, we use a rigid two-poster cervical orthosis, which has rigid lateral side pieces, or a halo cast. In patients with severe neurologic deficits and complete sensory loss, we do not use a halo cast or halo vest because of the significant complications of pressure sores. Following posterior arthrodesis and wiring using a separate wire through and around the spinous processes as well as additional wires through and around the iliac bone grafts, a halo cast is not necessary, and we use a rigid two-poster orthosis until healing has occurred.

COMPLICATIONS

Complications associated with the treatment of lower cervical spine fractures and dislocations are numerous and involve all organ systems. Many of these are iatrogenic and can be prevented as long as the physician is aware of them prior to institution of treatment.[6]

Gastrointestinal System Complications

In Bohlman's review of 300 cervical spine injuries, a common problem associated with these fractures was gastrointestinal hemorrhage, which occurred on or about the 10th or 14th day following injury. This was highly associated with the administration of steroids and exclusively in the spinal cord-injured patient. Of the 37 spinal cord injury patients who received steroids within 72 hours of injury, 15 developed gastrointestinal hemorrhage (40%); on the other hand, of 97 patients with cord injuries who did not receive steroids, only 9% had gastrointestinal hemorrhage. There was no difference in the recovery rate of neurologic function between the steroid and nonsteroid group of patients. Twelve percent of the quadriplegics in this group died of massive gastrointestinal hemorrhage proved at autopsy and all were treated with steroids (Fig. 6-75). Although there are other factors associated with this problem, such as gastric stasis, excessive gastric secretions, and immobilization of the patients, one cannot ignore the fact that steroids played an important role.

In addition, we have on occasion seen patients treated in halo casts develop superior mesenteric artery syndrome, secondary to duodenal obstruction. This may require repositioning of the patient and, in some cases, surgical intervention.

Pulmonary System Complications

As mentioned, pulmonary problems may occur in the cervical spine and spinal cord injury patient, and may become a major factor in patients with a higher level of paralysis. Initial hypoventilation is secondary to paralysis of intercostal muscles, and in the patient with the fourth cervical level of quadriplegia, diaphragmatic paralysis may occur, with resultant hypoxic state and the problems of atelectasis and pneumonia necessitating respiratory assistance and tracheostomy.

Central Nervous System Complications

Although very rare, ascending paralysis in the spinal cord injury patient can occur early or late after the injury. The etiology is usually secondary to ascending central necrosis of the gray matter with an enlarging central syrinx. Following the acute injury, this complication is usually fatal; however, it may also occur later after injury. Acute central necrosis can now be diagnosed by MRI.

Massive epidural hemorrhage has been previously mentioned in Bohlman's review article; however, it only occurred in the patient sustaining a fracture in the ankylosed spine.

Complications with Traction and Immobilization Devices

Although the Minerva plaster jacket was used quite extensively in previous years, we have found that

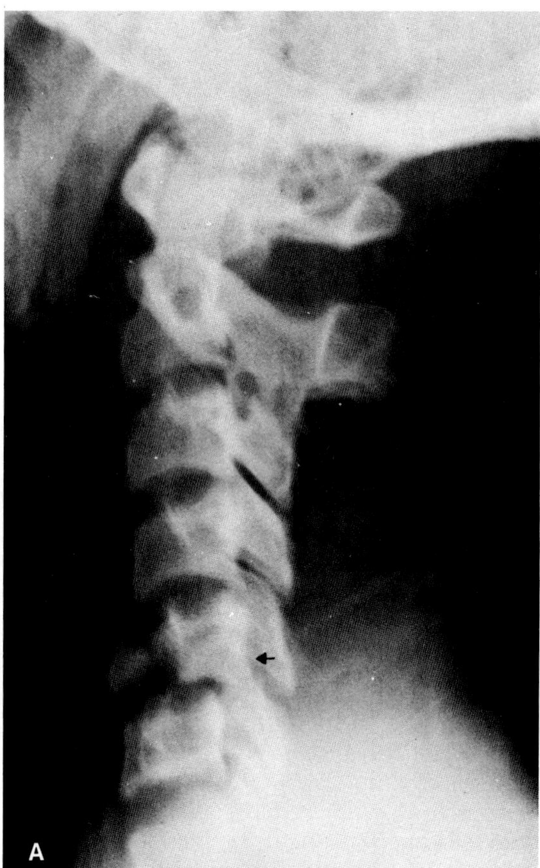

Fig. 6-75. (*A*) This compression fracture at C5 resulted in complete quadriplegia. The patient was treated by immediate laminectomy and steroids. (*B*) The patient died from massive gastrointestinal hemorrhage ten days postoperatively. The autopsy specimen shows the stomach with a probe in one of the many perforated ulcers. (Bohlman HH: Complications of Treatment of Fractures and Dislocations of the Cervical Spine. In Epps C (ed): Complications in Orthopaedic Surgery, 2nd ed, pp. 897–918. Philadelphia, JB Lippincott, 1985)

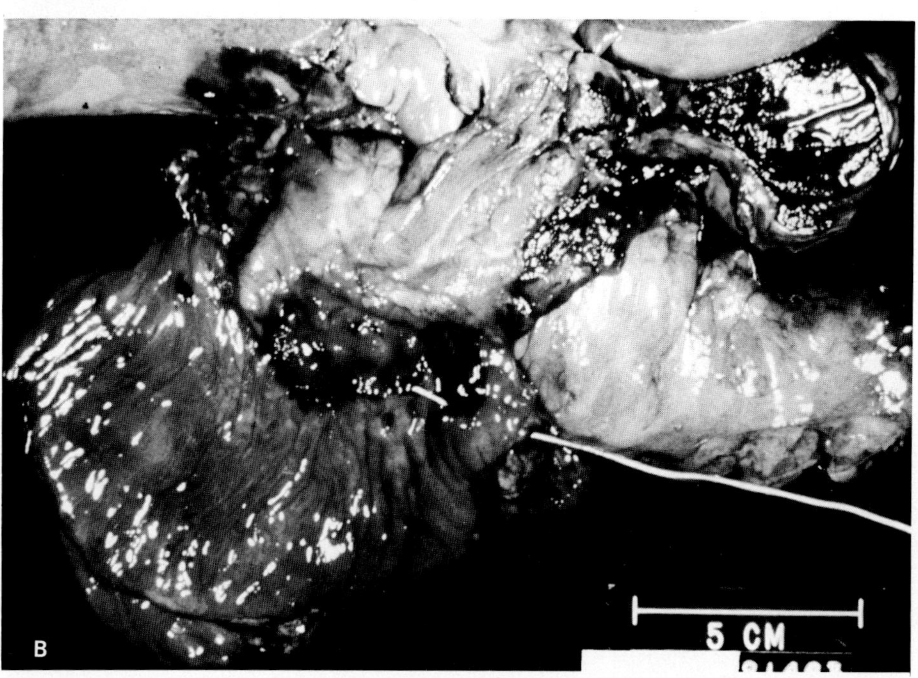

it is not a good immobilization device: it may allow recurring dislocations secondary to poor ligamentous healing. The halo cast is, therefore, preferred for the treatment of patients with very unstable cervical fractures who are going to be followed without operative treatment. On the other hand, as mentioned above, the halo cast may produce pressure sores in the asensory patient.[26]

Early Spinal Deformity

Dislocations of the lower cervical vertebrae should be reduced as soon as possible by skeletal traction or operative means. Unreduced dislocations may further compress spared nerve roots or impair radicular feeder arteries supplying the spinal cord; therefore, reduction and spinal stability should be achieved as soon as possible in relation to the other medical problems of the patient.

Overdistraction in skeletal traction can occur with cervical fracture-dislocations in which all of the ligament structures are torn anteriorly and posteriorly. This is more common in the patient with osteoarthrosis or ankylosing spondylitis. Ascending neurologic deficit has been reported in this situation. Generally, we do not apply more than 40 or 50 pounds of traction to lower cervical fractures; if reduction cannot be achieved by this method, open reduction and arthrodesis are carried out.

Operative Complications

As with any other operative procedure, sepsis may occur secondary to introduction of bacteria during the operation, but is rare. Contamination of posterior operations, especially in the upper cervical spine, may result in meningitis and death, and iatrogenic perforation of the esophagus with sharp retractors may occur with anterior operative procedures and create an esophageal cutaneous fistula and consequent osteomyelitis of the cervical vertebrae. The use of wires or screws for anchoring an anterior bone graft has been abandoned because of resultant perforations of the esophagus when the bone remodeling occurs. Methylmethacrylate has been used, as reported in the literature, to achieve posterior stabilization. We have reported the complications of its use including loosening, loss of stabilization, and infection.[34] Bone cement does not attach to cortical bone; wire fixation used in conjunction with this technique loosens, and loss of reduction occurs. We think the use of cement for fixation in cervical fractures should be abandoned.

Direct cord injury during laminectomy is the most common cause of increased neural deficit in the treatment of lower cervical fractures. In Bohlman's review series of 300 cervical spine injuries, 22% of the 55 patients who were treated by laminectomy had increased permanent loss of neural function immediately postoperatively. Permanent loss of neural function did not occur after anterior or posterior fusion or adequate nonoperative treatment. In addition, laminectomy causes increased instability and allows further subluxation or dislocation. At this point, it should be evident to most surgeons that laminectomy cannot accomplish decompression of the spinal cord or retrieval of bone and disc fragments that lie anterior to the spinal cord.

In rare instances, reduction of a dislocated lower cervical vertebra has resulted in retraction of an anteriorly ruptured disc, which may be pulled back against the spinal cord and produce further neural compression. This should be recognized immediately following a posterior surgical procedure, and an anterior decompression should be carried out.

Finally, open reduction of cervical dislocations and posterior wiring without arthrodesis is to be condemned; it only allows redislocation of the fracture, and not all cervical spine injuries fuse spontaneously.

REFERENCES

1. *Assemnacher DR, Ducker TB:* Experimental traumatic paraplegia: The vascular and pathological changes seen in reversible and irreversible spinal cord lesions. J Bone Joint Surg 53A:671, 1971
2. *Bailey RW, Badgley CE:* Stabilization of the cervical spine by anterior fusion. J Bone Joint Surg 42A:565, 1960
3. *Bohlman HH:* Surgical management of cervical spinal fractures and dislocations. In Stauffer ES (ed): Instructional Course Lectures, American Academy of Orthopaedic Surgery, Vol 34, pp 163–187, St. Louis, CV Mosby, 1985
4. *Bohlman HH:* The neck. In D'Ambrosia RD (ed): Regional Examination and Differential Diagnosis of Musculoskeletal Disorders, 2nd ed, pp 183–219, Philadelphia, JB Lippincott, 1985
5. *Bohlman HH:* Cervical spondylosis with moderate to severe myelopathy: A report of 17 cases treated by Robinson anterior cervical discectomy and fusion. Spine 2:151, 1977
6. *Bohlman HH:* Complications of treatment of fractures and dislocations of the cervical spine. In Epps CH (ed): Complications in Orthopaedic Surgery, 2nd ed, pp 897–918, Philadelphia, JB Lippincott, 1985

7. *Bohlman HH:* Acute fractures and dislocations of the cervical spine: An analysis of 300 hospitalized patients and review of the literature. J Bone Joint Surg 61A:1119, 1979
8. *Bohlman HH:* Late anterior decompression and fusion for spinal cord injuries: Review of 100 cases with long term results. Orthopaedic Transactions 4:42, 1980
9. *Bohlman HH:* Indications for late anterior decompression and fusion for cervical spinal cord injuries. In Tator CH (ed): Early Management of Acute Cervical Spinal Cord Injury. Seminars in Neurological Surgery, pp 315–333. New York, Raven Press, 1982
10. *Bohlman HH, Bahniuk E, Raskulinecz G, Field G:* Mechanical factors affecting recovery from incomplete cervical spinal cord injury: A preliminary report. Johns Hopkins Med J 145:115, 1979
11. *Bohlman HH, Bahniuk E, Field G, Raskulinecz G:* Spinal cord monitoring of experimental incomplete cervical spinal cord injury. Spine 6:428, 1981
12. *Bohlman HH, Ducker TB, Lucas JT:* Spine and spinal cord injuries. In Rothman RH, Simeone FA (eds): The Spine, 2nd ed, pp 661–756. Philadelphia, WB Saunders, 1982
13. *Bohlman HH, Eismont FJ:* Surgical techniques of anterior decompression and fusion for spinal cord injuries. Clin Orthop 154:57, 1981
14. *Bohlman HH, Rekate H, Thompson GH:* Problem fractures of the cervical spine in children. In Haughton G, Thompson G (eds): pp 101–124. Boston and London, Butterworth, 1983
15. *Bohlman HH, Riley L Jr, Robinson RA:* Anterolateral approaches to the cervical spine. In Ruge D, Wiltse LL (eds): Spinal Disorders, pp 125, Lea & Febiger, 1977
16. *Braakman R, Penning L:* Injuries of the Cervical Spine, p 262, Amsterdam, Excerpta Medica, 1971
17. *Burke DC:* Hyperextension injuries of the spine. J Bone Joint Surg 53B:3, 1971
18. *Burke DC, Berryman D:* The place of closed manipulation in the management of flexion–rotation dislocations of the cervical spine. J Bone Joint Surg 53B:165, 1971
19. *Catttell HS, Filtzer DL:* Pseudosubluxation and other normal variations in the cervical spine in children: A study of one hundred and sixty children. J Bone Joint Surg 47A:1295, 1964
20. *Cheshire DJE:* The stability of the cervical spine following the conservative treatment of fractures and fracture-dislocations. Paraplegia 7:193, 1969
21. *Crock HV, Yoshizawa H:* The Blood Supply of the Vertebral Column and Spinal Cord in Man. New York, Springer-Verlag, 1977
22. *Davis D, Bohlman H, Walker AE, Fisher R, Robinson R:* The pathological findings in fatal craniospinal injuries. J Neurosurg 34:603, 1971
23. *Ducker TB, Salcman M, Daniel HB:* Experimental spinal cord trauma III: Therapeutic effect of immobilization and pharmacologic agents. Surg Neurol 10:71, 1978
24. *Eismont FJ, Clifford S, Goldberg M, Green B:* Cervical sagittal canal size in spine injury. Spine 9:663–666, 1984
25. *Fried LC:* Cervical spinal cord injury during skeletal traction. JAMA 229:181, 1974
26. *Garfin SR, Botle MJ, Waters RL, Nickel VL:* Complications in the use of the halo fixation device. J Bone Joint Surg 68A:320–325, 1986
27. *Hinchey JE, Hreno A, Benoit PR, et al:* The stress ulcer syndrome. In Welch C (ed): Advances in Surgery, Vol 4, pp 325–393. Chicago, Year Book Medical Publishers, 1970
28. *Hohl M:* Soft tissue injuries of the neck in automobile accidents. J Bone Joint Surg 46A:1777, 1964
29. *Jellinger K:* Neuropathology of cord injuries. In Vinken PJ, Bruyn GW (eds): Handbook of Clinical Neurology, Vol. 25, pp 43–121. Amsterdam, North Holland Publishing Co, 1976
30. *Kobrine AI, Doyle TF, Rizzoli HV:* Spinal cord blood flow as affected by changes in systemic arterial blood pressure. J Neurosurg 44:12, 1976
31. *Kobrine AI, Evans DE, Rizzoli HV:* Experimental acute balloon compression of the spinal cord. J Neurosurg 51:841, 1979
32. *Lazorthes G, Gouzae A, Zadeh JO, et al:* Arterial vascularization of the spinal cord: Recent studies of the anastomotic substitution pathways. J Neurosurg 35:253, 1971
33. *Marar BC:* Hyperextension injuries of the cervical spine: The pathogenesis of damage to the spinal cord. J Bone Joint Surg 56A:1655, 1974
34. *McAfee PC, Bohlman HH, Ducker T, Eismont FJ:* Failure of stabilization of the spine with methylmethacrylate. J Bone Joint Surg 68A:1145–1157, 1986
35. *Rossier AB, Hussey RW, Kenzora JE:* Anterior fibular interbody fusion in the treatment of cervical spinal cord injuries. Surg Neurol 7:55, 1977
36. *Stauffer ES, Kelly EJ:* Fracture-dislocations of cervical spine: Instability and recurrent deformities following treatment by anterior interbody fusion. J Bone Joint Surg 59A:45, 1977
37. *Tarlov IM:* Acute spinal cord compression paralysis. J Neurosurg 36:10, 1972
38. *Turnbull IM:* Miscovasculature of the human spinal cord. J Neurosurg 35:141, 1971
39. *Verbiest H:* Anterolateral operations for fractures and dislocations in the middle and lower parts of

the cervical spine: Report of a series of forty-seven cases. J Bone Joint Surg 51A:1489, 1969

40. *White JB, Kneisley LW, Rossier AB:* Delayed paralysis after cervical fracture dislocation: Case report. J Neurosurg 46:512, 1977

41. *White AA, Southwick WO, Panjabi MM:* Clinical instability in the lower cervical spine. Spine 1:15, 1976

Internal Fixation of the Unstable Cervical Spine by a Posterior Osteosynthesis with Plates and Screws

RAYMOND ROY-CAMILLE, GERARD SAILLANT, AND CHRISTIAN MAZEL

This technique of fixation is based on the use of special plates with screws implanted into the cervical spine articular masses. It is simple, safe, and strong. The technique is used alone or is combined with an anterior stabilization of the cervical spine. In our practice, the anterior procedure includes a graft and a fixation with a special staple.

Cervical spine instability is mainly induced by injuries and tumors, and in some cases it results from a congenital malformation. The technique must be adapted to the various cases, depending on the pathology and on the level of injury to the lower cervical spine (C3–C7) or to the upper cervical spine (Occiput C1 and C2).

LOWER CERVICAL SPINE

Anatomy

The anatomy of the lower cervical spine is not commonly well known. When a posterior fixation is performed, one can only see the posterior aspect of the posterior arches. Their shape provides information about the anterior elements.

The vertebral posterior arch (Fig. 6-76) includes the spinous process in the middle with the laminae on both sides and the articular masses more laterally. A groove resembling a valley is located at the border between the lamina and the bulging articular mass, which can be compared to a hill. The cord is in front of the spinous process and the laminae. The vertebral artery is in front of the valley, which is an excellent landmark (Fig. 6-77). The roots at each level are exiting the canal through the foramina; they are lying at the level of the articular joints, which are their posterior datum lines. The plates will be placed over the articular masses and the screws implanted into these masses.

This anatomic knowledge and these landmarks make it easy to implant the screws into the articular masses. Because of their lateral position the screws avoid the cord, and, owing to their implantation into the articular masses and their length, they avoid the roots in the foramina. The screws also avoid the vertebral artery, being lateral to the valley in front of which it flows.

Experimental Study

A study was performed with the help of Rollin Johnson in New Haven at the Veterans Administration Hospital, in which we investigated the osteosynthesis mechanical properties in flexion and extension stress.

Two cervical vertebrae from a fresh cadaver were fixed together posteriorly with a symmetrical pair of two-hole plates, after removal of the whole ligaments and interbody disc material. The lower vertebra was firmly fixed, and stress was applied to the upper vertebrae. Displacements were analyzed during the stress with displacement gauges. The entire experiment was performed in a large glass chamber in order to keep a constant hygrometic level and to stay as close as possible to *in vivo* characteristics.

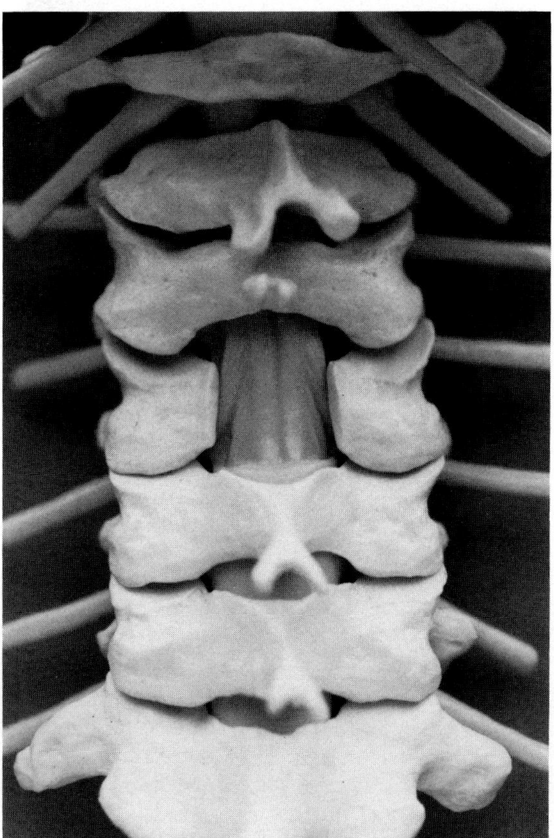

Fig. 6-76. The posterior aspect of the cervical spine.

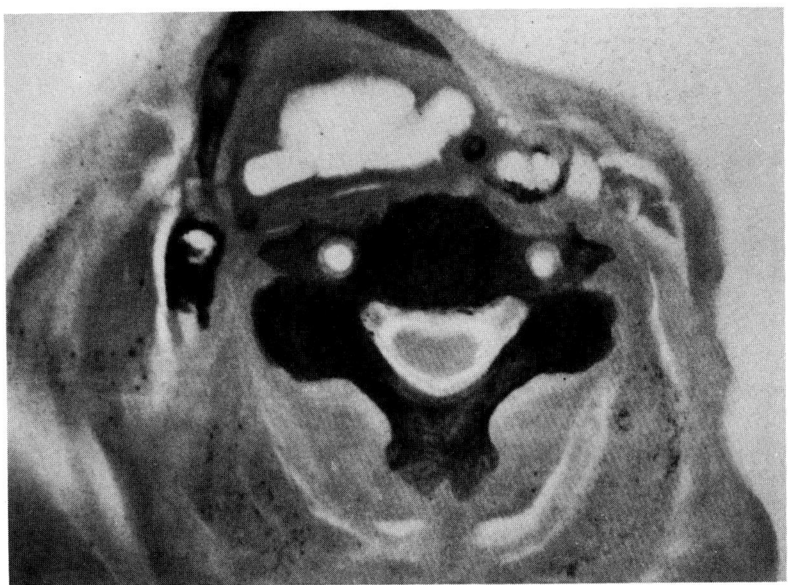

Fig. 6-77. Transverse cut demonstrating the place of the different elements. The arrow indicates the direction for the implantation of a screw in the articular mass.

Displacements were measured as well as radiographed. All the results were computerized.

The average breaking load in extension stress is 52.5 kg (515 N). This represents 60% of the load necessary to dislocate two normal cervical vertebrae. These results have been compared with the other methods of cervical posterior fixation. For an extension stress, a posterior wiring on the spinous processes or in the articular masses is inefficient for stabilizing the spine. Fixation using posterior plates increases the normal stability by 60%. A methyl methacrylate fixation on the spinous processes provides a 99% increase in stability.

For a flexion stress, the posterior wiring between the spinous processes results in a 33% increase in stability. The same wiring, but around a complementary bone graft, provides a 55% increase of stability, and the increase is 88% when the wiring is through the articular masses. The plate fixation gives a 92% increase in stability.

Surgical Procedure

Surgery is performed through a midposterior approach. The patient is in prone position and the head firmly fixed with a head holder that enables a flexion–extension range motion. A traction device, if necessary, can be fixed to the operating table. A local xylocaine and adrenaline infiltration helps to divide the muscles on the midline and diminishes the bleeding. The posterior approach is achieved primarily with an electrocautery down to the lateral side of the articular masses in order to locate exactly the reference marks.

The spot for drilling and implanting the screws is at the top of the articular mass hill, exactly in its middle (Fig. 6-78). The drilling is done with a 2.8 mm-drill when using a 3.6-mm screw. A special drill with depth gauge at 19 mm prevents going too far forward. A slow motor drill is necessary. The drilling direction is perpendicular to the vertebral plane or, better, 10° oblique laterally—but never medially. The lateral obliquity is to increase safety and to be sure to avoid the vertebral artery, which is medial in front of the valley. When the procedure is performed with the necessary care, we have not noted complications.

The screw diameter is 3.6 mm and the length is 16 or 19 mm. The plate is premolded to fit the cervical spinal lordosis. It is 2 mm thick and 1 cm wide, and the holes are positioned every 13 mm. Usually, two plates are symmetrically implanted with two, three, four, or five holes, depending on the number of vertebrae that have to be fixed (Fig. 6-79).

Posterior Plate Fixation in Lower Cervical Spine Injuries

Prevalent posterior lesions are better treated with a posterior technique, anterior lesions with an anterior one, and horizontal lesions of the mobile vertebral segment can be treated either posteriorly

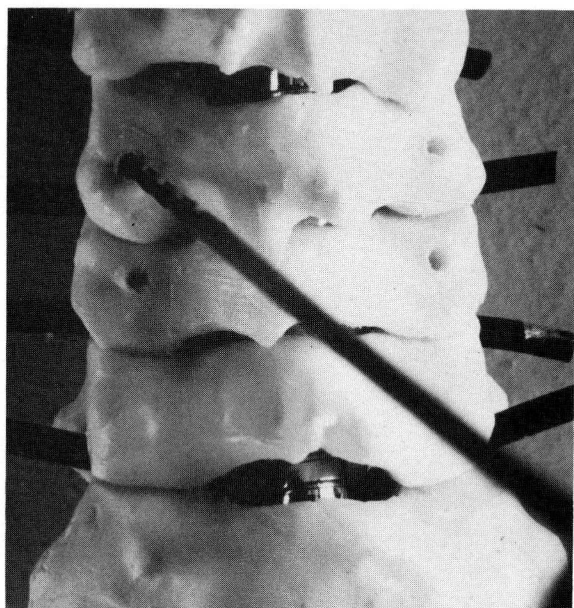

Fig. 6-78. Drilling in the articular mass starting at the top of the hill, driven 10 degrees oblique and outward.

or anteriorly. If there is any question about which to use, we prefer the posterior plate fixation.

Our surgical technique with plates and screws implanted into the articular masses is used to stabilize all cervical spine injuries with prevailing posterior lesions, as well as severe sprains. In trauma this technique is used very often, because most cervical injuries include a dislocation, a fracture, or a fracture dislocation of the articular masses. Under those conditions, the posterior approach is best for reduction, and the posterior plates stabilize the bony lesion as well as the associated disc and ligament injuries.

We must point out that this plate fixation over the articular masses induces a spontaneous fusion of the bridged facets. Therefore, no complementary grafting is necessary.

CERVICAL DISLOCATION. These dislocations can be unilateral or bilateral.

UNILATERAL DISLOCATIONS. In these cases, the reduction is achieved operatively with spatulae introduced between the laminae at the dislocated level. The first spatula is introduced near the midline close to the spinous process. While the first spatula is kept in place, a second one is introduced laterally; the first is then placed further on, between the dislocated articular facets. It is then possible with a tyre level maneuver to achieve the reduction by moving the upper articular facet backward over the lower one. The reduction is then stabilized by the table head holder positioned in extension. A first posterior two-hole plate is implanted on the dislocated side, and the fixation is completed with a second plate on the opposite side (Fig. 6-80).

BILATERAL DISLOCATIONS. The same maneuver is performed on both sides symmetrically. Once

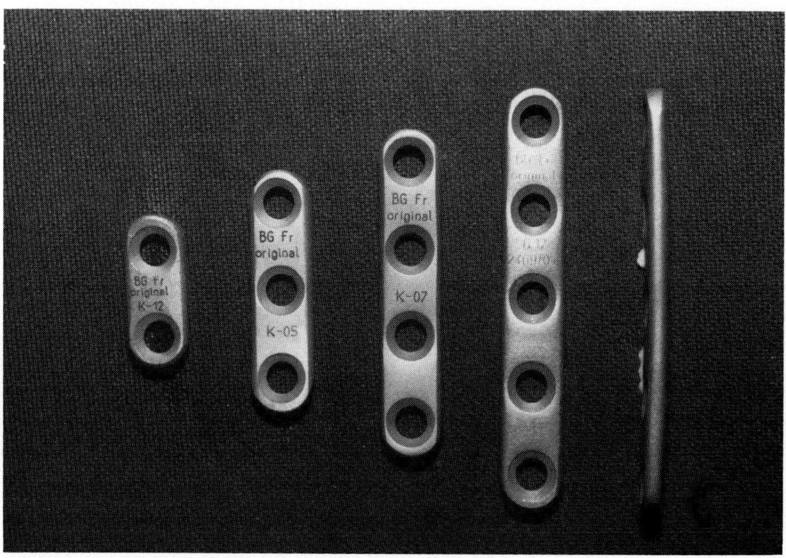

Fig. 6-79. The cervical plates, with their curvature and the 13-mm distant holes.

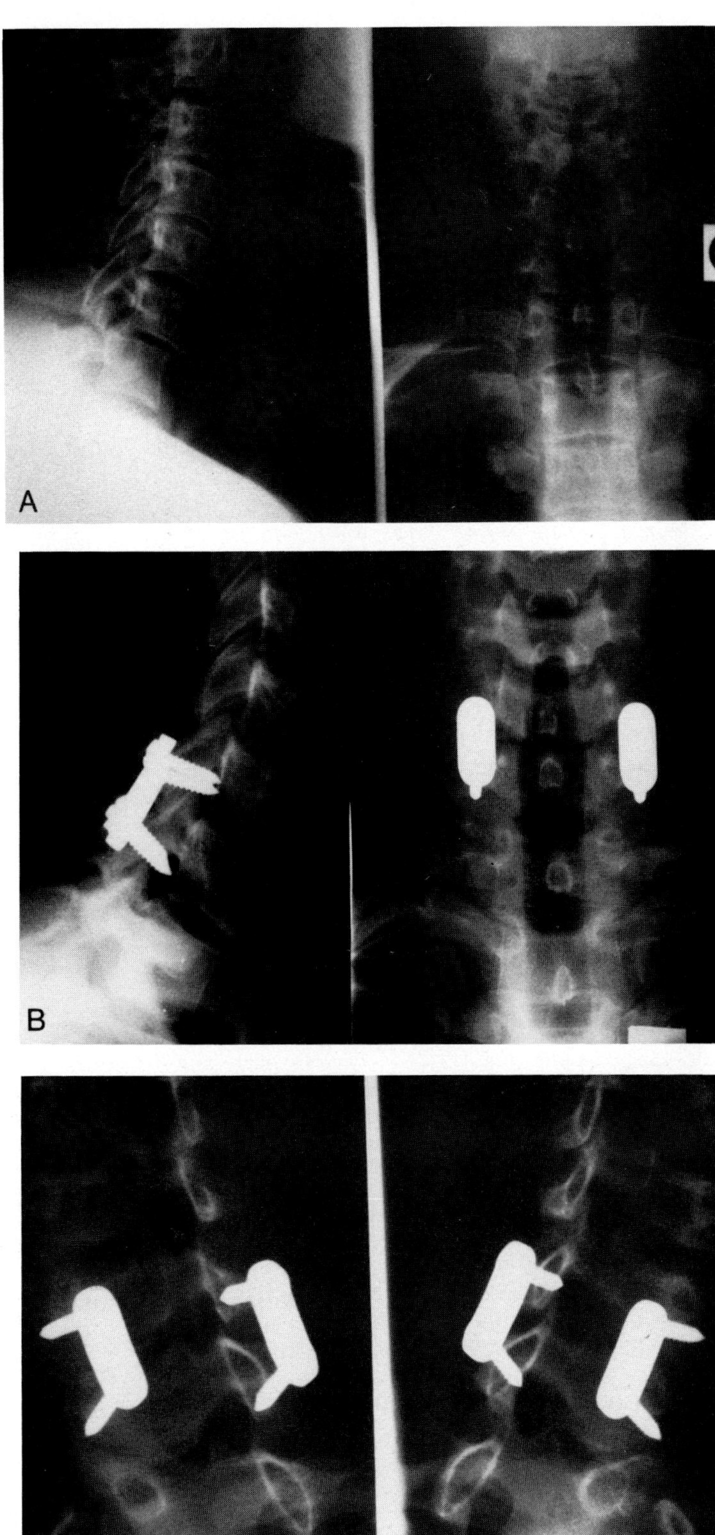

Fig. 6-80. Internal fixation of a cervical spine dislocation with two-hole plates: (*A*) C6–C7 dislocation; (*B*) A–P and lateral views of the reduction and fixation; (*C*) oblique views—the foramina are free.

again, the stabilization is achieved with two posterior two-hole plates.

The fixation of one-level dislocations with the two-hole plates is strong enough to prevent any secondary displacement. Postoperatively, the patient will wear a simple collar for 5 weeks.

We prefer to perform this surgical treatment on an emergency basis in the absence of previous traction. Furthermore, we prefer the open reduction with the direct visual control of the lesion. The maneuvers are precise and smooth, and the posterior fixation is achieved at the same time, shortening the period of postoperative care. Patients without neurologic involvement are usually discharged from the hospital on the fifth day after the operation.

FACET JOINT FRACTURE AND DISLOCATION. When a facet joint fracture is combined with a dislocation, it is usually a fracture of the upper articular facet (Fig. 6-81). Its displacement follows the upper vertebra, and the broken fragment pushed into the foramen can compress the homolateral cervical nerve root. Two problems must therefore be solved: (1) the cure of a possible cervicobrachialgia induced by the compression of the nerve root, and (2) the fixation, which is difficult because the stabilization from the articular facet is missing after reduction.

The displaced compressive fragment must be removed from the foramen before achieving the fixation. This can be performed only by a posterior approach through the facet joint.

The fixation is then achieved with a reconstruction of the renewed articular facet using a special tile-shaped plate (Fig. 6-82). This very precise technique is a real joint replacement. The upper part of the plate is oblique and is slipped beneath the facet of the upper rotated vertebra. The lower part of the plate is fixed in the articular mass with screws. At the beginning of our experience the plate was used alone. We now prefer to combine a tile plate with a standard two-hole plate. The normal plate is placed over the tile plate like a *porte-manteau.* The fixation is achieved with a lower screw driven through the holes of the two plates and an upper screw implanted into the articular mass of the vertebra above (Fig. 6-83).

In case of important instability, one may use the same *porte-manteau* fixation with a long tile plate, bridging three vertebrae (Fig. 6-84).

SEPARATION-FRACTURE OF THE ARTICULAR MASS. This fracture is difficult to stabilize. Two fracture lines separate the articular mass from the rest of the vertebra. The first one is on the pedicle, the second one is on the lamina on the same side. Thus, the articular mass is completely liberated from the vertebra and will rotate with the upper or the lower adjacent vertebra. On the lateral radiograph it appears horizontal and no longer parallel to the adjacent facets; this is pathognomonic. The fracture lines can be demonstrated on the lamina (A–P view), or on the pedicle (oblique view). The correct fixation of such fractures is a long *porte-manteau* on the side of the articular mass fracture and a simple three-hole plate on the other side. It provides both reduction and stabilization.

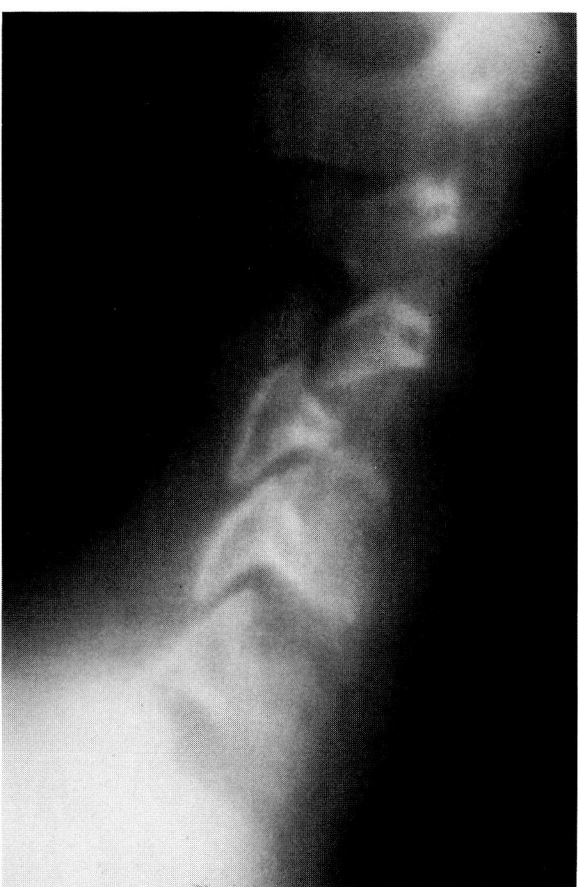

Fig. 6-81. Tomogram of a dislocation with fracture of an upper articular facet of C5.

TEARDROP FRACTURE. The teardrop fracture is more like a severe sprain than a fracture. The lesions are mainly on the disc and the ligaments, and the small broken bony fragment of the vertebral body is not important. Instability comes

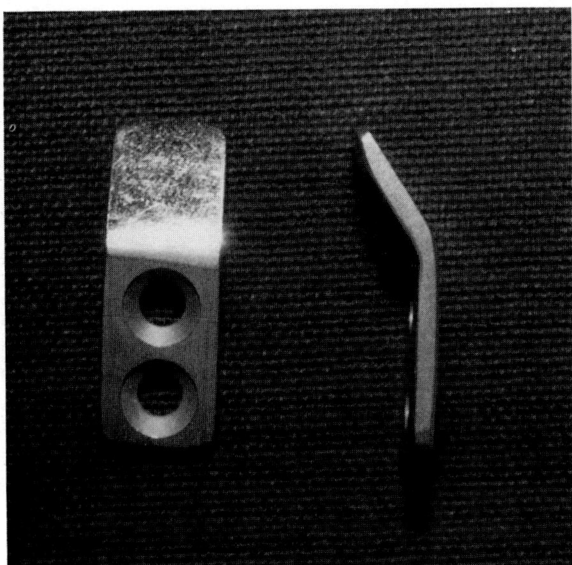

Fig. 6-82. Tile plates.

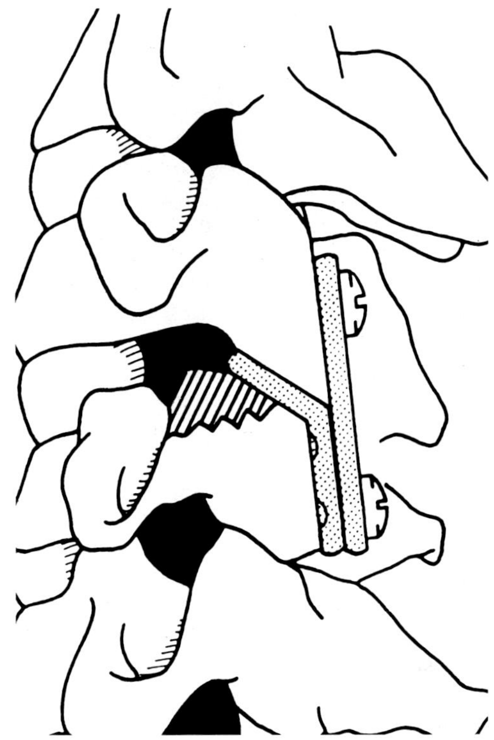

Fig. 6-83. A short *porte-manteau* fixation. Same patient as in Fig. 6-81.

from the severe sprain. When the injury is primarily posterior with demonstrable interspinous widening and facet joint posterior opening, the surgical treatment can be performed posteriorly with posterior plates.

SEVERE SPRAINS. Severe sprains need to be well understood because they are often misdiagnosed. The whole mobile vertebral segment is involved by the trauma without any bony lesion. This is the stage before the complete tear of a dislocation. Induced by the continuous mobilization of the neck, the displacement occurs a few weeks or months later and is characterized by the following: interspinous widening, facet joint subluxation, disc posterior opening, and anterior olisthesis of the upper vertebra. The fixation with posterior plates and screws is a simple and perfect technique for stabilization of these lesions.

FAILURE OF AN ANTERIOR STABILIZATION. The posterior fixation with plates and screws is a very simple and elegant method to achieve a fusion that does not succeed after an anterior technique has been tried. The posterior stable fixation induces the anterior fusion.

COMPLEMENTARY PROCEDURES. The posterior approach and the use of posterior plates and screws implanted into the articular masses enables different associated procedures. A laminectomy is easily performed when necessary because the plates are lateral to the laminae on the articular masses.

It was pointed out that grafting is not necessary in patients with pure dislocation, but in those with associated fractures a Hibbs fusion on the laminae is always possible, if desired.

The only contraindication to this plating method is a severe degree of osteoporosis.

POSTOPERATIVE CARE. Simple injuries such as unilateral dislocations are immobilized by a simple collar for 5 weeks. More unstable lesions with associated fractures are immobilized for 2 to 3 months by a light plastic Minerva jacket.

In case of cord injury with tetraplegia, the stable fixation induced by the plates facilitates nursing care.

RESULTS. The mechanical stability of this fixation is demonstrated by the study of a continuous series of 221 patients with lower cervical spine injuries treated by this technique. There is no secondary displacement in 85.2% of the patients, a displacement of less than 5 degrees in 8.8%, of 5 to 10

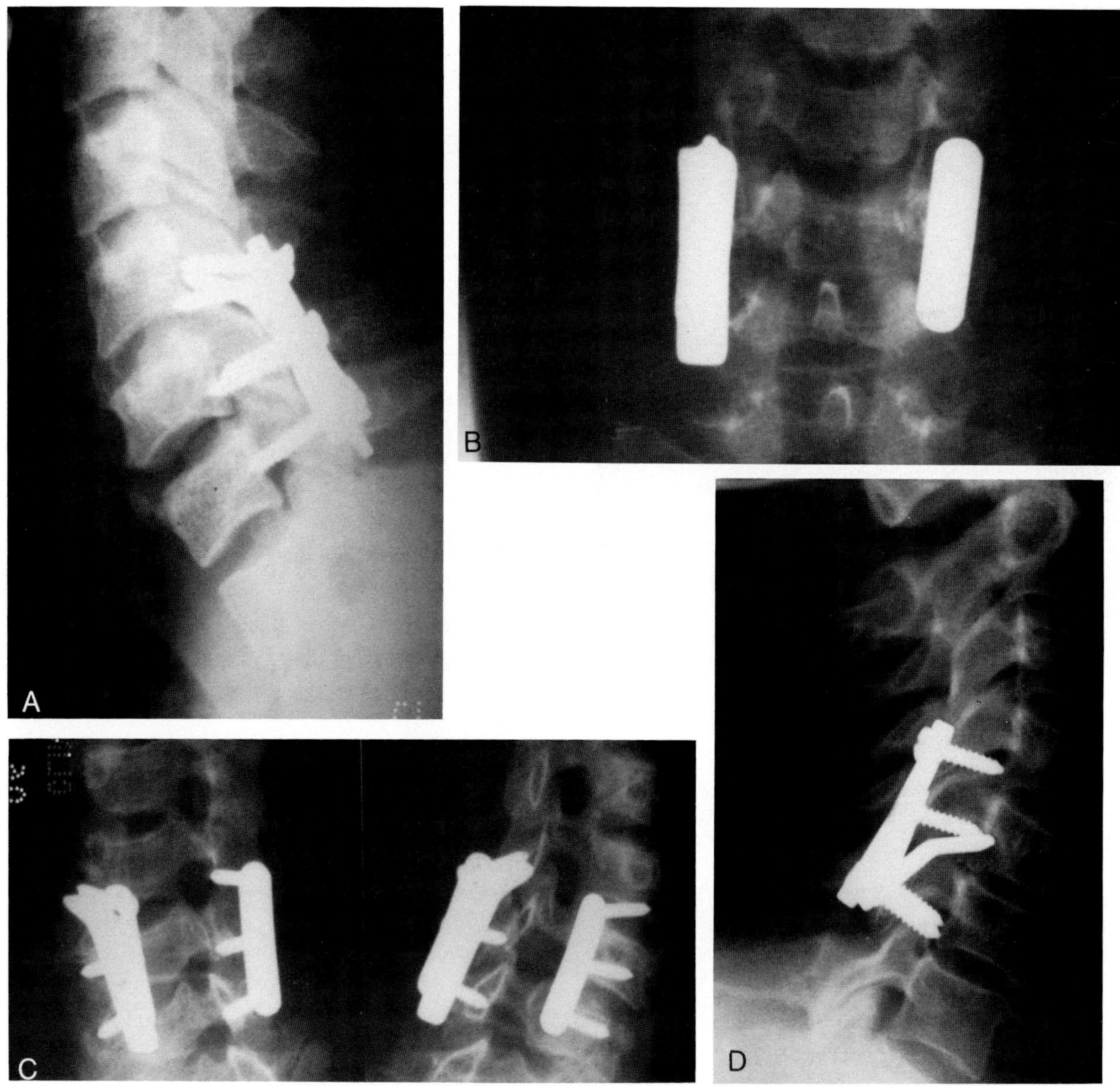

Fig. 6-84. A long *porte-manteau* fixation for a dislocation with an articular facet fracture: (*A*) lateral view. (*B*) oblique views of the reduction and fixation. (*C*) A–P view. (*D*) Lateral view showing alternative fixation technique.

degrees in 3%, and over 10 degrees in 3%. No breakage of plates or screws was observed.

Posterior Plate Fixation in Lower Cervical Spine Tumor Localization

The basic procedure of implantation is the same as described above. The tumor extension often leads to an extensive fixation using plates of three, four, and five holes.

The necessity of removing a tumor of the vertebral body is often an indication for two-stage surgery. The posterior stage may be imperative, in case of great instability, or it may be used for safety. It can be the first or the second stage.

We must point out that for the anterior stage we use an original stapling (Fig. 6-85). The staples have four "fish teeth" like feet. They are implanted on the midline of the vertebral bodies. The size is

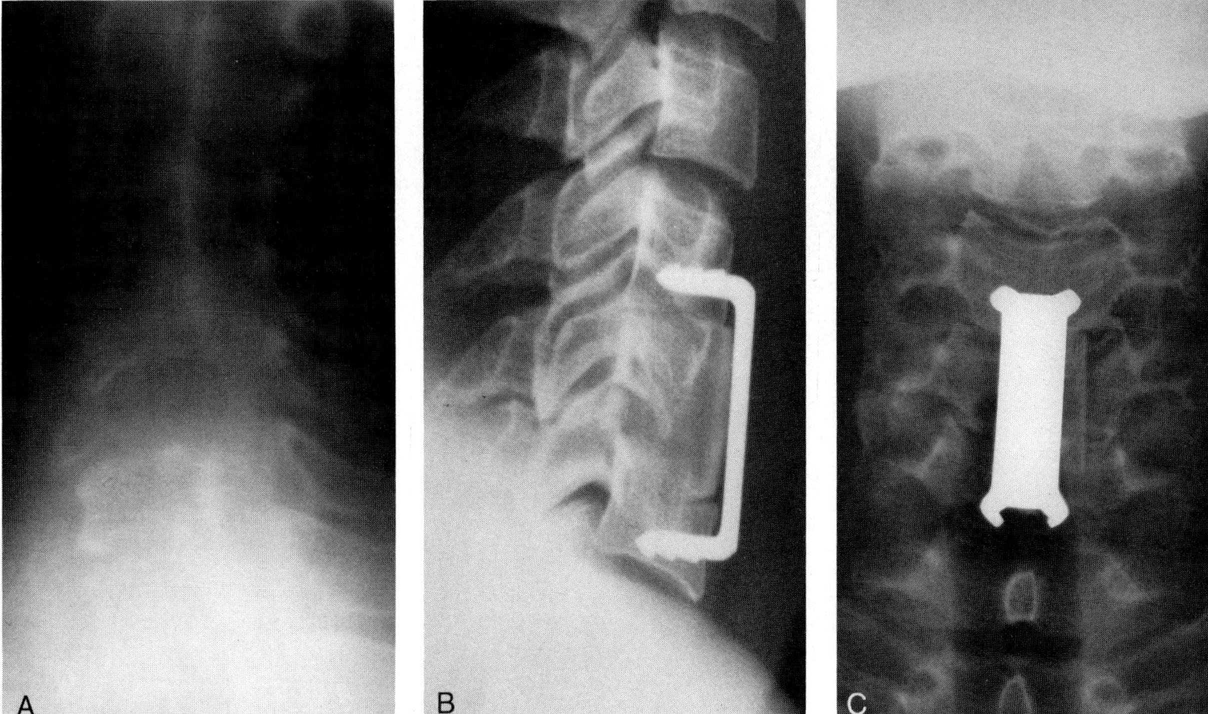

Fig. 6-85. Cervical tumor. Tumoral excision and fixation with a staple: (*A*) tomogram of C5 lytic tumor. (*B*) lateral view after the first anterior stage. (*C*) A–P view.

selected to bridge the graft and find a support for the four feet in the adjacent vertebral bodies. To prepare the implantation, a flat model of the adequate size is used with a hole in each corner corresponding to the position of the feet of the staple (Fig. 6-86). After drilling through these holes is performed, the staple, presented on a holder, is implanted by hammering on the handle.

UPPER CERVICAL SPINE

Plates and screws can also be used for the treatment of upper cervical spine instability in case of injuries, tumor localizations, congenital malformations, rheumatoid disease, among other conditions.

Anatomy

The normal occipitocervical angulation is 105 degrees, giving a normal horizontal direction to the eyes. An osteosynthesis with plates must maintain this angulation.

The longitudinal posterior venous sinus is on the midline of the occipital bone. Lateral to this sinus, the bone is about 10 to 12 mm thick with two cortices. It allows only a short screw implantation but is strong because of the two cortices.

When it is necessary to implant a screw into a C2 pedicle, it is important to know its direction and its relationships with the cord and the vertebral artery. A C2 pedicle is oblique 10 to 15 degrees upward and inward. A screw implanted into such a pedicle must have the same direction. The C1 ring is normally divided into three equal spaces: one for the odontoid process, one for the cord, and one that is empty. At C2 level, the ring is still large and there is no intimate contact between the cord and the pedicles.

The vertebral artery is included in the C2 articular mass following a loop like a horizontal S. The posterior aspect of the articular mass, which is discovered through a posterior approach, can be divided into four quarters. The vertebral artery occupies the two inferior quarters and the upper lateral quarter (Fig. 6-87). The upper medial quarter is free, and a screw can be implanted into it.

Surgical Procedures

To stabilize the occipitocervical junction, we use special premolded plates (Fig. 6-88). Their shape

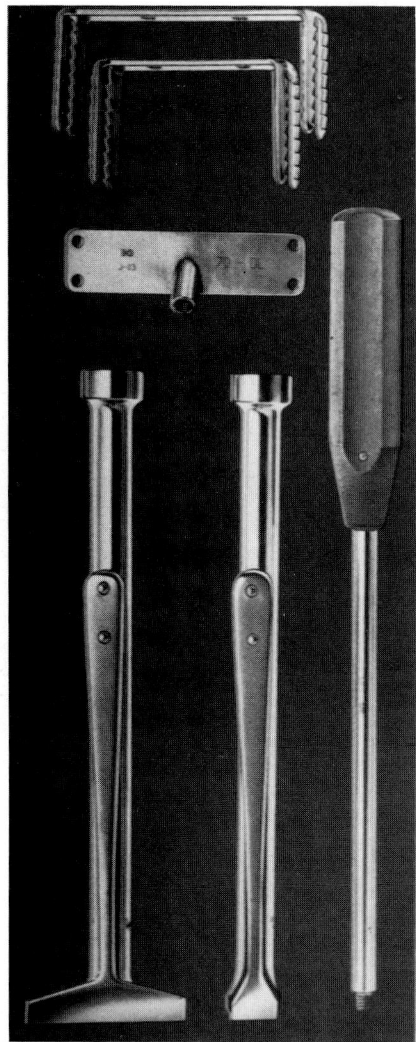

Fig. 6-86. Instrumental set for stapling here presented for cervical and lumbar spine.

is designed to restore the normal curve of the occipitocervical junction with a 105-degree angulation. They are reinforced in their middle at the top of the curve. The occipital part of the plates is flat to prevent skin scarring at this level. Two plates are placed, laterally and symmetrically. The fixation to the occiput is lateral and achieved with 13-mm-long screws. The drilling is performed with a depth gauge drill of 12 mm. The screw point penetrates into the skull without any neurologic damage because of the fluid protection. At the cervical level, the fixation is achieved with screws in the articular masses as usual. Some plates are short, extending down to C4, others are longer and extend to C5. Between the two plates there is a large place to put a corticocancellous bone graft. This one will be fixed with a 9-mm screw into the external occipital cortex at its upper extremity and with a wire into the C4 or C5 spinous process at its lower extremity (Fig. 6-89).

To implant a screw into a C2 pedicle is a difficult technique that demands very precise anatomic landmarks to prevent any vertebral artery injury. The superior border of C2 lamina is cleared. Then a slightly curved spatula is introduced into the large vertebral canal along the medial aspect of the pedicle. On the posterior aspect of the articular mass, the upper medial quarter is determined, and the point of penetration of the drill is prepared with an awl. This point is as high and medial as possible on the articular mass. From this point, with the control of the spatula in the vertebral canal, the drilling can be performed with an upward and inward obliquity of 10 to 15 degrees (Fig. 6-90). The drill must be as close as possible to the medial and to the upper cortex of the pedicle. The drilling will be 35 mm deep. The vertebral artery is lateral and inferior to the drill. A 35-mm-long screw can then be inserted.

Posterior Plate Fixation in Upper Cervical Spine Injuries

To our knowledge, the stabilization of the occipitocervical junction can be achieved only posteriorly. To ensure the fusion it is necessary to have a strong fixation which can be obtained by the implantation of two occipitocervical plates.

OCCIPITOCERVICAL DISLOCATION. This type of dislocation is usually immediately fatal. We have observed two patients who survived, one in whom the injury occurred 14 months before and one in whom it occurred recently. They needed a simple fusion with two plates and a graft for the chronic case and a reduction with a light traction followed by fixation with two plates for the fresh one. It is important to notice the difficulty of the diagnosis of this dislocation, and the interest in the anterior occipitocervical line (Fig. 6-91).

TEARDROP FRACTURE OF C2. If there is significant instability, these fractures have to be fixed by an occipitocervical fusion. In case of a lesser instability, a simple C2–C3 stabilization is sufficient. This fixation is then performed with two posterior plates, with the screws implanted into C2 pedicles and C3 articular masses.

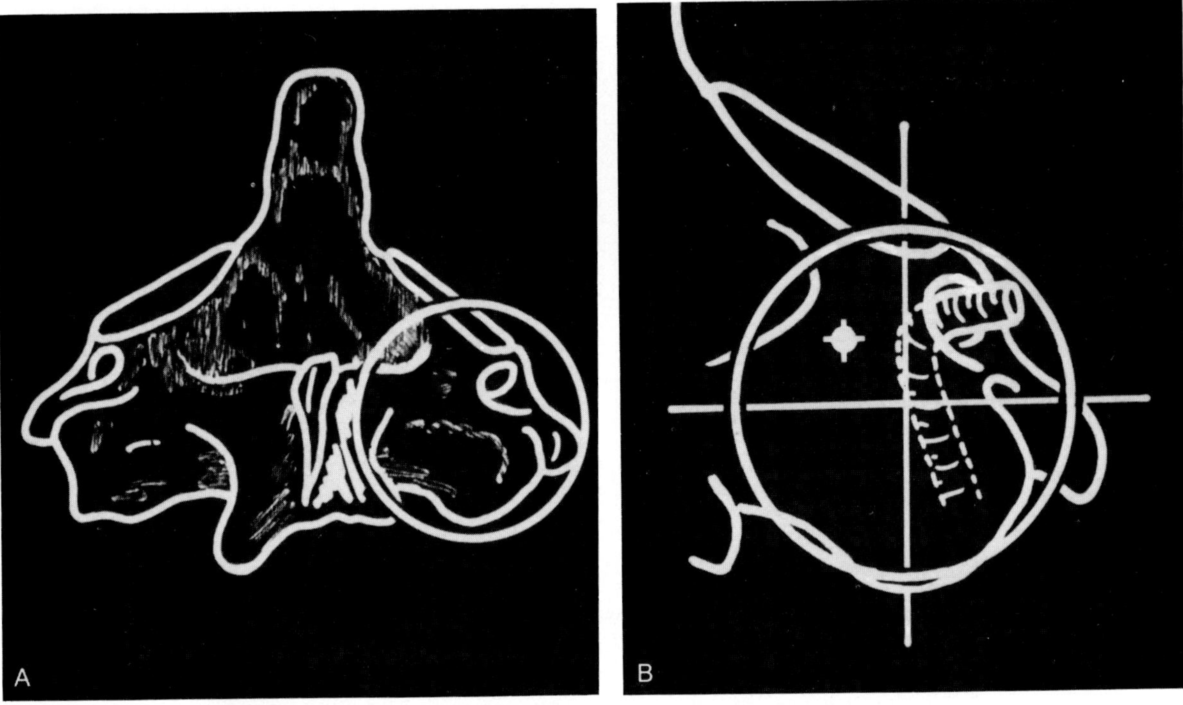

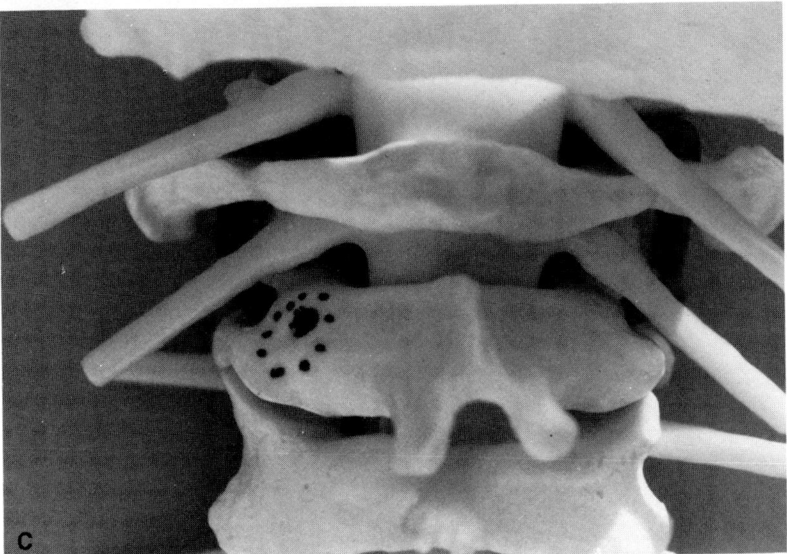

Fig. 6-87. (*A*) Posterior aspect of C2 articular mass. (*B*) the vertebral artery. (*C*) the point of penetration of a screw.

HANGMAN'S FRACTURE. When the fracture is stable or the displacement minimal, healing will occur with conservative treatment. But in case of an associated complete C2–C3 posterior dislocation (Fig. 6-92*A*), surgical treatment is necessary to reduce and to stabilize the lesion. The reduction is impossible with traction and it must be achieved by a posterior approach. Through the same approach, the fixation is performed with two-hole plates, which stabilize C2–C3 instability. The upper

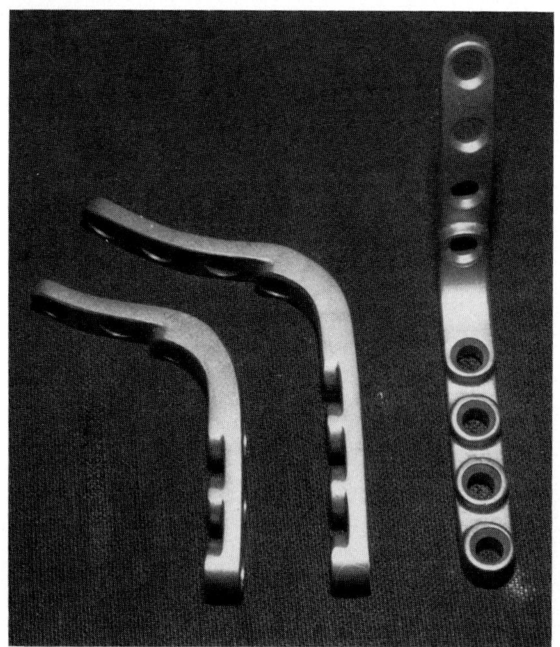

Fig. 6-88. Occipitocervical plates, one short, one long.

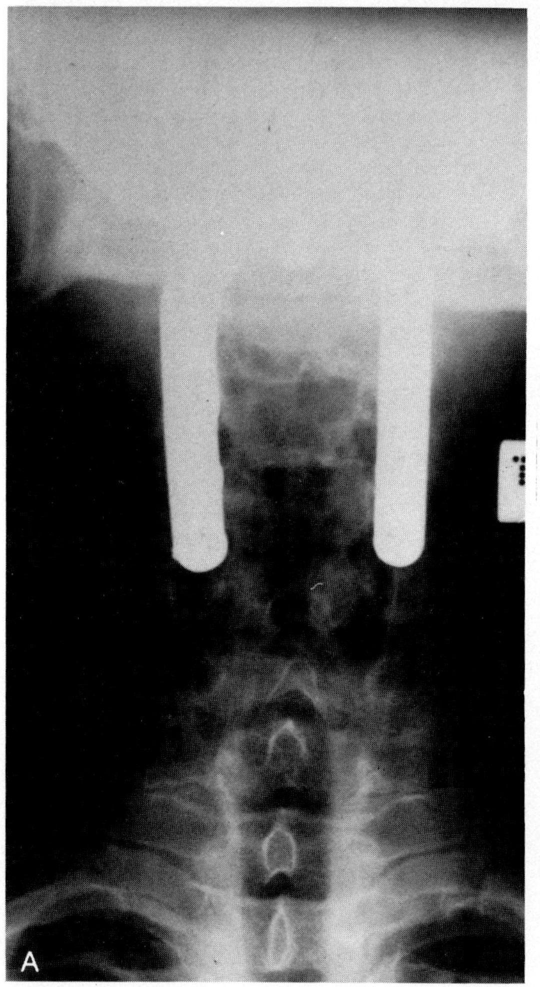

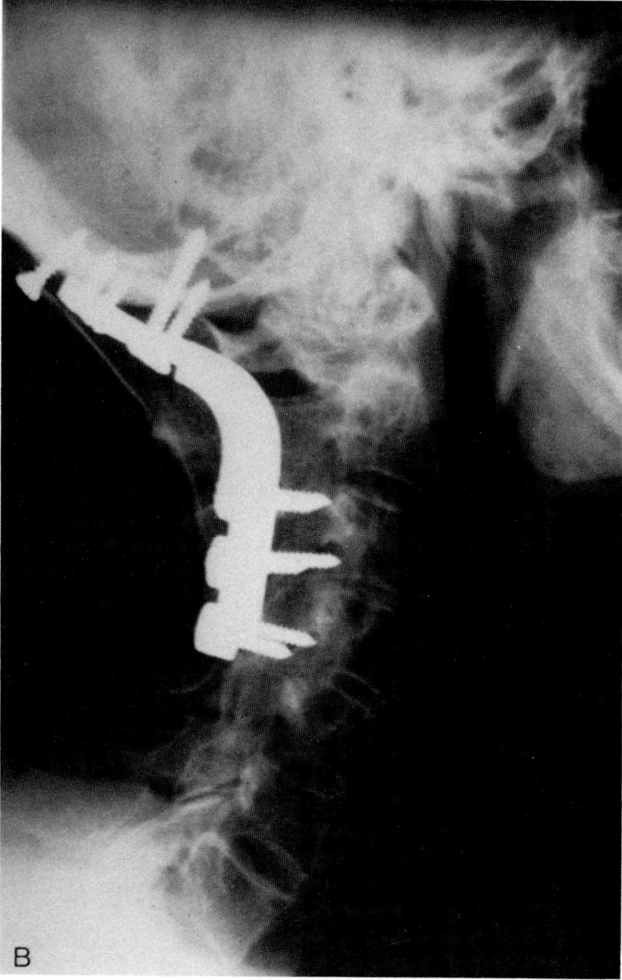

screws driven into the C2 pedicles achieve the direct fixation of the fracture lines (Fig. 6-92*B* and *C*).

Other Indications for the Posterior Plate Fixation in the Upper Cervical Spine

Tumor Localization. Tumor localization on C2 vertebral body is one of the best indications for the occipitocervical fixation with posterior plates. It restores the upper cervical spine stability with its normal curvature, permitting oncologic treatment including radiotherapy. A Minerva jacket is helpful postoperatively, up to the time of ossification of the vertebral body, which depends on the histologic type of the tumor. At any rate, the fixation allows immediate ambulation.

Congenital Malformations. These malformations are often localized in the upper cervical spine. Difficulty arises from instability with cord compression, usually by the odontoid process or by the posterior border of the foramen magnum. Posterior plate fixation restoring stability and normal curvature relieves cord compression, but it may be necessary, by the same posterior approach, to widen the foramen magnum posteriorly.

Rheumatoid Disease. In case of rheumatoid disease with progressive occipitocervical dislocation, a C1–C2 fusion is usually insufficient in our experience, and an occipitocervical fusion is necessary. In these steroid-dependent patients, skin healing is slow. These patients need care to prevent any local compression on the occiput at the fixation level. The large corticocancellous bony graft between the two plates fuses much better than a C1–C2 graft, which often disappears spontaneously.

Cord Compression. In some patients with cord compression caused by the odontoid process (malunion, congenital deformity, rheumatoid disease), it may be necessary to remove the dens and C2 vertebral body through an anterior approach. This induces great instability and the more stable fixation is then the posterior occipitocervical plating, achieved in a second stage. Skull traction is necessary between the two surgical stages.

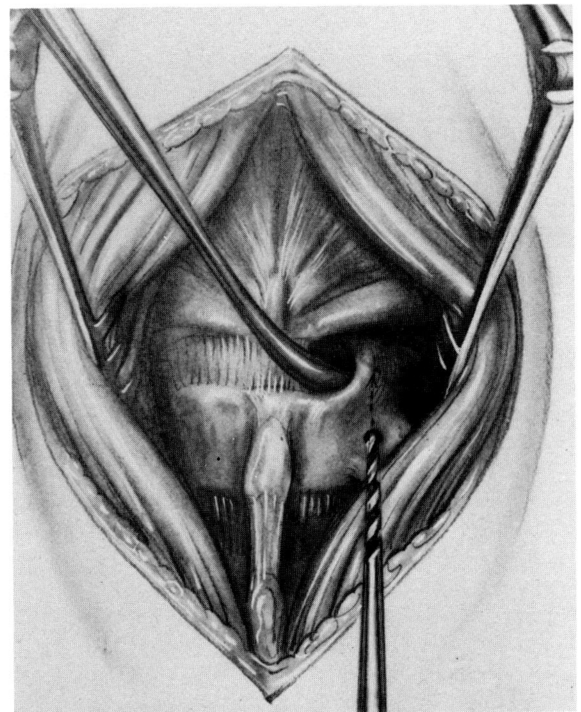

Fig. 6-90. Drilling of C2 pedicle.

Postoperative Care

A Minerva jacket is necessary postoperatively when the patient is able to walk. In patients with tetraplegia, the head and neck are left free, except for two lateral head supports.

CONCLUSION

In patients with posttraumatic cervical spine instability, a posterior approach is often necessary to reduce a facet locking. Posterior plating and fixation are easy and efficient, as demonstrated by the mechanical results. This fixation is also very helpful for tumor-related instability.

At the level of the upper cervical spine, the use of the special occipitocervical plates increases confidence in the immediate postoperative stability when an occipitocervical fusion is necessary.

←

Fig. 6-89. Occipitocervical fusion after failure of a C1–C2 fusion for rheumatoid disease: (*A*) A–P view; (*B*) lateral view.

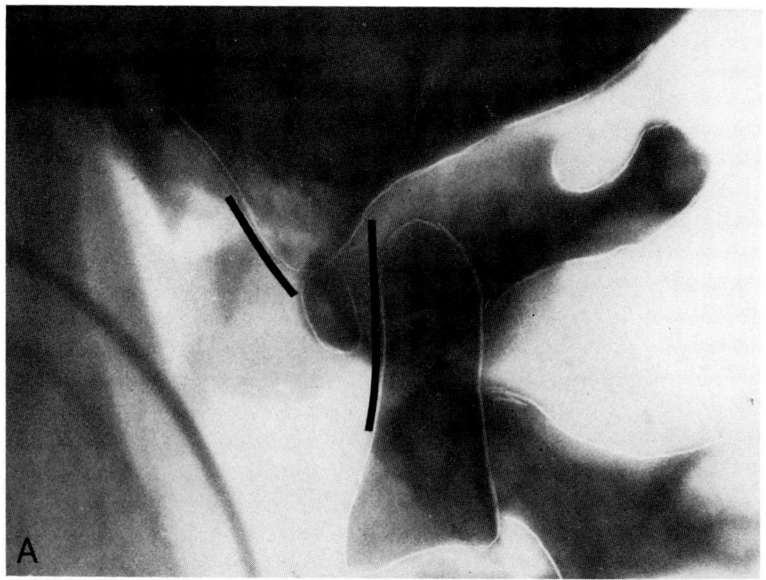

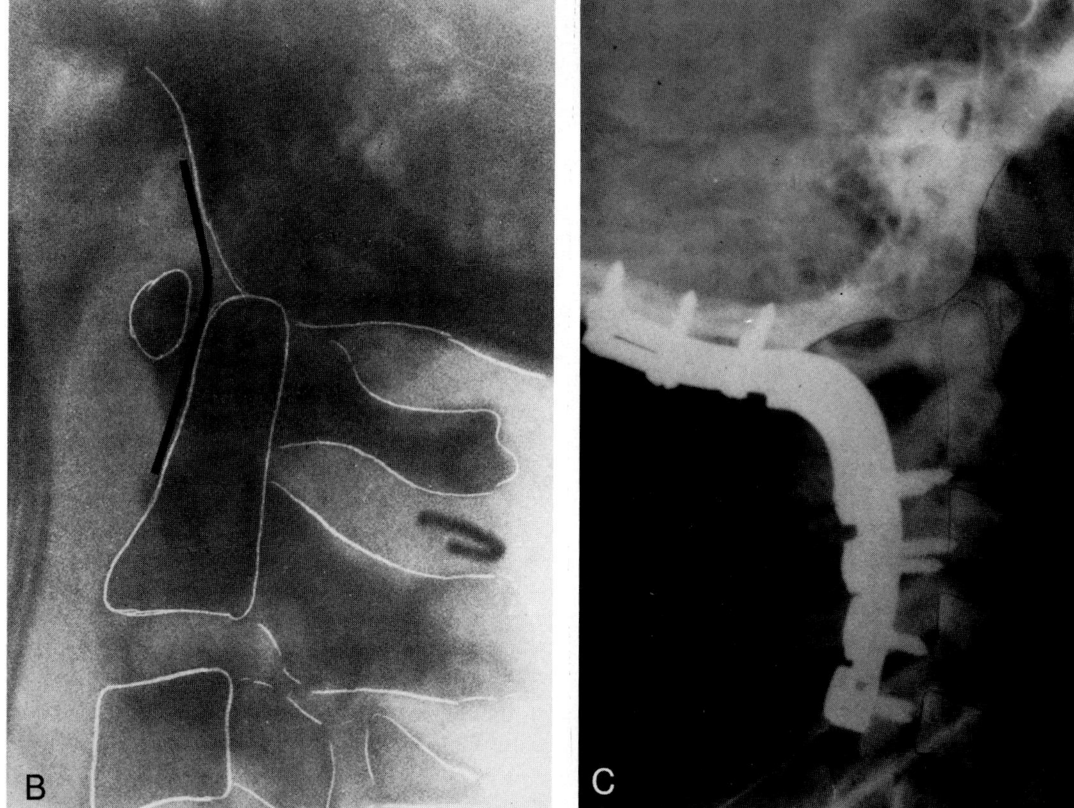

Fig. 6-91. Anterior occipitocervical line: (*A*) anterior occipitocervical dislocation. (*B*) reduction. (*C*) Lateral x-ray showing implant for occipitocervical stabilization.

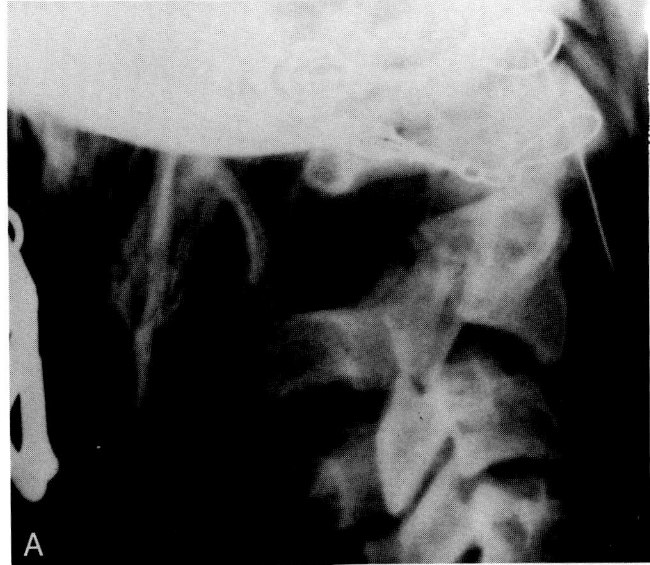

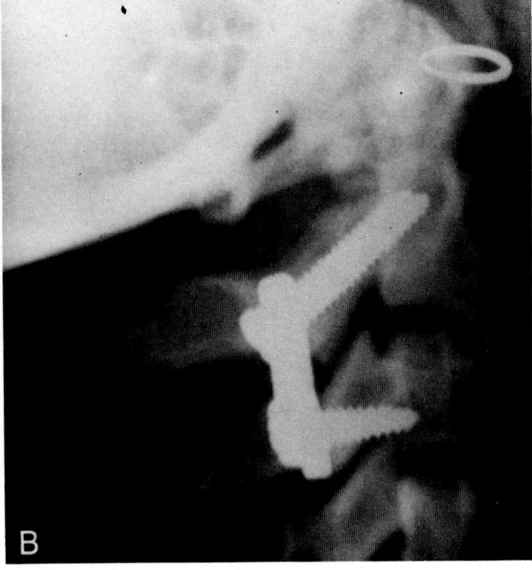

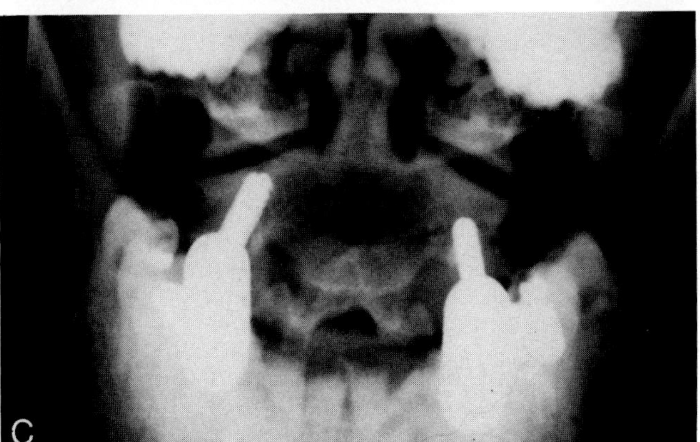

Fig. 6-92. (*A*) Hangman's fracture with a C2–C3 locked-facets dislocation. (*B*) Fixation with two plates, the pedicular screws of C2 achieved the direct fixation of the fracture (*C*) lines.

REFERENCES

1. *Roy-Camile R, Saillant G, Lazennec JY:* Chirurgie par abord postérieur du rachis cervical. In : Encyclopédie médico-chirurgicale. Paris, Techniques chirurgicales (Orthopédie) 44176:12
2. *Roy-Camille R, et al:* Rachis cervical traumatique non neurologique. In Roy-Camille (ed): Leres Journées d'Orthopédie de la Pitie, Masson 1979
3. *Roy-Camille R, Saillant G, Sagnet P:* Luxation fracture du rachis. In Detrie P (ed): Chirurgie d'urgence, pp 750–766. Masson, 1985
4. *Roy-Camille R, Bouchet T, Saillant G:* Décompression postérieure occipito-atloidienne par élargissement du trou occipital et laminectomie de C1. In Roy-Camille (ed): 5èmes Journées d'Orthopédie de la Pitie, Rachis Cervical Supérieur, pp 32–35. Masson, 1986
5. *Roy-Camille R, Gagna G, Lazennec JY:* L'arthrodése occipito-cervicale. In Roy-Camille (ed): 5êmes Journées d'Orthopédie de la Pitie. Rachis Cervical Supérieur, pp 49–51. Masson, 1986
6. *Roy-Camille R, Saillant G, Bouchet T:* Technique du vissage des pédicules de C2. In Roy-Camille (ed): 5émes Journées d'Orthopédie de la Pitie. Rachis Cervical Supérieur, pp 41–43. Masson, 1986

Internal Fixation with Metal Plates and Screws

ANDREAS WEIDNER

Instability or the loss of stability of the cervical spine is a pathologic state that can arise through trauma, degenerative changes, tumors, and infection, and also as a result of surgery (laminectomy). Instability limits the function of the spine, produces pain, and means that the spine is no longer in the position of being able to protect the spinal cord and nerve roots from mechanical damage. It is therefore essential to recover any stability lost in the spine.

Through the use of an external support a bone injury can be allowed to heal, or by means of a spondylodesis, to strengthen.[7,19] Discoligamentous injuries, however, require long-term support, which is often a great strain on the patient. External immobilization is especially a burden on patients whose life expectancy has already been curtailed through malignancy.

Absolute immobilization cannot be achieved by means of an external support such as a halo. Nor is it possible to restrict only one cervical segment, as external immobilization encompasses the whole cervical spine.[22,25,46]

Surgical techniques for stabilizing the cervical spine without metal plates have long been known and successfully implemented. Poly-methyl methacrylate (PMMA) has been used to provide immediate fixation in the cervical spine. Panjabi and colleagues[32] have reported biomechanical studies in which long-term results in 26 patients indicate that this procedure is safe and effective for both immediate and long-term stabilization of cervical spine fracture-dislocations. However, McAfee and coworkers[29] found that long-term results are not always satisfactory. They have 24 cases of significant complications (*e.g.,* delayed loosening or failure of fixation). Stabilization without metal plate fixation occasionally requires additional support externally to allow successful healing of the bone graft or PMMA. Biomechanical investigations in the healing of bone fracture have shown better results when total immobilization is achieved.[1,33] For this reason, internal fixation has been developed that can achieve immediate stabilization of the cervical spine. The essential principles for this have been adopted from long bone surgical techniques, which have world-wide acceptance. Spinal internal fixation has now been achieved with the use of metal plates and screws, in conjunction with autogenous bone grafts.

Even external immobilization has been shown to have its complications, although as a rule these are not serious.[14,16,17] However, complications associated with internal fixation, such as loosening of the plate, suggest that there was a false indication for surgery or that operative technique was poor, and liability cases are common as they are easily demonstrated by x-ray. This has understandably hindered more widespread use of these techniques.

In our own experience of over 180 cervical fusion operations using metal plates, we have only encountered two cases of screw loosening, both of which had no sequelae. The loosening of the screws was due to lack of care and attention to the principle of internal fixation and could have been avoided. More serious complications, such as loosening of the plate, increased neurologic damage, and esophageal or vascular injury were not encountered. Therefore, we are able to recommend this technique when autogenous bone grafts, or in special cases (metastases) bone cement, cannot achieve primary stability and when external immobilization is to be avoided.

INDICATIONS

The use of metal plates and screws on the spine is only an additional method that improves the stability of the spine. The indication for stabilizing interventions is thoroughly described elsewhere in this book. Basically, I see the indication for internal fixation in traumatic changes (Fig. 6-93), spondylectomies (Figs. 6-94 and 6-95), which are necessary for decompression of the spinal cord in cervical myelopathy, and in tumors (Figs. 6-96 and 6-97). In the usual ventral fusion at one level of a hard or soft disc, additional internal fixation with metal plates and screws is not necessary, in my opinion, since the instability risk is very low. However, if at the same time a structural disorder indicating ligamentous instability is present, internal fixation is to be considered (Fig. 6-98).

OSTEOSYNTHESIS OF THE MIDDLE AND LOWER CERVICAL SPINE

Specialized instruments are essential for cervical internal fixation. The originally used metal plates and screws were those that had been developed in

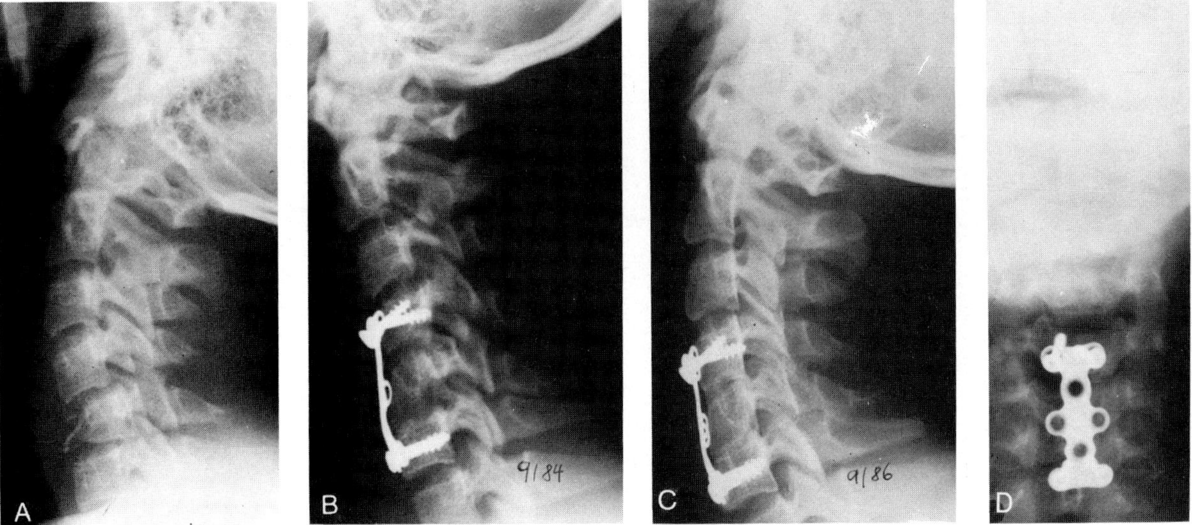

Fig. 6-93. A 16-year-old male patient. (*A*) Teardrop fracture of C5. No neurologic deficits. Immediate spondylectomy of C5 with decompression of the dura. Insertion of an iliac crest graft. AO plate from C4–C6. The right upper screw should have been better placed, because it does not reach the posterior margin of the vertebral body (*B*). Follow-up x-ray obtained 2 years postoperatively reveals consolidated spondylodesis. The plate has not loosened (*C* and *D*).

Fig. 6-94. Cervical myelopathy with narrow spinal canal. Myelographic block at C4–C5 (*A*). Partial spondylectomy of C5 with medial decompression of the dura. Insertion of a bone graft and securing with an AO plate from C4–C6 (*B*). X-ray obtained 6 days postoperatively. The screws do not reach the posterior margin. No signs of loosening are seen 2 years postoperatively.

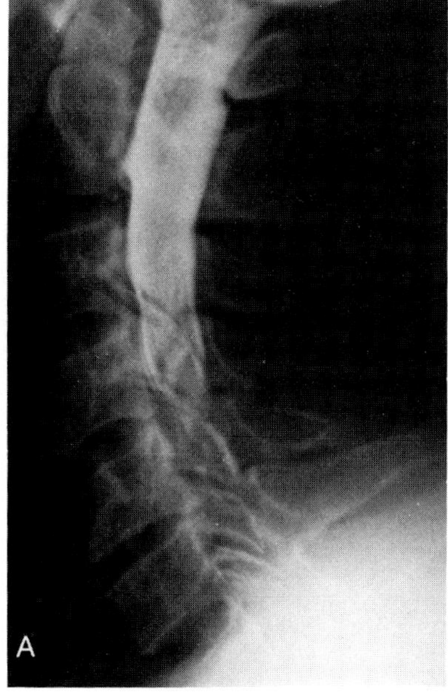

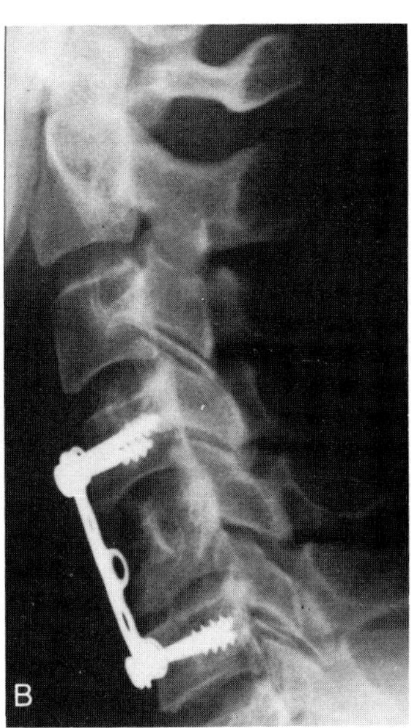

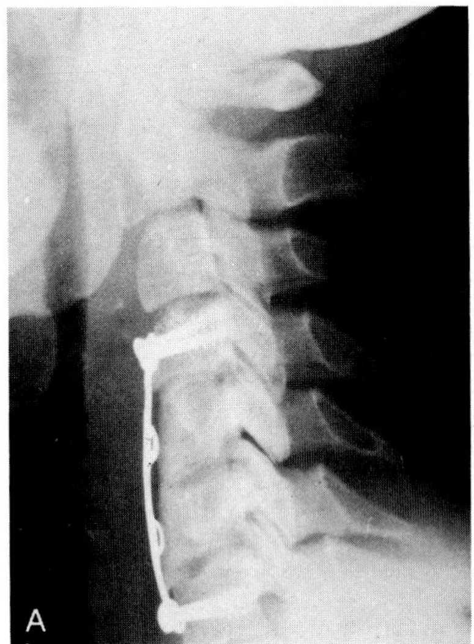

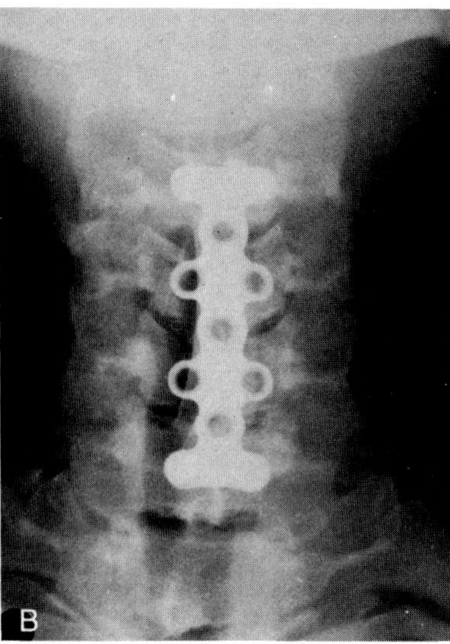

Fig. 6-95. Cervical myelopathy. For decompression of the dura, a partial spondylectomy of the vertebral bodies C5 and C6 was necessary. The vertebral bodies were replaced by an iliac crest graft. AO plate from C4–C7. (*A*) Lateral view. (*B*) A-P view.

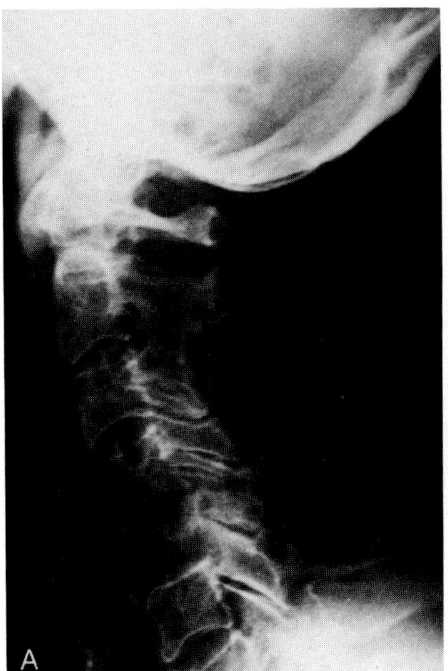

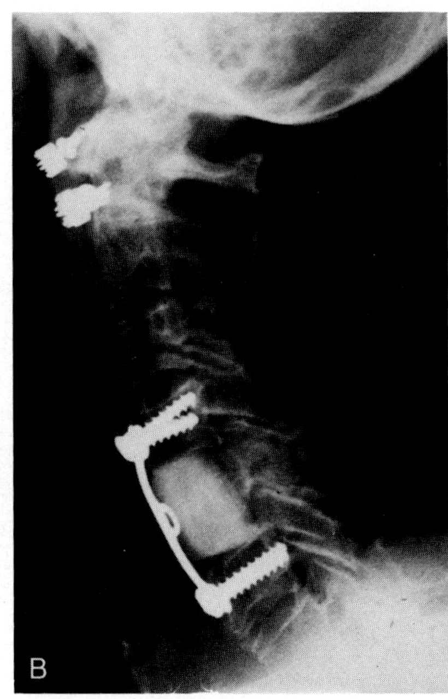

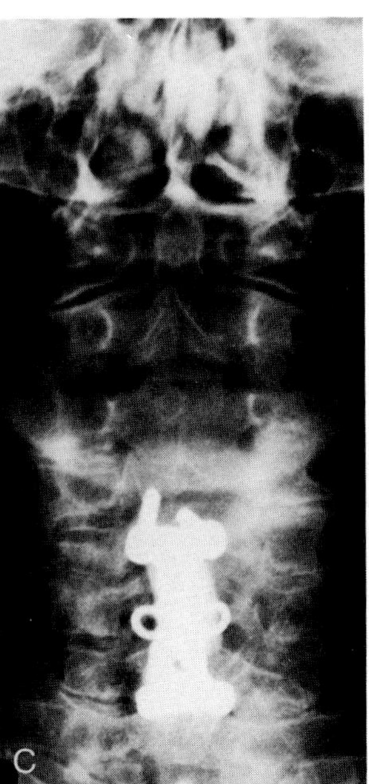

Fig. 6-96. Metastasis of a carcinoma of the breast within C5 with symptoms of instability (*A*). Removal of the metastasis and decompression of the dura. Insertion of a PMMA block and securing with AO plate was performed (*B* and *C*). Immediate postoperative mobilization is possible.

long-bone surgery.[2,18,43] Thus, the metal plates used in ventral spondylodesis had only one row of screw holes (Fig. 6-99*D*). These plates could not prevent rotation in the area of the spondylodesis and plate loosening occurred (Fig. 6-99*C*). The plates now used for ventral spondylodesis have generally two rows of vertical screw holes like the H-plate developed by ASFI[31] and this plate is now the standard method for ventral plating[4,8,15,20] (Figs. 6-93 to 6-96, 6-98, 6-100 to 6-102). Sene-

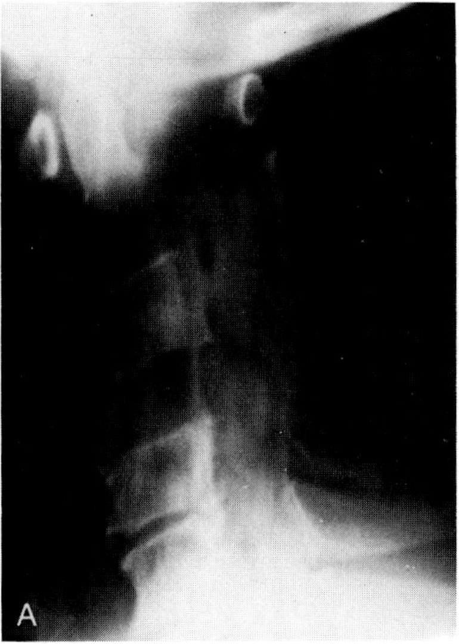

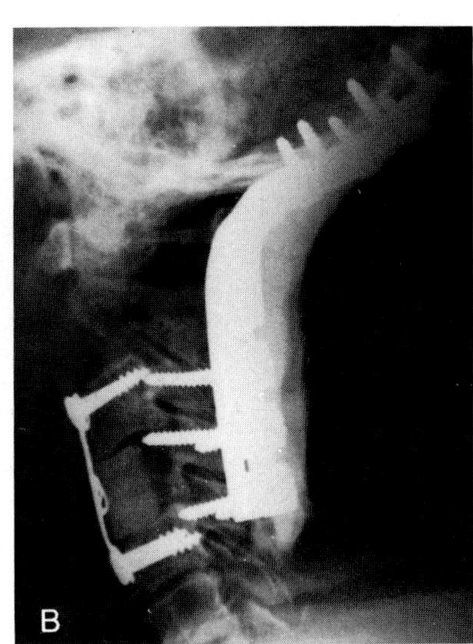

Fig. 6-97. Metastasis of the carcinoma of the prostate at C2 and C4 with therapy-resistant neck pain (*A*). Removal of metastasis at C4, PMMA block, securing with an AO plate. In the same surgery additional dorsal stabilization with two Roy-Camille occipital plates (*B*). Since this involved a malignant process, autogenous bone chips were not used, but a PMMA block was used instead. The patient was mobilized immediately postoperatively. Symptoms ,decreased.

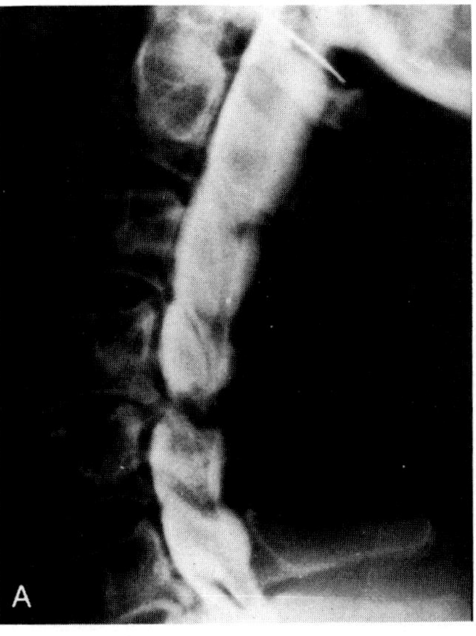

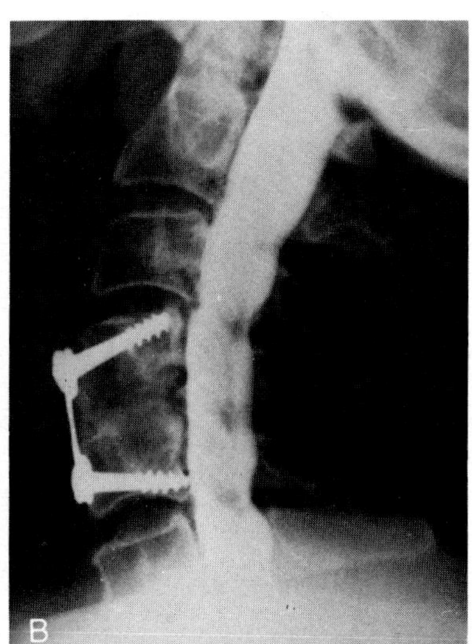

Fig. 6-98. C5–nerve root compression (*left*) and structural disorder at C4–C5 with compression of the spinal cord with retroflexion (*A*). Decompression takes place with discectomy at C4–C5, osteochondrosis is removed, and a bone block is inserted and secured with an AO plate, owing discoligamentous instability. Two years postoperatively, myelography shows a C6–nerve root compression (*right*): Spondylodesis is consolidated at the level of C4–C5, no loosening of the metal plate exists, and spinal cord compression is no longer detectable (*B*).

gas,[40] Strehli,[42] Fuentes,[12,13] and Caspar[5,6] have also developed plates that allow exact positioning of the screws. For dorsal spondylodesis, plates have been developed by Roy-Camille[36–38] (Figs. 6-97*B*, 6-99*E*, 6-103, 6-104*B*), Louis,[26] Fuentes,[13] and Magerl[27] (Fig. 6-105) that are specially tailored to the cervical spine.

In vitro biomechanical investigations have shown that the best stabilization is achieved using a combined hold, both ventral and dorsal fixation and that when used alone dorsal fusion produces higher stability than ventral fusion.[44,45] Clinical experience has shown, however, that ventral fixation using a metal plate is adequate biomechanically *in vivo.*[5,6,8,15,18]

In injuries that involve spinal cord compression or vertebral body tumors, it is essential to decompress the spinal cord. This is only possible through a ventral approach. The decision between ventral and dorsal fixation is therefore also dependent on the necessity of spinal cord decompression.

The disadvantage of the ventral approach is that

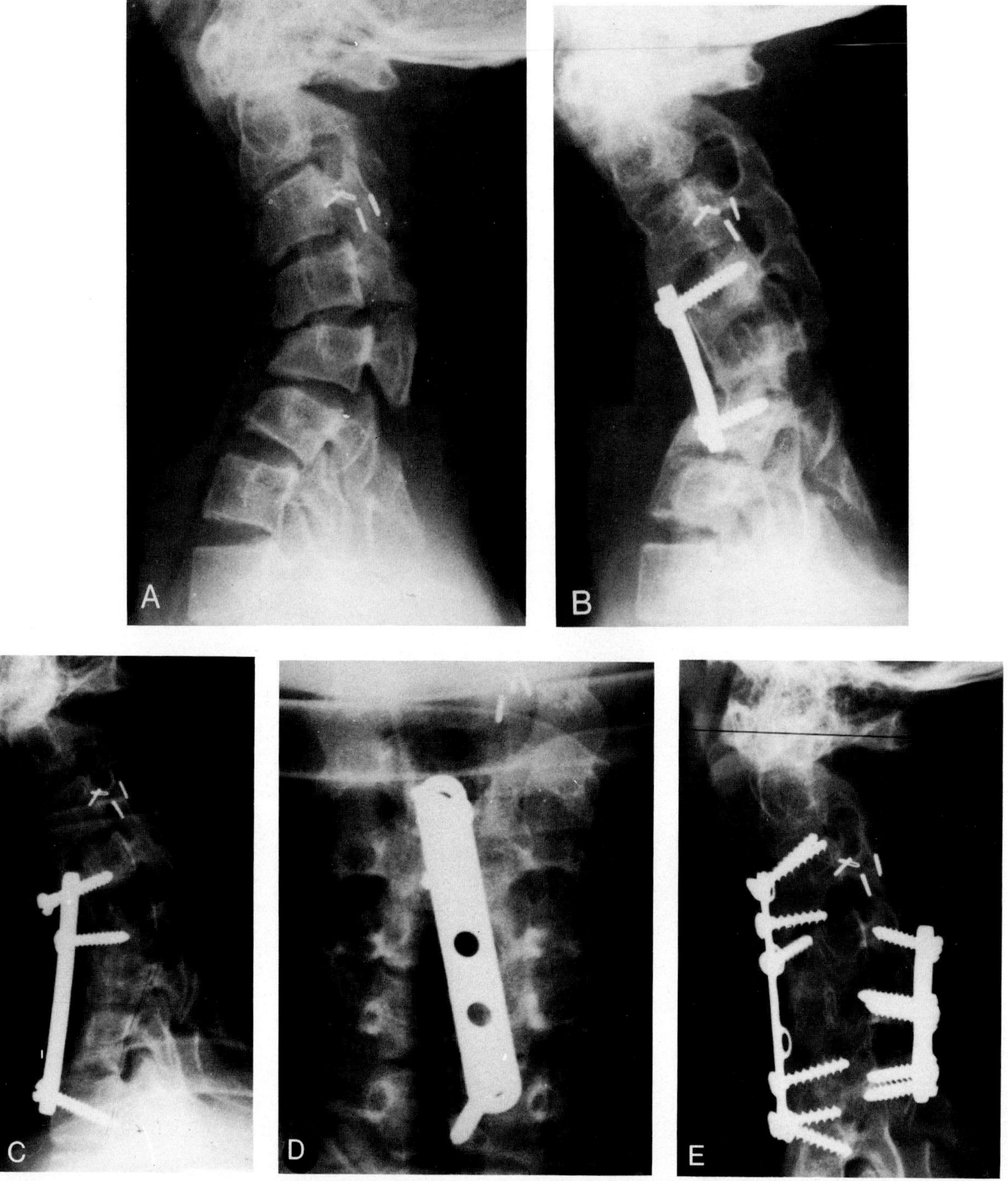

Fig. 6-99. Kyphosis after laminectomy (*A*). The metal plate C4–C6 is too short, resulting in increasing kyphosis with spinal cord compression (*B*). The metal plate was changed. This one-hole plate did not produce sufficient rotatory stability ventrally, and the upper screw loosened (*C* and *D*). The metal plate was changed again and a ventral AO plate with two rows of holes was inserted. In this case, the screws were also established into the bone block. This is not indicated with shorter fusion sections. To improve stability, dorsal Roy-Camille plates were applied bilaterally (*E*).

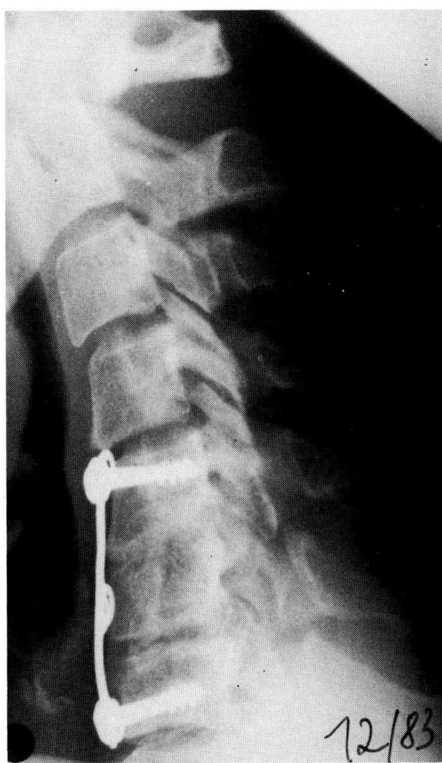

Fig. 6-100. Spondylectomy of C6 for cervical myelopathy. The applied AO plate is too long and impinges on C4 cranially, which produces irritation within this intervertebral segment. Because of these movements, loosening of the plate is possible.

it is not always possible to reposition locked facets. This is more easily achieved through a dorsal approach. It is also possible to decompress nerve roots through partial removal of the facet by means of the dorsal approach.

From personal experience, I favor the ventral approach, as the neck muscles, which are essential for stability, are not weakened.[41] Furthermore, in multiple injuries, especially unstable rib fractures, positioning of the patient is less a problem.[35] In pseudoarthrosis after ventral spondylodesis, I prefer the dorsal osteosynthesis (Fig. 6-103).

VENTRAL OSTEOSYNTHESIS

The operation is performed using lateral image intensification. However, A–P imaging does not appear necessary, as the midline can be marked preoperatively using the chin and the jugulum. The midline can also be determined intraoperatively (see below). When using the imager to visualize the lower cervical spine it is important to pull the shoulders caudally by means of a heavy bandage. Secure venous access is also extremely important, as it is very difficult for the anesthetist to gain access to the veins of the limbs during the operation. A nasogastric tube can also be helpful in allowing the position of the esophagus to be felt. Throughout the operation, the cervical lordosis should be maintained.

The approach to the ventral spine has often been described (see Chapter 13). After decompression of the spinal cord or removal of the tumor, disc, or vertebral body, an autogenous illiac bone graft is inserted in the normal fashion, for which purpose the Casper instruments[5,6] are particularly useful. Once the bone graft has been inserted and the retraction released, the correct length of plate can be determined. There are different sizes available (see Figs. 6-93*B*, 6-95, 6-98*B*). The metal plate should only cover the area to be fused and should not impinge either caudally or cranially onto the other vertebrae, as any movement of these vertebrae would cause movement of the plate, thereby loosening it (see Fig. 6-100).

The metal plate should lie exactly in the midline of the vertebral body. There are three methods by which the midline can be exactly determined.

1. Preoperatively, it is possible to draw lines using the chin and the jugulum, which can then be used intraoperatively to determine the midline. (Beware of distortion of the skin by traction and covering of the markings prior to operation.)
2. It is also possible to use the symmetrical lines formed by the longus colli muscles above and below the fusion area in order to estimate the midline.
3. In cases where destruction due to scarring or tumor prevents either *1* or *2* from being applicable, it is possible to estimate the midline intraoperatively by locating the uncinate processes both caudal and cranial to the fusion area, which lie to either side of the midline.

When the plate is correctly positioned on the midline, the cortex of the caudal vertebral body on the side of the surgeon is perforated. Using continuous image intensification, the passage for the screw is then drilled using an instrument 2 mm in diameter. While the surgeon is observing the intensifier image, the assistant surgeon observes the actual operative site to ensure that no vessels are damaged by the drill despite the safety cover. It is possible to use instruments with a predeter-

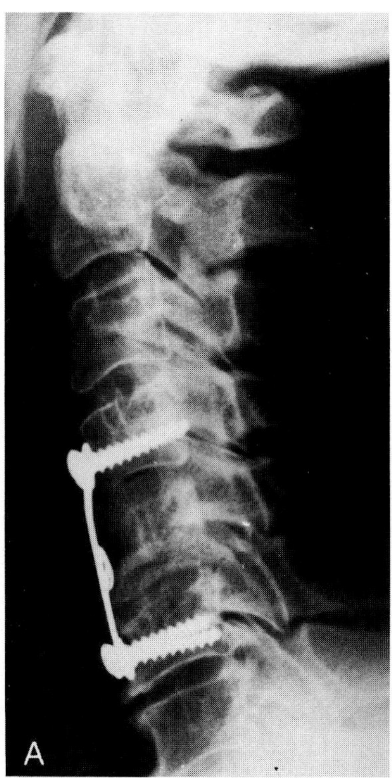

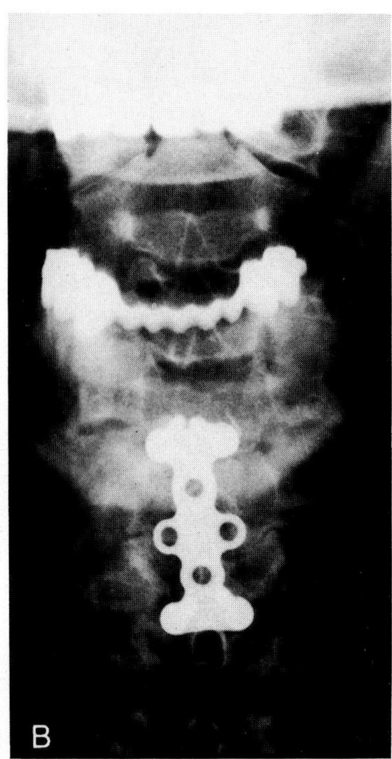

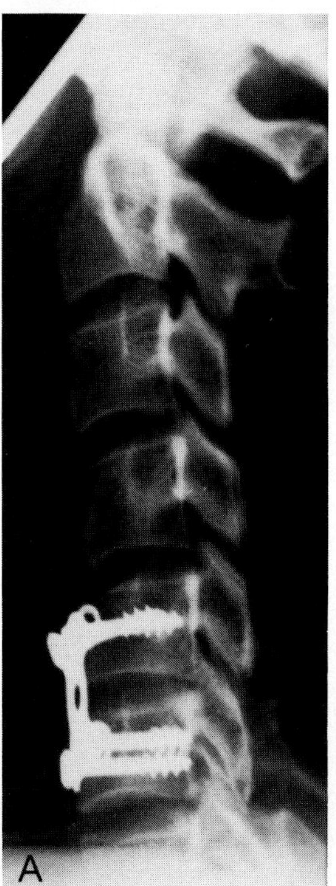

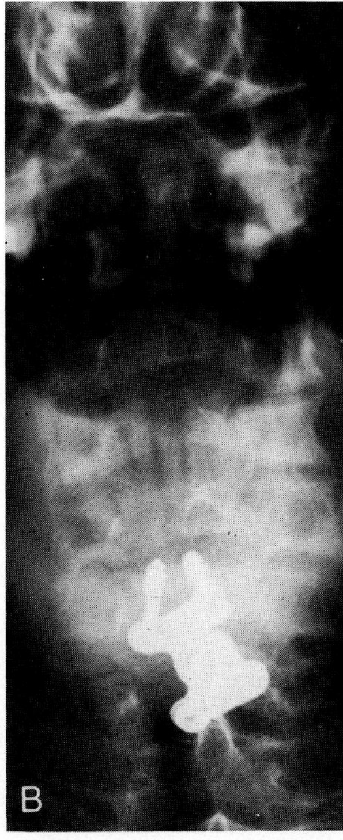

Fig. 6-101 and 6-102. Intraoperatively with lateral imaging (Figs. 101*A* and 102*A*), one can recognize if the metal plate lies within the bodily axis. If the upper or lower two holes of the plate are superimposed then the plate is placed correctly. If the drill holes are not superimposed as in Figure 102A, then the plate lies transversely to the bodily axis. Figures 6-101*B* and 6-102*B*, Anteroposterior views.

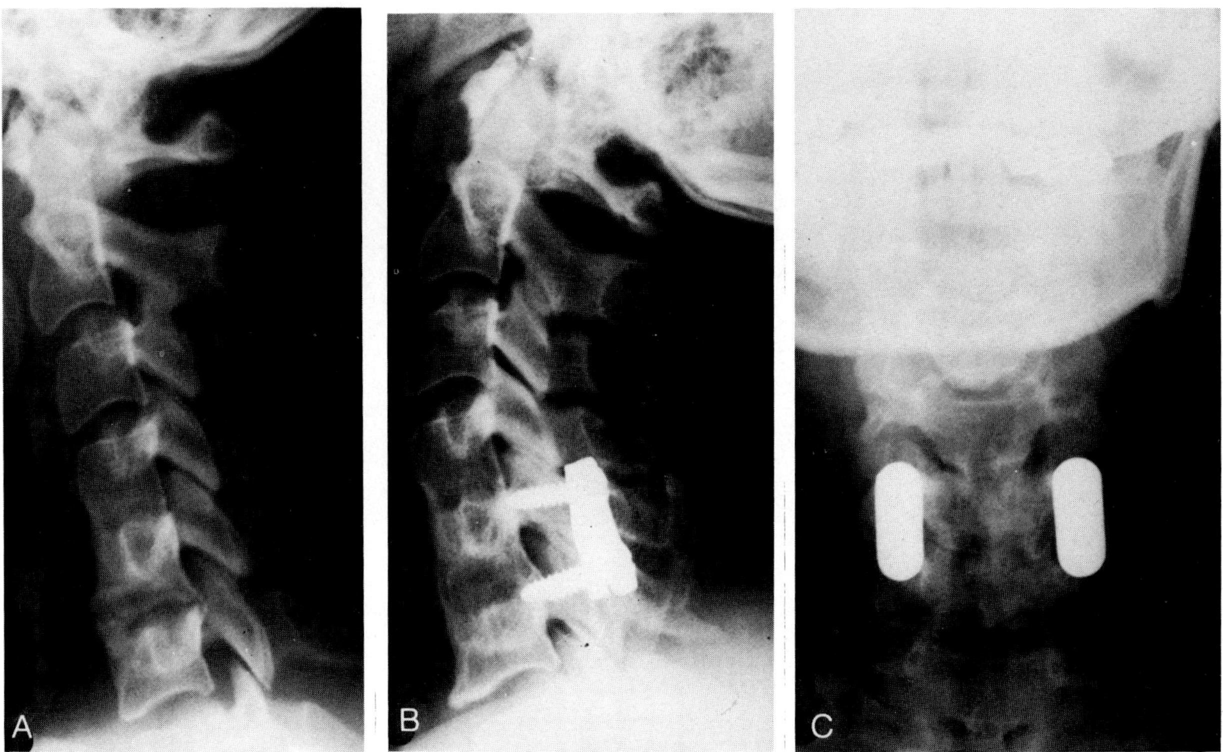

Fig. 6-103. Pseudoarthrosis at C5–C6 after ventral fusion of C4–C5 and C5–C6 (*A*). Healing of pseudoarthrosis with dorsal fusion with Roy-Camille plates to C5–C6 and additional interlaminar autogenous bone chips (*B* and *C*).

mined safety guard, which allow drilling to occur only to a certain depth. This can prevent possible damage to the spinal cord. From personal experience of 125 ventral fusion operations, I find that it is not necessary to puncture the dorsal vertebral body cortex with the drill. Using x-ray control drilling continues until just before the dorsal cortex is reached. The length of the screw is then measured. It is very important to ensure that the plate lies tight against the vertebral body to prevent even the slightest movement between the plate and the vertebral body (Figs. 6-98 and 6-101).

A screw, approximately 1 mm longer than the previously measured length, is then inserted and should reach the dorsal vertebral body cortex (Figs. 6-95, 6-96, and 6-101). The first screw is not fully tightened. At this point it is possible to ensure that the plate is lying directly on the midline by use of a lateral imager. If the plate is positioned correctly, the upper two screw holes will be superimposed on each other and will be seen as one hole (Fig. 6-101), whereas if the plate is tilted, two distinct holes will be visible (Fig. 6-102). Thus, it is possible to realign the plate before the top screw hole is drilled. The top screw on the same side is then similarly inserted.

The screws on the opposite side of the plate are inserted by the same method.

Initially, only screws with very short threads were available (Fig. 6-93, 6-94, and 6-100). Now preference is given to screws with a continuous thread of 3.5 mm diameter (Fig. 6-96 and 6-101). Using spongiosa screws, it is not necessary to cut a channel for the thread, as the freshly cut spongiosa provides a better grip for the screw. It is important that the screws be inserted only once into any screw hole, in order not to disrupt the spongiosa.

Only after all the screws have been inserted are they tightened fully so that they reach the dorsal cortex. The tips of the screws are rounded so that there is no danger of damaging the dura or spinal cord (Fig. 6-98). On the other hand, I have per-

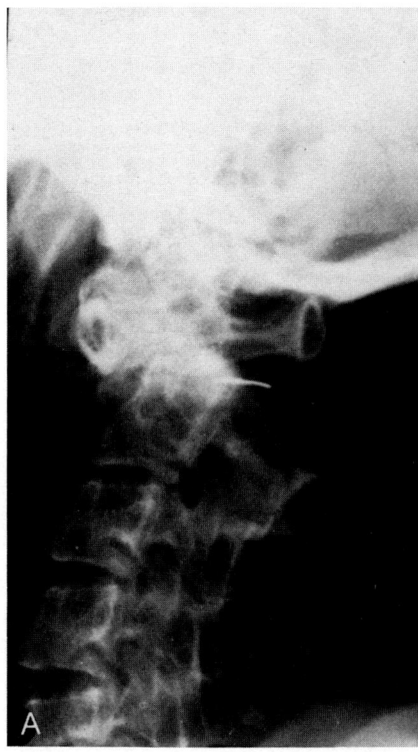

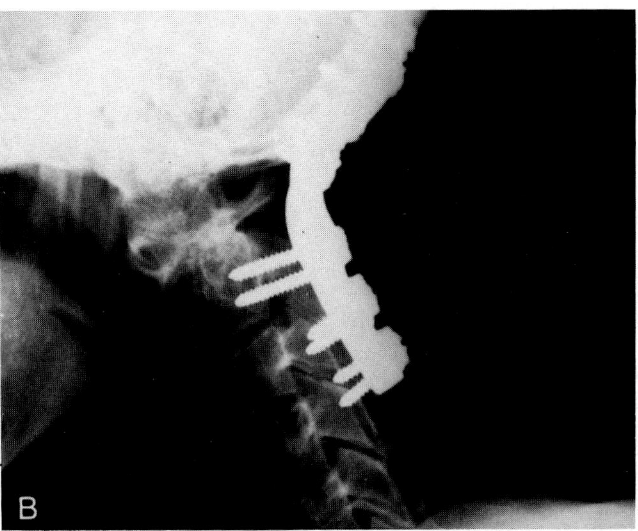

Fig. 6-104. Atlantodental instability with chronic polyarthritis and spinal cord compression (*A*). For decompression of the dura, the arch of C1 was removed. Stabilization with an occipital plate was developed by Roy-Camille. Additional autogenous iliac crest graft at occiput–C2 (*B*). The metal plate was removed after healing of the bone chip.

sonally never seen screw or plate loosening even when the screws have only been inserted into two thirds of the vertebral body (Fig. 6-93*B, C,* and 6-94). Because the front surface of the vertebral body is curved, it is possible that certain views on lateral imaging may give the false impression that the screws have not been fully inserted (Fig. 6-102).

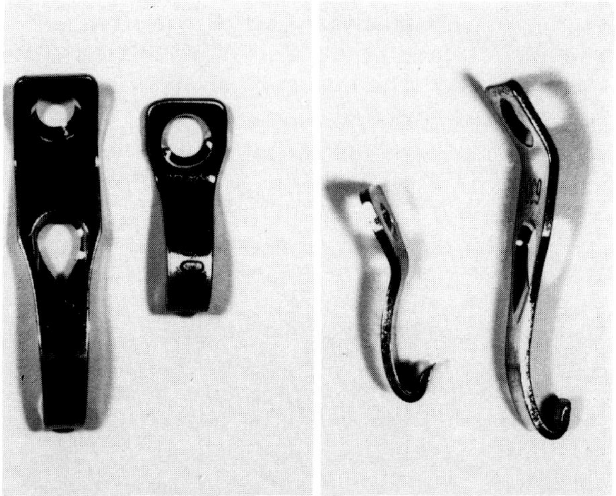

Fig. 6-105. Design of hook plates developed by Magerl. (Magerl F, Grob D, Seemann P: Stable dorsal fusion of the cervical spine [C2–Th1] using hook plates. In Kehr P, Weidner A [eds]: Cervical Spine I, p 217. Wien-New York, Springer Verlag, 1987)

Before completing the operation, the correct position of the plate and screws must be confirmed using lateral and finally A–P imaging. If even by correction the exact position cannot be achieved, it is best to remove the ventral plate and rely on postoperative halo immobilization. Severe complications are only encountered through lack of attention to these details.

POSTOPERATIVE CARE

There is no need for external immobilization postoperatively (Fig. 6-106), although patients find a cervical collar useful for the first 4 to 6 weeks. Isometric physiotherapy to strengthen the paravertebral muscles can begin 2 weeks postoperatively when the spondylodesis is stable.

Lateral x-rays are done routinely at 6 days and 6 weeks in order to detect any postoperative complications.

Removal of the plate is not indicated, if the spon-

Fig. 6-106. Patient 3 weeks after spondylectomy of C5 and internal fixation. Cervical support for 3 weeks (x-ray refers to Fig. 6-93). (*A*) Flexion. (*B*) Extension.

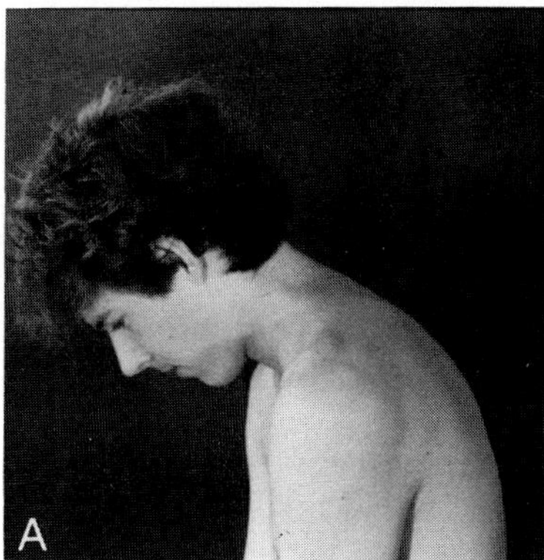

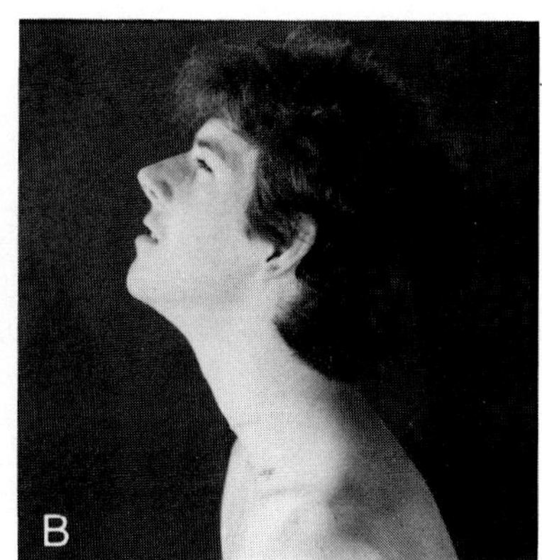

dylodesis has consolidated firmly and if the screws have not loosened.

INTRAOPERATIVE COMPLICATIONS

Even without considering the metal plate and screws, complications such as loosening of the bone graft or injury to the vertebral artery, the esophagus, or the spinal cord can occur during a fusion operation. Complications associated with attaching the metal plate are rarely encountered when intraoperative anatomic landmarks are used to position the plate correctly in the midline and continuous imaging is used during the insertion of the screws. One danger is that during drilling, vessels may become entangled in the drill if the safety cover fails to function properly. It is also possible to injure the esophagus should a fold lie between the vertebra and the metal plate. Both complications can be avoided if the retractors are correctly positioned around the drilling area when the screws are being fully tightened.

POSTOPERATIVE COMPLICATION

Using the above technique, I have never experienced loosening of the plate. In my clinical experience of 125 ventral spondylodeses involving metal plates, screw loosening has occurred only twice. Both of these were due to technical errors in which the screws were originally too loosely inserted, owing to vertebral sinuses. If a screw fails to grip the spongiosa of the vertebral body, then the screw should be reinserted in another direction. The screw must be inserted to the hilt so that scar tissue associated with the screw is avoided. If scar tissue does form on the screw, then movement of this tissue through swallowing and movement of the cervical spine will eventually loosen the screw. Thus, postoperative x-ray follow up is essential.

Severe osteoporosis is a contraindication to ventral plate fixation.

The danger of plate loosening arises more often with the use of artificial bone cement than with autogenous illiac bone grafts, as bone cement cannot form a solid bone spondylodesis and even the slightest bone movement can lead to plate loosening. For this reason we only use bone cement in conjunction with ventral metal plates in metastatic disease (Fig. 6-96 and 6-97). I have not experienced loosening of the plate, even in these patients, as the postoperative activities of these patients are of course more restricted than those of adolesscent motor bike riders who require internal fixation of their cervical injuries (Figs. 6-93 and 6-106).

Two patients out of about 180 spondylodesies involving metal implants developed infections, despite prophylactic perioperative antibiotics. In these patients, the implants were removed and halo immobilization offered. In our clinical experience this was necessary in only one case, while in the other the spondylodesis was already stable.

DORSAL OSTEOSYNTHESIS

Biomechanical investigations have shown that a dorsal plate spondylodesis produces better stability then a ventral plate approach.[44]

Studies using the dorsal plate developed by Roy-Camille show that in flexion stress the posterior wiring between the spinous processes provides a

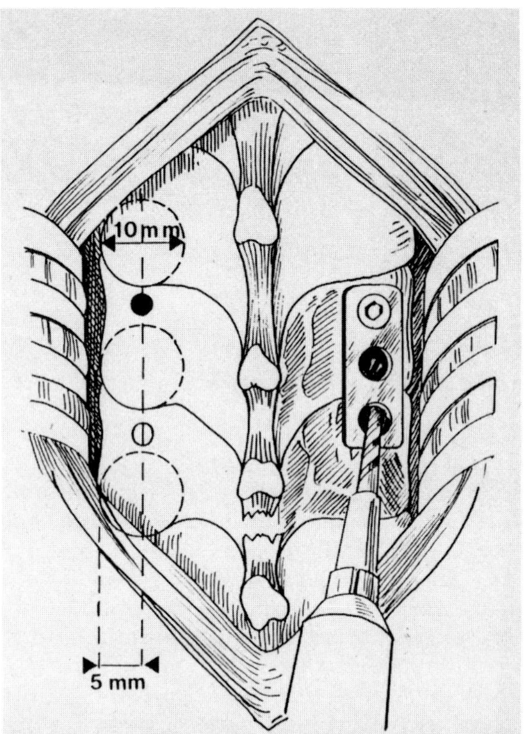

Fig. 6-107. The points of screw penetration are identified as follows: The projection of the articular surfaces on the vertebral arches is first identified by inscribing a 1-cm diameter circle beginning at the posteroinferior angle of the vertebral arches. The point of screw penetration lies halfway between two adjacent articular projections and 5 mm medial to the lateral margin of the articular pillars. (Louis R: Posterior Vertebral Bone Plates. Paris, Ceprime, 1982)

3% increase in stability, the same wiring around a complementary bone graft results in a 55% increase in stability, and the increase is of 88% when the wiring passes through the articular masses. The plate fixation provides a 92% increase in stability.[38]

Using this technique of plates and screws in the articular facets, it is possible to stabilize all dorsal cervical injuries. However, it is essential to preoperatively exclude ventral compression of the spinal cord or nerve root through a slipped disc or bone fragment. The operation is carried out with the patient in the prone position and the head firmly held in a device that allows a flexion–extension range of movement as well as the application of traction. Lateral image intensification should also be used as in the ventral approach. It is essential that the paraspinal muscles be well retracted laterally so that the facets are visible on both sides. A wide caudal–cranial approach is required so that the paraspinal muscles are not compressed through extreme tension.

There are exact anatomic points through which drill holes should be made (Fig. 6-107). Roy-Camille compares the dorsal aspect of the vertebra to a hilly landscape. The valley is the area between the lamina and the facets, and the articular mass is analogous to a hill. The vertebral artery is found in front of the valley and the plates are attached to the peak of the articular facets so that during drilling neither the vertebral artery nor the radicular nerve is encountered. The procedure is done with a 2.8 mm drill when a 3.5 mm screw is used. A special drill is used with a depth gauge to prevent drilling too far forward. The direction is perpendicular to the vertebral plane of 10° oblique laterally, but never medially to avoid damaging the vertebral artery. The screws are 16 or 19 mm long and are inserted under continuous imaging. It is easy to establish the position of the screw using lateral imaging.

Initially, autogenous bone chips were used in conjunction with the plates (Fig. 6-103), but further experience has shown that the plate alone is sufficient, as the facets themselves fuse together.

Severe osteoporosis is also a contraindication for dorsal-plate spondylodesis, as it is for ventral, because the screws are unable to achieve a firm hold.

Screw loosening does not produce the same problems in a dorsal approach as in a ventral approach, because there is no danger to either the esophagus or the trachea.

Postoperatively, Roy-Camille additionally applies a cervical collar for 6 weeks in patients with a unilateral dislocation, and for those with more unstable lesions immobilization is maintained with a Minerva cast for 4 to 6 weeks.[38]

In our own experience, we have found that a cervical collar worn 4 to 6 weeks provides sufficient immobilization.

In a series of 221 patients with lower cervical injuries, Roy-Camille has seen no secondary displacement in 85.2% of the cases.[38]

In cooperation with the ASFI (AO), Magerl[27] has described a method of dorsally stabilizing the spine from C2 to T1 by means of a hook plate (Figs. 6-105 and 6-108). He has used this technique since 1979. The principle is that a hook is placed beneath the lamina, so that a small notch prevents it from slipping laterally into the joint. The position of the hook is immediately medial to the facet joint. In the superior vertebra the plate is anchored with a screw, which is inserted as shown in Figure 6-108. In this way, damage to the vertebral artery or the nerve roots is easily avoided. A bone graft is applied as a buttress between the spinous processes to achieve a three-point fixation.

Between 1979 and 1984 Magerl operated on 40 patients with this method, and none experienced any pseudoarthrosis.[27]

In comparison with the method of Roy-Camille[36–38] and Louis,[26] if only a single drilling per side is required. From the biomechanical point of view, it is superior to all other fixation techniques.[44] However, compared with the technique of Roy-Camille, an additional bone graft is required. In the case of damaged lamina after laminectomy the hook plate can be used only by increasing the fusion area.

OSTEOSYNTHESIS OF THE UPPER CERVICAL SPINE

The craniocervical junction can be reached and stabilized both by a ventral or dorsal approach. The ventral decompression of the spinal cord is possible by a transoral approach (see Chapter 13).[9,39] However, this approach has the disadvantage of operating through a potentially infected area (the pharynx). A dens fixation can be carried out extrapharyngeally[23,24,30] through a ventrolateral approach using the technique described by Böhler[3] and Knöringer.[21]

Generally with ventral processes, especially in the case of rheumatoid arthritis, a transoral decompression of the medulla is carried out and followed by a dorsal fusion.[10]

VENTRAL DENS FIXATION

The fixation is carried out[3,21] with the patient in a supine position under traction. An anteromedial approach is made at the level of the cricoid cartilage. The skin is undermined and the platysma split longitudinally. The retropharyngeal space is reached medial to the neurovascular bundles, and a blunt dissection is carried out above the anterior longitudinal ligament up to the base of the second cervical vertebra. From there a 1.8-mm drill is inserted from the base into the dens under lateral and A–P imaging. A screw of appropriate length is inserted to the tip of the dens. As this does not achieve rotational stability, an additional screw is inserted parallel to the first in the same direction.

Knöringer[21] has developed a special instrumen-

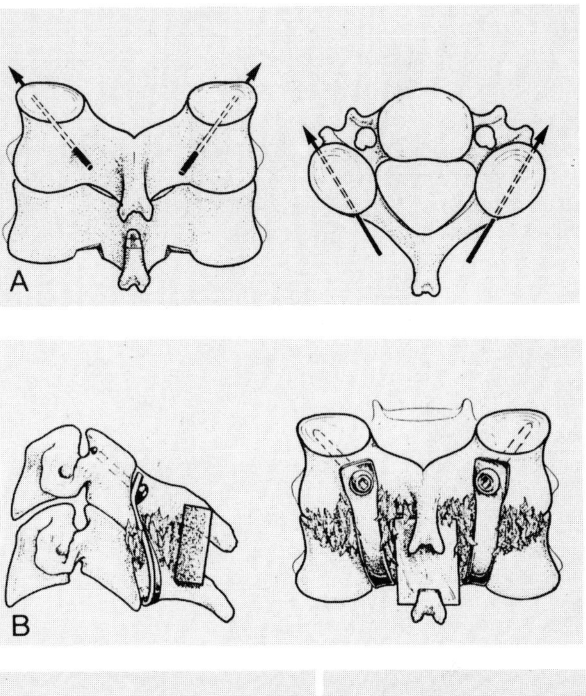

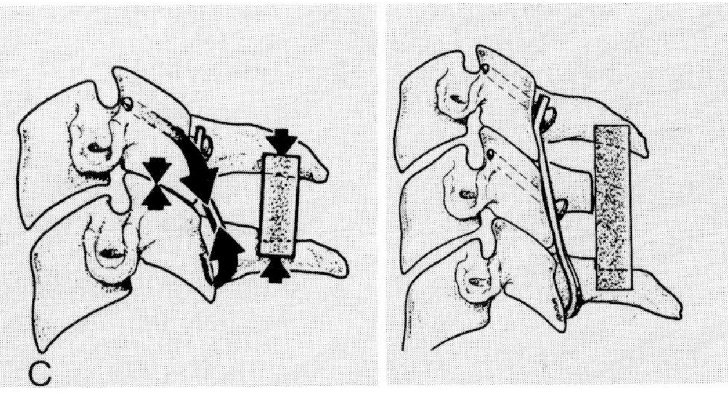

Fig. 6-108. (*Top*) Direction of the screws. The notches for the hooks in the lower lamina and for the H graft in the lower spinal process are shown. (*Middle*) Hook plate fixation. The screws lie parallel to the articular surfaces. The plates are twisted to adapt to the bone surface. An H graft is placed between the spinal processes. Cancellous chips are applied. (*Bottom left*) Biomechanics of the hook plate fixation. Since the resulting force vector created by the plates lies within this triangle, the fusion is stable in all directions. (*Bottom right*) Hook plate fixation over two intervertebral segments (cancellous chips are not shown). Magerl F, Grob D, Seeman P: Stable dorsal fusion of the cervical spine [C2–Th1] using hook plates. In Kehr P, Weidner A [eds]: Cervical Spine 1, p 217. Wein-New York, Springer Verlag, 1987)

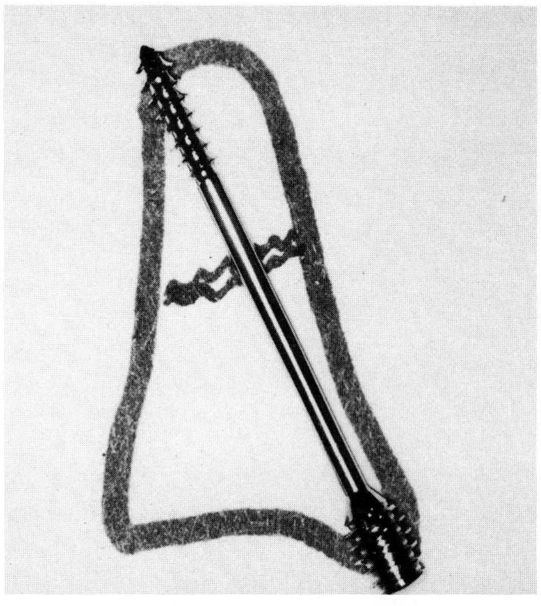

Fig. 6-109. Double-threaded compression screw developed by Knöringer.[21] The caudal screw thread is firmly anchored within the vertebral body of C2 and does not irritate the segment C2–C3. No threads lie within the fractured space. The dorsal cortex of the dens is utilized fully for anchorage.

tarium; the screws do not have any screw-heads, which could produce irritation to the intervertebral segment of C2–C3, but have a second thread that lies within the cortical substance of the second cervical vertebra. By the different pitch of both screw threads, compression of the fractured gap is produced. He also uses parallel-positioned screws so that rotational stability is achieved (Fig. 6-109 and 6-110).

The advantage of this method is that the range of motion of the craniocervical junction is not restricted postoperatively. Essential complications experienced with this method are not described by Böhler[3] and Knöringer.[21]

ATLANTOAXIAL SCREW FIXATION

This technique was developed by Magerl[28] (Fig 6-111) in 1979. He describes the surgical technique as follows: A midline approach is used and the neural arches are exposed from the occiput to C7. By careful subperiostal dissection, the cranial surface of the isthmus of C2 is exposed bilaterally to the facet joints. The facet joints of C1–C2 are opened, and the posterior surfaces of the inferior articular processes C1 are exposed by approximately 5 mm. K wires are inserted into these processes and used to retract the soft tissues containing the greater occipital nerve and its accompanying venous plexus. The C1–C2 joints are visible. Reduction may be verified visually, as well as the direction, entering C2 close to the lower edge of the caudal articular process of C2 (Fig. 6-111) crossing the isthmus close to its posterior surface and exiting C2 at the posterior rim of the upper articular surface. The screws are placed through

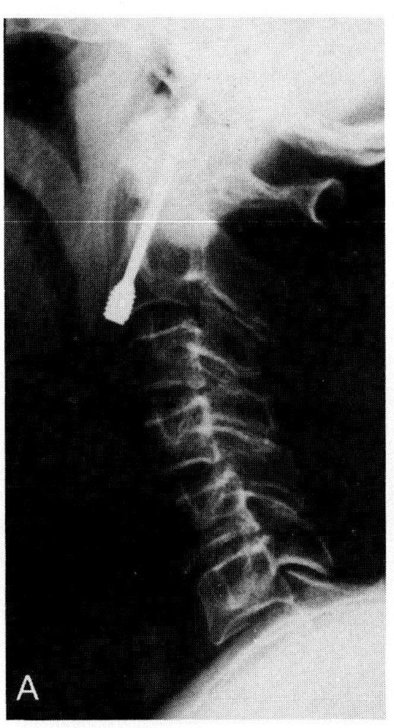

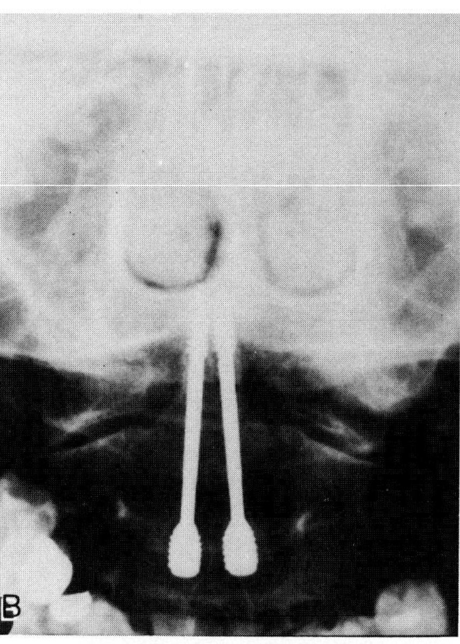

Fig. 6-110. Dens fracture, ventral dens fixation with two Knöringer screws (ref. 21). These x-ray pictures were received with thanks from P. Knöringer, M. D. (Neurosurgical Clinic, 8870 Günzburg, FRG).

the facet joints into the massae laterales. The length of the screws may be checked using an image intensifier. Following screw fixation, a Gallie-type posterior fusion is added (Fig. 6-111).

DORSAL OCCIPITAL CERVICAL INTERNAL FIXATION (Fig. 6-97*B* and 6-104*B*)

The indications for this technique are when fusion of C1 and C2 is insufficient or impossible. In our clinical experience, this is mostly seen in rheumatoid arthritic patients with pseudobasilar invagination, in which occiput support should prevent further collapse. Also in rheumatoid arthritic patients beyond cure, an atlas arch resection was necessary so that preference was given to the occipitocervical fusion (Fig. 6-104*B*).

Ransford and coworkers[34] described a rigid posterior fixation of the skull to the 3rd, 4th and 5th vertebral bones. An anatomically contoured steel loop was secured to occiput via small burr holes, and to the vertebra by sublaminar wiring. A more stable fixation is achieved by using the plate developed by Roy-Camille[38] (Figs. 6-97 and 6-104) and Fuentes.[13]

In these cases we have used a Roy-Camille occipital plate, which was placed from the occiput to the articular facets of C2 to C4, occasionally including C5. This technique corresponds to dorsal fusion of the lower cervical spine. Perforation of the skull is performed by step-by-step drilling using a thin diamond drill. The drilling is then continued using the normal drill. The screws are 10 to 11 mm long.

COMBINED VENTRAL–DORSAL PLATE OSTEOSYNTHESIS

The majority of cervical instabilities can be rectified by use of either a ventral or dorsal approach. In our clinical experience of 180 cervical fusions involving metal plates, we have only found it necessary in three cases to perform a combined operation. These are special cases such as multiple cervical metastases. Another special case is that of adolescent cervical kyphosis which is associated with a very high risk of instability.

Case 1 (Fig. 6-97*A* and *B*)

This 72-year-old male patient suffered from therapy-resistant neck pain. X-rays showed osteolysis in C2 and C4. The metastasis was first removed from C4 using a ventrolateral approach and a bone cement block inserted. C3–C5 were then fixed us-

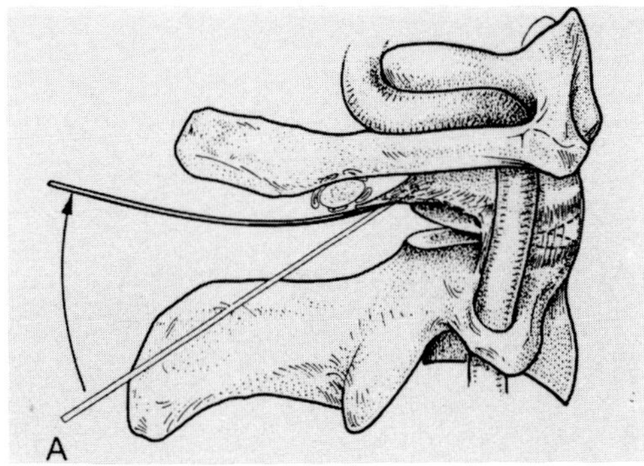

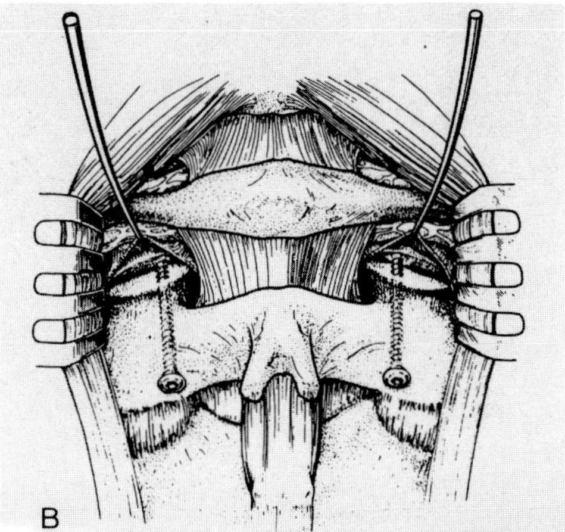

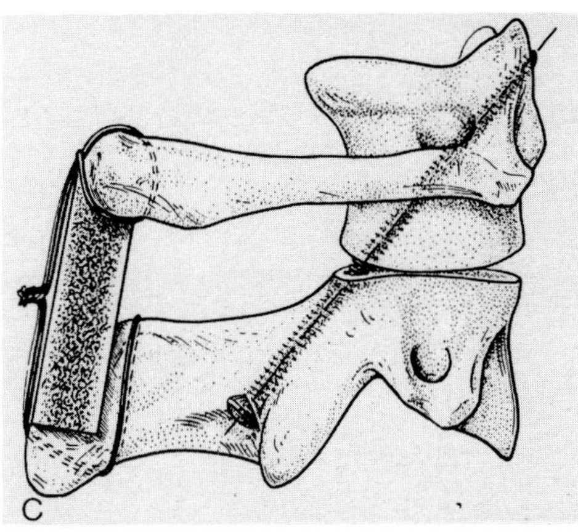

Fig. 6-111. (*Top*) Lateral view of C1 and C2 with the vertebral artery. The K wire reflects the soft tissue containing the occipital nerve and its accompanying venous plexus. (*Middle*) Dorsal view of C1 and C2. The K wire holds back the soft tissue permitting visualization of the C1–C2 joint. The screws are inserted sagittally and may be observed as they go through the joint. (*Bottom*) Lateral view of C1 and C2 with the transarticular screw in place and the standard posterior fusion using corticocancellous bone graft and wire loop. (Magerl F, Seemann P: Stable posterior fusion of the atlas and axis by transarticular screw fixation. In Kehr P, Weidner A [eds]: Cervical Spine I, p 322. Wien-New York, Springer Verlag, 1987)

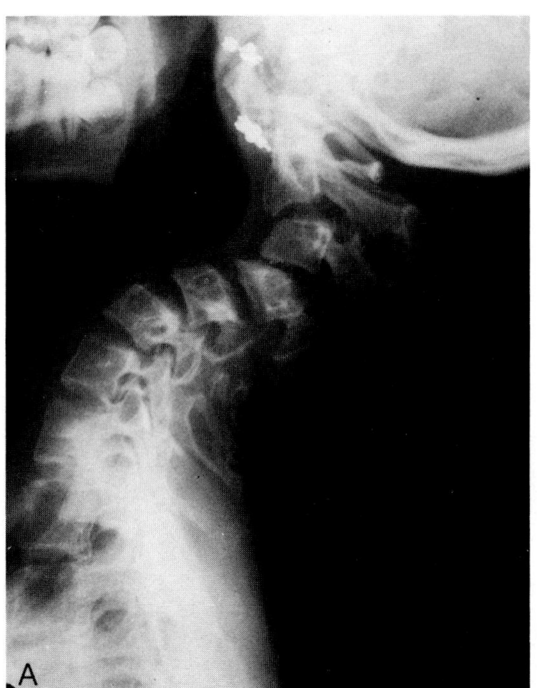

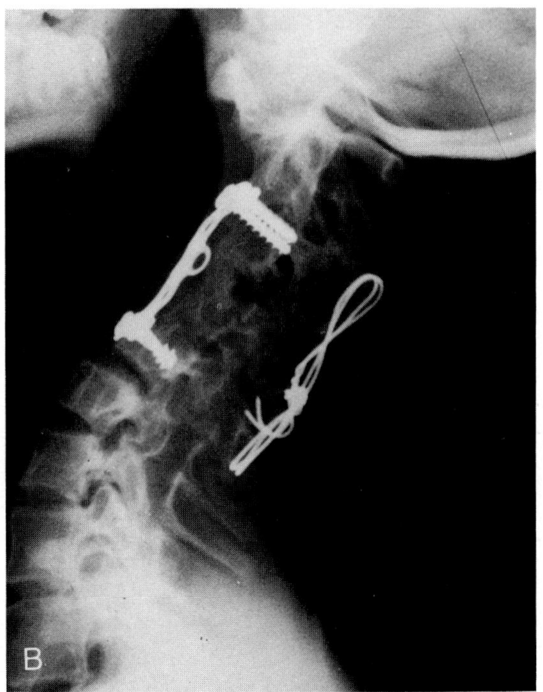

Fig. 6-112. A 13-year-old female with kyphosis at C3–C4. Correction with a halo was attempted and distraction remained unsuccessful; therefore, spondylectomy of C4 and correction of kyphosis with both ventral and dorsal internal fixation were performed. No neurologic deficits were seen postoperatively. The halo system was removed and a cervical collar was used for 4 weeks postoperatively. (*A*) Preoperative. (*B*) Postoperative.

ing an AO plate. Then the patient was turned over and the occiput and upper and middle cervical spine were exposed so that a Roy-Camille occipital plate could be fixed from the occiput to the facets of C3, C4, and C5. Bone cement was used to fix the plate. The patient was mobilized the next day with a cervical collar. Pain was significantly reduced.

Case 2 (Fig. 6-112*A* and *B*)
This 13-year-old female patient with cervical kyphosis at the level of C3 and C4 had been treated for 4 months with a halo extension without success. The fourth cervical vertebra was removed using a ventral approach, and the dura decompressed. A preformed block of bone cement was then inserted to maintain the space. The patient was repositioned in order to remove part of the locked facets. Posterior wiring and bone chips were also used. Then the patient was again repositioned, and the bone cement block was removed and replaced by an autogenous bone graft that was fixed with an AO plate. At the end of the operation the halo extension was removed.

Case 3 (Fig. 6-99*A* through *E*)
This 17-year-old male patient had already undergone laminectomy of C2 to C6 due to a neurinoma in another hospital, resulting in postlaminectomy kyphosis (see Fig. 6-99*A*). This caused increasing spinal cord compression. First, a ventral plate with only one row of screw holes was used. However, the plate was too short, so that a longer plate had to be fixed to the spine. This type of plate prevents rotatory instability, so that loosening of the plate does not occur. Finally spondylectomy of C4–C6 was used to decompress the spinal cord ventrally. An iliac bone graft was inserted and further stabilized using an AO plate held by two screws in the third and seventh cervical vertebrae. Additionally, three screws were used to fix the graft to the plate, and a dorsal osteosynthesis was performed using a Roy-Camille plate incorporating C4, C5, and C6. Neurologic symptoms improved, and the

patient regained mobility: Until now, there has been no loosening of the metal plates.

SUMMARY

In summarizing the procedure of internal fixation with metal plates and screws, the following points can be made:

1. Metal plates and screws can be used on the spine to obtain in a spondylodesis the anatomically correct position without the need for external immobilization (halo).
2. Healing of the bone graft can be improved by osteosynthesis. Once the bone has formed a firm spondylodesis, metal implants are no longer necessary.
3. Metal plates and screws should only be inserted under intraoperative imaging to prevent damage to the spinal cord.
4. No more should be fused than is absolutely necessary so as not to diminish postoperative spinal mobility.
5. A metal plate should not be placed over an intact vertebral disc, since the constant micromovements will cause loosening of the plate.
6. Only in cases of malignancy should bone cement (PMMA), as opposed to autogenous bone, be used to fix a ventral plate. It is then important to obtain particularly good positioning of the screws. With the use of bone cement, the danger exists of loosening of the plate through micromovements, owing to the absence of firm spondylodesis.
7. When loosening of the screws or plates occurs, the ventral metal implants should be removed at once to prevent eosphageal perforation.
8. The implantation of a foreign body in internal fixation produces a high risk of infection. For this reason perioperative antibiotics are indicated. If infection occurs, the metal plates should be removed.
9. The decision as to whether a ventral, dorsal, or even a combined approach should be attempted depends on where the instability is localized and whether the spinal cord and nerve roots need to be decompressed at the same time.
10. Severe spinal osteoporosis is a contraindication to the use of metal plates and screws.
11. For the future, it is important to develop materials that do not produce artifacts in CT scans and MRI studies.
12. With due attention to these guidelines and with correct surgical techniques, internal spinal fixation with metal plates and screws is an essential contribution to improving the quality of life for patients, since they can be immediately mobilized postoperatively and released earlier from inpatient treatment.

REFERENCES

1. *ALLGÖWER M, PERREN SM, MATTER P:* A new plate for internal fixation—the dynamic compression plate (DCP). Injury 2, No. 1, 1970
2. *BÖHLER J:* Operative Behandlung von Halswirbelsäulenverletzungen. Hefte Unfallheilk 108:132, 1971
3. *BÖHLER J:* Anterior stabilization for acute fractures and non-unions of the dens. J Bone Joint Surg 64A:18, 1982
4. *BRENNER A, ROOSEN K, WISSING HJ, GROTE W, SCHMIT-NEUERBURG KP:* Osteosynthesis with AO plates in the cervical and lumbal regions of the vertebral column in cases of spinal metastases. In Wenker H, et al (eds): Advances in Neurosurgery, Vol 14, p 133. New York, Springer Verlag, 1986
5. *CASPAR W:* Anterior cervical fusion and interbody stabilization with the trapezial osteosynthetic plate technique. Aesculap Wissenschaftl. Informationen, Aesculap-Werke AG, D-7200, Tuttlingen, West Germany, 1986
6. *CASPAR W:* Anterior stabilization with the trapezial osteosynethetic plate technique in cervical spine injuries. In Kehr P, Weidner A (eds): Cervical Spine I, p 198. Wien-New York, Springer Verlag, 1987
7. *COOPER PR, MARAVILLA KR, SKLAR FH, MOODY SF, CLARK WK:* Halo immobilization of cervical spine fractures. J Neurosurg 50:603, 1979
8. *CORREIA MARTINS MA:* Anterior cervical fusion—indications and results. In Kehr P, Weidner A (eds): Cervical Spine I, p 205. Wien-New York, Springer-Verlag, 1987
9. *CROCKARD HA, BRADFORD R:* Transoral transclival removal of a schwannoma anterior to the craniocervical junction. J Neurosurg 62:293, 1985
10. *CROCKARD HA, POZO JL, RANSFORD AO, STEVENS JM, KENDALL BE, ESSIGMAN WK:* Transoral decompression and posterior fusion for rheumatoid atlanto-axial subluxation. J Bone Joint Surg 68B:350, 1986
11. *DUFF TA:* Surgical stabilization of traumatic cervical spine dislocation using methyl methacrylate. J Neurosurg 64:39, 1986
12. *FUENTES JM:* Description d'une plaque d'ostéosynthèse cervicale antérieure. Neurochirurgie 5, 30: 351, 1984

13. *FUENTES JM, BENEZECH J:* Les ostéosynthèses rachidiennes en Neurochirurgie. Montpellier, France, Centre de Neurochirurgie, Clinique Rech, 1986
14. *GARFIN ST R, BOTTE MJ, WATERS RL, NICKEL VL:* Complications in the use of the halo fixation device. J Bone Joint Surg 68A:320, 1986
15. *GASSMANN J, SELIGSON D:* The anterior cervical plate. Spine 8:700, 1983
16. *GLASER JA, WHITEHILL R, STAMP WG, JANE JA:* Complications associated with the halo-vest. J Neurosurg 65:762, 1986
17. *GOODMAN ML, NELSON PB:* Brain abscess complicating the use of a halo orthosis. Neurosurgery 20:27, 1987
18. *HERRMANN HD:* Metal plate fixation after anterior fusion of unstable fracture dislocations of the cervical spine. Acta Neurochir 32:101, 1975
19. *JOHNSON RM, HART DL, SIMMONS EF, RAMSBY GR, SOUTHWICK WO:* Cervical orthoses. J Bone Joint Surg 59A:332, 1977
20. *KNÖRINGER P:* Osteosynthesis in patients with malignant tumors of the cervical vertebral column: indications, technique, and results. In Wenker H, et al (eds): Neurosurgery, Vol 14, p 125. New York, Springer Verlag, 1986
21. *KNÖRINGER P:* Double-threaded compression screws in osteosynthesis of acute fractures of the odontoid process. In Voth D, Glees O (eds): Disease in the cranio-cervical junction, p 217. Berlin-New York, de Gruyter, 1987
22. *KOCH RA, NICKEL VL:* The halo vest—an evaluation of motion and forces across the neck. Spine 3:103, 1978
23. *LESOIN F, JOMIN M, PELLERIN P, PRUVO JP, CARINI S, SERVATO R, ROUSSEAUX M:* Transclival transcervical approach to the upper cervical spine and clivus. Acta Neurochir 80:100, 1986
24. *LESOIN F, PELLERIN P, VILLETTE L, JOMIN M:* Anterior approach and osteosynthesis for recent fractures of the pedicles of the axis. Neurosurgery 19:374, 1986
25. *LIND B, SIHLBOM H, NORDWALL A:* Forces and motions across the neck in patients treated with halo-vest for unstable cervical spine fractures. In Kehr P, Weidner A (eds): Cervical Spine I, p 55. Wien-New York, Springer Verlag, 1987
26. *LOUIS R:* Posterior Vertebral Bone Plates. Paris, Ceprime, 1982
27. *MAGERL F, GROB D, SEEMANN P:* Stable dorsal fusion of the cervical spine (C2 - Th1) using hook plates. In Kehr P, Weidner A (eds): Cervical Spine I, p 217. Wien-New York, Springer Verlag, 1987
28. *MAGERL F, SEEMANN P:* Stable posterior fusion of the atlas and axis by transarticular screw fixation. In Kehr P, Weidner A (eds): Cervical Spine I, p 322. Wien-New York, Springer Verlag, 1987
29. *MCAFEE PC, BOHLMAN HH, DUCKER T, EISMONT FJ:* Failure of stabilization of the spine with methylmethacrylate. J Bone Joint Surg 68A:1145, 1986
30. *MURRAY J, SEYMOUR RJ:* An anterior extrapharyngeal, suprahyoid approach to the first, second and third cervical vertebra. Acta Orthop Scand 45:43, 1974
31. *OROZCO DELCLOS R, LLOVET-TAPIES J:* Osteosintesis en las fracturas de raquis cervical not de tecnica. Revista de Ortopedia y Traumatologica 14:285, 1970
32. *PANJABI MM, TECH D, GOEL VK, CLARK CH R, KEGGI K, SOUTHWICK WO:* Biomechanical study of cervical spine stabilization with methylmethacrylate. Spine 10:198, 1985
33. *RAHN BA, GALLINARO P, BALTENSPERGER A, PERREN SM:* Primary bone healing. An experimental study in the rabbit. J Bone Joint Surg 53A:783, 1971
34. *RANSFORD AO, CROCKARD HA, POZO JL, THOMAS NP, NELSON IW:* Craniocervical instability treated by contoured loop fixation. J Bone Joint Surg 68B:173, 1986
35. *REISS ST J, RAQUE GH, SHIELDS CH B, GARRETSON HD:* Cervical spine fractures with major associated trauma. Neurosurgery 18:327, 1986
36. *ROY-CAMILLE R, SAILLANT G:* Chirurgie du rachis cervical. Nouv Presse Med 1:2707, 1972
37. *ROY-CAMILLE R, SAILLANT G:* Les traumatismes du rachis sans complication neurologique. Int Orthop 8:155, 1984
38. *ROY-CAMILLE R, MAZEL CH, SAILLANT G:* Treatment of cervical spine injuries by a posterior osteosynthesis with plates and screws. In Kehr P, Weidner A (eds): Cervical Spine I, p 163. Wien-New York, Springer Verlag, 1987
39. *SCHMIDEK HH, SMITH DA, SOFFERMAN RA, GOMES FB:* Transoral unilateral facetectomy in the management of unilateral anterior rotatory atlantoaxial fracture/dislocation: A case report. Neurosurgery 18:645, 1986
40. *SENEGAS J, GAUZERE JM:* Traitement des lésions cervicales par voie anterieure. Rev Chir Orthoped 63:466, 1977
41. *SHERK HH:* Stability of the lower cervical spine. In Kehr P, Weidner A (eds): Cervical Spine I, p 59. Wien-New York, Springer Verlag, 1987
42. *STRELI R:* Double hole plate fixation of the lower cervical spine. In Kehr P, Weidner A (eds): Cervical Spine I, p 175. Wien-New York, Springer Verlag, 1987
43. *TSCHERNE H, HIEBLER W, MUHR G:* Zur operativen Behandlung von Frakturen und Luxationen der Halswirbelsäule. Hefte Unfallheilk 108:142, 1971
44. *ULRICH C, WOERSDOERFER O, CLAES L, MAGERL F:* Comparative stability of anterior or posterior cer-

vical spine fixation in vitro investigation. In Kehr P, Weidner A (eds): Cervical Spine I, p 65. Wien-New York, Springer Verlag, 1987

45. *WHITE AA, PANJABI MM:* Clinical biomechanics of the spine. Philadelphia, JB Lippincott Co, 1978

46. *WHITEHILL R, RICHMANN JA, GLASER JA:* Failure of immobilization of the cervical spine by the halo vest. J Bone Joint Surg 68A:326, 1986

Cervical Spine Injuries in Children

J. WILLIAM FIELDING

Injuries to the cervical spine are rare in children, and are most common from the occiput to C3 (in the adult, they are more common in the lower regions). Hasue and associates, in reviewing 228 cases of cervical spine or cord injury, mention only 10 cases under the age of 15. Lesions of the atlas and axis were noted in 70% of those under 15 but in only 16% of adults.[23]

Blount notes in *Fractures in Children* that "except in cases of extreme violence, fractures and dislocations of the cervical spine are rare and are less likely to cause cord transection than similar injuries in adults."[3] Rang states that the child's spine is more mobile than the adult's, and that force is dissipated more easily over a greater number of segments. In a 15-year period at the Hospital for Sick Children in Toronto, 75 children with skeletal spinal injuries at all levels were admitted (5 per year); 31 had associated cord damage, 19 in the cervical region.[40] These 19 represent an incidence of only 1.3 per year in a large children's hospital. Weber, Brunner, and Freuler state that "of all fractures of the vertebral column in children, those of the cervical spine occur less frequently." They reported 14 patients from 3 to 16 years of age, three of whom had fractures at C1–C2, eight at C2–C3, and three at C3–C4.[58] Becker notes the incidence of fractures and dislocations of the spine in children to be 0.2% of all children's fractures and dislocations, and 1.5% to 3.3% of all spine injuries in the literature.[2] Bohlman and Davis reviewed 300 patients hospitalized with acute fractures and dislocations of the cervical spine and found only 15 younger than 15 years of age, two of whom had cervical cord birth injuries.[4] Sherk and associates found only 12 odontoid fractures at the Children's Hospital in Philadelphia over a 20-year period.[45] In 631 neck injuries in all age groups reported from the Henry Ford Hospital in Detroit by Henrys and associates, only 12, or 1.9%, were in children under 15 years, mainly injured in the upper neck.[24]

From Rockwood CA Jr, Wilkins KE, King RE: Pediatric Fractures, Vol 3, Fractures, 2nd ed. Philadelphia, JB Lippincott (in preparation). Used with the permission of Charles A. Rockwood, Jr.

Neck injuries are often associated with trauma to other portions of the body such as the head. Aside from a bullet wound or similar penetrating injury, it is very difficult to injure the cervical spine by direct trauma. Most injuries are associated with head trauma with force transmission to the neck.[35] Bohlman reported neurologic deficit or death in 11 of 300 multiply injured patients with unrecognized cervical spine injury, because their necks were moved during the course of emergency management; he emphasized that serious neck injury can be overlooked, especially in patients with multiple injuries. Evidence of head or facial trauma, particularly in the comatose patient, might alert the physician to be on the lookout for "hidden" cervical spine injury.[4,5,*]

Aufdermaur demonstrated a discrepancy between roentgenogram and autopsy findings. He examined the autopsied spines (occiput to coccyx) of 12 juveniles who had spinal injury (7 cervical, 4 thoracic, and 1 lumbar). Clinically and radiologically, a fracture was suspected only once, yet in all 12 cases cartilage end-plates were split from the vertebral bodies in the zone of columnar and calcified cartilage. There was no extension into the bony vertebral body, nor was there evidence of tearing of the discs. Only roentgenograms at autopsy showed that the disruption was represented by a small gaping fissure, or apparent widening of the intervertebral space.[1]

Figures 6-113 through 6-119 illustrate the developmental anatomy of the cervical spine. Roentgenographic evaluation of the neck in children is different from that in adults because of the synchondroses and epiphyseal plates, as shown.

NEONATAL TRAUMA

Obstetric and neonatal trauma has been reported as the cause of serious, and occasionally fatal, cervical spine injury. Parrot, in 1870, 25 years before the introduction of the x-ray, described spinal cord injury after breech delivery.[38] By 1927, 150 cases had been recorded.[6] Shulman and associates reported atlantoocipital and atlantoaxial dislocation, odontoid fractures, and cord transection. Forcible breech extraction with angulation appears to be the commonest cause, but it also occurs in cephalic presentations.[47]

The cervical muscles and ligaments in the new-

* Henry H. Bohlman, personal communication

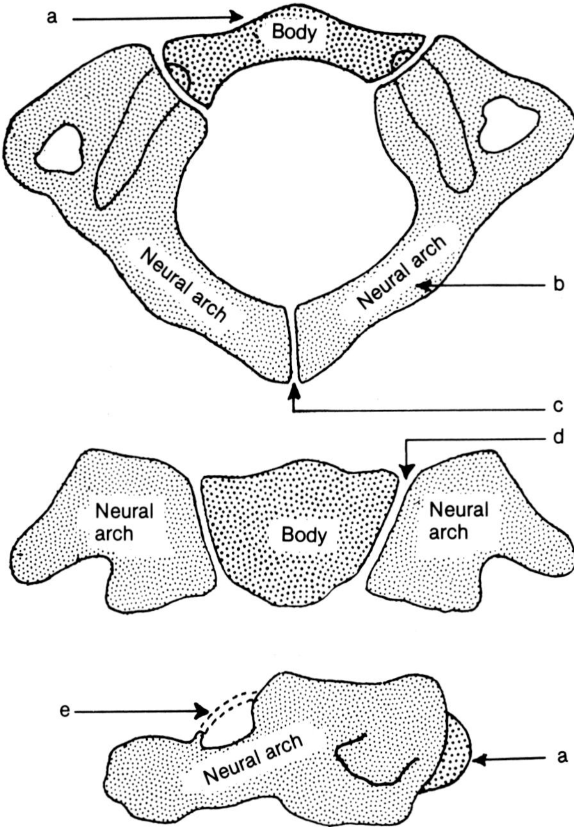

Fig. 6-113. Diagram of the first cervical vertebra (atlas). (*A*) Body. The body is not ossified at birth; the center occasionally two centers) appears during the first year after birth. The body may fail to develop, and forward extension of the neural arches may take its place. (*B*) Neural arches. These appear bilaterally at about the seventh fetal week. The most anterior portion of the superior articulating surface is usually formed by the body. (*C*) Synchondrosis of spinous processes. These unite by the third year. Union may rarely be preceded by the appearance of a secondary center within the synchondrosis. (*D*) Neurocentral synchondrosis. This fuses about the seventh year. (*E*) Ligament surrounding the superior vertebral notch. This may ossify, especially in later life. (After Bailey DK: Normal cervical spine in infants and children. Radiology 59:713–714, 1952)

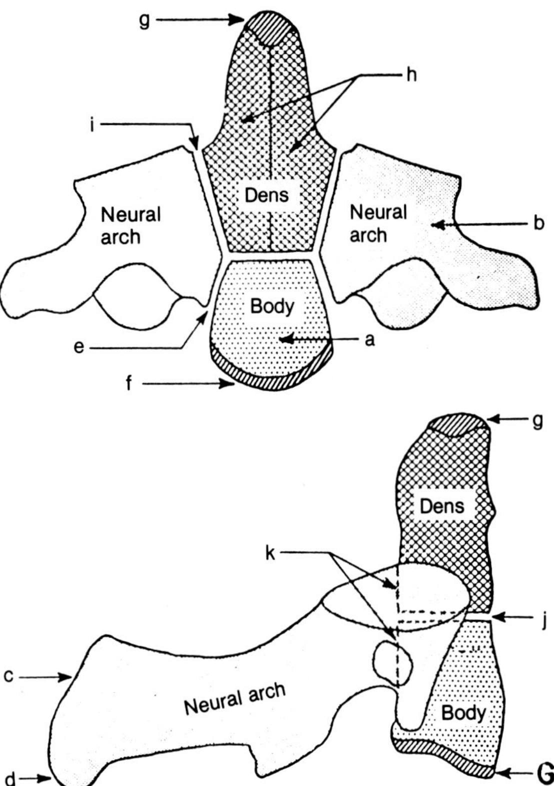

Fig. 6-114. Diagram of the second cervical vertebra (axis or epistropheus). (*A*) Body. One center (occasionally two) appears by the fifth fetal month. (*B*) Neural arches. These appear bilaterally by the seventh fetal month. (*C*) Neural arches. These fuse posteriorly by second or third year. (*D*) Bifid tip of spinous process (occasionally a secondary center is present in each tip). (*E*) Neurocentral synchondrosis. This fuses at 3 to 6 years. (*F*) Inferior epiphyseal ring. This appears at puberty and fuses at about 25 years. (*G*) "Summit" ossification center for the odontoid. This appears at 3 to 6 years and fuses with the odontoid by 12 years. (*H*) Odontoid (dens). Two separate centers appear by the fifth fetal month and fuse with each other by the seventh fetal month. (*I*) Synchondrosis between odontoid and neural arch. This fuses at 3 to 6 years. (*J*) Synchondrosis between odontoid and body. This fuses at 3 to 6 years. (*K*) Posterior surface of body and odontoid. (After Bailey DK: Normal cervical spine in infants and children. Radiology 59:713–714, 1952)

born are so weak that the average child is incapable of adequately supporting the head until about 3 months of age and, hence, incapable of protecting the cervical spine and cord against the excessive torsional and traction trauma that may occur in obstetrics.[36] These forces may exceed the stretch capability of the neck, or, according to Stern and Rand the lax ligaments of a child's neck may not be able to protect the less elastic cord, possibly explaining severe cord injuries that occur without skeletal injury.[49] Spinal cords removed from newborns who have died from obstetric trauma may

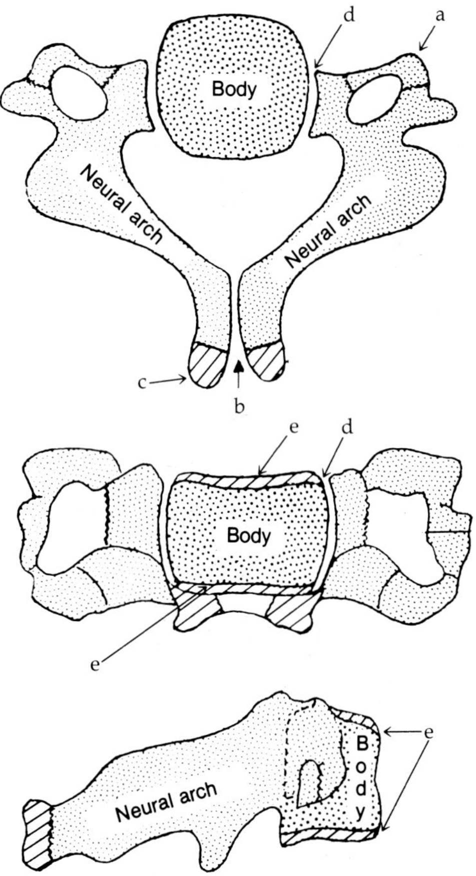

Fig. 6-115. Diagram of typical cervical vertebrae, C3 to C7. The body appears by the fifth fetal month. (*A*) Anterior (costal) portion of the transverse process. This may develop from a separate center which appears by the sixth fetal month and joins the arch by the sixth year. The neural arches appear by the seventh to ninth fetal week. (*B*) Synchondrosis between spinous processes. This usually unites by the second or third year. (*C*) Secondary centers for bifid spine. These appear at puberty and unite with the spinous process at 25 years. (*D*) Neurocentral synchondrosis. This fuses at 3 to 6 years. (*E*) Superior and inferior epiphyseal rings. These appear at puberty and unite with the body at about 25 years. The seventh cervical vertebra differs slightly because of a long, powerful, nonbifid spinous process. (After Bailey DK: Normal cervical spine in infants and children. Radiology 59:713–714, 1952)

show changes over long segments, suggesting the longitudinal traction was a major injuring factor, whereas in adults cord injury occurs over a shorter segment.[46,49]

Most publications on the subject of obstetric trauma stress injury to the cervical cord, nerve roots, brain, and vertebral arteries. One suggested that vertebral artery trauma at birth could cause cerebral palsy later in life.[64] Skeletal injury is rarely reported, probably because the infantile spine with its large percentage of cartilage is difficult to evaluate radiologically, especially if the lesion occurs through cartilage or at the cartilage-bone interface.[1] Furthermore, the spine may appear normal when the injuring force that produced the deformity (*e.g.*, rotation elongation) is removed, and there may be a discrepancy between severe soft-tissue damage and the absence of radiologically apparent bone injury.

Yates dissected 30 cervical spines randomly selected from 78 stillbirths and 114 neonatal deaths, and noted extradural, dural, subdural, and subarachnoid hemorrhages and tears and hemorrhages in the nerve roots and spinal ganglia.[64] Spinal cord lesions were evident in two cases; cord contusion in one case and bilateral necrosis of lateral columns in the other. In 19 cases there was evidence of hemorrhage around one or both vertebral arteries, either in the form of a crescentic adventitial hematoma or massive hemorrhage encircling the vessel.[64] Surprisingly, no mention was made of skeletal injury, which undoubtedly must have occurred to account for the extensive soft-tissue damage.

Bresnam and Abrams in 1971 noted that the presence of neck hyperextension *in utero* ("stargazing fetus") in breech presentation will result in an estimated 25% cord transection in vaginal delivery. This did not occur with cesarean section, which was recommended in such cases.[6]

Caffey in 1974 and Swischuck in 1969 described a form of child abuse called the "whiplash-shaken infantile syndrome," caused by excessive shaking.[7,52] Here the weak infantile neck cannot support the head, which is subjected to whiplash stresses. Intracranial and intraocular hemorrhages resulting in death, latent cerebral injury, retardation, or permanent visual or hearing defects have been reported, together with fractures of the spine and spinal cord injuries. Swischuck noted that the incidence of spinal trauma is not as high as that of trauma in the extremities and skull. He reported a case of cord injury in a 2-year-old girl, postulating that this was caused by violent shaking that

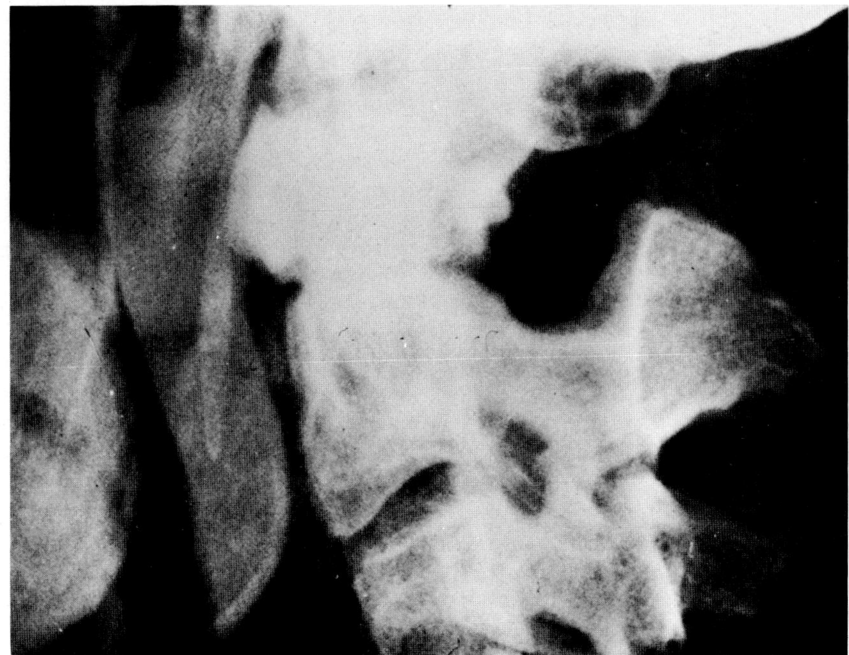

Fig. 6-116. The completely absent posterior arch of the C1 vertebra in this patient was an incidental finding. (Fielding JW: In Ahstrom JP Jr (ed): Current Practice in Orthopaedic Surgery, Vol 5. St. Louis, CV Mosby, 1973)

produced a cervical fracture dislocation with spontaneous reduction.[52]

OCCIPUT–C1 LESIONS

Occiput–C1 lesions occur infrequently, perhaps because the injury itself is infrequent in living patients or because the patient is "dead on arrival" owing to lethal cervicomedullary cord damage from an occiput–C1 dislocation that spontaneously reduced and was not identified. Davis and associates in 1971 reported that the occiput–C1 junction is commonly affected in fatal craniospinal injuries.[11] Bohlman reported two cases in 1979, one in an adult and the other in a 14-year-old child, in which the lesion was not discovered until an arteriogram was made that demonstrated stretching of the vertebral arteries.[4] Experimental studies on primates have demonstrated that this injury may be caused by an inertial phenomenon in "short stop" accidents. The head is inertially carried forward resulting in craniovertebral dislocation with immediate spontaneous reduction and, hence, normal roentgenographic findings. Autopsies of such experimentally produced injuries, however, revealed disruption of the craniovertebral joints, spinal cord, and vertebral arteries.*

Because of the potential for cord injury, it is suggested that these injuries be reduced by traction followed by craniovertebral fusion at an appropriate time.

ATLANTOAXIAL LESIONS

The three main lesions occurring at the atlantoaxial interval in children are (1) traumatic ligament disruption; (2) ligament laxity related to local inflammation, and (3) odontoid "epiphyseal" separation.

Stability at this joint is almost entirely dependent upon ligaments that must simultaneously protect the articulation and allow for its extensive mobility. Although the primary motion is rotation, flexion–extension, vertical approximation, and lateral slide also occur.[13] Approximately 50% of cervical rotation takes place between the first and second segments around the anteriorly eccentric odontoid process. Therefore, the lateral wall of the vertebral

* Ewing Channing, personal communication

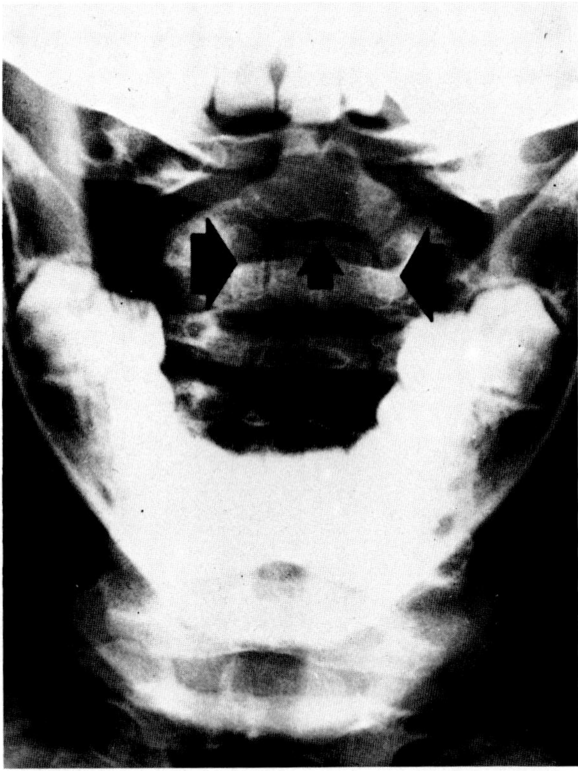

Fig. 6-117. The epiphysis at the base of the odontoid process (*small arrow*) is well below the level of the superior articular facet of the axis. The synchondroses between the body of the axis and the neural arches are shown by the large arrows. Just above this are the synchondroses between the odontoid process and the neural arches. The odontoid process, therefore, surmounts the body of the axis and is sandwiched between the neural arches. The epiphyseal line and synchondroses combine to form the letter H. (Fielding JW: In Ahstrom JP Jr (ed): Current Practice in Orthopaedic Surgery, Vol 5. St. Louis, CV Mosby, 1973)

foramen of C1 rotates to a considerable extent across the canal of C2, physiologically decreasing the opening of the spinal canal between the two segments.[13]

The spinal canal of C1 is large compared to its size in the other cervical segments and safely accommodates this degree of rotation and some degree of pathologic displacement without cord pressure. This has been expressed by Steel's rule of thirds. The canal of C1 is occupied equally by cord, odontoid, and free space. According to Steel, the cord moves into this free space when C1 displaces.[48] Therefore, anterior displacement of the atlas exceeding the thickness of the odontoid may place the adjacent segment of the cord in jeopardy.[48] The significance of trauma to this highly mobile articulation lies in the fact that it houses the vulnerable cervicomedullary portion of the spinal cord, which can be damaged by C1–C2 displacement. The vertebral arteries, which supply a significant amount of blood to the upper cord and a cerebellum, are fixed in the foramen transversarium of C1 and C2, and can be carried forward and compressed by an atlantoaxial shift with subsequent damage to neural tissue.[12,42]

Traumatic Ligamentous Disruption

It has been established in previous studies that displacement of C1 and C2 exceeding 3 mm in the adult represents ligamentous damage at the atlantoaxial articulation. It has been reported that the atlas–dens interval may measure up to 3 mm or more in children.[16] It can be reasonably assumed that displacements of over 5 mm in flexion are indicative of atlantoaxial ligamentous compromise, especially if there is documented history of trauma (Fig. 6-120).

Watson-Jones has stated that forward atlantoaxial displacement is more serious with an intact odontoid because of the great danger of the cord being compressed against it.[56] Studies on conservative treatment of acute ligamentous injuries in this area are infrequent. Suggested treatment is by reduction in extension maintained from 8 to 12 weeks in a Minerva or halo device, followed by stress films, with fusion if the displacement persists.

Displacement Due to Inflammation

In 1830, Bell first described spontaneous dislocation between the first and second cervical vertebrae. His observations were commendable since they were carried out 65 years before the introduction of roentgenograms.[36] Although the pathology of his case is controversial, and although roentgenography was not available, his patient did have an ulcer at the back of this throat that was believed to have caused destruction of the transverse ligament with resulting spontaneous dislocation.

Since that time there have been repeated reports of atlantoaxial displacement unassociated with trauma and secondary to chronic inflammatory disease in the neck or throat. Hess and coworkers[25] in 1935 reviewed 24 prior cases and added two of their own. The title of their article, "Atlantoaxial dislocation," does not appear to be accurate: the

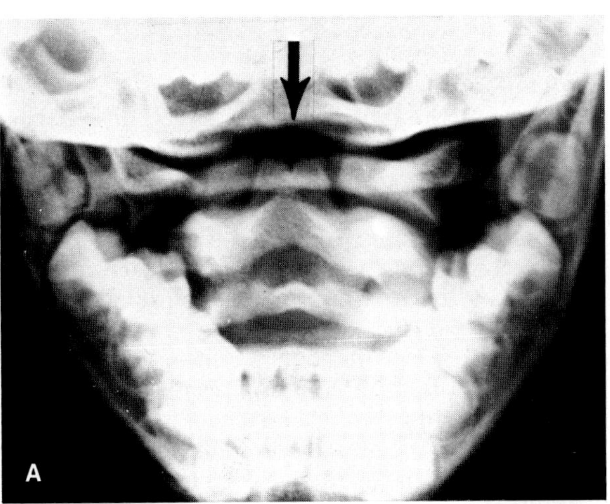

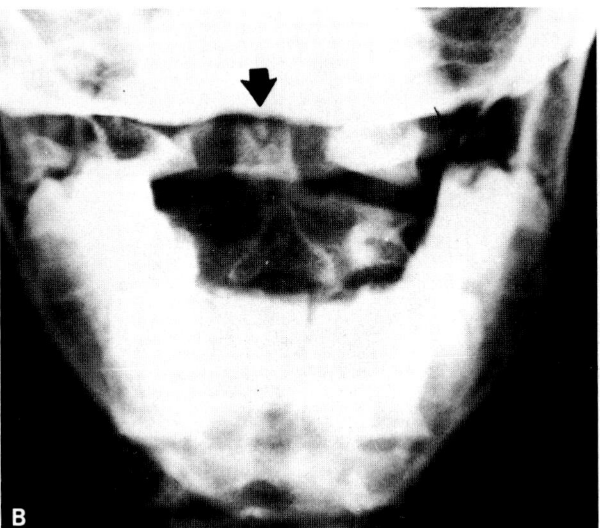

Fig. 6-118. (*A*) The bifid tip of the odontoid process in a 2-year-old child. (*B*) Terminal ossification center in a 5-year-old child. (*C*) The ossification center is fused with the odontoid process at age 12. (Fielding JW: In Ahstrom JP Jr (ed): Current Practice in Orthopaedic Surgery, Vol 5. St. Louis, C V Mosby, 1973).

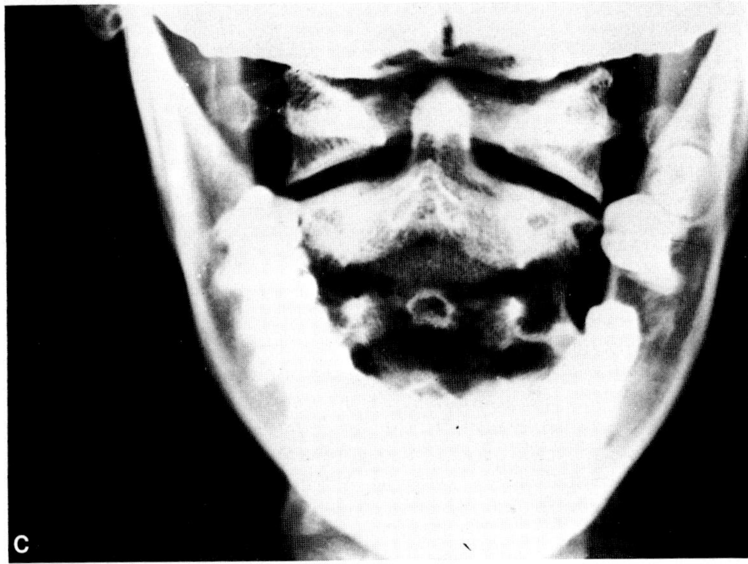

photographs show subluxation.[36] In 1930 Grisel described this phenomenon, resulting in the term "Grisel's syndrome." Various causes include rheumatoid disease, upper respiratory and throat infections, and tuberculosis.[21]

The pathogenesis is questionable but it has been hypothesized that it is caused by capsular distention with ligament softening similar to that seen in septic hip dislocations in children.[32] Watson-Jones in 1932 reviewed 21 cases and described decalcification of the bony structure secondary to hyperemia with resultant bone softening and weakening of the fibroosseous junction.[55] These conditions are complicated by muscle spasm holding the neck in flexion and aggravating the forward displacement.

Moran and Balachandran in 1973 reported it in only four patients, all of whom had a history of an upper respiratory infection.[34] This suggests a decreasing incidence with newer antibiotics and indicates a need to refer to earlier publications before the development of these more effective drugs.

Lippman in 1953 stated that there was no typical time schedule or clinical pattern; that there was no detectable relationship between the severity or in-

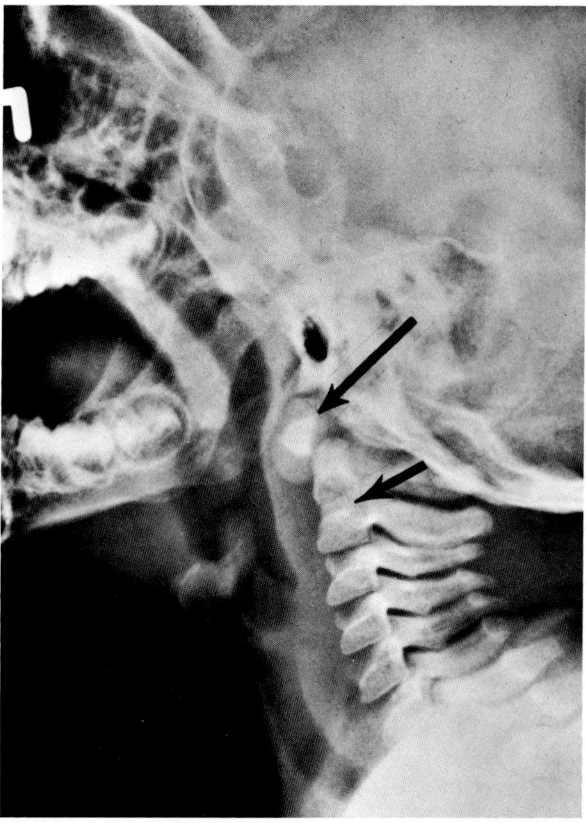

Fig. 6-119. In extension roentgenography of a very young patient, the anterior arch of the atlas may slide upward to protrude beyond the ossified part of the dens, giving the mistaken impression of odontoid hypoplasia. (Fielding JW, Hawkins RJ: Roentgenographic diagnosis of the injured neck. In the American Academy of Orthopaedic Surgeons: Instructional Course Lectures, Vol 25, p 156. St. Louis, CV Mosby, 1976)

tensity of the inflammatory process; that the cause may be primarily in the throat or due to drainage into the lymph nodes of the throat from a remote focus; that the condition starts during or shortly after subsidence of the original focus; that the pain may vary from mild discomfort to great agony; and finally that the lesion will heal firmly after reduction and immobilization, even if the causative inflammation continues.[32]

Evaluation may be difficult because of the frequently associated torticollis and atlantoaxial rotary deformity. Radiologic views should include a true lateral view of C1–C2 to determine the degree of anterior displacement of the atlas on the axis.[32]

Suggested treatment is by reduction, either by traction or neck extension, followed by a Minerva jacket or halo device for about 6 weeks.

Odontoid "Fractures"

Fractures of the odontoid process in children are in reality "epiphyseal slips" or, perhaps more correctly, "synchondrotic slips." The cartilage line at the base of the odontoid has more of the histologic appearance of a synchondrosis than an epiphysis, and it also closes much earlier than a normal epiphysis.[45] These injuries are frequently associated with head trauma, with force transmission to the upper cervical spine. Nachemson reports head injury to be the most common accompaniment of odontoid fracture.[35]

Sherk and associates reported severe falls or automobile accidents as the etiologic factor in all but 2 of 11 cases.[45] In a literature review of 24 fractures, they noted that the average age of the patient was 4, that the injury occurred at the cartilaginous plate, and that in every case the displacement was anterior. Twenty-three were treated conservatively either by skeletal or halter traction or manipulative reduction, and one by primary atlantoaxial fusion. It was noted that generally the results was good.[45] Growth disturbance was not noted in this group of 24 patients, probably indicating that the cartilage plate of the base of the odontoid contributes little to odontoid growth.[45]

A–P x-ray evaluation may be of little value since it may only show the normal synchondrotic line, and the displacement or angulation may only be apparent on the lateral view. Vigouroux and associates reported angulation of the odontoid process in approximately 4% of normal children, suggesting caution in interpretation of this particular feature (Fig. 6-121).[53] Prevertebral swelling can lead to the diagnosis in some cases, but changes in prevertebral shadows and inspiration can make these findings unreliable (Fig. 6-122).

The lack of complication and the generally good results in young children with synchondrotic slips contrasts sharply with the complications seen in adults, such as nonunion and the occasional late development of neurologic sequelae.[45]

Griffiths in 1972 reported four patients with this fracture whose average age was 31½ months. He noted that "the ease of reduction, certainty of union, [and] lack of persistent complications in this fracture are apparent from this small series and such has been the experience of others."[20] He suggested an intact hinge of soft tissue or periosteum

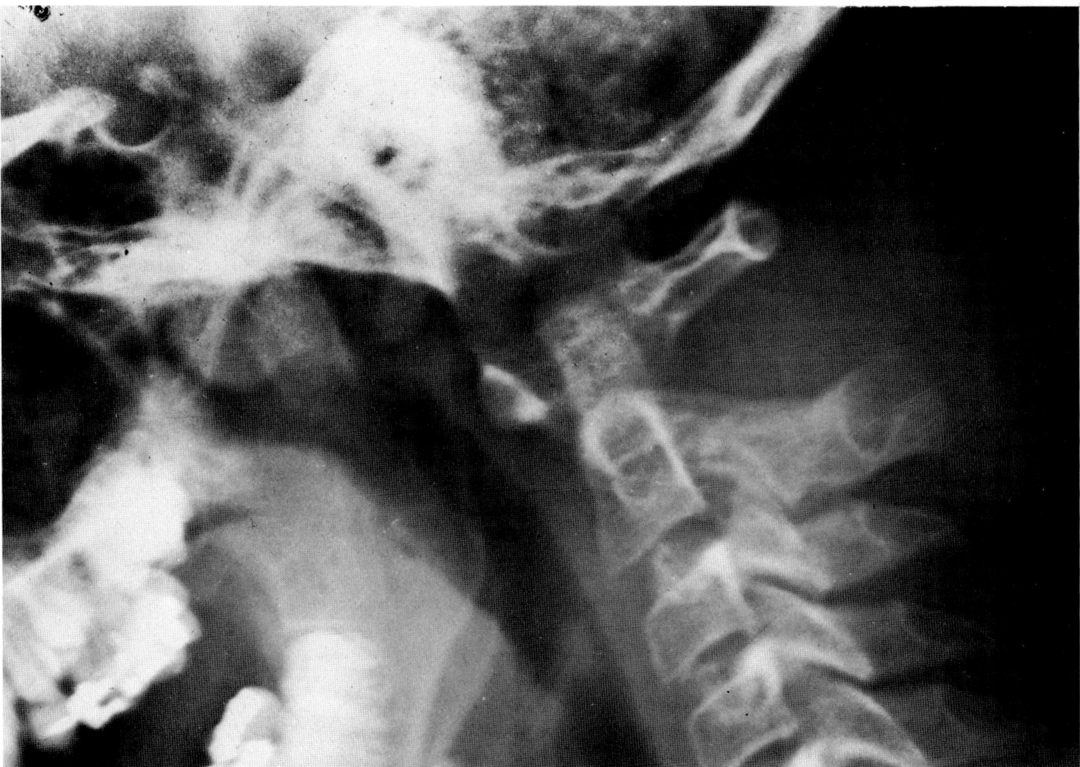

Fig. 6-120. Traumatic disruption of the transverse ligament with increased atlantal–dens interval.

might exist anteriorly, accounting for the apparent ease and stability of reduction in traction and the early appearance of callus anteriorly. Crutchfield tongs were used in three children, two of whom were 2 years of age; the fourth was treated by means of a Minerva jacket and manipulation under anesthesia. Immobilization was discontinued at 6 weeks or less with excellent results in all.[22] Sherk and coworkers, in reviewing their 11 cases, noted that the average age of patient was 3 and that there were relatively few associated injuries and no neurologic deficits attributable to the odontoid fracture.[45] Reduction was achieved in five patients by recumbency with hyperextension of the neck over the edge of a mattress from 1 to 12 days; in four by manipulation under sedation and general anesthesia; and in two by skull traction. The injury was immobilized after reduction for 6 to 16 weeks by Minerva jacket, halo cast, or in one case a soft collar. Thirteen years later follow-up roentgenograms failed to reveal growth disturbance.

In nine cases of os odontoideum, evidence is available of a previously normal odontoid. This suggests that injury to the soft tissues, an unrecognized fracture, or injury to the vascular supply of the developing odontoid process, rather than anomalous development, may be responsible for os odontoideum.[17] It also may suggest that treatment for some injuries to the odontoid may have less than satisfactory results.

Reduction of these lesions by recumbency in hyperextension, as suggested by Sherk, should be followed by a Minerva jacket for an average of 12 weeks depending upon the condition. Following removal of the jacket, stress films are recommended. If there is no motion, a soft collar should be worn for 1 to 2 weeks. If reduction cannot be obtained by recumbency and hyperextension, head halter traction is suggested. Skull tong traction and manipulation under general anesthesia should be reserved for those cases that are refractory to the more conservative treatment.

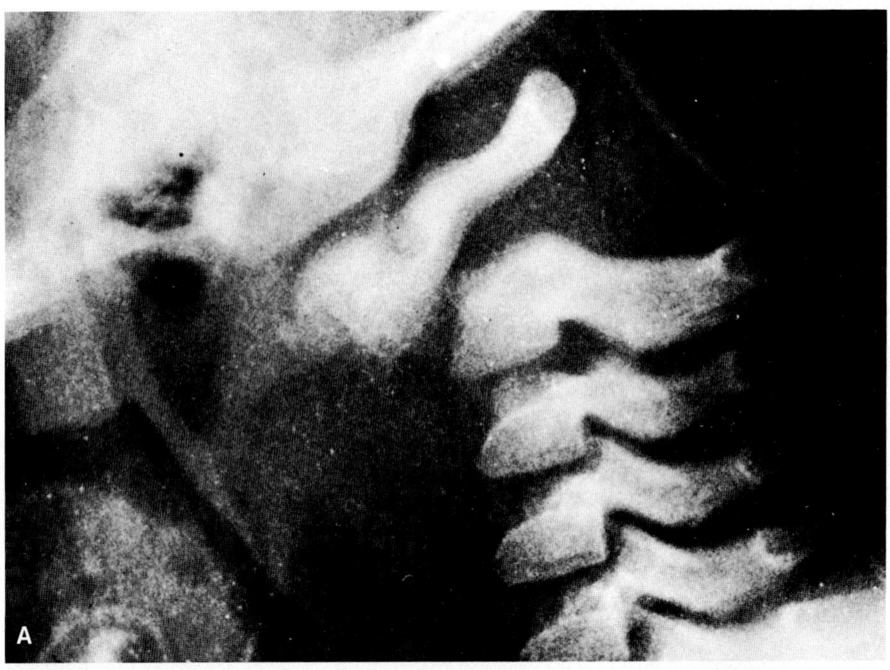

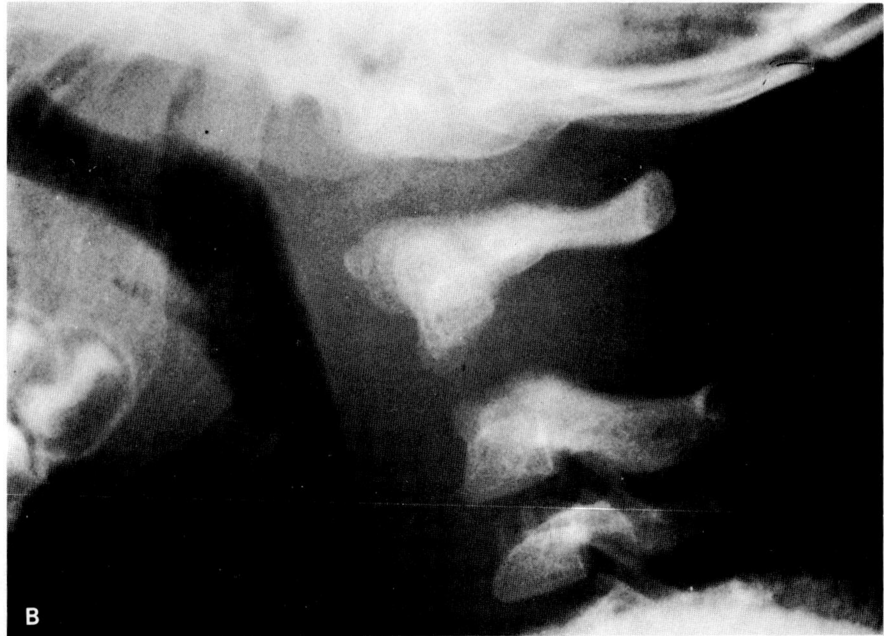

Fig. 6-121. (*A*) Anterior displacement of the odontoid at the epiphyseal line in a 17-month-old child. (*B*) Reduction with skull traction. Note the distraction of fragments. (*C*) Eight months later. The epiphyseal line is partially obliterated. (Ewald FC: J Bone Joint Surg 53A:1636–1640, 1971)

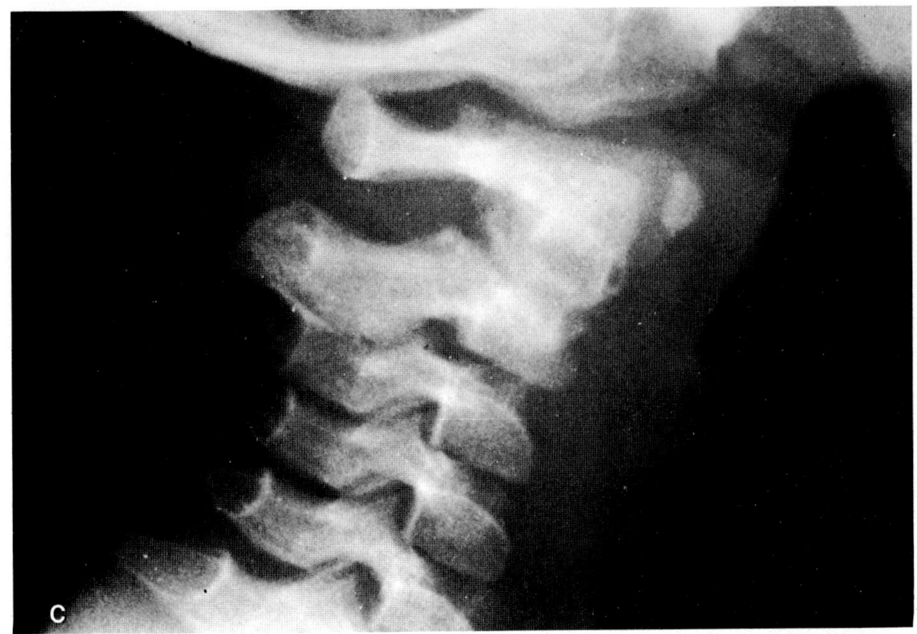

Fig. 6-121 continued.

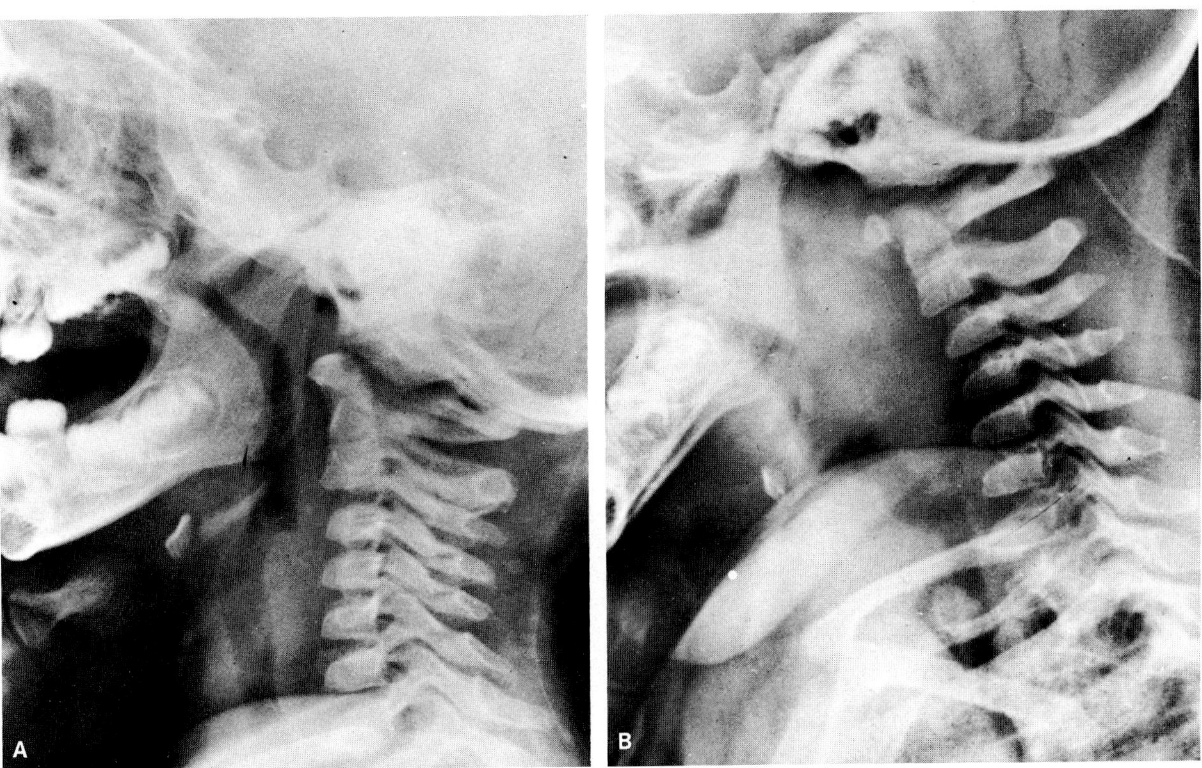

Fig. 6-122. (*A*) Roentgenogram of an 18-month-old girl taken at rest. Although the pharyngeal wall is farther forward than in an adult, it is relatively straight and normal. (*B*) Roentgenogram of 12-month-old girl showing widening of the retropharyngeal space, suggesting high-pitched cry at the end of expiration. (Ardran GM, Kemp FH: The mechanism of changes in form of the cervical airway in infancy. Med Radiogr Photogr 442), 1968. Published by Health Sciences Markets Division, Eastman Kodak Company, Rochester, New York.)

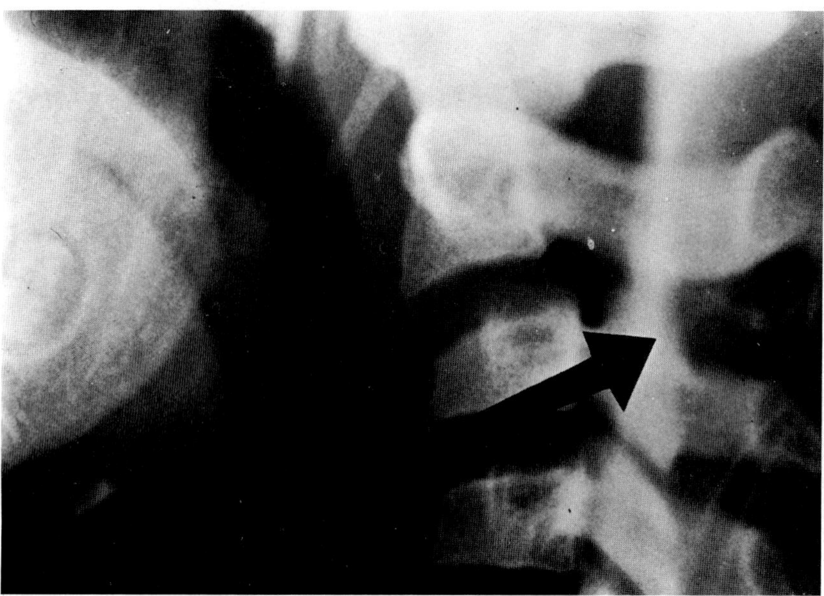

Fig. 6-123. Pathologic subluxation of C2 on C3. Note ossification in interspinous and posterior longitudinal ligaments. (Fielding JW: In Ahstrom JP Jr (ed): Current Practice in Orthopaedic Surgery, Vol 5. St. Louis, CV Mosby, 1973)

INJURIES BELOW C2

C2–C3 subluxation is one of the more difficult diagnostic problems in an injured child's neck since the x-ray findings may be identical to those in C2–C3 pseudosubluxation. The true nature of the lesion may only become apparent with the passage of time. The following suggestions are made to assist in the diagnostic dilemma:

1. Did the child sustain sufficient trauma, followed by pain, spasm, limited motion, tenderness, and so forth? Do the symptoms persist in spite of adequate conservative therapy?
2. Are there roentgenographically demonstrable abnormalities associated with the "subluxation," such as ossification of the posterior longitudinal ligament or avulsion fractures of the tips of the spinous processes?
3. Does the lower cervical spine gradually develop a compensatory lordosis, and does the "subluxation" fail to correct when the spine is placed in extension? Absent lordosis or reversal of lordosis may occur in normal subjects and is not always indicative of injury (Figs. 6-123 and 6-124).[15,31,59,*]

* D. C. Weir, personal communication

Injuries below C3 are very rare in the pediatric population, either because they seem to appear at cartilage-bone interface and are rarely seen on standard films or because the mobility of children's spines allow for dissipation of the force over a larger number of segments. There are a few cases from which to draw conclusions, as follows.[1]

Of the ten children with cervical spine injuries studied by Hasue, only two had injuries below C3; a 1-year-old with an oblique fracture at the level of C6 was lost to follow-up, and an 11-year-old who had a compression fracture of C3 and C4 became stable with conservative treatment.[23]

Henrys and coworkers, in reviewing 18 cases, had only four with injuries below C3: a case of C6–C7 quadriplegia from obstetric trauma; a C3–C4 fracture dislocation, also from obstetric trauma; a laminar fracture at C7; and a fracture dislocation at C3–C4 from diving, resulting in quadriplegia.[24]

In all probability, many serious injuries below C3 are those associated with ligamentous disruption. It is reasonable to assume that since the child's spine is extremely mobile, it may be even more so with a ligamentous disruption, with gradual displacement of one segment on the other and secondary adaptive changes occurring in the spine, making reduction difficult. If such lesions are sus-

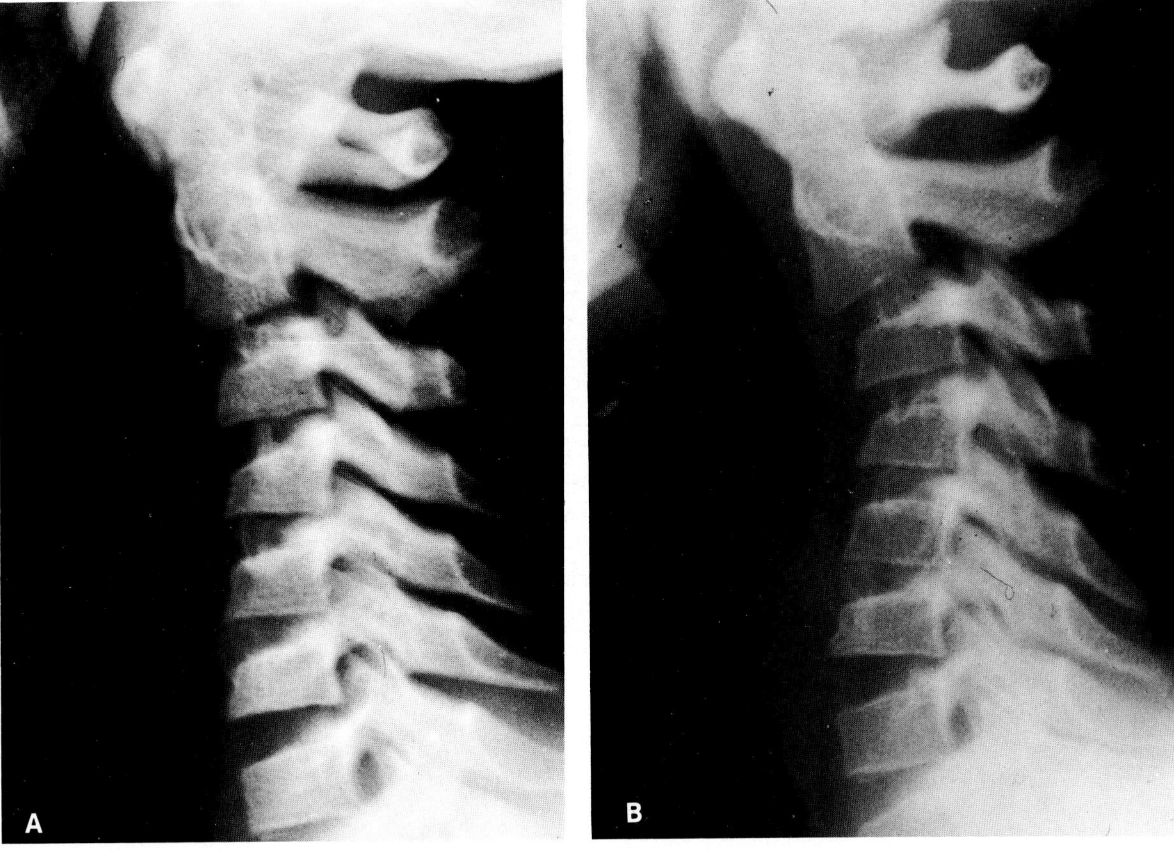

Fig. 6-124. (*A*) Subluxation of C2 on C3. (*B*) Six months later, the degree of subluxation increased and cannot be reduced in extension. Compensatory lordosis of the lower cervical spine is developing. (Fielding JW: In Ahstrom JP Jr (ed): Current Practice in Orthopaedic Surgery, Vol 5. St. Louis, CV Mosby, 1973)

pected, periodic observation is recommended, together with protection in an extension orthosis if necessary.

SURGERY

Surgery of the child's spine differs little from that of the adult, but on the average fusion occurs much more rapidly. Generally, children's spines fuse easily, and consequently it is prudent to expose only the area of the spine to be involved in the fusion. Extension of the dissection above or below the area will frequently result in an unwanted creeping fusion to the closely approximate lamina above and below. Atlantoaxial arthrodesis is performed essentially the same as in an adult, with care to avoid exposure of the occiput or C3 because of the great potential for involvement of these areas in the fusion mass. The vertebral arteries locking in a groove on the upper surface of the posterior arch of C1 are approximately 1 cm from the midline in the younger child, leaving a narrower margin of safety.* Skull tongs and halo devices have been used in young children as described by Griffiths, who used Crutchfield tongs in two children 2 years of age, but Minerva jackets might be more applicable.

REFERENCES

1. AUFDERMAUR M: Spinal injuries in juveniles: Neuropsy findings in twelve cases. J Bone Joint Surg 56B:513, 1971
2. BECKER F: Luxationsfranktur zwischen Atlas and Epistropheus im Kleinkindesaiter. Arch Orthop Unfallchir 55:682, 1963

3. *BLOUNT WP:* Fractures in Children. Baltimore, Williams & Wilkins, 1959
4. *BOHLMAN HH:* Acute fractures and dislocations of the cervical spine. J Bone Joint Surg 61A:1119, 1979
5. *BOHLMAN HH, DAVIS DD:* The pathology of fatal craniospinal injuries. In Brinkhous KM (ed): Accident Pathology: Proceedings of an International Conference, pp 154-159. Washington, DC, US Government Printing Office, 1970
6. *BRESNAM J, ADAMS F:* Neonatal spinal cord transection secondary to intrauterine hyperextension of the neck in breech presentation. Fatal Neonat Med 84(5):734, 1971
7. *CAFFEY J:* The whiplash shaken infant syndrome. Pediatrics 54(4):396, 1974
8. *CATTELL HS, FILTZER DL:* Pseudosubluxation and other normal variations in the cervical spine in children. J Bone Joint Surg 47A:1295, 1965
9. *CORNER ES:* Rotary dislocations of the atlas. Ann Surg 45:9, 1907
10. *COUTTS MB:* Atlanto-epistropheal subluxations. Arch Surg 29:297, 1934
11. *DAVIS D, BOHLMAN H, WALKER AE, FISHER R, ROBINSON R:* The pathological findings in fatal craniospinal injuries. J Neurosurg 34:603, 1971
12. *DOMMISSE GF:* The Arteries and Veins of the Human Spinal Cord from Birth. New York, Churchill Livingstone, 1975
13. *FIELDING JW:* Cineroentgenography of the normal cervical spine. J Bone Joint Surg 39A:1281, 1957
14. *FIELDING JW:* Normal and selected abnormal motion of the cervical spine from the second cervical vertebra to the seventh cervical vertebra based on cineroentgenography. J Bone Joint Surg 46A:1779, 1964
15. *FIELDING JW:* The cervical spine in the child. In Ahstrom JP Jr (ed): Current Practice in Orthopaedic Surgery, Vol 5. St. Louis, CV Mosby, 1973
16. *FIELDING JW, COCHRAN GVB, LAWSING JF III, HOHL M:* Tears of the transverse ligament of the atlas: A clinical and biomechanical study. J Bone Joint Surg 56A:1683, 1974
17. *FIELDING JW, HENSINGER RN, HAWKINS RJ:* Os odontoideum. J Bone Joint Surg 62A(3):375, 1980
18. *FIORANI-GALLOTTA G, LUZZATTI G:* Sublussazione Laterale e Sublussazione Rotatoria Dell-Atlanta. Arch Ortop 70:467, 1957
19. *GREELEY PW:* Bilateral (90 degrees) rotatory dislocation of the atlas upon the atlas. J Bone Joint Surg 12:958, 1930
20. *GRIFFITHS SC:* Fracture of the odontoid process in children. J Pediatr Surg 7:680, 1972
21. *GRISEL P:* Enucleation de l'atlas et torticollis nasopharyngien. Presse Med 38:50, 1930
22. *GROGONO BJS:* Injuries of the atlas and axis. J Bone Joint Surg 36B:397, 1954
23. *HASUE M, HOSHINO R, OMATA S, ET AL:* Cervical spine injuries in children. Fukushima J Med Sci 20:111, 1971
24. *HENRYS P, LYNE ED, LIFTON C, SALCICCIDI G:* Clinical review of cervical spine injuries in children. Clin Orthop, p 129, 1977
25. *HESS JH, ABELSON SM, BRONSTEIN IP:* Atlanto-axial dislocation unassociated with trauma and secondary to inflammatory foci of the neck. Am J Dis Child 49:1137, 1935
26. *HOHL M, BAKER HR:* The atlanto-axial joint: Roentgenographic and anatomical study of the normal and abnormal motion. J Bone Joint Surg 46A:1730, 1964
27. *HUNTER GA:* Non-traumatic displacement of the atlanto-axial joint. J Bone Joint Surg 50B:44, 1968
28. *JACKSON H:* Diagnosis of minimal atlanto-axial subluxation. Br J Radiol 23:672, 1950
29. *JACOBSON G, ADLER DC:* Examination of the atlanto-axial joint following injury with particular emphasis on rotational subluxation. Am J Roentgenol Rad Ther Nucl Med 76:1081, 1956
30. *JONES MD:* Cineradiographic studies of the normal cervical spine. California Medicine 93:293, 1960
31. *JUHL JH, MILLER SM, ROBERTS GW:* Roentgenographic variations in the normal cervical spine. Radiology 78:591, 1962
32. *LIPPMAN RK:* Arthropathy due to adjacent inflammation. J Bone Joint Surg 35A(4):1953
33. *MARTEL W:* The occipito-atlanto-axial joints in rheumatoid arthritis and ankylosing spondylitis. Am J Roentgenol Rad Ther Nucl Med 86:223, 1961
34. *MORAN BC, BALACHANDRAN N:* Non-traumatic atlanto-axial dislocation in children. Clin Orthop 92:220, 1973
35. *NACHEMSON A:* Fracture of the odontoid process of the axis: A clinical study based on 26 cases. Acta Orthop Scand 29:185
36. *NELSON'S TEXTBOOK OF PEDIATRICS.*
37. *PALANT DI, CARTER RL:* Klippel-Feil syndrome and deafness. Am J Dis Child 123:218, 1972
38. *PARROT J:* Rupture of the spinal cord in the newborn. J Union Med 9:137, 1870
39. *PAUL IW, MOIR WW:* Non-pathologic variations in relationship of the upper cervical vertebrae. Am J Roentgenol Rad Ther Nucl Med 62:519, 1949
40. *RANG M:* Children's Fractures. Philadelphia, JB Lippincott, 1974
41. *ROY-CAMILLE R, DE LA CAFFINIERE JY, SAILLANT G:* Traumatisines du Rochis Cervical Superieur C1–C2. Paris, Masson et Cie, 1973
42. *SCHNEIDER RC:* Head and Neck injuries in Foot-

ball: Mechanisms, Treatment and Prevention. Baltimore, Williams & Wilkins, 1973

43. *Sherk HH, Nicholson JT:* Rotary atlanto-axial dislocation associated with ossiculum terminale and mongolism. J Bone Joint Surg 51A:957, 1969
44. *Schneider RC, Schemm GW:* Vertebral artery insufficiency in acute and chronic spinal trauma. J Neurosurg 18:348, 1961
45. *Sherk HH, Nicholson JT, Chung SMK:* Fractures of the odontoid process in young children. J Bone Joint Surg 60A:921, 1978
46. *Sherk HH, Schut L, Lane JM:* Fractures and dislocations of the cervical spine in children. Orthop Clin North Am 7:593, 1976
47. *Shulman SI, Madden JD, Easterly JR, Shanklin DR:* Transection of spinal cord: A rare obstetrical complication of cephalic delivery. Arch Dis Child 46:291, 1971
48. *Steel HH:* Anatomical and mechanical consideration of the atlantoaxial articulation. Proceedings of the American Orthopaedic Association. J Bone Joint Surg 50A:1481, 1968
49. *Stern WE, Rand RW:* Birth injuries to the spinal cord: Report of 2 cases and review of the literature. Am J Obstet Gynecol 78:498, 1959
50. *Sullivan W:* Subluxation of the atlanto-axial joint. Sequel to inflammatory process of the neck. J Pediatr 35:451, 1949
51. *Sullivan RC, Bruwer AJ, Harris I:* Hypermobility of the cervical spine in children: A pitfall in the diagnosis of cervical dislocation. Am J Surg 95:636, 1958
52. *Swischuck LE:* Spine and spinal cord trauma in the battered child syndrome. Radiology 92:733, 1969
3. *Vigouroux RP, Baurand C, Choux M, et al:* Les traumatismes du rachis cervical chez. L'Ent Neurochinurgie 14:689, 1968
54. *Von Torklus D, Gehle W:* The Upper Cervical Spine. New York, Grune & Stratton, 1972
55. *Watson-Jones R:* Spontaneous hyperemic dislocation of the atlas. Proc Royal Soc Med 25:586, 1932
56. *Watson-Jones R:* Fractures and Joint Injuries, 4th ed, Vol 2. Baltimore, Williams & Wilkins, 1955
57. *Webb FWS, Hickman JA, Brew DS:* Death from vertebral artery thrombosis in rheumatoid arthritis. Br Med J 2:537, 1968
58. *Weber BG, Brunner CR, Freuler F:* Treatment of Fractures in Children and Adolescents. Berlin, Springer-Verlag, 1980
59. *Weir DC:* Roentgenographic signs of cervical injury. Clin Orthop 1099, 1975
60. *Werne S:* Spontaneous atlas dislocation. Acta Orthop Scand 25:32, 1955
61. *Werne S:* Studies in spontaneous atlas dislocations. Acta Orthop Scand (Suppl) 23:1, 1957
62. *Wilson MJ, Michele A, Jacobson E:* Spontaneous dislocation of the atlanto-axial articulation including a report of a case with quadriplegia. J Bone Joint Surg 22:698, 1940
63. *Wortzman G, Dewar FP:* Rotary fixation of the atlantoaxial joint: Rotational atlantoaxial subluxation. Radiology 90:479, 1968
64. *Yates PO:* Birth trauma to the vertebral arteries. Arch Dis Child 34:436, 1959

Soft-Tissue Neck Injuries

Mason Hohl

The terms *whiplash, hyperextension, acceleration injury, cervical strain,* and *cervical sprain* may also be called soft-tissue injury of the neck. The resulting syndrome is due to damage to cervical muscles, ligaments, discs, blood vessels, and nerves, as has been demonstrated experimentally. These experiments, as well as electroencephalograms on injured patients, have indicated varying degrees of brain dysfunction and damage.[13,24,26] The symptom complex resulting from these injuries is often so confusing both to the physician and his patient that the specter of psychosomatic illness and secondary gain is considered.[4,9,23] Fortunately, there is now a body of scientific knowledge that is helpful to the clinician in understanding injury production, the anatomic basis for many of the resulting symptoms, and prognosis for recovery.

MECHANISM OF INJURY

Motor vehicle collisions account for the vast majority of soft-tissue neck injuries. The rear-end automobile collision, occurring when a vehicle is struck from the rear, has produced most of the studied clinical material available in recent literature.[7,8,10,11,14,21] It has been established conclusively through documented experimental rear-end collisions, using volunteers for low velocity impact and anthropomorphic dummies for higher velocities, that the unsupported head and neck rapidly hyperextend until the back of the head strikes the seat, well beyond the normal range of allowable movement.[16,22] This violent motion occurs in the first quarter second after impact and is followed by a less rapid flexion of the neck as tissue elasticity and slowing of acceleration take effect. Thus, the actual injury to soft tissues occurs so rapidly that normal protective muscle reflexes cannot respond.

Today, head supports are provided in automobiles for the express purpose of preventing hyperextension and its associated injury. In one study, however, only 20% of adjustable head supports were found positioned at a level adequate to effectively prevent injury.[19] Research continues on alternate methods of prevention less dependent upon the occupant's position or size. A high back seat performs well to prevent hyperextension, but has other drawbacks.

Other mechanisms of injury include hyperflexion or lateral flexion as the result of automobile collision, athletics, or a falling object striking the head. Fortunately, these injuries are not usually as serious as those caused by hyperextension, owing to the fact that there is a natural restraint available to prevent the head from going beyond its normal range.[15] Hyperflexion is limited a the chin strikes the chest, and lateral flexion as the head strikes the shoulder. Nonetheless, injuries to soft structures do occur by these mechanisms and follow a similar clinical course.

EXPERIMENTAL INJURY PRODUCTION

The sometimes bizarre post-injury symptoms and signs in soft-tissue neck injuries have long been the subject of speculation over whether they were caused by organic injury or were psychological in origin. Unfortunately, no early direct observations of deep structure injury in humans have been possible since these injuries are neither fatal nor demanding of early operative treatment. However, several investigators constructed experiments that were designed to reproduce soft-tissue injuries in animals, usually small primates.[13,14,18,26] Many of these experiments were documented by high-speed photography, x-ray motion pictures, measurement of biomechanical forces generated, and continuous electroencephalographic observations. Direct tissue examinations at intervals following injury were obtained.

Macnab, Ommaya and associates, and Wickstrom and associates created experimental hyperextension injuries to animals. They found a variety of anterior neck injuries, including muscle hemorrhages and tears, ruptures of the anterior longitudinal ligament, intervertebral disc disruptions, and esophageal muscle hemorrhages.[14,18,26] Brain injury, long suspected, was substantiated by findings of superficial brain hemorrhages and electroencephalographic abnormalities. Much earlier, clinicians had noted frequent electroencephalographic changes in human victims of rear-end collisions.[24]

THE CLINICAL PICTURE

The typical patient with soft-tissue neck injury is a front seat passenger in a vehicle lacking head restraint that is struck without warning from the rear. Often the patient can recall being jolted backward and forward at the moment of collision. Occasionally a witness will describe the patient as having been unconscious for a moment to a few seconds following impact and confused for a period thereafter. Most patients are not aware of significant injury at that moment, but after a few minutes develop a feeling of discomfort in the neck associated with some degree of nausea. A feeling of increasing tightness and stiffness gradually ensues, most noticable in the early post-injury days.

Physical examination of the injured patient after only a few hours seldom results in significant finding of muscle tenderness, spasm, or restricted neck motion. However, after a few hours to a few days post-injury, when such patients are usually seen, there is tenderness and swelling in the anterior neck region and often palpable spasm in the trapezius muscles accompanied by variable restriction of neck movement. These symptoms and signs tend to change after the first few days, with the anterior soreness disappearing, and depending upon the severity of injury, either decreasing trapezius tightness with more movement or increased concentration of posterior symptoms with continued limitation of motion. The natural history of this injury in the absence of treatment is a few days to a few weeks of stiffness and restricted motion with gradual improvement in most patients. Many, however, continue to have some degree of neck symptoms on a permanent basis.

The soft-tissue injury syndrome is complicated by a wide variety of bizarre symptoms. These include headache, dizziness, visual disturbances, auditory abnormalities, pain in the interscapular area, shoulders, or arms, and numbness in the upper extremities. Special consultants frequently see patients with these complaints and seldom find significant abnormalities or offer help in clinical management. Fortunately, most of the complaints, such as blurred vision or buzzing or noises in the ear, gradually clear during the first months following injury. Unfortunately, when physicians cannot accurately define the causes of such symptoms and thus cannot suggest appropriate and effective treatment, the patient tends to distrust both doctors and his own perception of the symptoms. Thus, even if physicians do not label such symptoms neurotic in nature, the patient may unconsciously believe this.

Complaints of arm and hand pain or numbness are common at some time during the post-injury course and are not often typical of cervical radicular pain caused by nerve root compression, since they do not conform to anatomic pathways. Most such patients have areas of trigger tenderness in the periscapular region that produce a nonneurogenic, radiating, painful numbness into the arm with a lack of motor, reflex, or sensory changes. Autonomic nervous system impairment (Horner's syndrome) is occasionally seen, due to sympathetic ganglion damage around the sixth cervical level.

ROENTGENOGRAPHIC FINDINGS

Aside from showing alterations of the cervical curve and preexisting degenerative disc disease, routine x-ray examination is seldom revealing. Occult fracture and retropharyngeal soft-tissue swelling must always be suspected.[2] Older patients often show preexisting degenerative changes, including intervertebral disc narrowing, spurring, and facet arthritis.[5,6] Much has been said about alterations of the cervical curve from the normally expected lordosis.[10,12,20] The popular myth that loss of lordosis denotes muscle spasm has been subjected to scientific investigation. There is no question that a considerable number of rear-end collision victims have a cervical curve flattening or reversal. It does appear from studies that mere flattening is not necessarily indicative of any pathology or post-injury condition.[3,10,20] In fact, it is probably a normal variation in most cases. Dynamic studies, including flexion–extension views, are likely to persuade the careful observer, in cases of flattening or curve reversal, that no serious condition exists if the expected movement is demonstrated at each level.

The sharply reversed cervical curve appears to indicate a degree of structural damage, as shown in a long-term follow-up study.[10] When there is an existing sharp reversal, flexion–extension films usually fail to indicate normal mobility at the involved level. If the reversal occurs over more than one segment, it is termed a reversed curve and may show relatively normal flexion–extension at each level, and thus seems to represent a lesser degree of injury.

The abnormal cervical curve tends to persist rather than to revert to normal over a period of time. Alterations of the cervical curve without injury have been noted frequently in association with intervertebral disc degenerative narrowing and spur formation. In patients with disc degeneration, x-ray films showing reversal after soft-tissue injury are not particularly significant (Fig. 6-125).

Special roentgenograms to show the pillars and

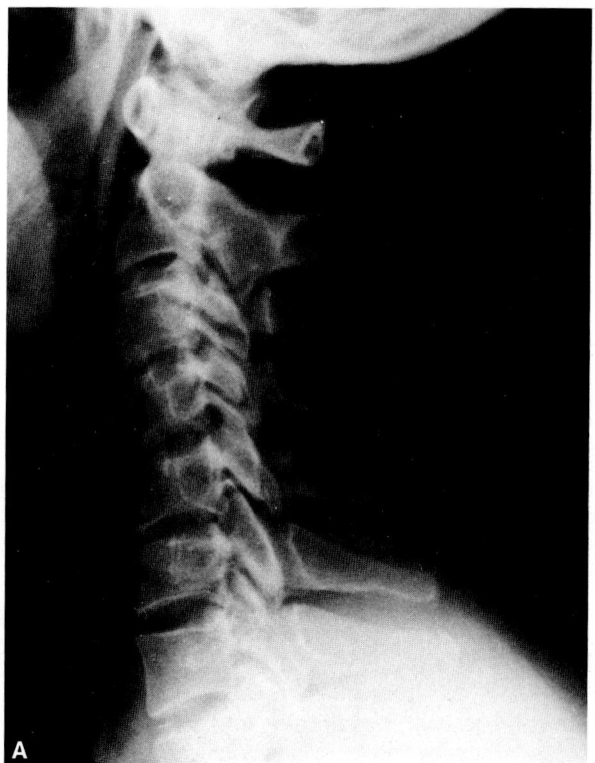

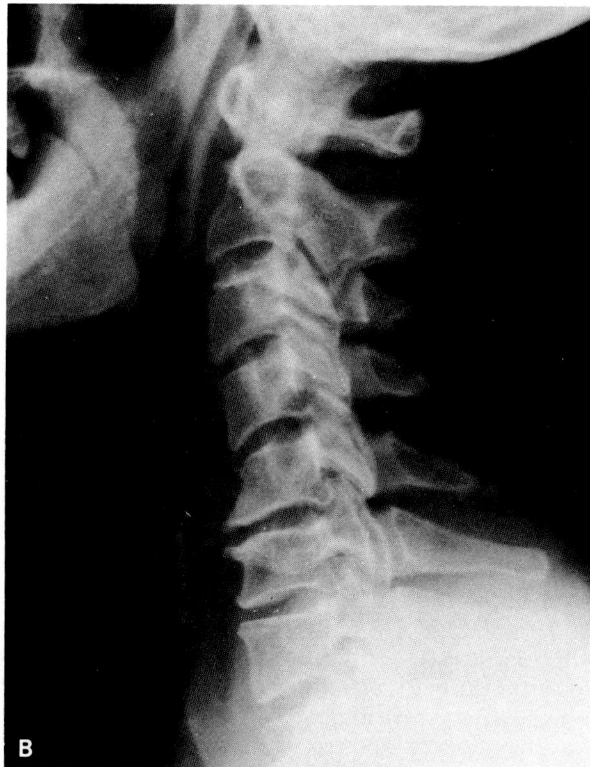

Fig. 6-125. Roentgenograms of a 29-year-old woman who sustained hyperextension neck injury after the rear of her car struck a wall during a spin-out. (*A*) Note the normal lordotic curve with the disc narrowing at C5–C6. (*B*) Seven years later, the patient experienced occasional stiff neck and discomfort. Further narrowing of C5–C6 has occurred.

articular processes are useful in patients experiencing more lasting symptoms and with findings of persistent restriction of neck movement, to rule out fractures not seen in routine views. Abel demonstrated so-called occult fractures after neck injury in some patients.[1] Bone scan studies screen for occult fractures and may be useful in patients with persisting symptoms. When the bone scan is positive, computed axial tomography may aid in the diagnosis of occult fracture.

TREATMENT

The basic treatment for overstretched muscle and ligament injury is protection and rest, depending somewhat upon the clinical presentation. Such an approach following thorough physical and x-ray examination gives the patient the confidence to trust his physician in the face of a disturbing degree of neck tightness associated with a variety of other puzzling symptoms. Moderate and severely symptomatic patients do better with bed rest and sedation for a few days until the initial spasm and symptoms improve.

Soft collars of felt, foam, or rubber seem to add comfort in many patients, allowing them to become more active soon after injury. Rigid collars have not been shown to be any more effective but may be better when there is evidence of ligament injury. Wearing the collar should not be allowed to become a habit and should be discontinued as soft-tissue healing occurs.

Heat from a heating pad or hot shower can relieve muscle tension and permit active exercise with less discomfort. However, the frequent or prolonged use of a heating pad, ultrasound, or diathermy tends to cause irritation and perpetuate symptoms. Exercises to stretch muscles and increase neck motion are generally encouraged within limits of comfort. Isometric neck exercises are advocated by some as a primary treatment soon after injury, continuing until recovery.[8]

Various forms of physical therapy are frequently used, including heat, massage, and traction. Traction performed manually or by machine is used by many who treat these injuries. It is difficult however, to rationalize traction in the early weeks after injury, since this would involve pulling and stretching on injured muscles and ligaments. Later, however, after fibrous healing of structures, traction may be a significant aid in restoring motion.

Medication can be quite helpful in relieving painful tension but should be cautiously administered, as pointed out by Macnab.[15] It is better to use physical measures such as rest, support, and heat for pain relief than to rely upon muscle relaxers or strong analgesics. Drugs and physical therapy both tend to impress patients with the seriousness of their injury.

Recent trends in soft-tissue injury management use rest and support early, with heat and range of motion and isometric exercises as initial discomfort subsides.[25] Isometric neck exercises have achieved some popularity as a substitute for formal physical therapy. Perhaps the most important advantage of exercises done regularly is the patient's participation in treatment and recovery.

RESULTS OF TREATMENT

Studies have pointed out clearly that a significant number of patients at various intervals after neck injury have continuing symptoms that they attribute to that injury.[7,8,10,11,14,17] The incidence varies between 20% and 90%, depending upon the series reviewed and the time of follow-up. These lasting symptoms were most often intermittent neck ache, stiffness, and headache, but a few patients had

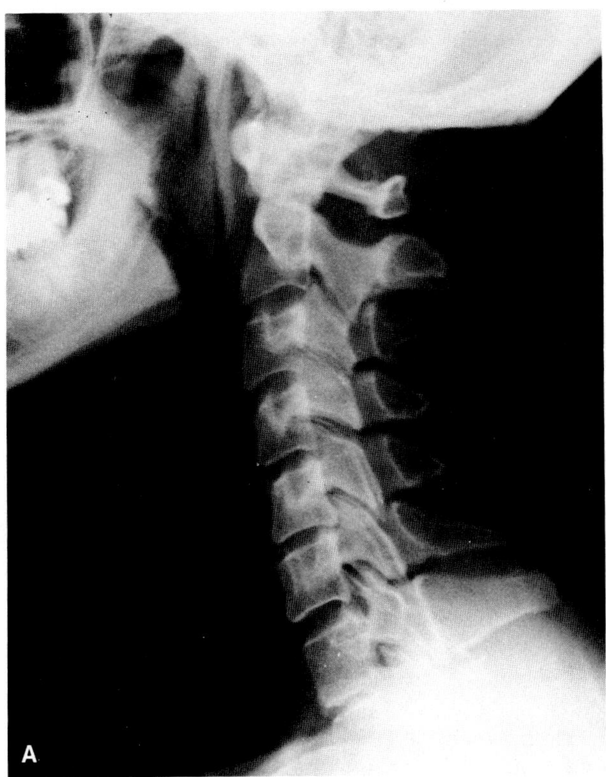

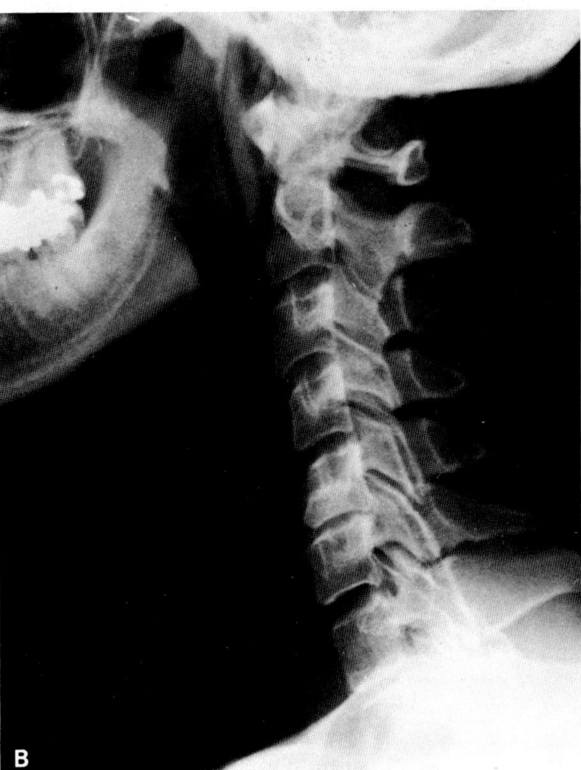

Fig. 6-126. Roentgenograms of a 28-year-old man who was involved in an automobile collision in which he was struck from the side. His head struck the car interior, producing a lateral flexion injury. (*A*) the initial roentgenogram a few days after injury indicates reversal of the cervical curve at C4–C5. (*B*) Eight years later. Note the C5–C6 disc degenerative change. The patient is often aware of clicking and discomfort in the neck.

radicular pain. In general there was little to be found in physical examination.

Follow-up roentgenograms taken an average of 7 years after injury in one series of patients without prior roentgenographic evidence of disc disease indicated that 39% had developed degenerative disc disease at one or more disc levels since injury.[10] It was pointed out that available evidence indicated an expected incidence of 6% degenerative change in a population with this mean age of 30 years.[10] Thus, it appeared that the injury had started the slow process of disc degeneration (Fig. 6-126).

In another follow-up study of patients with similar injuries but with preexisting degenerative changes in the neck, it was observed that after an average of 7 years 39% had residual symptoms, and roentgenographic evidence of new degenerative change at another level occurred in 55%.[11] Of considerable interest was the finding in both series that there was no statistical correlation between the development of degenerative changes and continued symptoms.[10,11]

Attempts have been made to determine which early symptoms or findings might provide a reliable index to the short-term or long-term prognosis. Greenfield and Ilfeld, who studied short-termprognostic factors in 179 consecutive soft-tissue injury patients, noted that shoulder pain and arm and hand pain indicated slower progress toward recovery, and that when upper back pain and interscapular pain were present, a longer and more intensive treatment program was needed.[8] The average length of treatment in this series was just over 7 weeks, at which time 37% of the patients were asymptomatic.

Norris and Watt grouped 61 patients into three groups after rear-end collision, depending upon initial symptoms and signs. After 2 years follow-up 44% of those initially presenting with only symptoms had residual complaints.[17] Eighty-one percent of those with initial symptoms and physical findings were symptomatic, while those with neurologic involvement were 90% symptomatic. A poorer prognosis resulted from early neurologic involvement, degenerative changes on original x-rays, or abnormal cervical curves.

Hohl and Hopp, in their long-term follow-up studies, found that complaints of interscapular pain, upper extremity pain and numbness, or findings of sharp cervical curve reversal or one-level restricted motion on flexion–extension x-ray films carried a poor prognosis.[10,11] They also noted that the incidence of symptomatic recovery was better in men, that degenerative changes developed more often in patients that had been unconscious, and that litigation or its absence did not appear to influence the long-term result.

REFERENCES

1. *Abel S:* Moderately severe whiplash injuries of the cervical spine and their roentgenographic diagnosis. Clin Orthop 12:189, 1958
2. *Birsner JW, Leask WH:* Retropharyngeal soft tissue swelling due to whiplash injury. Arch Surg 68:369, 1954
3. *Borden AGB, Rechtman AM, Gershon-Cohen J:* The normal cervical lordosis. Radiology 74:806, 1960
4. *Braaf MM, Rosner S:* Whiplash injury of neck: Fact or fancy? Int Surg 46:176, 1966
5. *Friedenberg ZB, Broder HA, Edeiken JE, Spencer HN:* Degenerative disc disease of the cervical spine: Clinical and roentgenographic study. JAMA 174:374, 1960
6. *Friedenberg ZB, Miller WT:* Degenerative disc disease of cervical spine: A comparative study of asymptomatic and symptomatic patients. J Bone Joint Surg 45A:1171, 1963
7. *Gotten N:* Survey of one hundred cases of whiplash injury after settlement of litigation. JAMA 162:865, 1956
8. *Greenfield J, Ilfeld FW:* Acute cervical strain: Evaluation and short term prognostic factors. Clin Orthop 122:196, 1977
9. *Hohl M:* Medical aspects of neck injuries. In Stumpf FF, Horwitz WS (eds): Medicolegal Aspects of Head, Neck and Back Injuries. Berkeley, University of California Press, 1955
10. *Hohl M:* Soft-tissue injuries of the neck in automobile accidents: Factors influencing prognosis. J Bone Joint Surg 56A:1675, 1974
11. *Hohl M, Hopp E:* Soft tissue injuries of the neck. II. Factors influencing prognosis (abstr). Orthop Transact 2:29, 1978
12. *Juhl JH, Miller SW, Roberts GW:* Roentgenographic variations in the normal cervical spine. Radiology 78:591, 1962
13. *Liu K, Chandran K, Heath R, Unterharnscheidt F:* Subcortical EEG changes in rhesus monkeys following experimental hyperextension-hyperflexion (whiplash). Spine 9:329–338, 1984
14. *Macnab I:* Acceleration injuries of the cervical spine. J Bone Joint Surg 46A:1797, 1964
15. *Macnab I:* Acceleration: Extension injuries of the cervical spine. In AAOS Symposium of the Spine, pp 10-17. St. Louis, CV Mosby, 1969
16. *McKenzie J, William J:* The dynamic behavior of the head and cervical spine during whiplash. J Biomech 4:477–490, 1971

17. *Norris S, Watt I:* The prognosis of neck injuries resulting from rearend vehicle collisions. J Bone Joint Surg 65B:608–611, 1983
18. *Ommaya AK, Faas F, Yarnell P:* Whiplash and brain damage. JAMA 204(4):285, 1968
19. *O'Neill B, Haddon W Jr, Kelley AB, Sorenson WW:* Automobile head restraints: Frequency of neck injury claims in relation to the presence of head restraints. Am J Public Health 62:399, 1972
20. *Rechtman AM, Borden AGB, Gershon-Cohen J:* The lordotic curve of the cervical spine. Clin Orthop 20:208, 1961
21. *Schutt CH, Dohan FC:* Neck injury to women in auto accidents. JAMA 206:2689, 1968
22. *Severy DM, Mathewson JH, Bechtol CD:* Controlled rear end collisions: An investigation of related engineering and medical phenomena. Can Servi Med J 11:727, 1955
23. *States JD, Korn MW, Massengill JB:* The enigma of whiplash injury. NY State J Med 70:2971, 1970
24. *Torres F, Shaprio SK:* Electroencephalograms in whiplash injury. Arch Neurol 5:40, 1961
25. *Wickstrom JK, LaRocca H:* Management of patients with cervical spine and head injuries from acceleration forces. Curr Pract Orthop Surg 6:83, 1975
26. *Wickstrom JK, Martinez JL, Rodriguez RP Jr, Haines DM:* Hyperextension and hyperflexion injuries to head and neck of primates. Dissertation, presented at Wayne State University, May 1969

Epidemiology, Pathomechanics, and Prevention of Athletic Injuries to the Cervical Spine

JOSEPH TORG

The specter of catastrophic cervical neurotrauma resulting from athletic participation, although infrequent, has been consistently associated with water sports,[1,16,25,35,38] football,[13,33,34,41–44,48–50] gymnastics,[17,18,20,22,29,36,46,53,54] rugby,[10,24,32] and ice hockey.[19,37,39,40] A review of the available literature reveals changing injury patterns as well as prevailing concepts regarding the mechanism responsible for most athletic injuries to the cervical spinal structures.[48,49] Accurate descriptions of the mechanism, or mechanisms, responsible for a particular injury transcend simple academic interest. In order that preventive measures be implemented, the manner in which an injury occurs must be accurately defined. The purpose of this section is to describe and clarify the concepts regarding pathomechanics of these injuries as they relate to prevention based on existing clinical, epidemiologic, and laboratory evidence. Specifically, we will consider these factors as they pertain to tackle football, gymnastics, water sports (diving and surfing), and ice hockey.

Athletic injuries to the cervical spine and brachial plexus cover the spectrum from cervical sprains and transient neuropraxia to fracture-dislocations with quadriplegia. Fortunately, the frequency of these injuries appears to be inversely proportional to the severity of the lesions. Clancy and coworkers documented the occurrence of brachial plexus neuropraxia among collegiate football players.[14] Specifically, 50% of all players at the United States Naval Academy and the University of Wisconsin sustained at least one significant injury during their playing careers. On the other hand, Clarke retrospectively surveyed (1973–1975) nonfatal, catastrophic spinal cord injuries among all high school and intercollegiate athletes and reported an average annual incidence of 1 per 7000 participants in men's gymnastics to 1 per 792,000 participants in men's basketball.[15] He further indicated that only football, gymnastics, and wrestling showed an annual persistence of such injuries, and of these only football and gymnastics displayed describable patterns. Other reports indicate the disquieting occurrence of cervical spine injuries with associated quadriplegia in nonorganized water sports and amateur Canadian ice hockey.

The classical concept of the mechanism responsible for sports-related cervical spine trauma has emphasized the role of hyperflexion (Fig. 6-127).[34] Whether it is a diving accident or one resulting from trampolining, rugby, or American football, injury has been assumed to occur, in most cases, in a hyperflexion mode. The subject is an unsuspecting victim of some untoward circumstance, such as an accidental fall, a dive into shallow water, an unexpected blow to the head, or, as in the case of the athlete, a poorly executed physical act in which the cervical spine is forced into hyperflexion with resulting injury. Recent observations, both in the laboratory and in the clinical setting, indicate that in the majority of instances athletically induced cervical spine trauma results from axial loading (Fig. 6-128).[11,23,42–45,47,49,50]

Roaf has published results of studies in which spinal units were subjected to forces differing in magnitude and direction, that is, compression, flexion, extension, lateral flexion, rotation, and horizontal shear.[30] He stated unequivocally that he had never succeeded in producing pure hyperflexion injuries in a normal, intact spinal unit and concluded that hyperflexion of the cervical spine is an anatomic impossibility. Of equal significance is the fact that Roaf was able to produce almost every variety of spinal injury by a combination of compression and/or flexion–rotation.

Bauze has reported the experimental production of forward dislocation of the cervical spine by subjecting it to pure vertical loads.[8] The spine in human cadavers was subjected to loads in a compression apparatus to simulate the clinical situation for dislocations. The movements were recorded by lateral cineradiography. The lower part of the spine was flexed and fixed, and the upper part extended and free to move forward. Vertical compression then produced bilateral dislocation of the facet joints without fracture. If lateral tilt or axial rotation occurred as well, a unilateral dislocation was produced. The maximum vertical loading required was 145 kg (319 lbs); this was accompanied by rupture of the posterior ligament and capsule and severing of the anterior longitudinal ligament prior to dislocation. The low vertical load indicates the peculiar vulnerability of the cervical spine in this position. Bauze concluded that this low load correlated well with the minor trauma often seen and associated with forward dislocation.

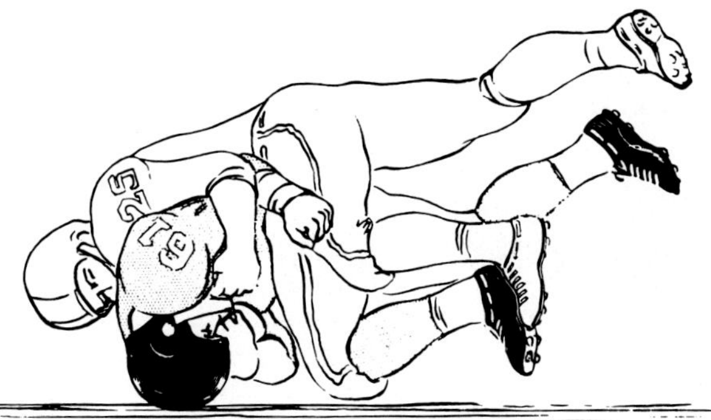

Fig. 6-127. Hyperflexion injury to the cervical spine occurs when it is forced beyond the limits of motion and the applied force exceeds the elastic capabilities of the involved structures. Recent evidence indicates that, contrary to past thinking, this mechanism is an infrequent cause of cervical spine injury in athletes. (Melvin WJS: The role of face guard in the production of flexion injuries to the cervical spine in football. Can Med Assoc J 93:1110, 1965)

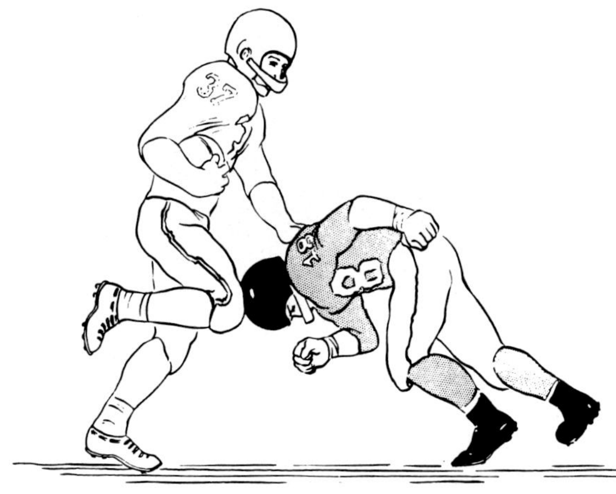

Fig. 6-128. Axial loading of the cervical spine due to impact on the crown of the head or helmet is responsible for most of the serious injuries that occur in football. The same mechanism is responsible for diving injuries. (Melvin WJS: The role of the face guard in the production of flexion injuries to the cervical spine in football. Can Med Assoc J 93:1110, 1965)

FOOTBALL

Various mechanisms have been proposed as being responsible for cervical spine injuries occurring in athletics, and more specifically, in tackle football. Two concepts have not survived close scrutiny: one implicates the face mask acting as a lever, forcing the head and neck into hyperflexion,[34] and the other implicates the posterior rim of the football helmet acting as a "guillotine."[34] When evaluated in the light of existing evidence, these two concepts must be dismissed as erroneous.

In regard to the first concept, that of the face mask acting as a lever causing cervical spine fracture or dislocation with or without quadriplegia: Of 209 severe injuries that occurred between 1971 and 1984,[49] in no instance has this been a factor. The suggestion that the upward sweep of a long-lever arm, the face guard, can cause a marked mechanical advantage as the posterior rim of the rigid helmet guillotines the cervical cord has been effectively refuted on the basis of radiographic, biomechanical, and epidemiologic data.[12,23,52]

Regarding the second concept, Virgin performed a cineradiographic study to evaluate the possible role of the posterior rim of the football helmet in causing neck injuries.[52] A series of lateral cineradiograms were taken to document the path and position of the posterior rim of the football helmet relative to the spinal column in 16 subjects as they moved their heads from the fully flexed to fully extended position under several loading conditions. Five different football helmets were used in the study. No contact occurred at any time between the posterior rim of the five helmets and the spinous processes of the cervical vertebrae. Virgin concluded that the notion of injury being caused by the posterior rim of the helmet striking the cervical spine above C7 is without foundation (Figs. 6-129 and 6-130).

Carter and Frankel studied the biomechanics of cervical spine hyperextension injuries in football players using quasistatic free-body analysis.[12] The study examined the guillotine mechanism of injury. The static free-body analysis was undertaken to determine the forces imposed on the cervical spine when the face guard was struck in such a manner as to create hyperextension of the cervical spine. Three situations that corresponded to the loading conditions created by three different helmet designs were examined. In the first situation, it was assumed that the helmet rim was cut high enough posteriorly that it did not impinge on the posterior cervical spine (Fig. 6-131). In the second situation, it was assumed that the helmet rim impacted at the level of the fourth cervical vertebra (Fig. 6-132). In the third case, it was assumed that the posterior rim of the helmet struck the shoulder pads (Fig. 6-133). The results of this analysis suggest that the most dangerous hyperextension occurs with the first condition, which leads to large forces and possible injury to the upper cervical

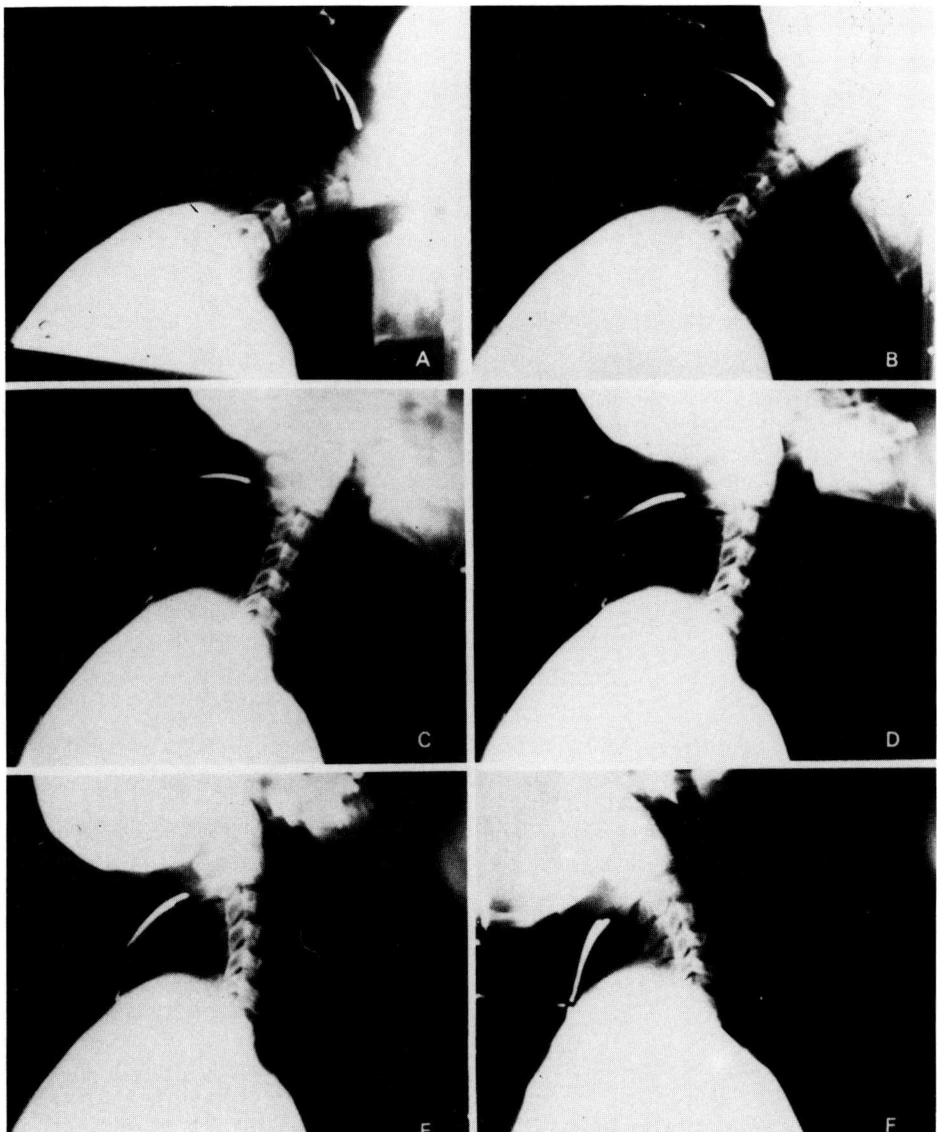

Fig. 6-129. A series of cineradiograms demonstrating the failure of the posterior rim of one of five different brand football helmets to impinge on the soft tissue overlying the spinous processes of C1 through C6. (Virgin H: Cineradiographic study of football helmets and the cervical spine. Am J Sports Med 8:310, 1980)

spine (Fig. 6-134). The impact of the posterior rim of the helmet at the fourth cervical vertebra significantly reduced these forces. This finding directly conflicts with the so-called guillotine concept of injury. The impact of the posterior rim of the helmet on the shoulder pads is the least hazardous of loading conditions.

Data related to the mechanism of cervical spine injuries, both with and without neurologic involvement, resulting from tackle football further refute the hyperextension-guillotine concept. Torg and coworkers identified only 3% of injuries that resulted in quadriplegia as resulting from hyperextension, whereas 8% of those resulting in fracture or dislocation without quadriplegia were due to this mechanism.[43,44] The concept of the posterior

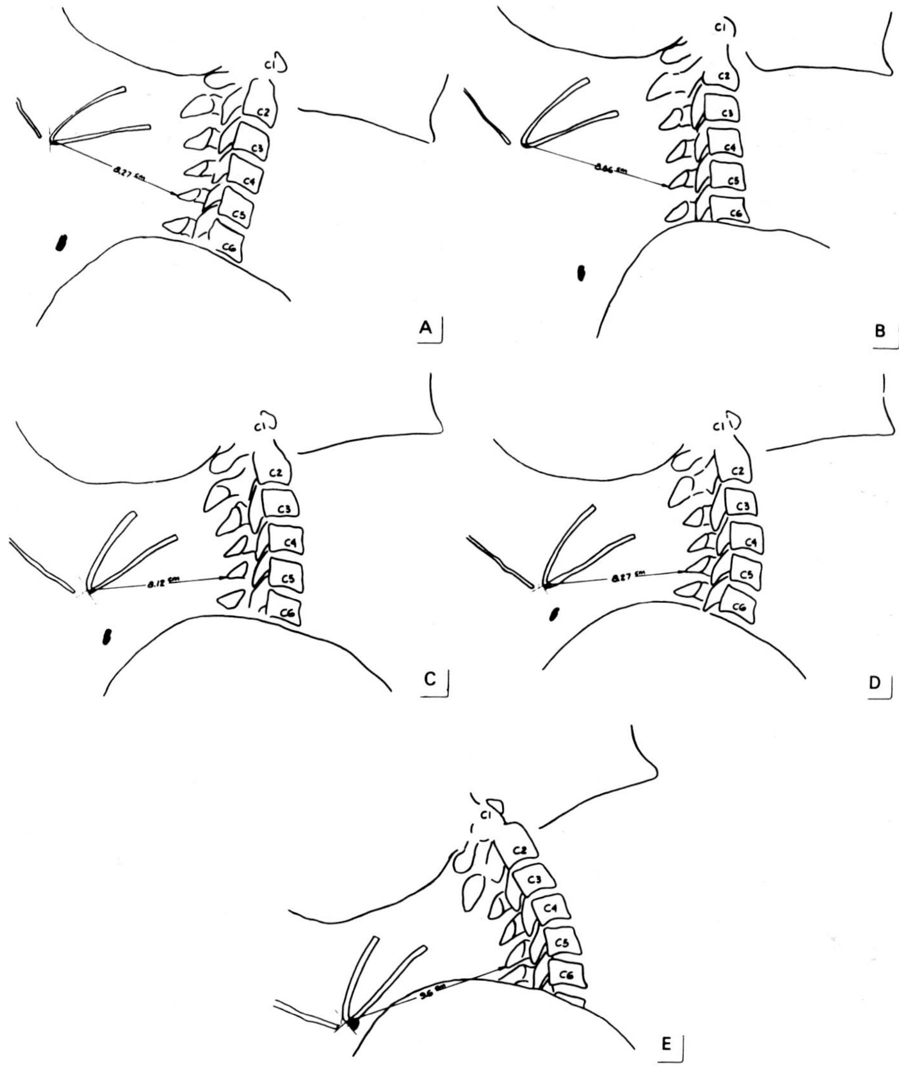

Fig. 6-130. Measurements of the distance from the posterior rim of the helmet to the spinous processes C5 from the neutral position to point of impingement: (*A*) 8.27 cm; (*B*) 8.06 cm; (*C*) 8.12 cm; (*D*) 8.27 cm; and (*E*) 9.6 cm. Determined from cineradiographic studies, these measurements refute the contention that the posterior rim of the football helmet can act as a guillotine in the extremes of forced cervical extension. (Virgin H: Cineradiogaphic study of football helmets and the cervical spine. Am J Sports Med 8:310, 1980)

rim of the football helmet acting as a guillotine and inflicting injury on the cervical cord in extreme forced hyperextension is without foundation.

Schneider has observed that "There is probably no better experimental or research laboratory for human trauma in the world than the football fields in our nation."[34] An analysis of available information about cervical spine injuries resulting in quadriplegia substantiates this statement.

The effect of axial loading of the cervical spine has been vividly demonstrated on a clinical level in American football. Epidemiologic and cinematographic analyses establish that most cases of cervical spine quadriplegia resulting from American football injuries are caused by direct compression

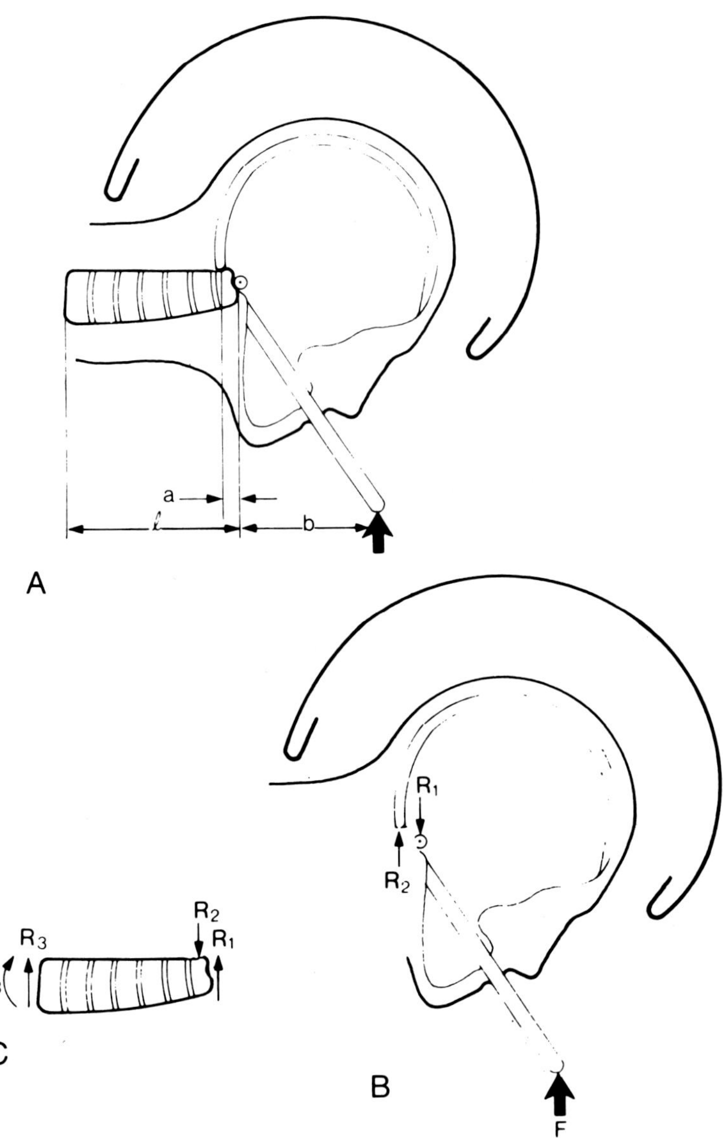

Fig. 6-131. (*A*) Loading condition of hyperextension limited by bony contact of occiput in the atlas. (*B*) Free body diagram of the head and helmet. (*C*) Free body diagram of the cervical spine. (Carter D, Frankel VH: Biomechanics of hyperextension injuries to the cervical spine in football. Am J Sports Med 8:302, 1980)

in head-on type collisions in which the initial contact is made with the top or crown of the helmet.[49,50] Thus, rather than an accidental, untoward event, a technique is used that places the cervical spine at risk of catastrophic injury.

During the 1975 football season, 12 severe cervical spine injuries occurred in Pennsylvania and New Jersey.[41] Determination of the mechanism of injury responsible for the cervical spine fractures and dislocations resulting in quadriplegia was revealing. Six of the eight players were rendered quadriplegic while playing defensive back and making a tackle. In each instance, the head was used as a battering ram in tackling by striking an opponent with the top of the helmet.

In order to document the extent of head and neck injury problems, the National Football Head and Neck Injury Registry was established in 1975.[43,44] Reportable injuries included cervical spine and head injuries that required hospitalization for a minimum of 72 hours; that involved a fracture, dislocation, or subluxation; or that resulted in paralysis or death.

Initially, the Registry collected information retrospectively from 1971 through the 1975 season.[43] Four parameters of severe head and neck injuries

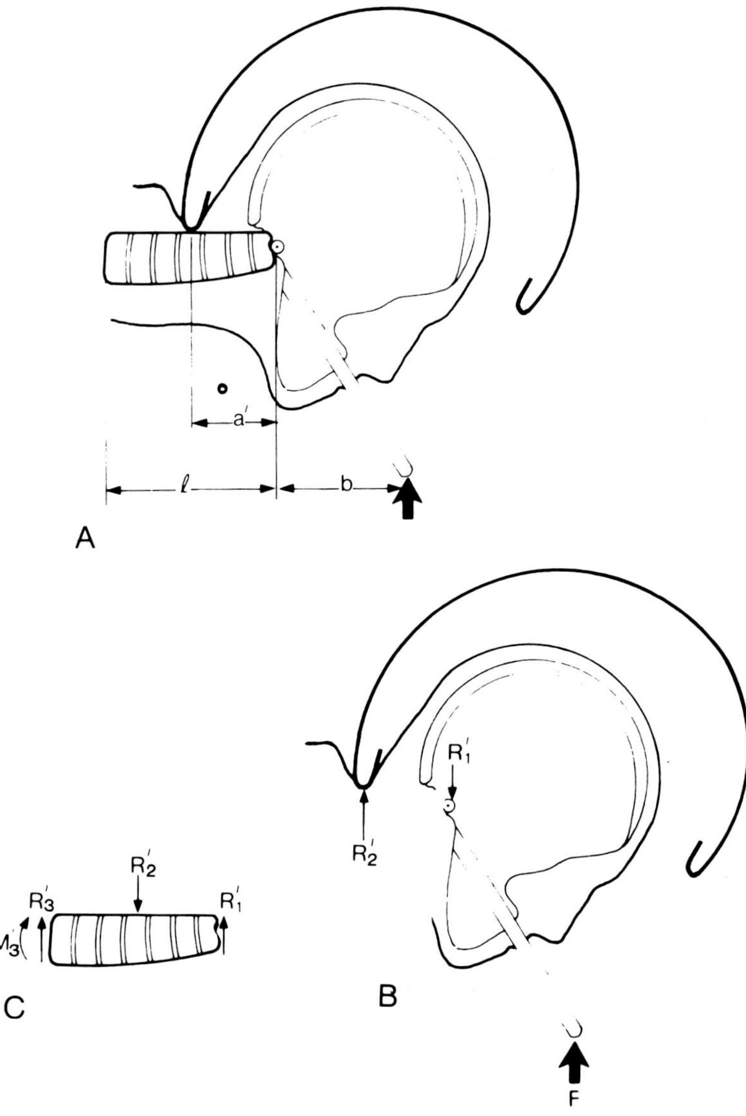

Fig. 6-132. (*A*) Loading condition with hyperextension limited by the impingement of the helmet rim at the fourth cervical vertebra. (*B*) Free body diagram of the head and the helmet. (*C*) Free body diagram of the cervical spine. (Carter D, Frankel VH: Biomechanics of hyperextension injuries to the cervical spine in football. Am J Sports Med 8:302, 1980)

were considered: (1) intracranial hemorrhage, (2) intracranial injuries resulting in death, (3) cervical fractures, subluxations, and dislocations, and (4) cervical spine fracture-dislocations with permanent quadriplegia. Available data allow a comparison of these four categories for two 5-year periods—1959 through 1963 and 1971 through 1975.[33,43]

During the 5-year period from 1959 to 1963 Schneider reported 139 (3.4 in 100,000) lesions in which intracranial hemorrhage was a component and 65 (1.6 per 100,000) deaths from intracranial injuries.[33] During this period, 820,000 athletes were exposed annually. The Registry reported 72 (1.2 per 100,000) intracranial lesions and 58 (0.9 per 100,000) intracranial deaths occurring between 1971 and 1975, with 1,250,000 individuals exposed annually (Table 6-2).[43]

Regarding cervical spine injuries, Schneider reported 56 (1.4 per 100,000) injuries that involved a fracture and/or dislocation and 30 (0.7 per 100,000) with associated permanent cervical quadriplegia occurring during the 5-year period of 1959 to 1963.[33] The Registry documented 259 (4.1 per 100,000) injuries involving a fracture and/or dislocation of the cervical spine and 99 (1.67 in 100,000) with associated permanent quadriplegia during the 1971 to 1975 seasons.[43] When com-

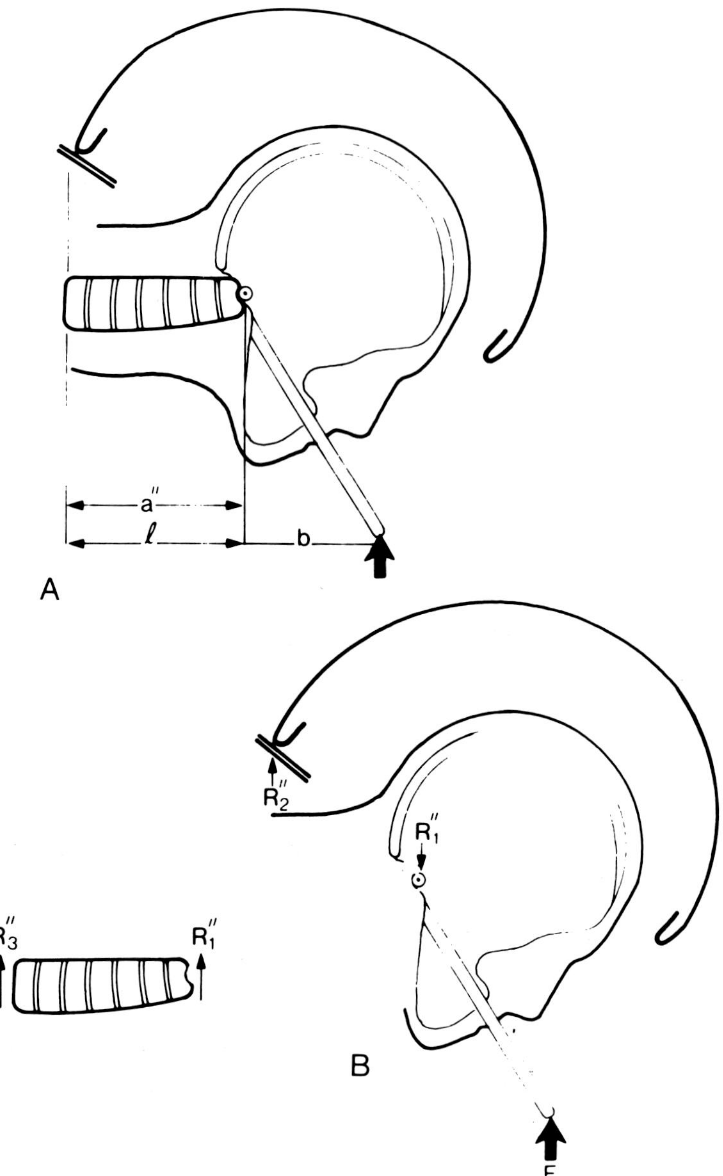

Fig. 6-133. (*A*) Loading condition for hyperextension limited by impingement of the helmet rim on the shoulder pad. (*B*) Free body diagram of the head and helmet. (*C*) Free body diagram of the cervical spine. (Carter D, Frankel VH: Biomechanics of hyperextension injuries to the cervical spine in football. Am J Sports Med 8:302, 1980)

pared on an exposure basis, these data indicate a decrease had occurred in intracranial lesions and deaths and, conversely, an increase in the number of individuals who were rendered quadriplegic while playing football during the latter 5-year period (Table 6-2).

These changes were attributed to the improved protective capabilities of the helmet–face mask unit that was developed during the 1960s and early 1970s and provided better head and face protection. As a result, the use of the head as the primary point of contact in blocking, tackling, and head-butting occurred. Fifty-two percent of the permanent cervical quadriplegias occurring between 1971 and 1975 were caused by "spearing" or direct compression, the injured player having made initial contact with the top of his helmet.[43] Seventy-two percent of high school players and 78% of college players were rendered quadriplegic while attempting to make a tackle. When injury by position was evaluated for the same period, at the high school level, 52% of the quadriplegics were defensive backs, 13% were on specialty teams, and 10% were linebackers; at the college level, how-

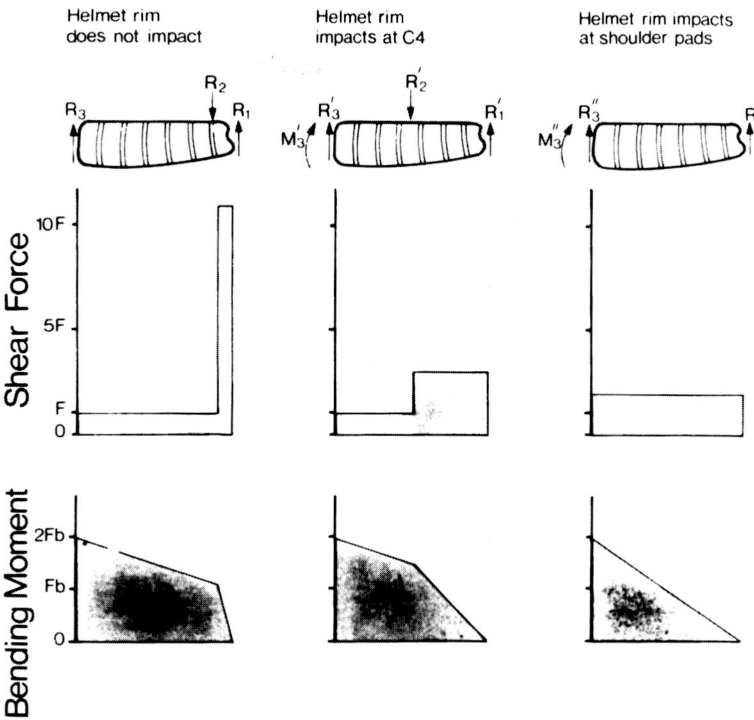

Fig. 6-134. Diagram showing the distribution of cervical spine shear forces and bending movements created in each of the three loading conditions examined. (Carter D, Frankel VH: Biomechanics of hyperextension injuries to the cervical spine in football. Am J Sports Med 8:302, 1980)

ever, 73% were defensive backs, and 7% were specialty team players.[43]

Clearly, defensive backs who make a tackle with the head as the initial point of contact are at greatest risk of sustaining a cervical spine injury resulting in permanent cervical quadriplegia.

As a result of The National Football Head and Neck Injury Registry findings, The NCAA and the NFSHAA adopted rule changes intended to control the "head first" techniques. The NCAA Football Rules Committee implemented the following rules beginning with the 1976 season: (1) No player shall intentionally strike a runner with the crown or top of the helmet; (2) spearing is the deliberate use of the helmet in an attempt to punish an opponent; (3) no player shall deliberately use his helmet to butt or ram an opponent (NCAA Football Rule Changes and/or Modifications, Jan. 23, 1976, rule 2, section 24; rule 9, section 1, article 2-1, 2-N).

In order to ascertain the effect of the new rules at both the college and high school levels, a prospective data collection mechanism was initiated.[44,50] Data were collected prospectively to identify injuries associated with (1) intracranial hemorrhage, (2) craniocerebral death, (3) fracture/

Table 6-2. Comparisons of the Occurrence of Injuries Reported by the National Football Head and Neck Injury Registry

	INTRACRANIAL HEMORRHAGES	INTRACRANIAL DEATHS	CERVICAL SPINE FRACTURES/SUBLUXATIONS DISLOCATIONS	PERMANENT CERVICAL QUADRI-PLEGICS
Schneider (1959 to 1963)	139 (3.39/100,000)*	65 (1.58/100,000)	56 (1.36/100,000)	30 (0.73/100,000)
H/N Registry (1971 to 1975)	72 (1.15/100,000)	58 (0.92/100,000)	259 (4.14/100,000)	99 (1.58/100,000)

* The annual injury rate per 100,000 participants is in parentheses.

dislocation/subluxation, and (4) cervical spine injuries with associated quadriplegia. Maintained at the University of Pennsylvania Sports Medicine Center as an ongoing registry, information was collected by several methods. At the conclusion of each season, a project description and injury report form were mailed to all members of the National Association of Secondary School Principals and the National Athletic Trainers Association. In addition, a newspaper clipping service was utilized to identify head and neck injuries reported in the press. Finally, when a catastrophic injury was reported, detailed information was obtained from the responsible physician, school administrator, and coach.

Analysis of the data demonstrated interesting trends with regard to the incidence of head and cervical spine injuries occurring in high school and college football.

When expressed as number of injuries per 100,000 participants, closed head injuries associated with intracranial hemorrhage generally increased over the 9-year period (1976 to 1984). At the high school level, these injuries ranged from a low of 0.55 per 100,000 participants in 1977 to a high of 1.88 per 100,000 participants in 1982. At the college level, the low was 1.3 per 100,000 in 1976, increasing to a maximum of 4.00 per 100,000 participants in 1984 (Table 6-3). Graphic representation of combined intracranial hemorrhages of all groups demonstrates an increase in the incidence from seven injuries in 1977 to 21 intracranial hemorrhages in 1984 (Fig. 6-135). This apparent increase is due to the advent of widespread use of computerized axial tomography (CT) and the resulting increase in the accuracy with which these lesions are diagnosed. This interpretation is substantiated by the relatively constant craniocerebral death rate over the same 9-year period (Table 6-3). Graphic representation of combined craniocerebral deaths during the period from 1975 to 1984 also reveals a relatively constant occurrence rate (Fig. 6-136).

Whether expressed as occurrences or injuries per 100,000 participants, fractures, dislocations, and subluxations of the cervical spine decreased at both the high school and college levels. In 1975, the season before the rule changes were initiated, the injury incidence was 6.5 per 100,000 and 29.3 per 100,000 at the high school and college levels,

Table 6-3. Nine-Year Data on Injuries for High School, College, and Recreational/Professional Levels of Participation

	1976	1977	1978	1979	1980	1981	1982	1983	1984
Intracranial Hemorrhage									
High school	10 (0.89)*	6 (0.55)	10 (0.93)	8 (0.85)	8 (0.85)	11 (1.15)	17 (1.88)	12 (1.30)	16 (1.73)
College	1 (1.33)	1 (1.33)	1 (1.33)	1 (1.33)	0	3 (4.00)	1 (1.33)	1 (1.33)	4 (4.00)
Other	1	0	0	2	4	3	1	0	1
Total	12	7	11	11	12	17	19	13	21
Craniocerebral Deaths									
High school	11 (0.98)	5 (0.46)	5 (0.46)	1 (0.10)	7 (0.74)	6 (0.63)	8 (0.88)	6 (0.65)	6 (0.65)
College	0	0	0	1 (1.33)	1 (1.33)	2 (2.66)	1 (1.33)	1 (1.33)	1 (1.33)
Other	1	0	0	2	3	1	1	0	2
Total	12	5	5	4	11	9	10	7	9
Cervical Spine Fx/Disl/Subl									
High school	86 (7.72)	76 (7.06)	40 (3.72)	42 (4.47)	52 (5.54)	49 (5.16)	46 (5.10)	60 (6.50)	36 (3.91)
College	23 (30.66)	15 (20.00)	8 (10.66)	7 (9.33)	9 (12.00)	8 (10.66)	6 (8.00)	7 (9.33)	5 (6.66)
Other	1	5	3	2	1	0	5	2	1
Total	110	96	51	51	62	57	57	69	42
Permanent Quadriplegia									
High school	25 (2.24)	14 (1.30)	14 (1.30)	8 (0.85)	13 (1.38)	7 (0.73)	7 (0.77)	9 (0.97)	4 (0.43)
College	8 (10.66)	2 (2.66)	0	4 (4.00)	2 (2.66)	2 (2.66)	1 (1.33)	1 (1.33)	0
Other	1	2	2	1	1	2	1	1	1
Total	34	18	16	13	16	11	10	11	5

* The injury rate per 100,000 participants is in parentheses.

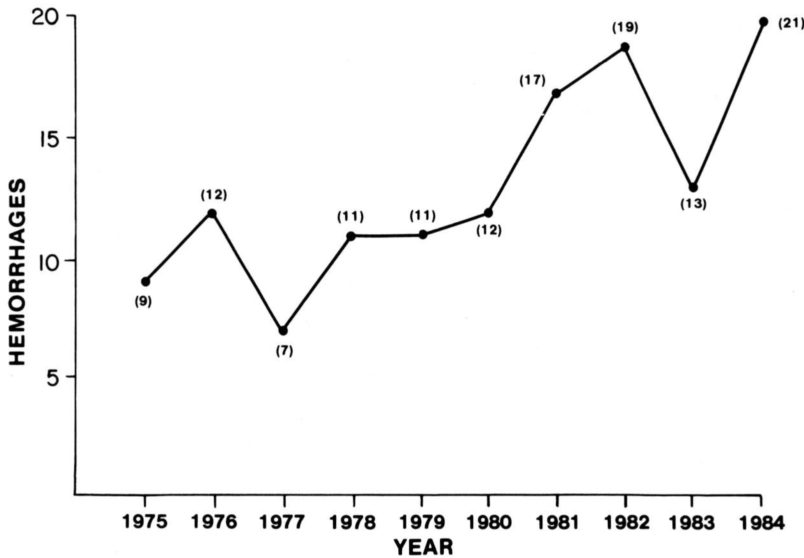

Fig. 6-135. The yearly incidence of intracranial hemorrhages for levels of participation demonstrates an increase during the 10-year period 1975–1984. (Torg JS, Vegso JJ, Sennett B: The National Football Head and Neck Injury Registry: 14-year report on cervical quadriplegia, 1971 through 1984. J Am Med Assoc 254:3439–3443, 1985)

respectively. In 1976, the first year of the rule changes, the incidence increased slightly to 7.2 per 100,000 and 30.6 per 100,000 at the high school and college levels, respectively. Subsequently, a gradual decrease in cervical spine injury rates occurred over the following 8 years; by 1984 these rates were 3.9 per 100,000 and 6.7 per 100,000 at the high school and college levels, respectively (Table 6-3). Graphic representation of the total number of cervical spine fractures, dislocations, and subluxations over the 10-year period demonstrates a dramatic decrease from 110 in 1976 to 51 in 1978, the third season after spearing was prohibited, with maintenance of the decrease at this level over the subsequent years (Fig. 6-137).

Cervical spine injuries resulting in permanent quadriplegia have also decreased dramatically over this 10-year period, In 1975, the season prior to the rules change, quadriplegia occurred in 2.2 per 100,000 high school players and 8.4 per 100,000 college players. In 1976, the injury rate rose to 3.2 per 100,000 and 10.7 per 100,000, respectively. A marked decrease occurred in 1977, the second year of the antispearing rules, when the rate dropped to 1.3 per 100,000 at the high school level and 2.7 per 100,000 at the college level. This downward trend continued over the subsequent 7 years. In 1984, 0.43 cases of cervical quadriplegia occurred per 100,000 players at the high school level, and none occurred at the college level (Table 6-3). The total of number of permanent cervical quadriplegias in high school, college, and recreational football during the 10-year survey period of 1975 to 1984 underwent a marked decrease from

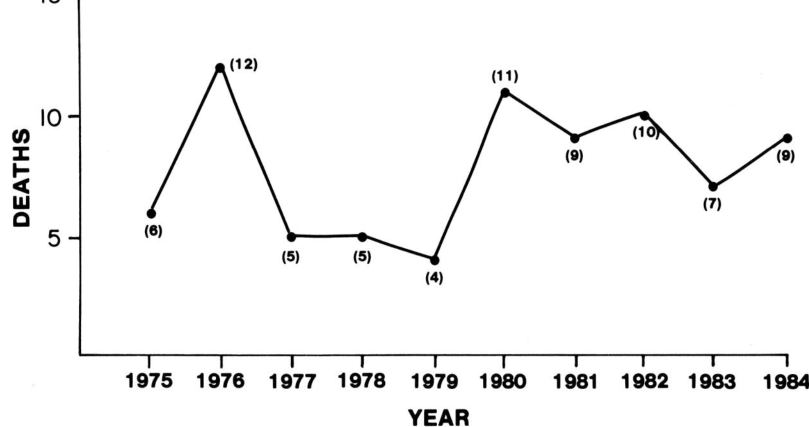

Fig. 6-136. The yearly incidence of craniocerebral deaths for all levels of participation is relatively constant during the 10-year period 1975–1984. (Torg JS, Vegso JJ, Sennett B: The National Football Head and Neck Injury Registry: 14-year report on cervical quadriplegia, 1971 through 1984. J Am Med Assoc 254:3439–3443, 1985)

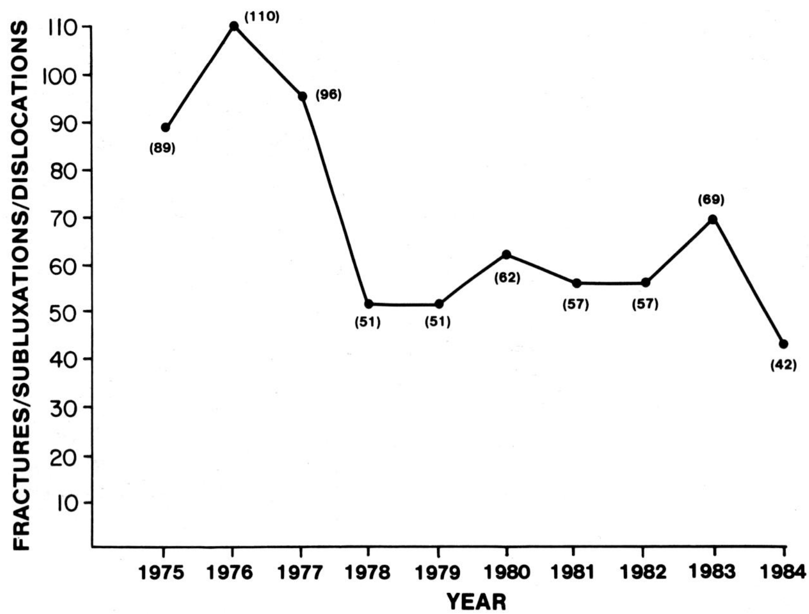

Fig. 6-137. The incidence of cervical spine fractures, subluxation, and dislocations for all levels of participation underwent a dramatic decrease from 1976, the first year of the rules change, to 1978. This decrease has been maintained since 1978. (Torg JS, Vegso JJ, Sennett B: The National Football Head and Neck Injury Registry: 14-year report on cervical quadriplegia, 1971 through 1984. J Am Med Assoc 254:3439–3443, 1985)

34 in 1976 to 18 in 1977, with a continued decline in subsequent years, until a low of five injuries was reached in the 1984 season (Fig. 6-138).

Compression or axial loading continues to be the mechanism causing the highest percentage of quadriplegias and cervical fractures/dislocations/subluxations. From 1971 to 1975, 78% of the quadriplegias were caused by this mechanism.[10] During the 9-year period from 1976 to 1984, 54% of the quadriplegias and 50% of the nonquadriplegic cervical spine injuries were caused by the same mechanism (Fig. 6-134).

Identifying the cause and subsequently preventing cervical quadriplegia from football involved four areas: (1) the role of the helmet–face mask protective system; (2) the concept of the axial loading mechanism of injury; (3) the effect of the 1976 rule changes banning spearing and the use of the top of the helmet as the initial point of contact in tackling; and (4) the necessity for continued research, education, and rules enforcement.

The protective capabilities provided by the modern football helmet have resulted in the advent of playing techniques that have placed the cervical

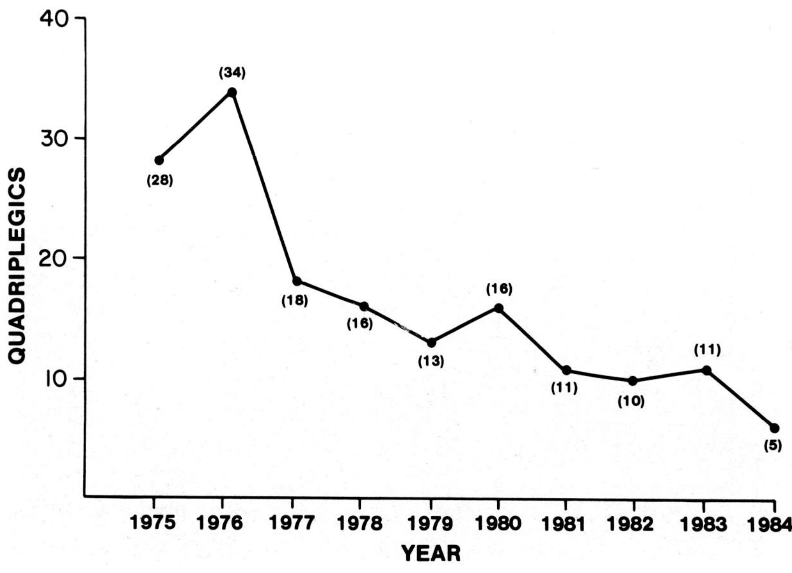

Fig. 6-138. The yearly incidence of permanent cervical quadriplegia for all levels of participation demonstrate a significant decrease in 1977, the first year after the rules change. Total quadriplegia has continued to decline to a low of 5 in 1984. (Torg JS, Vegso JJ, Sennett B: The National Football Head and Neck Injury Registry: 14-year report on cervical quadriplegia, 1971 through 1984. J Am Med Assoc 254:3439–3443, 1985)

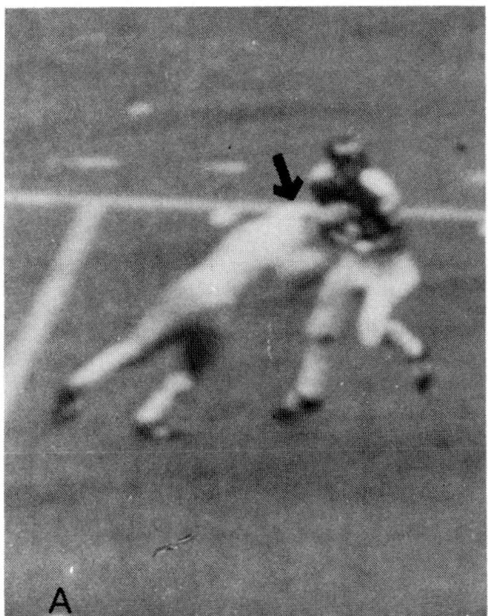
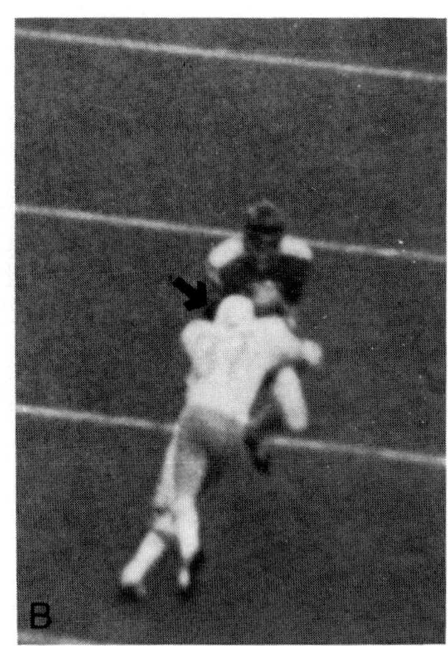

Fig. 6-139. Injured player (number 37) is observed attacking the ball carrier with his neck slightly flexed and his head down (*arrow*). This preload position straightens the cervical spine, obviating the ability to dissipate energy inputs by controlled cervical motion. (Torg JS, Truex RC, Marshall J, et al: Spinal injury at the level of the third and fourth cervical vertebra from football. J Bone Joint Surg 59A:1018, 1977). (*A*) Side view. (*B*) Back-to-front view.

spine at risk of injury with associated catastrophic neurologic sequelae. Available cinemetographic and epidemiologic data clearly indicate that cervical spine injuries associated with quadriplegia that occur as a result of football are not hyperflexion accidents. Rather, they are due to purposeful axial loading of the cervical spine as a result of "spearing" and head-first playing techniques.[47,49,50] The current helmet–face mask system is a secondary etiologic factor, contributing to these injuries only because it permits the head to be used as a battering ram, exposing the cervical spine to risk of injury.

Classically, the role of hyperflexion has been emphasized in cervical spine trauma due to a diving accident, trampolining, rugby, or American football. Epidemiologic and cinematographic analyses establish that most cases of cervical spine quadriplegia from football result from axial loading (Figs. 6-139, 6-140, and 6-141).[47,49,50] Deliberately used techniques, rather than accidental, untoward events, place the cervical spine at risk of catastrophic injury. Recent laboratory observations also indicate that athletically induced cervical spine trauma results from axial loading.[8,30]

In the course of a collision activity, such as tackle football, most energy inputs of the cervical spine are effectively dissipated by the energy-absorbing capabilities of the cervical musculature through controlled lateral bending, flexion, or extension motion. However, the bones, discs, and ligamentous structures can be injured when contact occurs on the top of the helmet with the head, neck, and trunk positioned so that forces are transmitted along the longitudinal axis of the cervical spine.[11]

With the neck in the anatomic position, normal

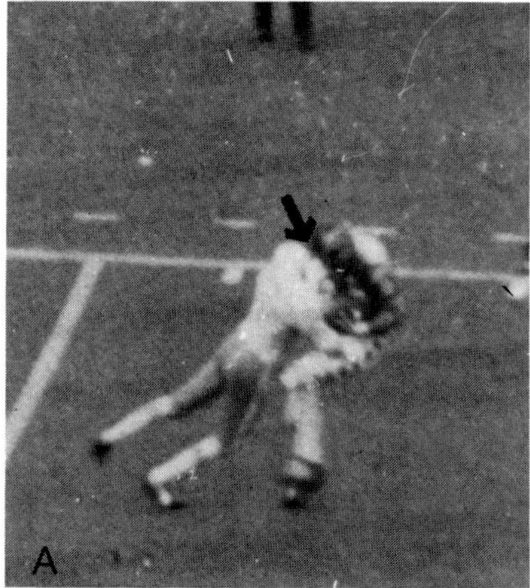
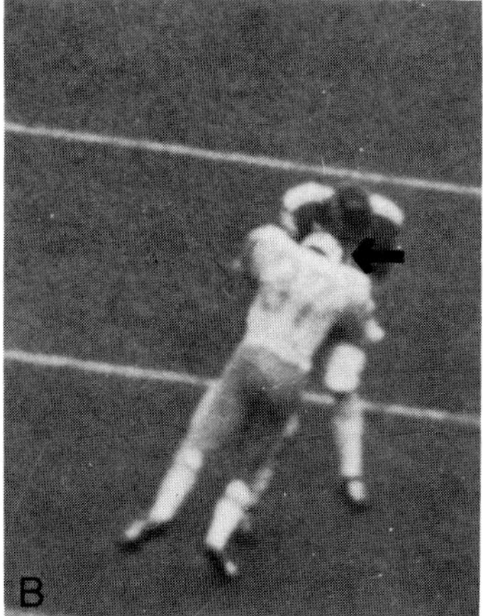

Fig. 6-140. Impact occurs; there is rapid deceleration of the player's head, and the cervical spine is compressed between the decelerated head and the continued momentum of the body. Failure occurred at the C3–C4 level in a compression flexion–rotation mode with a unilateral facet dislocation resulting. (Torg JS, Truex RC, Marshall J, et al: Spinal injury at the level of the third and fourth cervical vertebra from football. J Bone Joint Surg 59A:1018, 1977). (*A*) Side view. (*B*) Back-to-front view.

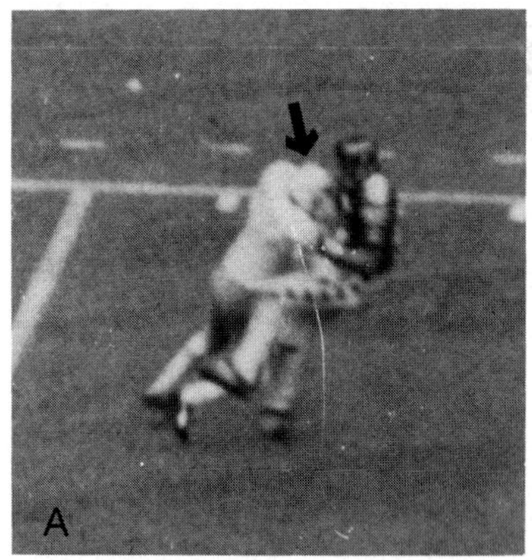

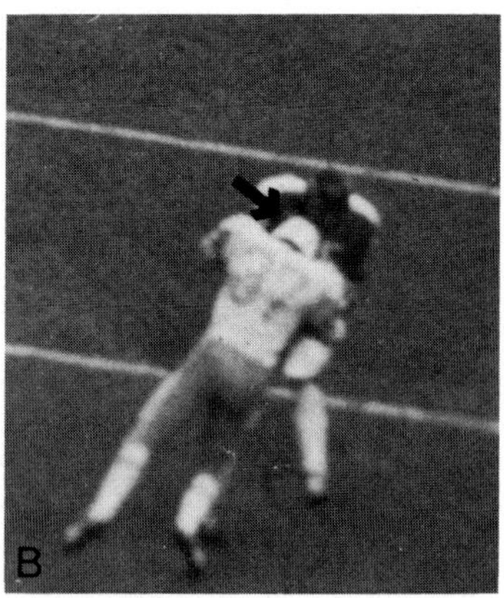

Fig. 6-141. Recoil occurs with maintenance of the axial relationship of the head and neck to the torso (*arrow*). The player has been rendered quadriplegic. Hyperflexion of the cervical spine did not occur; the mechanism of injury was axial loading. (Torg JS, Truex RC, Marshall J, et al: Spinal injury at the level of the third and fourth cervical vertebra from football. J Bone Joint Surg 59A: 1018, 1977).

cervical lordosis causes the cervical spine to be extended (Fig. 6-142). When the neck is flexed to 30 degrees, the cervical spine straightens (Fig. 6-143). In axial loading injuries, the neck is slightly flexed and normal cervical lordosis is eliminated, thereby converting the spine into a straight segmented column. Assuming that the head, neck, and trunk components are in motion, the head rapidly decelerates when it strikes another object, such as another player, a trampoline bed, or a lake bottom. This results in the cervical spine being compressed between the abruptly decelerated head and the force of the oncoming trunk (Fig. 6-144). When maximum vertical compression is reached, the straightened cervical spine fails in a flexion mode, and fracture, subluxation, or unilateral or bilateral facet dislocation can occur (Fig. 6-145).

The "freak accident" concept can be replaced by the more logical principle of cause and effect; this change has been most rewarding in regard to problems of football-induced cervical quadriplegia. Definition of the axial loading mechanism in which a football player, usually a defensive back, makes a tackle by striking his opponent with the top of his helmet, has been the key in this process (Fig. 6-139). Rule changes and coaching techniques eliminating the use of the head as a battering ram have resulted in a dramatic reduction in the incidence of quadriplegia since 1976. We believe that most athletic injuries to the cervical spine associated with quadriplegia also occur as a result of axial loading.

The National Football Head and Neck Registry has documented severe and catastrophic head and neck injuries that have occurred in football. On the basis of this information, axial loading of the cervical spine has been established as the mechanism of injury responsible for quadriplegia. Identification of this mechanism of injury and subsequent modifications of playing techniques have resulted in a significant decrease in football-induced cervical spine injuries. The necessity for continued research, education of coaches and players, and rules enforcement is essential. It is also suggested that axial loading of the cervical spine is responsible for catastrophic injuries in water sports (diving), rugby, ice hockey, and gymnastics. Appropriate changes in playing techniques and/or equipment might reduce the incidence of cervical spine injuries in these sports.

GYMNASTICS (TRAMPOLINE)

Cervical spine injuries resulting from participation in gymnastics have become synonymous with the trampoline and the minitrampoline. Numerous reports in the world literature document an alarming number of injuries resulting in cervical quadriplegia and indicate a real danger in the use of these devices.[17,18,20,22,28,36,53,54] A controversy has existed regarding whether or not these two devices should be banned from use in recreation, supervised physical education, and competition, or whether by means of manufacturing standards and enforcement of safety guidelines they can be made safe. A comprehensive review of the historical development of the use of the trampoline and minitrampoline, with particular regard to injury documentation, appears appropriate.

In 1956, Zimmerman was the first to mention cervical spine injuries that occurred on trampolines.[54] In a retrospective study, he reported two fractures of the cervical spine.

Four years later, Ellis and colleagues published a "communication designed to warn the medical profession of the hazards involving the use of the

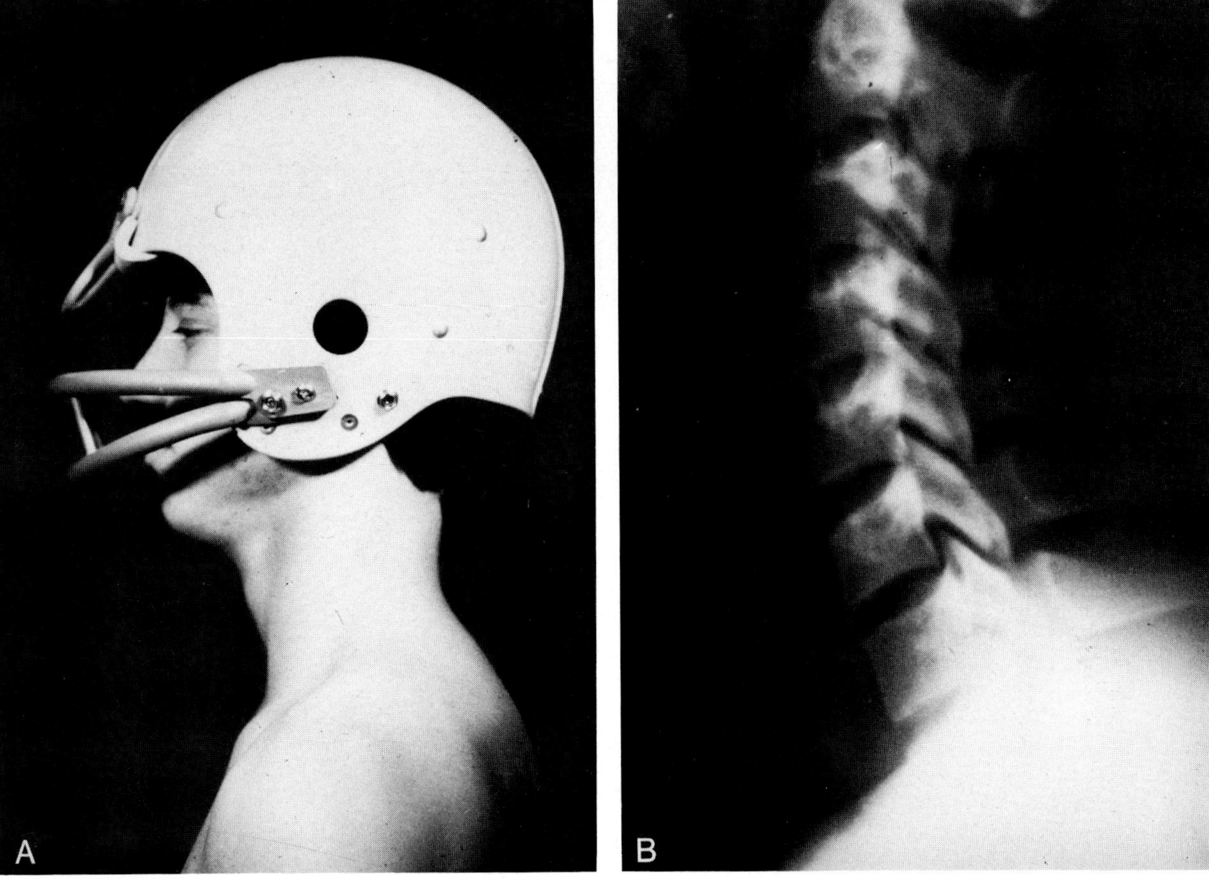

Fig. 6-142. With the head and neck held in the neutral position, because of normal cervical lordosis, the posture of the cervical spine is one of extension. (Torg J: National Football Head and Neck Injury Registry: Report on cervical quadriplegia from 1971 to 1975. Am J Sports Med 7:127, 1979). (*A*) Photograph. (*B*) Roentgenogram.

trampoline."[17] They reported on five patients who incurred neurologic injuries, three as a result of cervical spine injuries.

In 1969, Witthaut reported on six patients with trampoline injuries in the German literature.[53] The author pointed out that cervical spine injuries on the trampoline "either resemble those which occur when swimmers dive into shallow water or those which occur during high dives into deep water when the neck is forcefully hyperextended."

Three cervical spine injuries were reported in the Swedish literature by Frykman and Hilding in 1970.[20] The injuries have several points in common: (1) All occurred in young, well-trained gymnasts performing difficult stunts. (2) Although the nature and severity of the lesions differed somewhat in each case, lesions occurred at the C5–C6 level. (3) All three patients experienced a "blackout" or period of unconsciousness just prior to their injuries. The authors suggested that these blackouts might be due to brief concussions or pathologic conditions similar to Wallenberg's syndrome (occlusion of the posterior inferior cerebellar artery). They recommended that trampolining be banned from school gymnastics and that investigation into these injuries continue.

In the German literature, Steinbruck and Paeslack reported 25 cases of cervical quadriplegia due to trampoline and minitrampoline injuries between 1967 and 1977.[36] They treated eight of these patients personally at the Heidelberg Center for Spinal Cord Injuries.

In a letter to the British Medical Journal, R. F. Evans reported a fracture-dislocation of the cer-

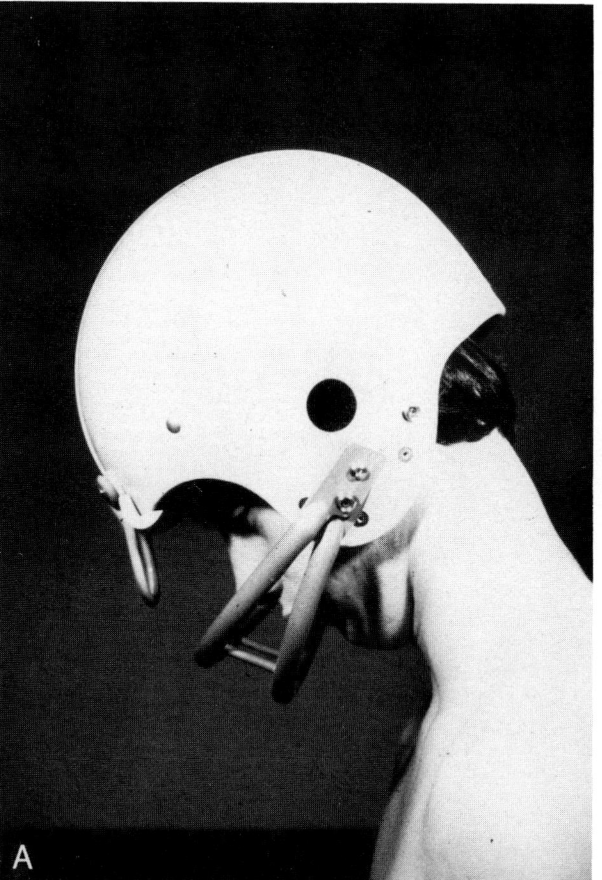

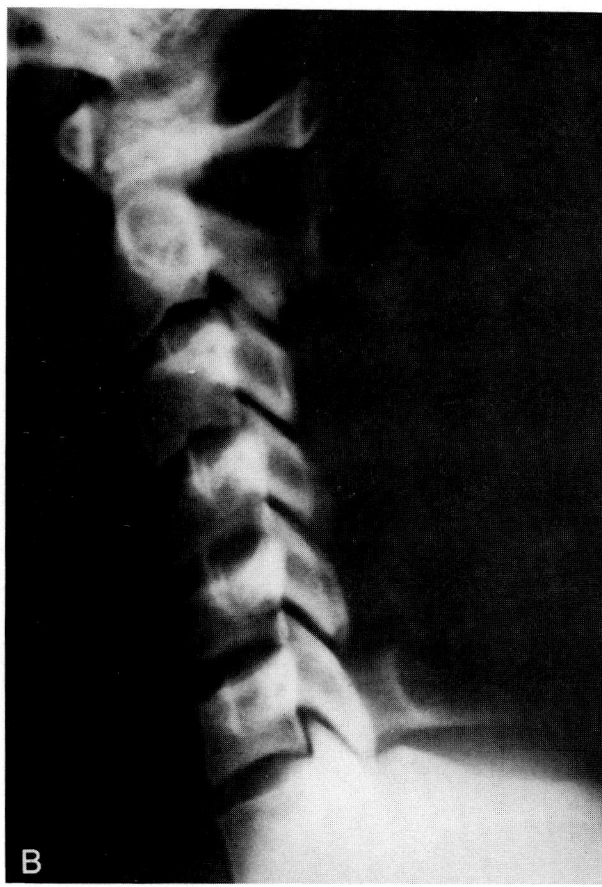

Fig. 6-143. When the neck is flexed approximately 30 degrees, the cervical spine becomes straight; from the standpoint of force, energy absorption, and the effect on tissue deformation and failure, the straightened cervical spine, when axially loaded, acts as a segmented column. (Torg J: National Football Head and Neck Injury Registry: Report on cervical quadriplegia from 1971 to 1975. Am J Sports Med 7:127, 1979). (*A*) Photograph. (*B*) Roentgenogram.

vical spine resulting in quadriplegia in a 13-year-old girl who had been trampolining.[18]

Hammer and colleagues reported eight trampoline accidents in Denmark that resulted in severe neurological damage between 1966 and 1981.[22] In seven cases the accidents occurred on minitramps, and four of the eight patients experienced momentary "black outs" immediately preceding their accidents.

During the early and middle 1970s, a number of reports appeared in the American literature on cervical quadriplegia resulting from trampoline injuries. The articles called attention to the trampoline as a possible cause of cervical spine injuries in the United States.[21,26,28,29]

In January 1976, Rapp and Nicely reported on 34 cases of quadriplegia, including three deaths, resulting from trampoline accidents.[28]

One of the most influential articles in the recent American literature is that of Clarke who, in 1975, retrospectively surveyed sports-related spinal cord injuries.[15] Questionnaires were sent to 18,085 high schools, 683 2-year colleges, and 1125 4-year colleges to ascertain the incidence of permanent paralysis resulting from sports participation that occurred during the period 1973 to 1975. Only eight sports accounted for all of these injuries. Football was first, accounting for 54%, and it was followed by gymnastics with 26%. There were 15 gymnastic injuries for which the activity is specified, eight of which occurred on the trampoline and one on the minitrampoline. Unlike football, however, not all

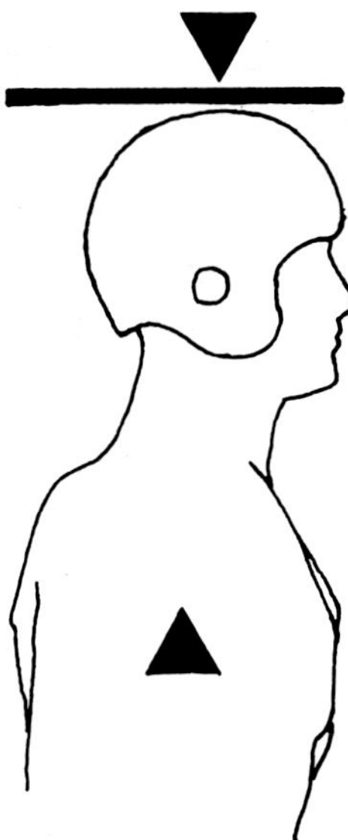

Fig. 6-144. The composite model of a trunk mass, a nonlinear spring cervical spine, a head and mass. The basic law of dynamics (F = MA) characterizes the system. The model, representing the axial loading injury condition, illustrates how the cervical spine is compressed between the abruptly decelerated head mass and the continued momentum of the body. (Burstein AH: Mechanisms and Pathomechanics of Athletic Injuries to the Cervical Spine. In Torg JS (ed): Athletic Injuries to the Head, Neck, and Face. Philadelphia, Lea & Febiger, 1982)

of these injuries were suffered by varsity athletes. From this study it was concluded that competent trampoline teachers are necessary to prevent gymnastic students from attempting maneuvers for which they are not prepared. He also advocated that a spotter be present for off-apparatus landings.

A result of this paper was the issuance of a policy statement in September 1977 by the Committee on Accident and Poison Prevention of the American Academy of Pediatrics:

> Trampoline accidents have resulted in a significant number of cases of quadriplegia. In many cases, these accidents have occurred while the victims were participating in supervised physical education activities. A recent national survey of sports injuries in high schools and colleges conducted by the National Athletic/Illness Reporting System (NAIRS) showed that between 1973–1975 spinal cord injuries with permanent paralysis resulted more frequently from trampolines that any other gymnastic sport. Next to football, trampolines were found to be the highest cause of permanent paralysis in this survey.
>
> Therefore, the Committee on Accident and Poison Prevention of the American Academy of Pediatrics recommends that trampolines be banned from use as part of the physical education programs in grammar schools, high schools and colleges, and also be abolished as a competitive sports.[2]

After the American Academy of Pediatrics issued its 1977 policy on trampolines, most, if not all, school districts eliminated trampolining from their physical education programs, either voluntarily, as a result of parental pressure, or because liability insurance became difficult or impossible to obtain.[3]

Because of this strong reaction against the use of the trampoline in schools, the United States Gymnastics Safety Association and a group of trampoline manufacturers sponsored the establishment of the National Gymnastic Catastrophic Injury Registry at the University of Illinois in 1978.[13] The purpose of this registry was to collect reliable data for accurate characterization of the patterns and relative frequency of catastrophic head, neck, and spinal injuries occurring in gymnastics and cheerleading. A secondary objective of the registry was estimation of national participation in gymnastics. Under the directorship of Kenneth Clarke and, more recently, Charlene Christensen, this registry has issued four annual reports that document 20 catastrophic gymnastics injuries, 14 of which occurred on this trampoline. The large trampoline was implicated in nine of these injuries, and the minitrampoline in five. Most of the maneuvers leading to these injuries were somersaults.[13]

From July 1978 through June 1983, the frequencies of cervical cord injuries due to the trampoline were as follows: 1978 to 79, 7; 1979 to 80, 1; 1980 to 81, 5; and 1981 to 82, 0. The authors comment that "In the four annual reports, the cases reported do not reflect annually persistent patterns" and caution against any generalization on the state of the problem from a single year's experience. However, a distinct drop was observed in all catastrophic gymnastics injuries occurring in United States schools and college programs since 1978 and, more specifically, a drop in those injuries resulting from trampolines and minitrampolines.[13]

From a study of trampoline-related head and neck injuries in children between 5 and 14 years of age who were treated in hospital emergency

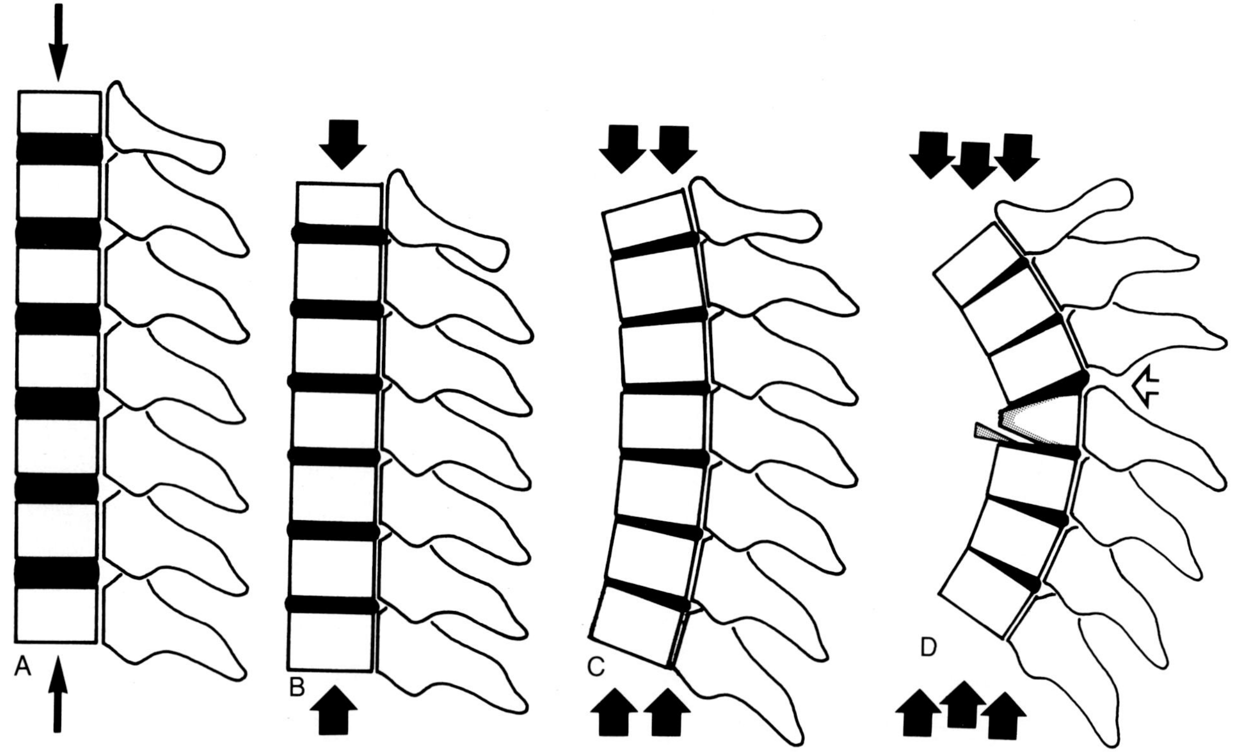

Fig. 6-145. (*A*) Diagrammatic representation of a segmented column. With 20 degrees of neck flexion the cervical spine is straightened and theoretically responds as a segmented column to energy inputs. (*B*) Application of an axial load on a segmented column first results in compressive deformation. (*C*) When energy input exceeds maximum possible compressive deformation, angulation of the column occurs. In instances of cervical spine injury, this is in the flexion mode. (*D*) With excessive energy input, buckling occurs at some point in the segmented column. In instances of cervical spine injury, this can result in disruption of the invertebral disc structures, ligamentous supporting structures, or bony elements. If structural instability results, the cord may be violated with the associated neurologic involvement.

rooms, the Consumer Product Safety Commission (CPSC) estimated the annual frequency of such injuries from 1975 through 1980.[31] Commenting on these statistics, Christensen and Clarke observed:

> Trampoline injuries for the 5 to 14 age group account for almost 50 percent of the total trampoline injuries treated in hospital emergency rooms each year. Head and neck injuries account for an average of 19 percent of those injuries incurred in the 5 to 14 age group. It should be noted, however, that the estimated frequency of head/neck injuries associated with trampolines reported through NEISS has declined by almost two thirds since 1978 (from 1,755 to 600). This may be a result of the removal of trampolines from many athletic programs in the schools. . . . Head and neck injuries due to other forms of gymnastics have not shown a similar decline: rather they have remained relatively constant showing a slight increase. In gymnastic activities (including trampolines) there is no specific protection for the head or neck. The participant must rely on his/her abilities and those of a spotter. The use of harnesses in teaching various stunts and techniques is essential to prevent impacts to the head or neck from falls.[13]

Presumably, on the basis of the CPSC report indicating an almost two-thirds decline in head and neck injuries resulting from the trampoline and a decline in catastrophic injuries resulting in quadriplegia observed by the National Gymnastic Catastrophic Injury Report, the American Academy of Pediatrics Committees on Accident and Poison Prevention and on Pediatric Aspects of Physical Fitness, Recreation, and Sports reassessed their position on the use of the trampoline. In 1981, they published their Trampolines II position paper.[6,7] Their statement is as follows:

> In September 1977, the American Academy of Pediatrics published a statement calling for a ban on the use of trampolines in schools because of the high number of quadriplegic injuries caused by this apparatus. A considerable amount of thought and action resulted. The Academy does not endorse trampoline use, but a revision of the Academy's position to allow for a trial period of limited and controlled use by schools seems appropriate. However, careful assessment of the incidence and severity of injury must continue during this trial period.
> The trampoline is a potentially dangerous apparatus, and its use demands the following precautions.
>
> 1. The trampoline should not be a part of routine physical education classes.
> 2. The trampoline has no place in competitive sports.
> 3. The trampoline should never be used in home or recreational settings.
> 4. Highly trained personnel who have been instructed in all aspects of trampoline safety must be present when the apparatus is used.
> 5. Maneuvers, especially the somersault, that have a high potential for serious injury should be attempted only by those qualified to become skilled performers.
> 6. The trampoline must be secured when not in use, and it must be well maintained.
> 7. Only schools or sports activities complying with the foregoing recommendations should have trampolines.[3]

It should be noted that the American Academy of Pediatrics presents no data or rationale to explain or justify its change in position "to allow for a trial period of limited and controlled use" of the trampoline.[7] Perhaps the committees responsible for this statement overlooked the well-documented cases in the European literature that clearly establish the unpreventable nature of these trampoline accidents. On the basis of available facts and observations, it appears that the advisability of permitting even limited use of the trampoline is to be seriously questioned.

Starting with the report of Ellis and coworkers, 23 years ago, this review of the world literature has identified 114 catastrophic cervical spine injuries with associated quadriplegia resulting from the trampoline and minitrampoline. Unfortunately, it is not possible to present these injuries on a rate or exposure basis. However, because of the magnitude of the human and economic consequences of quadriplegia, we firmly believe that that trampoline and minitrampoline have clearly been established as very dangerous devices, regardless of the number of athletes exposed.

Just prior to their injuries, all three of the Swedish and four of the eight Danish cases blacked out.[20,22] The pathophysiology of this brief interval of unconsciousness prior to the injury requires explanation.

Most noteworthy are observations on the skill levels of the athletes in well-documented cases.[13,20,22] Specifically, the Swedes reported that their cases involved experienced, expert, and elite trampolinists.[20] Of the eight Danish patients, five had from 1 to 8 years of experience, and one was a trampoline instructor.[22] As noted, Christensen and Clarke's 14 cases involved one expertly skilled, three highly skilled, and two skilled trampolinists and two skilled novices.[13] Most of these cases fall into a pattern. During performance of a forward or backward somersault, a highly skilled and experienced trampolinist sustains an injury to the cervical spine resulting in quadriplegia. This situation certainly challenges the widespread assumption that catastrophic trampoline injuries can be prevented with equipment standards, better-trained instructors and spotters, and safety harnesses.

Since the first trampoline position paper was published by the American Academy of Pediatrics in 1977, a decrease has occurred in both noncatastrophic head and neck injuries and in catastrophic neck injuries due to the use of the trampoline and minitrampoline. It appears that this decrease is the direct result of the effect of the statement on the use, manufacture, and distribution of these devices. Unfortunately, prompted by the success of its own efforts, the American Academy of Pediatrics has chosen to soften its stand on this matter. In item #5 of their Trampolines II position paper, they state that "Maneuvers, especially the somersault, that have a high potential for serious injury should be attempted only by those qualified to become skilled performers."[7]

Judging from well-documented evidence in the

literature cited above, it is the "skilled performer" attempting difficult maneuvers and somersaults who is at risk of sustaining a cervical spine injury resulting in quadriplegia.

On the basis of this review, it appears that the American Academy of Pediatrics was ill-advised in altering its position on the use of trampolines. Both the trampoline and minitrampoline are dangerous devices, even under the best circumstances, and they have no place in recreational, educational, or competitive gymnastics.

WATER SPORTS (DIVING) INJURIES

The incidence of cervical spine injuries due to diving in shallow water is unknown, and the potential dangers of this activity are little appreciated. Shields and associates[35] have indicated that the majority of athletic injuries to the cervical cord are a result of water-related activities. Between June 1, 1964, and December 31, 1973, 1600 patients were admitted to the spinal injury service at Rancho Los Amigos Hospital. Of these, 152 or 9.5% had been injured in recreational activities. Of this group, 118 or 78% were injured in water-related sports. Diving accidents were the leading cause of injury and occurred when the patients misjudged the depth and safety of the water at the time of the incident. Most of these patients were injured by diving into shallow water or striking a submerged object. The average depth of water in which the cervical spine injuries occurred in this group was 5 feet. Kewalramani and Thomas reviewed 126 cases of fresh spinal injuries admitted to the Sacramento Medical Center during the period January 1970 to October 1973.[25] Of this group, 23 or 18% were injuries secondary to diving accidents. Albrand and Walter reporting on a survey of 18 counties in Northern California with an estimated 5.8 million inhabitants found 619 cases of spinal cord injuries during a 2-year period.[1] Thirty-three or 5% were due to diving accidents. On the basis of these figures, they project a national incidence of over 1800 serious diving injuries each year. They also suggest that diving accidents rank fourth after auto accidents, falls, and firearms as a major cause of traumatic spinal cord injuries. Considering that many cases of death due to "accidental drowning" are secondary to paralysis resulting from diving injuries, the actual incidence may be somewhat higher.

In a retrospective study of 358 patients with acute spinal cord injuries who were admitted to two Toronto hospitals during the 25-year period 1948 to 1973, Tator and coworkers identified 38, or 11%, as being due to diving accidents.[37,38] The authors observed that "In most cases the cervical spine was fractured and the spinal cord crushed when the top of the head struck the bottom of the lake or pool."

Albrand and Walter have constructed deceleration curves for experienced athletes diving from various heights above water. They observed that experienced divers strive for a vertical entry into the water and streamline their bodies, protecting their heads by extending their arms over them.[1] On the other hand, inexperienced divers, often not knowing the depth of the water or diving techniques, leave their heads unprotected. They also recognize the danger of striking bottom with the top of the head and sustaining either hyperflexion or vertical compression injury. It is noteworthy that the velocities are not dissipated until the divers achieve a depth of 10 to 12 feet. The authors emphasize the dangers that rivers, lakes, and reservoirs with shifting depths hold for uneducated divers. Also, they observe that diving into an above-ground pool should be prohibited. In view of the potential for disaster associated with unsupervised water activities, education of the public to the following guidelines is in order:

1. Do not dive into water that is shallower than twice your height. A 6-foot individual requires 12 feet of depth for safe diving.
2. Do not dive into unfamiliar water. Know the depth and be sure the water is free of submerged objects.
3. Do not assume water is deep enough. Familiar rivers, lakes, bays, and swimming holes change levels. Remember that at low tide the depth is 6 to 8 feet less than at high tide.
4. Do not dive near dredging or construction work. Water levels may change, and dangerous objects may lie beneath the surface.
5. Do not dive until the area is clear of other swimmers.
6. Do not drink and dive. Alcohol distorts judgment.
7. Do not permit or indulge in horseplay while swimming and diving.
8. Do not dive into the ocean surf or lake-front beaches.

Diving is best confined to a properly maintained and supervised pool where the depth has been measured and marked.

ICE HOCKEY

Until recently, injuries to the cervical spine have not been identified as a problem associated with ice hockey.[19] Tator and coworkers[39] have reported treating six patients with cervical spine injuries due to hockey between 1974 and 1981; five were seen during a 13-month period from September 1980 to October 1981.[39] They contrast this experience to that occurring between 1948 and 1973, when no hockey players incurred acute cord injuries in a series of 55 such sports-related injuries treated at two Toronto hospitals. All six cases involved cervical vertebral body burst fractures with accompanying neurologic sequelae. Two patients had complete cord injury, three had complete motor loss but incomplete sensory loss at the level of the lesion, and one had a cervical root injury. The mechanism of injury in all six patients involved a collision of the helmet and head against the board with axial loading of the flexed neck in extension. The one player who escaped cord injury struck with the neck in extension. In response to the apparent dramatic increase in cervical spine injuries, a Canadian Committee on Prevention of Spinal Injuries due to hockey was formed to investigate the problem. Utilizing a national questionnaire survey, 42 injuries were reported, 28 of which involved the spinal cord; 17 of those resulted in complete paralysis. The injury mechanism involved a check from behind in most instances. All injuries resulted from a collision between the player's head and the boards with the neck flexed.[40]

In this series, the most common mechanism involves a push or check with the injured players striking the boards "with the tops of their heads while their necks were slightly flexed." In this group of 42 hockey-related spinal injuries, 39 involved the cervical spine and half of these consisted of vertebral body burst fractures.

The distribution of the injuries over the 7-year period from 1976 to 1982 was revealing. Two injuries occurred in 1976 and 1977, four in 1978, one in 1979, eight in 1980, 13 in 1981, and 10 in 1982. Although this distribution may be due to the retrospective nature of the survey, the possibility of a real increase in cervical spine injuries resulting from ice hockey is interesting. Thirty-seven of the 42 players were known to be wearing a helmet. Since most nonprofessional hockey leagues in Canada made the wearing of hockey helmets mandatory during the 1970s, the situation that emerged was analogous to that in American football: The number of catastrophic cervical injuries increased with the advent of an improved helmet–face mask protective system. It should be noted that most of the individuals in this series, when interviewed, were unaware of the dangers inherent in striking another player or object with their helmets.

On the basis of this study, the Canadian Committee on the Prevention of Spinal Injuries due to hockey recommended the following: (1) rules against boarding and cross-checking should be enforced and new rules against pushing and shoving from behind should be adopted; (2) players should be educated about the possibility of neck injuries and should avoid spearing and impact at the boards; (3) research and equipment design and the biomechanics of neck injuries should be pursued. The Committee concluded that the evidence strongly suggests that hockey is faced with a new problem. This observation appears to be well founded.[40]

SUMMARY

Athletic injuries to the cervical spine associated with quadriplegia most commonly occur as a result of axial loading. Whether it is a football player striking an opponent with the top or crown of his helmet, a poorly executed dive into a shallow body of water where the head strikes the bottom, or a hockey player pushed into the boards head first, the fragile cervical spine is compressed between the rapidly decelerated head and the continued momentum of the body. Appropriate rule changes have resulted in reducing football quadriplegia by two thirds. Presumably, informing the public of the dangers of diving would have a similar effect. The predominance of the axial-loading mechanism is not as clearly defined in trampoline and minitrampoline injuries. However, these devices are dangerous, even under the best circumstances, and they have no place in recreational, educational, or competitive gymnastics. Finally, severe cervical spine injuries resulting from ice hockey are a recognized emergency. Methods to modify the games based on sound scientific evidence are needed to prevent these injuries.

REFERENCES

1. *ALBRAND OW, WALTER J:* Underwater deceleration curves in relation to injuries from diving. Surg Neurol 4:461–465, 1975
2. *AMERICAN ACADEMY OF PEDIATRICS. COMMITTEE ON ACCIDENT AND POISON PREVENTION:* Policy

statement. Trampolines. Evanston, American Academy of Pediatrics, Sept 1977

3. *American Society for Testing and Materials:* Standard consumer safety specification for components, assembly, and the use of a trampoline. In Annual Book of ATSM Standards, F381-77, Part 46, pp 586–589, 1977
4. *American Alliance for Health, Physical Education, and Recreation:* The use of trampolines and minitramps in physical education. J Phys Educ Recreat. 49:14, 1978
5. *American Alliance for Health, Physical Education, and Recreation:* The use of the trampoline for the development of competitive skills in sports. J Phys Educ Recreat 49:14, 1978
6. *American Academy of Pediatrics:* Trampolines. Pediatrics 67:438, 1981
7. *American Academy of Pediatrics:* Trampolines II. Pediatrics 67:438–439, 1981
8. *Bauze RJ:* Experimental production of forward dislocations in the human cervical spine. J Bone Joint Surg 60B:239–245, 1978
9. *Blyth CS, Arnold CD:* Forty-Sixth Annual Survey of Football Fatalities—1931–1977. Read before the 55th Annual Meeting of the American Football Coaches Association, Atlanta, Jan 1978
10. *Burry HC, Gowland H:* Cervical injury in rugby football—A New Zealand survey. Br J Sports Med pp 56–59, 1981
11. *Burstein AH, Otis JC, Torg JS:* Mechanisms and pathomechanics of athletic injuries to the cervical spine. In Torg JS (ed): Athletic Injuries to the Head, Neck, and Face, pp 139–142. Philadelphia, Lea & Febiger, 1982
12. *Carter DR, Frankel VH:* Biomechanics of hyperextension injuries to the cervical spine in football. Am J Sports Med 8:302–309, 1980
13. *Christensen C (with the assistance of Clarks KS):* Fourth Annual National Gymnastic Catastrophic Injury Report 1981–82, pp 1–35. College of Applied Life Studies, Urbana-Champaign, University of Illinois, April 1982
14. *Clancy WG, Brand RC, Bergfeld JA:* Upper trunk brachial plexus injuries in contact sports. Am J Sports Med 5:209–216, 1977
15. *Clarke KS:* A survey of sports-related spinal cord injuries in schools and colleges, 1973–1975. J Safety Res 9:140–147, 1977
16. *Coin CG, Pennick M, Ahmad WD, Keranen VJ;* Diving-type injury to the cervical spine: Contribution of computed tomography to management. J Comput Assist Tomogr 3:363–372, 1979
17. *Ellis WG, Green D, Holzaepfel NR, Sahs AL:* The trampoline and serious neurological injuries. A report of five cases. J Am Med Assoc 174:1673–1676, 1960
18. *Evans RF:* Tetraplegia caused by gymnastics. Br Med J 2:732, 1979
19. *Feriencik K:* Trends in ice hockey injuries: 1965 to 1977. Phys Sportsmed 7:81–84, 1979
20. *Frykman G, Hilding S:* Hopp pa studsmatta kan orsaka allvarliga skador. [Trampoline jumping can cause serious injury.] Lakartidningen 67:5862–5864, 1970
21. *Hage P:* Trampolines: An "attractive nuisance." Phys Sportsmed 10:118–122, 1982
22. *Hammer A, Schwartzbach AL, Darre E, Osgaard O:* Svaere neurologiske skader some folge af trampolinspring. [Severe neurologic damage resulting from trampolining.] Ugeskr Laeger 143:2970–2974, 1981
23. *Hodgson VR, Thomas LM:* Mechanism of cervical spine injury during impact to the unprotected head. In Proceedings of the 24th Stapp Car Crash Conference, pp 15–42. Society of Automotive Engineers, Warrendale, PA, 1980
24. *Hoskins T:* Rugby injuries to the cervical spine in English schoolboys. Practitioner 223:365–366, 1979
25. *Kewalramani LS, Thomas RG:* Injuries to the cervical spine from diving accidents. J Trauma 15:130–142, 1975
26. *Kravitz H:* Problems with the trampoline. I. Too many cases of permanent paralysis. Pediatr Ann 7:728–729, 1978
27. *National Collegiate Athletic Association. National Collegiate Athletic Association Football Rules Changes and/or Modifications.* January 23, 1976. Rule 2, Section 24; Rule 9, Section 1, Article 2-L; Rule 9, Section 1, Article 2-N
28. *Rapp GF, Nicely PG:* Trampoline injuries. Am J Sports Med 6:269–271, 1978
29. *Rapp GF:* Problems with the Trampoline. II. Safety suggestions for trampoline use. Pediatr Ann 7:730–732, 1978
30. *Roaf R:* A study of the mechanics of spinal injuries. J Bone Joint Surg 42B:810–823, 1968
31. *Rutherford GW, Miles RB, Brown VR, et al:* Overview of sports-related injuries to persons 5–14 years of age, pp 1–47. US Consumer Product Safety Commission, Washington, DC, Dec 1981
32. *Scher AT:* Vertex impact and cervical dislocation in rugby players. S Afr Med J 59:227–228, 1981
33. *Schneider RC:* Serious and fatal neurosurgical football injuries. Clin Neurosurg 12:226–236, 1966
34. *Schneider RC:* Head and Neck Injuries in Football, pp 77–125. Baltimore, Williams & Wilkins, 1973
35. *Shields CL Jr, Fox JM, Stauffer ES:* Cervical Cord injuries in sports. Phys Sportsmed 6:71–76, 1978

36. *Steinbruck J, Paeslack V:* Trampolinspringen—ein gefahrlicher Sport? [Is trampolining a dangerous sports?] Munchen Med Wochenschr 120:985–988, 1978
37. *Tator CH, Edmonds VE*: Acute spinal cord injuries: Analysis of epidemiologic factors. Can J Surg 22:575–578, 1979
38. *Tator CH, Edmonds VE, New ML:* Diving: a frequent and potentially preventable cause of spinal cord injury. Can Med Assoc J 124:1323–1324, 1981
39. *Tator CH, Ekong CEU, Rowed CA, Schwartz ML, Edmonds VE, Cooper PW:* Spinal injuries due to hockey. Can J Neurol Sci 11:34–41, 1984
40. *Tator CH, Edmonds VE:* National survey of spinal injuries in hockey players. Can Med Assoc J 130:875–880, 1984
41. *Torg JS, Quedenfeld TC, Moyer RA, Truex R Jr, Spealman AD, Nichols CE III:* Severe and catastrophic neck injuries resulting from tackle football. J Am Coll Health Assoc 25:224–266, 1977
42. *Torg JS, et al:* Spinal injury at the level of the third and fourth cervical vertebrae from football. J Bone Joint Surg 59A:1015–1019, 1977
43. *Torg JS, Quedenfeld TC, Burstein A, Spealman A, Nichols C:* National Football Head and Neck Injury Registry report on cervical quadriplegia 1971–1975. Am J Sports Med 7:127–132, 1977
44. *Torg JS, Truex R Jr, Quedenfeld TC, Burstein A, Spealman A, Nichols C III:* The National Football Head and Neck Injury Registry. Report and conclusions 1978. J Am Med Assoc 241:1477–1479, 1979
45. *Torg JS, Yu A, Pavlov H, Vegso J:* Cervical quadriplegia resulting from axial loading injuries. Cinematographic, radiographic, kinematic, and pathologic analysis. Orthop Trans
46. *Torg JS, Das M:* Trampoline-related quadriplegia: Review of the literature and reflections on the American Academy of Pediatrics' position statement. Pediatrics 74:804–812, 1984
47. *Torg JS, Vegso JJ, Yu A, et al*: Cervical quadriplegia resulting from axial loading injuries: Cinematographic, radiographic, kinematic, and pathologic analysis. American Orthopaedic Society for Sports Medicine Interim Meeting abstracts, Atlanta, Feb 8–9, 1984, p 18. Chicago, American Orthopaedic Society for Sports Medicine, 1984
48. *Torg JS:* Epidemiology, pathomechanics, and prevention of athletic injuries to the cervical spine. Med Sci Sports Exer 17:295–303, 1985
49. *Torg J, Vegso JJ, Sennett B:* The National Football Head and Neck Injury Registry: 14-year report on cervical quadriplegia, 1971 through 1985. J Am Med Assoc 254:3439–3443, 1985
50. *Torg JS, Vegso JJ, Torg E:* Cervical quadriplegia resulting from axial loading injuries: cinematographic, radiographic, kinetic and pathologic analysis (movie). Am Acad Orthop Surg Film Library, 1987
51. *US Consumer Product Safety Commission. Fact Sheet 85:* Trampolines, pp 1–3. Y3, C76/3:11/85
52. *Virgin H:* Cineradiographic study of football helmets and the cervical spine. Am J Sports Med 8:310–317, 1980
53. *Witthaut H:* Verletzungen beim Trampolinturnen. [Injuries in trampolining.] J Monatschr Unfallheilk 72:25–29, 1969
54. *Zimmerman HM:* Accident experience with trampolines. Res Q 452–455, 1956

CHAPTER 7

Injuries to the Cervical Cord

Acute Spinal Cord Injuries: Experimental Therapy, Pathophysiological Mechanisms, and Recovery of Function

WISE YOUNG AND JOSEPH RANSOHOFF

For many years, acute spinal cord injury research has largely been predicated on one central hypothesis: Treatments that maximally preserve surviving axons from further damage provide the best chance for recovery from spinal cord injury. From a surgical point of view, the hypothesis has led to the belief that rapid alleviation of spinal cord compression will maximize preservation of surviving axons at the injury site. In the laboratory, this hypothesis has led to intense efforts to elucidate the pathophysiologic mechanisms and to identify treatments that can ameliorate these mechanisms. Several pharmacologic treatments have shown promise in animal spinal injury models. Two, in particular, naloxone and methylprednisolone, are now undergoing clinical trial. In the meantime, close parallels between pathophysiologic mechanisms in spinal injury and cerebral ischemia mechanisms are leading researchers toward a unified theory of neural injury involving Ca entry into cells and lipid peroxidation. The theoretical foundation established by this research has provided a rational basis for the selection of treatments to test.

In recent years, the goal of spinal cord injury research has expanded from prevention of secondary injury to include functional restoration. Three observations have especially contributed to this expansion. First, quantitative axon counts in animals that recovered locomotor function indicated that surprisingly few axons (less than 10% of the normal number) can support substantial recovery, suggesting that the spinal cord is capable of remarkable adaptation to losses of spinal tracts. Second, neurophysiologic studies have suggested that demyelination may play a major role in producing and maintaining the neurologic deficits in spinal cord injury. Third, some recent studies suggest that the mammalian spinal cord may be capable of limited regeneration. Combined, these findings have stimulated the search for therapeutic approaches to enhance survival of axons during the acute phase of spinal cord injury, to improve conduction in surviving axons, and to encourage regeneration in the spinal cord.

Advances in other fields are beginning to take acute spinal cord injury research into uncharted territories. For example, recent successes in neural transplantation research bring closer the day when cells containing specific neurotransmitters can be implanted to modulate spinal cord activity. The availability of programmable electrical stimulation devices that can be safely implanted may also allow specific manipulation of spinal cord activity in order to enhance function. Studies of axonal sprouting in injured brains are beginning to show that the central nervous system is capable of more plasticity and growth than hitherto believed. Although these advances in our understanding of the determinants of functional recovery have not yet had a direct impact on clinical care of spine-injured patients, they do provide a strong argument for aggressive care of acute spinal cord injury to maximize the chance that patients will benefit from future treatments.

Rational therapy of acute spinal cord injury requires a broad understanding of the mechanisms of injury and the determinants of recovery, which spans many disparate disciplines. The following four parts of this section provide a framework for understanding these mechanisms. The first part summarizes the principles of acute spinal cord injury care. The second describes our experience applying these principles to clinical patient care. The third reviews recent advances in our understanding of the pathophysiology of acutely injured spinal cords, emphasizing particularly the roles of blood flow changes, ionic derangements at the injury site, Ca entry into cells, lipid peroxidation, and free radicals in the injury process. The fourth discusses the determinants of functional recovery in spinal cord injury.

PRINCIPLES OF ACUTE SPINAL CORD INJURY CARE

Prevention of further damage is the primary goal of surgical care in acute spinal cord injury. The main causes of further damage to the spinal cord are instability of the spinal column and continued compression of the spinal cord. Therefore, the initial management of acute spinal cord injury should emphasize safe transport and interim stabilization of the spinal column until definitive evaluation and therapy can be undertaken. Continued compression of the spinal cord can be alleviated by either appropriate external traction or surgical reduction and decompression. Surgical intervention, however, carries risks that must be carefully weighed against potential benefits. Aggressive surgical intervention must go hand in hand with thorough neuroradiologic evaluations to identify surgically correctable causes of spinal cord injury. Every effort must be made to reduce the risks of intervention, including neurophysiologic monitoring of patients during procedures that pose the possibility of additional damage to the spinal cord and cytoprotective treatments to reduce damage to the spinal cord.

Initial Management

Initial management of acute spinal cord injury is aimed at stabilizing the patient until definitive radiographic and neurologic evaluation can be undertaken and an appropriate therapy can be applied. The value of early injury recognition should not be underestimated, particularly at the accident site allowing immediate and appropriate triage, atraumatic transport, and transfer to a spinal injury treatment center where neurosurgeons, anesthesiologists, radiologists, orthopedists, and neurologists can collaborate in the care of the patient. The increasing percentage of patients seen worldwide with partial preservation of function over the past decade attests to the importance of educational programs for personnel involved in emergency medical services. During its first year of operation nearly 20 years ago, only 12% of spinal injury patients at the NYU-Bellevue Medical Center were admitted with partial preservation of function below the lesion level. This contrasts with 25% in the second and third years. At the present time, ~40% of the patients admitted to the center have some preserved function below the lesion level. Such a trend supports our suspicion that proper initial management of patients can reduce the incidence of additional trauma.

The initial management for cervical, thoracic, and lumbrosacral spinal cord injuries differs in one respect. In the injuries of the cervical region, compromise of the respiratory system complicates the care of patients. Severe injuries to the spinal cord above C3, in particular, are almost invariably associated with respiratory paralysis. This factor dominates clinical decisions. Injuries to the C4–C7 segments involve the anterior horns subserving upper-extremity function and the long spinal white matter tracts controlling trunk, lower extremities, and sphincter functions. Although patients with lower cervical injuries usually do not show evidence of respiratory difficulties on admission, they may develop respiratory difficulties, often associated with pneumonia, within the first few days. By contrast, lower thoracic and lumbrosacral injuries rarely result in compromise of the respiratory system. Consequently, in cervical and upper thoracic injury, early and continuing evaluation and support of pulmonary function are essential.

A careful neurologic examination is critical for identifying the lesion site and determining the functional status of the spinal cord. Electrophysiologic studies such as somatosensory-evoked potentials (SSEPs) and segmental reflex testing may complement the information obtained by neurologic examination. Although patients are commonly classified as either neurologically "complete" or "incomplete," this determination should be made only if a 48 hour period has elapsed in which no motor or sensory function can be detected below the lesion level, total areflexia is present below the level of the lesion, and SSEPs are absent below the lesion level. The judgment of complete spinal cord injury often colors both surgical and medical decisions, delaying recognition of potentially treatable lesions in a small percentage of patients.

Immediate stabilization of the fracture site must be achieved. Initial x-ray examination should include computed tomographic (CT) scanning, even if no fracture is seen on routine anteroposterior and lateral films. The unwary clinician may be lulled into a false sense of security when a report of "no fracture" is received and may be misled by fracture being classified as "stable." Probably very few fractures are stable enough to allow the patient to ambulate or support the weight of the head in the immediate posttrauma period. Stability must be defined in terms of functional capacity. The fracture may be stable if the patient is kept at absolute bed rest, whereas weight bearing can produce progressive angulation and deformity. An unstable fracture requires immediate immobilization and usually definite fusion to protect the underlying spinal cord from secondary injury and to prevent eventual bony deformity.

Neuroradiologic Evaluation

Definitive neuroradiologic procedures should be performed shortly after admission. At present, the procedure of choice is high-resolution CT scan of the spinal column with myelography. Because of the potential for stress to the injured spinal cord during administration of intrathecal contrast material, the patient must receive a thorough pulmonary evaluation prior to the procedure and must be monitored during the procedure. Metrizamide or iopamidol myelography via lumbar puncture is used for thoracic and lumbar injuries. These agents are likely to be replaced by newer non-ionic radiographic contrast materials in the near future.[41,247,257] A C1 puncture may be preferred for cervical injuries. Contrast-enhanced CT scans may be more informative than standard myelography. A complete cervical myelogram can be achieved by means of a lateral C1 puncture with the patient in a recumbent position under skeletal traction, without manipulation or inherent mechanical risk to the spinal cord.

CT scanning provides excellent images of bony abnormalities, extruded disc material, and epidural hematomas. Injection of a contrast agent by way of a C1 puncture as a supplement to CT scanning will show the spinal cord profile. Metrizamide contrast placed in the subarachnoid space outlines the cord. Some contrast can occasionally be seen in the spinal cord, suggesting avulsion of the cord. Magnetic resonance imaging (MRI) provides superior images of soft tissues and has already become the definitive diagnostic tool for documenting the presence of late posttraumatic syrinx. The advent of ^{31}P-MRI spectroscopy offers many exciting theoretical possibilities for localizing injury sites and studying the metabolic status of the spinal cord.[29] In acute spinal cord injury, however, because of the need for definitive bone images, the CT scan provides the information required for surgical decisions.

Radiologic evaluations must identify or rule out conditions requiring surgical decompression. Also, the mechanical status of the injury site must be thoroughly assessed. Forces acting on the cervical spinal column in trauma can be categorized into four main vectors: compression, extension, flexion, and rotation. Compression trauma produces explosion fractures of vertebral bodies and ruptures sustaining ligaments. Extension injuries produce fractures of the posterior elements of the spinal column and disruptions of the anterior longitudinal ligaments. Flexion injuries are likely to compress vertebral bodies and disrupt posterior longitudinal ligaments and the intervertebral discs. Rotational injuries disrupt ligamentous structures, fracture or dislocate facets, and damage vertebral bodies. Rotational and flexion or extension injuries are often combined, particularly in the cervical region, producing extensive damage to the bony and ligamentous structures. Detailed localization and characterization of these possibilities must be achieved prior to further surgical intervention.

Surgical Approaches

There have been few well-organized efforts directed at defining indications for early surgical treatments of the injured spinal cord to improve or to restore cord function. The role of surgical decompression is still more controversial than the indications for stabilization. Both early exploratory laminectomy and no surgical treatments have been recommended.[30,123,239] Although progressive loss of function is relatively rare in our experience, it is clearly an indication for immediate surgical decompression and stabilization.[102,234,259] However, a number of patients with residual cord function have developed permanent paralysis after early laminectomy.[134,226] Why laminectomy may aggravate injury, apart from operative and instrument damage, is not well understood. Some animal studies suggest that laminectomy alone produces significant decreases in blood flow[7,236,237] and biochemical derangements[78] in the spinal cord. Laminectomy alone may certainly increase instability. Therefore, laminectomy performed early after trauma without specific attention to stabilization is hard to justify.[134,226,239]

Surgical decompression should be considered when compression of the spinal cord is found. Anterior osteoarthritic ridges in older patients may press against the spinal cord, compromising spinal cord function, even in the absence of fractures or dislocations and particularly in patients with narrow cervical canals. External compression of the dural sac by bony fragments, extradural hematomas, or extruded disc material and ruptured ligaments may call for an anterior, anterolateral, or a posterior operative approach. In the presence of a localized area of major spinal cord swelling, a laminectomy should be considered. Dural decompression, myelotomy for drainage of intramedullary hematoma and necrotic hemorrhagic gray matter, and insertion of a dural substitute may be necessary to provide adequate decompression. Note, however, that because of the risk of damage to residual pathways in the spinal cord, the more invasive procedures are probably applicable only in patients with total losses of function below the lesion level.

Surgical intervention must provide rapid and reliable stabilization of bony elements involved at the site of injury. The timing for surgical intervention clearly depends on the individual circumstances of each case. It is worthwhile pointing out that operative decompression and fusion months to years after injury may improve function in patients who are incomplete.[176] Late surgical intervention may also prevent or correct spinal deformities that might diminish rehabilitation potential. The cardinal principle, however, is that instability in the spinal column must be corrected in order to decrease the likelihood of secondary injury.[122] In the event that surgery is not possible or must be delayed, external traction must be maintained to reduce the likelihood of additional trauma to patients with unstable fractures. Finally, there is the consideration that ease of surgically correcting deformities decreases with time after trauma.

Considerable surgical judgment and close collaboration between neurosurgery and orthopedics are required in the selection of the appropriate surgical procedure. Stabilization can be achieved by both anterior and posterior surgical approaches. These include techniques for interbody fusion, internal fixation devices, external fixation devices, and endogenous bone grafts. External fixation devices, such as the halo, provide some degree of stabilization, allowing earlier mobilization of patients. Recently, new internal fixation techniques that utilize plates screwed either posteriorly or anteriorly to the vertebral column have been introduced, in some cases replacing older wiring techniques that require greater and more vigilant external traction to stabilize the injury site until it fuses. The major advantage of the new internal fixation devices is that they hasten mobilization of patients after spinal cord injury, eschewing the use of halo devices and increasing patient compliance. Experience with internal fixation devices is still relatively limited, and the actual contribution of these devices to improved recovery of patients has yet to be determined. However, the decrease in bed rest and possibility of reduced hospitalization time required with such devices more than justify research into their use.

Pharmacologic Therapy

The rationale for pharmacologic treatment of acute spinal cord injury stems from laboratory studies suggesting that spinal cord lesions produced by physical contusion progress over a period of several hours.[1,2,21,22,130,265] Many mechanisms of progressive injury in animal models of spinal injury have been proposed. These include posttraumatic falls in spinal cord blood flow,[5,33,92,139,140,187,230,236,237,265,274–276] ionic shifts,[182,265,268,273–275,278,279] metabolic derangements,[6,8,51,54,157] Ca ionic entry into traumatized axons,[23–26,145,146,246,266,267,272,275,281] and generation of free radicals.[79–82,116,117,200] Excessive Ca entry into cells activates proteinases[27,28,72,160] that digest cellular constituents and phospholipases[4,9,47,48] that break down membranes and generate toxic biological products, including lipid peroxides[4,50,78,135,138,142–145] and prostaglandins.[78,155,159] Lysosomal release adds to tissue and cellular autodestruction.[72] These mechanisms can act alone or in concert to enhance cell damage in the traumatized spinal cord.

Much research has been directed at identifying and testing drugs that can reduce putative secondary tissue damage. Two classes of drugs in particular have attracted much attention: glucocorticosteroids and opiate receptor blockers. A large body of literature suggests that corticosteroids exert beneficial effects in animal models of spinal cord injury. Positive effects of steroid administration on functional recovery and histologic appearance of injured animal spinal cords have been reported by many investigators.[5,61,35,80,93,95,110,133,137,141,174,196,217] Recent studies have focused on the biomechanical and physiologic effects of very high doses of methylprednisolone,[4,5,9,49–53,80,135–140,198,270,275] suggesting that the optimal dose range of cytoprotective effects is 15 to 30 mg/kg. Given the variety of models and methods utilized in these studies, it is not surprising that some workers in the field have found steroid therapy to be ineffective in spinal cord injury.[35,110,112,149] Most of these studies, however, utilized dexamethasone or relatively low doses of methylprednisolone (< 15 mg/kg).

High doses of naloxone (>2mg/kg) have been reported to improve blood flow in injured spinal cords[104,270,276] and to improve functional recovery[103–112,119,120,270,276] in animal models of spinal injury. Naloxone is a potent opiate receptor blocker with little agonist activity and a relative specificity for the μ class of opiate receptors.[168] Although capable of reversing exogenously applied opiates in doses of <0.1 mg/kg, naloxone is metabolized rapidly and has a half-life of approximately 30 minutes.[114] The mechanisms of action of naloxone in spinal cord injury are not known, although there have been reports that it affects cerebral metabolism,[132] produces vasodilation,[256] and alters immune responses.[194] Faden[104] has proposed that naloxone and thyrotropic-releasing hormone (TRH), a physiologic opiate receptor blocker with cytoprotective effects similar to naloxone, act through the kappa opiate receptors,[168] although the presence and roles of such receptors in central nervous system are uncertain.[150]

Although naloxone and methylprednisolone differ considerably in molecular structure and presumptive modes of action, they share two features. First, both have been reported by investigators to exert cytoprotective effects in cerebral ischemia[154,175,188,213] and other types of neural injuries,[55,137,194] although their effectiveness has been questioned by some workers.[153,161,189,214,215,231] Second, animal studies indicate that these two drugs have to be given in doses far in excess of those necessary for their normal mechanisms of blocking opiate receptors and activating glucocorticosteroid receptors. High-dose glucocorticosteroids have been used for many years to treat various neurosurgical disorders,[164,264] and the side-effects of prolonged administration are well known. Relatively less is known about the side-effects of high dose naloxone. Some researchers have reported that administration of high-dose naloxone can produce behavioral and mood changes,[73] hypertension,[10,13,190] cardiac arrythmias,[13,199] and pulmonary edema.[10,115,248]

Clinical Trials of Naloxone and Methylprednisolone

Despite the wealth of laboratory data suggesting that certain pharmacologic treatments are beneficial in animal models of acute spinal injury, no clinical data support the efficacy of any of these treatments in human spinal cord injury. One reason for this situation is the dearth of rigorously randomized clinical trials with sufficient numbers of spine-injured patients to afford definitive conclusions. For example, the first randomized clinical trial of a pharmacologic treatment of spinal cord injury was completed recently.[45,46] Administered by the National Acute Spinal Cord Injury Study (NASCIS), this trial compared the neurologic recovery patterns of patients treated with *high-dose* methylprednisolone (1 gm bolus initial dose, followed by 1 gm per day for 10 days) with *low dose* (100 mg bolus initial dose, followed by 100 mg per day for 10 days). No statistically significant differences ($p < 0.05$) between these two doses were found.

The first NASCIS trial was flawed for the following reasons. First, it did not compare treatment against placebo. Consequently, the results showed that there was no difference between two doses of methylprednisolone but did not rule out the possibility that the low dose may have an effect. Second, the so-called high-dose treatment may not have been adequate. Recent laboratory studies have strongly suggested that the optimal dose for methylprednisolone effects is 30 mg/kg. A gram of methylprednisolone given to a 70-kg person is approximately 14 mg/kg. This dose may not effectively raise blood flow,[139,140,265,270,275] inhibit lipid peroxidation,[47,50–53,135–138] and improve the metabolic state[51,54] of injured spinal cords. Third, the treatment protocol allowed patients admitted as late as 48 hours after injury to be randomized. Evidence from laboratory studies strongly suggests that the treatment must be applied within a few hours after injury to have an effect.

To correct these deficits, a second trial (NASCIS II) was initiated approximately 2 years ago. This trial incorporates new data from laboratory studies suggesting that higher doses of methylprednisolone are required and that maintenance of methylprednisolone levels requires continued administration of 50% of the initial dose per hour. The trial also emphasizes treating the patients as early as possible after injury and compares methylprednisolone against both placebo and high doses of naloxone. About 460 patients are being assigned to three treatment arms: methylprednisolone (~30 mg/kg initial dose and 15 mg/kg per hour for 24 hours), naloxone (~5.4 mg/kg initial dose and 75% of the initial dose every hour for 24 hours), and placebo. Only patients admitted within 12 hours after injury are randomized. The trial is due to be completed next year. Until trials such as NASCIS II show positive results, pharmacologic treatments of acute spinal cord injury must be considered experimental.

Many clinicians are already treating spine-injured patients with low doses of dexamethasone or 1 gm methylprednisolone per day. We do not recommend the use of these drugs at the present time and urge that the following be considered. First, no data from either animal or human studies support administration of small doses of naloxone (<1 mg/kg) or methylprednisolone (<15 mg/kg) to spine-injured patients. Second, high doses of methylprednisolone should not be given concomitantly with high doses of naloxone, as some laboratory data suggest that the combination may be deadly.[270] Third, animal studies indicate strongly that treatments are most effective when given early after injury or preferably before injury. Finally, no data from either animal or human studies indicate that long-term administration of naloxone or methylprednisolone is superior to short-term treatments (*i.e.*, <48 hours). In the case of methylprednisolone, treatments for more than 48 hours probably carry a higher risk of complications and should be avoided. In the case of naloxone, doses exceeding 1 mg/kg for periods longer than 48 hours have not been adequately tested for safety.

Spinal Cord Monitoring

Electrophysiologic monitoring of spinal cord conduction in patients who have partial preservation of function is often of assistance in the operating room or during aggressive external traction to reduce malalignments of the spinal column. Improvements of SSEPs or, more important, losses of SSEPs during manipulation of the spinal cord may help guide clinical decisions.[245,268,269,271] Although techniques have become available recently for monitoring spinal and subcortical components of somatosensory responses, as well as motor responses evoked by cortical stimulation, the cortical SSEP recorded from scalp electrodes and evoked by peripheral nerve stimulation has remained the standard in the field against which other methods of intraoperative monitoring are judged.

SSEPs, however, are imperfect indicators of spinal cord function and several caveats attend their use. First and most obviously, evoked potential monitoring is often useless in patients who are so severely injured that they do not have reproducible responses at the outset. Second, SSEPs reflect conduction in sensory tracts from peripheral nerve to the cortex. Any alteration in the excitability of the many neural structures represented by the long pathway mediating sensory responses results in SSEP changes. Therefore, causes of SSEP changes unrelated to manipulation of the lesion site must be carefully ruled out. Third, patients with severe neurologic dysfunction, may be abnormally sensitive to anesthesia and manipulations of the spinal cord. This is especially true when the SSEP responses are small (<10% of normal) and variable. Paradoxically, in some patients, especially those with abnormally long latency responses suggestive of conductive delays in the pathway, SSEPs may be relatively insensitive to manipulations of the spinal cord. Finally, because SSEPs primarily test sensory tracts, they may occasionally (although rarely, in our experience) fail to reflect motor losses.

At the present time, there is no well-documented clinical trial showing that SSEP monitoring improves outcome of spine-injured patients. Some studies claim high incidences (20% to 30%) of false correlations between SSEP and neurologic findings. However, such claims have usually been based on data collected from unselected and relatively small series of patients, in which the abovementioned caveats have not been consistently applied to the interpretation of SSEP changes. The benefits of SSEP monitoring cannot be easily detected statistically. If the incidence of iatrogenically caused deficits is low (*i.e.*, on the order of 1% to 2%), as it should be, very large series of patients must be evaluated before statistically significant results can be obtained. However, if SSEP monitoring can prevent further injury in even a small proportion of spine-injured patients, its use would be more than justified.

PATIENT EXPERIENCE

We describe below our experience applying the above principles of acute spinal injury care at the NYU-Bellevue Spinal Cord Center over the past 10 years (1977 to 1987). During this period, a variety of treatment protocols were tested. For example, from 1977 to 1983, we were involved with the first NASCIS trial, comparing the neurologic recovery of patients treated with 1 gm and 100 mg of methylprednisolone per day for 10 days after injury.[45,46] In the 1983 to 1984 period, Phase-I clinical trials of high-dose naloxone and methylprednisolone (30 mg/kg) were undertaken.[119] From 1985 to the present, we have randomized patients to the NASCIS II trial, comparing the neurologic recovery of patients treated with very high doses naloxone (5.4 mg/kg), methylprednisolone (30 mg/kg), and placebo.

Patient Population

Of 230 patients admitted to the NYU-Bellevue Spinal Cord Trauma Center over the 6-year period that encompasses the NASCIS I trial (1977 to 1983), 185 (80%) had cervical injuries; 14 of these were above C4 and the remainder were between C4–C7. Approximately 42% of the patients were "incomplete," that is, they had some preserved sensation or motor function below the lesion level on admission. A majority (59%) of the patients were between 15 and 40 years of age. The remainder were fairly evenly distributed up to the age of 75. A great preponderance of the cases were due to falls, vehicular accidents, and sports injuries. There were 35 gunshot injuries. Approximately 75% were admitted to the Center within 24 hours after injury, and 90% within 72 hours.

For comparison, Figures 7-1 and 7-2 show the distribution of 52 patients seen in 1986 segregated by injury levels, age, sex, and whether the injury was complete or incomplete. The percentage of patients with cervical spinal cord injuries (~69%) is slightly lower than before. A majority (~62%) continue to have complete spinal cord injuries. The population remains young: 67% of the patients were between 15 and 40 years old. As with virtually every survey of spinal injured patients in the world, young male patients dominated the population. Only 19% of the population were female. The causes of injuries likewise were very similar, with approximately 15% due to gunshot wounds and the remainder related to falls, vehicular accidents, and sports injuries.

The data presented in Figures 7-1 and 7-2 exclude patients admitted to the hospital more than 1 week after spinal cord injury, those with chronic compression of the spinal cord due to either extruded discs or tumors, and those with purely ischemic lesions of the spinal cord. The last category of patients includes about 100 cases of arteriovenous malformations of the spinal cord and paraplegia related to aortic aneurisms. Since 1980, the number of patients with tumors and extruded discs exceeds 200. Unlike the trauma cases, the majority of these patients had lesions located in the thoracic cord, and the population is equally divided between males and females. Thus, although trauma numerically dominates the causes of spinal cord injury, it is by no means the only cause.

Neurologic Evaluation

Independent neurologic evaluations were performed within 12 hours of admission to the hospital and at 1 week, 6 weeks, 6 months, and 1 year after injury (when possible). A total of 556 examinations were performed. The format for recording neurologic examination is a superset[269] of the one used by the National Acute Spinal Cord Injury Study (NASCIS[45,46]). Dermatome scores of both touch and pinprick sensation were obtained on a scale of 0 to 2 (0 = absent, 1 = abnormal, 2 = normal). All major muscle groups were scored on a scale of 0 to 5 (0 = absent activity, 1 = trace movement, 2 = definite movement, 3 = able to oppose gravity, 4 = able to oppose gravity and resistance, 5 = normal). In addition, superficial anal sphincter reflexes were assessed, as well as the ability of the patients to detect deep pressure stimuli to either legs.

SSEPs were monitored in these patients within 24 hours, at 6 weeks, and often at 6 months and at 1 year after injury.[268,271] In a rough assessment of the reliability of SSEP correlation with neurologic findings, we scored SSEP into categories of 0 (absent), 1 (trace), 2 (abnormal), 3 (normal) and compared these against averaged touch and pinprick sensory scores of three dermatomes supplied by the stimulated posterior tibialis nerve. On admission, approximately 83% of patients had SSEPs that predicted sensory preservation within 1 sensory score unit. Patients who had greater discrepancies of SSEP and sensory scores mostly had very long latency and bizarre SSEP responses. If we excluded these patients and only considered those

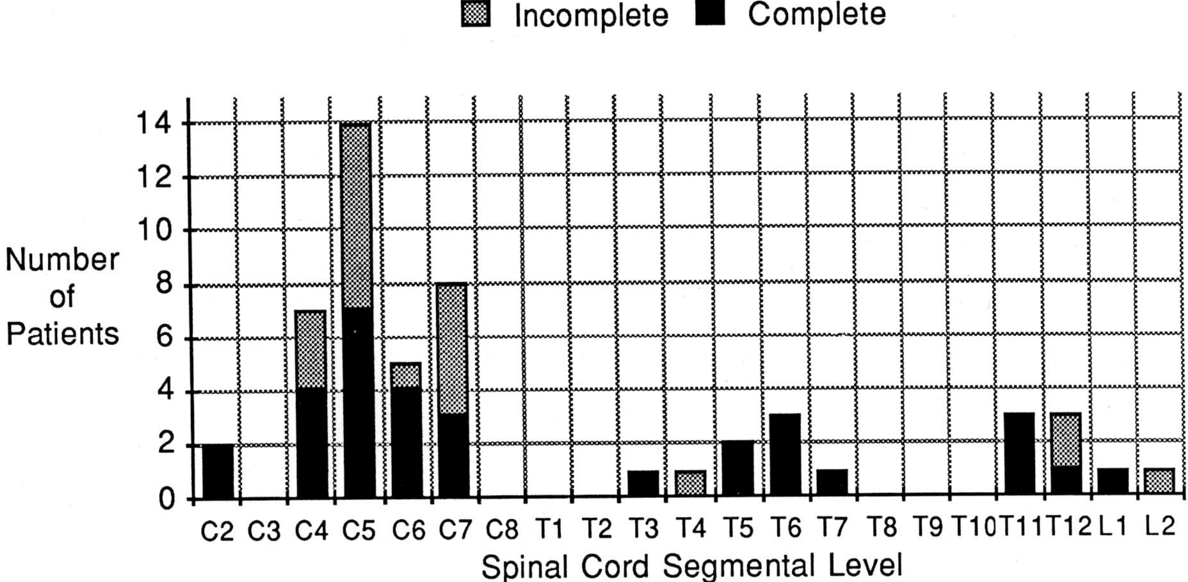

Fig. 7-1. The distribution of different segmental levels injury in patients admitted to treatment protocols at NYU-Bellevue Spinal Injury Center in 1986. A clear segregation of three groups of patients can be seen: cervical, midthoracic, and lower thoracic–lumbrosacral fractures. The proportion of patients that are "complete," *i.e.*, having no detectable sensory, motor, and reflex function below the lesion level for 48 hours after injury, is higher in the thoracic injuries, compared with the cervical injuries. Note the great preponderance of the injuries to the C4–C5 segments.

with early cortical responses (*i.e.*, <50 msec latency response), approximately 7% had SSEPs that did not predict touch and pinprick sensory scores within 2 category units. In no case did we observe a patient with normal sensation and no SSEP. Conversely, there were no cases of patients with normal SSEP and absent sensation in the appropriate dermatomes.

We began this study anticipating that SSEPs would detect residual function that might have been missed on neurologic examinations. For acute spinal cord injury, it became apparent that this occurred rarely, and usually when neurologic examinations were inadequate. In the few cases in which SSEPs were found in patients reported to have complete sensory loss, the patients almost always turned out to have some preserved sensation upon careful reexamination. Comparisons of SSEPs accurately predicted the most affected limb in >99% of the cases. Finally, we found that the incidence of false correlation between SSEP and neurologic examinations increased in chronic spinal cord injuries.[268] We found approximately 20% incidence of false negatives and false positives in patients studied at 6 weeks or longer after injury.

SSEP testing turned out to be most useful in two situations. First, when patients were unconscious, uncooperative, or malingering, SSEPs were often very useful for confirming the presence of spinal cord lesions. Second, when close monitoring of patients was called for, that is, during radiologic procedures and adjustment of traction, SSEPs provided an additional indicator of spinal cord function. For example, in patients with unstable fractures, it is possible to obtain almost continuous monitoring. The major advantage of SSEPs is that they are relatively free of subjective bias. Carried out by a properly trained technician and appropriately interpreted, SSEPs are beginning to achieve the reliability of electrophysiologic tests such as electrocardiography.

Surgical Therapy

We intervene early in patients with significant external cervical compression demonstrable on myelography after maximal reduction by skeletal traction. Surgery was by either the anterior or the

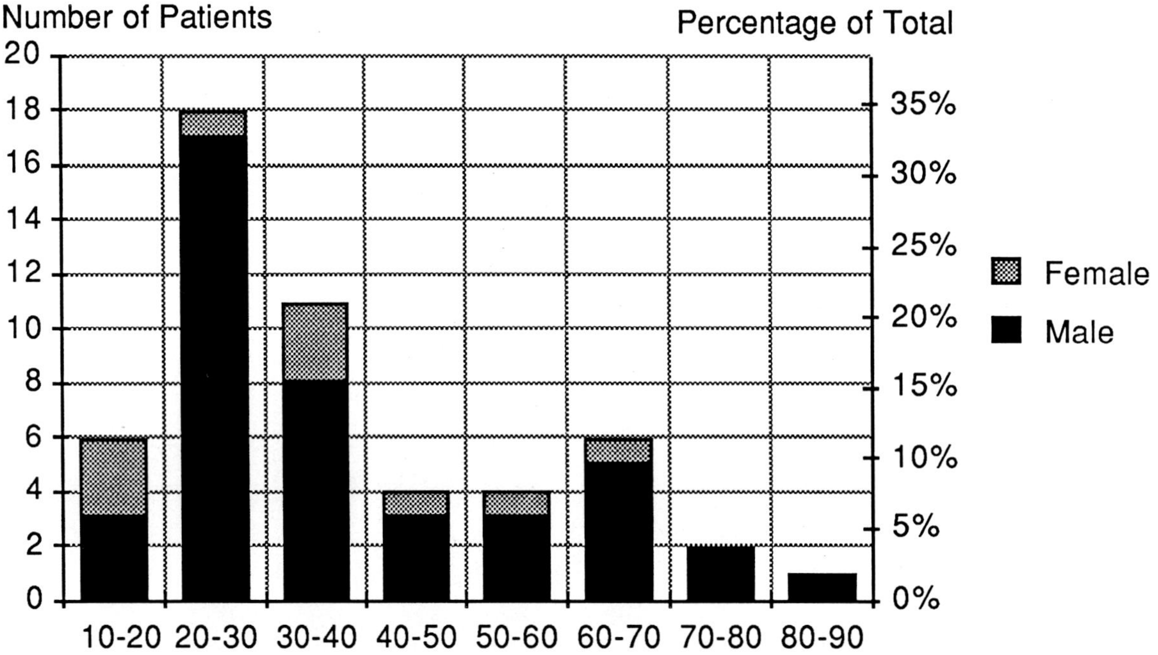

Fig. 7-2. The distribution of spinal injuries by age and sex. On the abscissa are the age categories of the patients by decades. Note the predominance of males at all age groups and high numbers of patients in the 20- to 30-year age group.

posterior approach, depending on the site of external compression. In patients with no external compression who had evidence of near or total myelographic block, we performed laminectomy and dural decompression below C3. Operating jointly with orthopedic surgeons, we stabilized fracture sites immediately and achieved long-term stability by bony fusions. These guidelines were followed, except when vasomotor or pulmonary instability, associated injuries, or medical problems contraindicated early surgical intervention.

One hundred and nine of 185 patients studied neuroradiologically had surgical decompression. Surgery was performed within the first 24 hours in 25% of cases, in an additional 50% within the first 5 days, and in the remaining 25% within 10 days of injury. The overall mortality rate within 30 days of injury was 9.5%. All deaths occurred in patients with high cervical injury from consequent pulmonary complications. No deaths occurred in patients with partial injuries. An analysis of the results of surgical versus nonsurgical management was restricted to improvement of motor function in the lower extremities and bladder function. As a rule, most patients recovered some function one to two segments immediately below the lesion level. Although an additional root can be important to the patient, it complicated the analysis of spinal cord function. In this analysis, we did not count the recovery of these one to two segments. According to our method of scoring motor function, 30 points are normal for each lower extremity; hence, a sum of 60 points is normal for both legs.

Evaluation of the results of surgical intervention in acute spinal cord injury requires the selection of a group in whom the risk of increased neurologic deficit can be weighed against possible benefits. For this reason, we chose to compare the results of surgery in those patients who had partial preservation of function prior to surgery. The indication for surgery was a significant myelographic defect, and surgery was tailored to the location of the defect (anterior or posterior). Surgery was carried out with stabilization (usually an external halo device) and fusion for long-term stability. A striking difference between the surgical and nonsurgical groups was seen in patients with motor scores of 0 to 20 in the lower extremities. Twenty-six of 30 patients who underwent surgery were ambulatory within 12 months (12 without crutches or braces) and 22 recovered bladder function. Seven of 18 patients with no myelographic defects and

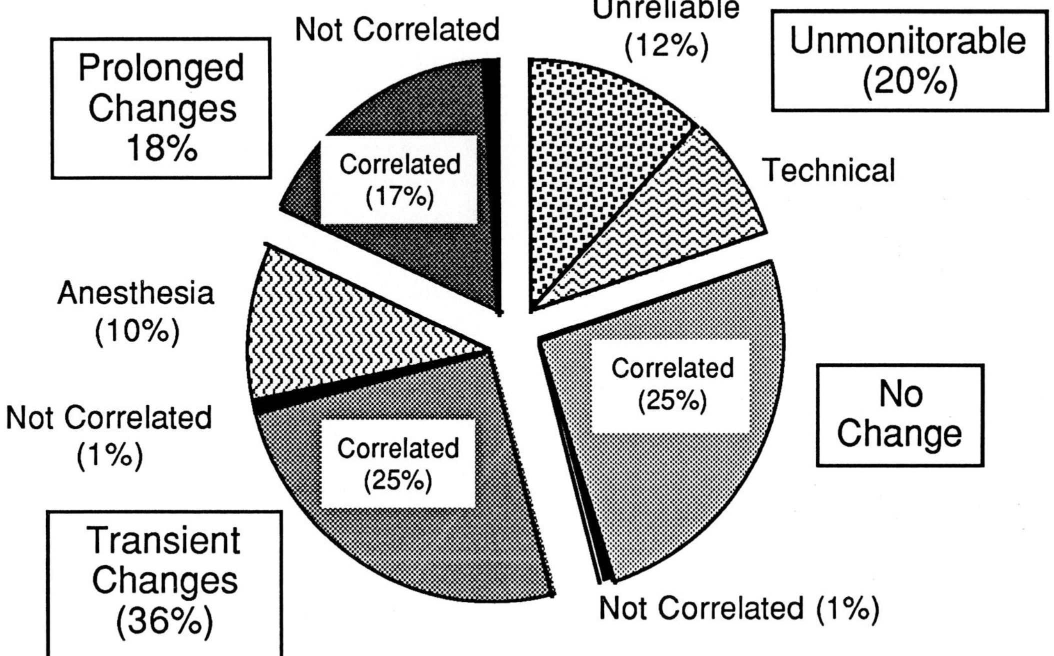

Fig. 7-3. Summary of 100 consecutive cases of intraoperatively monitored SSEPs. Four main categories of results are shown: Unmonitorable, No Change, Transient Changes, and Prolonged Changes of SSEP. The largest category is transient (36%) changes that resolved by the end of the cases, of which 69% were associated with manipulation of the spinal cord, 28% were due to changes in anesthesia levels, and 3% were unexplained. Note the relatively large proportion of unmonitorable cases (20%). A proportion of the cases (18%) had either improvement or reduction of SSEP amplitudes that lasted beyond the surgical procedure, of which 94% correlated with neurologic changes.

who, therefore, were not operated on became ambulatory and recovered bladder function.

Intraoperative SSEP Monitoring

In our experience, in patients with reproducible SSEPs that are >10% of normal amplitudes, prolonged losses in amplitudes exceeding 50% of preoperative amplitude that do not reverse by the end of operation and that cannot be explained by technical or anesthetic causes almost invariably are associated with postoperative sensory loss, and usually motor loss as well. To illustrate, we assessed the SSEP changes in 100 consecutive patients monitored intraoperatively between January, 1985, and June, 1986. Figure 7-3 shows the proportion of cases with and without SSEP changes and the causes. The data base includes patients with undergoing selective spinal angiography and embolization for spinal cord arteriovenous malformations and tumors. It does not include patients operated upon for correction of scoliosis.[101]

The compilation revealed several interesting points. First, although patients with no preoperative SSEPs were excluded from this data base, we were unable to record reproducible SSEPs after induction of anesthesia in about 20% of the cases. Most of these cases had SSEPs with amplitudes that were <10% of normal before surgery. Second, more patients showed SSEP changes than not. For example, 25% of the patients showed no change in SSEP during the operation, 36% showed transient changes, and 18% had definite SSEP changes that lasted beyond the operation. Third, we encountered false positive or false negative correlations with postoperative outcome in only 3% of the cases, that is, when the SSEP change or lack of change was not associated with neurologic sensory findings.

The most common error in intraoperative monitoring is over-reading of SSEP changes when the responses are small (<10% of normal) and variable before surgery. This is often true of SSEPs obtained from patients with severe neurologic dysfunction. In patients with severe spinal cord injury, SSEPs are often abnormally sensitive to anesthesia, such that even very low levels and slight changes of halogenated anesthesia alter them. The SSEPs may also be abnormally insensitive to manipulations of the spinal cord in some patients. Most of the cases of false negative and false positive correlations encountered in the study occurred in patients with small and variable SSEPs preoperatively. The other important principles are to repeat the SSEP and to rule out nonspecific causes of SSEP changes by monitoring a pathway not expected to change due to the surgical intervention. Careful adherence to these principles will reduce the incidence of false correlations. Misleading SSEPs are worse than no SSEP.

Methylprednisolone and Naloxone Therapy

On the basis of laboratory studies suggesting that high-dose naloxone (10 mg/kg) and methylprednisolone (30 mg/kg) significantly improved functional recovery in cats with severe spinal cord contusions, we embarked on a Phase-I trial to establish the feasibility of using these drugs in human spinal cord injury. We treated 59 consecutive patients with either naloxone or methylprednisolone. These patients do not overlap with the group of 230 patients described above. In the case of naloxone, since such huge doses have not been given to spinal injured patients before, we conducted an escalated dosage trial in the first 20 patients, starting with 0.14 mg/kg loading dose followed by 20% of the loading dose per hour for 48 hours. The dose was doubled every three to five patients when no side-effects were noted. When we reached the loading dose of 5.4 mg/kg, within the range in which some functional improvements were noted in animals, we altered the regimen. Four patients received 2.7 mg/kg, and five patients received 5.4 mg/kg loading doses, followed by 75% of the loading dose per hour for 24 hours. In the case of methylprednisolone, because we had considerable clinical experience giving 1-gm loading doses of methylprednisolone, we went directly to a 30 mg/kg loading dose followed by 50% of that dose every hour for 24 hours.

This Phase-I trial allayed two concerns. First, naloxone, an opiate receptor blocker, may enhance pain in patients who had just recently suffered trauma. This did not occur. Although 4 of the 29 patients treated with naloxone experienced pain, only one had to be withdrawn from the study. All four patients had some preserved sensation below the lesion level and a reason for pain (*e.g.*, fractured hip). However, because of the naloxone, opiate analgesics could not be used to alleviate pain. There was no relationship between the dose of naloxone and the incidence of pain. All the patients receiving loading doses of 5.4 mg/kg tolerated the treatment well.

Second, in the previous NASCIS trial involving 1 gm of methylprednisolone given daily for 10 days, there was a trend toward increased morbidity. Although this trend was not statistically significant, we were concerned that the higher 30 mg/kg doses of methylprednisolone might have greater adverse side effects. Likewise, some published reports suggest that high doses of naloxone can produce a variety of cardiorespiratory complications[10,13,190,199] and transient physiological changes.[73] Our study showed that morbidity and mortality in the 59 patients did not differ from historical controls. In the case of naloxone, there was no increase in morbidity and mortality associated with increased dosage. Finally, we found a significant improvement in the recovery of the ambulatory capabilities in the treated patients compared with historical controls. In the naloxone-treated group, there appeared to be a relationship between the recovery and dose. We concluded that these treatments did not prevent recovery and may have improved recovery.

PATHOPHYSIOLOGIC MECHANISMS

In the past decade, major advances have been made in our understanding of acute spinal injury mechanisms in the laboratory. Most of the laboratory research on spinal cord injury used the classic weight-drop contusion model first developed by Allen[1,2] in 1911. He described an intriguing pattern of progressive pathologic changes in spinal cords hit by a 20-gm weight falling 20 cm onto thoracic spinal cord exposed by laminectomy. Neglected for many decades, the model was revived in the 1960s, and the original findings have been confirmed.[21,22,91,95,130] The observation of progressive pathologic changes provided hope that injury processes may be amenable to treatments administered shortly after injury.

Primary Versus Secondary Injury

The hypothesis of secondary injury has played a major role in acute spinal cord injury research in the past decade. Prompted by the observations of progressive pathologic changes in contused spinal cords, this hypothesis emphasizes the cascade of events initiated by trauma. These include the release of toxic byproducts, alterations of the extracellular environment at the injury site, and secondary damage to axons that otherwise would have survived the injury.[265] Secondary injury is distinguished from the primary injury due to the mechanical disruption of the axons by the initial blow.[165,166,201] Although most extensively studied in the contusion model, the progressive pathologic events appear to be a universal accompaniment of all types of injuries to the spinal cord, including those produced by direct ischemic insults[156] and slow compression of the spinal cord.[250–253]

Much evidence has been gathered to support the possibility of secondary injury mechanisms in spinal cord trauma. Based on observations of endothelial damage and intravascular thromboses seen at the injury site shortly after trauma, several investigators[5,22,23,93,230] proposed that decreased blood flow secondarily damages the spinal cord after trauma. Subsequent studies indicated that blood flow falls rapidly in gray matter but with a delay of 1 to 2 hours in white matter at the lesion site.[33,92,139,140,187,230,236,237,265,274–276,279] Neurophysiologic monitoring of injured spinal cords revealed that although evoked potentials were immediately abolished by a contusion, they often recovered transiently, only to disappear again hours and sometimes even days afterwards.[265] Consequently, many investigators have sought to identify toxic factors in the injured spinal cord that may account for the vascular and neurophysiologic changes.

Many secondary injury mechanisms have been implicated in the spinal injury process. These include release of vasoactive and neurotoxic substances,[211,212] deranged ionic environment at the injury site,[265,273,278–280] edema,[182,265,268] entry of calcium ions (Ca^{+2}) into cells,[24–26,145,146,267,272,278,279] breakdown of lysosomes,[72] activation of phospholipases,[4,9,47,48] generation of membrane-damaging oxygen free radicals[79–82,116,117,200] lipid peroxidation and the resultant release of extremely potent vasoactive prostaglandins[78,155,159] and other lipid peroxides.[4,50,78,135,138]

Studies of these secondary injury processes have intensified with the increasing availability of pharmacologic tools for specifically manipulating biochemically and transmitter-mediated phenomena in injured spinal cords. Some of these studies have implicated hitherto unsuspected mechanisms of cell injury. For example, the finding in the early 1980s that high doses of naloxone improve functional recovery and blood flow in contused animal spinal cords[276] has linked the secondary injury processes to opiate receptors and immunologic mechanisms in spinal cord injury.[194] Some evidence suggests that similar mechanisms may play a role in the secondary tissue damage seen in cerebral ischemia[11,60,83,84,116,147,158,170,171,183,218,222,227,238,241–243,249,280] and other types of neural injury.[60,64–68,177,258]

The role of secondary tissue damage, however, needs to be critically assessed. Many phenomena that have been attributed to secondary tissue damage may be manifestations, rather than causes, of tissue death. In most experimental situations, cause–effect relationships are difficult to distinguish from the myriad of physiologic, biochemical, and morphologic changes that occur when cells die. In fact, in the contused spinal cord, necrotic changes dominate. The burden of proof cannot rest on correlation alone. Although many investigators have argued that the early appearance of an event indicates a causative role of the event, such arguments must be viewed skeptically. Ultimately, demonstrations of cause and effect have been most strongly supported by experiments showing that a treatment that eliminates a specific mechanism also produces significant functional recovery.

Posttraumatic Ischemia

Blood flow falls in severely injured spinal cords. For many years, this phenomenon was subject to intense scrutiny and controversy because of inadequacies of blood flow measurement methods and the variable presence of posttraumatic ischemia in different spinal injury models.[230,236,237] After a contusion or compression of the spinal cord, blood flow in the gray matter falls rapidly from 40 to 50 to < 20 ml/100gm/minute.[92,230] By contrast, white matter blood flow at the lesion site does not fall and may even be slightly elevated during the first 1 to 2 hours after trauma. By 2 to 3 hours, however, white matter blood flow falls from a normal range of about 12 to 15 to 6 to 7 ml/100gm/minute.[139,230,265,274–276,279] In moderate or mild injuries of the spinal cord, white matter blood flow may not fall at all.[165,187,236,237]

The causes of posttraumatic ischemia are not known. During the 1970s, much emphasis was placed on norepinephrine (NE) accumulation at the lesion site and its possible role in producing the posttraumatic ischemia in injured spinal cord.[211,212] Although the subject aroused much controversy, especially when claims of NE accumulation could not be confirmed by other laboratories,[235] the possibility that other neurotransmitters and substances may be responsible for posttraumatic secondary injury has not been ruled out. For example, cAMP[118] has been proposed as a cause of posttraumatic ischemia in spinal cord injury. Certain drugs that manipulate cAMP levels have been shown to improve posttraumatic spinal cord blood flow.[92] Other examples include the products of lipid peroxidation and especially arachidonic acid derivatives.[218] These compounds have been shown to be generated and released in injured spinal cords[78,155,159] and are capable of reducing blood flow.[67,167,218] Damage to endothelial cells,[21] similar to that described in cerebral ischemia[84] and head trauma[258] models, may result in thromboses and vascular occlusion vasoconstriction,[118] and breakdown of the blood–brain barrier. The gross metabolic depression that occurs in injured spinal cords,[6] lactoacidosis[8,54] and consequent pH shifts may also alter blood flow.[170,171]

Many pharmacologic treatments have been reported to improve blood flow in injured spinal cords. These include some that increase tissue cAMP (aminophylline and isoproterenol[92]), opiate receptor blockers (high doses of naloxone,[276] TRH,[103] kappa opiate receptor blockers[104]), free radical scavengers and lipid peroxidation inhibitors (high doses of methylprednisolone[5,139,275]), and others.[139] Posttraumatic decreases in blood flow, however, may simply be manifestations of injury, as opposed to being the cause of tissue damage.[265] Severe ionic derangements and metabolic depression are consequences of cellular disruption and may cause vascular constriction. Although many types of treatments have been shown to improve blood flow, these treatments may alter the course of pathophysiologic events in the injured spinal cord and therefore affect blood flow secondarily. Thus, the demonstration that a given treatment improves spinal cord blood flow and at the same time improves functional recovery does not necessarily mean that the two phenomena are causally linked. Both may be a result of an independent process.

Tissue Na and K Shifts and Edema

Total tissue Na ($[Na]_t$) and K concentrations ($[K]_t$) are normally 55 mM and 89 mM in the cat spinal cord.[273,278] Extracellular K ionic activity ($[K^+]_e$) is usually 3 to 4 mM[205,206,279] and extracellular Na ionic activity ($[Na^+]_e$) is ~150 mM.[206,273] If we assume that extracellular space occupies 20% of the tissue volume,[208] we can calculate that intracellular Na ($[Na^+]_i$) and K ($[K^+]_i$) concentrations are respectively 31 mM and 110 mM. Thus, large transmembrane ionic gradients motivate the movement of ions into and out of cells. Cellular disruption allowing equilibration of Na and K between the intracellular and extracellular space results in increases of $[K^+]_e$ and decreases in $[Na^+]_e$. Large ionic gradients consequently develop after injury between the lesion site and surrounding tissue, as well as across the blood–brain barrier.[131,220,228]

Complete cellular disruption and the consequent equilibration of intracellular contents with extracellular fluids should raise $[K^+]_e$ and lower $[Na^+]_e$ toward total tissue concentrations of 89 mM and 55 mM, respectively.[265] Using ion-selective microeletrodes, we showed that extracellular K ionic activity ($[K^+]_e$) rises from a normal level of 4 mM to a mean of 54 mM and as high as 87 mM within seconds after a contusion. The K ions clear with an exponential half-time of 31 to 38 minutes, depending on blood flow.[279] Figure 7-4 summarizes these data. In contrast, $[Na^+]_e$ falls from normal levels of 150 mM to <70 mM and remains <100 mM for more than 5 hours after injury.[273] The magnitudes of the K rise and Na fall suggest strongly that contusion of the spinal cord disrupts a majority of cells at the injury site.

These extracellular ionic derangements profoundly affect spinal cord function. Membrane potentials and activity depend on the Na and K transmembrane gradients.[205] Because $[K^+]_e$ is relatively low to begin with, even small increases of $[K^+]_e$ influence membrane resting potentials. For example, a 16-mM increase of $[K^+]_e$ represents a fourfold decrease in transmembrane K ionic gradient. This will depolarize axons sufficiently to block action potential conduction. Indeed, studies of evoked potential conduction across the lesion site showed that recovery did not occur until $[K^+]_e$ fell below 10 to 15 mM.[279] Note that disruption of 5% of cells in the spinal cord results in a rise of $[K^+]_e$ to >20 mM. In contrast, a decrease in $[Na^+]_e$ by >110 mM would be required to produce a fourfold decrease in transmembrane Na ionic gradient. This would necessitate disruption of 80% to 90% of the cells in order to lower $[Na^+]_e$ to this extent.

To ascertain the origin and destination of these ions, we measured total tissue Na, K, and water concentrations of spinal cords at 1 and 3 hours after being contused with a 20-gm weight dropped 20 cm.[278] The ions were measured by atomic absorption spectroscopy and the water by wet-tissue and dry-tissue weights. Figure 7-5 summarizes the data, expressed in μmol/gm wet tissue. By 1 hour,

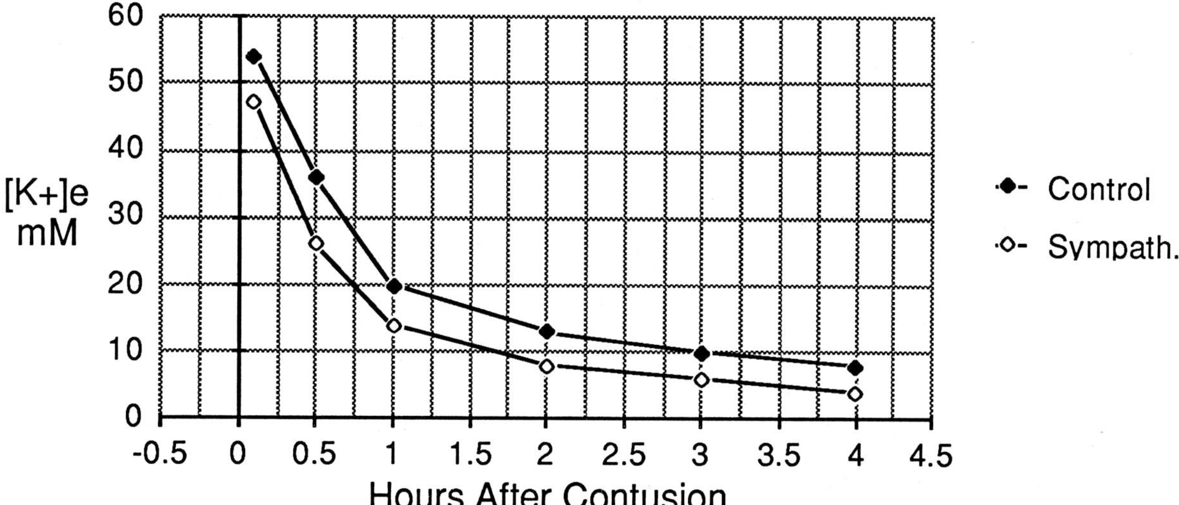

Fig. 7-4. Mean extracellular K ionic activity in white matter at the lesion site after 20 gm–20 cm contusion injury. The averaged half-time of clearance is about 38 minutes. Half-times averaged approximately 38 minutes (Control, n = 8). Paravertebral sympathectomy (Sympath, n = 6), which prevented posttraumatic decrease in blood flow, resulted in faster clearances with half-times of about 31 minutes.

tissue water concentration ($[H_2O]_w$) increased significantly from 0.662 ml/gm to 0.685 ml/gm at the lesion site and by 3 hours to 0.705 ml/gm. At 1 hour, $[Na]_w$ already increased at the lesion site by a mean of 40%, and 30% of tissue K was lost. By 3 hours, $[Na]_t$ levels at the lesion center were 100% greater than normal, whereas close to 70% of $[K]_t$ was gone.

These ionic shifts probably signify irreversible damage to cells at the lesion site. By 3 hours after injury, 70% of tissue K is gone from the tissue, not just shifted from cells into extracellular space. The loss of K parallels the loss of ascorbic acid, another soluble intracellular substance, measured in the same model.[78] In addition, the ionic shifts probably contribute to edema. The net ionic shift at the lesion site alone generates enough osmotic force to account for most of the observed water shift. The entry of water itself produces swelling of the spinal cord. This is evident in the rapid swelling of the tissue through any opening when dura and pia mater overlying a contused spinal cord are cut open. Significant pressures may be generated by the water entry and tissue swelling, possibly enough to reduce blood flow by the observed 50%. Treatment with methylprednisolone (15 mg/kg) shortly (45 minutes) after injury significantly reduces the amount of Na accumulation, K loss, and water entry at the lesion site. It also improves blood flow at the contusion site at 3 hours after injury.

Ca Shifts in Injured Spinal Cords

The large extracellular Na and K shifts observed in acutely injured spinal cords pale in comparison with the dramatic falls in extracellular Ca ionic activity ($[Ca^{+2}]_e$) Measured with ion-selective microelectrodes, $[Ca^{+2}]_e$ falls more than a hundredfold from a normal level of 1.2 mM[207] to <0.01 mM within a few seconds after a 20-gm to 20-cm weight drop contusion and remains depressed (<0.1 mM) at the lesion center for hours after injury.[246,281] As shown in Figure 7-6, $[Ca^{+2}]_e$ in white matter at the lesion site recovered during the first hour but declined between 1 to 3 hours to <0.1 mM. In the surrounding cord, $[Ca^{+2}]_e$ returned close to preinjury values by 3 hours.

Note that even if we assume that intracellular Ca activity ($[Ca^{+2}]_i$) is negligible,[20,89,90] the equilibration of extracellular with intracellular fluids should at most cause fivefold to tenfold fall in $[Ca^{+2}]_e$ (assuming that the extracellular volume fraction is 10% to 20%.)[181] The finding that $[Ca^{+2}]_e$ falls one order of magnitude or more below this expected level, while total tissue Ca concentration increases, can be explained only by precipitation of Ca ions at the lesion site. The

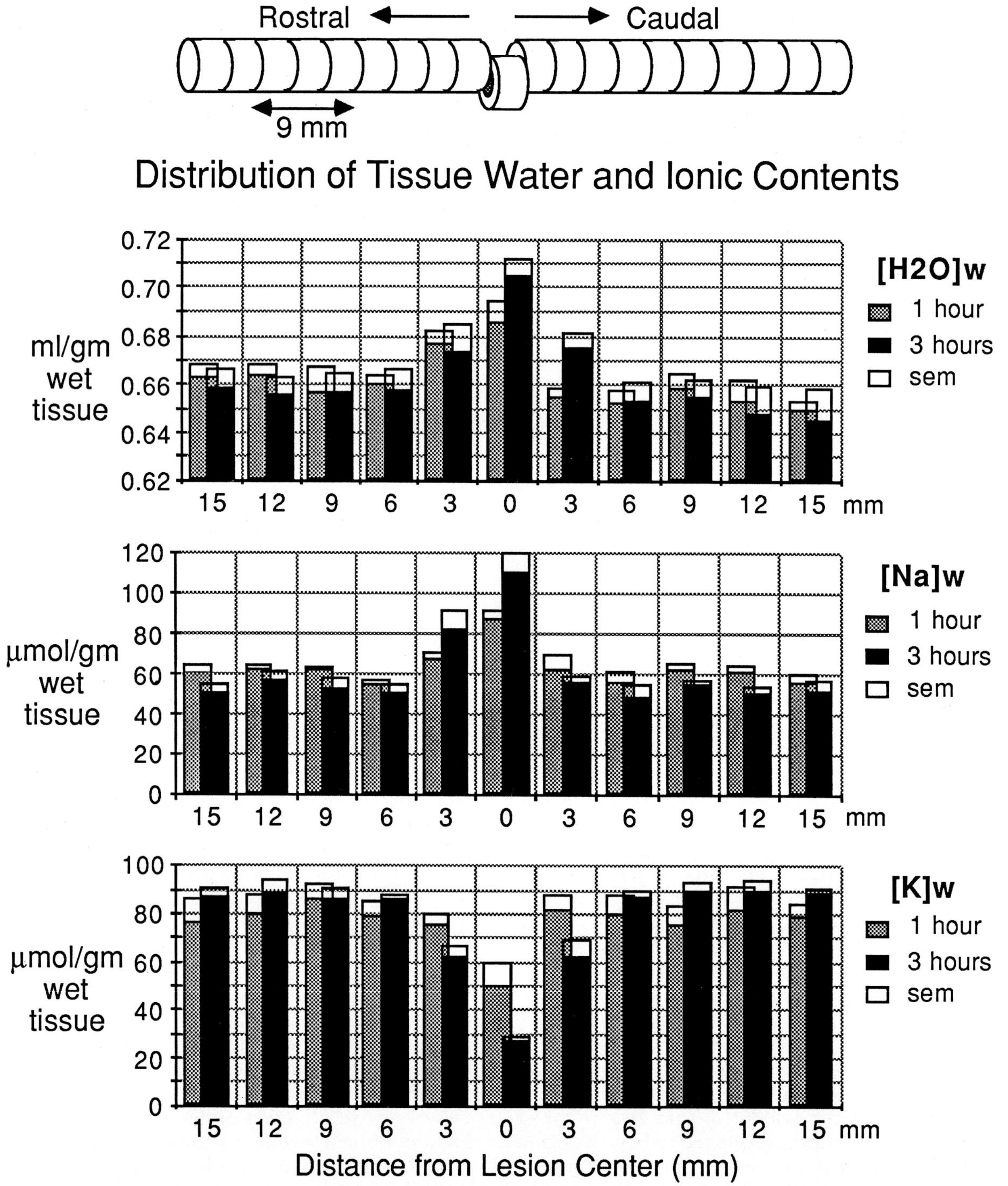

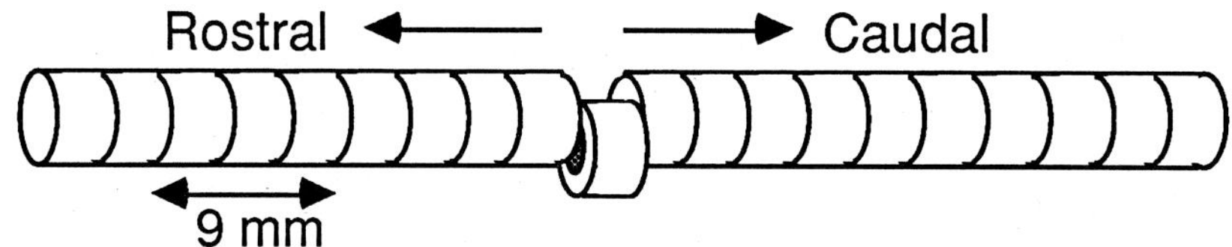

Fig. 7-5. Mean tissue water ($[H_2O]_w$), Na ($[Na]_w$), and K ($[K]_w$) concentrations. The spinal cords were cut into 3-mm segments centered on the impact site and the measurements made at 1 hour ($n = 5$) and 3 hours ($n = 8$) after a 20 gm–20 cm contusion, shown as a function of distance from the lesion site.

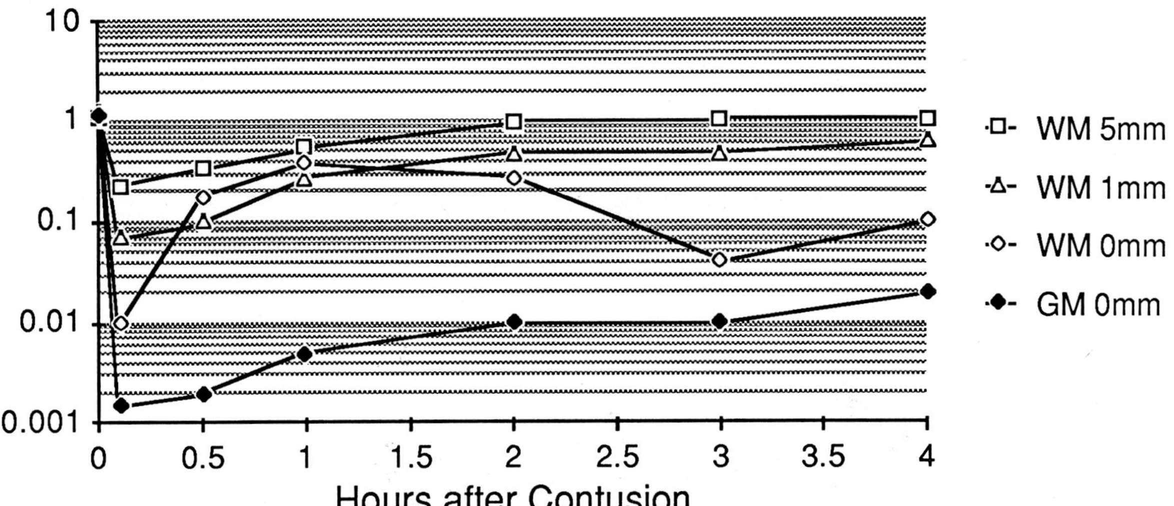

Fig. 7-6. Mean extracellular Ca ionic activities ($[Ca^{+2}]_e$) recorded from gray matter at the lesion center (GM 0 mm), white matter at the lesion center (WM 0 mm), 1 mm from the lesion edge (WM 1 mm), and 5 mm from the lesion edge (WM 5 mm). At the lesion site, $[Ca^{+2}]_e$ falls to <0.01 mM and remains <0.1 mM for >4 hours.

continued depression of $[Ca^{+2}]_e$ at the lesion center, despite the recovery of $[Ca^{+2}]_e$ in the surrounding cord to 1 mM and the presence of 1.2 mM of $[Ca^{+2}]_e$ in blood, indicates the presence of a remarkably effective mechanism for preventing Ca ionic diffusion to the lesion site.[267] Such a diffusion limitation probably results from a decrease in extracellular volume and an increase in the tortuosity of the extracellular space[169,208] produced by cellular edema.

Atomic absorption spectroscopy studies indicated that total tissue Ca concentration ($[Ca]_w$) increases from about 2 μmol/gm wet tissue before injury to 3 μmol/gm at 3 hours after injury.[278] Figure 7-7 summarizes these results. Although a 1 μmol/gm or 1-mM increase may seem small in comparison with the 50- to 100-mM changes of $[K]_t$ and $[Na]_t$ at the injury site, it actually represents a substantial increase of tissue Ca. Normally, $[Ca^{+2}]_e$ activity is about 1.2 mM. If the extracellular volume fraction is 20%, the amount of free Ca ions available in the extracellular to enter cells is ~0.24 μmol/gm wet tissue. A 1-μmol/gm increase of $[Ca]_t$ represents more than four times the amount of Ca ions present in the extracellular space before injury.[272] By 24 hours after injury, $[Ca]_t$ may be more than eight times normal.[145,146] Thus, a large amount of Ca enters and precipitates in injuried tissues.

Normally, neurons regulate intracellular Ca activity by binding Ca ions with mitochondria[57,58,62–63,69] or cytoplasmic substances[15–20,56] or by transmembrane transport.[152] We recently conducted a survey of biological substances present in sufficient quantity and with enough affinity for Ca to precipitate large amounts of Ca.[267] Only one class of substances qualified: phosphates. Several species of inorganic phosphate in tissues avidly bind Ca ions[12,191] and form insoluble Ca phosphate complexes.[59,162,233] Interestingly, the mammalian spinal cord (especially the human) has extraordinarily high levels of phosphates (exceeding 170 mM), higher than any other tissue and surpassed only by egg yolk, viruses, and bacterial particles.[3,267] Furthermore, Ca entry into cells powerfully activates phospholipases and phosphatases[113] that lead to the release of as much as 80% of tissue phosphates for binding Ca ions.

The Role of Ca in Spinal Cord Injury

Excessive entry of Ca ions has long been believed to be deleterious to cells. Driven by the steepest ionic gradient known in biology,[15,20,89,90] Ca ions disrupt the multitude of cellular processes that utilize Ca as a messenger. These include intracellular transport,[207] secretion,[186] metabolism,[71] and control of membrane ionic permeability.[173,192,197] In addition, Ca ions bind to mitochondria,[16–20,56–

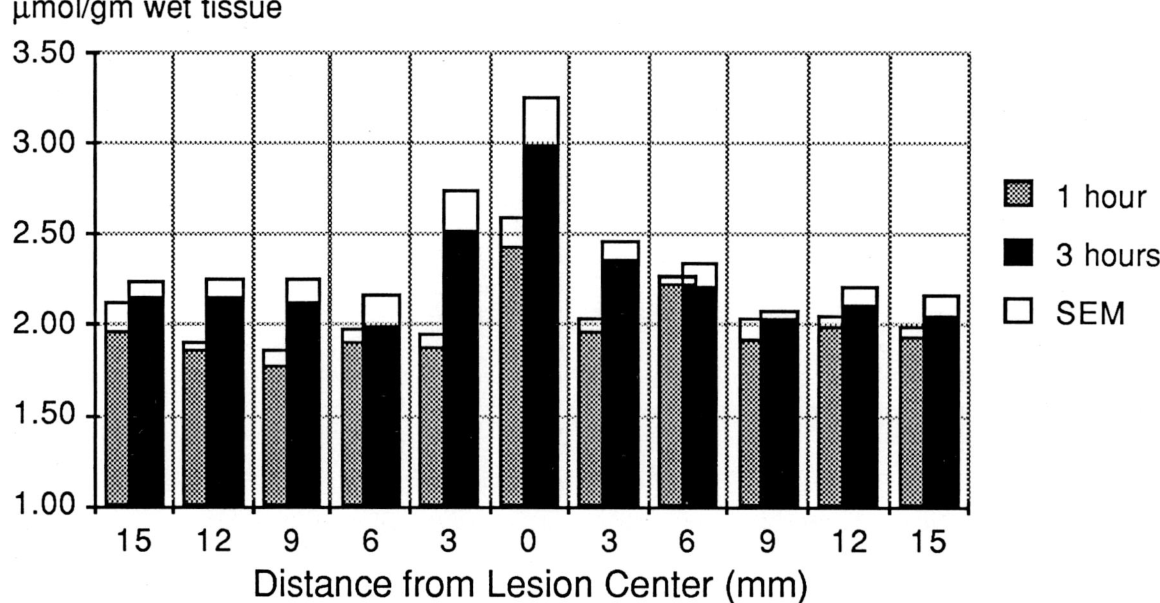

Fig. 7-7. Tissue Ca concentration ($[Ca]_w$) at and around the impact site. The mean values of $[Ca]_w$ at 1 hour (n = 5) and 3 hours (n = 8) in µmol/gm wet tissue weight after a 20 gm–20 cm contusion are shown as a function of distance from the lesion site.

[58,204] stopping electron transport,[69] releasing hydrogen ions,[62,63] and interrupting the generation of phosphorylated metabolic substrates.[71,172] Ca ions activate phospholipases in the cells, breaking down membrane phospholipids and releasing free fatty acids.[47,48] The latter, particularly free arachidonic acids, are enzymatically converted to eicosanoid products, such as prostaglandins. These, in combination with lipid peroxides generated by the membrane breakdown, are among the most potent vasoactive[262,263] and edema-causing agents[64–67] found in nature. Thus, there are many reasons to believe that Ca ions play a role in spinal cord injury.[272] As some have suggested, Ca ions may form a "final common pathway" for cell death.[232,242]

Much experimental evidence has been gathered to implicate a role of Ca ions in acute spinal cord injury. Ca ions enter and accumulate in injured cells at the lesion site of contused spinal cords.[145,146,278] Balentine and coworkers[23–28] have shown that application of Ca-containing solutions or Ca iontophores to the spinal cord can reproduce the pathologic changes resulting from trauma, including degradation of myelin and cytoskeletal proteins by Ca-activated proteinases.[27,28] Studies in other models of neuronal injury have shown that Ca entry into cells can release prostaglandins and toxic lipid peroxides that can initiate and aggravate cellular injury, as well as cause edema and ischemia.[64–67,79] We unfortunately do not know how to treat this situation. A steep ionic gradient drives Ca into cells and probably through a variety of membrane "holes," rather than through specific channels that can be blocked pharmacologically.

The observed profound and prolonged depression of $[Ca^{+2}]_e$ in injured spinal cords prompts an intriguing thought: The fall in $[Ca^{+2}]_e$ may reduce Ca entry into cells that survive the initial injury. In fact, cells of the spinal cord contain such excessive Ca buffering capacity that the death of 10% of the cells should release enough phosphate to bind many times all the extracellular Ca ions present in the tissue prior to injury. We recently suggested that this is the means whereby central nervous tissues protect cells against excessive Ca entry.[267] This mechanism essentially sacrifices a small proportion of severely damaged cells in order to protect the remaining cells.

The gross decline of $[Ca^{+2}]_e$ at the lesion site, however, may paradoxically contribute to the tissue injury. A large literature has accumulated on the effects of restoring extracellular Ca to isolated hearts exposed to Ca-free solutions.[14,148,282–284] During the Ca-free period, the tissue appears to be undamaged. However, upon restoring normal Ca ionic activity, the tissue dies. This phenomenon is called *Ca paradox.* We recently proposed that a similar mechanism may be present in injured brains and spinal cords.[266] In injured brains and spinal cords, regardless of injury mechanism, $[Ca^{+2}]_e$ invariably falls to very low levels. In contused spinal cords, for example, $[Ca^{+2}]_e$ falls more than a hundredfold from >1 mM to <0.01 mM within seconds and remains depressed below 0.1 mM for many hours. We proposed that secondary damage to surviving neurons occurs as $[Ca^{+2}]_e$ at the lesion site returns to normal, as it inevitably must, owing to diffusion from blood and surrounding tissues.

No amount of Ca binding at the lesion site is likely to be effective, if Ca diffusion to the lesion site from blood and surrounding tissues is not limited in some way. We therefore hypothesized that the edema and decreased blood flow at the lesion site that occurs after severe injury is a response evolved by the spinal cord to reduce extracellular Ca ionic diffusion to the lesion site.[267] One implication of the hypothesis is that rapid restoration of $[Ca^{+2}]_e$ should be deleterious to cells at the lesion site. Thus, care must be taken that treatments of spinal cord injury do not produce overly rapid restoration of blood flow and reduction of edema, causing paradoxically greater Ca entry into cells.

Lipid Peroxidation

One consequence of Ca entry into cells is the disruption of the mitochondrial electron transport mechanisms.[242] The interrupted transport chains, instead of passing electron ultimately to ATP and other phosporylated high energy compounds, will release free radical intermediates into cytosol. These free radicals attack surrounding membranes. Aided by Ca-activated phospholipases and metabolic acidosis,[241] free radicals break down membranes, producing more free radicals, prostaglandins, and lipid peroxides. After spinal cord injury, for example, as much as 50% of tissue phospholipids may be broken down within a few hours.[78] Several vasoactive prostaglandins and lipid peroxides have been measured recently and found to be elevated in injured spinal cords.[78,155,159] There is also evidence of free radical reactions in injured spinal cords.[79–82,116,117,200]

Lipid peroxidation occurs in dead and dying cells. Therefore, it is difficult to know whether free radical mechanisms and lipid peroxidation are causes or simply manifestations of cell death. Several characteristics of the lipid peroxidative reactions, however, strongly argue that lipid peroxidation in injured tissues is not simply a byproduct of cell death. First, lipid peroxidation is a complex phenomenon, mediated by a series of enzymes that are universally present in all neural tissues. Second, most of the enzymes participating in lipid peroxidation are activated by Ca. Many of these enzymes are activated by intracellular Ca activities of >1 μM whereas most of the enzymes mediating normal cellular functions such as transport and neurotransmitter release are activated at levels of <1 μM. Third, cells possess specific receptors for major products of lipid peroxidation. One major family of lipid peroxidation reaction products, the eicosanoids, possess some of the most vasoactive and edema producing agents known in biology. Lipid peroxidation therefore appears to be a highly evolved reaction of tissues to injury.

What adaptive advantage may be served by lipid peroxidation reactions? First, lipid peroxidation will rapidly clear out lingering dying cells that would otherwise consume valuable metabolites and oxygen better reserved for less injured cells. The use of Ca ions to trigger this reaction is particularly elegant. Given the powerful Ca buffering capacity of neuronal cytoplasm, prolonged increases of $[Ca^{+2}]_i$ above 1 μm represent a reliable indicator of irreversible cell damage. The reaction, once started, will allow more Ca into cells and rapidly stop any residual metabolic reaction within the cells. Second, as pointed out above, lipid peroxidation releases phosphates to bind Ca, lowering $[Ca^{+2}]_e$ and thereby reducing Ca entry into surviving cells. Third, the products of lipid peroxidation may serve specific purposes. As pointed out above, to prevent Ca paradox phenomena in the tissue, ionic diffusion to the lesion site must be slowed down. Lipid peroxidation generates powerful vasoconstrictatory substances. In addition, these substances mediate thrombosis of blood cells and increase cellular swelling. The combination of these actions will effectively reduce blood flow, hemorrhage, and ionic diffusion to the lesion site.

One reason for the current intense interest in lipid peroxidation mechanisms is the availability of several powerful pharmacologic approaches for reducing lipid peroxidation in tissues. For example, superoxide dysmutase (SOD) catalyzes the reaction of superoxide free radicals to hydrogen peroxide and catalase. These convert hydrogen peroxide to oxygen and water. Free-radical scavengers also may ameliorate free-radical processes. In particular, methylprednisolone[80] and vitamin E[9] are scavengers of free radicals and have beneficial effects in acute spinal cord injury. Cyclooxygenase and lipooxygenase enzymes that catalyze the production of prostaglandins can be blocked by specific pharmacologic agents.[138,139] Likewise, receptors to eicosanoid products can be blocked. Finally, methylprednisolone has been shown to be remarkably effective in suppressing lipid peroxidation.[47–55,135–138]

If lipid peroxidation reactions indeed are natural biological protective mechanisms, complete suppression of the reactions in injured tissues may not be desirable. Perhaps for this reason, certain drugs with powerful effects on lipid peroxidation reactions appear to produce beneficial effects with very narrow dose-response ranges. In order to inhibit lipid peroxidation, for example, methylprednisolone has to be given in doses of 15 to 30 mg/kg. Interestingly, at doses of 60 mg/kg, methylprednisolone can produce deleterious effects and greater tissue damage. The effective dose range many also vary depending on the severity of injury. This factor may account for the inconsistent results in clinical trials and laboratory studies of drugs that decrease lipid peroxidation.

RECOVERY OF FUNCTION

Ultimately, the measure of success in treatments of acute spinal cord injury must be recovery of function. Successful treatment of acute spinal cord injury requires an understanding of how and why functional recovery occurs. Functional deficits in spinal cord injury are usually attributed to loss of axons, and recovery of function to survival of axons in the spinal cord. Recent studies suggest that the situation is more complicated. These findings suggest new avenues of therapeutic approaches to spinal cord injury.

Complete Versus Incomplete Spinal Cord Injury

For centuries, clinicians have recognized the exceedingly poor prognosis of patients who suffer spinal cord injury of sufficient intensity to abolish neurological function below the lesion level. Many clinicians still equate these "complete" spinal cord injury with transections of the spinal cord, although physical severance of the spinal cord is exceedingly rare.[260] Studies by Dimitrijevic and colleagues[85–88] have shown that many patients with so-called complete spinal cord injuries have neurophysiologic evidence of preserved function below the lesion level, albeit subclinical evidence. Patients with even slight preservation of sensory or motor function below the lesion level often can recover substantial function. These patients are called "incomplete."

Why do spinal cord injuries segregate into complete and incomplete lesions? Several answers to this question should be considered. First, the physical trauma to the spinal cord may be all or none. Mechanical forces sufficient to penetrate the bony protection afforded by the vertebral column may be enough to produce major disruptions of the spinal cord. Second, extremely severe injuries may cause secondary injury to the lower spinal cord, preventing recovery. Third, a minimum number and type of axons may be required for clinically detectable function. Below this threshold, the patients may not be able to initiate movement. Fourth, the neurologic deficits of patients with spinal cord injury may be more graded than they appear.

Some truth probably attends all the answers proposed above. In the case of the first answer, trauma capable of breaking bone is likely to wreak severe mechanical disruption to the spinal cord. The dichotomy between complete and incomplete injuries is less applicable to chronic compression of the spinal cord by a slowly protruding disc or slow-growing tumor. The second answer raises an issue seldom considered in spinal cord injury. The lower lumbrosacral spinal cord may be subject to occult damage that is masked by injury to the thoracic or cervical spinal cord.[87] Indeed, enough exceptions to the rule of complete spinal cord injury have arisen that we now define complete spinal cord with the stipulation that all functional activity must be absent below the lesion for 48 hours, including segmental reflex activity. The third answer reminds us that a majority of the spinal pathways mediate inhibition and that motor function is composed of excitatory initiation and inhibitory modulation.[126,127,255] If the axons that produce motor initiation are lost, voluntary activity can no longer occur, even if the patients retain inhibitory modulatory control of movements initiated segmentally.[85,87,178–180] In contrast, if a small subpopulation of initiatory axons survive and most of the inhibitory pathways are lost, patients may be able to initiate movement but cannot control the movements well.[86,126,127,255] Since clinical examinations place much greater emphasis on motor initiation and strength, as opposed to coordination and control, voluntary motor function is likely to present as an all-or-none phenomenon.

Clinicians who take care of acute spinal cord injury seldom follow large populations of patients for long periods of time after injury. In contrast, clinicians who specialize in chronic spinal cord injury may not see patients in the initial acute phases. As a result, many so-called complete patients who recover significant function slowly over a period of many months and even years may be missed by the acute care specialist. Likewise, severely injured but incomplete patients who may seem to recover well within the first 6 weeks after injury are seen by the rehabilitation specialist as having a less steep improvement curve. For example, in the recently published follow-up results of the National Acute Spinal Cord Injury Study, significant improvement was observed in patients between 6 months and 1 year after injury.[46] Finally, the acute-care specialist, who relies on classic neurologic findings and grades motor function on the basis of strength and voluntary initiation, will see a very different picture compared with the rehabilitation specialist, who is much more concerned with actual functional capabilities such as locomotory coordination. This situation is resolvable with better and closer coordination of acute and chronic care of spine-injured patients.

Axon Number and Function

Animal studies have provided some insights into the determinants of recovery in spinal cord injury. In the 1950s, Windle and coworkers[260,261] reported that as much as 90% of the spinal tracts of cats can be sectioned without loss of locomotion. Eidelberg and associates showed that ferrets,[95] cats,[94,96,97,99,100] and monkeys[98] with 90% of their spinal cords sectioned often retained locomotory ability, as long as portions of the ventral column were preserved.[97] More recently, Blight and coworkers[37,40] systematically counted the axons of cats with severe spinal cord contusions, comparing those what walked with those that were paralyzed. They found that some cats could walk with as little as 10% of their original axon populations countable on light microscopy. There was a cutoff point (~5%) for axon counts below which no animal recovered. More important, they observed a substantial overlap in axon counts between some animals that could walk and others that remained paralyzed after severe spinal contusions. Upon further study,[36–38] Blight found that demyelination can account in part for the inability of some cats to recover, even though they had more axons than recovered cats. He concluded that axons can survive in paralyzing contusions of the spinal cord and that those axons have abnormal conduction properties that contribute to the overall functional deficits of spine-injured animals.

These findings indicate that mammalian spinal cords possess a remarkable capability of adapting to devastating axonal loss and, given time, many animals can learn to function on a small proportion of their original axons. Extrapolated to humans, these findings suggest that many patients who eventually recover function from apparently severe but incomplete spinal cord injuries may actually be functioning on relatively few axons. The presence of a threshold of axons required for recovery of function explains the clinical difference between complete and incomplete spinal cord injury. More important, the observations that demyelination may be an important factor in spinal cord injury opens up new possibilities of treating dysfunctions of axons in spinal cord injury.

Demyelination in the spinal cord is potentially treatable. First, unlike more general demyelinative disorders such as multiple sclerosis, in which the areas of demyelination are often scattered and can recur, demyelination in spinal cord injury is limited to a single region. It is thus more amenable to treatments such as transplantation of oligodendroglial or Schwann cells to the injury site. Second, local application of pharmacologic agents that improve conduction in demyelinated axons may work better for spinal cord injury than for general demyelinative disorders. Finally, many of the axons in spine-injured animals are severely demyelinated and have abnormal nodal structures, suggesting that improvement of the conduction in even a small proportion of these axons may result in significant functional recovery.

For many years, much of the pessimism surrounding spinal cord injury recovery stemmed from the belief that mammalian spinal cords do not regenerate effectively.[225] Some recent studies suggest that the mammalian spinal cord may be capable of limited regeneration[42,43] comparable to the degree of regeneration and axonal plasticity reported in lower vertebrates[44] and peripheral nerve bridges.[76] The finding that as little as 2% to 5% of the original axons in the spinal cord can support functional recovery provides hope that a limited amount of regeneration may be able to restore some function. In the coming years, methods will undoubtedly be developed to harness and direct the axonal growth that occurs in injured spinal cords.

Potential for Recovery from Spinal Cord Injury

The spinal cord can compensate for lost systems through a variety of mechanisms. Pyramidal tract ablations, for example, initially raise the threshold of tendon reflexes.[126,127,255,185] However, the reflexes will subsequently recover, probably as a result of collateral sprouting of dorsal root inputs in the spinal cord.[124,202] Although such sprouting does not strictly replace the descending influences, it appears to be able to compensate for the loss and thereby to produce apparent functional recovery. Conversely, deafferentation of a particular spinal segment abolishes the limb reflexes supplied by the particular segment. Responses to descending influences initially are depressed and then become grossly exaggerated.[164,193] Eventually, centrally patterned movements return partially, without the benefit of afferent inputs and probably as a result of increased excitation by corollary diffuse descending pathways in the spinal cord.[126,127]

Spinal cord pathways can be roughly categorized into two types: specific and diffuse. These two types of spinal influences may vicariously compensate for each other in injury. Destruction of the diffuse nontopographical projections to the spinal cord generally provokes generalized deficits from which the animal often recovers eventually but slowly as the remaining diffuse and specific projections take over.[126,127,185] Lesions of specific projections can be masked due to substitution by remaining specific projections and generalized projections increasing excitability of the target cells. In such cases, activity in remaining conducting axons provokes greater responses than normal.

Systems remaining after lesions may adversely affect recovery of function.[178] For example, bilateral deafferentation may paradoxically produce fewer motor deficits than unilateral lesions in monkeys.[164] Likewise, animals with bilateral pyramidotomies may show impressive functional recovery. The creation of a second lesion in the opposite hemisphere after an initial unilateral lesion of the motor cortex may also improve function.[126,127] Finally, Robinson and Goldberger[229] recently reported that interference with inhibition during the recovery may improve motor function after spinal cord injury. Many theories have been proposed to explain this phenomenon. These include the possibility that residual inhibitory systems may retard or prevent the recovery of some movements, that bilateral lesions may "force" alternative recovery strategies that would not otherwise come into play,[255] and that collateral sprouting may be enhanced not only in the spinal cord but in more proximal structures after more extensive lesions.

Clinical assessments of functional recovery in spinal cord injury often neglect basic neurophysiologic principles. For example, the majority of the synaptic connections of the corticospinal, rubrospinal, and vestibulospinal tracts act on inhibitory interneurons rather than motoneurons in the spinal cord.[126,127] Unfortunately, inhibition is not usually assessed in clinical examinations of patients. As Dimitrijevic and colleagues[85] found, patients may be unable to activate motor responses voluntarily but still may be able to suppress segmentally activated reflexes. Although inhibition may seem irrelevant if it does not contribute to voluntary motor recovery, we must remember that motor function is probably 90% inhibitory modulation and 10% excitatory initiation. The finding that a patient cannot voluntarily initiate movement should not predispose us to dismiss the case as hopeless. On the contrary, a patient who has lost the ability to initiate movement but can still inhibit responses in the spinal cord may be more easily helped than a patient who can excite but not inhibit motor activity. Provision of excitatory stimuli to the spinal cord is much easier than inhibitory modulation.

Plasticity of the Spinal Cord

Kirk and Denny-Brown[163] demonstrated a curious phenomenon of dermatome expansion in monkeys. They unilaterally cut three nerve roots above and three roots below a given thoracic root and then assessed the size of the dermatome supplied by the isolated nerve root over time. Over several weeks, the dermatome of the isolated root expanded to occupy dermatomes vacated by the cut roots. They also showed that the new dermatome borders were dynamic and rapidly shrank or expanded with additional sections or stimulation of roots on the contralateral side. This data clearly showed that determinants of sensory dermatome boundaries are complex and can be partially related to physiologic changes such as disinhibition.

Liu and Chambers[184] found with a similar isolated root preparation that changes in the anatomic substrate of the spinal cord may be in part responsible for such alterations of dermatomes. They demonstrated that axons entering through the isolated root will sprout. Goldberger and colleagues[124,125,128,129] expanded on early work of Liu and Chambers, showing that axons in the isolated root will proliferate as far as one to two segments above and below their normal distribution. As in the brain, where central axons have been shown to engage in proliferative innervation of denervated regions outside of their normal boundaries,[74,77,121,223,224] growth occurs in the spinal cord. Increasing evidence suggests that such growth influences and perhaps mediates spasticity[193] and motor recovery.[124,125,128,129,202]

Clinically, patients with severe spinal cord injury

almost invariably show some recovery of sensory and motor function one to two segments below the lesion level observed on admission. For example, >90% of patients seen at NYU showed >1-segment descent of the sensory level at 6-month follow-up. In fact, approximately 30% of the patients in our series showed >2-segment descent of the sensory levels. In patients with cervical spinal cord injuries, the recovery of one to two segments often represents a significant difference in the functional capabilities of the patient. Although the phenomenon is commonly attributed to "nerve root recovery," its uncanny resemblance to the findings in animal studies suggest strongly that the segmental recovery may be related to disinhibition and axonal sprouting.

Clinicians caring for acute spinal injured patients should be cognizant of these possibilities so that they do not unnecessarily preclude the future recovery of patients because of insufficiently aggressive action to preserve as much of the spinal cord as possible, even in patients with apparently complete spinal cord lesions. Many clinicians tend to be less aggressive with so-called complete spine-injured patients than with those who have some residual function. This attitude is paradoxical because patients with complete lesions have much less to lose and much more to gain then patients with incomplete lesions.

Therapeutic Approaches of the Future

The emphasis in experimental spinal cord injury research has expanded dramatically in the past 5 years beyond the traditional twin goddesses of prevention (of acute injury) and regeneration (of long spinal tracts) to more sophisticated manipulations of the physiology and recovery processes of the injured spinal cords. Two developments in particular will have a major impact on the way that spine-injured patients are viewed and treated in the coming years. First, electrical stimulation of both peripheral and central nervous systems has become feasible as a clinical treatment of spinal cord injury. Not only may it be useful to activate muscles to maintain their strength and reduce atrophy, it may be possible to use electrical stimulation to supply specific excitatory or inhibitory influences to the spinal cord to modulate spasticity and to restore function. Second, specific pharmacologic intervention and even transplantation of neurons and adrenal cells may supply neurotransmitters to spinal neuronal circuits to optimize the function of residual pathways.

Spasticity has long been regarded by clinicians as a disinhibitory phenomenon. The studies of Dimitrijevic,[85–88] however, provide a new perspective on this pathologic phenomenon, suggesting that spasticity may be a manifestation of residual pathways in the spinal cord, because patients and animals with very severe injuries to the spinal cord have less spasticity than those with less severe injuries. Most clinicians regard spasticity as an undesirable manifestation of spinal cord injury that should be suppressed by pharmacologic agents that inhibit interneural activity. These drugs have undesirable side effects and are often ineffective. A neglected possibility suggested by animal studies is early selective deafferentation to enhance or suppress the plastic response of the spinal cord to the injury. For example, selective rhizotomies performed during the acute phase may effectively alter the characteristics of spasticity that may develop later. Such therapeutic approaches, however, require greater understanding of the recovery processes in the injured spinal cord than we currently possess. Clearly, much work needs to be done.

Recent developments in neural transplantation techniques[32,34,75,209,210] for treating Parkinson's disease have suggested the exciting possibility of placing cells containing specific neurotransmitters into the spinal cord to enhance the function of surviving pathways in injured spinal cords. Unlike electrical stimulation and pharmacologic treatments, cell transplants provide the unique promise of a continuing supply of neurotransmitters. Whether the supply of these neurotransmitters is by synaptic connections, possible through implantation of fetal cells, or by release and diffusion of secreted neurotransmitters (such as adrenal medullary cells), the potential of such a therapeutic approach will undoubtedly have an impact on spinal cord injury care of the future.

REFERENCES

1. *Allen AR:* Remarks on histopathological changes in spinal cord due to impact: an experimental study. J Nerv Ment Dis 41:141–147, 1914
2. *Allen AR:* Surgery of experimental lesion of spinal cord equivalent to crush injury of fracture dislocation. J Am Med Assoc 50:941–952, 1911
3. *Altman PL, Dittmer DS:* Biology Data Book, 2nd ed, Vol II, pp 1206–1229. Washington DC, Federation of American Society for Experimental Biology, 1973
4. *Anderson DK, Means ED:* Iron-induced lipid peroxidation in spinal cord: Protection with mannitol and methylprednisolone. J Free Rad Biol Med 1:59–64, 1985
5. *Anderson DK, Means ED, Waters TR, Green*

BS: Microvascular perfusion and metabolism in injured spinal cord after methylprednisolone treatment. J Neurosurg 56:106–113, 1982

6. *ANDERSON DK, MEANS ED, WATERS TR, GREEN ES:* Spinal cord energy metabolism following compression trauma to the feline spinal cord. J Neurosurg 53:375–80, 1980
7. *ANDERSON DK, NICOLOSI GR, MEANS ED, HARTLEY LE:* Effects of laminectomy on spinal cord blood flow. J Neurosurg 48:232, 1978
8. *ANDERSON DK, PROCKOP LD, MEANS ED, HARTLEY LE:* Cerebrospinal fluid lactate and electrolyte levels following experimental spinal cord injury. J Neurosurg 44:715–722, 1976
9. *ANDERSON DK, SAUNDERS RD, DEMEDIUK P, DUGAN LL, BRAUGHLER JM, HALL ED, MEANS ED, HORROCKS LA:* Lipid hydrolysis and peroxidation in injured spinal cord: Partial protection with methylprednisolone or vitamin E and selenium. CNS Trauma 2:257–267, 1985
10. *ANDREE RA:* Sudden death following naloxone administration. Anesth Analg 59:782–784, 1980
11. *ASTRUP J, REHNCRONA S, SIESJO BK:* The increase in extracellular potassium concentration in the ischemic brain in relation to the preischemic functional activity and cerebral metabolic rate. Brain Res 199:161–174, 1980
12. *AYLWARD GH, FINDLAY TJV:* Chemical Data Book, 2nd ed, p 12. New York, John Wiley & Sons, 1966
13. *AZAR I, TURNDOFF H:* Severe hypertension and multiple atrial premature contractions following naloxone administration. Anesth Analg 59:524–525, 1979
14. *BAKER JE, BULLOCK GR, HEARSE DJ:* The temperature dependence of the calcium paradox: enzymatic, functional, and morphological correlates of cellular injury. J Mol Cell Cardiol 15:293–411, 1983
15. *BAKER PF:* The regulation of intracellular calcium in giant axons of Loligo and Myxicola. Ann N Y Acad Sci 207:250–268, 1978
16. *BAKER PF:* The regulation of intracellular calcium. Soc Exper Biol Symp 30:67–88. Cambridge, Cambridge University Press, 1976
17. *BAKER PF:* Transport and metabolism of calcium ions in nerve. Prog Biophys Molec Biol 24:177–223, 1972
18. *BAKER PF, CRAWFORD AC:* Mobility and transport of magnesium in squid giant axons. J Physiol (London) 227:855–874, 1972
19. *BAKER PF, HODGKIN AL, RIDGEWAY EB:* Depolarization and calcium entry into squid giant axons. J Physiol (London) 218:709–755, 1971
20. *BAKER PF, UMBACH JA:* Calcium buffering in axons and axoplasm of Loligo. J Physiol (London) 383:369–394, 1987
21. *BALENTINE JD:* Pathology of experimental spinal cord trauma. I. The necrotic lesion as a function of vascular injury. Lab Invest 39:236–253, 1978
22. *BALENTINE JD:* Pathology of experimental spinal cord trauma. II. Ultrastructure of axons and myelin. Lab Invest 39:254–255, 1978
23. *BALENTINE JD, DEAN D:* Calcium-induced spongiform and necrotizing myelopathy. Lab Invest 47:286–295, 1982
24. *BALENTINE JD, GREEN W:* Ultrastructural pathology of axons and myelin in calcium induced myelopathy. J Neuropathol Exp Neurol 43:500–510, 1984
25. *BALENTINE JD, HOGAN EL, BANIK NL, PEROT PL:* Calcium and the pathogenesis of spinal cord injury. In Dacey RG Jr, Winn HR, Rimmel RW, Jane JA (eds): Trauma of the Central Nervous System, pp 285–295. New York, Raven Press, 1985
26. *BALENTINE JD, SPECTOR M:* Calcification of axons in experimental spinal cord trauma. Ann Neurol 2:520–523, 1977
27. *BANIK NL, HOGAN EL, POWERS JM, WHETSTINE LJ:* Degradation of cytoskeletal proteins in experimental spinal injury. Neurochem Res 7:1465–1475, 1982
28. *BANIK NL, HOGAN EL, WHETSTINE LJ, BALENTINE JD:* Changes in myelin and axonal proteins in $CaCl_2$-induced myelopathy in rat spinal cord. CNS Trauma 1:131–138, 1984
29. *BARANY M, GLONEK T:* Identification of disease states by phosphorus-31 NMR. In Gorenstein DG (ed): Phosphorus-31 NMR. Principles and Applications, pp 512–545. New York, Academic Press, 1984
30. *BENES V:* Spinal Cord Injury. Baltimore, Williams & Wilkins, 1968
31. *BERENSTEIN A, YOUNG W, RANSOHOFF J, BENJAMIN V, MERKIN H:* Somatosensory evoked potentials (SEP) during spinal angiography and therapeutic transvascular embolization. J Neurosurg 60:777–785, 1984
32. *BERNSTEIN JJ, UNDERBERGER D, HOOVLER DW:* Fetal CNS transplants into adult spinal cord: techniques, initial effects, and caveats. CNS Trauma 1:39–46, 1984
33. *BINGHAM WG, SIRINEK L, CRUTCHER L, MOHNACKY C:* Effect of spinal cord injury on cord and cerebral blood flow in monkey. Acta Neurol Scand (Suppl 64) 56:132, 1977
34. *BJÖRKLUND A, STENEVI U:* Reconstruction of the nigrostriatal dopamine pathway by intracerebral nigral transplants. Brain Res 17:555–564, 1981
35. *BLACK P, MARKOWITZ RS:* Experimental spinal cord injury in monkeys: comparison of steroids and local hypothermia. Surg Forum 22:409–411, 1971
36. *BLIGHT AR:* Axonal physiology of chronic spinal

cord injury in the cat: intracellular recording in vitro. Neuroscience 10:1471–1486, 1983

37. *Blight AR:* Cellular morphology of chronic spinal cord injury in the cat: Analysis of myelinated axons by line sampling. Neuroscience 10:521–543, 1983
38. *Blight AR:* Delayed demyelination and macrophage invasion: a candidate for "secondary" cell damage in spinal cord injury. CNS Trauma 2:299–315, 1985
39. *Blight AR:* Motor evoked potentials in CNS trauma. CNS Trauma 3:207–214, 1986
40. *Blight AR, DeCrescito V:* Morphometric analysis of experimental spinal cord injury in the cat: the relation of injury intensity to survival of myelinated axons. Neuroscience 19:321–341, 1986
41. *Block BB, Ginocchio AV:* Local and systemic subarachnoid toxicity of metrizamide in mice and monkeys. Acta Radiol (Suppl) 335:14, 1973
42. *Borgens RB, Blight AR, Murphy DJ:* Axonal regeneration in spinal cord injury: a perceptive and new technique. J Comp Neurol 250:157–167, 1986
43. *Borgens RB, Blight AR, Murphy DJ, Stewart L:* Transected dorsal column axons within the guinea pig spinal cord regenerate in the presence of an applied electric field. J Comp Neurol 250:168–180, 1986
44. *Borgens RB, Roederer E, Cohen MJ:* Enhanced spinal cord regeneration in lamprey by applied electrical fields. Science 213:611–617, 1981
45. *Bracken MB, Collins WF, Freeman DF, et al:* Efficacy of methylprednisolone in acute spinal cord injury. J Am Med Assoc 251:45–52, 1984
46. *Bracken MB, Shepard MJ, Hellenbrand KG, et al:* Methylprednisolone and neurological function 1 year after spinal cord injury. J Neurosurg 63:704–713, 1985
47. *Braughler JM, Duncan LA, Chase RL:* Interaction of lipid peroxidation and calcium in the pathogenesis of neuronal injury. CNS Trauma 2:269–283, 1985
48. *Braughler JM, Duncan LA, Goodman T:* Calcium enhances in vitro free radical-induced damage to brain synaptosomes, mitochondria, and cultured spinal cord neurons. J Neurochem 45:1288–1293, 1985
49. *Braughler JM, Hall ED:* Acute enhancement of spinal cord synaptosomal (Na^+-K^+)-ATPase activity in cats following intravenous methylprednisolone. Brain Res 219:464–469, 1981
50. *Braughler JM, Hall ED:* Correlation of methylprednisolone pharmacokinetics in cat spinal cord with its effect on (Na^+-K^+)-ATPase, lipid peroxidation and motor neuron function. J Neurosurg 56:838–844, 1981
51. *Braughler JM, Hall ED:* Effects of multi-dose methylprednisolone sodium succinate administration on injured cat spinal cord neurofilament degradation and energy metabolism. J Neurosurg 61:290–295, 1985
52. *Braughler JM, Hall ED:* Pharmacokinetics of methylprednisolone in cat plasma and spinal cord following a single intravenous dose of sodium succinate ester. Drug Metab Dispos 10:551–552, 1983
53. *Braughler JM, Hall ED:* The uptake and elimination of methylprednisolone from the contused cat spinal cord following an intravenous injection of the sodium succinate ester. J Neurosurg 58:538–542, 1983
54. *Braughler JM, Hall ED:* Lactate and pyruvate metabolism in the injured cat spinal cord before and after a single large intravenous dose of methylprednisolone. J Neurosurg 59:256–261, 1983
55. *Braughler JM, Lainer MJ:* The effects of large doses of methylprednisolone on neurologic recovery and survival in the Mongolian gerbil following three hours of unilateral carotid occlusion. CNS Trauma 3:153–161, 1986
56. *Brinley FJ:* Calcium buffering in squid axons. Ann Rev Biophys Bioengin 7:363–392, 1978
57. *Brinley FJ, Tiffert T, Scarpa A:* Mitochondria and other calcium buffers of squid axon studied in situ. J Gen Physiol 72:101–127, 1978
58. *Brinley FJ, Tiffert T, Scarpa A, Mullins LJ:* Intracellular calcium buffering capacity in isolated squid axon. J Gen Physiol 70:355–384, 1977
59. *Brown WE:* Solubilities of phosphates and other sparingly soluble compounds. In Griffith EJ, Beeton A, Spencer JM, Mitchell DT (eds): Environment Phosphorus Handbook, pp 203–240. New York, John Wiley & Sons, 1972
60. *Bruce DA, Langfitt TW, Miller JD, Schultz H, Vapalahtl MP, Staner A, Goldberg HI:* Regional cerebral blood flow, intracranial pressure and brain metabolism in comatose patients. J Neurosurg 38:131–144, 1973
61. *Campbell JB, DeCrescito V, Tomasula JJ, Demopoulos HB, Flamm ES, Ortega BD:* Effect of antifibrinolytic and steroid therapy on contused cords of cats. J Neurosurg 55:726–733, 1974
62. *Carafoli E, Crompton M:* The regulation of intracellular calcium by mitochondria. Ann NY Acad Sci 307:269–284, 1978
63. *Carafoli E, Lehninger AL:* A survey of the interaction of calcium ions with mitochondria from different tissues and species. Biochem J 122:681–690, 1971
64. *Chan PH, Fishman RA:* Brain edema: Induction in cortical slices by polyunsaturated fatty acids. Science 201:358–360, 1970
65. *Chan PH, Fishman RA:* Transient formation of superoxide radicals in polyunsaturated fatty acid

induced brain swelling. J Neurochem 35:1004–1007, 1980

66. *Chan PH, Fishman RA, Lee JL:* Arachidonic acid induced swelling incubated rat brain cortical slices. Effect of bovine free serum albumin. Neurochem Res 5:629–640, 1980
67. *Chan PH, Schmidley JW, Fishman RA, Langar SM:* Brain injury edema and vascular permeability changes induced by oxygen-derived free radicals. Neurology 34:315–320, 1984
68. *Chan PH, Yurko M, Fishman RA:* Phospholipid degradation and cellular edema induced by free radicals in brain cortical slices. J Neurochem 38:525–531, 1982
69. *Chance B:* The energy-linked reaction of calcium with mitochondria. J Biol Chem 240:2729–2748, 1965
70. *Chughtai AR, Marshall R, Nancollas GH:* Complexes in calcium phosphate solutions. J Phys Chem 72:208–211, 1968
71. *Cittadini A, Boss D, Wolf F, Dani AM:* The role of intracellular Ca/Mg ratio in bioenergetic reactions. In Anghileri LJ, Tuffet-Anghileri AM (eds): The Role of Calcium in Biological Systems, pp 189–200. Boca Raton, Florida, CRC Press, 1982
72. *Clendenon NR, Allen N, Ito T, Gordon WA, Yashon D:* Response of lysosomal hydrolases of dog spinal cord and cerebrospinal fluid to experimental trauma. Neurol 28:78–84, 1978
73. *Cohen MR, Cohen RM, Pickar D, et al:* High-dose naloxone infusions in normals. Dose-dependent behavioral, hormonal, and physiological responses. Arch Gen Psychiatr 40:613–619, 1983
74. *Cotman CW, Nieto-Sampedro M, Harris EW:* Synapse replacement in the nervous system of adult vertebrates. Physiol Rev 61:684–784, 1981
75. *Das GD:* Neural transplantation in the spinal cord of the adult mammal. In: Kao C, Reier P (eds): Spinal Cord Reconstruction, pp 367–396, New York, Raven Press, 1983
76. *David S, Aguayo AJ:* Axonal elongation into peripheral nervous system "bridges" after central nervous system injury in adult rats. Science 214:931–933, 1981
77. *Davis JN:* Neuronal rearrangements after brain injury: A proposed classification. In Becker DP, Povlishock JT (eds): NIH Central Nervous System Trauma Status Report, 1986 pp 491–501. NIH, NINCDS, 1986
78. *Demediuk P, Saunders RD, Anderson DK, Means ED, Horrocks LA:* Membrane lipid changes in laminectomized and traumatized cat spinal cord. Proc Natl Acad Sci USA 82:7071–7075, 1985
79. *Demopoulos HB, Flamm ES, Pietronigro DD, Seligman MC, Tomasula J, DeCrescito V:* The free radical pathology and the microcirculation in the major central nervous system disorders. Acta Physiol Scand 492:91–119, 1980
80. *Demopoulos HB, Flamm ES, Seligman MC, Pietronigro DD, Tomasula J, DeCrescito V:* Further studies on free radical pathology in the major central nervous system disorders: Effect of very high doses of methylprednisolone on the functional outcome, morphology and chemistry of experimental spinal cord impact injury. Can J Physiol Pharmacol 60:1415–1424, 1982
81. *Demopoulos HB, Milvy P, Kakari S, Ransohoff J:* Molecular aspects of membrane structure in cerebral edema. In Reulen HJ, Schurmann K (eds): Steroids and Brain Edema, pp 29–39. Vienna, Springer-Verlag, 1972
82. *Demopoulos HB, Yoder M, Gutman E, et al:* The fine structure of endothelial surfaces in the microcirculation of experimentally injured feline spinal cords. Scan Electron Miscrosc 2:677, 1978
83. *Dienel GA:* Regional accumulation of calcium in post-ischemic rat brain. J Neurochem 43:913–925, 1984
84. *Dietrich WA, Ginsberg MD, Busto R, Watson BD, Yoshida S:* Vascular aspects and hemodynamic consequences of central nervous system injury. CNS Trauma 3:265–280, 1986
85. *Dimitrijevic MR, Dimitrijevic M, Faganel J, Sherwood AM:* Suprasegmentally induced motor unit activity in paralyzed muscles of patients with established spinal cord injury. Ann Neurol 16:216–221, 1984
86. *Dimitrijevic MR, Faganel J, Gregoric M, Nathan PW, Trontelj, JK:* Habituation: effects of regular and stochastic stimulation. J Neurol Neurosurg Psychiatr 35:234–242, 1972
87. *Dimitrijevic MR, Faganel J, Lehmkuhl D, Sherwood A:* Motor control in man after partial or complete spinal cord injury. In Desmedt JE (ed): Motor Control Mechanisms in Health and Disease, pp 915–926. New York, Raven Press, 1983
88. *Dimitrijevic MR, Spencer WA, Trontelj JV, Dimitrijevic M:* Reflex effects of vibration in patients with spinal cord lesions. Neurology 27:1078–1086, 1977
89. *DiPolo R, Requena J, Brinley FJ, Mullins LJ, Carpa A, Tiffert T:* Ionized calcium concentration in squid axons. J Gen Physiol 67:433–467, 1976
90. *DiPolo R, Rojas H, Vergara J, Lopez R, Captuo C:* Measurements of intracellular ionized calcium in squid giant axons using calcium-selective microelectrodes. Biochim Biophys Acta 728:311–318, 1983
91. *Dohrmann GJ, Panjabi MM:* 'Standardized' spinal cord trauma: biomechanial parameters and lesion volume. Surg Neurol 6:263–267, 1976

92. *Dow-Edwards D, DeCrescito V, Tomasula JJ, Flamm ES:* Effect of aminophylline and isoproterenol on spinal cord blood flow after impact injury. J Neurosurg 56:350–358, 1982
93. *Ducker TB, Hamit HF:* Experimental treatments of acute spinal cord injury. J Neurosurg 30:693–697, 1969
94. *Eidelberg E, Nguyen L, Deza L:* Recovery of locomotor function after hemisection of the spinal cord in cats. Brain Res Bull 16:507–515, 1986
95. *Eidelberg E, Staten E, Watkins LJ, Smith JS:* Treatment of experimental spinal cord injury in ferrets. Surg Neurol 6:243–246, 1976
96. *Eidelberg E, Story JL, Walden JG, Meyer BL:* Anatomical correlates of return of locomotor function after partial spinal cord lesions in cats. Exp Brain Res 42:81–88, 1981
97. *Eidelberg E, Straehley D, Erspamer R:* Relationship between residual hindlimb assisted locomotion and surviving axons after incomplete spinal cord injuries. Exp Neurol 56:312–322, 1977
98. *Eidelberg E, Walden J, Nguyen L:* Locomotor control in macaque monkeys. Brain 104:647–663, 1981
99. *Eidelberg E, Yu J:* Effects of corticospinal lesions upon treadmill locomotion in cats. Exp Brain Res 43:101–103, 1981
100. *Eidelberg E, Yu J:* Effects of vestibulospinal lesions upon locomotor function in cats. Brain Res 22:179–183, 1981
101. *Engler GH, Spielholz N, Bernhard W, et al:* Somatosensory evoked potentials during Harrington instrumentation for scoliosis. J Bone Joint Surg 60A:528, 1978
102. *Erickson DL, Leider LL, Brown WE:* One stage decompression stabilization for thoracolumbar fractures. Spine 2:53, 1977
103. *Faden AI:* Opiate antagonists and thyrotropin-releasing hormone. II. Potential role in the treatment of central nervous system injury. J Am Med Assoc 252:1452–1454, 1984
104. *Faden AI:* Pharmacologic therapy in acute spinal cord injury: experimental strategies and future directions. In Becker DP, Povlishock JT (eds): Central Nervous System Trauma Status Report, NINCDS/NIH, pp 481–485. Bethesda, Maryland, NIH, NINCDS, 1986
105. *Faden AI, Holaday JW:* Opiate antagonists: a role in treatment of hypovolemic shock. Science 205:317–318, 1979
106. *Faden AI, Jacobs TP, Holaday JW:* Comparison of early and late naloxone treatment in experimental spinal injury. Neurology 32:677–681, 1982
107. *Faden AI, Jacobs TP, Holaday JW:* Opiate receptor antagonist improves neurologic recovery after spinal injury. Science 211:493–494, 1981
108. *Faden AI, Jacobs TP, Holaday JW:* Thyrotropin-releasing hormone improves neurologic recovery after spinal trauma in cats. N Engl J Med 305:1063–1067, 1981
109. *Faden AI, Jacobs TP, Mougey E, Holaday JW:* Endorphins in experimental spinal injury: therapeutic effect of naloxone. Ann Neurol 10:326–332, 1981
110. *Faden AI, Jacobs TP, Patrick DH, Smith MT:* Megadose corticosteroid therapy following experimental traumatic spinal injury. J Neurosurg 60:712–717, 1984
111. *Faden AI, Jacobs TP, Smith MT:* Thyrotropin-releasing hormone in experimental spinal injury: Dose response and late treatment. Neurology 34:1280–1284, 1984
112. *Faden AI, Jacobs TP, Smith MT, et al:* Comparison of thyrotropin-releasing hormone (TRH), naloxone, and dexamethasone treatments in experimental spinal injury. Neurology 33:673–678, 1983
113. *Feder J:* The phosphatases. In Griffith EJ, Beeton A, Spencer JM, Mitchell DT (eds): Environment Phosphorus Handbook, pp 475–508. New York, John Wiley & Son, 1972
114. *Fishman J, Hahn EF, Norton BI:* Comparative in vivo distribution of opiate agonists and antagonists by means of double isotope techniques. Life Sci 17:1119–1126, 1975
115. *Flacke JW, Flacke WE, Williams GD:* Acute pulmonary edema following naloxone reversal of high-dose morphine anesthesia. Anesthesiology 47:376–378, 1977
116. *Flamm ES, Demopoulos HB, Seligman ML, et al:* Free radicals in cerebral ischemia. Stroke 9:445, 1978
117. *Flamm ES, Demopoulos HB, Seligman ML, et al:* Ethanol potentiation of central nervous system trauma. J Neurosurg 46:328, 1977
118. *Flamm ES, Viau AT, Ransohoff J, et al:* Experimental alterations in cyclic adenosine monophosphate concentration in the cat basilar artery. Neurology 26:664, 1976
119. *Flamm ES, Young W, Collins WF, Piepmeier J, Clifton GL, Fischer B:* A Phase I trial of naloxone treatment in acute spinal cord injury. J Neurosurg 63:390–397, 1985
120. *Flamm ES, Young W, Demopoulos HB, DeCrescito V, Tomasula JJ:* Experimental spinal cord injury: Treatment with naloxone. Neurosurgery 10:227–231, 1982
121. *Forester AP:* Spontaneous regeneration of cut axons in adult rat brain. J Comp Neurol 210:335–356, 1982
122. *Forsythe HF, Alexander E Jr, Davie C Jr, Un-*

DERAL R: The advantages of early spinal fusion in the treatment of fracture dislocation of the cervical spine. J Bone Joint Surg 41A:17, 1969

123. *FRANKEL HL, HANCOCK DO, HYSLOP G, ET AL:* The value of postural reduction in the initial management of closed injuries of the spine with paraplegia and tetraplegia. Paraplegia 7:179, 1969

124. *GOLDBERGER ME:* Different patterns of recovery of motor function associated with different patterns of post lesion axonal growth. In Seil F (ed): Nerve, Organ and Tissue Regeneration: Research Perspectives, pp 124–138. New York, Academic Press, 1983

125. *GOLDBERGER ME:* Restitution of function and collateral sprouting in the cat spinal cord: The deafferented animal. Anat Rec 175:329, 1973

126. *GOLDBERGER ME:* The extrapyramidal systems of the spinal cord: II. Results of combined pyramidal and extrapyramidal lesions in the macaque. J Comp Neurol 135:1–12, 1972

127. *GOLDBERGER ME:* The extrapyramidal systems of the spinal cord: results of combined spinal and cortical lesions in the macaque. J Comp Neurol 124:161–174, 1965

128. *GOLDBERGER ME, MURRAY M:* Recovery of movement and axonal sprouting may obey some of the same laws. In Cotman CW (ed): Neuronal Plasticity, pp 73–96. New York, Academic Press, 1978

129. *GOLDBERGER ME, MURRAY M:* Restitution of function and collateral sprouting in the cat spinal cord: the deafferented animal. J Comp Neurol 158:37–54, 1981

130. *GOODKIN R, CAMPBELL JB:* Sequential pathological changes in spinal cord injury. Surg Forum 20:430–432, 1969

131. *GOTOH O, ASANO T, KOIDE T, TAKAKURA K:* Ischemic brain edema following occlusion of the middle cerebral artery in the rat. I. The time courses of brain water, sodium, and potassium contents and blood brain barrier permeability to ^{125}I-albumin. Stroke 16:101–109, 1985

132. *GRANDISON L, BUCHWEITZ E, WEISS HR:* Effect of naltrexone on regional brain oxygen consumption in the cat. Brain Res 233:367–379, 1982

133. *GREEN BA, KAHN T, KLOSE KJ:* A comparative study of steroid therapy in acute experimental spinal cord injury. Surg Neurol 13:91–97, 1980

134. *GUTTMANN L:* Spinal Cord Injuries. Oxford, Blackwell Scientific Publications, 1976

135. *HALL ED, BRAUGHLER JM:* Acute effects of intravenous glucocorticoid pre-treatment on the in vitro peroxidation of cat spinal cord tissue. Exper Neurol 72:321–324, 1981

136. *HALL ED, BRAUGHLER JM:* Effects of methylprednisolone on spinal cord lipid peroxidation and $(Na^+$-$K^+)$-ATPase activity: dose response analysis during the first hour after contusion injury in the cat. J Neurosurg 57:247–253, 1982

137. *HALL ED, BRAUGHLER JM:* Glucocorticoid mechanisms in acute spinal injury: A review and therapeutic rationale. Surg Neurol 18:320–327, 1982

138. *HALL ED, BRAUGHLER JM:* Role of lipid peroxidation in post-traumatic spinal cord degeneration—a review. CNS Trauma 3:281–294, 1986

139. *HALL ED, WOLF DL:* A pharmacological analysis of pathophysiological mechanisms of posttraumatic spinal cord ischemia. J Neurosurg 64:951–961, 1986

140. *HALL ED, WOLF DL, BRAUGHLER JM:* Effects of a single large dose of methylprednisolone sodium succinate on experimental posttraumatic spinal cord ischemia. J Neurosurg 61:124–130, 1984

141. *HANSEBOUT RR:* A comprehensive review of methods of improving cord recovery after acute spinal cord injury. In Tator CH (ed): Early Management of Acute Cervical Spinal Cord Injury pp 181–186. New York, Raven Press, 1982

142. *HANSEN AJ:* The extracellular potassium concentration in juvenile and adult rat brain cortex during anoxia. Acta Physiol Scand 99:412–420, 1978

143. *HANSEN AJ, GJEDDE A, SIEMKOWICZ E:* Extracellular potassium and blood flow in the post-ischemic rat brain. Pfluegers Arch 389:1–7, 1980

144. *HANSEN AJ, OLSEN CE:* Brain extracellular space during spreading depression and ischemia. Acta Physiol Scand 108:355–365, 1980

145. *HAPPEL RD, BANIK NL, BALENTINE JD, HOGAN EL:* Tissue calcium levels in $CaCl_2$-induced myelopathy. Neurosci Lett 49:279–283, 1984

146. *HAPPEL RD, SMITH K, POWERS JM, BANIK NL, HOGAN EL, BALENTINE JD:* Ca^{+2} accumulation in experimental spinal cord trauma. Brain Res 211:476–479, 1983

147. *HARRIS RJ, SYMON L, BRANSTON NM, BAYHAN M:* Changes in extracellular calcium activity in cerebral ischaemia. J Cereb Blood Flow Metabol 1:203–209, 1981

148. *HEARSE DJ, HUMPHREY SM, BULLOCK GR:* The oxygen paradox and the calcium paradox. J Mol Cell Cardiol 10:641–668, 1978

149. *HEDEMAN LS, SIL R:* Studies in experimental spinal cord trauma. Part 2. Comparison of treatment with steroids, low-molecular weight dextran and catecholamine blockade. J Neurosurg 40:44–51, 1974

150. *HILLER JM, SIMON EJ:* Specific, high affinity [^{3}H]-ethylketocyclazocine binding in rat central nervous system: lack of evidence for κ receptors. J Pharmacol Exp Ther 214:516–519, 1980

151. *HIRATA F, SCHIFFMAN E, VENKATASUBRAMANIAN K, SALOMAN D, AXELROD J:* A phospholipase A2 inhibitory protein in rabbit neutropils induced by

glucocorticoids. Proc Natl Acad Sci USA 77:2533–2536, 1980

152. *HODGKINS AL, KEYNES RD:* Active transport of cations in giant axons from Sepia and Loligo. J Physiol (London) 128:28–60, 1957
153. *HOLADAY JW, D'AMATO RJ:* Naloxone or TRH fails to improve neurological deficits in gerbil models of "stroke." Life Sci 31:385–392, 1982
154. *HOSOBUCHI Y, BASKIN OS, WOO SK:* Reversal of induced ischemic neurologic deficit in gerbils by the opiate antagonist naloxone. Science 215:69–71, 1982
155. *HSU CY, HALUSHKA PV, HOGAN EL, BANIK NL, LEE WA, PEROT PL:* Alterations of thromboxane and prostacyclin levels in experimental spinal cord injury. Neurology 35:1003–1009, 1985
156. *HUKUDA S, WILSON C:* Experimental cervical myelopathy: Effect of compression and ischemia on the canine cervical cord. J Neurosurg 37:631–652, 1972
157. *ITO T, ALLEN N, YASHON D:* A mitochondrial lesion in experimental spinal cord trauma. J Neurosurg 48:434–442, 1978
158. *JARROTT DM, DOMER FR:* A gerbil model of cerebral ischemia suitable for drug evaluation. Stroke 11:203–209, 1980
159. *JONSSON HT, DANIELL HB:* Altered levels of PGF in cat spnial cord tissue following traumatic injury. Prostaglandins 11:51–61, 1976
160. *KAMAKURA K, ISHIURA S, SUZUKI K, SUGITA H, TOYOKURA Y:* Calcium-activated neutral protease in the peripheral nerve, which requires μM order Ca^{+2}, and its effect on the neurofilament triplet. J Neurosci Res 13:391–403, 1985
161. *KASTIN AJ, NISSEN C, OLSON RD:* Failure of MIF-1 or naloxone to reverse ischemia-induced neurological deficits in gerbils. Pharmacol Biochem Behav 17:1083–1085, 1982
162. *KERST AF:* Dissociation constants of phophorus-containing chelating agents. In Griffith EJ, Beeton A, Spencer JM, Mitchell DT (eds): Environment Phosphorus Handbook, pp 265–280. New York, John Wiley & Son, 1972
163. *KIRK EJ, DENNY-BROWN D:* Functional variation in dermatomes in the macaque monkey following dorsal root lesions. J Comp Neurol 139:307–320, 1952
164. *KNAPP HD, TAUB E, BERMAN AJ:* Movements in monkeys with deafferented limbs. Exp Neurol 7:305–315, 1963
165. *KOBRINE AI:* The neuronal theory of experimental traumatic spinal cord dysfunction. Surg Neurol 3:261, 1975
166. *KOENIG C, DOHRMAN GJ:* Histopathological variability in "standardized" spinal cord trauma. J Neurol Neurosurg Psychiatr 40:1203, 1977
167. *KONTOS HA, WEI EP, ELLIS EF, POVLISHOCK JT, DIETRICH WD:* Prostaglandins in physiological and in certain pathological responses of the cerebral circulation. Fed Proc 40:2326–2330, 1981
168. *KOSTERLITZ HW, LESLIE FM:* Comparison of the receptor binding characteristics of opiate antagonists interacting with μ- or κ-receptors. Br J Pharmacol 64:607–614, 1978
169. *KRAIG RP, NICHOLSON C, PHILLIPS JM, GARDNER-MEDWIN, AR:* Diffusion from an iontophoretic source in the brain: Role of tortuosity and volume fraction. Brain Res 169:580–584, 1979
170. *KRAIG RP, PETITO C, PULSINELLI WA, PLUM F:* Lactoacidosis and brain injury during severe or complete ischemia. In Battastini N, Fiorini P, Courbier R, Plum F, Fieschi C (eds): Acute Brain Injury: Medical and Surgical Therapy, pp 35–40. New York, Raven Press, 1986
171. *KRAIG RP, PULSINELLI WA, PLUM F:* Hydrogen ion buffering during complete brain ischemia. Brain Res 342:280–290, 1985
172. *KRETSINGER RH:* Calcium in neurobiology: A general theory of its function and evolution. In Schmitt FO, Worden FG (eds): The Neurosciences—Fourth Study Program, pp 617–622. Cambridge, MIT Press, 1979
173. *KRNJEVIC K, LISIEWICZ A:* Injection of calcium ions in spinal motoneurones. J Physiol 225:363–390, 1972
174. *KUCHNER EF, HANSEBOUT RR:* Combined steroid and hypothermia treatment of experimental spinal cord injury. Surg Neurol 6:371–376, 1976
175. *LAHA RK, DUJOVNY M, BARRIONVEVO PF, DECASTRO SC, HELLSTROM HR, MAROON JC:* Protective effects of methylprednisolone and dimethylsulfoxide in experimental middle cerebral artery embolectomy. J Neurosurg 49:508–516, 1978
176. *LANDAU B, RANSOHOFF J:* Late surgery for incomplete traumatic lesions of the conus medullaris and cauda equina. J Neurosurg 28:25, 1980
177. *LANGFITT TW, OBRIST WD:* Cerebral blood flow and metabolism after intracranial trauma. Prog Neurol Surg 10:14–48, 1981
178. *LASHLEY KS:* Factors limiting recovery after central nervous system lesions. J Nerv Ment Dis 88:733–755, 1938
179. *LAWRENCE DG, KUYPERS HGJM:* The functional organization of the motor system in the monkey. I. The effects of bilateral pyramidal lesions. Brain 91:1–14, 1968
180. *LAWRENCE DG, KUYPERS HGJM:* The functional organization of the motor system in the monkey. II. The effects of lesions of the descending brainstem pathways. Brain 91:15–36, 1968
181. *LEVIN VA, FENSTERMACHER JD, PATLAK CS:* Sucrose and inulin space measurements of cerebral

cortex in four mammalian species. Am J Physiol 219:1528–1533, 1970

182. *Lewin MG, Hansebout RR, Pappius HM:* Chemical characteristics of traumatic spinal cord edema in cats. Effects of steroids on potassium depletion. J Neurosurg 56:106–113, 1974

183. *Little JR, Kerr FWL, Sundt TM:* The role of lysosomes in the production of ischemic nerve cell changes. Arch Neurol 30:448–455, 1974

184. *Liu C-N, Chambers WW:* Intraspinal sprouting of dorsal root axons. Arch Neurol Psychiatr 79:46–61, 1958

185. *Liu C-N, Chambers WW:* An experimental study of the corticospinal tract of the monkey. J Comp Neurol 123:257–284, 1964

186. *Llinàs R:* The role of calcium in neuronal function. In Schmitt FO, Worden FG (eds): The Neurosciences—Fourth Study Program, pp 555–572. Cambridge, MIT Press, 1978

187. *Lohse DC, Senter JH, Kauer JS:* Spinal cord blood flow in experimental transient paraplegia. J Neurosurg 52:335–345, 1980

188. *Lombard JH, Loegering DJ, Stekiel WJ:* Prevention by methylprednisolone of norepinephrine depletion in vascular tissue during severe hemorrhage in dogs. Blood Vess 17:276–280, 1980

189. *Long JB, Martinez-Arizala A, Petras JM, Holaday JW:* Endogenous opioids in spinal cord injury: A critical evaluation. CNS Trauma 3:295–316, 1986

190. *Martin WR, Eades CG, Thompson JA, et al:* The effects of morphine and nalorphine like drugs in the nondependent and morphine dependent chronic spinal dog. J Pharmacol Exp Ther 197:517–532, 1976

191. *Matheja J, Degens ET:* Structural Molecular Biology of Phosphates, pp 2–6. Stuttgart, Gustav Fischer Verlag, 1971

192. *Maury JF:* Effect of Ca on membranes. Fed Proc 25:1804–1810, 1966

193. *McCouch GP, Austin GM, Liu CN, Liu CY:* Sprouting as a cause of spasticity. J Neurophysiol 21:205–216, 1958

194. *McNicholas LF, Martin WR:* New and experimental therapeutic roles for naloxone and related opioid antagonists. Drugs 27:81–93, 1984

195. *McNicholas LF, Martin WR, Sloan JL, Nozaki M:* Innervation of the spinal cord by sympathetic fibers. Exp Neurol 69:383–394, 1980

196. *Means ED, Anderson DK, Waters TR, Kalaf L:* Effect of methylprednisolone in compression trauma to the feline spinal cord. J Neurosurg 55:200–208, 1981

197. *Meech RW:* Intracellular calcium and the control of membrane permeability. Symp Soc Exp Biol 30:161–191, 1976

198. *Metz R, Giebler C, Forster W:* Evidence for a direct inhibitory effect of glucocorticoids on the activity of phospholipase A2 as a further possible mechanism of some actions of steroid anti-inflammatory drugs. Pharm Res Commun 12:817–827, 1980

199. *Michaelis LL, Hickey PR, Clark TA, et al:* Ventricular irritability associated with the use of naloxone hydrochloride. Two case reports and laboratory assessment of the effect of the drug on cardiac excitability. Ann Thorac Surg 28:608–614, 1974

200. *Milvy P, Kakari S, Campbell JB, Demopoulos HB:* Paramagnetic species and radical products in cat spinal cord. Ann NY Acad Sci 222:1102–1111, 1973

201. *Molt JT, Nelson LR, Poulos DA, Bourke RS:* Analysis and measurement of some sources of variability in spinal cord trauma. J Neurosurg 50:784–791, 1979

202. *Murray M, Goldberger ME:* Restitution of function and collateral sprouting in the cat spinal cord: the partially hemisected animal. J Comp Neurol 158:19–36, 1974

203. *Naylor WG, Perry SE, Elz JS, Daly MJ:* Calcium, sodium, and the calcium paradox. Circ Res 55:227–237, 1984

204. *Nicholls D, Akerman K:* Mitchondrial calcium transport. Biochim Biophys Acta 805:393–404, 1982

205. *Nicholson C:* Dynamics of the brain cell microenvironment. Neurosci Res Prog Bull 18:177–322, 1980

206. *Nicholson C:* Measurements of extracellular ions in the brain. Trends Neurosci 3:216–218, 1980

207. *Nicholson C:* Modulation of extracellular calcium and its functional implications. Fed Proc 39:1519–1523, 1980

208. *Nicholson C, Phillips JM:* Ion diffusion modified by tortuosity and volume fraction in the extracellular microenvironment of the rat cerebellum. J Physiol 321:225–257, 1981

209. *Nornes H, Björklund Å, Stenevi U:* Reinnervation of the denervated adult spinal cord of rats by intraspinal transplants of embryonic brain stem neurons. Cell Tissue Res 230:15–35, 1983

210. *Nornes, H, Björklund Å, Stenevi U:* Transplantation strategies in spinal cord regeneration. In Sladek J Jr (ed): Neural Transplants, pp 407–421. New York, Plenum Press, 1984

211. *Osterholm JL:* Noradrenergic mediation of traumatic spinal cord autodestruction. Life Sci 14:1363, 1974

212. *Osterholm JL:* The pathophysiological response in spinal cord injury. J Neurosurg 40:5–33, 1974

213. *Palmer GC, Taylor MD, Callahan A:* Thera-

peutic protection of adenylate cyclase systems following bilateral stroke in gerbils. Fed Proc 42:1367, 1983

214. *Pappius HM:* Dexamethasone and local cerebral glucose utilization in freeze-traumatized rat brain. Ann Neurol 12:157–162, 1982
215. *Pappius HM:* Effect of drugs on local cerebral glucose utilization in traumatized brain: Mechanisms of action of steroids revisited. In Go KG, Baethmann A (eds): Recent Progress in the Study and Therapy of Brain Edema, pp 11–26. New York, Plenum Press, 1984
216. *Pappius HM:* The therapeutic effects of drugs in injured central nervous system. CNS Trauma 2:93–98, 1985
217. *Parker AJ, Smith CW:* Functional recovery from spinal cord trauma following dexamethasone and chlorpromazine therapy in dogs. Res Vet Sci 21:246–247, 1976
218. *Pickard JD:* Role of prostaglandins and arachidonic acid derivatives in the coupling of cerebral blood flow to cerebral metabolism. J Cereb Blood Flow Metab 1:361–384, 1981
219. *Pietronegro DD, DeCrescito V, Tomasula JJ, Demopoulos HB, Flamm ES:* Ascorbic acid: A putative biochemical marker of irreversible neurologic functional loss following spinal cord injury. CNS Trauma 2:85–92, 1985
220. *Povlishock JT, Becker DP, Sullivan HG, Miller JD:* Vascular permeability alterations to horseradish peroxidase in experimental brain injury. Brain Res 153:223–239, 1978
221. *Pryor WA:* The role of free radical reactions in biological systems. In Pryor WA (ed): Free Radicals in Biology, pp 1–49. New York, Academic Press, 1976
222. *Pulsinelli WA, Kraig RP, Plum F:* Hyperglycemia, cerebral acidosis, and ischemic brain damage. In Cerebrovascular Diseases (14th Princeton-Williamsburg Conference), pp 201–205. New York, Raven Press, 1985
223. *Raisman G:* Neuronal plasticity in the septal nuclei of the adult rat. Brain Res 14:25–48, 1969
224. *Raisman G, Field PM:* A quantitative investigation of the development of the collateral reinnervation after partial deafferentation of the septal nuclei. Brain Res 14:25–48, 1971
225. *Ramon y Cajal S:* Degeneration and Regeneration of the Nervous System. London, Oxford University Press, 1928
226. *Ransohoff J:* Lesions of the cauda equina. Clin Neurosurg 17:331, 1970
227. *Rappaport ZH, Young W, Flamm ES:* Regional brain Ca changes in the rat middle cerebral artery occlusion model of ischemia. Stroke 18:760–764, 1987
228. *Rinder L, Olsson Y:* Studies on vascular permeability in experimental concussion. II. Duration of altered permeability. Acta Neuropathol 11:200–214, 1968
229. *Robinson GA, Goldberger ME:* Interfering with inhibition may improve motor function. Brain Res 346:100–104, 1985
230. *Sandler AN, Tator CH:* Review of the effects of spinal cord trauma on vessels and blood flow in the spinal cord. J Neurosurg 45:638–646, 1976
231. *Sapolsky RM, Pulsinelli WA:* Glucocorticoids potentiate ischemic injury to neurons: therapeutic implications. Science 229:1397–1400, 1985
232. *Schanne FA, Kane AB, Young EE, Farber JL:* Calcium dependence of toxic cell death: a common pathway. Science 206:700–702, 1979
233. *Schmidt G:* The biochemistry of inorganic pyrophosphates and metaphosphates. In McElroy WD, Glass B (eds): Phosphorus Metabolism, pp 442–476. Baltimore, Johns Hopkins University Press, 1953
234. *Schneider RC:* Trauma to the spine and spinal cord. In: Kahn EA, Crosby EC, Schneider RC, Taren JA (eds): Correlative Neurosurgery, pp. 597. Springfield Illinois, Charles C Thomas, 1969
235. *Schoultz TW, DeLuca DC, Reding DL:* Norepinephrine levels in traumatized spinal cord of catecholamine depleted cats. Brain Res 109:367–374, 1976
236. *Senter HJ, Venes JL:* Altered blood flow and secondary injury in experimental spinal cord trauma. J Neurosurg 49:569–578, 1978
237. *Senter HJ, Venes JL:* Loss of autoregulation and posttraumatic ischemia following experimental spinal cord trauma. J Neurosurg 50:198–206, 1979
238. *Shibata S, Hodge CP, Pappius HM:* Effect of experimental ischemia on cerebral water and electrolytes. J Neurosurg 41:146–159, 1974
239. *Shields CG, Stauffer ES:* Late instability in cervical spine fractures secondary to laminectomy. Clin Orthop 119:144, 1976
240. *Siemkowicz E, Hansen AJ:* Brain extracellular ion composition and EEG activity following 10 minutes ischemia in normo- and hyperglycemic rats. Stroke 12:236–240, 1981
241. *Siesjo BK, Bendek G, Koide T, Westerberg E, Wieloch T:* Influence of acidosis on lipid peroxidation in brain tissues in vitro. J Cereb Blood Flow Metab 5:253–258, 1985
242. *Siesjo BK:* Cell damage in the brain: a speculative synthesis. J Cereb Blood Flow Metab 1:155–181, 1981
243. *Siesjo BK:* Cerebral circulation and metabolism. J Neurosurg 60:883–908, 1984
244. *Sillén LG, Martell AE:* Stability Constants of Metal-Ion Complexes. Chemical Society of London, Special Publication 17, p 182, 1964

245. *SPIELHOLZ N, BENJAMIN V, ENGLER G, RANSOHOFF J:* Somatosensory evoked potentials and stabilization of the spine. Methods and findings. Spine 4:500–505, 1979

246. *STOKES BT, FOX P, HALLINDEN G:* Extracellular calcium activity in the injured spinal cord. Exp Neurol 80:561–572, 1983

247. *SVARE A, TALLE K:* Lumbar myelography with metrizamide: An evaluation of 15 cases. Acta Radiol (Suppl)335:387, 1973

248. *TAFF RH:* Pulmonary edema following naloxone administration in a patient without heart disease. Anesthesiology 59:576–577, 1983

249. *TAKAHASHI H, TANAKA S, SANO K:* Changes in extracellular potassium concentration in cortex and brain stem during the acute phase of experimental closed head injury. J Neurosurg 55:708–717, 1981

250. *TARLOV IM:* Acute spinal cord compression paralysis. J Neurosurg 36:10–20, 1972

251. *TARLOV IM, KLINGER H:* Spinal cord compression studies: II. Time limits of recovery after acute compression in dogs. Arch Neurol Psychiatr 71:271–290, 1954

252. *TARLOV IM:* Spinal Cord Compression, Mechanisms of Paralysis and Treatment. Springfield, Illinois, Charles C Thomas, 1957

253. *TATOR CH:* Actue spinal cord injury in primates produced by inflatable extradural cuff. Can J Surg 16:222–231, 1973

254. *TORNHEIM PA, MCLAURIN RL:* Effect of dexamethasone on cerebral edema from cranial impact in the cat. J Neurosurg 48:220–227, 1978

255. *TOWER SS:* Pyramidal lesions in the monkey. Brain 63:36–90, 1940

256. *TURNER DM, KASSELL NF, SASAKI T, COMAIR YG, BECK DO, BOARINI DJ:* High dose naloxone produces cerebral vasodilation. Neurosurgery 15:192–197, 1984

257. *TVENTEN L, SALVESEN S:* Histology of the central nervous system of the rabbit about suboccipital injection of metrizamide. Acta Radiol (Suppl)335:166, 1973

258. *WEI EP, DIETRICH WD, POVLISHOCK JT, NAVARO RM, KONTOS HA:* Functional, morphologic and metabolic abnormalities of the cerebral microcirculation after concussive injury in cats. Circ Res 46:37–47, 1980

259. *WHITESIDES TW, SHAH SGA:* On the management of unstable fractures of the thoraco-lumbar spine. Spine 1:99, 1976

260. *WINDLE WF:* Concussion, contusion, and severance of the spinal cord. In Windle WF (ed): The Spinal Cord and Its Reactions to Traumatic Injury pp 205–217. New York, Marcel Dekker, 1980

261. *WINDLE WF, SMART JO, BEERS JJ:* Residual function after subtotal spinal cord transection in adult cats. Neurology 8:518–521, 1958

262. *WOLFE LS:* Eicosanoids: Prostaglandins, thromboxanes, leukotrienes, and other derivatives of carbon-20 unsaturated fatty acids. J Neurochem 38:1–14, 1982

263. *WOLFE LS, COCEANI F:* The role of prostaglandins in the central nervous system. Ann Rev Physiol 41:669–684, 1979

264. *WOODBURY DM, VERNADKIS A:* Effects of steroids on the central nervous system. Methods Horm Res 5:1–56, 1966

265. *YOUNG W:* Blood flow, metabolic and neurophysiological mechanisms in spinal cord injury. In Becker D, Povlishock JT (eds): Central Nervous System Trauma Status Report, pp 463–473. Bethesda, NIH, NINCDS, 1985

266. *YOUNG W:* Ca paradox in neural injury: A hypothesis. CNS Trauma 3:235–251, 1986

267. *YOUNG W:* Cellular defenses against excessive calcium entry in trauma and ischemia. Critical Care: State of the Art, Vol 8. FB Cerra, WC Shoemaker (eds). The Society of Critical Care Medicine pp 71–98. (251 E. Imperial Highway, Suite 480, Fullerton, CA 92635), 1987

268. *YOUNG W:* Correlation of somatosensory evoked potentials and neurological findings in clinical spinal cord injury. In Tator CH (ed): Early Management of Cervical Spinal Injury, pp 153–166. New York, Raven Press, 1981

269. *YOUNG W, MEYER P:* Neurological and neurophysiological evaluations of spinal cord injury. In Standards for Evaluation of Spinal Cord Injury. In: Illis L (ed): Spinal Cord Dysfunction-Assessment, pp 148–165. Oxford, Oxford University Press

270. *YOUNG W:* Pharmacological treatments of acute spinal cord injury: a review of naloxone and methylprednisolone. Clin Neurosurg. 34:675–679, 1988

271. *YOUNG W:* Somatosensory evoked potential (SEPs) in spinal cord injury. In Schramm J, Jones SJ (eds): Spinal Cord Monitoring, pp 127–142. Berlin-New York, Springer Verlag, 1985

272. *YOUNG W:* The role of calcium in spinal cord injury. CNS Trauma 2:109–114, 1985

273. *YOUNG W, DECRESCITO V:* Sodium ionic changes in injured spinal cords: Mechanisms of edema (absrt). Proc Soc Neurosci 16:267, 1986

274. *YOUNG W, DECRESCITO V, TOMASULA JJ:* Role of the sympathetic nervous system in spinal cord blood flow autoregulation and traumatic ischemia. J Neurosurg 56:706–710, 1982

275. *YOUNG W, FLAMM ES:* Effect of high dose corticosteroid therapy on blood flow, evoked potentials, and extracellular calcium in experimental spinal cord injury. J Neurosurg 57:557–673, 1982

276. *Young W, Flamm ES, Demopoulos HB, DeCrescito V, Tomasula JJ:* Effect of naloxone on posttraumatic ischemia in experimental spinal contusion. J Neurosurg 55:209–219, 1981
277. *Young W, Hadani M, Rappaport H, DeCrescito V, Flamm ES, Cornu P:* Tissue Na, K, and Ca changes in regional cerebral ischemia: Their measurement and interpretation. CNS Trauma 3:215–234, 1986
278. *Young W, Koreh I:* Potassium and calcium changes in injured spinal cords. Brain Res 365:42–53, 1986
279. *Young W, Koreh I, Yen V, Lindsay A:* Effect of sympathectomy on extracellular potassium activity and blood flow in experimental spinal cord contusion. Brain Res 253:115–124, 1982
280. *Young W, Rappaport ZH, Chalif DJ, Flamm ES:* Regional brain Na, K, and water changes in the rat middle cerebral artery occlusion model of ischemia. Stroke 18;751–759, 1987
281. *Young W, Yen V, Blight A:* Extracellular calcium ionic activity in experimental spinal cord contusion. Brain Res 253:105–113, 1982
282. *Zimmerman ANE, Hulsmann WC:* Paradoxical influence of calcium ions on the permeability of the cell membranes in the isolated rat heart. Nature 211:646–647, 1966
283. *Zimmerman V, Hossman KA:* Resuscitation of the monkey brain after one hour's complete ischemia. II. Brain water and electrolytes. Brain Res 85:1–12, 1975
284. *Zivin JA, DeCirolami U:* Spinal cord infarction: A highly reproducible stroke model. Stroke 11:200–202, 1980

Evaluation and Treatment of Acute Cervical Spinal Cord Injury

SANFORD J. LARSON

The radiologic and electrophysiologic aspects of the evaluation of patients with acute spinal cord injury have been presented in preceding chapters. As far as the clinical evaluation is concerned, it is important to remember that in patients with spinal cord injury the symptoms of associated visceral and musculoskeletal injuries may be masked by altered sensory perception. Consequently, a physical examination more extensive than usual and a roentgenographic evaluation are required. Although hypotension may be secondary to peripheral vasodilatation associated with acute myelopathy, this occurs in a minority of patients,[16] and loss of circulating volume should be suspected and excluded as a cause.

Because of its segmental early development, and because of the segmental character of the spinal column and spinal nerves, the spinal cord is customarily considered segmentally. Functionally, however, the spinal cord is a continuum, with its rootlets emerging in an almost unbroken line and with the anterior horn cell columns for the individual muscles extending over two or more levels. The posterior portions of the head, the neck, and the upper limbs are supplied by nine spinal, eight cervical, and one thoracic nerve, leaving the spinal cord from C1 through the midportion of the body of T1. Therefore, the vertebral segments do not corresponds one-to-one to the cord and root segments (Fig. 7-8). The portions of the spinal cord supplying various muscles are shown in Figure 7-9, the relationship to the vertebral levels in Figure 7-10, and the corresponding functional relationships in Figures 7-11 and 7-12. It is evident that patients with a complete myelopathy secondary to fracture dislocation at C3 will be ventilator dependent and without function in the upper limbs. Those with a fracture of C4 will also have hypoventilation but should eventually be able to breathe without assistance and have weak abduction of the shoulder. Abduction of the shoulder and elbow flexion should be present in patients with C5 fractures, and those with C6 fractures should also be able to flex and extend at the wrist, in addition to having extension at the elbow. Patients with complete myelopathy secondary to C7 fracture should have flexion and extension of the fingers, and those with lesions as low as T1 may have intrinsic hand muscle function. This correspondence among vertebral level, cord level, and function is subject to individual variation but, nevertheless, is a useful approximation. For sensory perception, the outer aspect of the arm is supplied by C5 and the radial portion of the forearm and hand, including the thumb and index finger, by C6. Because of overlap, the C7 representation is limited to the middle finger and middle portion of the hand. The eighth root supplies the ulnar aspect of the hand and distal forearm. The ulnar portion of the forearm and arm are supplied by T1 and T2, respectively. The level of the clavicle is the approximate boundary between C4 and T2.

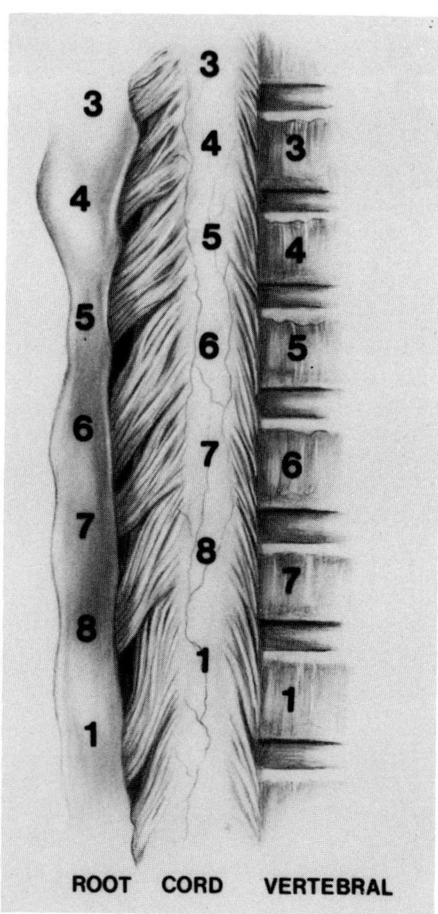

Fig. 7-8. Relationship between cervical root (left), cord (center), and vertebral (right) segments.

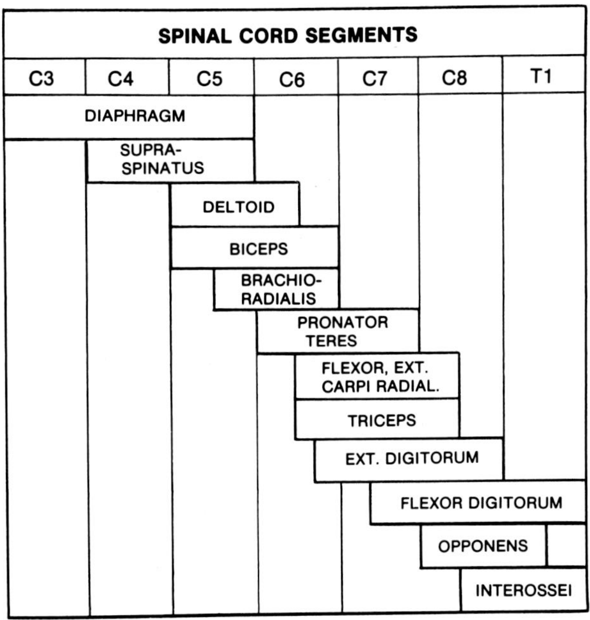

Fig. 7-9. Spinal cord segments and related muscles. (Adapted from Haymaker W, Woodhall B: Peripheral nerve injuries, 2nd ed. Philadelphia, WB Saunders Co, 1953)

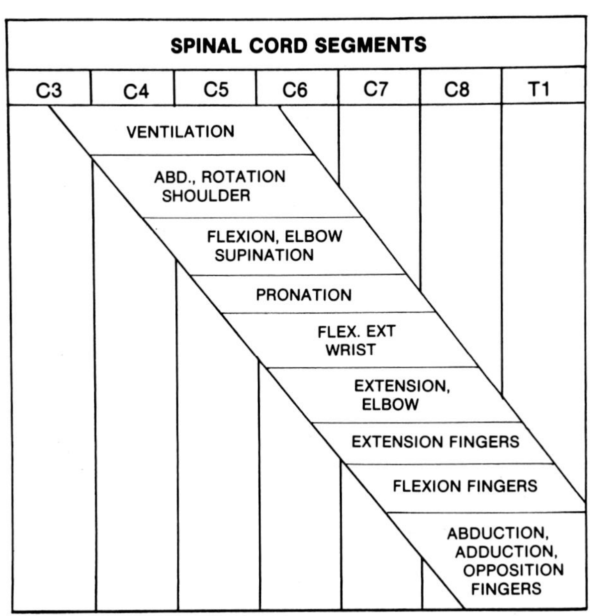

Fig. 7-11. Correspondence between cervical cord segments and function.

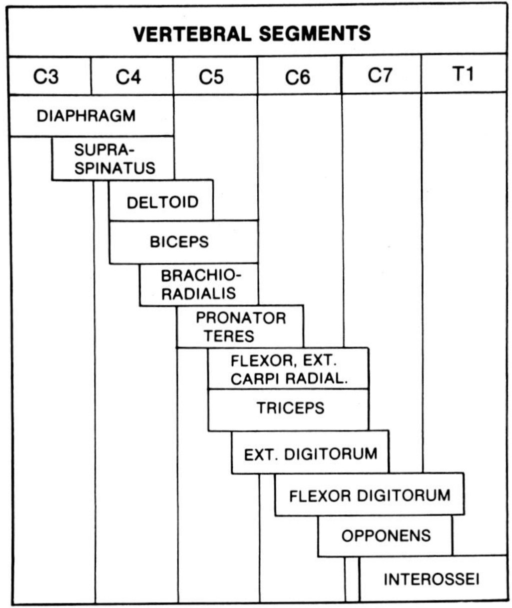

Fig. 7-10. Vertebral segments and related muscles.

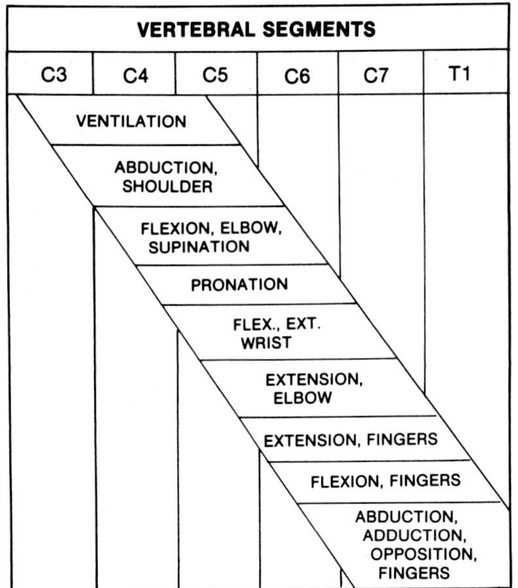

Fig. 7-12. Correspondence between vertebral segments and function.

In the case of complete myelopathy, the loss of function is usually bilaterally symmetrical. However, in many patients with incomplete myelopathy the functional deficit is asymmetrical, with loss of proprioception and muscle strength greater on the side of the more severely damaged cord and with loss of both pain and temperature perception greater on the opposite side. A true Brown-Séquard syndrome, with strictly ipsolateral loss of strength and proprioception, and only contralateral loss of pain and temperature perception, is seen only with hemisection of the cord resulting from stab wounds (Fig. 7-13).

In the central cord syndrome, usually associated with a stenotic spinal canal and hyperextension injury, functional loss is greater in the upper limbs than in the lower. This reflects the greater sensitivity to trauma of cell bodies and synapses, as compared with that of axons. Although an ischemic cause of the central cord syndrome has been suggested, this explanation appears unlikely because loss of function is immediate with the syndrome. Even with abrupt and complete interruption of cerebral blood flow in humans, consciousness is retained for at least 4 seconds[29] and neurologic deficit secondary to traumatic occlusion of the vertebral arteries does not appear for several hours or more.[32]

TREATMENT

Impaired function of the spinal cord following trauma is related to transfer of energy to the spinal cord at impact and to persisting deformity of the spinal cord by displaced tissue.[10,24,27,34] Nothing can be done to affect the transfer of energy once it has occurred. In spite of the great interest in treating the secondary effects of energy transfer, such as edema and vascular and ionic changes, there is little evidence that these effects cause significant additional deficits. As far as the long tracts are concerned, function either remains the same or improves following injury. If the secondary changes are significant, deterioration should occur in some patients, but this does not happen unless mechanical factors are introduced such as overdistraction, progressive angulation, or additional displacement of tissue.[26] Although in some patients the segmental level may rise in the days immediately following injury, for example, decrease or loss

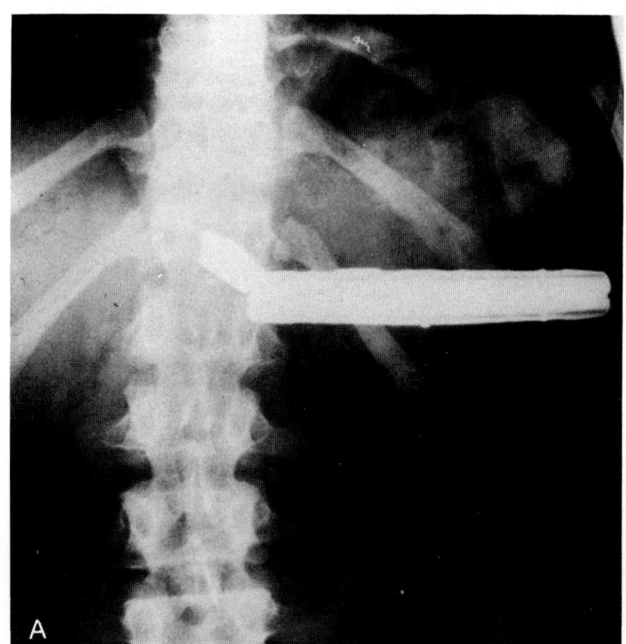

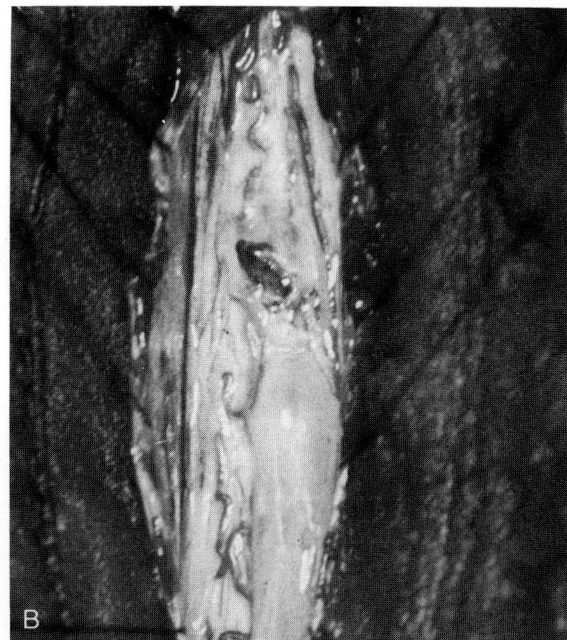

Fig. 7-13. (*A*) A–P radiograph of patient with Brown-Séquard syndrome. The knife blade was imbedded in the vertebral body. (*B*) Surgical exposure in the same patient. Despite apparent hemisection of the cord, this patient was eventually able to walk without assistance.

of intrinsic hand muscle function that had been initially present in a C7–T1 lesion, the lost function returns without specific treatment. Despite their extensive use in ever-increasing dosages over a period of many years, steroids have been shown to be effective only in increasing the incidence of infection[9,13] and gastrointestinal bleeding.[4,5,17] Other measures such as hyperbaric oxygen and naloxone are currently being evaluated, but from the natural history of complete and incomplete traumatic myelopathy it appears unlikely that these agents will significantly improve long-tract function.

The goal of treatment is return of the patient to the best possible function in the shortest possible time, with the least mortality and morbidity. For patients with cervical cord injury, this requires the restoration of normal anatomic relationships between the spinal cord and its roots, and the spinal canal and foramina. While skeletal traction is useful, it must be used judiciously.[4,11,14,20] For example, in the case of bilateral locked facets, the disc and ligaments are completely disrupted, and only the cervical muscles maintain apposition of the vertebrae at the level of injury. If muscle spasm is overcome, overdistraction may occur with disastrous results (Fig. 7-14). Because patients with bilateral locked facets usually require a fusion to permit early mobilization and rehabilitation, open reduction at the time of fusion is preferable to overly enthusiastic attempts at closed reduction. Similarly, patients with distraction injuries should not be placed in traction, but instead the head should be immobilized. When muscle contractions have restored normal relationships, fusion can be performed (Fig. 7-15).

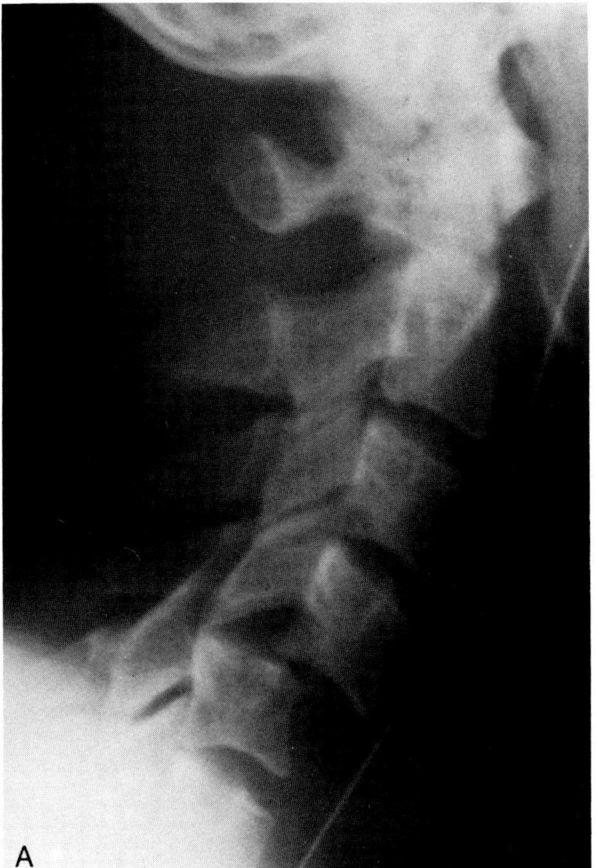

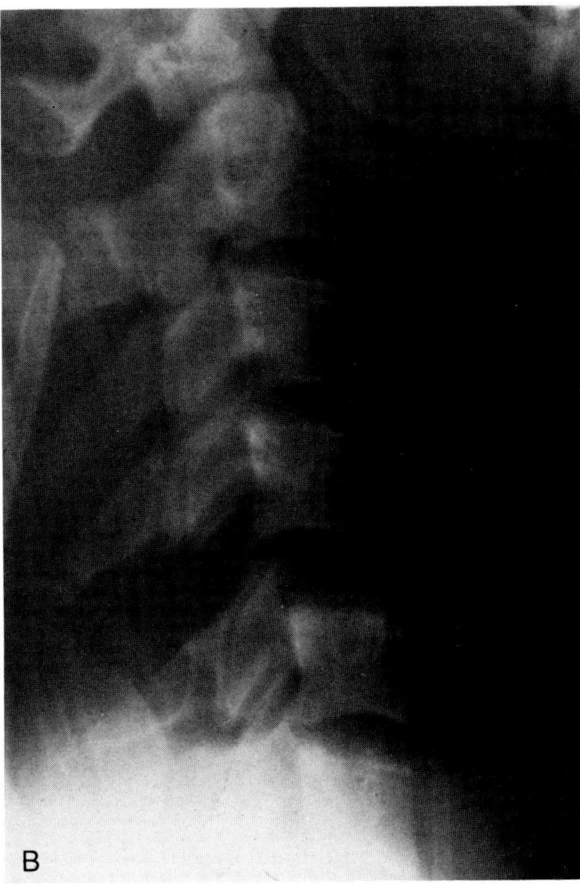

Fig. 7-14. (*A*) Bilateral locked facets in a quadriplegic patient with independent ventilation. (*B*) Film taken after apnea had developed during skeletal traction (Reproduced with permission of Neurosurgery[2])

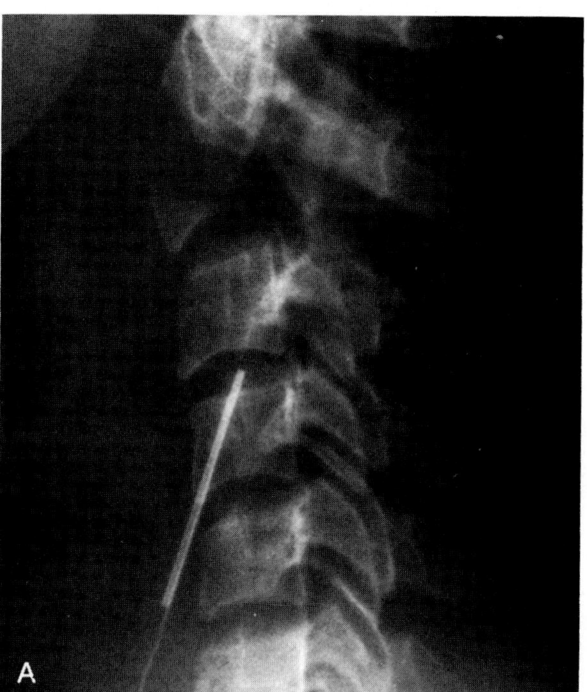

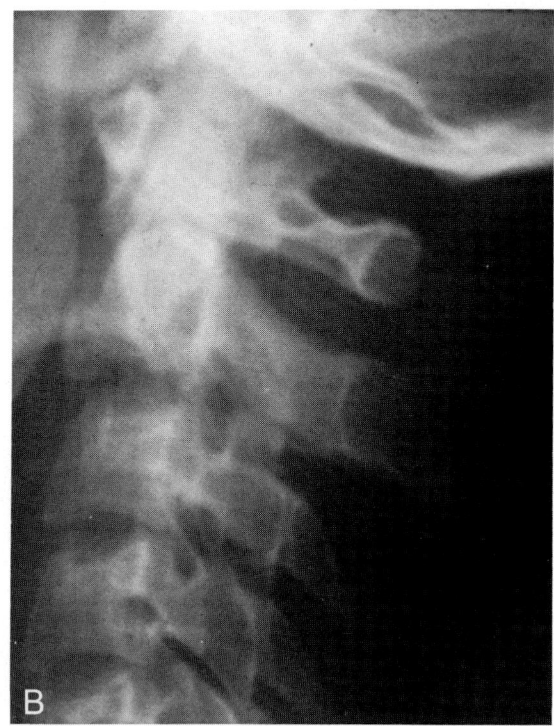

Fig. 7-15. (*A*) Lateral films from a patient who was quadriparetic after a vehicular-pedestrian accident. (*B*) Film from the same patient several days later. The head had been immobilized without traction. A C2–C3 posterior fusion was subsequently performed.

Certain areas of treatment remain controversial. With the recognition that laminectomy is largely useless and frequently harmful unless the pathologic process is posterior to the spinal cord, some of the controversy regarding surgical versus nonsurgical treatment has subsided. Nevertheless, advocates of nonsurgical management claim results that are at least equal to those obtained with surgical treatment.[1,12,21] When allowances are made for the level of injury and the time at which the patient enters the spinal cord injury unit, there is little difference in morbidity and mortality between patients operated upon and those treated nonsurgically.[5] If normal relationships between the spinal cord and canal can be restored by nonsurgical means, again the difference in the functional results between the two groups is small.[19] However, if normal relationships and stability cannot be restored by postural methods, this can be achieved surgically.[15] Consequently, the functional results are better, overall, in patients who are operated upon.[6,7,23] Even with complete myelopathy in patients who were neurologically stable, the segmental level has been shown to drop following surgery.[2] This is not surprising, because, for example, tissue deforming the cord at C6–C7 may also deform the C7 root, which originates from an uninjured portion of the cord. Restoration of normal root-canal-foramen relationships allows recovery of root function. Furthermore, immediately above the level of permanent functional transection, there may be a zone in which the spinal cord is reversibly impaired, and reconstruction of the canal could allow this portion to recover. Since the part of the cord supplying the diaphragm and upper limbs is only about 8 cm long, recovery of even a few millimeters of spinal cord can be functionally significant. In addition, surgical treatment permits earlier mobilization of the patient[18,28] with decreased opportunity for recumbency-related complications.

Different opinions also exist regarding the timing of surgery. Intuitively, early correction of deformity appears desirable but in practice does not prove necessary. Although the evidence is not conclusive, it seems that results of late operation are at least as good as are seen when surgery is performed immediately after the injury.[3,6,23,25,30] Fur-

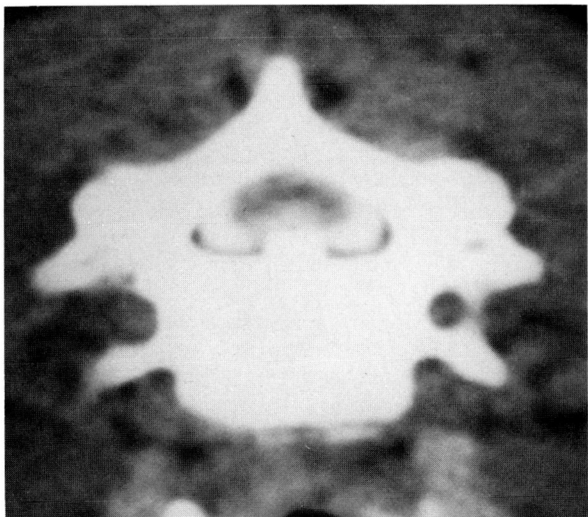

Fig. 7-16. Metrizamide enhanced CT scan in a patient who had complete recovery from a central cord syndrome.

ther support for this contention is provided by the results of nonsurgical management, in which restoration of normal relationships may take days or weeks, but which, when achieved, is as good as results with surgical methods.[19] Many patients have associated injuries that take precedence over treatment of the spinal cord injury and that can be safely attended to, once the spinal column has been adequately immobilized.

The management of central cord injury is another controversial area. Although some patients may recover substantially, or even completely, without specific treatment, others have a persistent and significant residual deficit. Although some authors have suggested that nonsurgical treatment is preferable,[31] others have demonstrated that in the patient whose spinal cord is persistently deformed and in whom neurologic recovery has reached a plateau, surgical treatment can be followed by significant functional improvement.[8] Since plain films do not demonstrate any change in diameter of the spinal canal in patients who improve as compared with those who do not, and because disc herniation is an uncommon cause of the central cord syndrome, it is possible that the persistent deficit in patients who recover function following surgery may be related to persistent thickening of the soft tissues lining the spinal canal. For example, the patient whose contrast-enhanced CT scan is shown in Figure 7-16 was completely quadriplegic following a water skiing injury. Recovery of function appeared first in the lower limbs and then in the upper limbs with return to a functionally normal condition within a few hours. Paresthesias persisted for several days and then disappeared, except during flexion of the cervical spine. In contrast, the patient whose gas myelogram is shown in Figure 7-17 had severe weakness of the upper

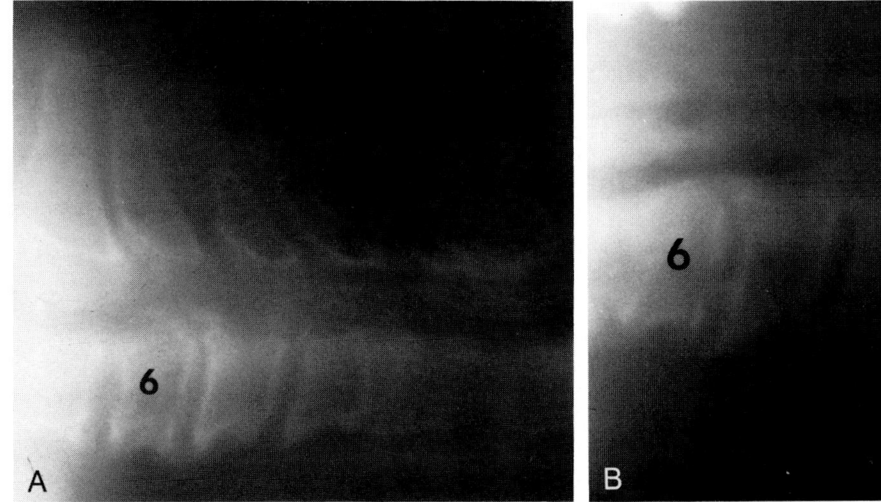

Fig. 7-17. (*A*) Gas myelogram in a patient with central cord syndrome. (*B*) Gas myelogram following laminectomy and dentatotomy in the same patient. The spinal canal was flat to inspection and palpation from C5 rostrally. The space between the posterior surface of the vertebral bodies and the dura is abnormally wide from C5 rostrally.

limbs and less pronounced weakness of the lower limbs following a hyperextension injury. Neurologic function improved slightly during the first week and then remained stable. Gas myelopathy was performed 3 weeks after injury, followed by laminectomy with division of the dentate ligaments from C3 to C7. Except at C5–C6, the floor of the spinal canal was flat. The patient recovered substantially and was able to walk without assistance but had persistent significant impairment of hand function. Consequently, another myelogram was obtained. Although the spinal cord was not deformed, the space between the vertebral bodies and the dura was abnormally wide above C6. The thickened soft tissue appears to have contributed to the spinal stenosis and related myelopathy, and was presumably a posttraumatic event.

The management of penetrating wounds involving the spinal cord is also being reevaluated. Based on the military experience with high-velocity missile wounds, surgical débridement with dural closure has been the standard treatment. However, extensive soft-tissue damage is not present with the low-velocity missile wounds encountered in civilian practice. Nonsurgical treatment has not been complicated by infection,[35] and some reports have suggested that the incidence of infection is greater in patients treated surgically.[33,35] It is possible that, because of the thick cervical musculature, the missiles are wiped clean of cutaneous bacteria before reaching the subarachnoid space. However, if the missile penetrates clothing, the possibility exists that fabric may be carried into the canal. In stab wounds, the knife itself must be considered contaminated and surgical treatment should be considered. Unless the missile or tissue displaced by it is deforming the spinal cord and the patient has incomplete myelopathy, the only rationale for surgical treatment is prevention of infection.

REFERENCES

1. *Bedbrook GM:* Stability of spinal fractures and fracture dislocations. Paraplegia 9:23–32, 1971
2. *Benzel EC, Larson SJ:* Recovery of nerve root function after complete quadriplegia from cervical spine fractures. Neurosurgery 19:809–812, 1986
3. *Bohlman HH:* Late, progressive paralysis and pain following fractures of the thoracolumbar spine. J Bone Joint Surg 58A:728, 1976
4. *Bohlman HH:* Complications of treatment of fractures and dislocations of the cervical spine. In Epps CH Jr (ed): Complications in Orthopaedic Surgery, Vol 2, pp 611–641. Philadelphia, JB Lippincott Co, 1978
5. *Bohlman HH:* Acute fractures and dislocations of the cervical spine: An analysis of 300 hospitalized patients and review of the literature. J Bone Joint Surg 61A:1119–1142, 1979
6. *Bohlman HH:* Late anterior decompression for spinal cord injury: Review of 100 cases with long term results. Orthop Trans 4:42–43, 1980
7. *Bohlman HH, Ducker TB, Lucas JT:* Spine and spinal cord injuries. In Rothman RH, Simeone FA, (eds): The Spine. Philadelphia, WB Saunders Co, 1982
8. *Bose B, Northrup BE, Osterholm JL, Cotler JM, DiTunno JF:* Reanalysis of central cervical cord injury management. Neurosurgery 15:367–372, 1984
9. *Bracken MB, Shepard MJ, Hellenbrand KG, et al:* Methylprednisolone and neurological function 1 year after spinal cord injury: Results of the National Acute Spinal Cord Injury Study. J Neurosurg 63:704–713, 1985
10. *Breig A:* Adverse Mechanical Tension in the Central Nervous System. Stockholm, Almquist and Wiksell, 1978
11. *Burke DC, Berryman D:* The place of closed manipulation in the management of flexion–rotation dislocations of the cervical spine. J Bone Joint Surg 53B:165–182, 1971
12. *Cheshire DJE:* The stability of the cervical spine following the conservative treatment of fractures and fracture–dislocations. Paraplegia 7:193–203, 1969
13. *Collins WF:* A review and update of experiment and clinical studies of spinal cord injury. Paraplegia 21:204–219, 1983
14. *Crutchfield WG:* Skeletal traction in treatment of injuries to the cervical spine. JAMA 155:29–32, 1954
15. *Dorr LD, Harvey JP Jr, Nickel VL:* Clinical review of the early stability of spine injuries. Spine 7:545–550, 1982
16. *Elias Z, Rosner MJ, Coley IB:* Cardiopulmonary monitoring in the spinal cord injured patient. Proc 3rd Annu Meet Joint Section Spinal Disorders AANS/CNS, pp 28–29, 1987
17. *Epstein E, Hood DC, Ransohoff J:* Gastrointestinal bleeding in patients with spinal cord trauma. J Neurosurg 54:16–20, 1981
18. *Forsyth HF, Alexander E Jr, Davis C Jr, Underdal R:* The advantages of early spine fusion in the treatment of fracture-dislocation of the cervical spine. J Bone Joint Surg 41A:17–36, 1959
19. *Frankel HL, Hancock DO, Hyslop G, Melzak J, Michaelisw S, Ungar GH, Vernon S, Walsh JJ:* The value of postural reduction in the initial management of closed injuries of the spine with paraplegia and tetraplegia. Paraplegia 7:179–192, 1969

20. *Fried LC:* Cervical spinal cord injury during skeletal traction. JAMA 229:181–183, 1974
21. *Guttman L:* Spinal deformities in traumatic paraplegics and tetraplegics following surgical procedures. Paraplegia 7:38–49, 1969
22. *Heiden JS, Weiss MH, Rosenberg AW, Kurze T, Apuzzo MLH:* Penetrating gunshot wounds of the cervical spine in civilians. Review of 38 cases. J Neurosurg 42:575–579, 1975
23. *Larson SJ, Holst RA, Hemmy DC, Sances A Jr:* The lateral extracavitary approach to traumatic lesions of the thoracic and lumbar spine. J Neurosurg 45:628–637, 1976
24. *Larson SJ, Walsh PR, Sances A Jr, Cusick JF, Hemmy DC, Mahler H:* Evoked potentials in experimental myelopathy. Spine 5:299–302, 1980
25. *Maiman DJ, Larson SJ, Benzel EC:* Neurological improvement associated with late decompression of the thoracolumbar spinal cord. Neurosurgery 14:302–307, 1984
26. *Marshall LF, Knowlton S, Garfin SR, Klauber MR, Eisenberg HM, Kopaniky D, Miner ME, Tabbador K, Clifton GL:* Deterioration following spinal cord injury. A multicenter study. J Neurosurg 66:400–404, 1987
27. *McAfee PC, Bohlman HH, Yuan HA:* Anterior decompression of traumatic thoracolumbar fractures with incomplete neurological deficit using a retroperitoneal approach. J Bone Joint Surg 67A:89–104, 1985
28. *Norton WL:* Fractures and dislocations of the cervical spine. J Bone Joint Surg 44A:115–139, 1962
29. *Rossen R, Kabat H, Anderson JP:* Acute arrest of cerebral circulation in man. Arch Neurol Psychiatry 50:510–528, 1943
30. *Schmidek HH, Gomes FB, Seligson D, et al:* Management of acute unstable thoracolumbar (T-11–L-1) fractures with and without neurological deficit. Neurosurgery 7:30–35, 1980
31. *Schneider RC:* Surgical indications and contraindications in spine and spinal cord trauma. Clin Neurosurg 8:157–183, 1960
32. *Schneider RC, Gosch HH, Noreau H, Jerva M, Combs LW, Smith RA:* Vascular insufficiency and differential distortion of brain and cord caused by cervicomedullary football injuries. J Neurosurg 33:363–375, 1970
33. *Stauffer ES, Wood RW, Kelly EG:* Gunshot wounds of the spine: The effects of laminectomy. J Bone Joint Surg 61A:389–392, 1979
34. *Tarlov IM:* Acute spinal cord compression paralysis. J Neurosurg 36:10–20, 1972
35. *Yashon D, Jane JA, White RJ:* Prognosis and management of spinal cord and cauda equina bullet injuries in sixty-five civilians. J Neurosurg 32:163–170, 1970

Nonsurgical Treatment

BRUCE E. NORTHRUP AND JOHN L. ALDERMAN

Although the primary goal in the treatment of the spinally injured patient is to preserve or restore function to the injured cord tissue and mechanical stability to its coverings, much of the current nonoperative therapy has been directed toward extraneuronal complications of spinal cord injury (SCI). As a consequence, the management of the extraneuronal complications has improved dramatically, whereas essentially no progress has been made toward alleviating the attending motor deficits.

There has, on the other hand, been a resurgence of interest in the nonoperative treatment of the injured neuronal tissue *per se* at the research level. This resurgence has been stimulated by a number of factors:

1. The delineation of a significant delay between wounding and development of the hemorrhagic necrosis within the cord indicated that immediate axonal disruption is an important mechanism in a minority of patients.
2. A unified theory of spinal cord injury based upon ischemia was developed. This theory proposes that paralyzing SCI initiates a severe ischemic condition that contributes significantly to the overall posttraumatic pathophysiologic condition of the injured cord. The initiation of severe ischemia at early time points within the injured cord has been confirmed by most but not all of those investigating this phenomenon (Fig. 7-18).[8,9,31,42,53,56,58]
3. The efficacy of a variety of pharmacologic agents in animal models of SCI was postulated.

It is the third factor, the pharmacologic treatment of SCI (including hypothermia and hyperbaric oxygen), that this section explores.

Obviously, many variables interact in man to make the clinical study of SCI extremely difficult: the interval between injury and treatment, the severity of injury, the degree of instability, the presence of continued compression, age, associated injuries, and variability of areas of involvement within the cord, among others. Clearly, then, the demonstration of efficacy is best carried out in the laboratory where the multiplicity of variables can be controlled to the extent that the effect of a therapeutic maneuver or agent can be properly evaluated. Possibly the most important variable to control is that relating to the degree of injury; an injury that is mild will improve markedly regardless of therapeutic intervention, whereas too severe an injury may mechanically render the cord incapable of therapeutic response. The current thinking is that a threshold injury yields a condition that best allows a given drug or treatment to express its therapeutic potential. The injury model must, of course, be highly reproducible.

Finally, the efficacy of a nonoperative or pharmacologic treatment in SCI can be evaluated according to various end points. Considering the relatively primitive state of our knowledge concerning SCI, as well as the fact that few, if any, nonoperative studies have been completed to date, it would be optimistic if not naive to believe we would be fortunate enough to observe significant functional motor gains very often. Hence, end points of therapeutic success that fall short of motor function must also be considered. Different investigators have measured efficacy in terms of histologic preservation of the cord tissue, improved regional spinal cord blood flow (rSCBF), impulse conduction (sensory evoked potential, SEP), a reduction in edema, biochemical indices, and, finally, motor function.

The overall body of evidence indicates that the outlook for nonoperative intervention in the pathogenesis of SCI is promising, but by no means well established. Before any nonoperative approaches can be properly and completely tested, the very nature of SCI pathogenesis must be better understood, and before pharmacologic intervention can be rationally entertained, the influence of the pathogenic environment on drug delivery and response must be ascertained (Table 7-1).

HYPOTHERMIA

One of the most effective agents studied experimentally has been hypothermia of the cord, which results in reduction in O_2 demand secondary to a slowdown in tissue metabolism. A reduced O_2 demand is specifically desirable in light of the ischemic condition of the injured tissue. Negrin, the first to apply cooling in an acute cord injury, perfused locally injured human spinal cords with saline precooled with a refrigeration compressor pump.[40,41] The subarachnoid and epidural spaces were perfused by means of a variable speed per-

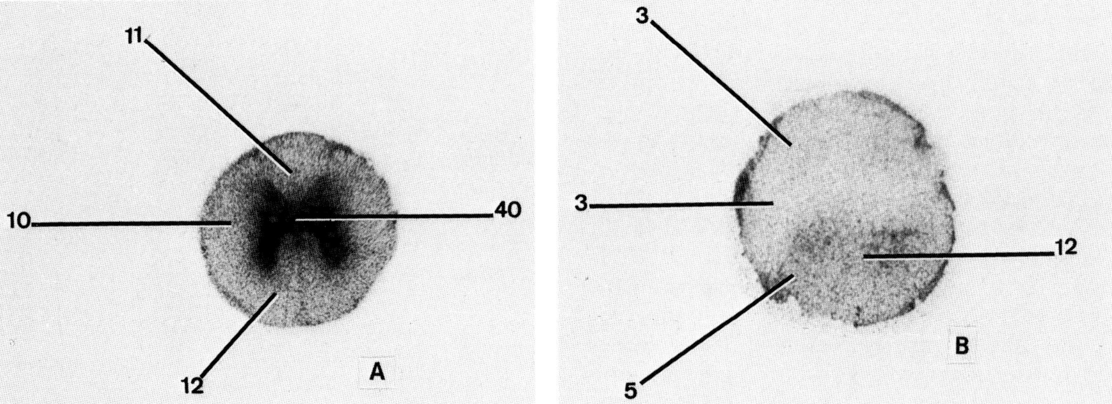

Fig. 7-18. C^{14} antipyrene autoradiogram in control (*A*) and spinally injured cat (*B*). Spinal injury at 5 min has induced a severe ischemia in this animal in both the white and the gray matter.

fusion pump following laminectomy. Negrin concluded that the cooling was beneficial, although a limited patient population was cited. Subsequently, Albin, White, and others investigated the phenomenon intensively in the laboratory and found a protective effect of cooling that they attributed, in part, to a hypothermia-induced reduction in edema.[1,2,63,64] They also postulated that the cooling increased local blood flow in addition to reducing O_2 demand. Recent studies have bolstered the rationale for hypothermia. Wells and Hansebout[62a] demonstrated that hypothermia resulted in the preservation of functional activity in dogs, although it was emphasized that appropriate temporal conditions must be fulfilled.

A number of laboratory studies have demonstrated significant improvement following SCI after hyperthermia treatment.[1,2,14,21,28,31,35,59–62] It seems, however, that the positive effect of hypothermia is most evident following injuries of limited severity, and that in this setting hypothermia is effective in promoting recovery of the moderately injured cord, a situation analogous to the human with incomplete spinal injury. Clearly, according to Albin, the requirements for successful hypothermia therapy are quite specific. For example, the rate of perfusion of coolant must be high (2000 cc/min), and cooling must be initiated within an 8-hour period of injury and carried out for a period of 8 hours for the treatment to be effective.

At the same time, clinical trials of local hypothermia generally failed to demonstrate a positive effect, largely because each study included only a small number of highly heterogenous patients, and no uniform treatment program or uniform criteria for case selection was used; thus, no relationships could be formulated between studies.[10,15]

A striking feature of the clinical hypothermia studies is that in each small group of patients there are one or two distinctly unusual patients. One would predict these patients would be extremely unlikely to do as well as they did. It was this kind of patient that stimulated the interest in hypothermia.

An inherent drawback to hypothermia is that it involves laminectomy, which in itself may adversely affect stability of the cervical spine. Ducker has shown that stabilization procedures improve neurologic outcome following a laminectomy and standard injury. Thus, hypothermia remains a highly provocative but unsolved issue.[31]

Table 7-1. Summary of the Effect of Pharmacologic Treatments on Spinal Cord Injury

Hypothermia	+
Hyperbaric oxygen	+
Steroids	+
Vasodilators	±
Adrenergic antagonists	±
Antihistamines	+
DMSO	±
Enzymes	−
Dilantin	+
Mannitol	+

+ Effective in laboratory setting
± Remains controversial or weak effect

HYPERBARIC OXYGEN

Following the observation of Assenmacher and Ducker of diminished vascularity in the injured tissue, Kelly demonstrated a dramatic decrease in oxygen tension in the injured tissue, and showed that hyperbaric oxygen (HBO) greatly improved neurologic outcome in the dog.[6,32] Yeo demonstrated similar findings in sheep, and found an improvement in histology following HBO.[67] Yeo has used HBO for specially injured patients with good success, particularly in the partially injured. Gainer was able to improve tissue O_2 using crocetin, and found this improved neurologic outcome following spinal injury.[23]

PHARMACOLOGIC APPROACHES

In theory there are appropriate pharmacologic agents available to correct or attenuate almost all of the pathophysiologic defects that accompany and probably contribute to the functional demise of the traumatized spinal cord. Unfortunately, the nature of the pathophysiologic defects themselves contributes to certain problems that in turn complicate a rational pharmacologic approach to SCI therapy. One of the most significant of these problems is obviously associated with the ischemic nature of the lesion. The vascular avenue of therapy is not only compromised, but the degree of compromise is unpredictable and especially difficult to assess in the human. Even if the flow conditions could be assessed, the heterogeneity of flow patterns among and within the various injured cord regions would make appropriate dosage delivery impossible to all regions of the injured cord. The cerebrospinal (CSF) has been used as a therapeutic route by a number of investigators, but tissue penetration is largely limited to superficial surfaces in direct contact with the CSF. Cord swelling often complicates CSF flow dynamics in the vicinity of the injured cord, and to further complicate matters, agents that can significantly influence normal central nervous system (CNS) physiology (such as reserpine) may be transported to the brain and there exhibit significant untoward effects. Osterholm has had some success with both microinjections of pharmacologic agents directly into the injured region, and perfusion by the exposed laminectomized or myelotomized cord.[43] On the other hand, if therapeutic agents could be delivered to the ischemic area, their half-lives would most probably be extended owing to slow perfusion washout.

A second problem exists because of the lower cord *p*H secondary to excessive lactate accumulation within the injured cords. The tissue *p*H environment strongly influences drug-receptor binding and the normally resultant pharmacologic effects. Therefore, even if predictable routes of delivery were present, the usually effective dosage regimens may be totally inappropriate.

These are but two of the problems that at present render normal pharmacologic approaches potentially inadequate for the therapeutic treatment of cord injury; doubtless, others exist. In spite of these problems, some success has been made with pharmacologic treatment in spinal cord injuries, at least in the laboratory, and these are discussed below.

Steroids

Because steroids were initially found to be dramatically effective in the treatment of cerebral edema, they were later applied to the treatment of spinal cord injury. Experimental animals receiving steroids following spinal cord injury consistently demonstrate more cord-related protection than do untreated controls.[9,26,28,47] A variety of dosage schedules and routes were examined by Green and coworkers and found to be equivalent in effect.[26] These investigators also noted that after an initial rise (0 to 8 hrs) in endogenous cortisol levels of injured but otherwise untreated animals, the cortisol response was greatly muted. This suggests still another reason why the completely paralyzed patient should be supported by an exogenous steroid. In this context, Alderman and associates found that total adrenal gland removal prior to SCI significantly aggravates the early pathophysiologic environment of the injured cord, suggesting that the endogenous steroids may exert an ameliorating influence when they are released in adequate concentrations.[3] Currently, proposed mechanisms by which the steroids may offer protection include the ability of these agents to maintain the integrity of the parenchymal and vascular membranes, thereby reducing edema and electrolyte abnormalities. The steroids can also prevent the release of lysosomal enzymes and interfere with tissue perioxidase reactions.

Agents Altering Blood Flow

A number of attempts have been made to pharmacologically influence the reduced blood flow attendant upon spinal injury. Dolen and Tator found that altering systemic arterial blood pressure to normotensive or hypotensive levels had no effect on motor behavior.[19] Autoregulation is lost in the injured segment. Rawe and coworkers think that the degree of hemorrhage in the spinal cord tissue is directly related to blood pressure variations, but according to Alderman it is independent of transient trauma-induced increases in blood pressure.[4,49,50] Authors Rivlin and Tator investigated the effect of topical papaverine, intravenous nitroprusside, or myelotomy, treatments they speculated might affect local blood flow to the injured tissue.[52] They observed no effect in the injured tissue. They also found that there was no effect on the recovery of neurologic function with either drug, but that myelotomy substantially improved the chances of recovery. Dow-Edwards and coworkers demonstrated that aminophylline and isoproterenol abolished the alterations in white matter blood flow and reduced the injury-related flow changes in the gray matter.[20] The effect on neurologic function could not be evaluated in their experiments because of the techniques used. Senter, Venes, and Kauer were unable to verify the findings of Dow-Edwards and associates but showed that γ-hydroxybutyrate, a CNS depressant, could abolish traumatically induced ischemia.[57] Both haloperidol and apomorphine dopamine receptor blockers had no effect.

Catecholamines and Other Vasoactive Agents and Their Pharmacologic Antagonists

The hypothesis that catecholamines (CA) might be involved in the etiology of at least some of the adverse events that follow SCI was first proposed by Osterholm and Mathews.[45] Their hypothesis was an attractive one because it offered an explanation of the mechanisms that underlie the initiation of the severe ischemia that in turn is almost certainly responsible for a majority of the additional pathophysiologic findings associated with SCI. Osterholm proposed that the CA norepinephrine (NE), which is stored in both noradrenergic nerve endings supplying the spinal cord parenchyma and portions of the vasculature, was released in abnormally large amounts immediately following cord trauma. The released NE could then act upon adrenergic receptors in the microvasculature to induce severe vasoconstriction and hence ischemia. Although the extent to which NE is involved in SCI, if at all, has yet to be conclusively determined, the hypothesis has stimulated researchers to investigate the potential involvement of not only this agent but others as well.[5] Investigators have since proposed a number of endogenous vasoactive agents (serotonin, histamine, the prostaglandins, and others) that might be involved in the response to SCI.[11,30,36,69] The evidence supporting these agents is too complicated an issue to discuss properly in this chapter, but it is theoretically possible that any or all of the above-mentioned agents could be involved in SCI. It is upon this premise that attempts have been made to pharmacologically antagonize their actions.

Phenoxybenzamine. If NE is acting to constrict the microvasculature of the injured spinal cord, the adrenergic blocker phenoxybenzamine (PB) should provide some protection in SCI. PB has the advantage of being covalently bound to its receptor sites, thereby being less susceptible to displacement by significant environmental *p*H changes. It can also block vascular constriction due to serotonin.

When experimental animals were treated with PB prior to SCI, dogs responded with improved motor function and cats with reduced cord necrosis and reduced cord hemorrhaging.[29,43,49] Rawe feels that this drug probably exerts its protective influence at the peripheral level by blocking the transient systemic pressor response that follows trauma.[49] Yet there is no evidence to contradict the argument that PB is exerting a protective effect at the local level by preventing the occurrence of vascular constriction. This issue could be easily resolved by simply determining the effect of PB in regional spinal cord blood flow after experimental SCI. It should be emphasized that these studies involved pretreatment with the drug; the drug does not show the same effect if given after the injury, possibly because of posttrauma receptor binding problems.

Other studies of agents designed to interfere with NE function have been both promising and equivocal. Depletion of NE stores with reserpine (also known to deplete stores of other bioamines such as 5HT) has been reported to offer some functional protection in studies by two laboratories and a clinical veterinary study.[9,38,43] Depletion of NE stores with the synthesis inhibitor α-methyltyrosine has yielded both positive and negative reports.[29,43,66]

Serotonin, like NE, is contained in the parenchyma and microvasculature of the mammalian spinal cord, is a powerful vasoconstrictor, and is an edematogenic agent. As mentioned above, both PB and reserpine may exert protection through their antiserotonin effects. In addition, Brodner reported a significant degree of protection in spinal injuries with the serotonin synthesis inhibitor parachlorophenylalanine.[12]

Prompted by a report of elevated histamine (H) levels in the traumatized spinal cord segment, Kobrine and Doyle treated rhesus monkeys with antihistamines of both the H_1 (chlorpheniramine) and H_2 (metiamide) receptor-blocking classes prior to injury and measured their effect on posttraumatic blood flow.[34,39] These authors, in contrast to others, had previously reported a hyperemic response in the lateral funiculus of injured but otherwise untreated animals (see above). After combined antihistamine pretreatment, the hyperemic response was abolished. Although the blood flow response to SCI originally described by these authors does not agree with the findings of most other authors, their observation is limited to the lateral funiculus, and may be indigenous to their specific model and experimental protocol. Nonetheless, a clear-cut interference of the posttraumatic response was noted with the antihistamine treatment, indicating some trauma-related histamine activity. No experiments were conducted to determine whether these agents actively exert a protective effect on the injured cord.

DIMETHYL SULFOXIDE. Dimethyl sulfoxide (DMSO) has been studied in a variety of CNS traumatic insults by de La Torre and associates.[17,18] They showed that intravenous DMSO significantly improved neurologic outcome following impact injury to the spine. Using the reduction in cytochrome oxidase attendant upon spinal injury as an index, Goodenough and coworkers were unable to show any beneficial effect of DMSO.[25] Similar negative results were obtained by Parker and Smith and by Alderman.[48,*]

ENZYMES. Matinian and Andreasian employed a number of proteolytic and mucolytic enzymes in an attempt to inhibit glial–connective tissue scar formation following trauma.[36] It has been proposed that local tissue scar formation that occurs following cord injury may present a physical barrier to endogenous attempts of axonal regeneration.[16] Matinian and Andreasian reasoned that if the scar were eliminated or otherwise compromised, axonal or vascular elements might be able to penetrate this barrier and increase the potential for cord regeneration.[7,36] Although these authors reported affirmative results, others have been unsuccessful using the transected model.[22,27,37]

Other agents that are reputed to offer some degree of protection to the injured spinal cord include osmotic diuretics (used for the antiedema activity), Dilantin, and antifibrinolysin.[13,24,39,46,51] Other drugs have been employed as well with controversial or borderline results, and numerous others have been postulated.

* J. L. Alderman, unpublished observations

REFERENCES

1. *ALBIN MS, WHITE RJ, LOCKE GS ET AL:* Localized spinal cord hypothermia. Anesth Analg 46:8, 1967
2. *ALBIN MS, WHITE RJ, YASHON D, HARRIS LS:* Effects of localized cooling on spinal cord trauma. J Trauma 9:1000, 1969
3. *ALDERMAN JL, OSTERHOLM JL, D'AMORE BR, IRVIN JD:* The influence of the adrenal glands upon acute spinal cord injury. Life Sci 26:1627, 1980
4. *ALDERMAN JL, OSTERHOLM JL, D'AMORE BR ET AL:* Influence of arterial blood pressure upon central hemorrhagic necrosis after severe spinal cord injury. Neurosurgery 4:53, 1979
5. *ALDERMAN JL, OSTERHOLM JL, D'AMORE BR, WILLIAMS HD:* Catecholamine alterations attending spinal cord injury: A reanalysis. Neurosurgery 6:412, 1980
6. *ASSENMACHER DR, DUCKER TB:* Experimental traumatic paraplegia: The vascular and pathological changes seen in reversible and irreversible spinal cord lesions. J Bone Joint Surg 53A:671, 1971
7. *BERNSTEIN JJ, WELLS MR, ZANAKIS MF:* Effects of puromycin on incorporation of [^{3}H] lysine into protein following hemisection of rat spinal cord. Exp Neurol 61:537, 1978
8. *BINGHAM WG, GOLDMAN H, FRIEDMAN SJ ET AL:* Blood flow in normal and injured monkey spinal cord. J Neurosurg 43:162, 1975
9. *BLACK P, MARKOWITZ RS:* Experimental spinal cord injury in monkeys: Comparison of steroids and local hypothermia. Surg Forum 22:409, 1971
10. *BRICOLO A, DALLE ORE G, DAPIAN R, FACCIOLI F:* Local cooling in spinal cord injury. Surg Forum 6:101, 1976
11. *BRODNER RA, DOHRMANN GJ, ROTH RH, RUBIN RA:* Elevated cerebrospinal fluid levels of 5-hydroxytryptamine following experimental spinal cord trauma. Brain Res 118:348, 1976
12. *BRODNER RA, DOHRMANN GJ, ROTH RJ, RUBIN RN:* Correlation of cerebral spinal fluid serotonin and spinal cord blood flow in experimental trauma. Surg Neurol 13:337, 1980
13. *BRODNER RA, VANGILDER JC, COLLINS WF:* The effect of antifibrinolytic therapy in experimental spinal cord trauma. J Trauma 17:48, 1977
14. *CAMPBELL JB, DECRESCITO V, TOMASULA JJ ET AL:* Experimental treatment of spinal cord contusion in the cat. Surg Neurol 1:102, 1973

15. *Cawthon DF, Senter HJ, Stewart WB:* Comparison of hydrogen clearance and ^{14}C-Antipyrine autoradiography in the measurement of spinal cord blood flow after severe impact injury. J Neurosurg 52:801, 1980
16. *Clemente CD:* Structural regeneration in the mammalian central nervous system and the role of neuroglia and connective tissue. In Windle WF (ed): Regeneration in the Central Nervous System, pp 147–161. Springfield, IL, Charles C Thomas, 1955
17. *De La Torre JC, Johnson CM, Goode DJ, Mullan S:* Pharamacologic treatment and evaluation of permanent experimental spinal cord trauma. Neurol 25:508, 1975
18. *De La Torre JC, Kawanaga HM, Rowed DW et al:* Dimethyl sulfoxide in central nervous system trauma. Ann NY Acad Sci 242–243:363–389, 1975
19. *Dolan EJ, Tator CH:* The treatment of hypotension due to acute experimental spinal cord compression injury. Surg Neurol 13:380, 1980
20. *Dow-Edwards D, DeCrescito V, Tomasula JJ, Flamm ES:* Effect of aminophylline and isoproterenol on spinal cord blood flow after impact injury. J Neurosurg 53:385, 1980
21. *Ducker TB, Hamit HF:* Experimental treatments of acute spinal cord injury. J Neurosurg 30:693, 1969
22. *Feringa ER, Kowalski TF, Vahlsing HL, Frye R:* Enzyme treatment of spinal cord transected rats. Ann Neurol 5:203, 1976
23. *Gainer JV:* Use of Crocetin in experimental spinal cord injury. J Neurosurg 46:58–360, 1977
24. *Gerber AM, Olson WL, Harris JH:* Effect of phenytoin on functional recovery after experimental spinal cord injury in dogs. Neurosurg 7(5):472, 1980
25. *Goodenough J, Allen N, Nesham ME, Clendenon NR:* The effect of dimethyl sulfoxide on gray matter injury in experimental spinal cord trauma. Surg Neurol 13:273, 1980
26. *Green BA, Kahn T, Klose KJ:* A comparative study of steroid therapy in acute experimental spinal cord injury. Surg Neurol 13:91, 1980
27. *Guth L, Albuquerque EX, Deshpande SS et al:* Ineffectiveness of enzyme therapy on regeneration in the transected spinal cord of the rat. J Neurosurg 52:73, 1980
28. *Hansebout RR, Kuchner EF, Romero-Sierra C:* Effect of local hypothermia and of steroids upon recovery from experimental spinal cord compression injury. Surg Neurol 4:531, 1975
29. *Hedeman LS, Sil R:* Studies in experimental spinal cord trauma. Part 2: Comparison of treatment with steroids, low molecular weight dextran, and catecholamine blockage. J Neurosurg 40:44, 1974
30. *Jonsson HT, Daniell HB:* Altered levels of PGF in cat spinal cord tissue following traumatic injury. Prostaglandins 11:51, 1976
31. *Kelly DL, Lassiter KRO, Calogero JA et al:* Effects of local hypothermia and tissue oxygen studies in experimental paraplegia. J Neurosurg 33:554, 1970
32. *Kelly DL, Lassiter KRL, Vongsvivut A et al:* Effects of hyperbaric oxygenation and tissue oxygen studies in experimental paraplegia. J Neurosurg 36:425, 1972
33. *Kobrine AI, Doyle TF, Martinez AN:* Local spinal cord blood flow in experimental traumatic myelopathy. J Neurosurg 42:144, 1975
34. *Korbine AI, Doyle TF, Rizzoli HV:* The effect of antihistamines on experimental post-traumatic edema of the spinal cord. Surg Neurol 5:307, 1976
35. *Kuchner EF, Hansebout RR:* Combined steroid and hypothermia treatment of experimental spinal cord injury. Surg Neurol 6:371, 1976
36. *Matinian LA, Andreasian AS:* Enzyme therapy in organic lesions of the spinal cord. Tanasexcu, E (trans). Los Angeles, Brain Information Service, University of California, 1976
37. *Matthews MA, St Onge MF, Faciane CL, Gelderd JB:* Spinal cord transection: A quantitative analysis of elements of the connective tissue matrix formed within the site of lesion following administration of Piromen, Cytoxan, or Trypsin. Neuropathol Appl Neurobiol 5:161, 1979
38. *Mendenhall HV, Litwak P, Yturraspe DJ et al:* Aggressive pharmacologic treatment of spinal cord injuries in dogs and cats. J Am Vet Med Assoc 168:1026, 1976
39. *Naftchi NE, Demeny M, DeCrescito V et al:* Biogenic amine concentrations in traumatized spinal cords of dogs and cats: Effect of drug therapy. J Neurosurg 40:52, 1974
40. *Negrin J:* Spinal cord hypothermia in the neurosurgical management of the acute and chronic post-traumatic paraplegic patient. Paraplegia 10:336, 1973
41. *Negrin J:* Spinal cord hypothermia: Neurosurgical management of immediate and delayed post-traumatic neurologic sequelae. NY State J Med 75:2387, 1975
42. *Northrup BE, Goldstein R, Alderman JL et al:* Presented at the Annual Cervical Spine Meetings, December 1979
43. *Osterholm JL:* The Pathophysiology of Spinal Cord Trauma. Springfield, IL, Charles C Thomas, 1975
44. *Osterholm JL, Hirtz D, Hill HF:* Successful

treatment of severe experimental spinal cord injuries by intracisternal 3-a-Dimethyltyrosine. Surg Forum 2:440, 1973

45. *Osterholm JL, Mathews GJ:* Altered norepinephrine metabolism following experimental spinal cord injury. Part 1: Relationship to hemorrhagic necrosis and post-wounding neurological deficits. J Neurosurg 36:386, 1972
46. *Parker AJ, Park RD, Stowater JL:* Reduction of trauma-induced edema of spinal cord in dogs given Mannitol. Am J Vet Res 34:1355, 1973
47. *Parker AJ, Smith CW:* Functional recovery from spinal cord trauma following dexamethazone and chlorpromazine therapy in dogs. Res Vet Sci 21:246, 1976
48. *Parker AJ, Smith CW:* Lack of functional recovery from spinal cord trauma following dimethylsulphoxide and epsilon amino caprioc acid therapy in dogs. Res Vest Sci 27:253, 1979
49. *Rawe SE, Lee WA, Perot PL:* The histopathology of experimental spinal cord trauma: The effect of systemic blood pressure. J Neurosurg 48:1002, 1978
50. *Rawe SE, Perot PL:* Pressor response resulting in experimental contusion injury to the spinal cord. J Neurosurg 52:58, 1979
51. *Reed JE, Allen WE, Dohrmann GJ:* Effect of Mannitol on the traumatized spinal cord: Microangiography blood flow patterns and electrophysiology. Spine 4:391, 1979
52. *Rivlin AS, Tator CH:* Effect of vasodilatators and myelotomy on recovery after acute spinal cord injury in rats. J Neurosurg 50:349, 1979
53. *Sandler AN, Tator CH:* Review of the effect of spinal cord trauma on the vessels and blood flow in the spinal cord. J Neurosurg 45:638, 1976
54. *Sandler AN, Tator CH:* Effect of acute spinal cord compression injury on regional spinal cord blood flow in primates. J Neurosurg 45:660, 1976
55. *Selker RG:* Icewater irrigation of the spinal cord. Surg Forum 22:411, 1971
56. *Senter HJ, Venes JL:* Loss of autoregulation and post-traumatic ischemia following experimental spinal cord trauma. J Neurosurg 50:198, 1979
57. *Senter JH, Venes JL, Kauer JS:* Alteration of post-traumatic ischemia in experimental spinal cord trauma by a central nervous system depressant. J Neurosurg 50:207, 1979
58. *Smith AJK, McCreery DB, Bloedel JR, Chou SN:* Hyperemia, CO_2 responsiveness, and autoregulation in the white matter following experimental spinal cord injury. J Neurosurg 48:239, 1978
59. *Smith CW, Parker AJ;* Functional recovery from spinal cord trauma following normothermic irrigation in dogs. Res Vet Sci 19:224, 1975
60. *Tator CH:* Spinal cord cooling and irrigation for treatment of acute cord injury. Neural Trauma 363, 1979
61. *Thienprasit P, Bantli H, Bloedel JR, Chou SN:* Effect of delayed local cooling on experimental spinal cord injury. J Neurosurg 42:150, 1975
62. *Tsubokawa T, Nakamura S, Hayashi N et al:* The circulatory disturbance of spinal cord injury and its response to local cooling therapy. Neurol Med Chir (Tokyo) 87, 1975

62a. *Wells JD, Hansebout RR:* Local hypothermia in experimental spinal cord trauma. Surg Neurol 10:200–204, 1978

63. *White RJ:* Current status of spinal cord cooling. Clin Neurosurg 20:400, 1979
64. *White RJ, Albin MS:* The localized vasomotor and permeability changes at the site of injury which determine the second development of permanent damage: The physical approach (cord cooling). Proceedings 19th VA Conference 19:113, 1977
65. *White RJ, Albin MS, Harris L, Yahon D:* Spinal cord injury: Sequential morphology and hypothermic stabilization. Surg Forum 20:432, 1969
66. *Yeo JD, Payne W, Hinwood B, Kidman A:* The experimental contusion injury of the spinal cord in sheep Paraplegia 12:275, 1975
67. *Yeo JD, Stabback S, McKenzie B:* A study of the effects of hyperbaric oxygen on the experimental spinal cord injury. Med J Aust 2:145, 1977
68. *Zielonka JS, Wagner FC, Dohrmann GJ:* Alterations in spinal cord blood flow during local hypotherma. Surg Forum 25:434, 1974
69. *Zivin JA, Doppman JL, Reid JL et al:* Biochemical and histochemical studies of biogenic amines in spinal cord trauma. Neurology 26:99, 1976

Surgical Treatment

PAUL R. COOPER AND JOSEPH RANSOHOFF

Optimal management of patients with fractures or subluxations of the cervical spine who do not have neurologic deficit consists of immobilization, reduction of fractures and subluxations, and stabilization. When spinal cord injury is present in addition to ligamentous disruption, subluxations, or vertebral fractures, the management is rendered more complex. In this situation, the surgeon must not only take action to ensure the immediate and long-term stability of the cervical spine and to reduce any subluxations that are present; he must also prevent additional spinal cord injury and remove spinal cord compression caused by bone, disc, or hematoma.

The preoperative management and the timing and choice of the operation are controversial. Moreover, statistical data on the effects of various operative procedures on the natural history and outcome of spinal cord injury provide little guidance in instituting therapy.

In this section, we attempt to review the most relevant literature to provide a rational guide to the management of patients with injuries of both the spinal cord and the surrounding supportive structures. The details of the various operative approaches to the cervical spine are discussed in detail elsewhere in this volume. This section emphasizes timing, operative decision making, and the simultaneous management of both the neural and bony injuries.

DIAGNOSIS AND PREOPERATIVE MANAGEMENT

The clinical diagnosis of cervical spinal cord injury is generally obvious and is usually made by the emergency room physician or emergency medical technicians before the neurosurgeon or orthopedic surgeon is called in for consultation. The details of the examination are discussed in another section. It is important, however, that the initial examination be detailed and accurately recorded so that it can serve as a baseline for judging whether the patient is improving, stabilizing, or deteriorating. This clinical course has a significant bearing on the timing and choice of therapy.

The patient is initially kept immobile by a wooden board with head strap or cervical collar applied at the scene of the injury. If the head has not been immobilized, this may be achieved by placing adhesive tape across the patient's forehead to either side of the stretcher, or by placing sandbags at the sides of the head.

After immobilization, but before x-ray films are obtained, all patients should have an assessment of the adequacy of ventilation. Arterial blood gases confirm decreased ventilatory exchange. Clinical observation also provides important clues of respiratory insufficiency. Tachypnea, shallow respirations, and cyanosis are all indications for respiratory assistance. Sometimes mask or nasal oxygen is sufficient. Often, however, endotracheal intubation and assisted ventilation are necessary to maintain adequate gas exchange. The neck should never be manipulated during intubation. Fiberoptic endotracheal intubation is safe and generally possible without manipulation of the neck. If fiberoptic intubation is not feasible, a relatively small endotracheal tube should be introduced through the nose. If attempts at intubation are not successful, a tracheostomy is indicated.

Hypotension and bradycardia often result from sympathetic denervation that accompanies spinal cord injury. The hypotension is generally of little clinical consequence and may be corrected by administration of appropriate crystalloid solutions. Following these resuscitative efforts, a lateral roentgenogram of the entire cervical spine should be taken without moving the patient from the stretcher. Complete visualization of the cervical spine may be achieved by pulling the patient's arms caudally or by obtaining a swimmer's view.

Stabilization, Reduction, and Further Assessment of the Injury

Once the fracture or subluxation is identified, the patient is moved, with the neck immobilized, from the stretcher to a hospital bed and is placed in cervical traction. A number of traction apparatuses have been described, and most are satisfactory. Our current preference is a halo ring secured to the patient's head and connected to appropriate weights over a pulley apparatus. The halo ring may subsequently be connected to a plaster or plastic molded vest. Gardner-Wells tongs, which may also be used, are easily inserted into the skull after the scalp is shaved, prepared, and anesthetized. We no longer use Crutchfield tongs because they are time consuming to insert and frequently become disengaged.

The goal of cervical traction in the patient with spinal cord injury is to achieve satisfactory positioning of bone fragments and to "decompress the spinal cord by restoring the anteroposterior diameter of the cervical spinal canal."[35] Initially, traction is begun with 3 to 4 kg of weight. The neck is kept in a neutral or slightly extended position, and traction is applied in the direction of the long axis of the body. After 30 minutes, a lateral cervical spine roentgenogram is taken; if the subluxation is reduced, the patient is maintained with this amount of weight. If the subluxation is not reduced, the weight is increased in 2-kg increments every 2 to 3 hours until reduction is achieved.

The maximum weight that is safe to apply is a matter of controversy, although 23 kg, 30 kg, and 35 kg have been suggested.[11,13,15,36] Fried emphasized that these estimates may have to be revised downward for elderly patients. He presented two cases of neurologic deterioration after weights well within these guidelines were applied.[15] If distraction between the vertebral bodies is seen, the weights should be reduced (Fig. 7-19). We emphasize that frequent neurologic examination is mandatory as weights are being added or removed in order to document changes in neurologic functioning.

If the subluxation cannot be reduced because of locking facet joints, muscle relaxants such as diazepam may be given intravenously. Before giving muscle relaxants, the weights should be reduced and then slowly increased over a period of several

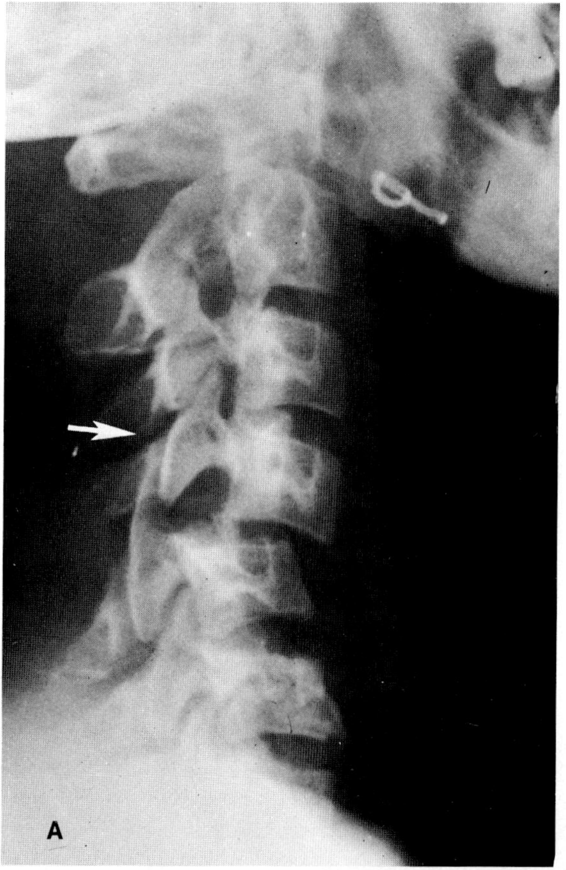

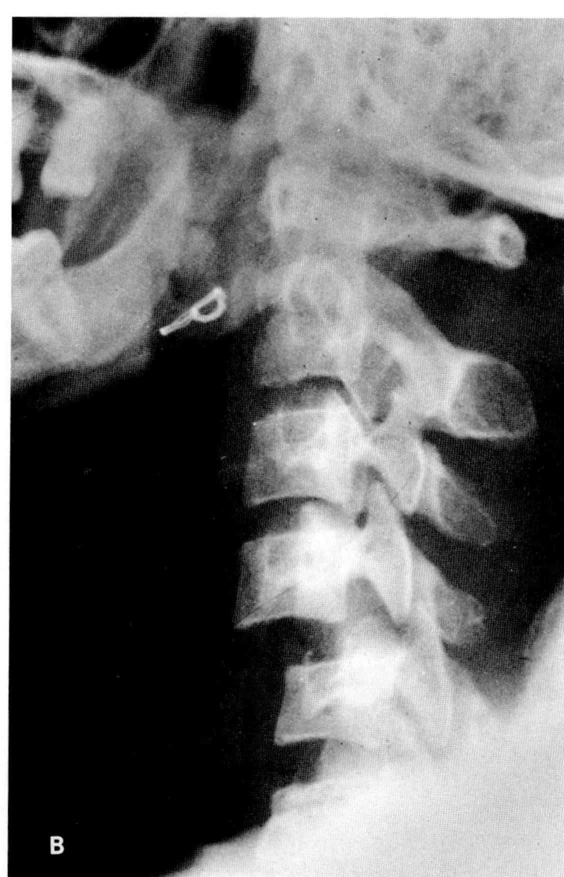

Fig. 7-19. (*A*) Lateral cervical spine roentgenogram of a patient with C4–C5 fracture subluxation and a jumped facet (*arrow*). (*B*) Lateral cervical spine roentgenogram after application of 15 kg of traction. The facet remains locked with persistent subluxation. There is some distraction at the C4–C5 interspace. Facetectomy was necessary to achieve reduction.

hours. The subsequent management of patients who remain subluxed in spite of all attempts at reduction is discussed under the section on facetectomy.

In patients with incomplete loss of neurologic function below the level of injury, myelography is performed as soon after admission as is practicable. Patients are placed on the myelography table in the supine position, and contrast material is introduced into the subarachnoid space through a lateral C1–C2 puncture. We now use 6 to 10 ml of iopamidol (Omnipaque-180) as the contrast agent. It is preferred to metrizamide because it provides greater contrast and has low toxicity. Oil-soluble agents, such as Pantopaque, are no longer used.

After contrast material is introduced, x-ray films are taken in both the frontal and lateral projections without moving the patient. The patients are then moved in traction to the computed tomography (CT) scanner, where attention is directed to the level of spinal cord compression seen on myelography. Scanning should also include areas of suspected bone and ligamentous injury. All imaging should be performed with both bone and soft-tissue windows.

Those patients with incomplete neurologic deficit and anterior (or less frequently, posterior) extradural compression are candidates for operative decompression and stabilization. The management of patients with cervical spinal cord swelling without extrinsic compression rarely includes operation (Fig. 7-20) and is only considered in the occasional instance of progressive loss of function (see General Indications for Early Operation).

Discography has been used as a preoperative diagnostic procedure in patients with severe injuries of the cervical spine.[26] Although it will show any leakage of contrast material from an injured disc, it cannot reliably delineate the site and severity of spinal cord compression. For this reason we believe it adds little to the diagnostic evaluation of these patients.

In the past, hypocycloidal tomography was used to define the anatomy of fractures and subluxations. Extensive use of tomography revealed that less than one half of all fractures were identified on plain films.[19] In spite of the usefulness of polytomography for the identification of bony abnormalities, high-resolution CT scanning is now the preferred diagnostic procedure in evaluating the bony injuries. Routine CT scanning clearly demonstrates fractures and subluxations (Fig. 7-21). With water-soluble contrast agents such as iopamidol in the subarachnoid space, one may simultaneously visualize the spinal cord and its relationship to surrounding structures in far greater detail than is achieved by conventional myelography. Thus, with CT evaluation the entire examination can be conducted with this single technique (Fig. 7-22).

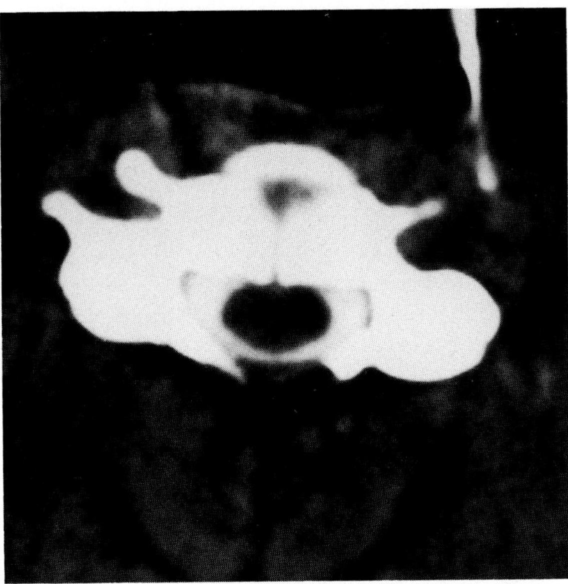

Fig. 7-20. CT/myelogram of patient with complete neurologic deficit following cervical spine injury. Fracture is seen in the vertebral body. The spinal cord is swollen, but there is no extrinsic compression of the dural tube.

INDICATIONS FOR AND CONTRAINDICATIONS TO OPERATION

There are two separate (but related) considerations in selecting the operative strategy for the patient with cervical spinal cord injury. The surgeon must first ask whether the spinal cord is being extrinsically compressed and whether anything can be done to relieve the compression. The surgeon must also determine whether the bony spine is unstable and how best to maintain stability for both the short and the long term (Fig. 7-23).

Operation shortly after admission is rarely needed for providing long-term stability of the cervical spine. In general, urgent operative intervention is reserved for patients with extrinsic cer-

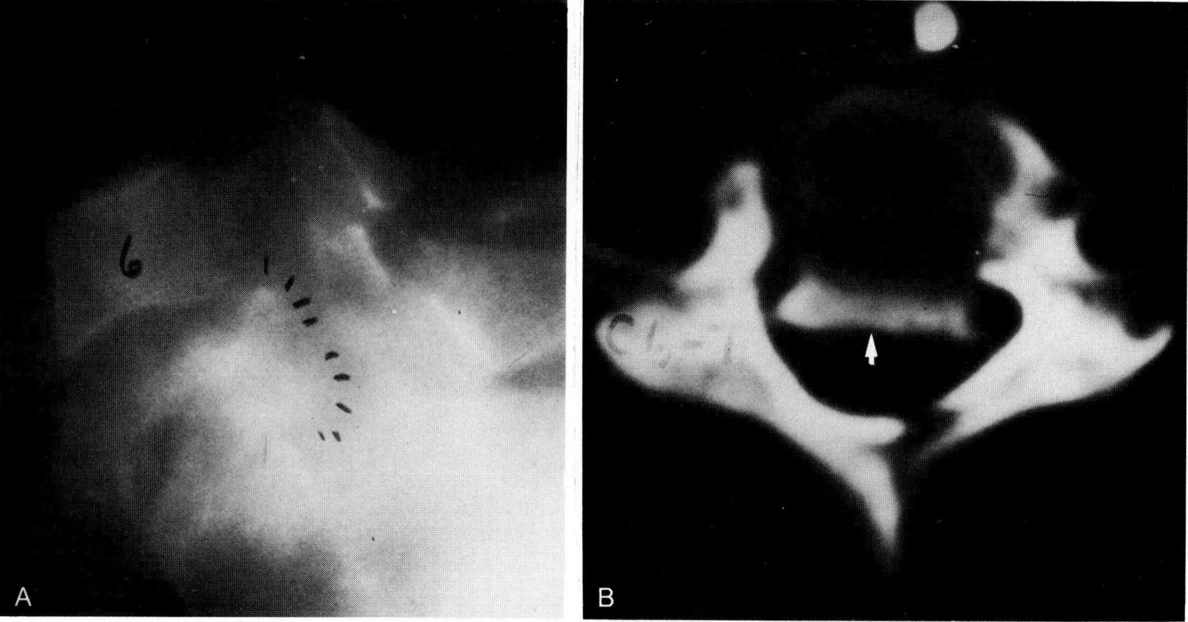

Fig. 7-21. (*A*) Lateral tomogram of the cervical spine demonstrating fragments of the C7 vertebral body retropulsed into the spinal canal in a patient with incomplete neurologic deficit. (*B*) CT scan of a patient with an injury similar to that seen in (*A*). Arrow delineates retropulsed body. Note also fracture at junction of lamina and spinous process. CT scan is clearly superior to polytomogram in clarifying the relationship of the spinal canal to surrounding bony structures.

vical spinal cord compression who also have progressive neurologic deterioration, in spite of adequate immobilization. The timing of decompression in patients with extrinsic spinal cord compression and partial neurologic deficit who are not deteriorating is controversial. At first glance, it seems that early decompression would be beneficial. However, Marshall and colleagues,[23] in an analysis of data from a multicenter study, showed that neurologic deterioration occurred exclusively in patients operated on within 5 days after injury.

In view of these data and those of Heiden and colleagues,[18] which also showed an increase in morbidity with early operation, and considering the absence of a controlled study showing improved outcome as a result of early operation, it seems that early operation is not indicated in neurologically stable patients with partial neurologic deficit. Indeed, experimental data exist to confirm the correctness of this approach. Bohlman and associates showed that complete recovery occurred in dogs if spinal cord compression was relieved as long as 8 weeks after the initial compression injury.[3]

Perhaps the major contraindication to operation is the complete loss of motor and sensory function below the level of the patient's spinal cord injury, regardless of the presence of neural compression.[7,18,29,33,34] Patients with preservation of motor or sensory function (no matter how slight) sometimes have return of useful motor function. In these patients, no therapeutic alternative should be overlooked.

In contrast, patients with complete sensory and motor loss do not regain useful function, regardless of the treatment, except in the rarest circumstances. Although Gillingham reported six patients with complete motor and sensory deficit who recovered "to a greater or lesser extent" after traction was applied,[16] he did not state that any of these patients were able to walk.

In summary, early operation in the first few days after injury is, in our opinion, indicated only in patients who experience neurologic deterioration

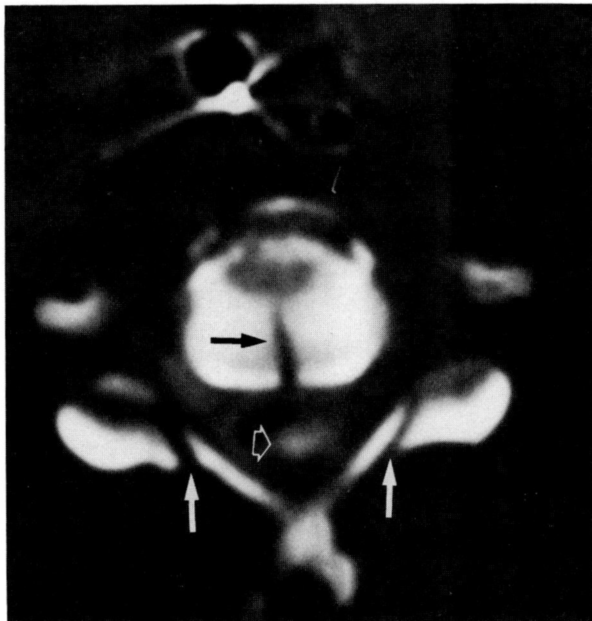

Fig. 7-22. CT/myelogram with bone windows of a patient with a severe spine and spinal cord injury. Black arrow demonstrates fracture of vertebral body. White arrows show bilateral laminar fractures. Open arrow shows contrast which has passed from the subarachnoid space to the center of the spinal cord, a sign of severe irreversible spinal cord injury.

in spite of adequate immobilization. In particular, we believe that there is no evidence that operative decompression in patients with *total* loss of neurologic functioning below the level of their injury has any significant beneficial effect on outcome. Regardless of the presence of neurologic deficit, operative stabilization of fractures and subluxations is indicated in patients who cannot be adequately reduced in cervical traction or safely immobilized in a halo vest.

CHOICE OF OPERATIVE PROCEDURE

Anterior Approach

In the vast majority of patients with spinal cord compression, neural structures are compressed anteriorly by bone or disc fragments. The anterior approach to the cervical spine as described by Smith and Robinson allows these fragments to be removed anterior to the spinal cord.[32] In contrast, the posterior approach (by means of a laminectomy) requires the surgeon to retract or work around an already injured, compromised spinal cord, with generally disastrous consequences.

Although the details of the operative approach are described in Chapter 13, several comments on the procedure as it pertains to patients with trauma to both the spinal column and spinal cord may be helpful. We believe that the anterior approach to the spine as described by Smith and Robinson[32] has several advantages over the Cloward procedure.[8] First, the Smith and Robinson procedure allows the surgeon to tailor a bone plug to fit the exact shape of the resected vertebral body fragments without compromising the fit of the bone plug. With the Cloward procedure, the surgeon is committed to removing a preselected round plug of bone from two adjacent vertebral bodies. In addition, the Cloward drill pushes down on the vertebral bodies and disc and theoretically (and perhaps actually) can push loose bone or disc fragments posteriorly to produce additional compression of the spinal cord.

The treatment of the posterior longitudinal ligament in patients who are undergoing anterior operation for cervical spinal cord and spinal column injury is controversial. Bohlman has stated that the surgeon "should not intentionally violate the posterior longitudinal ligament" simply to inspect the dura.[2] In patients who have sustained trauma and whose myelogram shows anterior extradural compression, the posterior longitudinal ligament must be removed to visualize any bone or disc fragments that may have extruded into the spinal canal between the ligament and the dura.[25,34] The absence of a visible tear in the ligament does not mean that bone or disc has not herniated posterior to the ligament; disc herniations may remain occult until much of the ligament is removed, even when microsurgical techniques are used.

In general, there is less urgency about operating to produce stability than to decompress the spinal cord. Cervical traction almost always provides excellent immobilization until the patient is in optimum condition for operation, 1 or 2 weeks, or even longer, after injury. Although the anterior approach with interbody bone grafting is essential to removing masses that compress the ventral aspect of the spinal cord, using the procedure to produce stability in the spinal-cord-injured patient without spinal-cord compression is questionable. In these circumstances, anterior cervical fusion is indicated in extension injuries involving disc dis-

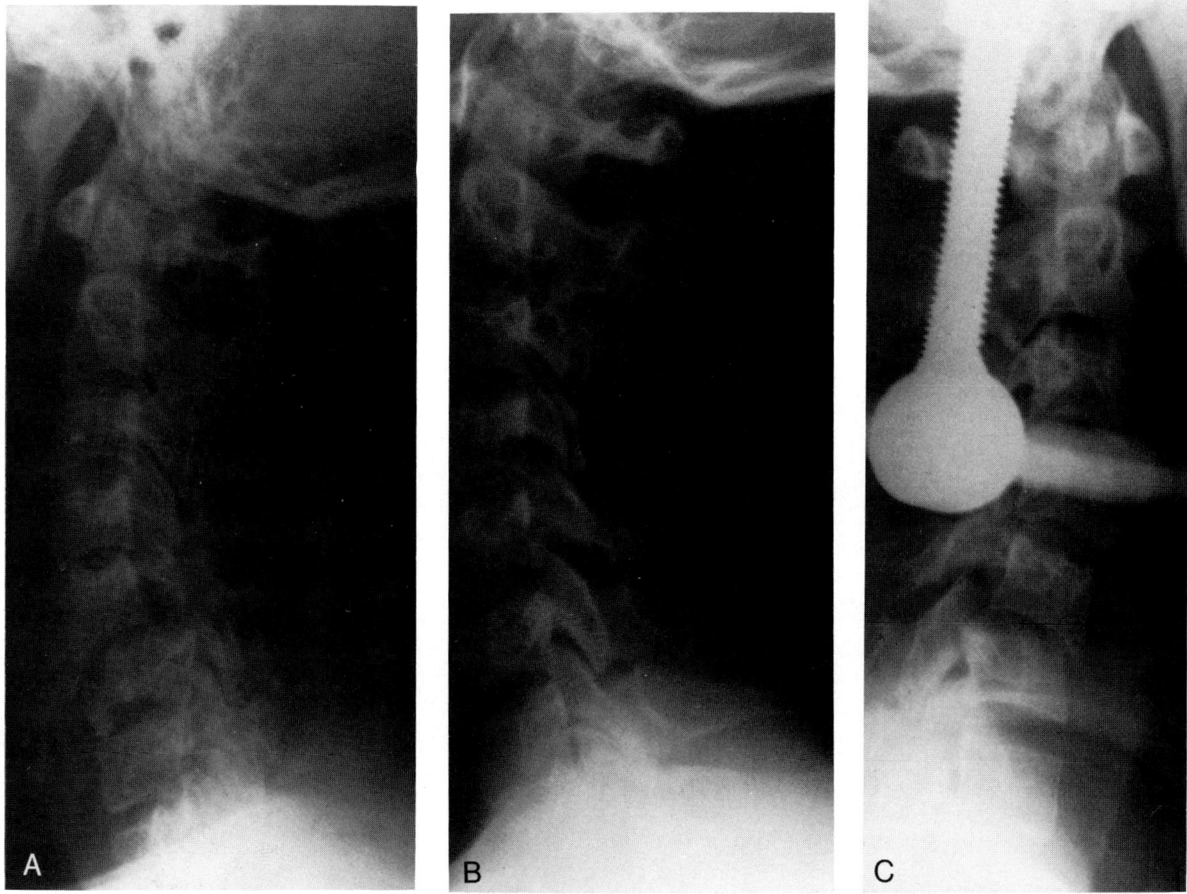

Fig. 7-23. (*A*) Lateral cervical spine roentgenogram of a patient with a C5–C6 subluxation and both anterior and posterior ligamentous instability. (*B*) Alignment is excellent after reduction in traction. (*C*) The patient was placed in a halo vest, but subluxation recurred. Such patients with severe ligamentous instability frequently cannot be held in reduction with orthosis. For the most part, they are no longer managed with external immobilization but are treated primarily with posterior cervical fusion.

ruption and injury to the anterior longitudinal ligament.[2]

Patients with flexion injuries that disrupt the posterior longitudinal ligament and facet joints are best approached by means of a posterior cervical fusion.[2,13,28] An anterior approach in these patients necessitates removal of the anterior longitudinal ligament and disc, both of which may result in additional instability in spite of the insertion of an interbody bone graft. We have seen some of these patients sublux in the postoperative period even when immobilized with the halo vest. The application of the anterior plate described by Kaspar[21] stabilizes the vertebral bodies above and below the graft and prevents this problem from occurring.

Laminectomy

In most circumstances laminectomy has nothing to offer the patient with a cervical spinal cord injury. It is indicated only in those rare instances of fracturing of the posterior elements of the cervical spine with dorsal compression of the spinal cord (most often occurring as a result of direct blows). In spite of this, as recently as 1975, laminectomy was performed in over 10% of patients with cervical spine injuries treated by neurosurgical practitioners in the Greater Los Angeles area.[18]

When the spinal cord is compressed anteriorly by bone or disc fragments, laminectomy by itself will not result in decompression of the dural tube. Attempts at removal of anteriorly placed fragments from a posterior approach is fraught with danger and has a high risk of exacerbating neurologic deficit. Laminectomy has also been performed to decompress a swollen spinal cord and has been advocated as a means of treating patients with a complete spinal block.[9] A swollen spinal cord or one that is posteriorly displaced by disc or bone fragments makes laminectomy a risky procedure because there is little or no room between the laminae and the already-injured spinal cord. Comarr, a proponent of laminectomy, was unable to show improvement in patients who had this procedure compared with those who had no operative intervention.[9] Indeed, his data seem to indicate that a higher percentage of nonlaminectomized patients had neurologic improvement.

Although some data indicate that patients having laminectomy improve after the procedure, there is no evidence that laminectomy *caused* the improvement.[24] Most likely, the patients would have improved, even if left untreated. The data of Morgan and coworkers[24] indicated that almost one quarter of all patients who had laminectomy within 48 hours of their injury and two thirds who had operation more than 48 hours after injury deteriorated. Because the percentage of patients deteriorating is so much higher than expected in patients managed without operation, it is likely that the operative procedure caused the deterioration. Bohlman and coworkers reviewed 300 cervical spine injuries and also concluded that laminectomy should be avoided.[2] Of 64 patients undergoing laminectomy, 10 suffered permanent loss of motor function.

Laminectomy in patients with cervical spinal cord injury and an unstable spine has an additional disadvantage: It may increase instability, result in late deformity, and make subsequent posterior cervical fusion difficult or impossible.

Facetectomy

Excision of the facet joints is indicated in patients with locked facets and subluxation that cannot be reduced by cervical traction. Special care must be taken during induction of anesthesia, intubation, and turning of the patient to the prone position to avoid manipulation of the neck. When anesthesia is induced, traction is reduced to 2 kg to 3 kg. The overriding facet or facets are exposed and are easily identified because the lower facet is seen to be posterior to the upper one. We use the high-speed air drill with a small burr to remove the overriding facet or facets. Often, only a portion of the facet must be removed before operative manipulation results in restoration of normal alignment and anatomic relationships. Nevertheless, these patients are very unstable and need posterior fusion (see below) at the time of facetectomy to assure both short-term and long-term stability.

Posterior Cervical Fusion

Posterior cervical fusion is indicated in patients who have flexion injuries with disruption of the posterior ligamentous complex.[2] These patients should not be stabilized by means of the anterior approach for the reasons presented earlier in this section.

A number of techniques have been described for the stabilization of the cervical spine by a posterior approach.[14,20,31] We now prefer to use the Roy-Camille plates for posterior stabilization of the middle and lower cervical spine.[27] They are easy to insert and provide immediate stability of the spine, without the need for bone grafting. These plates are screwed bilaterally into the articular masses of the involved vertebrae. They may be used to stabilize two or three vertebrae (one or two joints) and are particularly advantageous when fractures of the laminae or spinous processes preclude interspinous wiring.

If the Roy-Camille plates are not used, we stabilize the spine posteriorly with interspinous wiring and bone grafting, using a technique similar to that described by Johnson and Southwick.[20] Cahill and associates[4] have described a bilateral fusion of facet to spinous process, which has the theoretical advantage over the fusion of spinous process to spinous process of preventing rotational movement. Sublaminar wires should not be used below the C2 level in the cervical spine; the space between the spinal cord and lamina is small, and spinal cord injury may easily result from passage of wire beneath the laminae.

A fusion utilizing methylmethacrylate has been performed by some and has been described by Six and Kelly.[31] Acrylic adds little strength to wire fusion, is an organic foreign body capable of being infected, and is never incorporated into living tissue. Except for patients with pathologic fractures due to cancer, it is inferior to the bony fusion and should probably not be used. Indeed, experimental evidence suggests that acrylic progressively loses strength, providing less than bone fusion after 3 months."[35]

Myelotomy and Duroplasty

Myelotomy has been advocated in patients with spinal cord injury who have myelographic block without evidence of extrinsic spinal cord compression and in whom "the appearance of the exposed spinal cord suggests intramedullary hematoma and/or necrotic cord tissue."[30] The goal is removal of intramedullary hematoma and necrotic spinal cord tissue to prevent progressive hemorrhagic spinal cord infarction. Decompression of the swollen spinal cord may also be achieved by duroplasty, with fascia lata or synthetic materials. Unfortunately, no clinical data suggest that myelotomy or duroplasty beneficially influences the course or outcome of patients with spinal cord injury who do not have progressive neurologic deficit. We have already cited evidence that laminectomy in spinal cord–injured patients may result in exacerbation of the neurologic deficit. Because laminectomy must be performed to gain the exposure needed for posterior myelotomy and duroplasty, it is possible that the condition of certain patients may be poorer as a result of this procedure.

Spinal Cord Irrigation

Ice-water irrigation of the spinal cord has been proposed as a treatment for the amelioration of spinal cord injury.[1,30] There is no evidence that this procedure results in neurologic improvement in patients. Because exposure of the spinal cord for this procedure is accomplished by performing a laminectomy, it has the same risks as that procedure.

GUNSHOT WOUNDS

The objectives of the operative treatment of penetrating spine wounds have been summarized by Heiden and associates: (1) débridement of the missile tract and removal of missile and bone from the spinal canal, (2) dural closure to eliminate cerebrospinal fluid fistulas, (3) decompression of the injured spinal cord, and (4) visual identification of spinal cord injury to determine the prognosis.[19] Traditionally, laminectomy has accomplished these objectives.

We believe that laminectomy is indicated in patients with penetrating wounds who do not have immediate and total loss of neurological function. Removal of foreign bodies and bone fragments and repair of dural tears provide the optimal environment for recovery of function. Other data, however, indicate that operative exploration has no effect on the prognosis of patients with low-velocity missile wounds (whether their spinal cord injuries are total or partial) and that the only indication for operation is progressive neurologic deficit. Visual inspection of the spinal cord (unless it is transected) is not helpful in determining prognosis. In addition, patients with low-velocity civilian wounds who are managed nonoperatively do not have an increased incidence of infectious complications when compared with patients who are operatively treated.[19]

NONOPERATIVE TREATMENT

Nonoperative treatment of patients with spinal cord injuries is an acceptable management alternative in patients who have complete neurologic injury and in those with partial injury who do not have extrinsic spinal cord compression. Where compression is not present, the primary goal of therapy is stabilization of the spinal column. Indeed, Guttmann believes that there are rarely indications for operative intervention and that virtually all patients are best served by conservative treatment consisting of skull traction for reduction of subluxations and healing of unstable areas.[17] It is likely that Guttmann overstated his case and that the truth lies somewhere between his point of view and that of Norell and Wilson, who advocated anterior fusion for virtually all patients.[25]

Many patients with unstable spines can be successfully managed with external immobilization. Cervical traction and bed rest, advocated by Guttman, are now infrequently used; the majority of patients can be managed using a halo vest.[10] Originally, it was thought by some that patients with spinal cord injury and lack of sensation might not be candidates for the halo because of their propensity to develop skin breakdown at pressure points; however, more recent data show that the incidence of this complication is low. Moreover, patients whose fractures are stabilized with the halo vest can be immediately immobilized and can receive early rehabilitation therapy.

External immobilization in the halo vest is specifically contraindicated in patients with unsatisfactorily reduced fracture dislocations and should probably be avoided in those who have ligamentous instability without bone injury.[10] Patients in the latter group have a high incidence of instability after halo treatment or other forms of immobilization, and cervical fusion should be their primary treatment modality.[2,10] Instability, in spite of external immobilization, is also seen in patients who have disruption of both anterior and posterior elements.[9] Overall, late instability after external immobilization (either by the halo or cervical traction) has been reported to range from 5.4% to 15%.[2,5,6,10]

REFERENCES

1. *ALBIN MS, WHITE RJ, LOCKE GS, ET AL:* Localized spinal cord hypothermia: Anesthetic effects and application to spinal cord injury. Anesth Analg 46:8, 1967
2. *BOHLMAN HH:* Complications of treatment of fractures and dislocations of the cervical spine. In Epps CH Jr (ed): Complications in Orthopaedic Surgery, pp 611–641. Philadelphia, JB Lippincott Co, 1978
3. *BOHLMAN HH, BAHNIUK E, RASKULINECZ G, FIELD G:* Mechanical factors affecting recovery from incomplete cervical spinal cord injury: A preliminary report. Johns Hopkins Med J 145:115, 1979
4. *CAHILL DW, BELLEGARRIQUE R, DUCKER TB:* Bilateral facet to spinous process fusion: a new technique for posterior spinal fusion after trauma. Neurosurgery 13:1, 1983
5. *CHAN RC, SCHWEIGEL JF, THOMPSON GB:* Halothoracic brace immobilization in 188 patients with acute cervical spine injuries. J Neurosurg 58:508–515, 1983
6. *CHESHIRE DJE:* The stability of the cervical spine following the conservative treatment of fractures and fracture-dislocations. Paraplegia 7:193, 1969–1970
7. *CLAWSON DK, GUNN DR, FRY LR, ET AL:* Letter to the Editor: Early anterior fusion for cervical spine injury. JAMA 215:2113, 1971
8. *CLOWARD RB:* Treatment of acute fractures and fracture dislocations of the cervical spine by vertebral body fusion: A report of eleven cases. J Neurosurg 18:201, 1961
9. *COMARR AE:* Laminectomy in patients with injuries of the spinal cord. J Int Coll Surg 31:437, 1959
10. *COOPER PR, MARAVILLA KR, SKLAR FH, ET AL:* Halo immobilization of cervical spine fractures: Indications and results. J Neurosurg 50:603, 1979
11. *CRUTCHFIELD WG:* Skeletal traction in treatment of injuries to the cervical spine. JAMA 155:29, 1954
12. *DUCKER TB, BELLEGARRIGUE R, SALCMAN M, WALLECK C:* Timing of operative care in cervical spinal cord injury. Spine 9:525–531, 1984
13. *FEUER H:* Management of acute spine and spinal cord injuries: Old and new concepts. Arch Surg 111:638, 1976
14. *FORSYTH HF, ALEXANDER ED JR, DAVIS C JR, UNDERDAL R:* The advantages of early spine fusion in the treatment of fracture dislocation of the cervical spine. J Bone Joint Surg 41A:17, 1959
15. *FRIED LC:* Cervical spinal cord injury during skeletal traction. JAMA 229:181, 1974
16. *GILLINGHAM J:* Letter to the Editor: Early Management of spinal cord trauma. J Neurosurg 44:766, 1976
17. *GUTTMANN L:* Spinal Cord Injuries: Comprehensive Management and Research. Oxford, Blackwell Scientific Publications, 1973
18. *HEIDEN JS, WEISS JH, ROSENBERG AW, ET AL:* Management of cervical spinal cord trauma in Southern California. J Neurosurg 43:732, 1975
19. *HEIDEN JS, WEISS JH, ROSENBERG AW, ET AL:* Penetrating gunshot wounds of the cervical spine in civilians. Review of 38 cases. J Neurosurg 42:575, 1975
20. *JOHNSON RM, SOUTHWICK WO:* Surgical approaches to the spine. In Rothman RH, Simeone FA (eds): The Spine, pp 69–156. Philadelphia, WB Saunders, 1975
21. *KASPER W:* Anterior cervical fusion and interbody stabilization with the trapezial osteosynthetic plate technique. Aesculap Scientific Information 12:1, 1985
22. *MARAVILLA KR, COOPER PR, SKLAR FH:* The influence of thin-section tomography on the treatment of cervical spine injuries. Radiology 127:131, 1978
23. *MARSHALL LF, KNOWLTON S, GIRFIN SR, ET AL:* Deterioration following spinal cord injury. A multicenter study. J Neurosurg 66:400, 1987
24. *MORGAN TH, WHARTON GW, AUSTIN GN:* The results of laminectomy in patients with incomplete spinal cord injuries. Paraplegia 9:14, 1971
25. *NORRELL H, WILSON CB:* Early anterior fusion for injuries of the cervical portion of the spine. JAMA 214:525, 1970
26. *RAYNOR RB:* Severe injuries of the cervical spine treated by early interbody fusion and ambulation. J Neurosurg 28:311, 1968
27. *ROY-CAMILLE R, SAILLANT G, BERTEAUX, SERGE MA:* Early management of spinal injuries. In McKibben B (ed): Recent Advances in Orthopaedics, pp 57–87. Edinburgh, New York, London, Churchill Livingstone, 1979
28. *SAN GIORGI SM:* Orthopaedic aspects of the treatment of injuries to the lower cervical spine. Acta Neurochir 22:227, 1970
29. *SCHNEIDER RC, CROSBY EC, RUSSO RH, GOSCH HH:* Traumatic spinal cord syndromes and their management. Clin Neurosurg 20:424, 1972

30. *Selker RG:* Ice water irrigation of the spinal cord. Surg Forum 22:411, 1971
31. *Six E, Kelly DS Jr:* Technique for C-1, C-2, C-3 fixation in cases of odontoid fracture. Neurosurgery 8:374, 1981
32. *Smith GW, Robinson RA:* The treatment of certain cervical spine disorders by anterior removal of the intervertebral disc and interbody fusion. J Bone Joint Surg 40A:607, 1958
33. *Suwanwela C, Alexander E Jr, Davis CH Jr:* Prognosis in spinal cord injury with special reference to patients with motor paralysis and sensory preservation. J Neurosurg 19:220, 1962
34. *Verbiest H:* Anterolateral operations for fractures and dislocations in the middle and lower parts of the cervical spine: Report of a series of forty-seven cases. J Bone Joint Surg 51A:1489, 1969
35. *Whitehill R, Bany J:* Evolution of stability in the cervical spine. Constructs using either autogenous bone graft or methylmethacrylate cement: a follow-up report on a canine in vivo model. Spine 10:32, 1985

Rehabilitation of Posttraumatic Cervical Spinal Cord Quadriplegia and Pentaplegia

E. SHANNON STAUFFER

The first question the patient and his family want answered following an injury to the cervical spinal cord is, "What are the chances of recovery?" The decisions about medical and surgical management and the rehabilitation potential depend on an accurate assessment of the degree and level of the injury to the spinal cord. It is of primary importance to ascertain whether the spinal cord injury is complete or incomplete. Incomplete injuries have a good prognosis for progressive recovery of spinal cord function, depending upon the degree of injury, and the area of the spinal cord affected. In complete injuries that demonstrate no recovery of cord function, specific rehabilitation goals are dictated by the segmental level of the spinal cord injury and the associated injury to the nerve roots innervating the upper extremities. Rehabilitation has assumed an increasingly important role in the management of patients with permanent pentaplegia and quadriplegia during the past 2 decades.[1] With the advent of intensive emergency care for patients with fractures of the spine and the improvement in management of pulmonary complications and urologic infections, the survival rate of patients with cervical spinal cord injuries has vastly improved over the past 10 years. Experience reveals that there is a high incidence of mortality in the first 2 to 3 months postinjury. The mortality depends upon the severity of coexisting injuries, the age of the patient, and the level of the spinal cord injury. The survival statistics indicate that 80% of the quadriplegic patients who survive the first 3 months survive at least 10 years.[3]

The primary responsibility of the physician during the first examination is to document the extent of the spinal cord injury. The preservation of any long-tract function of the spinal cord indicating a partial or incomplete injury must be noted. If the patient has a complete spinal cord injury that persists for 24 hours with evidence of reflex activity recurring in the sacral areas, he can be classified as a "complete injury" patient in whom no distal recovery will occur.[4] If, however, the patient has any signs of "sacral sparing," which are elicited by examining the areas of sacral nerve innervation (*i.e.*, sensation around the anus and the perineum as well as motor control of the rectal sphincter and toe flexor muscle), the patient is classified as having an "incomplete injury" and may show progressive recovery. The incomplete spinal cord injury can be subclassified as a Brown-Séquard (hemisection) injury, a central cord syndrome, or an anterior cord syndrome, depending upon the degree and location of the injury. Each of these syndromes has a specific statistical prognosis. The examination for sacral sparing is very important because if any fibers are still intact transmitting spinal cord function distally in the apparently complete injury, they will be along the periphery of the spinal cord. The most peripheral fibers of the long tracts, the spinothalamic sensory and corticospinal motor fibers, innervate the sacral segments. Therefore, the fine difference between the complete versus the incomplete injury often rests on the presence or absence of sacral innervated perineal sensation alone.

INCOMPLETE CORD INJURIES

The patient with Brown-Séquard syndrome, in which the injury lateralizes to one half of the spinal cord, has the best prognosis. His motor paralysis is distal to the injury on the same side as the injury, and his loss of sensation is distal to the injury on the opposite side of the body. Therefore, he has greater motor strength associated with less sensation on one side of the body and greater weakness but better sensation on the opposite side. Most patients with this syndrome are able to ambulate and recover bowel and bladder control.

The central cord syndrome is an apparent complete motor paralysis distal to the level of injury but with preservation of a small amount of sensation, allowing sharp–dull discrimination around the sacral area. Since the motor tracts are near the spinothalamic tracts, the ability to discriminate pinprick stimuli around the rectum indicates the patient is likely to show progressive recovery of motor power of the sacral segments. Patients with central cord syndrome usually show progressive return of motor power, first toe flexors, then toe extensors, and then lumbar innervative muscles (*i.e.*, plantar flexors and extensor and dorsal flexors of the ankle, then flexors–extensors of the knee and hip). These patients have a 50% chance of recovery of enough muscle power and sensation to be independently ambulatory. However, their lower extremity muscles retain significant spasticity owing to the upper motor neuron injury in the cervical long tracts. The return of upper extremity function to the arms and hands is very limited owing to the central gray matter damage, that is, lower motor neuron paralysis of the muscles of the hands, which remains profound and permanent. Therefore, the typical patient with a central cord syndrome regains bowel and bladder control and is able to walk with a spastic gait but has poor recovery of fine motor function of the upper extremities.

Anterior cord syndrome patients have complete motor paralysis and retain only deep pressure sensation and proprioceptive sense in the lower extremities without the ability to discern sharp–dull discrimination. These patients have the poorest prognosis for motor recovery. They may gain some increased protective sensation, but only 10% to 20% regain functional motor control.

Therefore, as a rule of thumb, the incomplete cervical spinal cord injury patient with Brown-Séquard syndrome has a 90% chance of good functional recovery; the central cord syndrome patient has a 50% chance of good functional recovery; and the anterior cord syndrome patient has only a 10% chance of good functional recovery.[2]

COMPLETE CORD INJURIES

Approximately 3% of the patients who demonstrate a complete spinal cord injury initially demonstrate some recovery within 24 hours. However, if the patient experiences an immediate complete paralysis and anesthesia below the level of injury, and if this persists for 24 hours, he can be diagnosed as having a complete lesion and will make no progressive recovery. Following a severe injury to the spinal cord, the patient enters into a period of spinal shock. Spinal shock is the condition of absent reflexes below the level of injury, and this may persist for hours or days. However, complete spinal shock rarely persists longer than 24 hours. In 99% of the cases, the emergence from spinal shock as evidenced by the return of bulbocavernosus reflex can be detected within 6 to 24 hours postinjury. As long as the patient is in spinal shock, one cannot diagnose definitively that he has a complete spinal cord injury. However, when the patient demonstrates the return of the bulbocavernosus reflex and still has no sign of sacral sparing or other motor power or sensation below the level of injury, it can then be safely diagnosed that he has a complete spinal cord injury from which he will no functional motor recovery.

The rehabilitation goals of the quadriplegic or pentaplegic depend upon an accurate assessment of the neurologic function present following an injury.

Quadriplegia is defined as paralysis of all four extremities. Posttraumatic quadriplegia is due to an injury to the spinal cord in the cervical region. The most common cause of the spinal cord injury is a fracture–dislocation of the cervical spine or a gunshot wound to the neck. Patients with complete lesions manifest no motor or sensory function in the lower extremities and varying amounts of sensation and voluntary muscle control in the upper extremities, depending upon the level of the lesion in the cervical spine. The level is determined by the sensory and motor physical examination. The most critical functional determination is whether the lesion is above or below the fourth cervical cord segment.

In a complete lesion below the C4 level of the spinal cord, the voluntary control of the innervation of the diaphragm is preserved and the patient is able to breathe without the assistance of external mechanical ventilation. A complete lesion above the C4 level of the spinal cord produces diaphragmatic paralysis, and therefore the patient is dependent upon external mechanical respiratory assistance for survival. A respiratory quadriplegic is a patient with a complete lesion of the cervical spinal cord with C3 as the lowest voluntarily controlled functioning segment. This patient is respirator dependent but has head and neck control.

A pentaplegic is a patient with a complete lesion with C1 or C2 as the lowest voluntarily controlled functioning segment of the spinal cord. This patient is not only respirator dependent, but has also lost complete control of the position of the head and neck on the trunk—thus the term pentaplegia.

C1 Injuries

The patient with a neurologic functional level of C1 has sensation and motor control over the cranial nerve innervation of his head only. He is able to perceive sensation over the face only, and his motor control extends only to the facial muscles. He needs permanent respiratory assistance with a volume respiratory through a tracheostomy. Medically and surgically he requires stabilization from C2 to the thorax, that is, stabilization of the head and neck so that he can sit upright in a wheelchair. This patient is a good candidate for a phrenic nerve pacemaker implant to provide reciprocal stimulation of the phrenic nerves, which allows breathing without the necessity of the mechanical respirator. The successful use of a phrenic nerve stimulator depends upon an intact lower motor neuron innervation of the diaphragm by way of the phrenic nerve. The injured area of the cord must be above C4 and must not include the central gray matter of C4 or the nerve roots of C4 or C5. Transcutaneous stimulation of the intact lower motor neuron by surface electrodes over the phrenic nerve in the neck will cause diaphragm contraction as observed by fluoroscopy. Noncontraction of the diaphragm with stimulation of the phrenic nerve means the phrenic nerve is not functional and a phrenic nerve pacemaker will not be effective.

C2 Injuries

The sensory level of a patient with no neurologic function below C2 includes sensation over the back of the head and scalp. His motor power includes only capital flexors and extensors with inadequate neck control. This patient is also dependent upon the mechanical respirator for breathing, is also a good candidate for phrenic nerve stimulator implants, and may require a surgical spinal stabilization for head control.

C3 Injuries

The patient with a C3 injury has sensation over the entire head and neck and has motor control of the strap muscles and cervical extensors and flexors. He does not need a surgical stabilization of his cervical spine but remains dependent upon external ventilation for breathing, and therefore he requires a respirator at least at night. He may be able to breathe independently for short periods during the day with neck accessory muscles of respiration or glossopharyngeal breathing techniques. This patient also may be a candidate for an internal phrenic nerve pacemaker if the phrenic nerve is found to have the lower motor neuron intact and reacting to external stimulation. This patient has better head and neck control and can propel an electric wheelchair in the upright position using a chin control mechanism.

C4 Injuries

The patient with a C4 functional level has the all important innervation of the diaphragm under voluntary control and also has sensation over the upper part of the shoulders and chest. The area of sensation is capelike in distribution, from the point of one shoulder down over the chest halfway to the nipple line up to the point of the opposite shoulder.

Midcervical Injuries

Patients suffering from complete injuries to the spinal cord demonstrate no recovery of distal lower extremity or trunk sensation or motor power transmitted across the injured area of the spinal cord; however, 80% of patients recover one additional nerve root level of function. The nerve root that exists the neuro-foramen at the level of the fracture or dislocation emanates from normal spinal cord above the level of the spinal cord injury and suffers a peripheral nerve injury. It can therefore be expected to show some recovery of motor function. The patient who suffers a fracture of the C4 vertebra on C5 will usually present in the emergency room with the C4 nerve root as the lowest functioning nerve root. One can elicit sensation over the anterior capelike chest distribution. The patient is able to control his head and shoulders with the trapezius and sternocleidomastoid muscles and is able to breathe with the diaphragm, but has no upper extremity function. We expect his fifth nerve root to recover within 6 to 12 weeks. If he remains at a complete C4 functional level without any voluntary motor control of the upper extremity, his rehabilitation potential will consist of complete dependency in transfers, but he will be able to sit up in a wheelchair, breathe on his own, propel an electric wheelchair with a tongue or chin control, and use a mouthstick for writing, typing, communicating, and manipulating environmental controls of such functions as elevation of the head of the bed, turning on electric modalities (radios, television), opening doors, turning on alarms and call bells, and so forth.

Recovery of the fifth nerve root is evidenced by increased sensation over the upper arm and voluntary control of the deltoid, biceps, and perhaps brachioradialis muscles. A patient with fifth nerve root recovery is able to abduct his shoulder and flex his elbow, but is unable to move his wrist or hand voluntarily. His necessary equipment includes an electrically driven motorized wheelchair with mobile arm supports for his weak arm control and an externally powered hand splint for prehension. The hand splint can be powered by electric motors or carbon dioxide motors, or it can be a passive "ratchet hand splint." This patient will continue to be dependent upon others for positioning and mobility in bed, transfer activities, feeding, and hygiene. There are some new advances in both externally powered hand orthoses with myoelectric controls, and implant electrodes for the electrical stimulation of nerves and muscles. However, these are not functional at the present time for the typical C5 quadriplegic. The realistic functional goals for the C5-level quadriplegic are assisted swivel bar transfers from bed to wheelchair, an electric wheelchair for mobilization (even though the patient may be able to propel a manual wheelchair for short distances with quad pegs), and ratchet hand splint for prehension.

The next level of fracture–dislocation, that of the C5 vertebra on the C6 vertebra, produces a patient who presents with an initial C5 functional level whom we expect to recover his C6 nerve root. The C6 nerve root provides sensation over the forearm, thumb, index, and long fingers, and the very important wrist extensor motor power control. The presence of the extensor carpal radialis and longus provides stronger upper extremity function and the ability to be independent in sliding board transfers from bed to wheelchair, in propelling the manual wheelchair, and in the use of the wrist-driven flexor-hinge hand splint for prehension. Propelling a manual wheelchair may require quad pegs on the hand rims or a plasticized hand rim. The patient is able to perform range of motion of upper and lower extremities, independent ischial pressure relief in the wheelchair, and independent upper extremity dressing; with the use of the hand splint he is able to feed himself, button upper extremity clothing, take care of his personal hygiene (shaving, combing hair, brushing teeth), cook, write with a pen or pencil, and use a typewriter with typing sticks. The C6 functional level patient is usually able to transfer independently in and out of an automobile and to drive an automobile with adapted hand controls.

The C7 functional level, which usually results from a C6–C7 dislocation with progressive recovery of the C7 nerve root, includes not only discriminatory sensation over the ring and part of the small finger of the hand, but also voluntary control of the triceps for elbow extension, the flexor carpal radialis for wrist flexion, and the extensor digitorum communis for voluntary finger extension. A patient with C7-level function still has no voluntary control of the finger flexors or thumb muscles, and is still considered a quadriplegic, but he has much more control and strength in the upper extremity than does the C6-level quadriplegic. C7 functional level patients are the so called super quads who can, with the addition of elbow extensors and wrist flexors, transfer much more easily independently, dress their lower extremities independently, balance their wheelchairs on the back wheels, transfer in and out of automobiles, and drive automobiles much more effectively.

The patient who has the C8 nerve root intact has finger flexors under voluntary control to provide hand grasp, grip, and prehension. His only paralysis is of the intrinsic muscles. This is an uncommon level of quadriplegia. The patient who has the T1 nerve root function intact also has intrinsic muscle control, and is therefore technically and functionally classified as a paraplegic patient rather than a quadriplegic patient.

In summary, patients with high cervical lesions of the C1–C2 area are respiratory dependent and have no neck control. Their rehabilitation goals are limited to sitting in the upright position in an electric wheelchair, and they have the potential for breathing with implanted phrenic nerve stimulators. The C3 functional level patient is respiratory dependent, has functional neck control, and may be a candidate for phrenic nerve implants. The C4 functional level allows the patient to breathe on his own, but his rehabilitation goals also include only the ability to sit upright in the electric wheelchair, propel the electric wheelchair with chin control, and communicate by speaking or by writing with a mouthstick. The C5 functional level patient has deltoid and biceps function and requires mobile arm supports, an electric wheelchair, and an externally powered hand splint. He will always be dependent on an attendant for most of the activities of daily living. The C6 functional level patient who has strong wrist extensors is able to propel a manual wheelchair, transfer independently in and out of bed, and use a wrist-driven flexor-hinge hand splint for voluntary prehension, and may be independent in most activities of daily living. The C7, or "low quad," has strong control of shoulder muscles, both flexion and extension voluntary control of the elbow, both flexion and extension voluntary control of the wrist, and control of the finger extensors. Even though he has no voluntary grip, he is able to use the flexor hinge hand splints much more efficiently, and is able to transfer in and out of bed, wheelchair, and car. He is also able to drive a car with hand controls. This patient also has a greater potential to benefit from tendon transfers of wrist flexion and extension muscles to provide finger and thumb flexion and prehension.

PSYCHOLOGICAL REHABILITATION AND READAPTATION

Even though the functional goals can be well delineated and listed for each level of incomplete and complete quadriplegics, the devastating psychological effects of permanent paralysis and alteration of body image are difficult to document and quantitate.

During the first 1 to 2 months following an injury, the patient is in a state of denial. Even though he realizes that he is unable to control his body, he cannot consciously believe that he is going to remain this way permanently, no matter what he is told by the doctor or rehabilitation team. Realistic functional rehabilitation goals are emphasized. The family is helped to overcome this initial period of loss and grief. As the patient moves to the wheelchair and proceeds with his functional rehabilitation, he begins to realize that not all patients recover and that he may be this way forever. During the third and fourth months postinjury, the patient becomes very belligerent. He begins to "bargain" with the nurses and therapists. He is grieving for his former self that he has now lost, and he becomes a "bad patient." During the fifth and sixth months postinjury, the patient is out of the initial life-threatening situation and functioning at his maximum capacity in the wheelchair. He realizes that he has reached maximum recovery and enters a period of depression. Unfortunately, at about this time he has reached his maximum rehabilitation hospital program goals and is ready to be discharged. Psychologically, he is at the depth of greatest depression. During the sixth to twelfth month postinjury, the patient learns to cope with his new life-style as an outpatient living at home with his family. It takes at least 1 year before a patient can realistically plan vocational, avocational, social, and family aspirations for the future. Some patients never cope with the situation, allow their medical condition to deteriorate, and are repeatedly admitted to the hospital for medical complications of pressure sores, urinary tract infections, joint contractures, and so forth. They deny that their state is permanent and await the miracle cure or "medical research breakthrough" that will repair their spinal cords.

The goal of the rehabilitation team, which consists of physician, rehabilitation nurse, physical therapist, occupational therapist, medical social worker, orthotist, and medical psychologist, is to have the patient at 1 year postinjury complication free, functioning upright in the wheelchair at the maximum potential for the level and degree of his injury, at home with his family, knowledgeable about his condition, and prepared for the future.

REFERENCES

1. *Bosch AE, Stauffer ES, Nickel VL:* Incomplete traumatic quadriplegia: A ten-year review. JAMA 216:473, 1971
2. *Mesard L:* Survival after spinal cord trauma. Arch Neurol 35:78, 1978
3. *Stauffer ES, Bell GD:* Traumatic respiratory quadriplegia and pentaplegia: Symposium on the upper cervical spine. Orthop Clin North Am 9(4):1081, 1978

BIBLIOGRAPHY

Stauffer ES: Diagnosis and prognosis of acute cervical spinal cord injury. Clin Orthop 112:9, 1975

Stauffer ES: Fractures and dislocations of the cervical spine. In Rockwood CA, Green DP (eds): Fractures. Philadelphia, JB Lippincott, 1975

Stauffer, ES: Long-term management in traumatic quadriplegia. In Pierce DS, Nickel VL (eds): The Total Care of Spinal Cord Injuries. Boston, Little, Brown & Co, 1977

Stauffer ES: Rehabilitation of the spinal cord injured patient. In Rothman R (ed): The Spine, 2nd ed. Philadelphia, WB Saunders, 1981

CHAPTER 8

Cervical Cord Tumors

DONLIN M. LONG

Though tumors affecting the cervical spinal cord have been known and described for centuries, it was not until 1887 that Sir Victor Horsley first carried out successful removal of a thoracic tumor.[29] McEwen had successfully performed laminectomies for other spinal cord compressive problems, but operation for spinal cord tumor was generally held to be impossible and the prognosis considered hopeless.[48] Following Horsley's surgical feat, operations upon spinal cord tumors rapidly became routine. Thirty-seven years later, Elsberg was able to write a definitive monograph that remains a standard reference. Over his long career, Elsberg successfully removed seven intramedullary tumors.[22] However, it was not until 1954 that Greenwood was able to remove an intramedullary spinal cord tumor in a patient who was normal neurologically before and after operation.[30] Recent advances, including bipolar coagulation, the operating miscroscope, and improved microsurgical tools, have greatly improved the prognosis for patients with cervical spinal cord tumors of all types, but the intramedullary lesions remain challenging management problems and many of them cannot be satisfactorily treated by any known mechanism.[46,50]

Intraspinal tumors are not as common as tumors of the brain. Kernohan reports that only about 15% of primary central nervous system tumors are intraspinal, and their incidence appears to be approximately 1.3 per 100,000 people per year. Spinal cord tumors are rare in children. They are generally of the congenital type, though intramedullary gliomas do occur. Spinal tumors in adults are more likely to be metastatic tumors, meningiomas, neurofibromas, or intramedullary gliomas. Cervical tumors account for about 17% of all spinal cord tumors, and cervicothoracic tumors another 3% or so; about 20% of all spinal cord tumors occur in the cervical area.[2,4]

Spinal cord tumors are traditionally classified as extradural, intradural-extramedullary, and intramedullary. Some tumors may have unique characteristics, but in general the clinical syndromes are more dependent upon their location and their relationship to neural structures than on tumor type. The differential diagnosis is extensive in the extradural tumors and quite restricted for the others.[44]

IMAGING SPINAL CORD TUMORS

Plain x-ray, myelography, CT, and MRI are among the armamentarium of neuroradiologic imaging modalities used in the work-up for cervical spine tumors. With a high-field-strength magnet, MRI appears to be the only imaging modality to provide the most conclusive informations. However, in some cases intrathecal enhanced CT can be complementary. Because MRI is not yet widely available, CT still plays an important role in diagnosis. Intrathecal enhanced CT surpasses myelography in providing information such as the presence of subtle cord enlargement, syringohydromyelia, and paraspinal pathology.

Computed tomography (CT) has been employed as an imaging modality for spinal, intraspinal, and paraspinal neoplasms of the cervical region.[5] Unenhanced spinal CT is valuable in outlining the entire extent of tumors, including the bony, extradural, and paraspinal involvement. However, detailed visualization of intrathecal abnormalities cannot be achieved without introducing water-soluble contrast agents into the subarachnoid space.[38] Hydrosoluble, nonionic intrathecal enhanced CT usually allows epidural lesions to be clearly differentiated from intradural lesions. With intravenous contrast agents, some vascular neoplasms—even those located intradurally—can be visualized.[38] Occasionally, a specific tissue diagnosis such as lipoma can be made based on CT attenuation values. Accurate analysis of the circumferential and craniocaudal extent of the tumor can be accomplished by obtaining the axial CT, the computer-reformatted images, and the localization scout digital radiography.

Magnetic resonance imaging (MRI), the latest imaging modality, is capable of providing clear visualization of the bony, extradural, intrathecal, and paraspinal tumor involvement. This technique obviates the need for adding an intrathecal contrast agent. Images in axial, sagittal, and coronal views can be obtained in all cases, if desired. By choosing the correct pulse sequence and different combinations of TR (repetition time) and TE (echo delay time), the signal intensity of various tissues can be generated and characterized.

The vertebral bodies have a high intensity signal because of fat in the bone marrow. Tumor invasion into the cervical spine, which alters the bone marrow fat content, will have a relatively low signal intensity.[52,53] The liagmentous structures adjacent to the cortical surface of vertebral bodies cannot be differentiated because the signal intensities are similar. Images of the intervertebral disc distinguish a central region of high intensity (nucleus pulposus) with a circumferential surrounding ring of low signal intensity (anulus fibrosus). The degenerated disc (desiccated disc) and herniated and extruded disc fragments can be readily identified[52] by its low intensity signal and its morphology.

Cerebrospinal fluid has low intensity with small TR and TE values (i.e., T1-weighted images). However, with increased TR and TE (i.e., T2-weighted images), the intensity of CSF is augmented, preventing the discrimination of CSF from the adjacent spinal cord. Epidural compression on the thecal sac is clearly appreciated. The spinal cord is clearly delineated in axial, sagittal, and coronal planes on T1-weighted images; epidural, intradural, and intramedullary lesions are readily apparent. The different signal intensities in the spinal cord on T2-weighted images usually differentiate the normal neural tissue from neoplasm. Arnold-Chiari malformation and syringohydromyelia are also vividly demonstrated.[47,56,63]

EXTRADURAL TUMORS

Extradural tumors represent about 22% of the total number of primary spinal cord tumors. Of course, this figure changes considerably when metastatic disease is involved, in which case the percentage relates entirely to the frequency of cancer incidence. The majority of extradural tumors are metastatic; the most frequent primary disease is carcinoma of the lung, but carcinoma of the breast, prostate, gastrointestinal tract, thyroid, and kidney also metastasize to the spine.[23] The differential diagnosis also includes sarcoma, chordoma, and lymphoma.[2,24,54,62] Less frequently giant cell tumors, aneurysmal bone cysts, osteogenic sarcoma, osteogenic chondroma, giant osteoid osteoma, and Ewing's sarcoma are found.[9,28,44,45] All of these lesions must be differentiated from rheumatoid spondylitis and from inflammatory lesions.[13] Spontaneous epidural hemorrhage from a blood dyscrasia and severe cervical osteoarthritis may also mimic an extradural tumor.[39] A massively herniated cervical disc should also be considered in the differential diagnosis.[7,42]

Symptoms

Symptoms of extramedullary lesions may include local tissue destruction, radicular involvement either by tumor or by bony compression, or spinal cord compression secondary to bony collapse or tumor.[51] Radicular pain is common and the spinal cord level is usually discrete.[6] The sensory loss is uniform and motor loss is also frequently uniform. Bladder dysfunction occurs early in the course of the disease. Symptoms frequently are precipitous in onset and spinal block occurs early in the symptomatic course. The usual history begins with pain, first apparent locally in the neck and then radicular in character. Frequently there is rapid onset of transverse myelopathy with early involvement of bowel and bladder, and progressive sensory and motor deficit, often rapid in nature. In high cervical cord tumors, respiratory distress and diaphragmatic paralysis may occur early. The specific neurologic sensory deficits depend upon the level of the lesion. Simple guidelines for a rapid localization are as follows: If the deltoid muscle is spared, the lesion is likely to be at C4–C5. If the biceps are spared, the lesion is likely to be at C5–C6. If the triceps is spared, the level is likely to be C6–C7, and if the hands are spared, the level is likely to be C7–T1 or below. Radicular complaints follow the roots involved and are not different from those found with disc herniation.

Diagnosis

The first and most important diagnostic aid following a complete physical examination is a set of plain spine roentgenograms. Virtually all of the extramedullary lesions show a nondescript pattern of bony destruction. Inflammatory disease usually begins in the disc, whereas metastatic tumors usually begin in the vertebral body (Fig. 8-1). Furthermore, the plain films usually allow one to differentiate Paget's disease, rheumatoid spondylitis, and severe spondylosis from these lesions. Aneurysmal bone cysts and giant cell tumors have specific characteristics. The absence of plain film change makes an extradural lesion extremely unlikely. Much has been made of the spinal fluid protein in the differential diagnosis, but with the radiographic techniques now available, a lumbar puncture no longer seems to be of value. The definitive study is a myelogram. The newest techniques use water soluble dyes, often placed at the C1–C2 level, and the CT scan may show dramatic changes that are diagnostic. The CT scan also demonstrates the levels of compression and the structures compressing the spinal cord more effectively than any other technique. The myelographic picture of extradural block is usually typical, and the combination of plain films, CT scan, and myelogram is diagnostic in most instances (see Fig. 8-1).[55]

The MRI scan is not as useful for extradural lesions as it is for intradural abnormalities, but much can be learned about the soft-tissue masses. The CT scan is superior for demonstrating bony abnormalities. The three-dimensional CT scan is the most useful available technique for accurate assessment of changes in the bone.

Pathology

The pathology of the tumors found in the cervical region does not differ from the pathology of tumors found anywhere else in the body. The tumors have no special characteristics and there is no need to describe them separately.

Treatment

The treatment of the extradural lesion in the cervical area is considerably different from the treatment of spinal cord compression from extradural lesions in the thoracic or lumbar spine. Basically, the aim of treatment is threefold: relief of compression of neural structures, stabilization of the spine, and relief of pain. In the thoracic and lumbar regions of the spine, surgical therapy usually requires only posterior decompressive laminectomy. Internal stabilization is rarely necessary and major bony deformities are not common. The cord compression is nearly always from soft tumor. There is no agreement on the necessity for surgery in many of these patients and there is no good evidence indicating that the results of surgical therapy are superior to those of radiotherapy or chemotherapy directed at the tumor.

The problem in the cervical region is quite different. Virtually all extradural cervical spine lesions begin in the vertebral body so that the compression on the cord is from the front. Furthermore, collapse of the spine with angulation is common so that spinal cord compression is bony rather than tumorous. Instability is obviously a greater problem and poses an ongoing threat to the spinal cord.[16] These factors all mean that surgical intervention is much more likely to be necessary with extradural cervical spine tumors.[36,66] Direct therapy of the tumor without decompression of the spinal cord is unlikely to reverse neurologic symptoms, since the cord compression is often bony and the prevention of further injury of the spinal cord by stabilization of the spine is mandatory in many instances. Because the bony compression is anterior, it is unlikely that a posterior laminectomy will be satisfactory, and anterior approaches with radical removal of tumor and bone are indicated. This means that anterior stabilization is also usually necessary.

In making decisions about therapy, the most important factor is the identification of the extent of spinal cord compression, the degree of instability, and the risk of dislocation. If there is marked instability and spinal cord compression due to this instability, the first step should be reduction of the abnormality, if possible. If the abnormality is serious and acute, the patient should be placed in skeletal tongs and traction applied, the same as for spinal fracture. If the problem is less acute, correction in a halo vest is the best choice. If no apparent angulation or instability exists prior to surgery, it is only necessary to choose the method of stabilization that will be used postoperatively; either skeletal tong fixation or a halo device may be employed. Currently, the usual choice at Johns Hopkins is to place the patient in the headpiece of the halo vest and to use this for traction during surgery. In the immediate postoperative period, after the patient has stabilized and there is no longer a concern for the airway, the complete halo can be applied for immobilization of the patient.

When operative decompression using the anterior approach is planned, the fixation devices are generally applied in the operating room if they have not been required for stabilization prior to surgery. Endotracheal anesthesia is used, and great care must be taken not to move the spine, further compressing the spinal cord. The patient is positioned as for standard anterior cervical fusion and the traction applied to a light weight, usually no more than 5 pounds. A lateral roentgenogram is taken to verify the patient's position and the amount of reduction of any spinal deformity that may be present. Heavier weights may be used in order to obtain optimal reduction. The approach is usually made through the left side, though this is personal choice. A horizontal incision is used unless the bony decompression is going to involve more than two segments. The approach is made between the midline structures medially and the carotid sheaths laterally. The perivertebral space is entered, and self-retaining tractors are used to expose the entire area of abnormality; the Cloward self-retaining instruments are very valuable in obtaining this adequate exposure. Standard techniques are used to remove the compressive tumor and bone. Complete removal of abnormal tissue that may be compressing the spinal cord or interfering with stabilization is necessary. Lateral spine films are taken to assure that the decompression is adequate and that proper cervical alignment is obtained. Once decompression and alignment are achieved, the problem is stabilization. With nonmalignant tumors such as giant cell tumors or aneurysmal bone cysts, it is possible to fuse with autogeneous or bank bone; because of the size of the graft, autogeneous bone is preferable. The entire thickness of the iliac crest makes a convenient graft. Bony surfaces are well exposed above and below and an appropriately sized graft is cut and placed. Large grafts that cover even two or three vertebral segments are tolerated well. However, these grafts are quite unstable and there is a significant tendency to dislodgment. It is necessary that the patient be absolutely immobilized for whatever period of time is required for solid fusion of the graft. A minimum of 3 months is usually necessary, and it may take 6 months before such a graft can be considered solid. In the face of malignancy, it is not possible to use autogeneous bone in most circumstances. A number of ingenious techniques, mostly using methacrylate, have been employed. In all of these techniques, the missing vertebral bodies are replaced with methacrylate, which is allowed to fill the surgical defect and then fastened in place with some form of fixation. The techniques described by Galicich result in close approximations of the original anatomy and appear to be the best of all of the methacrylate stabilization procedures yet employed.[17,26,59]

When extensive bony removal is necessary anteriorly, the patient remains at risk for a significant period of time. With benign processes and tumors that have a reasonable chance of responding to therapy, it is wise to carry out a posterior fusion a few weeks after the anterior procedure. These fusions are more reliable in terms of eventual bony union and provide immediate stability and safety for the patient. With malignant processes, the additional surgery is not indicated unless the prognosis for the malignancy is good.

Following the operative procedures, subsequent therapy depends upon the underlying histologic type and may include x-ray treatment, chemotherapy, or both. There is nothing about the location that influences the choice of treatment. X-ray therapy potentially is complicated by transverse myelopathy if not carefully administered, and the patient should be warned of this possibility.

INTRADURAL-EXTRAMEDULLARY TUMORS

Of the intradural tumors, 71% are extramedullary. Thirty-two percent of these are meningiomas and 38% are schwannomas. The remaining tumors found in this location are sarcomas, angiomas, chordomas, lymphomas, lipomas, epidermoids, melanomas, and neuroblastomas. Other kinds of lesions occur very rarely. Virtually any kind of tumor may metastasize to the intradural space, but such spread is distinctly unusual.[51]

Symptoms

It is fortunate that the neurofibromas and meningiomas, which are benign tumors and usually curable, frequently announce themselves by radicu-

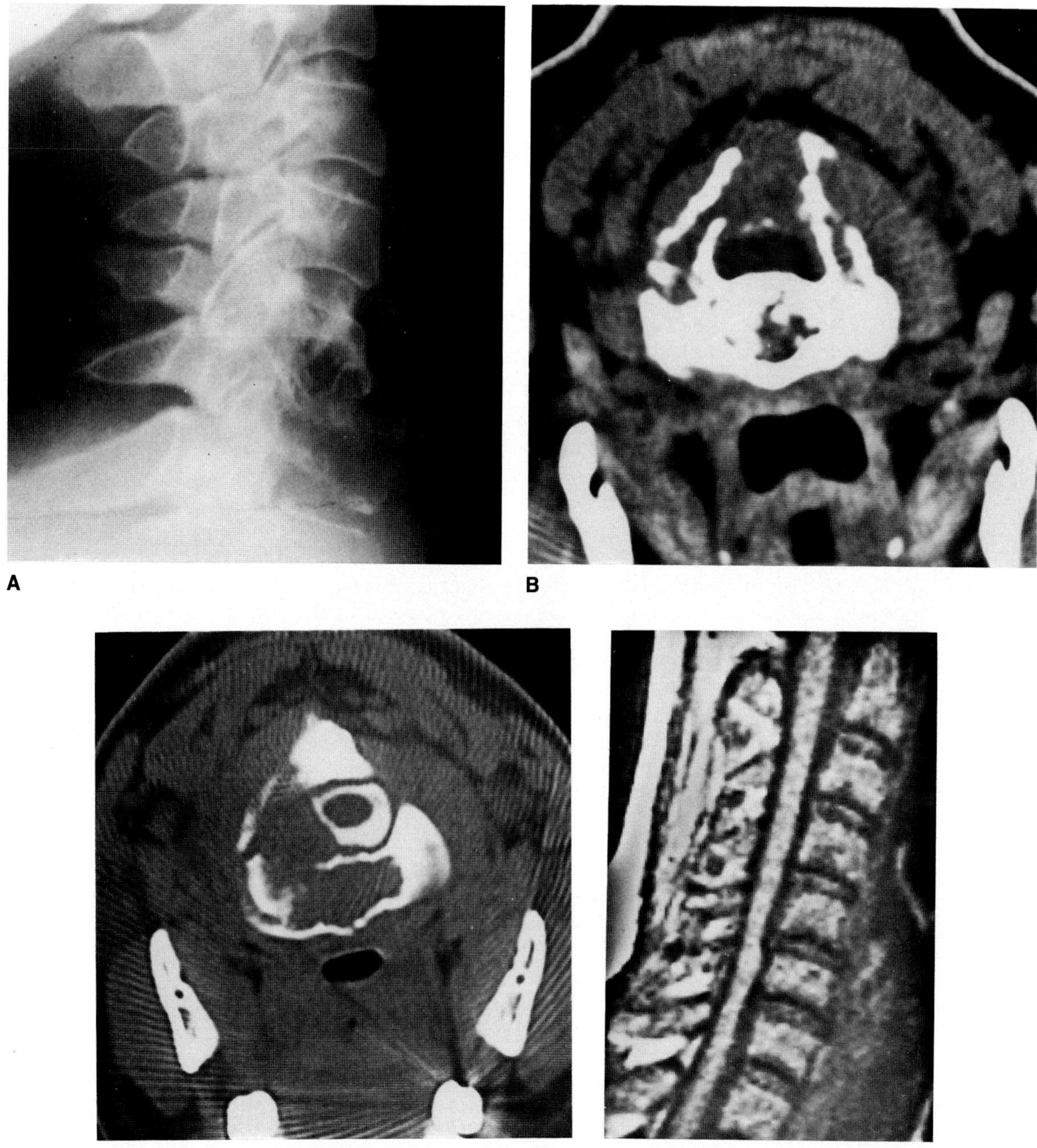
A
B
C
D

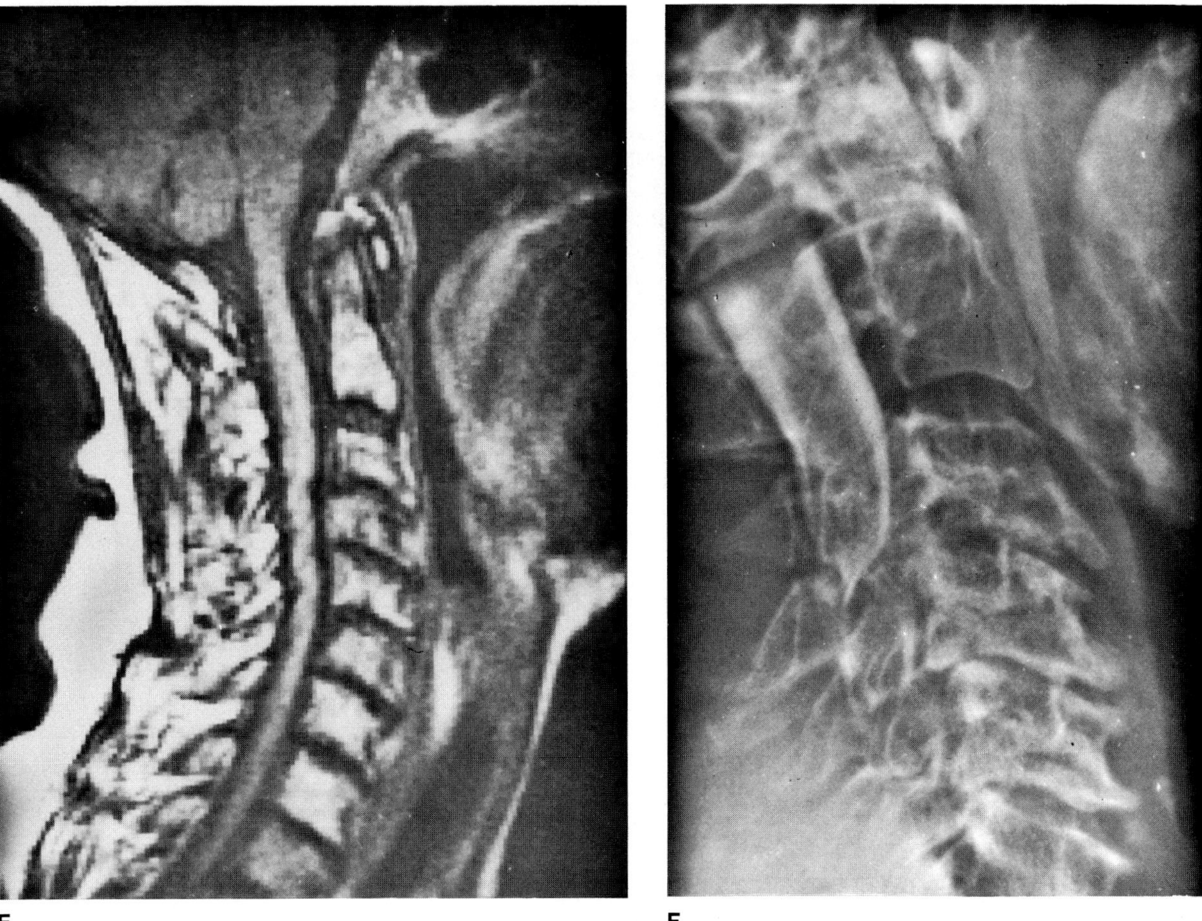

Fig. 8-1. (*A*) A destructive lesion involving the bodies of C5 and C6 with destruction of the C6 disc space. This proved to be metastatic myeloma. (*B*) Plain axial CT of C2 vertebra showed lytic destructive bony process involving the vertebral body as well as the posterior elements. Soft-tissue mass invading the posterior aspect of the spinal canal with compression on the thecal sac in a patient with plasmocytoma. (*C*) Intrathecal metrizamide enhanced CT of C2 level revealed an expansile lytic bony lesion involving the body of C2 vertebra, the large epidural tumor component compressing and displacing the cord and the thecal sac to the right. Histologic diagnosis is osteosarcoma. (*D*) Midsagittal view T1-weighted MRI of the cervical spine showed a protruded disc at C5–C6 level with impingement of the ventral aspect of the cervical cord. Postoperative diagnosis is herniated nucleus pulposus (HNP) C5–C6. (*E*) Midsagittal view MRI of the cervical spine demonstrates marked stenosis of the spinal canal with no discernible cerebrospinal fluid flow signals at C3, C4, C5 levels. Associated spondylosis involving the corresponding vertebrae, narrowed disc spaces with cord impingement noted. (*F*) Metrizamide cervical myelogram via lateral C1–C2 approach showed nearly total block to the CSF flow beginning at C3–C4 level by marked spondylosis.

lar pain. The pain is most commonly continuous, increased by straining, and characteristically worse at night.[6] Root compression is also accompanied by the appropriate muscle atrophy, loss of reflexes, and sensory loss. Anterior horn cell compression may also lead to focal fasciculations. When spinal cord compression signs occur, they are rarely symmetrical. There is often impaired motor function on the side of the tumor and pain and temperature loss on the opposite side. Motor loss is usually spastic and greater in flexors than in extensors. Touch is most commonly defective in a patchy fashion. Sensory loss becomes less evident near the level of the lesion. Sweating may be decreased below the level of the lesion and bowel and bladder dysfunction occur commonly. However, it is usually difficult to distinguish intradural–extramedullary lesions from extramedullary tumors on the basis of the physical examination.[11,27] The clues that the lesion may be intramedullary are the radicular pain, the Brown-Séquard syndrome, and a long history suggesting a benign process.[48]

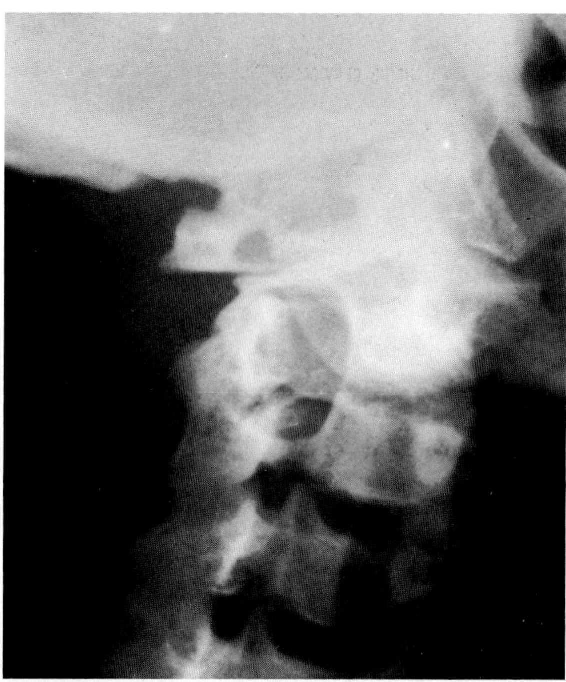

Fig. 8-2. The C2 neural foramen is significantly enlarged. This plain film finding is typical of neurofibroma.

X-ray Diagnosis

The plain x-ray films may be normal. Schwannomas characteristically demonstrate symmetrical enlargement of one neural foramen, and any of these tumors may lead to bony erosions (Fig. 8-2). CT scan and myelography are usually necessary to establish diagnosis. Intradural–extramedullary tumors are sharply circumscribed and separate from the spinal cord (Fig. 8-3). MRI is particularly useful in assessing the intradural extramedullary tumors around the cervicomedullary junction (Figs. 8-4 and 8-5*A* to *C*). A lumbar puncture no longer serves any purpose in the diagnosis, and such ancillary tests as electromyography are rarely indicated when the suspicion of spinal cord tumor is high. Spinal cord angiography is indicated only when a hemangioma or arteriovenous malformation is suspected.[10,40]

Treatment

The only therapy available for most extramedullary lesions is surgery, and verification of the histology is mandatory. These operations are carried out through standard laminectomy. The sitting position is advantageous. The operations are done under general anesthesia with all the precautions required for the sitting position. A midline incision is preferred, with laminectomy carried out to expose the spinal cord at least one segment above and one below the suspected tumor. Such lesions almost never cause instability, and postoperative fusion is rarely required. Some large lesions that erode bone significantly may destroy an apophyseal joint. In this situation, the fusion can be carried out immediately at the time of primary surgery or may be delayed until a later date. The type of fusion depends upon the bony defect and the nature of the instability. This decision is not usually made preoperatively but rather depends upon the operative findings. The tumors are removed totally and there is nothing unique about the techniques employed. When significant spinal cord compression exists, the use of spinal evoked potentials for intraoperative monitoring is of real value to ascertain that the spinal cord is not being compromised during tumor removal. Total removal is required for virtually all of the kinds of lesions found in this location. Most are benign and can be cured by adequate surgical removal.[57] The dura is closed in a watertight fashion whenever possible and it is rarely necessary to provide any form of postoperative stabilization. If necessary, simple lateral fusion can be carried out at the time of the tumor removal if the laminectomy is not too extensive. However, it is usually preferable to wait and carry out the fusion at a second procedure. Schurmann has recently described an intriguing technique for individual fusion of apophyseal

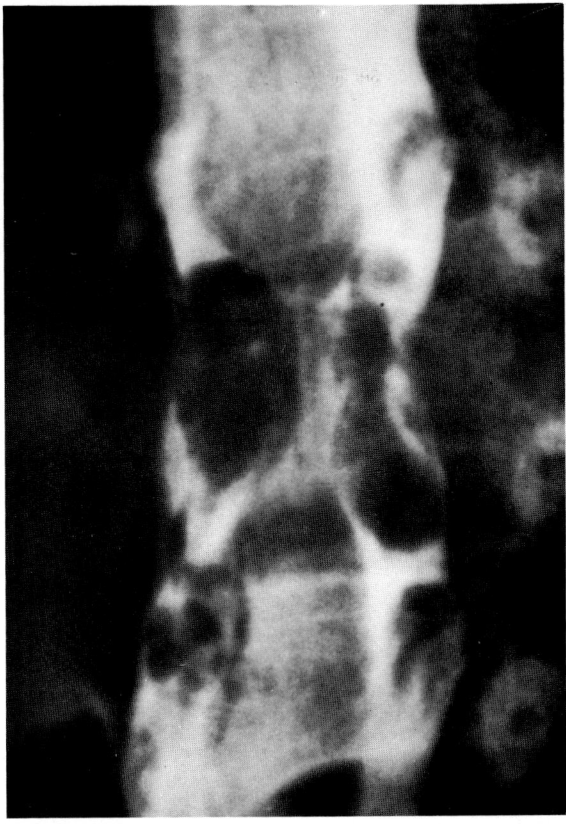

Fig. 8-3. Roentgenogram of a patient with neurofibromatosis. The classical picture of the intradural extramedullary lesion is repeated several times. The most obvious lesions are the two bilateral neurofibromata that are markedly compressing the cord. Multiple small neurofibromata on nerve roots above and below the obvious lesions are present. The characteristics of the smooth, well-defined, rounded intradural lesions suggestive of neurofibroma or meningioma are well demonstrated.

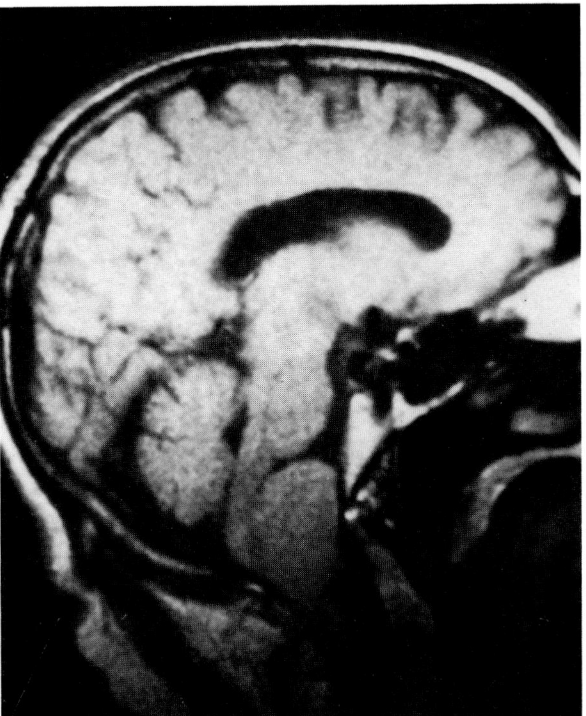

Fig. 8-4. MR scan of the craniocervical junction (obtained by spin-echo pulse sequence, T1 weighting). Midsagittal view showed a large extraaxial tumor, having signals isointense with brain and spinal cord, located ventral to the lower brain stem, and the upper cervical cord producing marked compression and displacement of the neural tissue. Surgical pathology is meningioma.

joints. This would seem to have real advantage with tumors in which a single joint is compromised, but only a few procedures have been carried out and the results over the long term have not been described.[45]*

ARTERIOVENOUS MALFORMATION

There is one extramedullary intradural problem that is somewhat different than the tumors described above. The ateriovenous malformation of the cervical cord may be intramedullary, extramedullary–intradural, or a combination of the two. However, the majority appear to be extramedullary. They may present with any of the radicular or compressive syndromes seen with any other lesions, but they have one special physical characteristic that may help distinguish them: the syndrome of exercise claudication, in which patients experience the gradual onset of quadriparesis with vigorous exercise. This is thought to be a steal of blood, but the exact pathophysiology remains unproven. The syndrome of exercise-induced quadriparesis is so typical that it should always suggest arteriovenous malformation. Of course, such malformations may hemorrhage; the presence of subarachnoid hemorrhage with the syndrome of cervical cord compression should always suggest an arteriovenous malformation. Other tumors may present with a similar syndrome, particularly melanoma, and such a syndrome may occur with blood dyscrasias as well.[3]

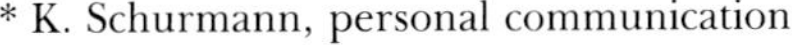

* K. Schurmann, personal communication

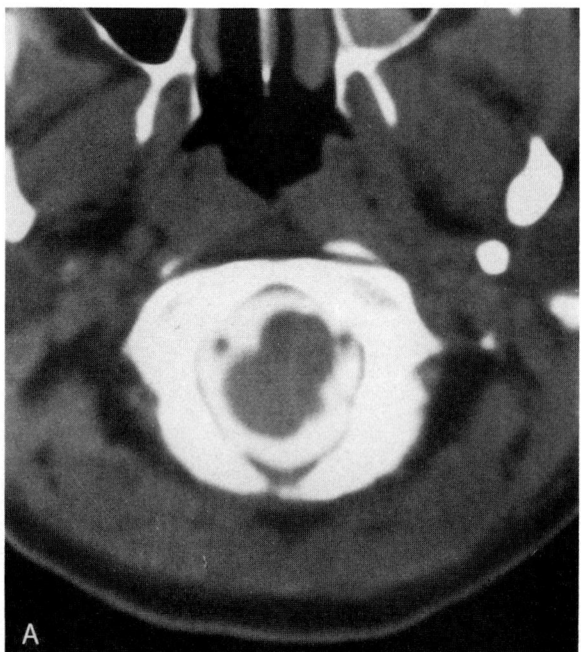

Fig. 8-5. (*A* to *C*) Intrathecal enhanced CT of the craniocervical junction. Axial, reformatted sagittal and coronal views showed an abnormally enlarged brain stem and upper cervical cord without evidence of syringohydromyelia. An extramedullary mass posterior and lateral to the upper cervical cord on the right causing compression and displacement of the neural axis. Surgical pathology is subpial intramedullary and extramedullary melanoma.

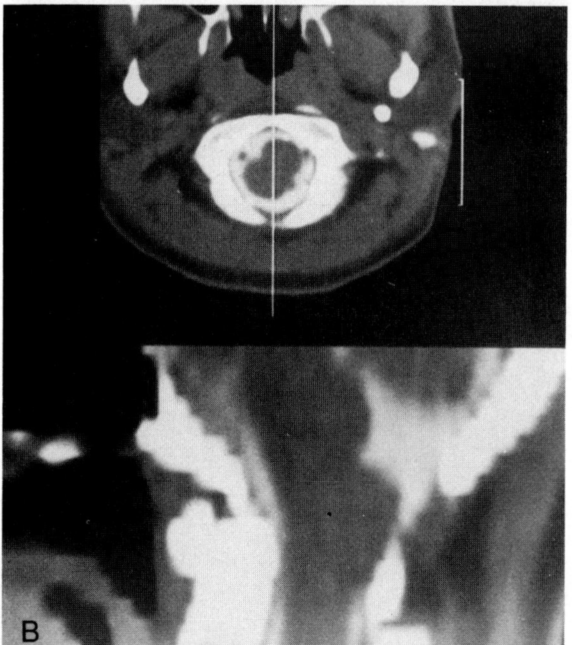

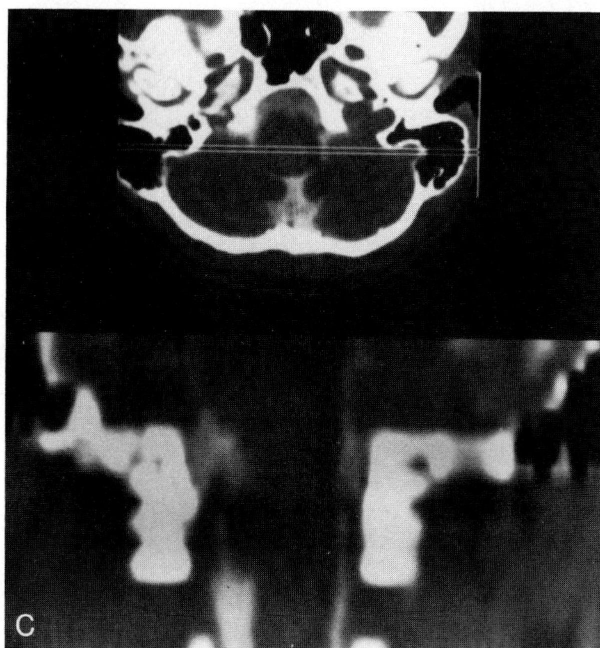

The diagnosis of arteriovenous malformation is usually made from the myelogram. Careful spinal angiography to define the extent of the malformation and its feeding vessels is necessary.[17,18]

The treatment of the symptomatic malformation is surgical. Those that are extramedullary in location can generally be removed safely without neurologic deficit. The use of bipolar coagulation, the operating microscope, and microsurgical techniques as pioneered by Krayenbuhl and Yasargil has led to the successful removal of many of these lesions in the past 10 years.[46]

INTRAMEDULLARY TUMORS

Intramedullary tumors are of two major histologic types. Approximately 28% are ependymomas and 34% are astrocytomas. No other single type of tumor is found a significant percentage of the time, but virtually any other glioma type may be intramedullary. Glioblastoma, polar spongioblastoma, mixed gliomas, oligodendroglioma, lipoma, teratoma, carcinoma and melanoma, and hemangioblastoma have all been described in the intramedullary position. However, these other groups rarely account for more than 2% each of intramedullary lesions. For all practical purposes of diagnosis and therapy, we can concentrate upon the ependymoma and the benign astrocytoma.[20,21,41,54,61,64]

History and Clinical Course

It is usually possible to differentiate the intramedullary lesion from extramedullary compression. Pain is common at the level of the lesion but is not radicular. A local band of hyperesthesia characteristically occurs. Sensory and motor loss are routinely worse at the level of the lesion than distally, the reverse of the extramedullary tumor. Perianal sensory sparing is common. The anterior horn cells are often involved with segmental fasciculations. Cortical spinal tract involvement with quadriparesis and spasticity is late in onset, and bowel and bladder dysfunction occur quite late. Spinal block is rare and does not occur until the tumor is extensive.

Diagnosis

Plain roentgenograms may show widening in the spinal canal with erosion of pedicles and increase in interpedicular distance (Fig. 8-6). The myelogram or myelogram-CT combination is diagnostic. However, these techniques usually do not define the nature of the problem. MRI scanning now allows cysts to be differentiated from tumor and an estimate of the character of the tumor can be obtained as well. The characteristic finding is a symmetrical widening of the cord that is usually fusiform (Fig. 8-7*A* and *B*). Lumbar puncture prior to myelography is not indicated, though cytology of the spinal fluid may be helpful in obtaining an appropriate histologic diagnosis. There are no diagnostic characteristics that define the astrocytoma from the ependymoma. Surgical exploration is required for verification of histology.[4]

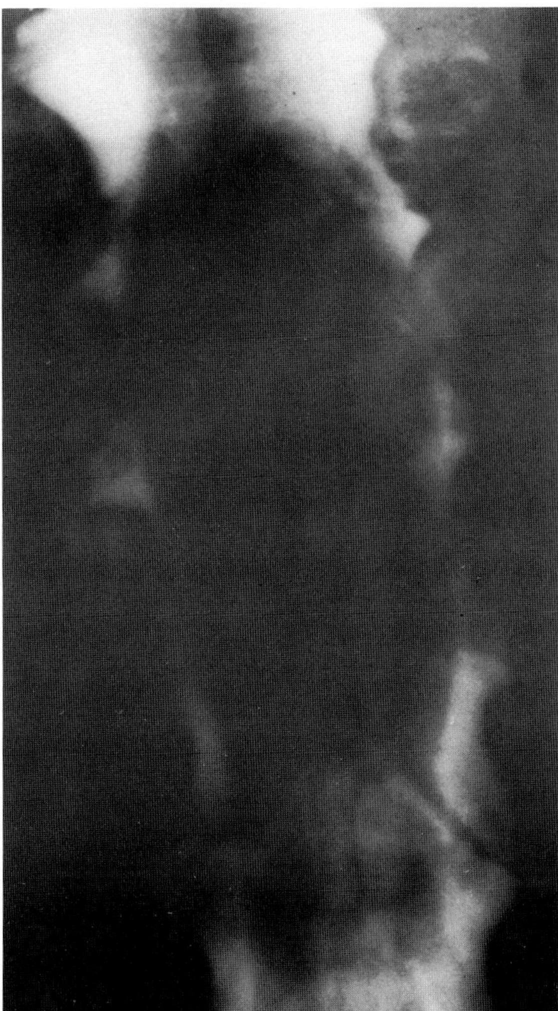

Fig. 8-6. This cervical myelogram demonstrates the classical picture of the intramedullary cervical cord tumor. Note the diffuse widening of the cord, which virtually obliterates the cervical subarachnoid space. The cord above and below the lesion rapidly assumes a normal shape. This proved to be a cervical astrocytoma.

Therapy

The most impressive advance in the therapy of spinal cord tumors in the recent past has occurred in the management of the intramedullary lesions. Greenwood first removed one of these tumors with complete preservation of neurologic function in 1954. With the advent of the operating microscope and greatly improved microsurgical tools, the removal of lesions has now become commonplace. The ependymoma is curable, easily separable from

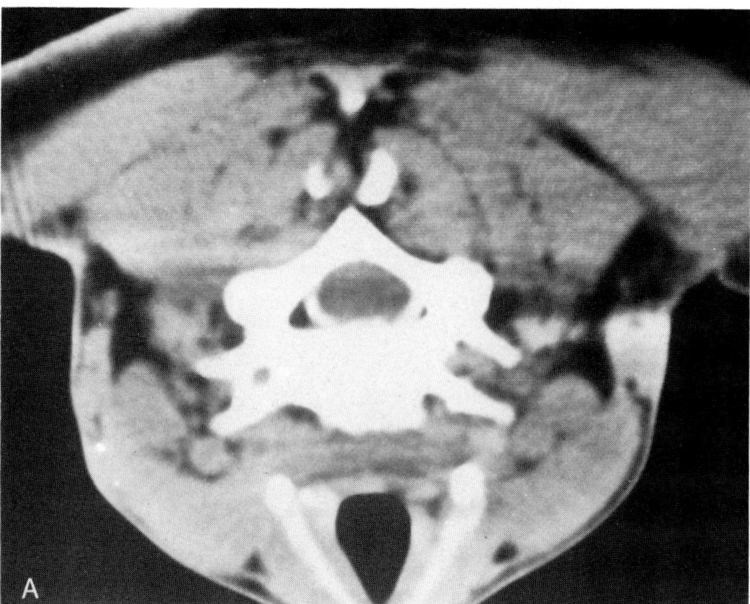

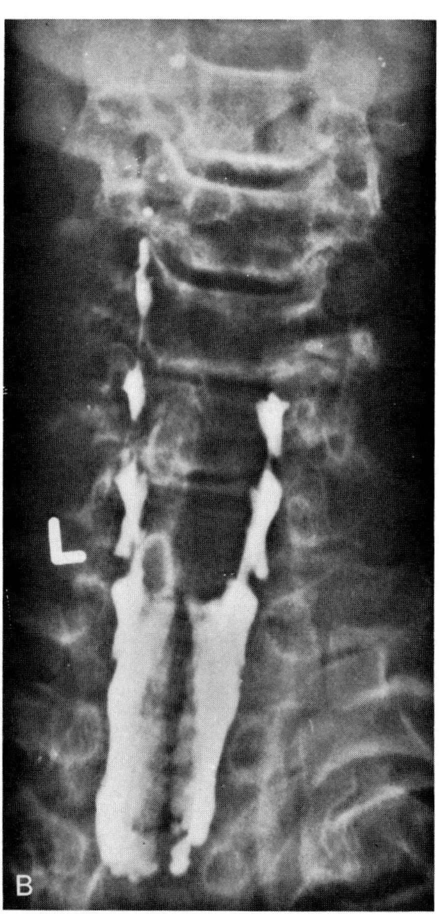

Fig. 8-7. (*A* and *B*) Pantopaque cervical myelogram from lumbar approach. The A–P film showed a nearly complete block to the flow of contrast material at the lower midcervical region by an intramedullary cord lesion. Post-metrizamide myelogram CT scan of C5 level demonstrated an abnormally enlarged cord causing thinning of the subarachnoid space. Postoperative diagnosis is astrocytoma, Grade II.

the surrounding spinal cord, and usually can be removed without serious increase in deficit. The astrocytoma is rarely curable because of its diffuse involvement of the spinal cord, but an occasional pseudoencapsulated astrocytoma may be successfully removed.[31–34]

The surgical procedure for removal of the intramedullary tumors is straightforward posterior cervical laminectomy. General anesthesia is employed, and all the precautions for the sitting position utilized, if that position is used. Prone positioning obivates the risk of air embolism. Spinal monitoring with spinal evoked potentials throughout the procedure is worthwhile. Standard laminectomy is performed. The exact localization of the tumor is important because it is very important to open the dura promptly from above the tumor downward so the herniation of the tumor or cord through a small dural opening does not occur. The spinal cord is carefully inspected, but in general a midline posterior approach to the intradmedullary lesion is desirable. The tumor is identified through a very small posterior midline myelotomy and categorized histologically. If it is an ependymoma, a midline posterior myelotomy exposing the entire tumor is used. It is usually possible to free the tumor capsule from the surrounding spinal cord without serious injury to the spinal cord; removal is usually accomplished without difficulty unless the tumor is an astrocytoma, in which case it cannot usually be totally removed. The tumor should be inspected because an occasional pseudoencapsulated astrocytoma may be removed partially with real benefit to the patient.

The laser and ultrasonic dissector have radically changed the surgeon's ability to manage intramedullary tumors. If there is a nodule within a cyst or if the tumor is even reasonably differentiated from surrounding cord, it is possible to obtain total or near-total removal. Physiologic monitoring is important during these maneuvers. The tumor can be carefully excised using the ultrasonic dissector, or coagulated and vaporized with the laser. When physiologic monitoring suggests cord embarrassment, the procedure can be changed and resumed when the cord recovers. Using this technique, it is possible to remove tumors much more completely and with greater safety than has ever been possible in the past. An older technique sometimes employed particularly with astrocytomas when no plane of cleavage exists is to carry out an extensive midline myelotomy posteriorly over the entire length of the tumor, then to close the wound loosely and return in 7 to 10 days for a second attempt at removal. The tumor will often herniate significantly through the myelotomy defect, and a significant amount of tumor can be removed without further injury to the spinal cord.

The unusual tumors that occur in the intramedullary position can frequently be removed successfully, but of course the prognosis depends entirely on the histology of the lesion itself.

Postoperative irradiation is employed for intramedullary gliomas except ependymomas, and for all of the malignant tumors.

Any of these tumors may be attended by extensive cyst formation. It may be necessary to drain the cyst separately. However, removal of the tumor is usually satisfactory treatment for the cyst. Many of these tumors also extend up and down the spinal cord. Multilevel laminectomy or staged procedures may be necessary to remove the entire tumor; this judgment must be made by the physician at the time of surgery.[41,43]

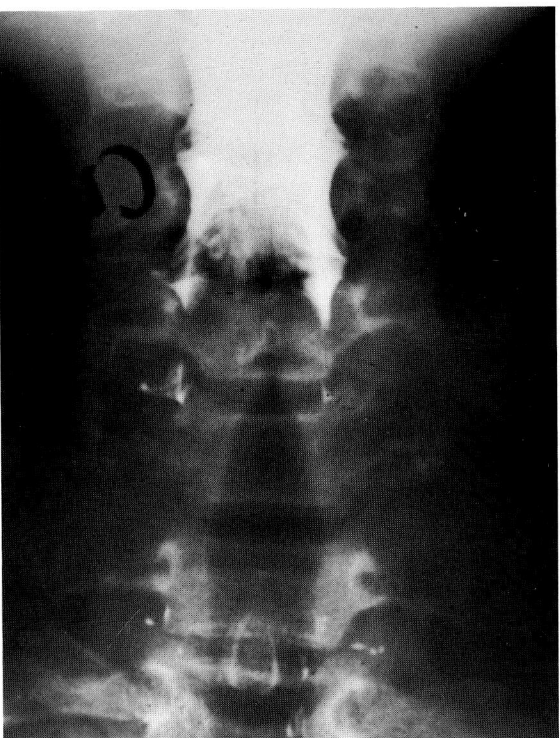

Fig. 8-8. This cervical myelogram demonstrates a complete block at C4. The correct diagnosis of intramedullary tumor is suggested by the relatively normal cord that suddenly bulges with smooth shoulders at the beginning of the cervical enlargement. It would not be possible from a single film to differentiate this from massive cord compression by an anteriorly placed lesion. However, the cord's sudden enlargement is highly suggestive of an intramedullary lesion. This proved to be an ependymoma with a sizable intramedullary cyst.

SYRINGOMYELIA

The presence of a cyst within the spinal cord unrelated to tumor is common. The syrinx is important because it mimics an intramedullary tumor and must be differentiated. Findings from the physical examination are characteristic, though not always diagnostic. The patient usually has low motor neuron findings in the upper extremities with atrophy and fasciculation, spasticity, and weakness in the lower extremities, and a dissociated capelike sensory loss involving the upper extremities and upper chest, in which pain and temperature sensation are lost with preservation of light touch in posterior columns. Diagnostic studies show only an intramedullary lesion. Sometimes air myelography is diagnostic when collapse of the cord can be demonstrated radiographically. The association of the Chiari malformation certainly suggests that a syrinx exists (Figs. 8-8, 8-9, 8-10).

The therapy of syringomyelia is still a matter of some discussion. Some favor simple decompression of the Chiari malformation with obliteration of a connection between the fourth ventricle and syrinx, if it exists. Others suggest direct attack upon the syrinx with creation of a syringostomy to the cervical subarachnoid space. There are no definitive papers that clearly state that one technique is better than another, and therapy still must be individualized according to the patient's abnormalities and the most important symptoms.[48]

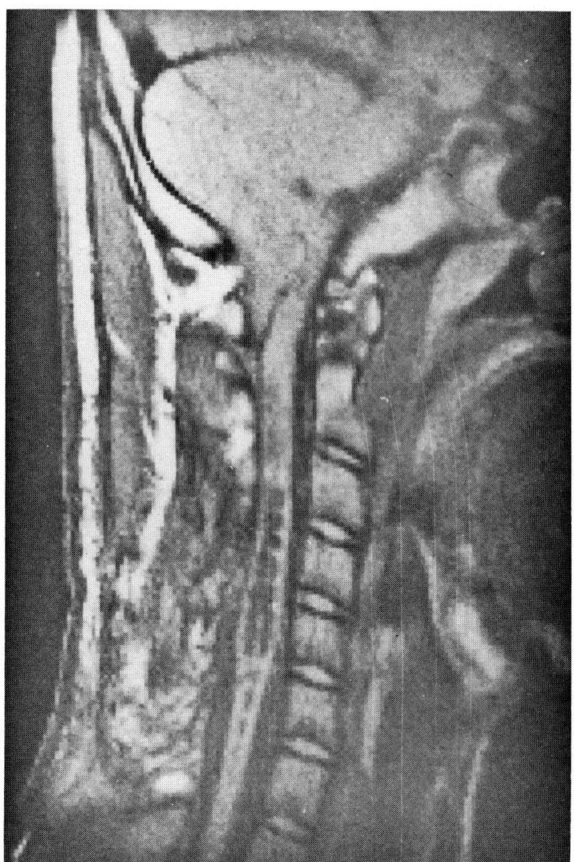

Fig. 8-9. MR scan of the cervical spine demonstrating Chiari Type I malformation with associated cervical syringohydromyelia.

SPECIFIC TUMORS OF THE SPINAL CORD

Three major groups of tumors make up the majority of spinal cord neoplasms. Schwannomas represent about 29%, meningiomas 25%, and gliomas 22% of all lesions. Therefore, more extensive discussion of these tumors is worthwhile.[15,54]

Schwannomas

One third of schwannomas are extradural and two thirds are intradural; a small group occupy both locations. They are least likely to be found in the cervical region. The schwannoma is a firm, encapsulated, rounded mass with a typical histologic appearance that has been extensively described. These tumors arise from the spinal root and frequently compress the root at the foramen (Fig. 8-2). Localized root symptoms are characteristic of their early course. Eventually, additional roots may be involved and spinal cord compression is common. The neurologic findings are not characteristic, but most commonly in advanced cases there is pyramidal tract and posterior column involvement below the level of the lesion, with local atrophy and sensory loss because of the root involvement. A Brown-Séquard symptom may commonly develop as well. These tumors are commonly seen in the syndrome of multiple neurofibromatosis, an inherited disorder in which multiple neurofibromas involving cranial nerves and spinal nerves, often associated with intracranial tumors of all types, are present (Fig. 8-3). Mutiple tumors may be present with this syndrome and it is frequently impossible to remove them all. The diagnosis is usually made on myelography; otherwise it is confirmed at the time of surgery. Since it is usually not possible to remove all tumors, surgical excision of symptomatic lesions is the preferable choice.[49]

Meningiomas

Fifteen percent of meningomas are completely extradural or both intradural and extradural. Eighty-five percent are intradural and extramedullary. They are found in the cervical region in about 13% of cases. The tumors are usually nodular, well circumscribed, and less well encapsulated than neurofibromas. The histology is not different from that for meningomas elsewhere, and malignant tumors are very rare. Most characteristically, the tumors originally grow at the dorsal root entry zone and are clinically not distinguishable from neurofibromas. The pain is less commonly localizing. An unusual meningoma that involves the upper cervical area as well as the intracranial cavity is the so-called foramen magnum tumor. Tumors in this area are very difficult to diagnose and are most commonly meningiomas. Symptoms are bizarre and often variable, and patients with these tumors are often dismissed as psychiatric. Nondescript headache is an early problem. Weakness and paresthesias in the lower extremities may occur but often are variable from examination to examination. Muscular atrophy and fibrillation in the hands and forearms are common, probably secondary to compression of the anterior spinal arteries. A mistaken diagnosis of lower motor neuron disease in the cervical region is common. The course of the illness is relentlessly progressive and the nature of the disease frequently becomes ap-

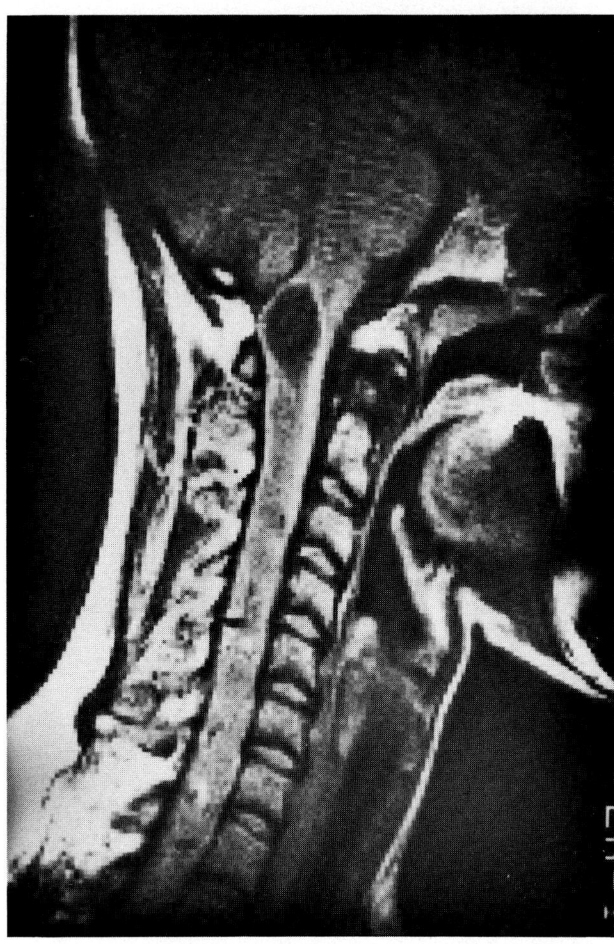

Fig. 8-10. MR scan of cervical spine spin-echo pulse sequence. T1-weighted sagittal view shows the entire cervical cord abnormally enlarged. There is a diffuse low-signal intensity as compared with normal spinal cord. The level of the foramen magnum focal dilatation of a cavity is seen. The cerebellar tonsils are in normal position. Postoperative diagnosis is syringobulbomyelia.

parent only when quadriparesis is evident. The treatment is surgical removal.[42]

Intramedullary Gliomas

Intramedullary gliomas are about equally divided between astrocytomas and ependymomas. All other tumors are extremely rare. Even so, gliomas are least likely to occur in the cervical region. These relatively benign tumors have clinical symptoms slow in onset. They rarely are diagnosed until a long period of time has elapsed after the onset of symptoms. Chronic pain is a common initial symptom, frequently followed by spasticity often initially described by the patients as gait disturbance. Sensory loss appears relatively late and usually is dissociated, with local loss of pain and temperature predominating. Eventually the patient becomes quadraplegic, but this occurs quite late. All of these tumors progress slowly, and while long survivals have been reported, the majority of patients left untreated or ineffectively treated will eventually succumb with quadriplegia secondary to the disease. Both astrocytomas and ependymomas appear as elongated fusiform swellings of the spinal cord (see Figs. 8-6 and 8-8). Cysts are present in about one third of astrocytomas. It may be extremely difficult to be certain about the pathology; the abnormal cells are few and very similar in appearance to normal astrocytes. Ependymomas are more likely to be well encapsulated with a clearer line of cleavage between the spinal cord and the tumor. It is not possible to differentiate the various kinds of gliomas on the basis of diagnostic studies or the physical examination.[50]

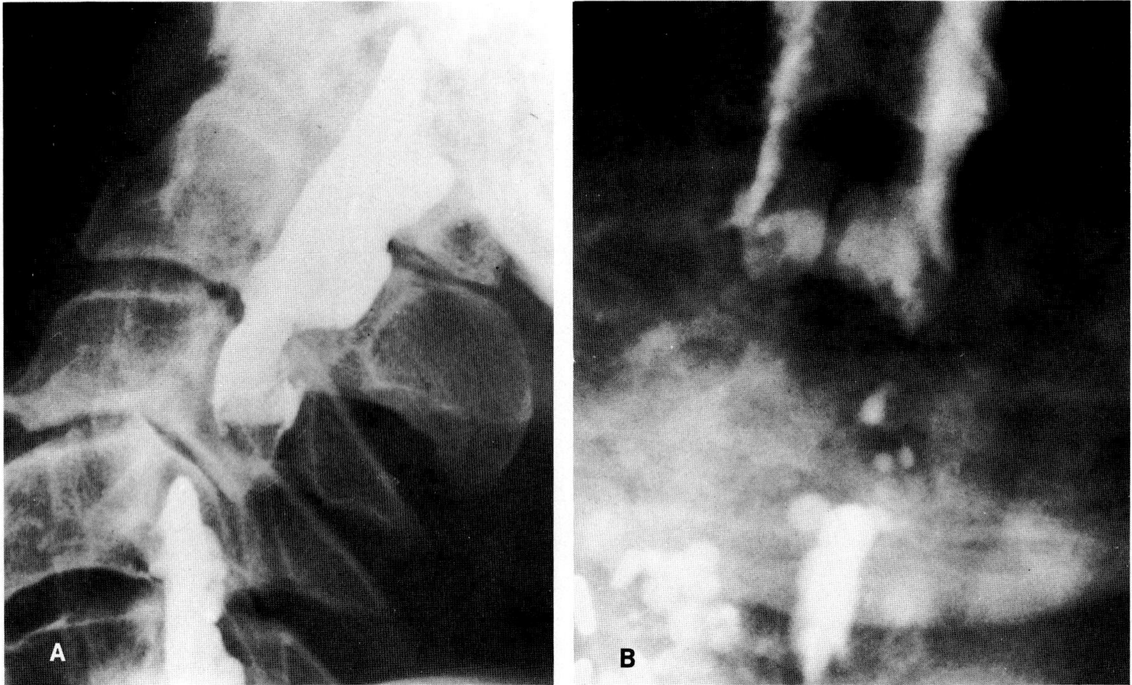

Fig. 8-11. (*A*) Lateral and (*B*) A–P views of a large, anteriorly placed extradural mass centered at the C3–C4 interspace. There is a virtually complete block of spinal fluid flow at this level. The cord is markedly widened over an anteriorly placed bony ridge, a condition typical of severe cervical spondylosis.

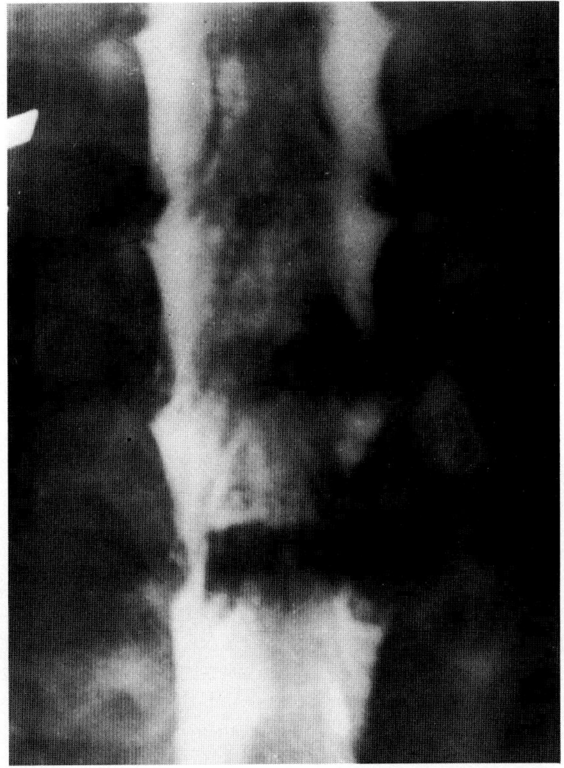

Fig. 8-12. The cervical myelogram demonstrates a large smooth defect indenting the sac without significant spinal cord displacement. The extradural lesion was proven to be an osteochondroma originating from the lamina and lateral masses.

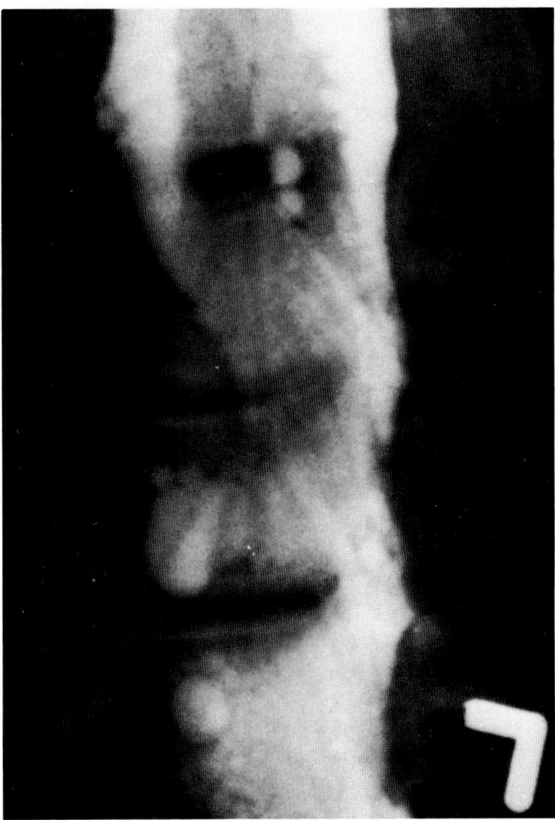

Fig. 8-13. The cervical myelogram demonstrates a large extradural defect smoothly compressing the dural sac and obliterating the root sleeve at C7–T1. This proved to be a herniated free-fragment disc still contained by the posterior longitude in the ligament.

ARACHNOID CYSTS

Cysts of the arachnoid are often seen in myelography. Although most occur in the thoracic region, a cyst occasionally appears in the cervical area. Most do not give rise to symptoms, but an occasional patient will have symptoms from such a lesion. Pain is the earliest common symptom, often exaggerated by physical activity, and arteriovenous malformation is often the suspected diagnosis. The pain is frequently relieved by lying down. The patient may develop signs of spinal cord compression, but these are not characteristic. Films are usually normal. The myelogram demonstrates an extramedullary lesion and the diagnosis is made at the time of surgery. Histologically these cysts do not show any difference from normal arachnoid and they require no special therapy.[1]

DIFFERENTIAL DIAGNOSIS

The most common confusion between spinal cord tumors and another disease state arises from the lack of recognition of an inflammatory process. Pyogenic abscess may occur in the epidural space. Tuberculous abscess is possible and tuberculomas may occur intradurally.[13,65] Syphilis may occasionally present with a gumma, but this is now an extremely rare disease. Fungal infections and parasites have also been reported; schistosomiasis and echinococciasis occur in areas where these diseases are common.[12,14] Occasionally a massively herniated intervertebral disc mimics an extradural spinal cord tumor (Figs. 8-11, 8-12, and 8-13). It may sometimes be difficult to differentiate the congenitally narrow spinal canal with a normal spinal cord from an enlarged spinal cord with a normal canal; careful measurements will usually settle this question. The number of diseases that can be mistaken for spinal cord tumors includes everything that may present with radicular symptoms or signs of myelopathy. Infectious myelitis, toxic myelopathy, intrinsic spinal cord vascular disease, demyelinating diseases, developmental defects at the craniocervical junction, and degenerative diseases all must be considered, but an extensive review of these conditions is beyond the scope of this publication.[8,35]

REFERENCES

1. *Adams RD, Wegner W:* Congenital cyst of the spinal meninges as cause of intermittent compression of the spinal cord. Arch Neurol Psychiatr 58:57, 1947
2. *Alexander E Jr, Davids CH Jr, Field CH:* Metastatic lesions of the vertebral column causing cord compression. Neurology 6:103, 1956
3. *Aminoff MJ, Logue V:* Clinical features of spinal vascular malformation. Brain 97:197, 1974
4. *Arseni CH, Simionescu MD, Horwath L:* Tumors of the spine: A follow-up study of 350 patients with neurosurgical considerations. Acta Psychiatr Scand 34:398, 1959
5. *Aubin ML, Jardin C, Bar D, Vignaud J:* Computerized tomography in 32 cases of intraspinal tumor. J Neuroradiol 6:81–82, 1979
6. *Austin GM:* The significance and nature of pain in tumors of the spinal cord. Surg Forum 10:782, 1959
7. *Barron KD, Hirano A, Araki S, et al:* Experiences with metastatic neoplasms involving the spinal cord. Neurology 9:91, 1959
8. *Bucy PC, Oberhill HR:* Intradural spinal granulomas. J Neurosurg 7:1, 1950

9. *BUCY PC:* The treatment of malignant tumors of the spine: Review. Neurology 13:939, 1963
10. *BULL JWD:* Spinal meningiomas and neurofibromas. Acta Radiol 40:283, 1953
11. *BUNTS AT:* The mimicry of tumors of the spinal cord. Am Surg 26:630, 1960
12. *CARREA R, MURPHY G:* Primary hydatid cyst of the spinal cord. Acta Neurol Lat Am 10:308, 1964
13. *CHADDUCK WM:* Intraspinal tuberculous abscess simulating lumbar disc disease. Va Med 99:968, 1972
14. *CHÜRAÜ JS:* Two cases of Echinococcus disease of the spinal cord. Bulletin Faculte Medecine d'Ankara 1:73, 1947
15. *COHEN DM, DAHLIN DC, MACCARTY CS:* Tumors of the vertebral column (apparently solitary). Mayo Clin Proc 39:509, 1964
16. *COHEN DM, SVIEN HJ, DAHLIN DC:* Long-term survival of patients with myeloma of the vertebral column. JAMA 187:914, 1964
17. *CROSS GO, WHITE HL, WHITE LP:* Acrylic prosthesis of the fifth cervical vertebra in multiple myeloma. J Neurosurg 35:112, 1971
18. *DICHIRO G, DOPPMAN JL, OMMAYA AK:* Selective arteriography of arteriovenous aneurysms of spinal cord. Radiology 88:1065, 1967
19. *DOPPMAN JL, WIRTH FP, DICHIRO G, ET AL:* Value of cutaneous angiomas in the arteriographic localization of spinal cord arteriovenous malformations. N Engl J Med 28:1140, 1969
20. *DUTTON JEM, ALEXANDER GL:* Intramedullary spinal abscess. J Neurol Neurosurg Psychiatr 17:303, 1954
21. *EDELSON RN, BECK MDF, POSNER JB:* Intramedullary spinal cord metastases. Neurology 22:1222, 1972
22. *ELSBERG CA:* Surgical diseases of the spinal cord, membranes, and nerve roots: Symptoms, diagnosis, and treatment. New York, Hoeber, 1941
23. *FORNASIER VL, HORNE JG:* Metastases to the vertebral column. Cancer 36:490, 1975
24. *FRIEDMAN M, KIM TH, PANAHON AM:* Spinal cord compression in malignant lymphoma. Cancer 37:1485, 1976
25. *FURNARI S:* Contribution to the study of intramedullary angiomas of the spinal cord. Minerva Chir 9:944, 1954
26. *GALICICH JH, SUNDARESAN N, BAINS M:* Surgical management of paravertebral thoracic tumors with intraspinal extension (abstr). Proc Neurosurg Soc Am, 1981
27. *GAUTIER-SMITH PC:* Clinical aspects of spinal neurofibromas. Brain 90:359, 1967
28. *GESCHICKTER CF, COPELAND MM:* Tumors of Bone, pp 489–562. Philadelphia, JB Lippincott, 1936
29. *GOWERS WR, HORSLEY V:* A case of tumor of the spinal cord: Removal, recovery. Medical-Chirugical Transactions (London) 71:377, 1888
30. *GREENWOOD J:* Total removal of intramedullary tumors. J Neurosurg 11:616, 1954
31. *GREENWOOD J:* Intramedullary tumors of spinal cord: A follow-up study after total surgical removal. J Neurosurg 20:665, 1963
32. *GREENWOOD J:* Surgical removal of intramedullary tumors. J Neurosurg 26:275, 1967
33. *GUIDETTI B:* Intramedullary tumours of the spinal cord. Acta Neurochir (Wien) 17:7, 1967
34. *GUIDETTI B, FORTUNA A:* Surgical treatment of intramedullary hemangioblastoma of the spinal cord and report of six cases. J Neurosurg 27:530, 1967
35. *HAFT H, RANSOHOFF J, CARTER S:* Spinal cord tumors in children. Pediatrics 23:152, 1959
36. *HALL AJ, MACKAY NNS:* The results of laminectomy for compression of the cord or cauda equina by extradural malignant tumour. J Bone Joint Surg 55B:497, 1973
37. *HACHEN HJ:* Computed tomography of the spine and spinal cord; limitations and applications. Paraplegia 19:155–163, 1981
38. *HANDEL S, GROSSMAN R, SARWAR M:* Computed tomography in the diagnosis of spinal cord astrocytoma. J Comput Assit Tomogr 2:226–228, 1978
39. *HEISKANEN O:* Benign extramedullary tumors in the high cervical region. Ann Chir Gynaecol Fenn 57:59, 1968
40. *HOLT JF, WRIGHT EM:* The radiological features of neurofibromatosis. Radiology 51:647, 1948
41. *HORRAX G, ANDERSON DG:* Encapsulated intramedullary tumor; Whole spinal cord from medulla to conus. Surg Gynecol Obstet 68:814, 1939
42. *HOWE JR, TAREN JA:* Foramen magnum tumors: Pitfalls in diagnosis. JAMA 225:1060, 1973
43. *JENKINS DHR:* Extensive cervical laminectomy: Long-term results. Br J Surg 60:852, 1973
44. *KEPLINGER JE, BUCY PC:* Giant cell tumors of the spine. Ann Surg 154:148, 1961
45. *KRAUS HI:* Malignant tumors of the vertebral column and the spinal cord. Wien Klin Wochenschr 64:867, 1952
46. *KRAYENBUHL H, YASARGIL MD, MCCLINTOCK HG:* Treatment of spinal cord vascular malformation by surgical excision. J Neurosurg 30:427, 1969
47. *LEE BCPO, ZIMMERMAN RD, MANNING JJ, DECK MDF:* MR imaging of syringomyelia and hydromyelia. AJNR 6:221–228, 1985
48. *LONG DM:* Spinal cord compression secondary to neoplasms. Minn Med 51:1239, 1968
49. *LOVE JG, DODGE HW:* Dumbbell (hourglass) neurofibromas affecting the spinal cord. Surg Gynecol Obstet 94:161, 1952

50. *Malis LI:* Intramedullary spinal cord tumors. Clin Neurosurg 25:512, 1977
51. *McAlhany HJ, Netsky MG:* Compression of the spinal cord by extramedullary neoplasms. J Neuropathol Exp Neurol 14:276, 1955
52. *Modic MT, Pavlicek W, Weinstein MA, et al:* Magnetic resonance imaging of intervertebral disk disease. Radiology 152:103–111, 1984
53. *Modic MT, Weinstein MA, Paulicek W, Boumphrey F, Starnes D, Duchesneau PLM:* Magnetic resonance imaging of the cervical spine: Technical and clinical observations. AJNR 5:15–22, 1984
54. *Mulder DW, Dale AJD:* Spinal cord tumors and disks. In Baker AB, Baker LS (eds): Clinical Neurology. New York, Harper & Row, 1978
55. *Nakawa H, Huang YP, Malis LI, Wolf BS:* Computed tomography of intraspinal and parapsinal neoplasms. J Comput Assist Tomogr 1:377, 1977
56. *Norman D, Mills CM, Brant-Zawadzki M, Yeates A, Crooks LE, Kaufman L:* Magnetic resonance imaging of the spinal cord and canal: Potentials and limitations. AJNR 5:9–14, 1982
57. *Poole JL:* The surgery of spinal cord tumors. Clin Neurosurg 17:310, 1970
58. *Sartor K:* Computed tomography of the cervical spine and spinal cord. Ann radiol 23:245–247, 1980
59. *Scoville WB, Palmer AH, Samra K, Chong G:* The use of acrylic plastic for vertebral replacement of fixation in metastatic disease of the spine. J Neurosurg 27:274, 1965
60. *Skalpe IO, Sortland O:* Cervical myelography with metrizamide (Amipaque) comparison between conventional and computer-assisted myelography with special reference to the upper cervical and foramen magnum region. Neuroradiology 16:275–278, 1978
61. *Slooff JL, Kernohan JW, MacCarty S:* Primary intramedullary tumors of the spinal cord and filum terminale a, pp 10–11; b, pp 194–237. Philadelphia, WB Saunders, 1964
62. *Snyder LJ, Wilhelm SK:* Multiple myeloma with spinal cord compression as the initial finding. Ann Intern Med 28:1169, 1948
63. *Spinous E, Laster DW, Moody DM, Ball MR, Witcofski RL, Kelly DL:* MR evaluation of Chiari I malformations at 0.15T. AJNR 6:203–208, 1985
64. *Thomas JE, Miller RH:* Lipomatous tumors of the spinal canal: A study of their clinical range. Mayo Clin Proc 48:393, 1973
65. *Torre M:* Solitary tuberculoma of the spinal cord with terminal secondary myelitis. Riv Neurol 19:285, 1959
66. *Vieth RG, Odom GL:* Extradural spinal metastases and their neurosurgical treatment. J Neurosurg 23:501, 1965

CHAPTER 9

Infections

Tuberculosis

LOUIS C. S. HSU AND ARTHUR C. M. C. YAU

Although the vertebral column is the most common site of skeletal tuberculosis, Pott's disease involving the cervical spine is relatively uncommon. In a series of over 1000 cases we reviewed, the incidence of cervical involvement was 3.5%. Disease involving the atlantoaxial joint is rare and occurred in 0.5% of the cases. In the past, tuberculous spondylitis was a disease of early childhood. With improved public health measures, the age incidence has changed and adults are more frequently affected. The number of vertebrae involved in each case has also lessened with improved general health care.

PATHOLOGY

The mode of spread of tubercle baccilli to the spine is by way of infected abdominal or pelvic organs at the level of the spine and then through the spine, up and down the spinal canal by way of the Batson's venous plexus. This explains the relative rarity of cervical involvement, the high association between tuberculosis of the kidney and of the thoracolumbar junction of the spine, and also the multiple levels of involvement that often occur.[8]

Two types of disease are recognized: that usually seen in younger children (the "child" type) and that which usually occurs in older children or adults (the "adult" type).[12] The child type is characterized by more diffuse and extensive involvement, the formation of the large abscesses, and a lower incidence of Pott's paraplegia or tetraplegia (Fig. 9-1, 9-2). The adult type is more localized and produces less pus, but it has a higher incidence of paraplegia (Fig. 9-3).

The disease usually involves only the anterior elements of the spine. The posterior elements or transverse processes are rarely affected. In children the focus of infection begins in the center of the vertebral body, whereas in adults the disease often begins as a paradiscal infection. In children, because of their relatively lower immunity to the disease, there is a tendency to spread to adjacent vertebral bodies, usually by extension beneath the

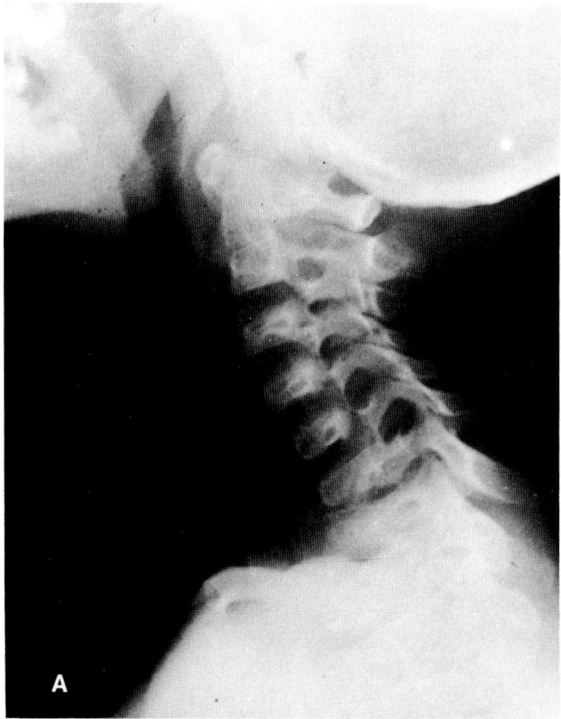

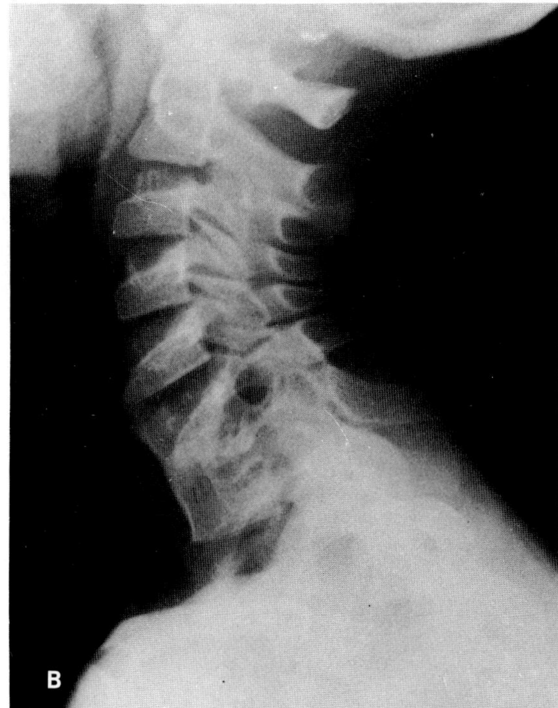

Fig. 9-1. (*A*) Roentgenogram of a 3-year-old boy who presented with stiffness of his neck that had lasted for 3 months. Note complete destruction of the C7 vertebral body and partial involvement of C5 and C6, prevertebral soft tissue swelling, and kyphosis. (*B*) Roentgenogram 7 months after anterior radical excision and grafting. Fusion was solid and soft tissue swelling had disappeared. (*C*) Roentgenogram 10 years after surgery. Note reconstitution of cervical lordosis. The patient is asymptomatic and has a full range of neck movements.

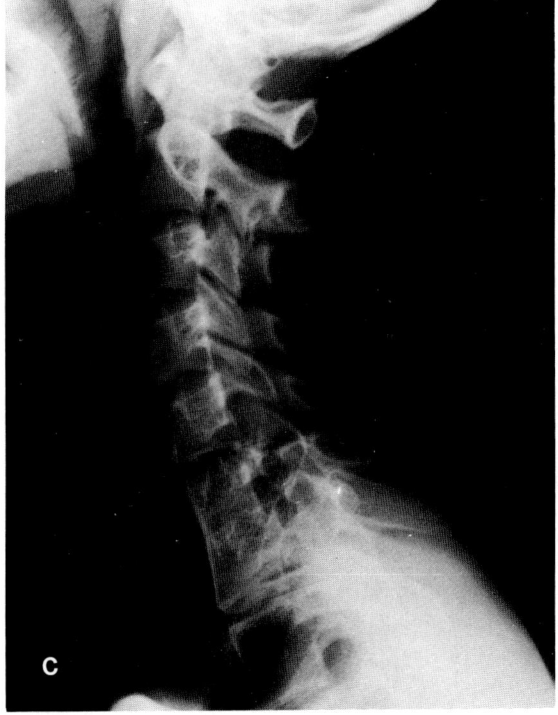

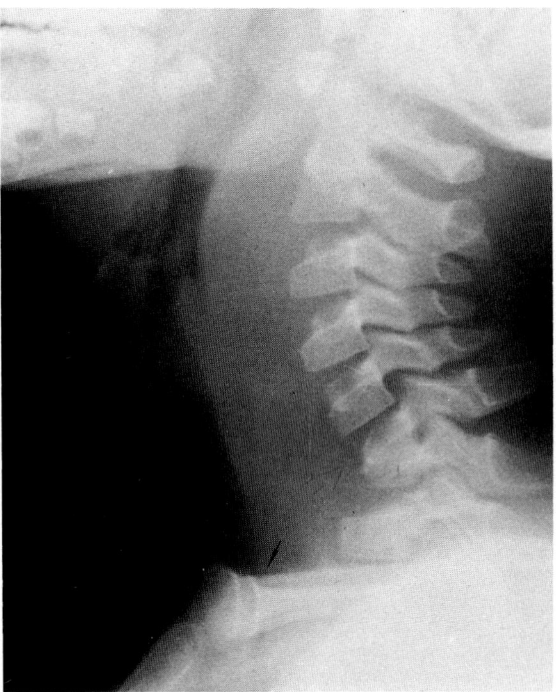

Fig. 9-2. Roentgenogram of a 5-year-old boy with tuberculous involvement of the C6 and C7 vertebral bodies. Note the large prevertebral shadow and narrowing of the trachea just behind the sternal notch. He presented with inspiratory stridor.

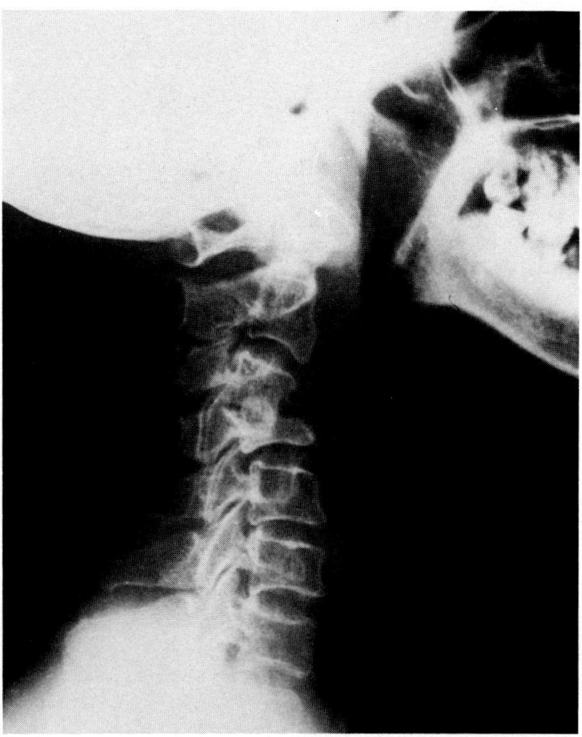

Fig. 9-3. Roentgenogram of a 38-year-old woman presenting with disease involving mainly C3–C4 and early tetraplegia. Note localized involvement and marginal soft tissue swelling.

anterior longitudinal ligaments or directly across the intervertebral disc, which eventually sequestrates. With vertebral destruction, tuberculosis granulation tissue, slough, caseous matter, and necrotic bones are extruded, forming a cold abscess. The prevertebral fascia in the cervical spine limits this abscess and allows it to collect in the retropharyngeal region. As its gathers, it displaces the pharynx, larynx, trachea, and esophagus forward. This displacement may be severe enough to cause asthma Millari, a condition first described by Millar in the 19th century in patients with cervicodorsal tuberculosis complicated by cyanosis, suffocation, and death due to pressure on the trachea. Fortunately this condition is rare. The cold abscess tract is often lateral behind the strong prevertebral fascia, pointing to the posterior triangle of the neck. Sinus formation, however, is not a prominent feature as compared with tuberculosis of the lumbar spine. Rupture of the cold abscess into the pharynx is rare but has been described.

In adults, because of their relative immunity to the disease in endemic countries, the disease is more localized and seldom spreads as it does in children. Often, it presents as a lesion of a single disc space or of a vertebral body (Fig. 9-3).

The pathologic process weakens the vertebral body, which eventually collapses, producing a mild kyphosis or loss of lordosis. Unlike the thoracic or thoracolumbar spine, severe kyphotic deformity seldom occurs in the cervical spine unless three or more vertebral bodies are involved, because most of the weight of the head is borne through the articular process, rather than the vertebral body. However, when disease in the lower cervical spine spreads down to the upper dorsal region, forward subluxation or dislocation of the cervical spine may occur on the thoracic spine so that the undersurface of the lowest remaining cervical vertebra comes to rest on the anterior surface of the uppermost thoracic vertebra.[8] This produces a severe kyphosis associated with cord compression.

Healing occurs by initial fibrosis followed by gradual calcification of the granulomatous tuber-

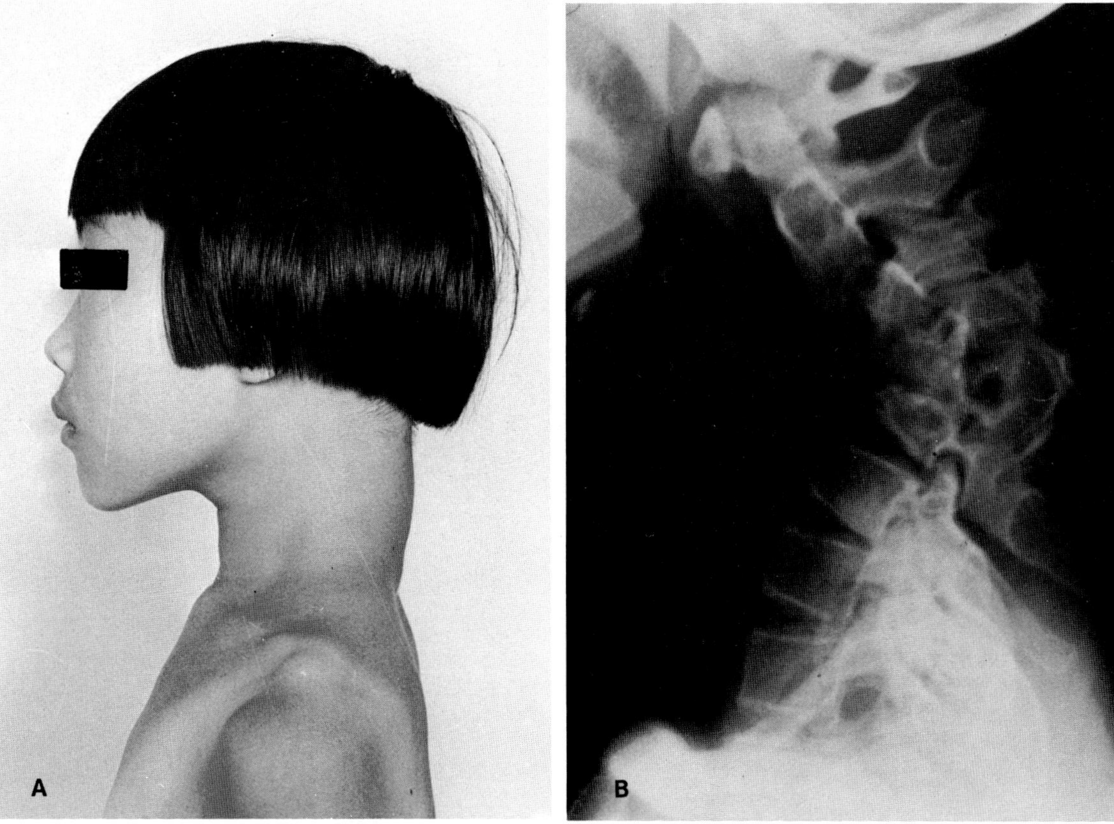

Fig. 9-4. A possible end result of conservative treatment. (*A*) This girl of 13 had tuberculosis of her cervical spine at the age of 5 years, which was treated by chemotherapy and Minerva jacket. (*B*) The disease has healed with significant kyphosis. Note the spontaneous posterior fusion.

culous tissue. Eventually, ossification and bony ankylosis occur. These are invariably accompanied by spontaneous fusion of the posterior facet joints (Fig. 9-4).

Quadriplegia or quadriparesis may appear at various stages of the disease and is particularly common in the adult type. In a series of 40 patients reported by Hsu and Leong in 1984, 13 of the 16 patients presenting with tuberculosis of the lower cervical spine over the age of 10 years had cord compression, whereas only 4 of 24 patients under age 10 had cord compression. The main reasons for the higher incidence with increasing age are progressive narrowing of the spinal canal from degenerative disease, loss of flexibility of the spine, and inelasticity of the prevertebral fascia.[12]

In the active disease, compression of the cord is usually due to tension of the abscess, to the posteriorly extruded sequestrated intervertebral disc of sequestra, tuberculous granulation tissue in the spinal canal, or subluxation and dislocation of the vertebrae. This is called quadriplegia of active disease. Very rarely the tuberculous disease involves the cord and meninges, producing tuberculous meningomyelitis. The prognosis of this type of quadriplegia is poor. In the healed disease, quadriparesis can still occur as a result of fibrosis of the meninges or mechanical compression by the healing internal kyphus.[9]

CLINICAL FEATURES

The commonest local symptoms are progressive pain and stiffness in the neck, often preceded by initial general symptoms of malaise, easy fatigability, loss of appetite and weight, lethargy, night sweats, and fever. The pain in the neck may be referred to the shoulders and arms. In the upper

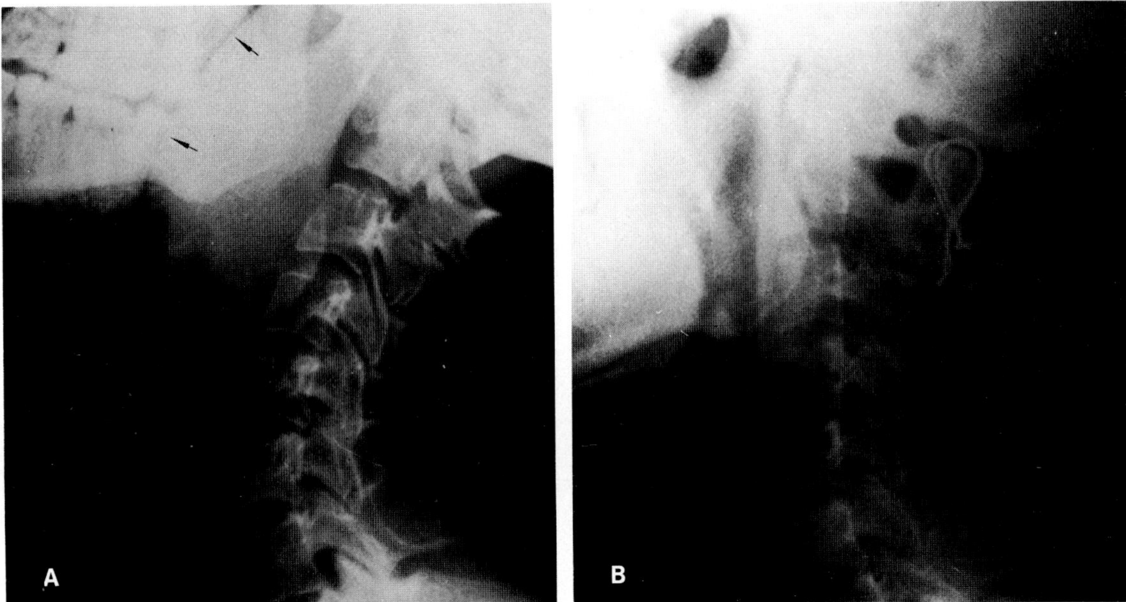

Fig. 9-5. (*A*) Roentgenogram of a 25-year-old man with disease in the atlantoaxial joint. Note the large retropharyngeal abscess and the subluxation of the joint. He had weakness of all four limbs and extensor Balinski. (*B*) Roentgenogram 6 months after transoral incision and drainage, halo traction with neck in extention, and posterior C1–C2 fusion with wiring.

cervical spine, the referred pain may be to the occiput or the forehead. The stiffness is due to spasm of the muscles around the neck, which is held rigid, and motion is limited in all directions. Occasionally young patients with a significant abscess may present with inspiratory stridor.

Flattening of the normal cervical lordosis is often the initial finding; gentle percussion or palpation over the spinous process of the affected vertebrae invariably produces tenderness. Fluctuant swelling in the posterior triangle of the neck may indicate a cold abscess, but it must be distinguished from a suppurative tuberculous lymph node.

Disease in the upper cervical spine may present with discomfort in the throat, often leading to a change of tone in the voice, and a swelling that may be seen or palpated behind the oropharynx (Fig. 9-5).

If quadriplegia or quadriparesis develops, there will be a lower motor neuron lesion of the dermatome at the level of the spinal lesion and an upper motor neuron lesion below the level of the spinal lesion. There will be varying degrees of muscle weakness, loss of sensation, and disturbance of bladder and bowel function. The deep tendon reflexes of the lower limbs will be hyperactive and the Babinski response will be extensor.

The sedimentation rate is invariably raised and there may be moderate lymphocytosis and anemia. The Mantoux or Tine test is usually positive but may be negative in the active phase of the disease. In endemic countries, the test is often positive because of the previous exposure to the bacilli and must be interpreted with discretion.

RADIOLOGIC FEATURES

In tuberculous spondylitis, the radiologic features are often characteristic in the young child, but in the elderly differentiation from pyogenic spondylitis or secondary deposits from malignant tumors is often difficult. In countries where the disease is endemic, an enlarged soft tissue shadow in front of the cervical spine coupled with destruction of vertebral bodies in a child is almost pathognomonic of the disease (Figs. 9-1 and 9-2). In the elderly, the changes are more subtle because the pathologic process tends to be more chronic. The involved vertebral body or bodies become rarified and lose their bony trabecular patterns. The intervertebral disc space may be preserved for a long time but eventually becomes narrow and later is obliterated. As the lesion in the vertebral body expands, its borders become indistinct and may eventually collapse. Soft tissue swelling in front of the cervical spine may be unremarkable despite the presence of cord compression.

Disease involving the atlantoaxial joint is invariably accompanied by subluxation of that joint (Fig. 9-5).

DIFFERENTIAL DIAGNOSIS

In the differential diagnosis one should consider suppurative spondylitis, pyogenic retropharyngeal abscess, metastatic tumorous deposits, eosinophilic granuloma, osteoclastoma, and chordoma. All these conditions may cause destruction or collapse of the vertebral body, narrowing and obliteration of the intervertebral disc space, and paraspinal soft tissue swelling.

Occasionally a cervical spinal deformity associated with neurofibromatosis or a congenital anomaly such as block vertebra may present like a healed tuberculous infection of the cervical spine.

Radiologically, tuberculosis involving the atlantooccipital and atlantoaxial joints may be difficult to differentiate from rheumatoid arthritis.

TREATMENT

The history of treatment of Pott's disease dates back to the 17th century when the only available method of treatment was prolonged recumbency and rest. With the advent of anesthesia, various surgical procedures were used, including posterior spinal fusion, posterior decompression by means of a laminectomy, and, in the thoracic region, anterolateral decompression or debridement through a costotransversectomy approach. None of these has been proved to be of real value in the management of the disease. Posterior fusion and laminectomy have actually been proved to be harmful since they both can cause further instability and dislocation.[16,23]

The introduction of specific antituberculous chemotherapy agents in 1945 provided the main breakthrough in the treatment of tuberculosis, and for some years chemotherapy together with immobilization or inpatient bed rest was a classical form of treatment. In 1958, Konstam and Konstam advocated a policy of ambulant outpatient chemotherapy treatment and reported good results.[15] This policy is most appealing, particularly in developing countries where hospital beds and surgical facilities are scarce.[1,13–15]

On the other hand, Hodgson and Stock in 1956 proposed a radical approach to the treatment of this disease. Under cover of antituberculous chemotherapy, the diseased spine was exposed by way of an anterior route that provided good exposure, the abscess was evacuated, and the infected and avascular or sequestrated bone and intervertebral disc were completely excised. The defect created was then filled by bony struts. The results on 412 cases treated by this method (the Hong Kong radical operation) were reported in 1960. A fusion rate of 93% was seen and complete recovery from the spinal disease was obtained in almost every case.[5–7]

The diversity of opinions on the treatment of tuberculosis of the spine led the medical research working party on tuberculosis of the spine to carry out in 1964 a large-scale controlled trial of the various methods of treatment. Over 600 patients with similar pretreatment factors were involved in the trial, which was carried out in various centers throughout the world. The analyses were made by independent assessors. The study, unfortunately, involved only the thoracic and lumbar spine. The cervical spine was excluded because of statistical reasons, but the published results and conclusions could be applied, with slight modification, to the cervical spine.[17–22]

The trial concluded that the best method of treating spinal tuberculosis was chemotherapy combined with the Hong Kong radical operation. This combination of anterior resection, grafting, and chemotherapy relieved patient's pain quickly, stopped their discharging sinuses earlier, produced early bony union, and prevented the development of kyphosis. The working party, however, felt that this operation should only be done if surgical expertise, adequate anesthetic facilities, and skilled nursing are readily available. The latter factor is perhaps not as important when applied to the third to seventh cervical vertebral bodies because the surgical approach to this region is certainly much easier and postoperative nursing care is less demanding than it would be after surgery of the thoracic, thoracolumbar, or lumbar spine. Surgery has the added advantage of evacuating the abscess and preventing the complications of Millar's asthma, which is not seen in the rest of the spine. It also eliminates all possibilities of early or late onset quadriplegia.

The trial also concluded that chemotherapy alone produced reasonable results, and that inpatient bed rest and plaster immobilization did not confer any added advantage. We do not doubt that chemotherapy alone can also produce favorable results in the cervical spine, but the process is much slower and allows the development of kyphosis, which is cosmetically deforming even if it is mild; it is certainly not the ideal form of treatment and should be used only when surgical facilities are not available. If implemented, some form of splintage should be used in conjunction to relieve pain and muscle spasm in the initial phase of treatment. In contrast to the thoracic and lumbar spine, the cervical spine is more mobile and therefore more painful when affected with the disease. Inpatient treatment is certainly unnecessary unless the patient develops reaction to the chemotherapy.

Some patients with quadriplegia from active disease do respond to conservative treatment, but the process is slow and often takes months or years. Surgical removal of the compressing agent by the Hong Kong operation allows the paralysis to resolve in a couple of days or weeks. It is therefore certainly unfair to treat the patient conservatively when he presents with quadriplegia. Again, laminectomy must be strongly condemned. In the active disease the compression element is always anterior; not only is the posterior approach a bad route, but removal of the laminae also may destroy the only stable element in the cervical spine.

The Hong Kong operation is usually done by way of a Southwick-Robinson approach between the carotid sheath and the esophagus.[24] The bulging abscess wall is incised longitudinally and the pus evacuated. Radical excision is done by removing from the front of the spinal canal all disease tissue, which may include bony sequestra, sequestrated disc, granulation tissue, slough, and avascular bone. Avascular bone is particularly hard and may be difficult to remove. The posterior longitudinal ligaments form the posterior limit of the abscess cavity just in front of the spinal cord. If the patient presents with quadriplegia, this ligament must be removed by making linear cuts, using a small-bladed scapel and then removing the ligament piecemeal by means of pituitary rongeurs. This will display the shiny dura, which should be pulsating. The excision is carried upward and downward until healthy, bleeding cancellous bone is exposed. If the affected bodies were so extensively diseased that healthy and bleeding cancellous bony surfaces are not available, the normal disc and end-plate in the adjacent body will have to be removed to obtain a suitable graft surface.[10] Graft is taken from the iliac crest in one block cut to the required length and inserted with an assistant applying longitudinal traction to the cervical spine. When the traction is released, the graft should be impacted firmly. The postoperative immobilization technique depends on the length and stability of the inserted graft. For grafts transversing one or two disc spaces, a thick soft collar is used for approximately 6 to 8 weeks. For longer grafts, a Minerva jacket or halo cast may have to be used for 12 to 16 weeks.

If the anterior fusion has bridged more than two disc spaces or if the anterior graft has slipped during the postoperative period, a posterior fusion is done 6 to 8 weeks after the anterior spinal fusion. It may also be considered in a growing child if progressive kyphosis develops following the anterior operation.[3] It should only be done when one is certain about the stability of the spine.

Disease in the occipitoatlantoaxial region is extremely rare but poses a challenging problem in management. Although the anterior elements of this region could be approached transorally as described by Fang and Ong in 1962, the exposure is generally limited and the lack of substance of the anterior elements makes grafting an unrewarding proposition.[2] In the presence of cord compression and significant abscess formation, disease in this region is best dealt with by initially draining and debriding by way of the transoral route. The atlantoaxial subluxation should then be reduced by halo traction with the neck in extension; this will relieve the cord compression. A posterior fusion with wiring should then be done, followed by immobilization either by a Minerva jacket or a halo cast for 12 to 16 weeks (Fig. 9-5).

Chemotherapy

It must be emphasized that drugs and not surgery remain the most important weapons in antituberculous therapy. The decision of which drug to be used should be made in consultation with an expert in chemotherapy. It is also vital that such chemotherapy be given and taken regularly and not haphazardly. Uncontrolled chemotherapy will lead not only to failure of the prescribed treatment but also to the development of acquired drug resistance.

We now use streptomycin, isoniazid (INAH), and rifampin routinely as our "first-line" drugs. Ethambutol and pyrazinamide are occasionally used, but only on consultation with an expert.

Streptomycin sulphate is used in doses of 20 mg per kg of body weight up to a maximum of 1 g per day and for a maximum period of 2 to 3 months, or a total dose of 50 g. It may produce a serious toxic effect on the vestibular nerve.

INAH is given in doses of 10 mg per kg body weight up to a maximum of 300 mg per day for a total period of 6 to 9 months. Side effects are rare but hypersensitivity reactions may develop.

Rifampin has now been substituted for para-aminosalicylic acid (PAS) as our first-line drug because the former has a greater bactericidal effect than any other antituberculous drug. It is used in doses of 15 mg per kg body weight up to a maximum of 600 mg daily for a total period of 6 to 9 months. Side effects are uncommon, the most serious of which is thrombocytopenia.

REFERENCES

1. *Dickson JAS:* Spinal tuberculosis in Nigerian children: A review of ambulant treatment. J Bone Joint Surg 49B:682, 1967
2. *Fang HSY, Ong GB:* Direct anterior approach to the upper cervical spine. J Bone Joint Surg 44A:1588, 1962
3. *Fang D, Leong JCY, Fang HSY:* Tuberculosis of the upper cervical spine. J Bone Joint Surg 65B:47, 1983
4. *Fountain SS, Hsu LCS, Yau ACMC, Hodgson AR:* Progressive kyphosis following solid anterior spinal fusion in tuberculosis of the spine in children. J Bone Joint Surg 57A: (8):1104, 1975
5. *Hodgson AR, Stock FE:* Anterior spinal fusion. Br J Surg 44:266, 1956
6. *Hodgson AR, Stock FE:* Anterior spinal fusion for the treatment of tuberculosis of the spine: The operative findings and results of treatment in the first one hundred cases. J Bone Joint Surg 42A:295, 1960
7. *Hodgson AR, Stock FE, Fang HSY, Ong GB:* Anterior spinal fusion. Br J Surg 48:172, 1960
8. *Hodgson AR, Wong W, Yau ACMC:* X-Ray Appearances of Tuberculosis of the Spine. Springfield, IL, Charles C Thomas, 1969
9. *Hodgson AR, Yau A:* Pott's paraplegia: A classification based upon the living pathology. Paraplegia 5 (1):1, 1967
10. *Hodgson AR, Yau ACMC:* Anterior surgical approaches to the spinal column. In Apley AG (ed): Recent Advances in Orthopaedics. London, Churchill Livingstone, 1969
11. *Hodgson AR, Yau A, Kwon JS, Kim D:* A clinical study of 100 consecutive cases of Pott's paraplegia. Clin Orthop 36:128, 1964
12. *Hsu LES, Leong JEY:* Tuberculosis of the lower cervical spine (C2–C7) J Bone Joint Surg 66B: 1984
13. *Konstam PG:* Spinal tuberculosis in Nigeria. Ann R Coll Surg Engl 32:99, 1963
14. *Konstam PG, Blesovsky A:* The ambulant treatment of spinal tuberculosis. Br J Surg 50:26, 1962
15. *Konstam PG, Konstam ST:* Spinal tuberculosis in Southern Nigeria. J Bone Joint Surg 40B:26, 1958
16. *McKee GK:* A comparison of the results of spinal fixation operations and non-operative treatment in Pott's disease in adults. Br J Surg 24:456, 1937
17. *Medical Research Council Working Party on Tuberculosis of the Spine:* A controlled trial of ambulant out-patient treatment and in-patient rest in bed in the management of tuberculosis of the spine in young Korean patients on standard chemotherapy: A study in Masan, Korea. J Bone Joint Surg 55B:678, 1973
18. *Medical Research Council Working Party on Tuberculosis of the Spine:* A controlled trial of plaster-of-Paris jackets in the management of ambulant out-patient treatment of tuberculosis of the spine in children on standard chemotherapy. A study in Pusan, Korea. Tubercule 54:261, 1973
19. *Medical Research Council Working Party on Tuberculosis of the Spine:* A controlled trial of debridement and ambulatory treatment in the management of tuberculosis of the spine in patients on standard chemotherapy: A study in Bulawayo, Rhodesia. J Trop Med Hyg 77:72, 1974
20. *Medical Research Council Working Party on Tuberculosis of the Spine:* A controlled trial of anterior spinal fusion and debridement in the surgical management of tuberculosis of the spine in patients on standard chemotherapy: A study in Hong Kong. Br J Surg 61:853, 1974
21. *Medical Research Council Working Party on Tuberculosis of the Spine:* A five-year assessment of controlled trials of in-patient and out-patient treatment and of plaster-of-Paris jackets for tuberculosis of the spine in children on standard chemotherapy: Studies in Masan and Pusan, Korea. J Bone Joint Surg 58B:399, 1976
22. *Medical Research Council Working Party on Tuberculosis of the Spine:* Five-year assessments of controlled trials of ambulatory treatment: Debridement and anterior spinal fusion in the management of tuberculosis of the spine: Studies in Bulawayo (Rhodesia) and in Hong Kong. J Bone Joint Surg 60B:163, 1978
23. *Seddon HJ:* Treatment of tuberculous disease of the spine. Proceedings of the Royal Society of Medicine 31:951, 1938
24. *Southwick WO, Robinson RA:* Surgical approaches to the vertebral bodies in the cervical and lumbar regions. J Bone Joint Surg 39A;631, 1957

Other Infectious Diseases

S. HENRY LA ROCCA AND FRANK J. EISMONT

EPIDEMIOLOGY AND BACTERIOLOGY

Clinical cases of infections in the cervical spine occur only rarely, yet they can result in problems of such gravity that an index of suspicion must be constantly maintained when attending any patient with cervical complaints. Forsythe and Rothman describe a young patient who presented with neck pain and malaise, but whose initial radiographs were entirely normal.[6] Nonspecific management was instituted, and 1 month later the patient returned in septicemia, with destructive changes in the cervical spine. Although the ultimate bacteriologic result of treatment was a cure, the spinal residuum was a three-segment spontaneous fusion with localized kyphotic deformity and an anatomic arrangement that can reasonably be expected to give rise to additional problems with spondylosis. Although not stated specifically, the authors imply that the possible diagnosis of sepsis was not entertained, and the delayed recognition produced an unnecessarily complex management problem with an anatomic outcome that was compromised from the beginning of specific therapy. No one can state how frequently such events occur, and for this reason more intensive educational efforts about this particular disease appear to be required.

Reported studies indicate that spinal sepsis constitutes only about 1% of all cases of skeletal infection due to pyogenic organisms.[19] Of these, 3% to 4% occur in the cervical spine.[6] Spinal involvement in skeletal tuberculosis is far more frequent than in pyogenic infections, but the frequency of tuberculosis of the cervical spine in any given geographic region of the world is obviously a function of the frequency of the disease itself in that region. The greater the epidemiologic problem, the more frequently will cervical involvement occur.

Further, there are host populations more susceptible to spinal sepsis; these include both children and the elderly as well as persons with chronic medical disorders, including diabetes, addiction to injectable drugs, and renal dysfunction requiring hemodialysis.[8,12,16] Persons with penetrating neck wounds and those undergoing pharyngeal surgery have developed cervical vertebral sepsis, and a case of osteomyelitis following lodging of a foreign body in the hypopharynx has been described. Other potential victims are those undergoing cervical angiography, discography, and cervical spine surgery.[1,6]

A wide spectrum of organisms has been cultured from septic vertebral foci, but the commonest organism encountered in all series is the staphylococcus. Gram-negative organisms also account for appreciable numbers of cases, and *Pseudomonas* appears to have a particular association with heroin addiction.[12] Nonbacterial agents responsible for the rare case include a variety of fungi and parasites.

PATHOLOGY

The primary route of bacterial access to the spine is hematogenous, owing to the abundant vascular supply to vertebral bone. Because of pressure gradient phenomena, the venous access route is less likely than the arterial, although the valveless internal venous system would favor intraspinal spread once infection becomes established.[22] Other routes of access include direct inoculation from traumatic or surgical wounds and lymphatic spread, which is common in tuberculosis. The initial deposit may be in either vertebral bone or intervertebral disc.[14]

The most common initial site of infection is the vertebral metaphysis, where an abscess begins as an organism localizes in the capillary sinusoidal space of cancellous bone. If the abscess is not checked by host response or by appropriate chemotherapy, its enlargement leads to bone destruction and extension to adjacent vertebrae or into the intervertebral disc. Neural arch involvement may develop from the extending metaphyseal lesions or from primary hematogenous inoculation.

A hyperemic response occurs as the abscess becomes established, leading to osteopenia in the region. This bone softening in association with direct bone destruction leads to bone collapse and deformity. Pyogenic abscesses evolve more rapidly than tuberculous ones, and these changes appear more quickly. Pyogenic lesions also tend to promote a hypertrophic response early in their development and bone excrescences form. Should extension into the disc occur, narrowing and collapse develop, along with sclerosis and surface irregularity along the vertebral margins. Sequestra of bone and disc may become isolated and can impinge upon neural elements. Carious lesions filled with purulent debris may cause further weakening of vertebral architecture, and angular deformity may develop. Anterior collapse of vertebral bone leads to the familiar kyphotic deformity of spinal sepsis.

Depending on the site of inoculation, three different localizations of infection can occur: paradiscal, anterior, and central.[3] The paradiscal lesion appears immediately adjacent to the vertebral end-plate of the adjacent vertebral body. The anterior lesion locates in the bone beneath the anterior longitudinal ligaments, forming shallow ulcers. Extension beneath the ligament may lead to involvement of multiple levels, sparing the intervening discs. The central lesion arises from metaphyseal involvement and may have normal discs above and below; the end-plates of the adjacent bodies may be normal. The paradiscal infection is the most common presentation in cases of pyogenic vertebral osteomyelitis. In a review of 64 patients with tuberculous vertebral osteomyelitis treated in the United States, 68% had paradiscal infections, 26% had anterior, and 6% had central.[7]

Although bone infection is more common, primary disc inoculation has been reported in the absence of associated vertebral osteomyelitis.[9] Generally, the disc is considered to be an avascular structure, thus prohibiting hematogenous introduction of organisms. However, in children as well as in many adults, there may be peripheral functioning blood vessels that can extend to the anulonuclear junction.[14] Furthermore, as disc degeneration advances, vascular routes into the disc are reestablished. Hence, there are persons in whom hematogenous discitis may develop.

Besides extension within the vertebral column, abscesses may dissect through the peripheral cortical bone to form paravertebral masses, enlarging the retropharyngeal space and leading to the formation of draining sinuses. Inferior dissection may induce a mediastinitis. Penetration of posterior vertebral wall or anulus will allow purulent spread to the epidural space, which can ultimately lead to meningitis. Tuberculous granulation may, in addition, induce cord ischemia and resultant neurologic deterioration.

The rapidity and extent of development of the changes described depend upon the virulence of the causative organism and the effectiveness of the host response. In general, bony lesions progress more rapidly than disc lesions, and pyogenic organisms provoke a more florid presentation than tuberculous ones.[14] On the other hand, because tuberculous spondylitis develops slowly over a protracted time period, stimulating little hypertrophic host response, resulting destruction and deformity are likely to be more pronounced upon initial evaluation.

Because no discs are present between the occiput and the axis in the upper cervical spine, pure osteomyelitis occurs. Depending upon the degree of hyperemia and the effect of destructive changes, ligamentous laxity and instability may develop, occasionally with devastating consequences. In children, altantoaxial instability may arise in response to infectious processes in the nasopharynx without any direct skeletal sepsis in the spine. This problem is known clinically as Grisel's syndrome, in which otorhinolaryngologic sepsis produces torticollis as atlantoaxial subluxation or dislocation occurs.[20] The mechanism involved is one of hyperemia and decalcification, which induce joint effusion and ligamentous laxity that result in the instability. Management requires orthopedic techniques (traction) in conjunction with specific antimicrobial therapy, and the spinal outcome is usually restoration of normalcy.

CLINICAL PRESENTATION

Septic cervical spondylitis may induce little systemic reaction, and because of this the patient may not develop the standard symptoms and signs of toxicity. Instead, the primary complaint is likely to be axial cervical pain with radiation into the shoulder girdles associated with occipital headache. Dysphagia may be reported. Neurologic symptoms of radiculopathy or even myelopathy may be added to the skeletal complaints. Physical examination discloses mechanical irregularities in the neck with restricted range of motion; paravertebral muscle spasm; tenderness in the occiput, the cervical midline, and the shoulder girdles; and pain intensification with head compression. The fullness of an anterior abscess may be palpable on the front of the neck. Radicular or cord involvement will give rise to neurologic deficits of varying degree, either confined to an upper extremity or generalized as in a myelopathy.

DIAGNOSIS

The sequence of events in any case of cervical osteomyelitis or discitis is one of steady progression modified by host response. Early in the disease—that is, before 3 weeks have elapsed—the diagnosis is often not apparent and will probably be missed unless there is a high index of suspicion. Later, after 3 to 6 weeks, the changes on radiography become distinct enough to permit recognition. Disc infections in patients with advanced cervical spondylosis probably stand as an exception to the rule and may prove to be diagnostic challenges even late in their evolution.

The greater the systemic reaction, the more likely will there be a leukocytosis with anemia. The erythrocyte sedimentation rate, although nonspecific, is apt to be elevated even early in the disease and provides circumstantial diagnostic evidence. It also provides a useful monitor for following response to management. No other hematologic or chemical assay is of particular relevance. Blood culture is useful in only a small percentage of cases, mainly in those patients who have a toxic response to bacteremic episodes.

Radiographic changes are slow to develop, and no abnormality is usually detected before 4 weeks with standard roentgenograms and 2 weeks with tomograms. During this interval the bone scan with technetium or gallium often allows identification of cellular hyperactivity in the cervical spine, which permits a presumptive diagnosis. Reactive scans are nonspecific and hence provide only corroborative information, but this may be extremely useful.

When radiographic changes do appear, they usually begin with decreased bone density in the area of involvement, arising from both osteolysis and reactive hyperemia. Involvement is most commonly paradiscal and less frequently anterior or central. As the disease progresses and bony collapse occurs, areas of increased density due to the presence of impacted or necrotic bone appear. Retropharyngeal space enlargement is apparent when there has been anterior extension. In pyogenic lesions, reactive new bone formation is commonly seen by the third month; such a finding will be greatly delayed in the usual tuberculous case. This new bone will be detected as increased regional density within the involved vertebra, progressive osteophyte development, or both. Disc involvement results in narrowing and collapse of the space, with reactive irregularities along the vertebral margins, both lytic and sclerotic. These findings may follow either disc infection or paradiscal vertebral osteomyelitis (Fig. 9-6).

Anterior lesions are detected as anterior ulcerations of one or more vertebral bodies. Central lesions ultimately produce reduction in vertebral height and consequent sagittal angular deformity, with or without disc collapse.[11] As time advances, particularly in pyogenic disease, spontaneous arthrodesis may develop.

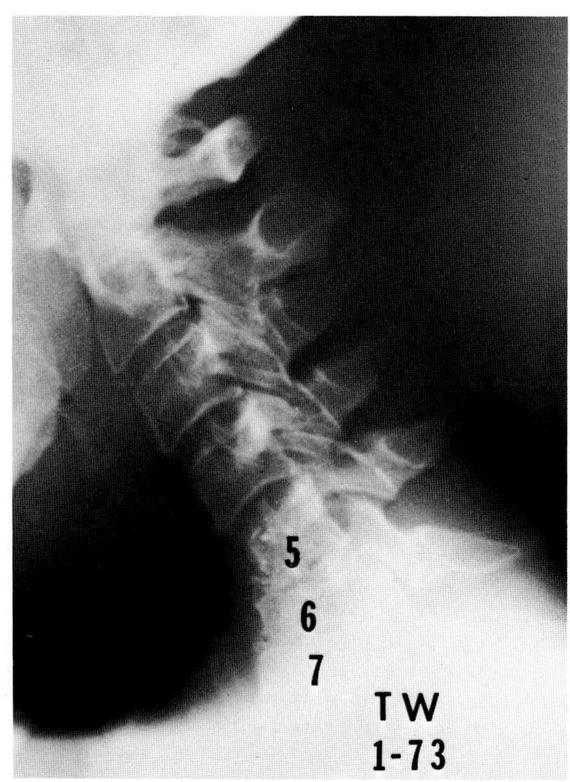

Fig. 9-6. Roentgenogram of a patient with esophageal carcinoma who underwent esophageal dilatation and subsequently developed a retropharyngeal abscess and vertebral osteomyelitis involving the fifth, sixth, and seventh cervical vertebrae. Air can be seen in the retropharyngeal abscess (*arrows*).

Diagnosis demands bacteriologic confirmation. A presumptive diagnosis may be accepted as indication for specific therapy when the clinical and radiographic presentations are characteristic and positive blood cultures are obtained. In such cases the organism grown on blood culture may be used to guide therapeutic decisions. On the other hand, when the presentation is not typical or when blood cultures are negative, a tissue diagnosis from the involved area must be made. Should there be a retropharyngeal collection, needle aspiration may provide material for staining and for culture and sensitivity studies. Trocar aspiration from bone is theoretically a source of vertebral tissue, but the risk of damaging adjacent structures such as the eosphagus or vertebral artery is significant. Open vertebral biopsy is a safe method and will provide tissue for pathologic and bacteriologic study. It will also permit definitive surgical treatment in appropriate cases. Open biopsy is even more necessary in the more bizarre fungal and parasitic disorders.

MANAGEMENT

The goals of therapy for septic cervical spondylitis include bacteriologic cure, minimization of instability or deformity, and neurologic protection or salvage. The ideal result would of course be a perfectly normal cervical spine, but destructive disease rarely permits this. Instead, some measure of compromise must usually be accepted.

Bacteriologic cure or control requires accurate identification of the organism, determination of its sensitivities, and administration of appropriate antimicrobial drugs in adequate dosage for a sufficient length of time. Securing material for culture is thus a critical step in initiating management, and whether this is done by blood cultures, needle biopsy, or open biopsy is determined by the features of the case. In patients with enlarged retropharyngeal spaces and little or no vertebral bony destruction, needle aspiration will probably suffice. However, in patients with impending or actual deformity resulting from vertebral sequestration and bony collapse, open biopsy through a standard anterior approach is preferred, since this will allow simultaneous debridement of necrotic and septic debris as well as definitive reconstruction, as discussed below.

In pyogenic infections, once the sensitivity of the organism is known, intravenous drug therapy with an appropriate agent should be instituted for 6 weeks. One hopes that before the culture is obtained there would be no antibiotic given to mask the organism's identity. After culture, while awaiting the sensitivity profile, broad-spectrum coverage against both gram-positive and gram-negative organisms must be employed, again intravenously. In a review of 65 patients with vertebral osteomyelitis, 25% had relapses indicated by recurrent fevers, meningitis, abscess formation, and markedly accelerated bone destruction. All who were treated for less than 28 days with antibiotics had relapses.[4] None of the patients treated with the prolonged course of antibiotics described here has had a relapse. Patients treated with antibiotics for intermediate periods of time have had intermediate recurrence rates. Relapses after 6 weeks of appropriate levels of parenteral antibiotics have been described before, and a long course of antibiotics as advocated here have been previously recommended in an attempt to reduce complications of this disease.[2,21]

In tuberculous disease, not only must vertebral material be obtained, but also a primary focus must be sought. Histologic identification of the organism is usually quickly available, but culture and sensitivity studies usually require 4 to 6 weeks. During this period triple drug therapy must be maintained, preferably using some of the newer and more effective agents such as ethambutal and rifampin. Once sensitivity studies are available, more specific drug choices may be made. Antimicrobial therapy must continue for a year or more. Consultation with appropriate specialists in infectious disease is particularly necessary in the overall management of patients with tuberculous or fungal spondylitis.

The second goal of management is the minimization of instability and deformity, either of which may be present at the initial examination. The general principles of management for cervical spine traumatic lesions apply, and spinal immobilization using the halo orthosis, skull tongs, or another cervical orthosis is necessary to supplement the antimicrobial program. Under the heading of discal or paradiscal lesions, there is a spontaneous tendency toward the establishment of a stable fibrous or bony ankylosis. If such lesions are confined to one segment, cervical immobilization may be relatively simple and will function largely to control pain and prevent additional trauma. Anterior lesions treated early will produce neither instability nor deformity as long as bone resorption remains minimal. However, because of the multiple segment involvement, more advanced lesions may be mechanically devastating, and surgical approaches to secure stability with arthrodesis will be required.[11] The same approach applies to central lesions, whether single or multiple, because of their tendency to produce kyphotic deformities. In such cases, external spinal stabilization must be secured before, during, and after surgical reconstruction. The surgery itself is most effectively an anterior debridement removing all septic material back to the posterior longitudinal ligament. Posterior approaches to address anterior septic deposits are not only inadequate and ineffective, but they also violate the principle of minimization of instability and deformity. The disastrous results of laminectomy to treat vertebral osteomyelitis have been well described (Fig. 9-7).[5,15,17]

(*Text continues on p. 559*)

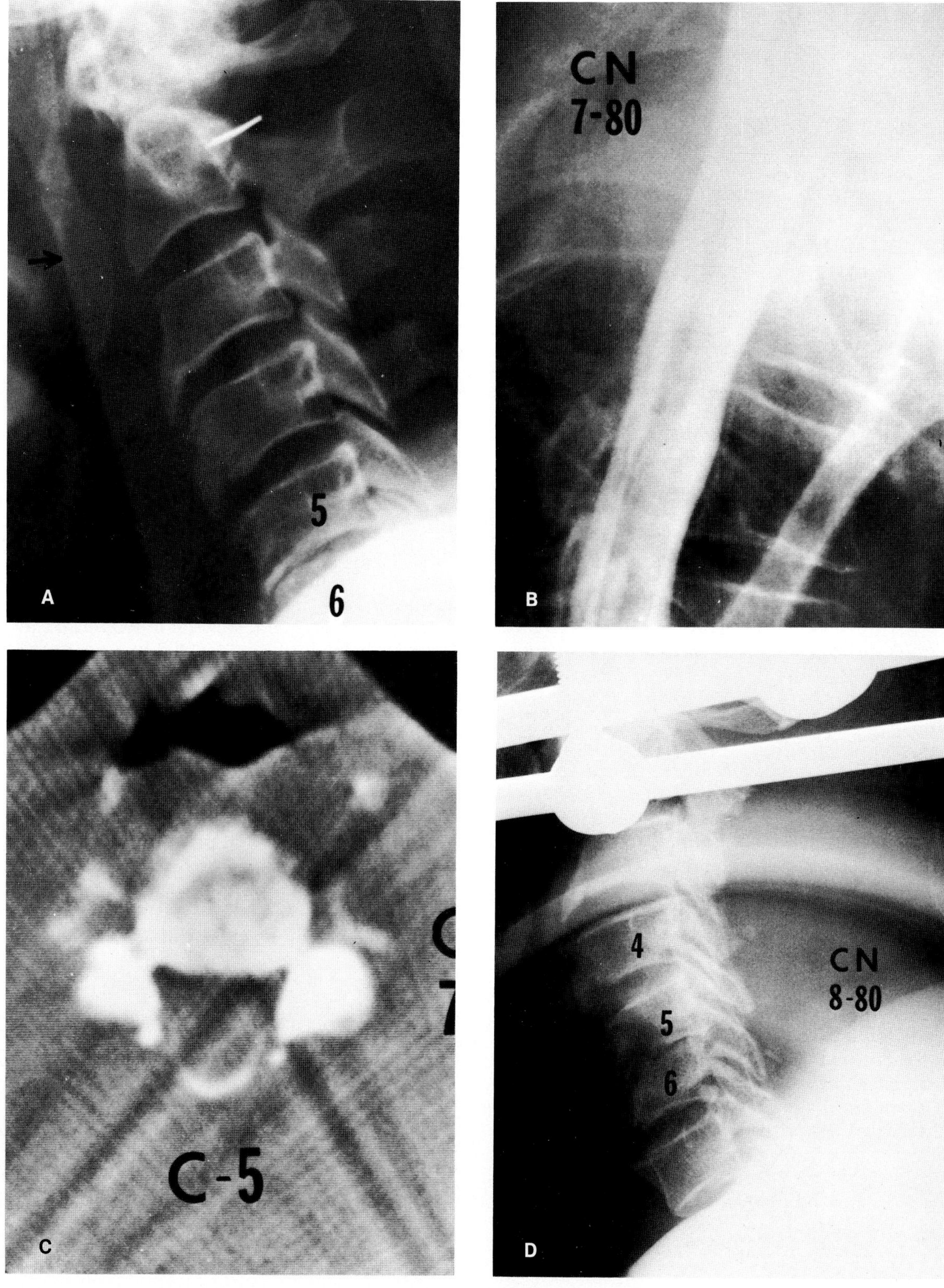
A
5
6
B
CN
7-80
C
C-5
D
4
5
6
CN
8-80

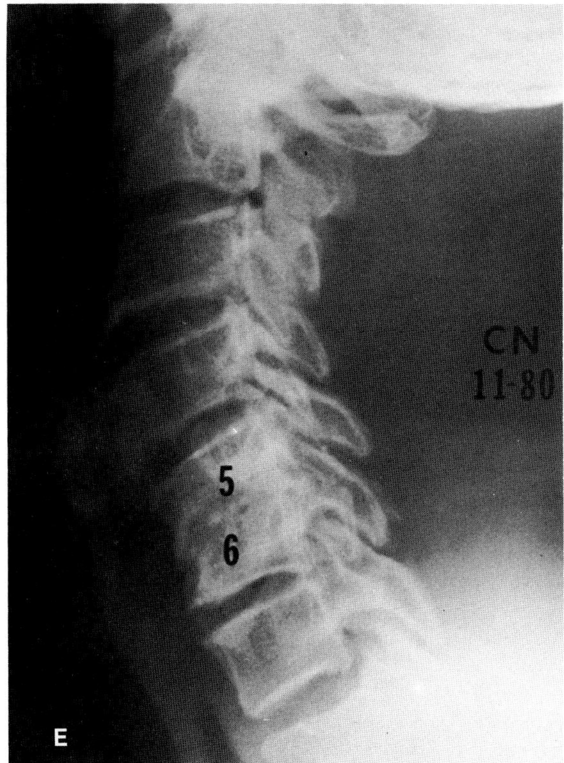

Fig. 9-7. A patient was admitted to the hospital with the complaint of fever, lethargy, and diffuse weakness. This was initially thought to be related to old head trauma. After 2 weeks of hospitalization, cervical spine roentgenograms and myelogram were performed. At this time the patient was severely quadriparetic, with only trace motor function in his legs and no motor function in the seventh and eighth cervical roots and the first thoracic root. He had fair motor function in the fifth and sixth cervical nerve roots. A myelogram from below showed a complete block at the first thoracic vertebra and a lateral C1–C2 myelogram demonstrated a complete block behind the second cervical vertebra. An extensive cervical epidural abscess was suspected and a posterior cervical laminectomy from the second cervical to the second thoracic levels was performed. No purulent material was found. Review of the roentgenograms disclosed increased retropharyngeal soft tissue swelling in front of the third cervical vertebra and decreased disc height at the C5–C6 interspace suggestive of a disc space infection with early adjacent vertebral osteomyelitis. The patient was placed in a halo vest postoperatively. He was remyelogramed and underwent a CT scan after 3 weeks, and this showed rapid flow of agent with no obstruction. If this had shown spinal cord compression at the level of infection, he would have undergone anterior cervical debridement and iliac graft fusion. He was treated with parenteral antibiotics for 6 weeks, followed by oral antibiotics for 4 additional months. He was kept immobilized in a halo vest for 3 months. He began to improve neurologically 1 month after laminectomy and he was ambulatory with no aids 5 months after onset of his infection. His finger strength returned to good levels after 1 year.

Critically reviewing this case, we decided that the anterior spine infection should have been recognized earlier and treated with a two-level cervical vertebrectomy and iliac graft fusion. Laminectomy is generally contraindicated in the face of anterior infection, but, considering the extensive myelographic block from the second cervical to the second thoracic levels, there was no way to differentiate preexisting disease, such as spondylosis, from a large posterior epidural abscess. The main factors allowing the patient to be satisfactorily treated were the use of a halo vest to prevent complete dislocation of the spine at the level of infection and the use of antibiotics for a long enough time to eradicate the infection.

(*A*) A lateral roentgenogram piror to the lateral C1–C2 myelogram shows increased soft tissue swelling in the retropharyngeal space (*arrows*) and decreased disc height at the C5–C6 interspace. At this time, the vertebral end-plates showed minimal destruction. A later myelogram showed a complete block behind the second cervical vertebra. (*B*) A lateral roentgenogram shows a complete block at the first thoracic level. (*C*) A CT scan 4 weeks after onset of infection shows erosion of the fifth cervical vertebral body. There is also a thin margin of metrizamide myelogram dye around the spinal cord. Streak artifact due to the halo vest metal uprights limits the resolution of the CT scan. (*D*) The anterior destruction of the fifth and sixth cervical vertebrae is now obvious 5 weeks after onset of infection. There is also erosion of the anterior aspect of the fourth cervical vertebra. The posterior laminectomy can also be seen, and the only thing to prevent complete spine dislocation at the level of infection is the halo vest. (*E*) A lateral roentgenogram 4 months after onset of infection demonstrates spontaneous anterior fusion of the C5–C6 interspace and resolution of the osteomyelitis. The retropharyngeal space in front of the third cervical vertebra is now normal.

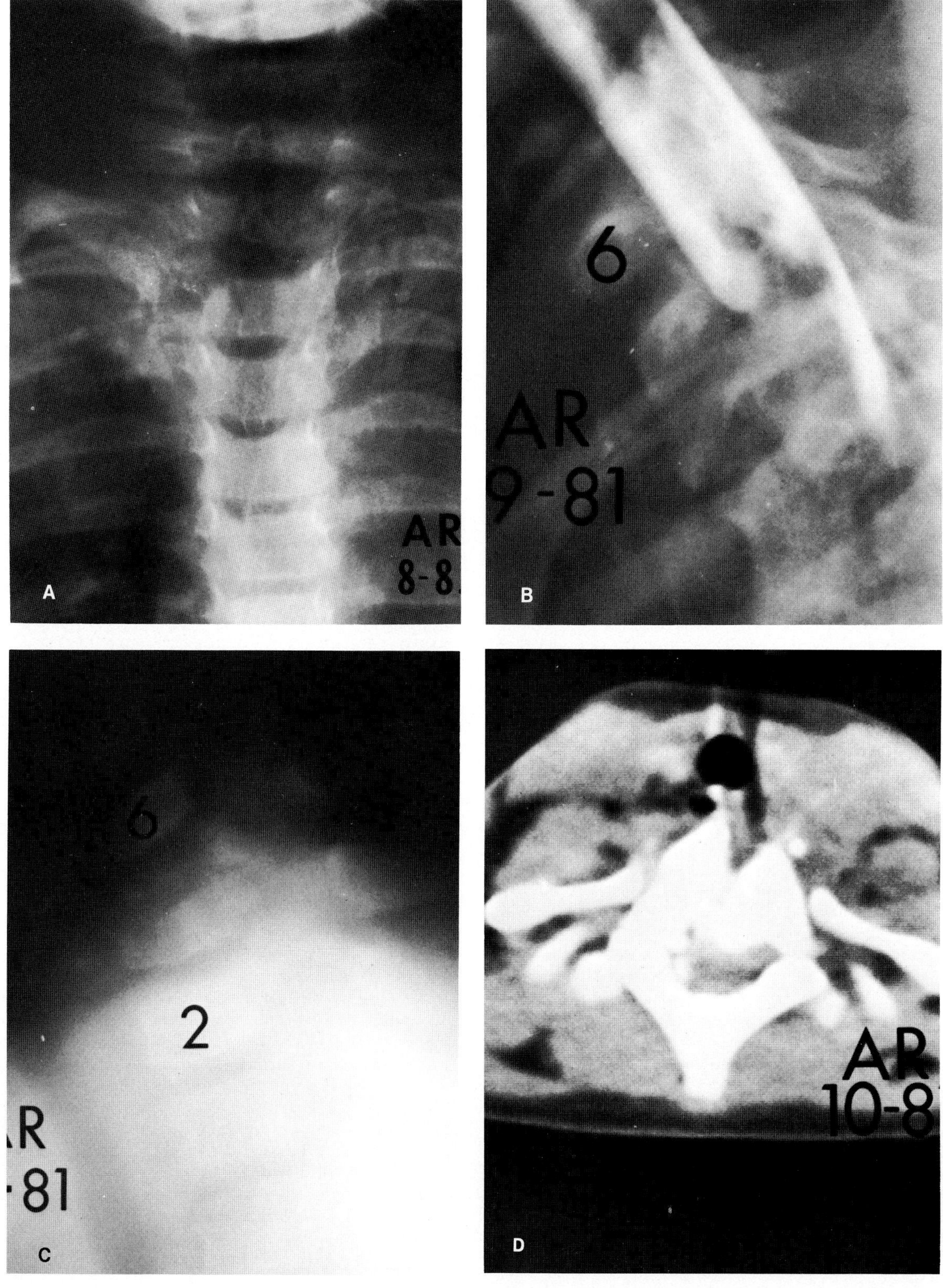
AR
8-8.
A
6
AR
9-81
B
6
2
AR
81
C
AR
10-8
D

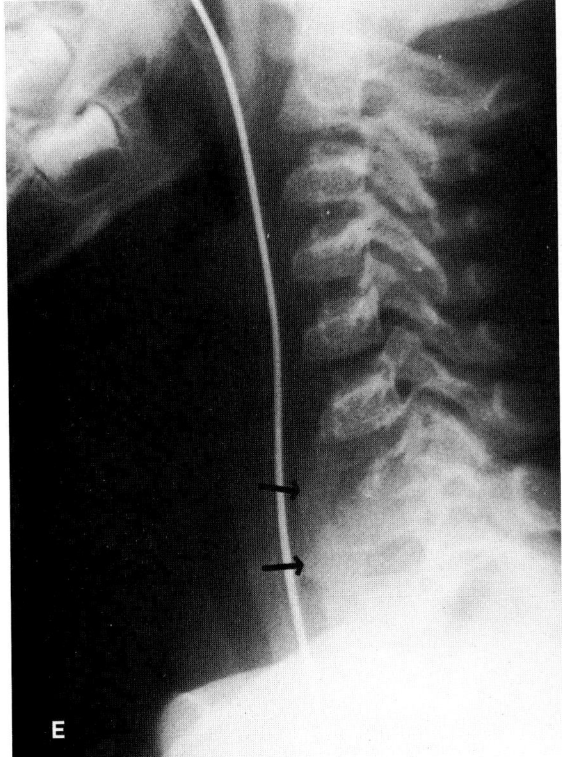

Fig. 9-8. A 4-year-old boy was shot through the neck, resulting in a complete paralysis below the T2 level. He was taken to surgery after an aortic arch arteriogram showed no damage to the neck vessels; a tear in the esophagus was repaired, a feeding gastrostomy was inserted, and his wounds were debrided. After a febrile course for several weeks, he was taken back to surgery and a streptococcus abscess in the retropharyngeal space was drained. He underwent several 10- to 14-day courses of antibiotics and remained febrile. At 3 months after injury he underwent an anterior vertebrectomy with resection of the seventh cervical and first thoracic vertebral bodies, which grew enterococcus from all surgical specimens. A primary iliac corticocancellous strut graft was inserted and he was immobilized in a halo vest. He was kept on appropriate parenteral antibiotics for 6 weeks, at the end of which time he was afebrile. The halo vest was removed after 6 weeks.
(*A*) The original A–P roentgenogram shows fractures of the bases of the right second and third ribs. (*B*) A lateral myelogram shows a complete block behind the seventh cervical vertebra with a suggestion of bone protruding into the spinal canal. (*C*) Lateral tomograms show severe destruction of the seventh cervical and first thoracic vertebral bodies with bone protruding into the spinal canal. The adjacent end-plates have remained intact. (*D*) A CT scan 2 months after injury shows bone protruding into the spinal canal, but it does not give any indication of the presence of vertebral osteomyelitis. (*E*) A lateral roentgenogram after a two-level vertebrectomy and iliac bone graft procedure shows satisfactory alignment of the spinal column. The arrows mark the anterior aspect of the iliac bone graft.

After adequate debridement, an inlay or strut bone graft sets the stage for fusion of the affected segments to secure permanent stability. Although bone grafting in a septic bed in the appendicular skeleton poses serious problems, this is not the case in the spine, where abundant vascularity makes such grafting safe and effective (Fig. 9-8).[10,13] Also, unlike reconstructions in the appendicular skeleton, spinal reconstructions for sepsis do not require prolonged drainage or suction–perfusion techniques. Wounds may usually be closed fully and without packings. Recurrent sepsis is not a problem if these principles are strictly followed. Only in some cases will supplementary posterior cervical fusion be necessary to secure permanent stability.

Much of what has been written thus far pertains to the lower cervical spine. The upper region with, for example, sepsis in the odontoid, or occipitoatlantal or atlantoaxial instability will require posterior stabilization with wiring and fusion techniques, protected by halo immobilization. Special techniques for anterior stabilization are not yet generally applied, although much progress has been made, as indicated elsewhere in this volume.

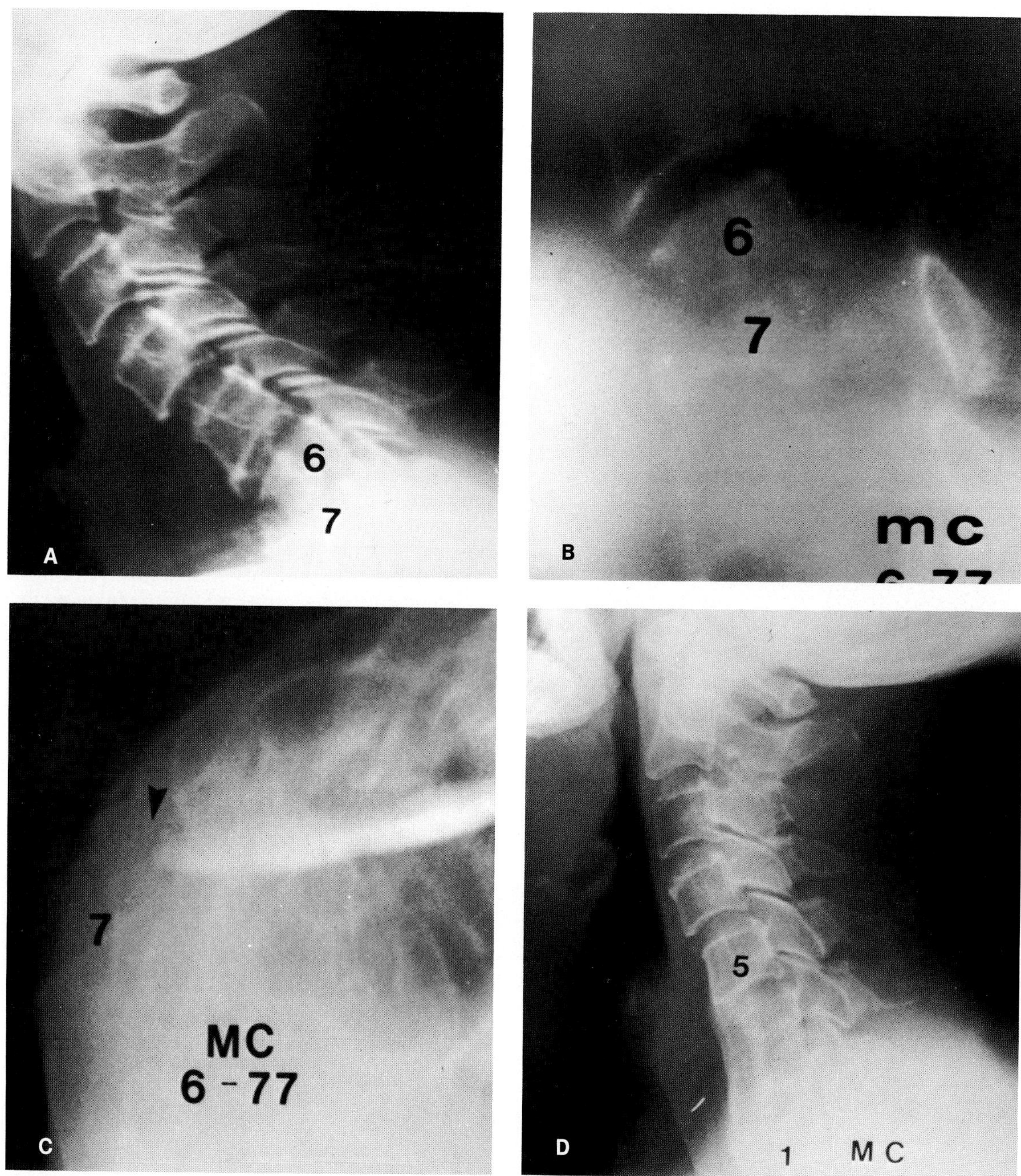
6
7
A
6
7
mc
B
7
MC
6 - 77
C
5
1 MC
D

Extirpation of the odontoid process through a transoral route has been described in the literature on trauma and is applicable to a case of odontoid sequestration, in conjunction with posterior stabilization.[18]

The management goal of neurologic protection or salvage follows what has been written regarding instability and deformity. Neurologic compromise in septic disease of the cervical spine is primarily the result of vertebral instability or deformity. Preservation or reconstruction of mechanical and architectural integrity will almost always protect or liberate the neural elements from compressive lesions. Whether recovery of the neurologic deficit is possible is a function of the length of time during which compression has been maintained. The special cases in spondylitis, however, arise when there has been invasion of the epidural space or penetration of the meninges by purulent material, or when granulomatous space-occupying masses (generally tuberculous) have induced vascular thrombosis and myeloradicular ischemia. In these events, timing is obviously an essential feature in salvage, with adequate and appropriate antimicrobial therapy along with the full application of current neurosurgical care (Figs. 9-9 and 9-10). The degree and extent of recovery depend upon the permanent loss already present at the time treatment is inaugurated. In tuberculous spinal cord deficits, particularly in children, response to antimicrobial therapy and neural decompression may be quite surprising.

←

Fig. 9-9. A 64-year-old woman entered the emergency room complaining of fever and neck pain. She had had an upper respiratory tract infection 2 weeks earlier. Examination now elicited bilateral ankle clonus and positive Babinski signs with seventh cervical root weakness in both arms. Radiographs indicated a sixth and seventh cervical nerve root weakness in both arms. Radiographs indicated a sixth and seventh cervical vertebral osteomyelitis, which was treated with open debridement, resection of the sixth and seventh cervical vertebral bodies, and iliac strut graft fusion. Specimens from surgery grew *Staphylococcus aureus*. The patient was placed in a halo cast for 8 weeks postoperatively. Signs of compression of the spinal cord resolved over 2 weeks. She was treated with parenteral antibiotics, as outlined in the text. At the 2-year follow-up she was asymptomatic. This case illustrates the correct treatment of cervical myelopathy due to cervical vertebral osteomyelitis.

(*A*) A lateral roentgenogram shows destruction of the inferior sixth cervical and superior seventh cervical vertebral end-plates. The soft tissue swelling anterior to the sixth cervical body far exceeds the normal 18 mm at this level. (*B*) Lateral tomograms better display the vertebral body destruction and the slight retrolisthesis of the sixth on the seventh cervical vertebral bodies. (*C*) A lateral myelogram demonstrates a complete block from below at the seventh cervical level. A lateral C1–C2 myelogram should then have been done to delimit the upper extent of neural compression. (*D*) Ten months after two-level vertebrectomy and iliac graft fusion, the patient is neurologically normal and has a solid anterior cervical fusion.

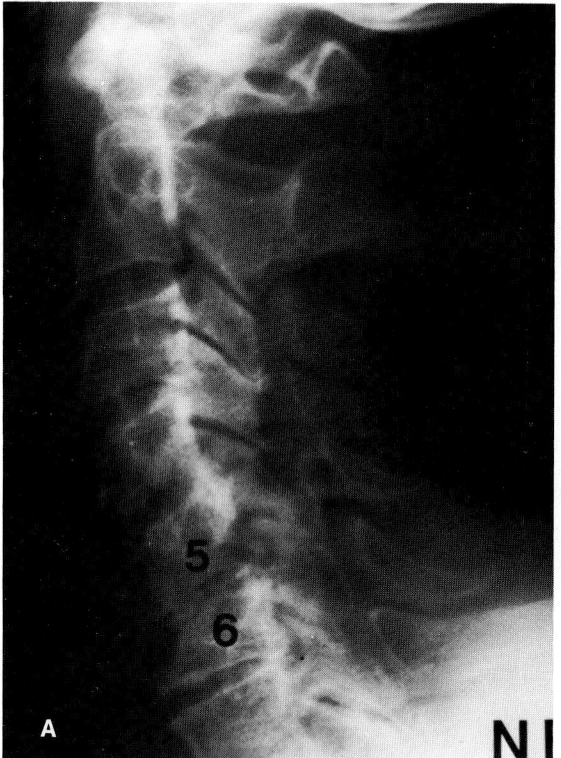

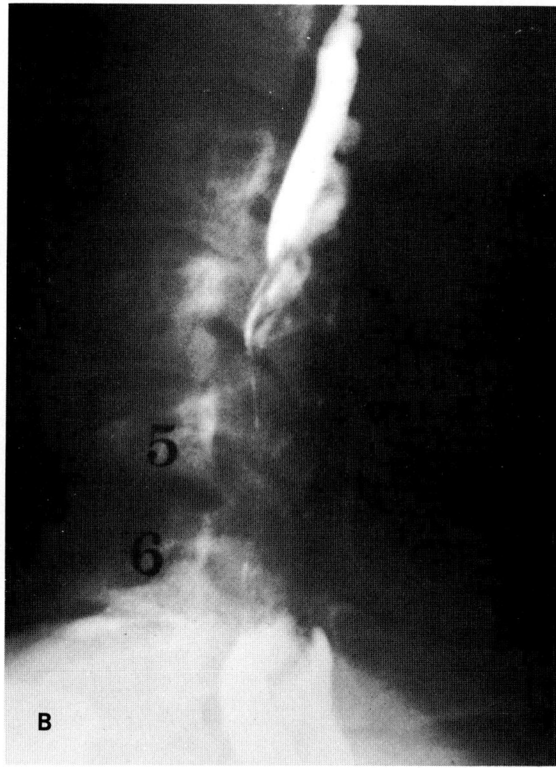

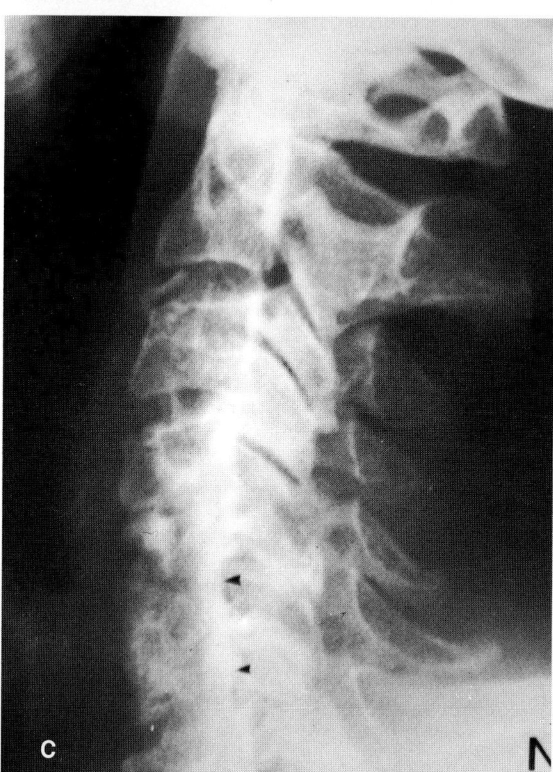

Fig. 9-10. A 74-year-old diabetic patient presented with fever, *Staphylococcus aureus* infection, neck pain, and severe arm weakness. There was no evidence of long tract signs. Roentgenograms displayed marked osteomyelitis of the fifth and sixth cervical vertebrae. Despite treatment with parenteral antibiotics for 3 weeks and immobilization in a halo vest, there was no neurologic improvement. The patient then underwent a myelogram followed by a two-level anterior cervical vertebrectomy and iliac graft fusion. His arm strength improved over 3 weeks. His course of antibiotics was as described in the text, and his halo was removed after 6 weeks. His neurologic examination was normal at 6-month follow-up, and his spine was stable and well aligned. This case illustrates the correct treatment of persistent cervical nerve root deficit due to cervical vertebral osteomyelitis that has not responded to treatment with the appropriate antibiotics, or to immobilization in a halo vest.
(*A*) A lateral roentgenogram exhibits complete destruction of the C5–C6 interspace, consistent with a disc-space infection with adjacent vertebral osteomyelitis. (*B*) A lateral cervical myelogram indicates a markedly thickened posterior longitudinal ligament, which corresponds with the marked reaction found at surgery with prolific granulation tissues. No attempt was made to remove this posterior longitudinal ligament, but once all the anterior infected bone was removed, this ligament bowed forward dramatically. (*C*) Three months after anterior cervical vertebrectomy and iliac strut grafting, the spine was well aligned and stable, and the infection was eradicated. The arrows show the posterior cortex of the iliac strut graft and show that the canal has been widened at this level.

REFERENCES

1. *Cloward RB:* Metastatic disc infection and osteomyelitis of the cervical spine. Spine 3:194, 1978
2. *Digby JM, Kensley JB:* Pyogenic non-tuberculous spinal infection. J Bone Joint Surg 61B:47, 1979
3. *Doub HP, Badgley CE:* The roentgen signs of tuberculosis of the vertebral body. AJR 27:827, 1932
4. *Eismont FJ, Bohlman HH, Goldberg UM, et al:* Pyogenic and Fungal Vertebral Osteomyelitis: A Review of Sixty-Five Cases. Unpublished data, VA Hospital Spine Center, Cleveland, Ohio
5. *Fellander M:* Paraplegia in spondylitis: Results of operative treatment. Paraplegia 13:75, 1975
6. *Forsythe M, Rothman RH:* New concepts in the diagnosis and treatment of infections of the cervical spine. Orthop Clin North Am 9:1039, 1978
7. *Friedman B:* Chemotherapy of tuberculosis of the spine: J Bone Joint Surg 48A:451, 1966
8. *Garcia A, Grantham SA:* Hematogenous pyogenic vertebral osteomyelitis. J Bone Joint Surg 42A:429, 1960
9. *Ghormley RK, Bickel WH, Dickson DD:* A study of acute infectious lesions of the intervertebral discs. South Med J 33:347, 1940
10. *Hodgson AR, Stock FE:* Anterior spinal fusion. Br J Surg 44:266, 1956
11. *Hodgson AR, Wong W, Yau ACMC:* X-Ray Appearance of Tuberculosis of the Spine. Springfield, IL, Charles C Thomas, 1969
12. *Holzman RS, Bishko F:* Osteomyelitis in heroin addicts. Ann Intern Med 75:693, 1971
13. *Kemp HBS, Jackson JW, Jeremiah JD, et al:* Anterior fusion of the spine for infective lesions in adults. J Bone Joint Surg 55B:715, 1973
14. *Kemp HBS, Jackson JW, Jeremiah JD, et al:* Pyogenic infections occurring primarily in intervertebral discs. J Bone Joint Surg 55B:698, 1973
15. *Kemp HBS, Jackson JW, Shaw NC:* Laminectomy in paraplegia due to infective spondylosis. Br J Surg 61:66, 1974
16. *Leonard A, Comty CM, Shapiro FL, et al:* Osteomyelitis in hemodialysis patients. Ann Intern Med 78:651, 1973
17. *Seddon HJ:* Pott's paraplegia: Prognosis and treatment. Br J Surg 22:769, 1935
18. *Spetzler RF, Selman WR, Nash CL, et al:* Transoral microsurgical odontoid resection and spinal cord monitoring. Spine 4:506, 1979
19. *Stone DB, Bonfiglio M:* Pyogenic vertebral osteomyelitis. Arch Intern Med 112:491, 1963
20. *Sullivan AW:* Subluxation of the atlantoaxial joint: Sequel to inflammatory processes of the neck. J Pediatr 35:451, 1949
21. *Wiesseman GJ, Wood VE, Kroll LL:* Pseudomonas vertebral osteomyelitis in heroin addicts. J Bone Joint Surg 55A:1416, 1973
22. *Wiley AM, Treuta J:* The vascular anatomy of the spine and its relationship to pyogenic vertebral osteomyelitis. J Bone Joint Surg 41B:796, 1959

CHAPTER 10

Rheumatoid Arthritis and Other Noninfectious Inflammatory Diseases

Rheumatoid Arthritis of the Cervical Spine

S. ASHBY GRANTHAM AND STEPHEN J. LIPSON

PATHOLOGY

Rheumatoid synovitis in the cervical spine causes pathologic changes in the ligaments with distention and rupture, articular cartilage destruction, and, in bone, osteoporosis, cyst formation, and erosion. The specific deformity caused is dependent on the structure destroyed. The inflammatory cells involved in rheumatoid inflammation have been identified in biopsy specimens at the atlantoaxial junction and reflect the same cell types as found peripherally.[23] Atlantoaxial subluxation (Fig. 10-1) is ascribed to erosive synovitis in the atlantoaxial, atlantoodontoid, and atlantooccipital joints as well as the synovium-lined bursa between the odontoid and the transverse ligament. Atlantoaxial impaction (upward translocation of the odontoid, pseudobasilar invagination, cranial settling, vertical subluxation) describes the settling of the skull on the atlas, and the atlas on the axis, resulting from erosion and bone loss in the occipitoatlantal and atlantoaxial joints (Fig. 10-2). Subaxial destruction occurs via the facets, interspinous ligaments, and intervertebral discs (spondylodiscitis) (Fig. 10-3). Ball and Sharp[1] argue that subaxial subluxation results from synovitic destruction of the discs originating in the synovially lined uncovertebral joints, with extension to adjacent disc and bone. Martel[28] contends that instability is secondary to facet and ligamentous destruction causing a traumatic discopathy. Interspinous bursae have also been shown to be involved in synovitis.

Cervical instability has been shown to have an early onset in the course of the disease. In a prospective series of 100 patients with new-onset rheumatoid arthritis, 83% of the 12 patients who developed anterior atlantoaxial subluxation did so in the first 2 years of the disease.[51] The severity of rheumatoid cervical disease has been shown to correlate strongly with the severity of peripheral erosive disease.[52]

ATLANTOAXIAL SUBLUXATION

Atlantoaxial subluxation is the most common and significant manifestation of rheumatoid involvement of the cervical spine. Conlon, Isdale, and

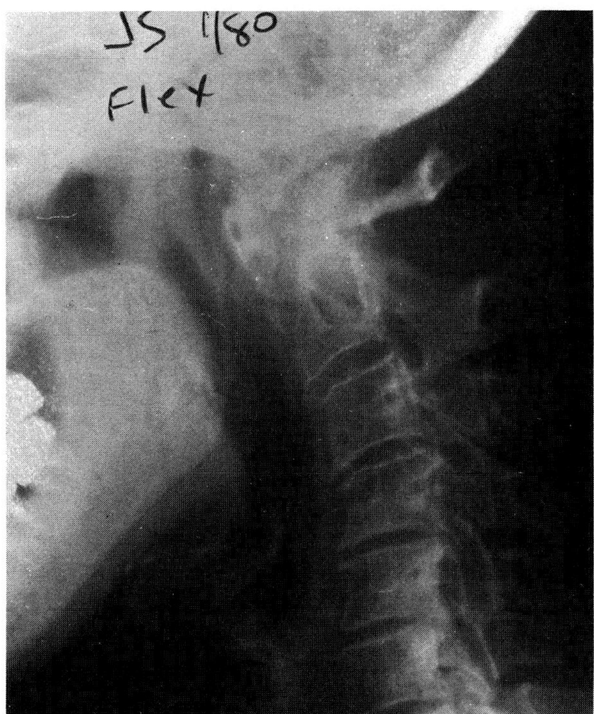

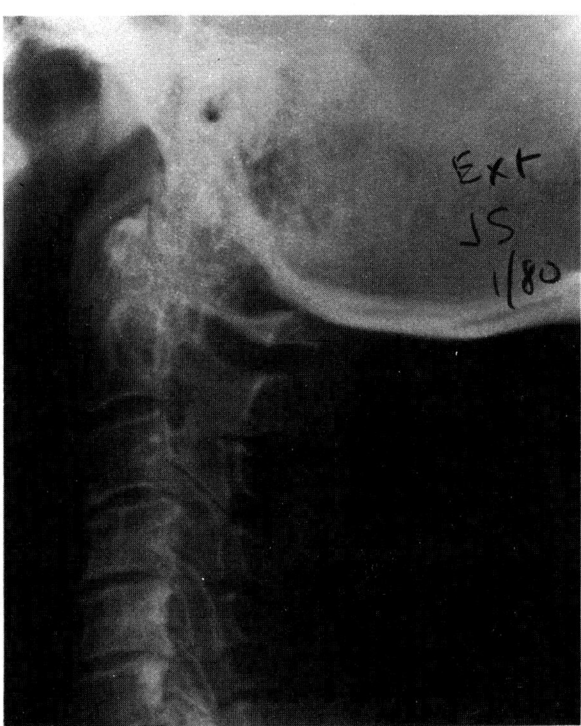

Fig. 10-1. Anterior atlantoaxial subluxation in flexion and extension. The increased atlantodental distance is noted.

Rose found a 25% incidence of radiographic C1–C2 subluxation in a hospital rheumatoid population of 333 patients, and in a study of 845 rheumatoid patients, 60% had signs and symptoms of neck involvement.[8] Eighty-six percent of 100 patients with classic rheumatoid arthritis were reported by Bland to show radiographic cervical spine involvement.[2] Sharp and Purser estimated the incidence of rheumatoid atlantoaxial instability to be 1 in 30 in patients with any evidence of rheumatoid disease, 1 in 15 in patients with clinical disease, and 1 in 5 in patients hospitalized for rheumatoid disease.[41] Martel found that 34 of 100 unselected rheumatoid arthritic clinic patients demonstrated subluxation, with higher figures for patients with neck symptoms or severe disease.[27] Long duration of disease, greater age of the patient, and peripheral joint erosive instability forms of the disease are usually reported to be associated with more frequent and severe C1–C2 instabilities. Conversely, Smith and associates in a prospective type study of 962 patients hospitalized for rheumatoid arthritis reported the incidence and severity of anterior subluxation found in 150 patients to be unrelated to the age of the patient or the duration of disease.[47] Upward migration of the odontoid, however, was found to be related to these factors. The use of steroids is thought by many to be another significant adverse association.

Garrod first described clinical involvement of the cervical spine in rheumatoid arthritis in 1890. Davis and Markley[12] in 1951 first documented death due to medullary compression caused by atlantoaxial subluxation. Survival in patients with cervical rheumatoid arthritis has been studied further. A postmortem study of 104 patients with rheumatoid arthritis estimated a 10% rate of fatal medullary compression.[33] Smith and coworkers[47] reported that survival among patients with rheumatoid arthritis is not influenced by cervical spine disease. Patients in that series died earlier, but not because of cervical spine lesions. Pellicci and colleagues[36] reported a 17% mortality rate in rheumatoid patients over 5 years, 10% higher than in the general population, but altantoaxial subluxation was not causal, although 80% of the subluxations progressed, and 27% of the patients acquired new atlantoaxial subluxations. Neurologic progression existed in 36%. Progression of existing radiologic subluxation over time is supported in

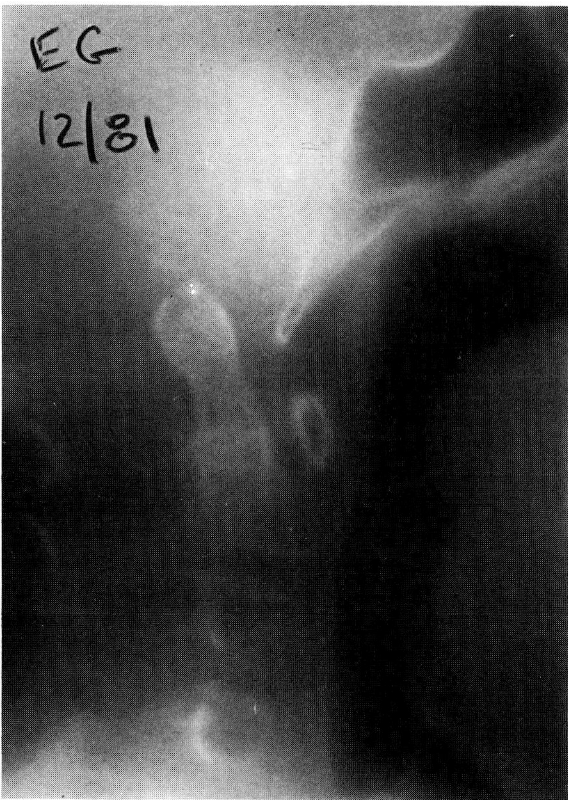

Fig. 10-2. Atlantoaxial impaction as seen on lateral tomography. The dens is noted above the clivus and is circumferentially eroded by synovitis. The ring of the atlas lies low on the body of C2.

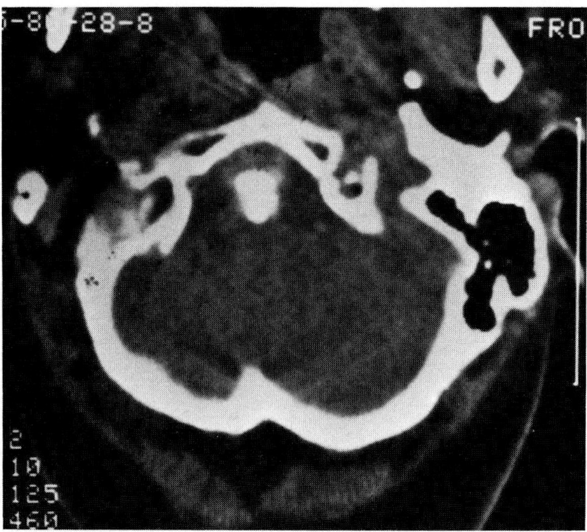

Fig. 10-3. A transverse CT section in atlantoaxial impaction demonstrates the dens within the foramen magnum.

the literature[20,47,49] and ranges from 39% to 41% for anterior atlantoaxial subluxation.[47,48] Neurologic progression is less marked, ranging from 2%[47] to 14%.[49] Once cervical myelopathy is established, Marks and Sharp[26] found that more than 50% of the patients died if they were not stabilized. Neurologic deaths occurred much earlier than death from nonneurologic causes. Patients with cervical rheumatoid arthritis, therefore, are at risk of a premature death, but not necessarily from neurologic causes. Subluxation can become worse over time, but neurologic progression is much less common. In an attempt to identify risk factors which predisposed patients to spinal cord compression, Weissman and associates[49] found that in anterior atlantoaxial subluxation and atlantoaxial impaction (AAI) risks included being male, an atlantodental distance of greater than 9 mm, and the presence of AAI.

The instability pattern of rheumatoid involvement of the atlantoaxial joint complex is usually one of two types: anterior atlantoaxial subluxation or vertical subluxation of the odontoid (also referred to as superior migration, upward translocation, atlantoaxial impaction, downward location of the atlas on the axis, and cranial settling).

Posterior atlantoaxial subluxation occurs infrequently. It accounted for 6.7% of all atlantoaxial subluxations in one series[49] and usually was not associated with cord compression. Odontoid fracture or erosion is usually found to be associated with this deformity. A recent report[25] indicates that this is not a benign subluxation and can cause myelopathy. Posterior kinking of the spinal cord at the cervicomedullary junction may be responsible for the myelopathy.

Anterior subluxation is considerably more common than upward migration, although the two patterns usually coexist. Isolated superior migration is very rare. Ranawat and associates, reporting on 33 rheumatoid patients surgically treated for cervical spine deformity, found 70% had atlantoaxial subluxation and 16% had superior migration of the odontoid (60% has subaxal subluxations).[39]

Rotatory atlantoaxial dislocations are reported by Sherk to occur in early rheumatoid disease, but this must be uncommon or poorly recognized.[45] Lateral atlantoaxial subluxation can be visualized on a frontal view when the lateral masses of C1 lie

2 mm or more laterally on those of C2. Rotation is difficult to assess, and, although it is reported, its incidence is probably underestimated. Lateral atlantoaxial subluxation was found to account for 21% of all atlantoaxial subluxations and is found more commonly in patients with cord compression than in those without it.[48]

MEASUREMENT OF INSTABILITY

Anterior atlantoaxial subluxation is assessed by measurement of the radiographic interval from the midposterior margin of the anterior ring of C1 to the anterior surface of the odontoid. Flexion–extension views identify the freedom of motion or degree of fixation. A measurement of this interval of more than 3 mm in the adult and 4 mm in children is accepted as pathologic or as a threat to cord function.[21,27] The anteroposterior diameter of the adult atlas is about 3 cm and by Steel's rule of thirds provides 1 cm for the odontoid, 1 cm for the cord, and 1 cm of free space.

The upper tip of the odontoid process normally lies 1 cm below the anterior margin of the foramen magnum (0.5 cm in children). Vertical migration of the odontoid can be radiographically assessed several ways (Fig. 10-4). McRae's line connects the front of the foramen magnum to the back (basion to opisthion), and the odontoid should not project above this plane. Chamberlin's line is drawn from the posterior margin of the hard palate to the posterior margin of the foramen magnum. The tip of the odontoid should not project more than 3 mm above this line with 6 mm being definitely pathologic. Commonly, however, the margins of the foramen magnum are difficult to precisely identify. McGregor's line connects the posterior margin of the hard palate to the most caudal point of the occiput and is easier to use. The tip of the odontoid should not project more than 4.5 mm above this line.

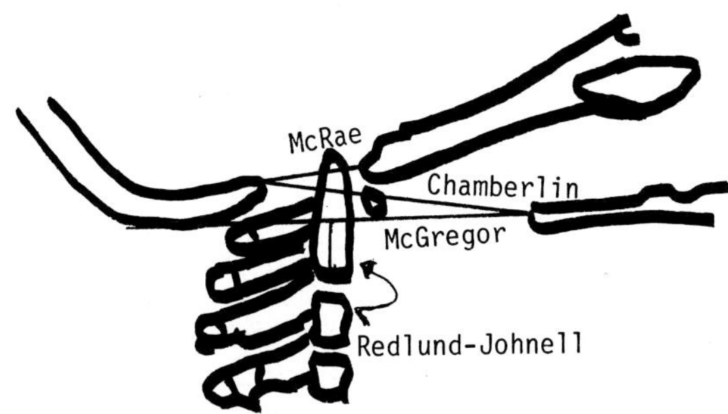

Fig. 10-4. Methods by which to judge odontoid displacement on the lateral x-ray.

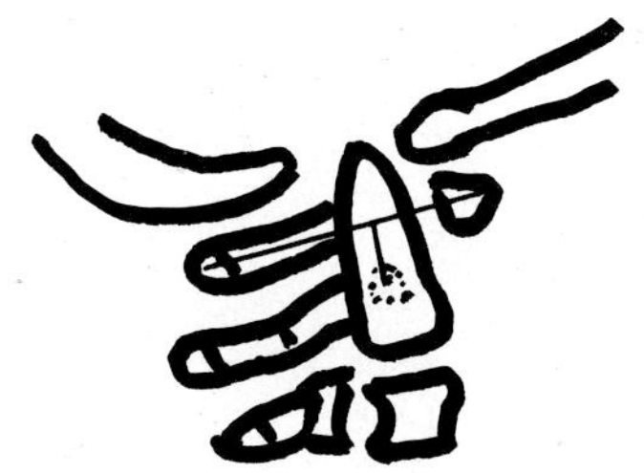

Fig. 10-5. Ranawat baseline measurement to quantify vertical migration of the odontoid.

Ranawat and associates in 1979 suggested another measurement for vertical odontoid migration because of the difficulty identifying the hard palate on cervical spine x-rays (Fig. 10-5).[39] On a lateral projection of the cervical spine, the coronal axis of C1 is marked by connecting the center of the anterior arch of C1 with the center of the posterior arch of C1. A second line starts at the center of the sclerotic ring of C2 (the pedicles) and extends superiorly along the midaxis of the odontoid until it intersects the first line. Measurement of less than 13 mm is abnormal. Similarly, Rana and associates noted earlier that a position of the body of the axis immediately behind the arch of the atlas seen on lateral x-ray to be a useful sign of vertical instability.[38]

Because the hard palate or foramen magnum may be difficult to see, or may be independently distorted or deformed, it may be worthwhile to consider the Fischgold and Metzger measurement (Fig. 10-6).[14] On an A–P open-mouth view of the odontoid (preferably a tomogram), the digastric lines should be connected from side to side. (The digastric line is where mastoid process joins the base of skull.) The tip of the odontoid should be 1 cm or more below this line.

Because the odontoid tip may be difficult to identify, particularly with rheumatoid deossification or destruction, another measurement has been proposed by Redlund-Johnell and Pettersson (Fig. 10-4).[40] On a neutral head position lateral x-ray, the McGregor palatooccipital line is drawn. Then one should measure the distance to the lower end-plate of the C2 vertebral body. Less than 34 mm in men, and 29 mm in women, defines the extent of vertical migration of the odontoid.

All of these measurements attempt to identify

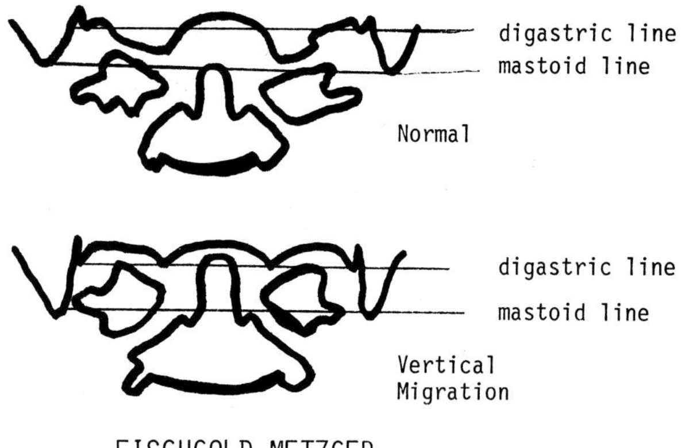

Fig. 10-6. Craniocervical A–P tomogram technique to evaluate odontoid position.

and quantitate the degree of odontoid competition with spinal cord and brain stem for space that is limited.

CLINICAL PRESENTATION

The clinical presentation of rheumatoid atlantoaxial instability results from a combination of (1) local arthritic and mechanical instability and pain, (2) neurologic dysfunction of brain stem, cord, and peripheral nerve (root), and (3) vertebral artery insufficiency. When one considers that many peripheral joints are often severely functionally compromised and painful, that peripheral nerve entrapment problems are common, and that tendons may be ruptured or tenosynovitic, in addition to the associated medical problems typical of this age group, recognition and definition of the significance of cervical instability may be difficult. Physical examination of these severely affected patients is difficult and requires considerable skill to interpret the multifactorial elements. A detailed study of sensibility is probably the most reliable means of diagnosing cord compression in these patients.[48]

Pain in the cervical area is common, usually of moderate severity. Many studies emphasize appropriately, however, that considerable instability and threat to cord function may exist with minimal pain complaints.[47] The poor correlation of neurologic signs and symptoms in some patients with considerable radiographic changes and demonstrable instability has suggested there are other sources of neurologic pathology.[30,43] Local circulatory changes related to obstructive proliferative rheumatoid granulation tissue have been suggested.

Subjective sensory symptoms of parethesias in hands, "electric shock" body sensation (Lhermitte's sign), and transient feeling of weakness are commonly noted. True weakness and spasticity may ensue as the cord becomes slowly progressively or acutely compromised. Dizziness, tinnitus, suboccipital headache, dysphagia, blurring of vision, vertigo, and nystagmus may reflect vertebral artery insufficiency due to kinking or brain-stem involvements by upward migration of the odontoid. Urinary dysfunction (frequency or retention) is an important warning sign.[38] Some loss of proprioception and vibratory sensibility is occasionally reported but not common. Trigeminal nerve tract involvement may produce facial sensory impairment.

Joint crepitation and instability may be felt on palpation of the upper cervical spine, in the form of a "clunk" as C1 moves forward subluxing on C2 producing an increased prominence of C2 posteriorly. This "clunk test," or Sharp and Purser test, is probably best undertaken gingerly.

RADIOLOGIC STUDIES

Radiographic studies of the rheumatoid cervical spine are often particularly difficult to interpret with confidence. Deossification, obliteration of joints, and deformities may require tomographic studies in addition to dynamic flexion–extension lateral roentgenograms. Vertebral artery abnormalities have been pinpointed by angiographic studies in a few patients.[1,9] Cineradiography may help show the degree of instability in a dramatic fashion. Computerized axial tomography (CT) of the spine has given us a new perspective to and more direct appreciation of spinal canal encroachment.[16] As it becomes more refined, it will allow more direct measurements of the threat to cord function in these patients. Whether or not to perform a myelogram depends on the degree of neurologic involvement and confidence in localization of the lesion, since simultaneous problems may also be arising from midcervical instability. Usually, it seems that the patient most likely to benefit from myelographic study is the one on whom it would be most difficult to perform safely and adequately.

Kaufman and Glenn strongly commend CT with multiplanner reconstruction when surgery is being considered and in place of myelography for the compromised rheumatoid spine.[22]

Magnetic resonance imaging (MRI) studies also appear to be an excellent method to appreciate nuances of soft-tissue reaction.[24,34] Rheumatoid granulation tissue posterior to the dens, for example, can be depicted as responsible for some of the spinal cord pressure.

TREATMENT

The natural history of atlantoaxial subluxation is such that treatment is controversial. According to some authors, most patients tolerate C1–C2 subluxation without neurologic changes, perhaps owing to rheumatoid general debility and peripheral joint crippling deformities that coexist.[47] Conversely, a 5-year study of 54 patients with atlantoaxial instability found that long tract signs developed in one third of those with anterior subluxation and one half of those with vertical subluxation.[29] Protective soft collars or firm collars or braces may safely provide some help but are not always well tolerated, and compliance rates are low. The Philadelphia collar is sometimes of particular help. Temperomandibular joint arthritis, skin sensitivity and fragility, and shoulder pain may be troublesome.

The indications for surgical intervention are significant progressive neurologic deficits, intractable pain, and perhaps severe instability.[9,13,30,39] Unfortunately, surgery in these patients is not always safe, predictable, and free of complications. Perioperative mortality rates of 27% to 42% have been reported, although more recent studies have been much more encouraging.[9,13,30,39] Failure of bone fusion may run as high as 50%, but, again, more recent reports show better results.[13] A tendency for resorption of bone graft has been suggested. Infection rates are higher in these debilitated patients with the use of corticosteroids and immunosuppressive agents are a complicating factor. The postoperative management and protection of the spine is difficult. Halo vest (or casts) have been useful but are far from being a panacea. Deossification of the skull may contribute to pin tract loosening or local infection. These debilitated patients may find it difficult, if not impossible, to cope with mobile secure fixation devices. Prolonged bed rest and traction have well-known deficiencies.

Successful surgery predictably relieves pain, provides stability, and halts the progression of neurologic dysfunction, with neurologic improvement seen in 30% to 40% of patients.[39] If surgery is elected, problems attendant upon anesthesia arise. Nasal intubation in an effort to minimize manipulation of a stiff or unstable neck with impaired mouth opening may be necessary. Tracheostomy may be preferable in the face of impaired respiratory function.

Posterior fusion (Fig. 10-7) of C1 to C2 with wiring and autogenous iliac bone graft may be adequate for treatment of anterior atlantoaxial instability.[39] Bone graft material may also be obtained from other anatomic sites or from a bone bank when the pelvis is too osteoporotic. The wire size used by most is #20 or #18. The fusion should extend to the occiput and perhaps include C3 for the patient with superior migration of the odontoid. Occipitalization of C1 or bony deficiency of the posterior arch of C1 may in addition require occipitocervical fusion.[18] Ferlic and associates have recommended evaluation of the occipitoatlantal joint for degree of mobility, with inclusion of this joint in the fusion when motion is severely restricted.[13] Extending the fusion beyond C1–C2 introduces some increase in morbidity and mortality rates, however, and is technically more difficult to perform and to control effectively after surgery. The indication for suboccipital bony decompression with removal of the posterior arch of C1 or enlargement of the posterior margin of the foramen magnum is not clear, and performance of dural release with the application of fascial graft

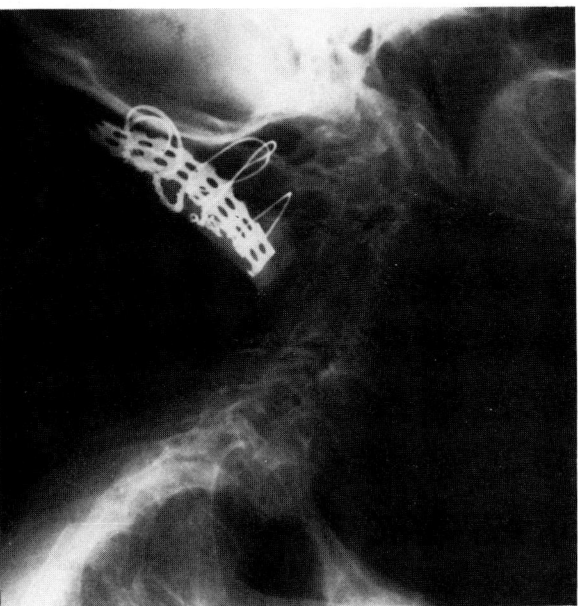

Fig. 10-7. A posterior atlantoaxial subluxation stabilized with an occipitocervical fusion utilizing metal mesh and methylmethacrylate backing to enhance the properties of the bone graft. (Lipson SJ: Cervical myelopathy and posterior atlanto-axial subluxation in patients with rheumatoid arthritis. J Bone Joint Surg 67A:593, 1985)

is even more controversial.[13] Following posterior stabilization with persistent fixed anterior subluxation or superior migration, transoral anterior decompression of the cord by removal of the odontoid has been suggested as beneficial.[3,11,37] Crockard and associates favorably report on 14 patients with cervical myelopathy treated by transoral removal of part of the C1 arch, odontoid, and pannus tissue immediately followed by occiput-to-C2 posterior wiring and bone graft.[10] Traction is avoided before or after surgery, and a preformed collar is used when the patient is mobilized on the fifth day. Although it is a rational approach, the fear of infection and technical requirements have put off most surgeons. Extrapharyngeal lateral exposures of the base of the skull, C1, and C2 have been devised by Simmons, Whitesides, and others; they are particularly useful in tumor surgery and trauma but probably have little or no application to the rheumatoid patient.[46,50] Supplemental fixation of a posterior fusion with methylmethacrylate has been tried with definite improvement in immediate surgical construct fixation and, more significantly, easier postoperative management avoiding prolonged traction and rest and cumbersome external immobilization devices. Attendant complications and difficulties related to the use of cement may, however, become evident as series are reported in the future.

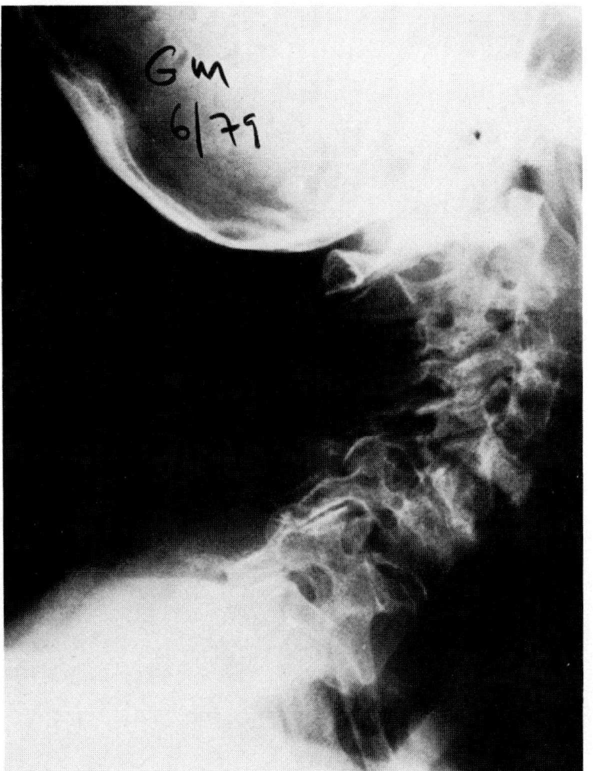

Fig. 10-8. Subaxial rheumatoid disease with spondylodiscitis and anterior subluxation.

SUBAXIAL SUBLUXATION

Subaxial subluxations tend to be located at multiple levels in a given patient,[32,35] producing a "stepladder" or "staircase" deformity (Fig. 10-8). Endplate erosions may be found in 12% to 15% of rheumatoid patients[8,32,42] and subluxations in 10% to 20%.[1,32,42] Lack of osteophyte formation is typical for rheumatoid arthritis, and narrowing and subluxation at higher levels than normally found in degenerative disease is characteristic for rheumatoid arthritis. Surgical intervention for subaxial subluxations usually involves wired posterior fusion. The role of anterior fusion is unclear and has not been strongly recommended.[39] Anterior fusion may be accompanied by graft resorption and collapse. Laminectomy has had a dubious role[7] and should always be accompanied by fusion. Fusion alone may be adequate treatment for subaxial subluxation, but to date the lack of extensive series indicates that the surgery selected for such cases must be individualized.

JUVENILE RHEUMATOID ARTHRITIS

Juvenile rheumatoid arthritis (JRA) does not commonly cause a serious clinical problem in the cervical spine. Facet ankylosis is a hallmark of this disease, particularly at C2–C3. Neck pain and stiffness are common, but problematic subluxations and myelopathy are not. In a study of 92 patients with JRA,[15] 29 had cervical involvement—14 with pain and stiffness, 2 with torticollis, and 5 with anterior atlantoaxial subluxation, 2 of whom had myelopathy. No AAI or subaxial subluxation was identified. Another series identified four out of eight JRA patients with anterior atlantoaxial subluxation, one of whom showed AAI.[6] Surgical intervention in JRA for cervical spine abnormalities is therefore uncommon and needs to be individualized.

OTHER CONDITIONS

Basilar invagination (upward translocation of the odontoid) can be identified in some patients with Paget's disease of bone, osteogenesis imperfecta, and rickets.[44] Fortunately, rarely does the question arise of the need for or wisdom of operative intervention in these patients.

The high incidence of odontoid dysplasia and atlantoaxial instability in a variety of congenital complex deformities (Morquio's syndrome, Hurler's syndrome, Larsen's syndrome, Down's syndrome, and Conradi's syndrome) is covered elsewhere in this text.

REFERENCES

1. *BALL J, SHARP J:* Rheumatoid arthritis of the cervical spine. In Hill AGS (ed): Modern Trends in Rheumatology, Vol 2, p 117. London, Butterworth, 1971
2. *BLAND JH:* Rheumatoid arthritis of the cervical spine. J Rheumatol 1:319, 1974
3. *BRATTSTROM H, ELNER A, GRANHOLM L:* Case report: Transoral surgery of myelopathy caused by rheumatoid arthritis of the cervical spine. Ann Rheum Dis 32:578, 1973
4. *BRAUNSTEIN EM, WEISSMAN BN, SELTZER SE, SOSMAN JL, WONG A, ZAMANI A:* Computed tomography and conventional radiographs of the craniocervical region in rheumatoid arthritis. Arth Rheum 27:26, 1984
5. *BYWATERS EGL:* Rheumatoid and other diseases of the cervical interspinous bursae, and changes in the spinous processes. Ann Rheum Dis 41:360, 1982
6. *CABOT A, BECKER A:* The cervical spine in rheumatoid arthritis. Clin Orthop 131:130, 1978
7. *CONATY JP, MONGAN ES:* Cervical fusion in rheumatoid arthritis. J Bone Joint Surg 63A:1218, 1981
8. *CONLON PW, ISDALE IC, ROSE BS:* Rheumatoid arthritis of the cervical spine: An analysis of 333 cases. Ann Rheum Dis 25:120, 1966
9. *CRELLIN RQ, MACCABE JJ, HAMILTON EB:* Severe subluxation of the cervical spine in rheumatoid arthritis. J Bone Joint Surg 52B:244, 1970
10. *CROCKARD HA, POZO JL, RANSFORD AO, KENDALL BE, ESSIGMAN WK:* Transoral decompression and posterior fusion for rheumatoid atlanto-axial subluxation. J Bone Joint Surg 68B:350, 1986
11. *DAVIDSON RC, HORN JR, HERNDON JH, ET AL:* Brain stem compression in rheumatoid arthritis. JAMA 238:2633, 1977
12. *DAVIS FW, MARKLEY HE:* Rheumatoid arthritis with death from medullary compression. Ann Intern Med 35:451, 1951
13. *FERLIC DC, CLAYTON ML, LEIDHOLT JD, ET AL:* Surgical treatment of the symptomatic unstable cervical spine in rheumatoid arthritis. J Bone Joint Surg 57A:349, 1975
14. *FISCHGOLD H, METZGER J:* Étude radiographic de l'impression basilaire. Rev Rheum 19:261, 1952
15. *FRIED JA, ATHREYA B, GREGG JR, DAS M, DOUGHTY R:* The cervical spine in juvenile rheumatoid arthritis. Clin Orthop 179:102, 1983
16. *GEEHR RB, ROTHMAN SL, KIER EL:* The role of computed tomography in the evaluation of upper cervical spine pathology. Comput Tomogr 2:79, 1978
17. *GLYNN MK, SHEEHAN JM:* Fusion of the cervical spine for instability. Clin Orthop 179:99, 1983
18. *GRANTHAM SA, DICK HM, THOMPSON RC, ET AL:* Occipito cervical arthrodesis: Indications, technic, and results. Clin Orthop 65:118, 1969
19. *GROKOEST AW, SNYDER AI, SCHLAEGER R:* Juvenile Rheumatoid Arthritis. Boston, Little, Brown & Co, 1962
20. *ISDALE IC, CONION PW:* Atlanto-axial subluxation. A six year follow-up report. Ann Rheum Dis 30:387, 1971
21. *JOHNSON JS, VAUGHAN JH, HENCH PK, ET AL:* Rheumatoid arthritis, 1970–1972. Ann Intern Med 78:937, 1973
22. *KAUFMAN RL, GLENN WV:* Rheumatoid cervical myelopathy: evaluation by computerized tomography with multi-planar reconstruction. J Rheumatol 10:42, 1983
23. *KONTINNEN Y, SANTAVIRTA S, BERGROTH V, SANDELIN J:* Inflammatory involvement of the cervical spine ligaments in rheumatoid arthritis. Acta Orthop Scand 57:587, 1986
24. *LEE BCP, DECK MDF, KNEELAND JB, CAHILL PT:* MR imaging of the craniocervical junction. AJNR 6:209, 1985
25. *LIPSON SJ:* Cervical myelopathy and posterior atlanto-axial subluxation in patients with rheumatoid arthritis. J Bone Joint Surg 67A:593, 1985
26. *MARKS JS, SHARP J:* Rheumatoid cervical myelopathy. Quart J Med 50:307, 1981
27. *MARTEL W:* The occipito-atlanto-axial joints in rheumatoid arthritis and ankylosing spondylitis. Am J Radiol 86:223, 1961
28. *MARTEL W:* Pathogenesis of cervical discovertebral destruction in rheumatoid arthritis. Arthr Rheum 20:1217, 1977
29. *MATHEWS JA:* Atlanto-axial subluxation in rheumatoid arthritis. Ann Rheum Dis 28:260, 1969
30. *MEIJERS KA, VAN BEUSEKAM GT, DUIJFJES F, ET AL:* Treatment of dislocations in the cervical spine in rheumatoid arthritis and ankylosing spondylitis complicated by signs of compression. Ann Rheum Dis 32:88, 1973
31. *MEIJERS KAE, VAN BEUSEKAM GT, LUYENDIJK W, DUIJFJES F:* Dislocation of the cervical spine with cord compression in rheumatoid arthritis. J Bone Joint Surg 56B:668, 1974

32. *Meikle JA, Wilkinson M:* Rheumatoid involvement of the cervical spine. Ann Rheum Dis 30:154, 1971
33. *Mikulowski P, Wollheim FA, Rotmil P, Olsen I:* Sudden death in rheumatoid arthritis with atlantoaxial dislocation. Acta Med Scand 198:445, 1975
34. *Modic MT, Weinstein MA, Pavlicek W, Boumphrey F, Starnes D, Duchesneu PM:* Magnetic resonance imaging of the cervical spine. Am J Radiol 141:1129, 1983
35. *Park WM, O'Neill MO, McCall IW:* The radiology of rheumatoid involvement of the cervical spine. Skel Radiol 4:1, 1979
36. *Pellicci PM, Ranawat CS, Tsairis P, Bryan WJ:* A prospective study of the progression of rheumatoid arthritis of the cervical spine. J Bone Joint Surg 63A:342, 1981
37. *Phonprasert C, Suwanwela C:* Management of chronic atlanto-axial dislocation. Surg Gynecol Obstet 149:534, 1979
38. *Rana NA, Hancock DO, Taylor AR, et al:* Upward translocation of the dens in rheumatoid arthritis. J Bone Joint Surg 55B:471, 1973
39. *Ranawat CS, O'Leary P, Pellicci P, Tsairis P, Marchisello P, Dorr L:* Cervical fusion in rheumatoid arthritis. J Bone Joint Surg 61A:1003, 1979
40. *Redlund-Johnell I, Pettersson H:* Radiographic measurements of the cranio-vertebral region. Acta Radiol Diagn 25:23, 1984
41. *Sharp J, Purser DW:* Spontaneous atlanto-axial dislocation in ankylosing spondylitis and rheumatoid arthritis. Ann Rheum Dis 20:47, 1961
42. *Sharp J, Purser DW, Lawrence J:* Rheumatoid arthritis of the cervical spine in the adult. Ann Rheum Dis 17:303, 1958
43. *Shaw DA, Cartlidge NE:* Cervical myelopathy in rheumatoid arthritis. Acta Neurol Belg 76:279, 1976
44. *Sherk HH:* Lesions of the atlas and axis. Clin Orthop 109:33, 1975
45. *Sherk HH:* Atlanto-axial instability and acquired basilar invagination in rheumatoid arthritis. Orthop Clin North Am 9:1053, 1978
46. *Simmons EH, de Toit Jr, Guillaume:* Lateral atlanto-axial arthrodesis. Orthop Clin North Am 9:1101, 1978
47. *Smith PH, Benn RT, Sharp J:* Natural history of rheumatoid cervical luxations. Ann Rheum Dis 31:431, 1972
48. *Van Beusekom GT:* The neurological syndrome associated with cervical luxations in rheumatoid arthritis. Acta Orthop Belg 58:38, 1972
49. *Weissman BNW, Aliabadi P, Weinfeld MS, Thomas WH, Sosman JL:* Prognostic features of atlantoaxial subluxation in rheumatoid arthritis patients. Radiol 144:745, 1982
50. *Whitesides TE, McDonald AP:* Lateral retropharyngeal approach to the upper cervical spine. Orthop Clin North Am 9(4):1978
51. *Winfield J, Cooke D, Brook AS, Corbett M:* A prospective study of the radiological changes in the cervical spine in early rheumatoid disease.

The Surgical Correction of Flexion Deformity of the Cervical Spine in Ankylosing Spondylitis

Edward H. Simmons

Ankylosing spondylitis of the Marie-Strümpell type, or a variant such as that associated with psoriasis, is a different disease from rheumatoid arthritis. Although it has often been described as "rheumatoid" spondylitis, it is a different disease with a different serology. It is more common in males, with a predilection for affecting the spine and major joints, whereas rheumatoid arthritis is more in females, with a predilection for smaller joints of the appendicular skeleton. In ankylosing spondylitis, the spine becomes inflamed, painful, and osteopenic, and later proceeds to ossification. If it ossifies with the spine in normal alignment the affliction is not too severe, but all too frequently the spine may bend and become ossified in a deformed position. There is a significant incidence of the disease, which on a clinically active basis is two to three patients per 1000 population.

The problems of major concern to the orthopedic surgeon are atlantoaxial instability, atlantooccipital disability, spondylodiscitis, and the presentation of gross flexion deformities of the trunk.

INDICATIONS FOR SURGICAL CORRECTION OF FLEXION DEFORMITY

The indications for surgical correction of deformity related to the spine are variable and depend on the extent of the deformity, the degree of functional embarrassment, the age and general condition of the patient, the feasibility of correction, and, perhaps above all else, the morale and the earnest desire of the patient to accept the risks and rehabilitative measures required for correction.

ASSESSMENT OF PATIENTS FOR CORRECTION

In assessing patients for possible correction, it is important to recognize the primary site of the deformity. We may occasionally compensate for deformity in one area by correction carried out in an area slightly removed from it. However, if any major correction is to be obtained, it must be performed in the area of main deformity. The main deformity in patients who present with apparent spinal deformity may be in the hip joints. It may be primarily in the lumbar spine, the thoracic spine, or in the cervical spine. The patient should be carefully assessed, and the main area or areas of deformity should be identified. Figure 10-9 illustrates a young man who could see to walk by going backward, with a chin-brow to vertical angle of 134 degrees. Assessment of his deformity indicated that he had some flexion deformity of his cervical spine and his thoracic spine. However, the major spinal deformity was in the lumbar region, with a loss of his normal lordosis of 45 degrees and a superimposed kyphosis of 54 degrees, resulting in a combined deformity of 94 degrees. It was also evident that he had a major flexion deformity of his hip joints. These were solidly fused in flexion and required bilateral total replacement arthroplasties, performed at the same sitting under combined epidural and local anesthesia. This mobilized his hip joints and corrected their deformities, but he then could see neither backward nor forward on walking. He required a resection–extension osteotomy correction of 104 degrees to his midlumbar spine under local anesthesia. This corrected his major deformities, and although he still has some residual flexion deformity of his neck and knees, he has been restored to a reasonably normal functional life at home with his family.

A few patients in whom the main deformity is in the thoracic region have maintained a normal cervical and lumbar lordosis. Patients with deformity restricted to the thoracic area require combinations of multiple anterior and posterior procedures in that area, depending on the rigidity of the deformity. Figure 10-10 illustrates this type of deformity in a general surgeon who suffered increasing thoracic kyphosis to the point at which he could no longer perform his surgery. He had a rigid thoracic kyphosis of 106 degrees with an associated area of spondylodiscitis. He required anterior resections of his ossified discs and the area of spondylodiscitis with bone grafting, followed by multiple posterior resection osteotomies with Harrington compression instrumentation and fusion. This corrected his major deformity, allowing him to stand and look ahead and to return to the practice of surgery.

Finally, a few patients with ankylosing spondylitis have flexion deformity of the spine occurring primarily in the cervical region. This deformity can be severely disabling with restriction of field

(*Text continues p. 580*)

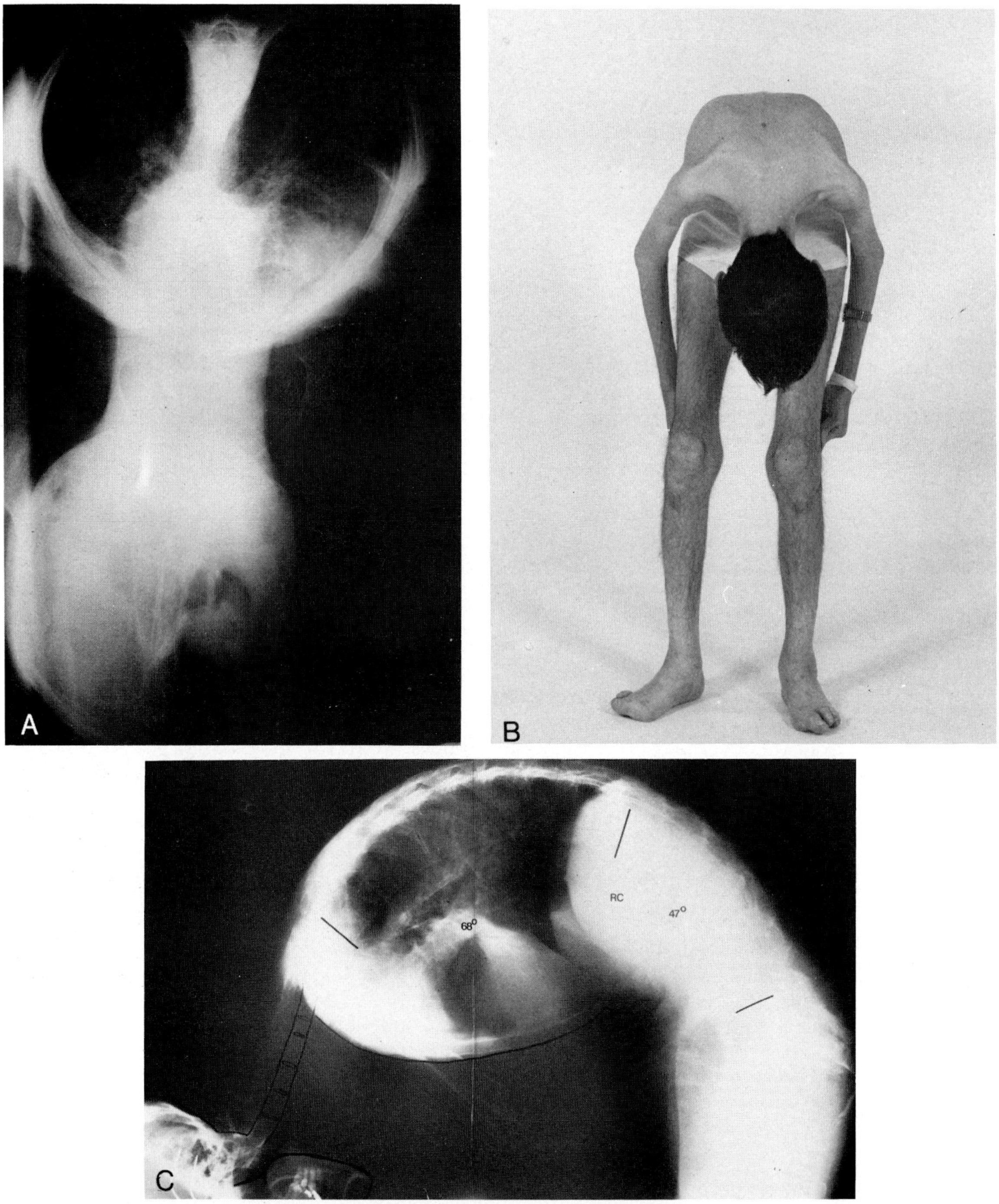

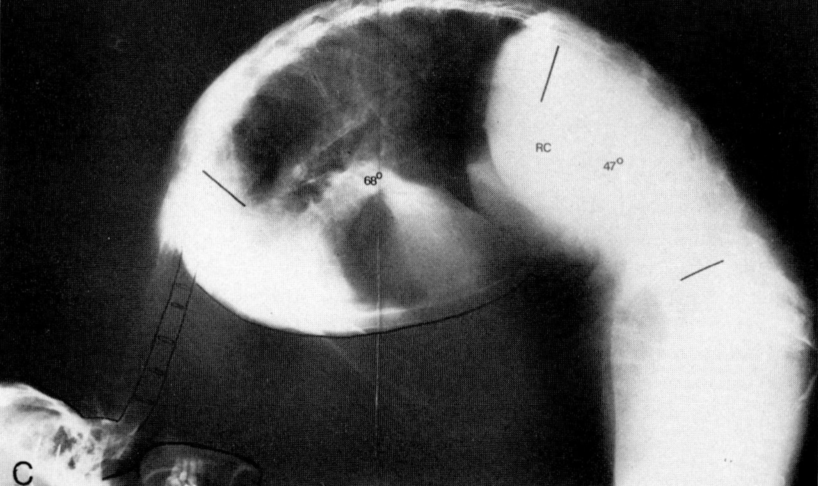

Fig. 10-9. (*A*) Standing A–P radiograph of spine of male patient with severe trunk deformity. The A–P film of the thoracic area resembles a CT axial view. (*B*) Anterior standing view of patient showing severe restriction of field of vision. The patient could only see backward, and walked going backward. (*C*) Standing lateral radiograph showing combination of severe flexion deformities, with thoracic kyphosis of 68 degrees, complete loss of lumbar lordosis with 47 degrees of kyphosis, and hip flexion deformities.

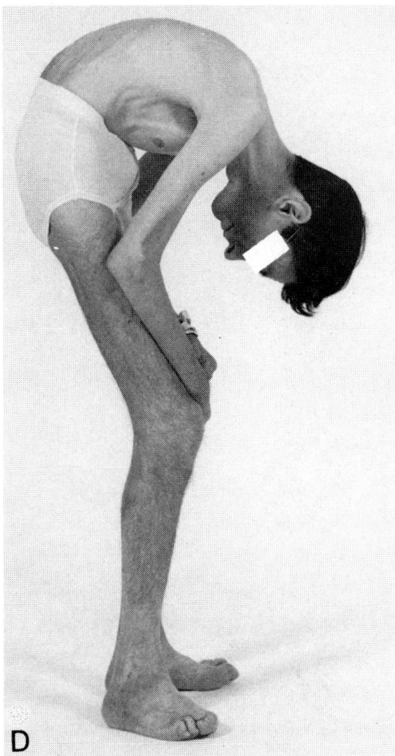

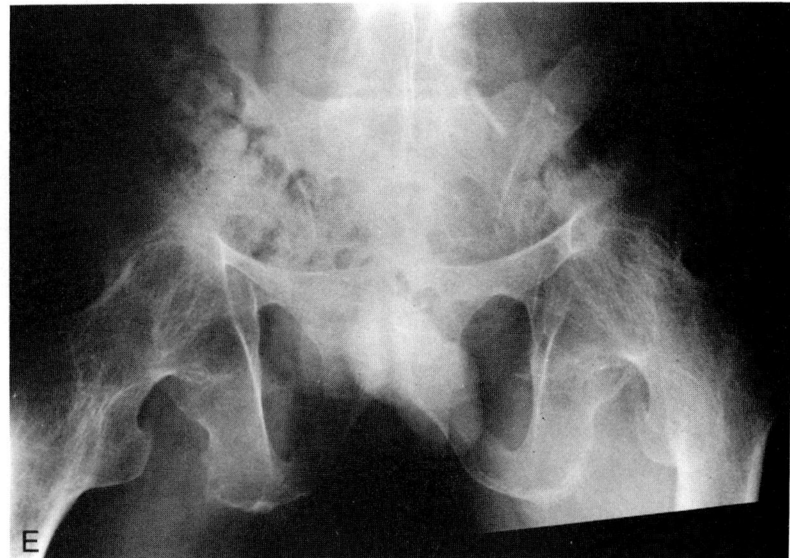

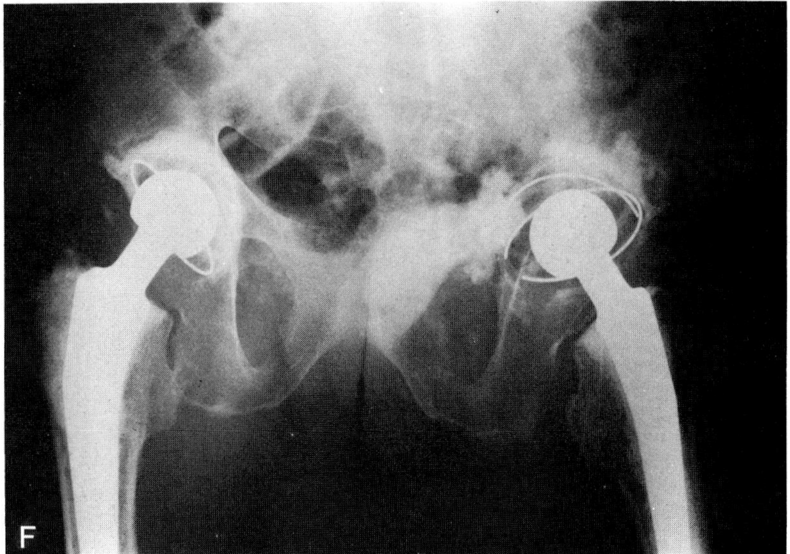

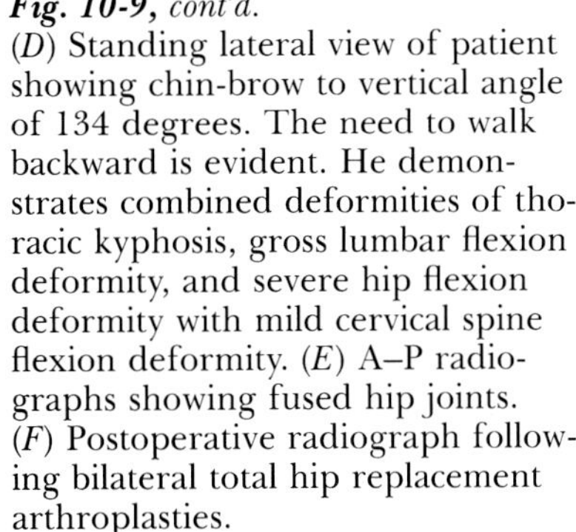

Fig. 10-9, *cont'd.*
(*D*) Standing lateral view of patient showing chin-brow to vertical angle of 134 degrees. The need to walk backward is evident. He demonstrates combined deformities of thoracic kyphosis, gross lumbar flexion deformity, and severe hip flexion deformity with mild cervical spine flexion deformity. (*E*) A–P radiographs showing fused hip joints. (*F*) Postoperative radiograph following bilateral total hip replacement arthroplasties.

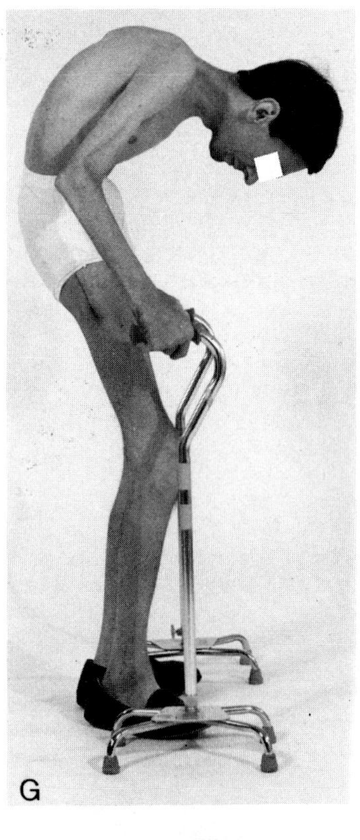

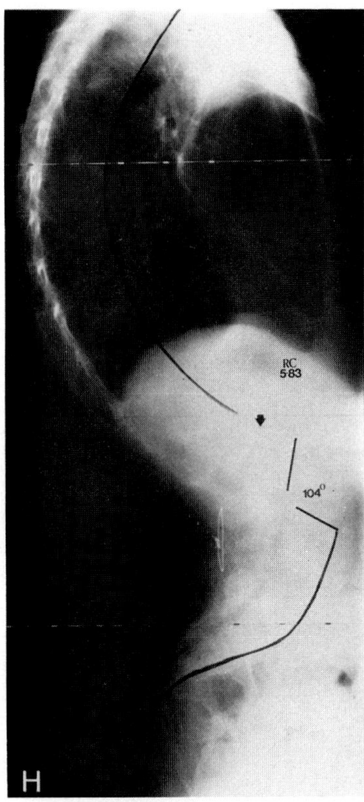

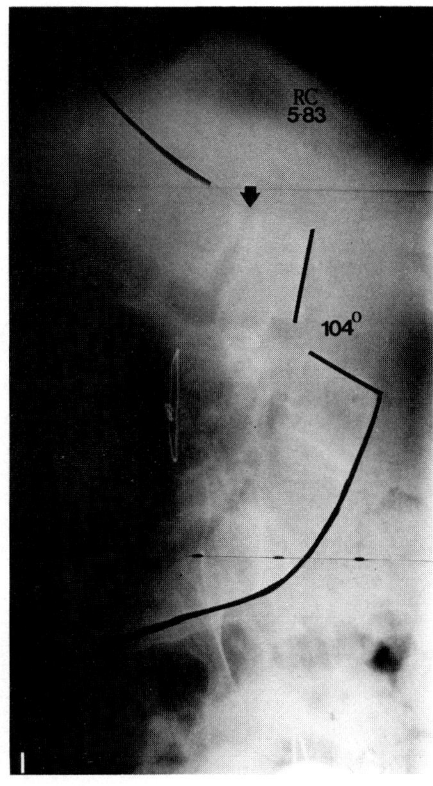

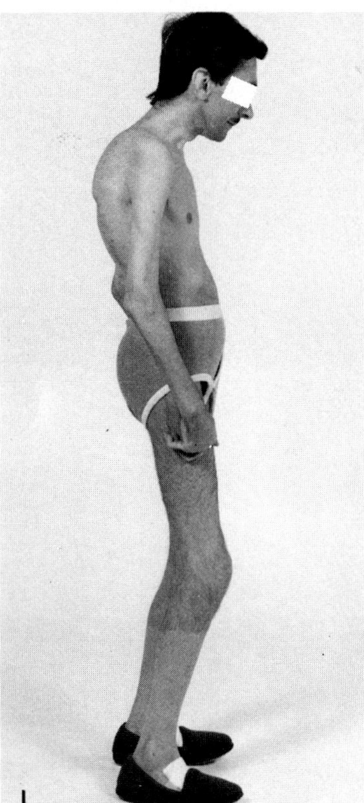

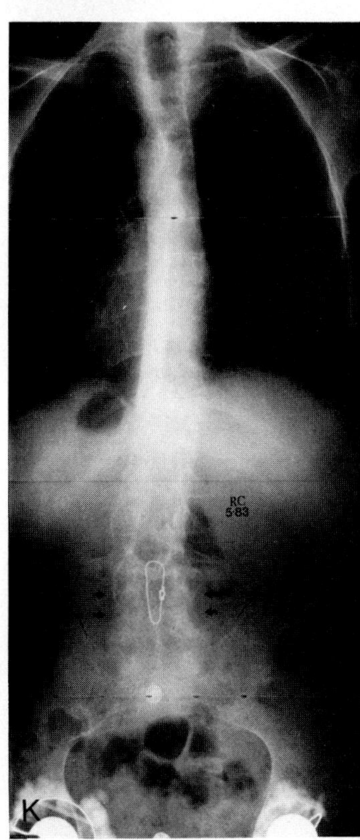

Fig. 10-9, *cont'd.*
(*G*) Standing lateral view of patient following correction of hip flexion deformities with bilateral total replacement arthroplasties. His deformity is improved, but the patient can now see neither backward nor forward for walking. (*H*) Standing lateral 3-foot radiograph of spine following lumbar resection–extension osteotomy of 104 degrees performed under local anesthesia. Note that the weight-bearing line has been shifted posterior to the osteotomy site. The arrow marks a previous area of spondylodiscitis, which has gone on to healing. (*I*) Lateral radiograph of lumbar spine showing healing of osteotomy with weight-bearing line posterior to it. (*J*) Postoperative standing lateral view of patient showing correction of his major deformities. He still has some flexion deformity of the knees and neck but is able to stand, look ahead, and walk in a relatively normal fashion. (*K*) Postoperative standing A–P 3-foot film of spine showing dramatic comparison to preoperative film (*A*).

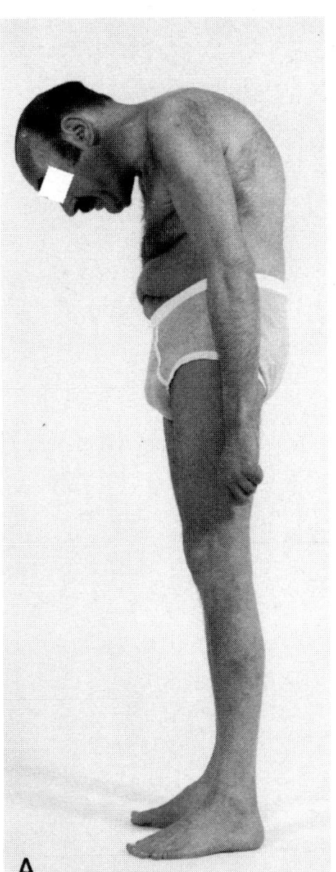

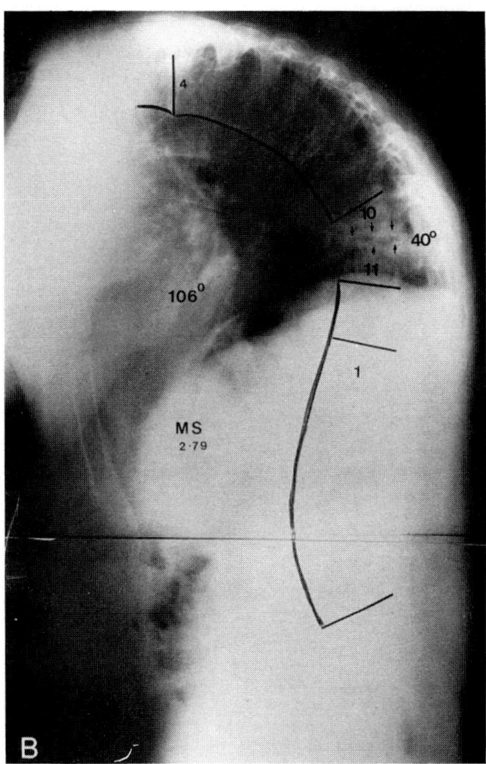

Fig. 10-10. (*A*) Lateral view of 48-year-old surgeon suffering a primarily thoracic deformity with normal cervical and lumbar lordosis. (*B*) Standing lateral 3-foot radiograph of spine showing fixed thoracic kyphosis of 106 degrees with normal lordosis. Despite a localized area of spondylodiscitis, the deformity was rigid with no correction on halo-dependent traction. He required combined anterior and posterior osteotomies with posterior instrumentation. (*C*) Postoperative standing lateral 3-foot radiograph of spine showing correction of thoracic kyphosis from 106 degrees to 69 degrees. This is balanced by his lordosis of 65 degrees. The area of spondylodiscitis has gone on to healing. (*D*) Postoperative lateral view of patient showing correction of his deformity. He was able to return to a normal lifestyle and the practice of surgery.

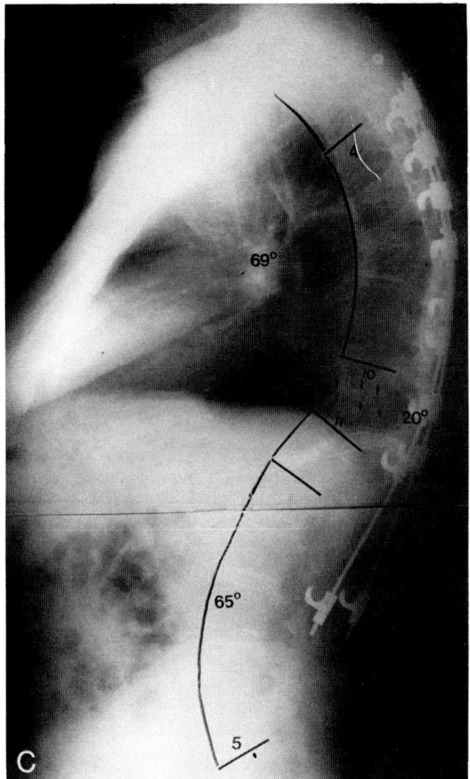

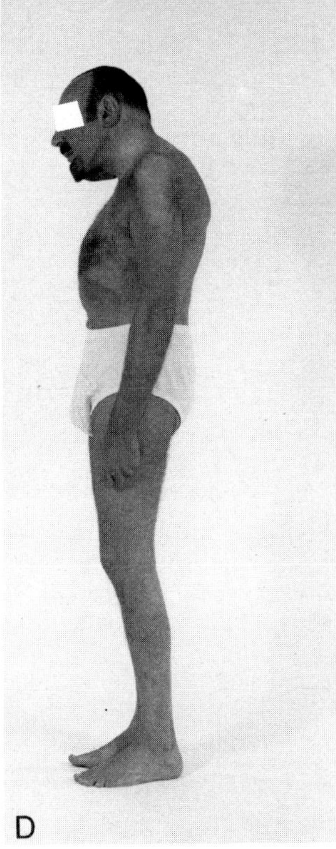

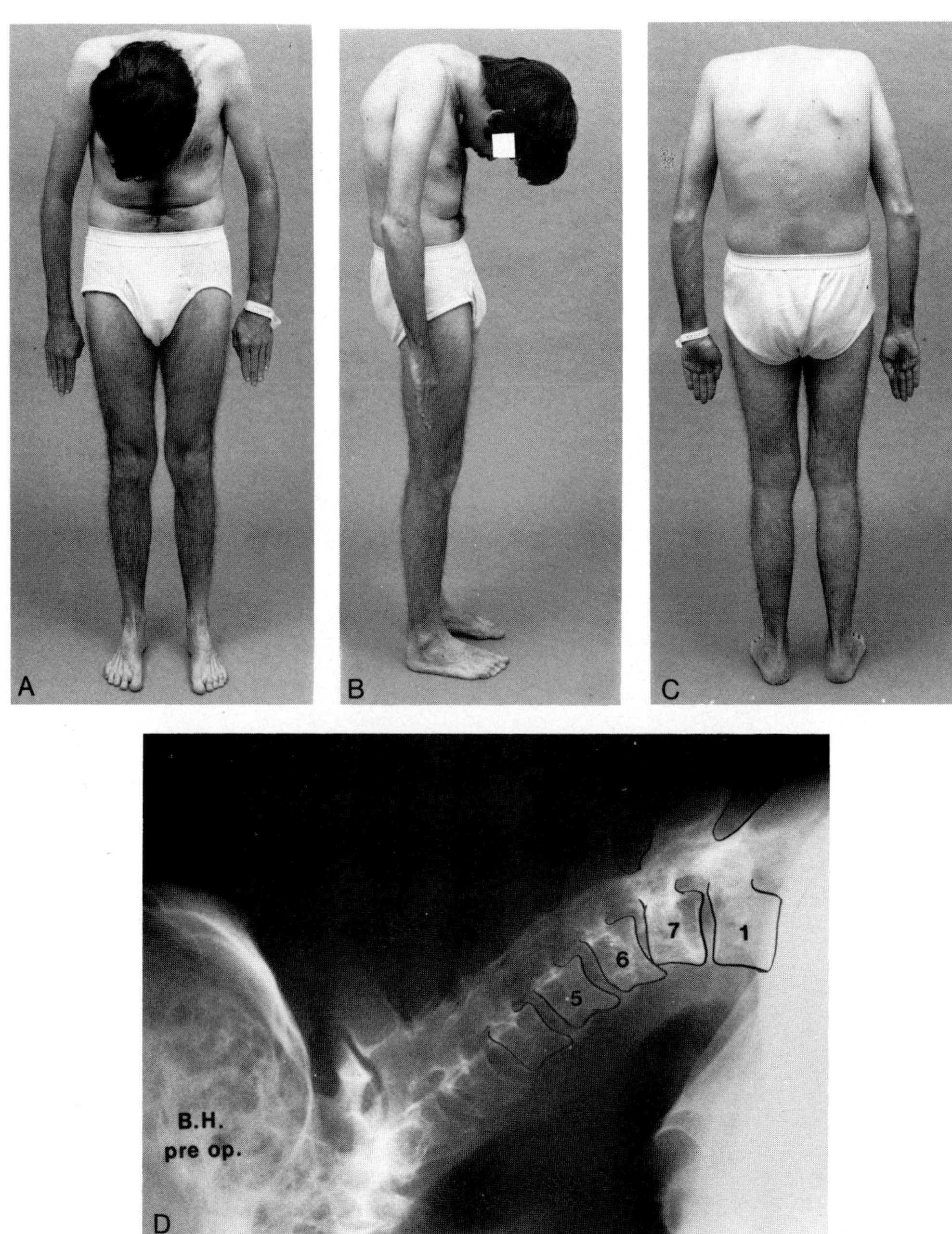

Fig. 10-11. (*A*) Anterior view of male patient with severe rigid flexion deformity of the cervical spine showing extreme restriction of field of vision. (*B*) Lateral view of patient further demonstrating marked restriction of field of vision, as well as difficulty opening the mouth, due to the chin being rigidly fixed against the chest. (*C*) Posterior view of patient showing apparent absence of head due to severe flexion deformity. (*D*) Preoperative lateral radiograph showing flexion deformity with fused cervical spine and previous subluxation of C6–C7.

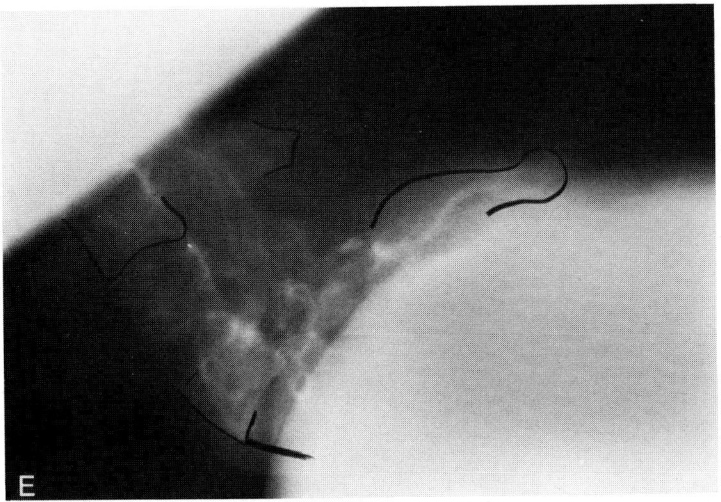

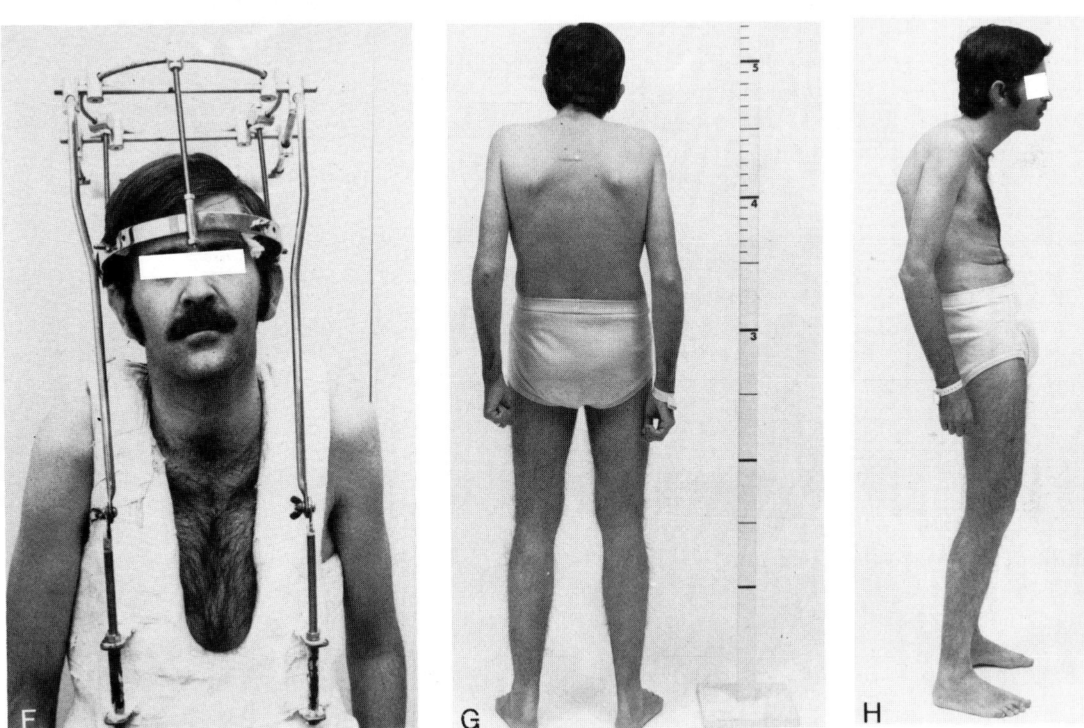

Fig. 10-11, *cont'd.*
(*E*) Postoperative lateral radiograph of cervical spine showing resection-extension osteotomy correction. (*F*) Postoperative anterior view of patient in halo cast showing correction of deformity with restoration of normal field of vision. (*G*) Posterior view of patient following union of osteotomy, showing restoration of head to trunk alignment. (*H*) Lateral postoperative view of patient showing complete correction of deformity with restoration of normal chin-brow to vertical angle.

of vision and interference with skin care under the chin and shaving in the male. It may progress to the point of interfering with opening the mouth (Fig. 10-11).

Regardless of what area of the spine is involved, including the hip joints, an accurate measurement of the deformity is required to indicate its significance and to allow comparison of results, as is done with other types of surgery. The most effective and reliable measure of the deformity is the chin-brow to vertical angle. This is a measure of the angle formed by a line from the brow to the chin through the vertical, when the patient stands with his hips and knees fully extended and the neck in a neutral or its fixed position (Fig. 10-12).

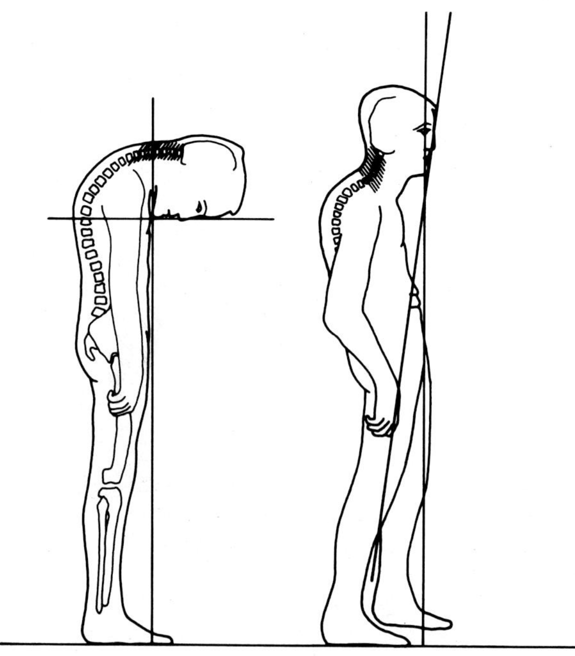

Fig. 10-12. Diagrammatic illustration of chin-brow to vertical angle as a measure of the degree of flexion deformity of the spine in ankylosing spondylitis. The angle is measured from the brow to the chin to the vertical, with the patient standing with the hips and knees extended, and the neck in its fixed or neutral position.

SELECTION OF PATIENT FOR CERVICAL OSTEOTOMY

It is very important to recognize that not all patients with a "chin-on-chest" deformity in ankylosing spondylitis require a cervical osteotomy. Those who present with a painful flexion deformity probably do not require osteotomy. A patient with ankylosing spondylitis whose spinal alignment has been relatively unchanged over a significant interval in a relatively pain-free state, and who then sustains minimal or ever minor trauma with subsequent painful progressive flexion deformity, can be considered as having a fracture of the cervical spine until proven otherwise. The fracture is usually at the base of the neck at the cervicothoracic junction. Fractures of the spine in ankylosing spondylitis resemble a fracture of an osteoporotic tubular bone with a transverse shear pattern. The fracture is difficult to recognize radiographically, being obscured by the shoulders and by the fact that it may vary in its location from C6 to T2, most commonly in the area of C7 or T1. The pain is often attributed to the patient's disease. The fracture undergoes gradual erosion, with compression and collapse anteriorly and the chin approaching the chest. The patient is aware that the position of his head varies during the day, being more elevated on waking in the morning and approaching the chest more after being ambulatory during the day. The patient, on presentation to the physician, may attempt to hold the head with their hands to ease the distress. It is important to recognize the fracture through the use of lateral tomography at the cervicothoracic junction. These patients do not require a cervical osteotomy. They should be treated with the application of a cranial halo and traction initially applied along the line of the neck, slowly restoring normal alignment with careful observation until the head is restored to its normal functional position. This is best accomplished with the patient supported on a circoelectric bed. A fairly normal chin-brow to vertical angle can usually be obtained. When this is achieved, the patient should be immobilized in a well-molded halo cast for 4 months. A halo cast, rather than a halo vest, is essential, as a halo vest will not supply adequate immobilization. In our experience, if rigid immobilization is provided in this fashion, union occurs almost consistently over that interval and is to be followed by a shorter period of bracing (Fig. 10-13).[6] In the rare or unusual instance in which spontaneous healing does not occur, then anterior cervical fusion using a keystone strut graft[7] or posterior fusion fixation may be required.

Although shear fractures occur most commonly at the base of the neck, they may occur at any level. The initial displacement may be sufficient that patients present with evidence of spinal cord injury when first seen, or this may occur relatively rapidly or suddenly during the course of their early management as a result of displacement. It is to be emphasized that patients with this problem are at a major risk and are prone to disastrous results with conventional methods of treatment, as are used for fracture–dislocations in patients without ankylosing spondylitis. These patients present with a rigid spine above and below. Any movement of the trunk translates all the force or motion to the fracture site. A common observation of the relatives of patients who are admitted to the emergency department with a fracture of the cervical spine is the fact that "the neck is straight," whereas prior to the injury the patient had a well-known forward flexion alignment. Those in emergency attendance should recognize that this means the patient has an extension displacement at the fracture site when lying flat. As an initial measure, information should be obtained from the patient or his relatives as to the preinjury alignment of his neck, and attempts should be made to simulate this position with the application of a halo and gentle traction along what was believed to be his normal alignment. The patient should be protected with a halo vest at this stage before any radiographic studies are carried out that might cause displacement. A lateral tomogram is the most valuable radiographic diagnostic aid as to the alignment at the fracture site, along with routine x-ray studies.

Where major but incomplete spinal cord injury with incomplete reduction has occurred, open reduction and internal fixation may be required to protect the cord from any further injury caused by motion induced by the solid segments above and below, and to allow decompression by the accuracy of reduction. It is important to recognize that the dangers of attempting this procedure under general anesthesia can be catastrophic. The movement of the neck required for intubation with a rigid upper cervical spine can cause further major spinal cord injury. Moving the patient to the operating table and positioning the patient can have a major deleterious effect. The patient is most safely operated on while awake and in the sitting position. After the patient has been stabilized with a halo jacket, which is firmly applied, he can be operated on in the sitting position, with traction applied along the line of the neck assisting immobilization. The posterior cervical spine can be exposed under local anesthesia, and the fracture accurately reduced and fixed internally, with methylmethacrylate applied to the segments above and below; threaded Compere wires are passed percutaneously through the bases of the spinous processes with an encircling stainless steel wire (Fig. 10-14). This provides an "instant fix," relieving the patient's pain, and it maintains accurate alignment of the spinal canal until healing occurs anteriorly. Subsequent to the surgery, the patient should be fitted in a well-molded halo cast that will supply more rigid and accurate immobilization than a halo vest. This must be well molded below the costal cage and over the iliac crest to prevent any upward or downward motion. The patient is immobilized for 4 months. In more longstanding cases with residual displacement, decompression can be accomplished by removing the adjacent arches at the fracture site. Similar immobilization is placed laterally on each side, using a bridge of methylmethacrylate on each side from the segments above and below.

The other area of the cervical spine where lesions may occur which cause patients to present with painful flexion deformity is the craniocervical junction. Erosive fractures through the posterior arch of C1 and subluxation at C1–C2 may present with painful flexion deformity with or without neurologic symptoms. Destructive arthritis at the atlantooccipital joints may cause the patient to flex the neck at these joints with the chin held downward. The lateral radiograph of the cervical spine is the clue to recognition of these abnormalities. It usually shows a relatively normal lordosis, indicating that the flexion deformity is at the craniocervical junction. These lesions should be recognized and the deformity corrected by graduated halo traction, restoring a normal chin-brow to vertical angle, and then by posterior stabilization. If reduction can be obtained for C1–C2 dislocation, then posterior atlantoaxial arthrodesis, such as the Gallie technique, may be all that is required. For occipitocervical destruction and erosive fractures through the arch of C1, occipitocervical fusion is required, and, where necessary, excision of the posterior fragmented arch of C1 (Fig. 10-15).[6]

Unrecognized and untreated fractures at the base of cervical spine proceed to gradual erosion and compression until the chin reaches the chest. The fractures ultimately heal, at which time the pain disappears, leaving the patient with a painless, fixed, flexion deformity. At this stage, osteotomy is required for correction.

In patients in whom I have performed cervical osteomy, 36% have shown evidence of previous cervical fracture. In 31%, the fracture contributed significantly to the final deformity. In only 14% of those who presented with evidence of cervical frac-

(*Text continues p. 586*)

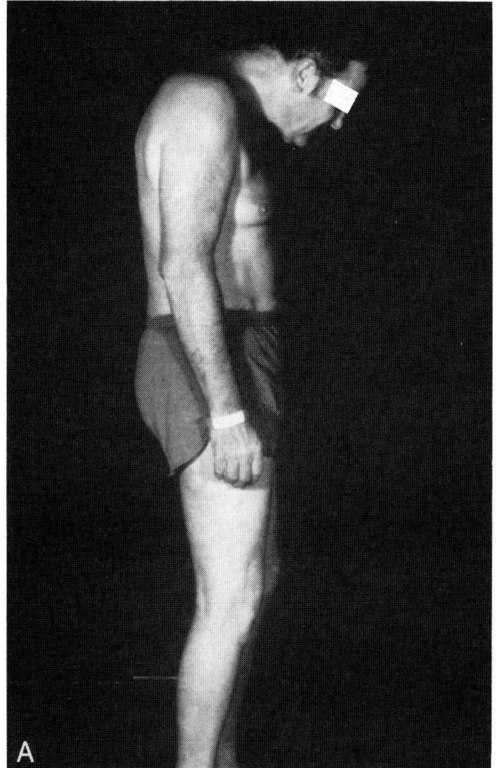

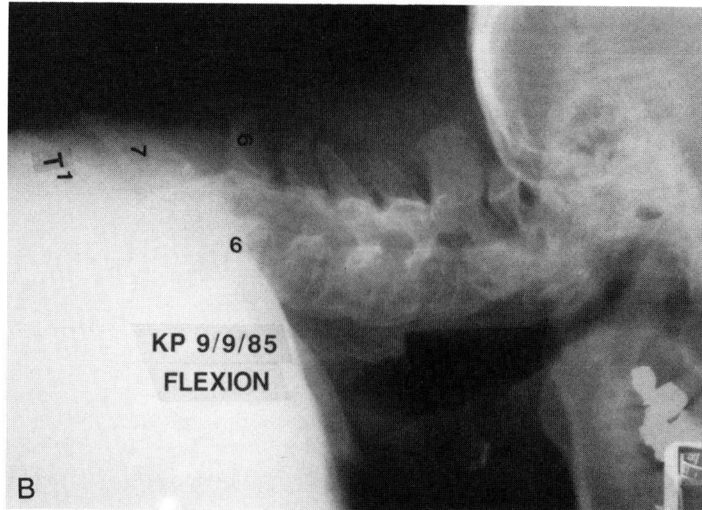

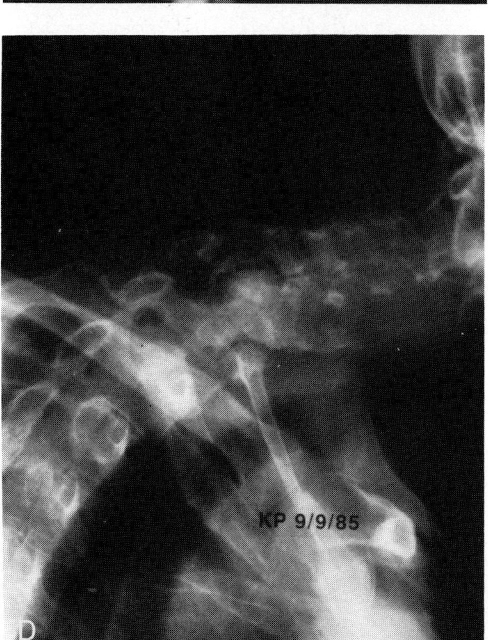

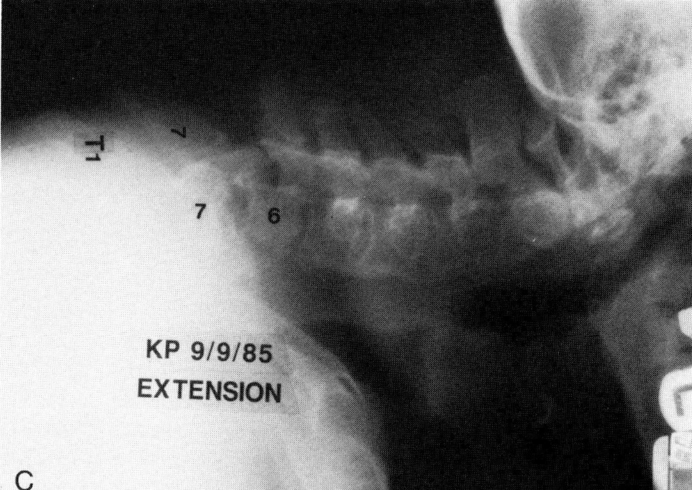

Fig. 10-13. (*A*) Lateral view of 54-year-old male presenting with painful flexion deformity of the cervical spine with a chin-brow to vertical angle of 55 degrees. He had suffered known ankylosing spondylitis for 17 years. Nine months previously he had sustained a mild injury that was initially not believed to be significant. He had been assessed and treated by medicine, psychiatry, neurosurgery, and finally orthopedic surgery. He had noted a painful increasing flexion deformity of his cervical spine. (*B*) Lateral radiograph of the cervical spine in flexion showing changes of ankylosing spondylitis above C6 but without satisfactory visualization below. Separation of the spinous processes of C6–C7 is noted. (*C*) Lateral radiograph of cervical spine in extension showing little change, but with suggestion of new bone formation anteriorly. (*D*) Oblique view showing area of fracture erosion and angulation of cervicothoracic spine.

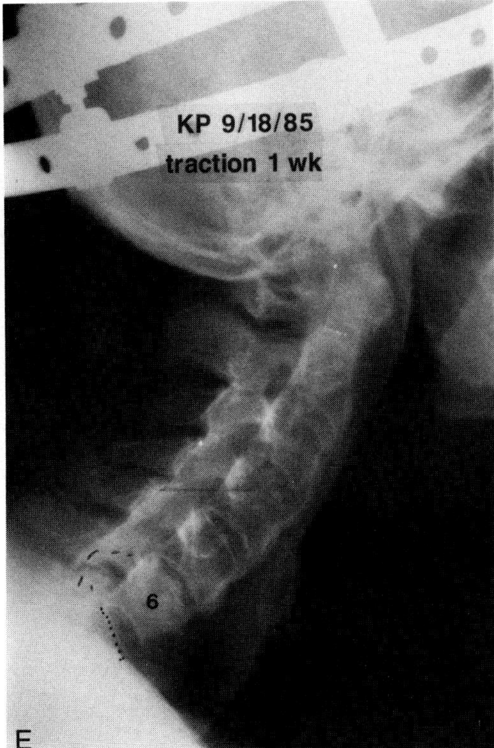

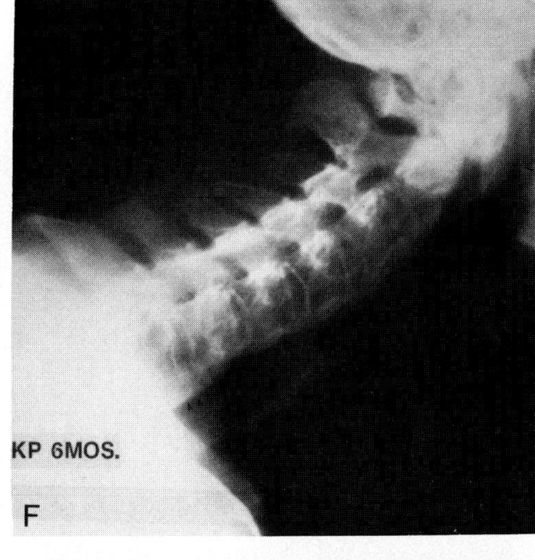

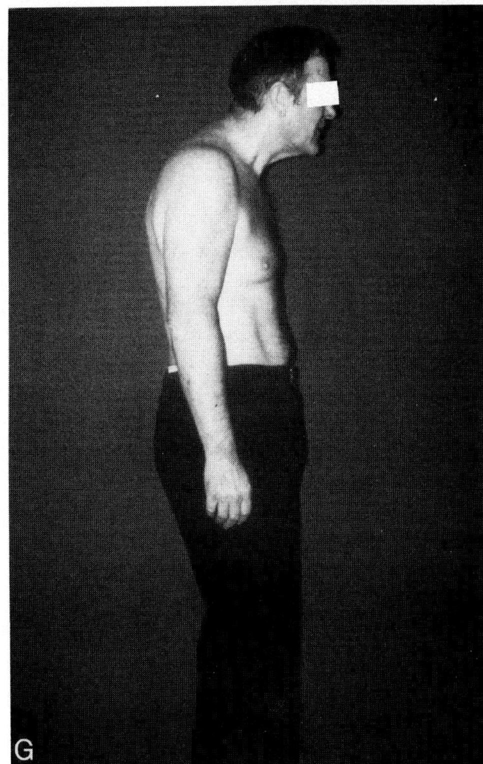

Fig. 10-13, *cont'd.*
(*E*) Lateral radiograph of cervical spine following 1 week of halo traction, initially along the line of the patient's neck, with gradual restoration of normal alignment. (*F*) Lateral radiograph of cervical spine 6 months following reduction of deformity and 2 months after removal of halo cast showing healing of fracture site with mature bone formation, despite the 9-month duration of the deformity. (*G*) Lateral view of patient following solid union showing correction of deformity. The patient is free of pain and has a normal field of vision. His chin-brow to vertical angle has been reduced to a normal of 3 degrees. No surgical operative procedure was required for correction of his deformity.

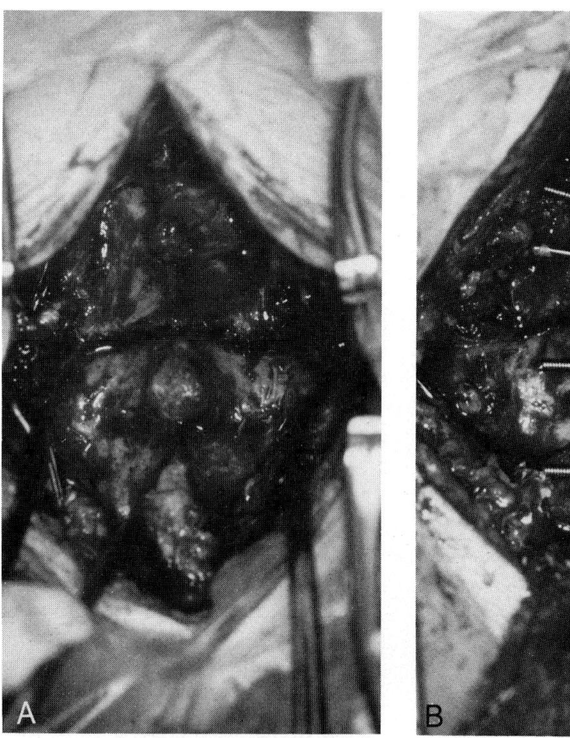

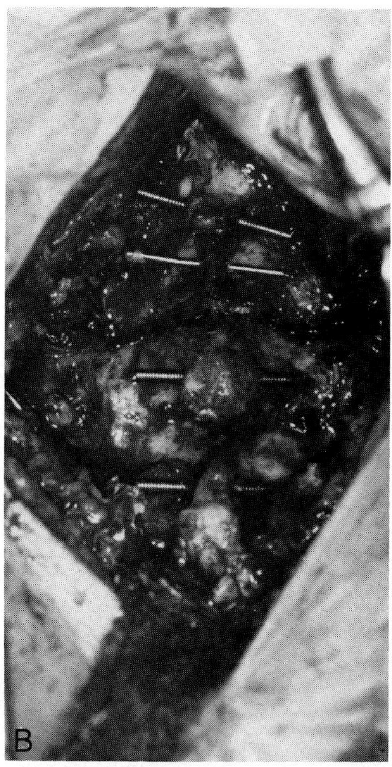

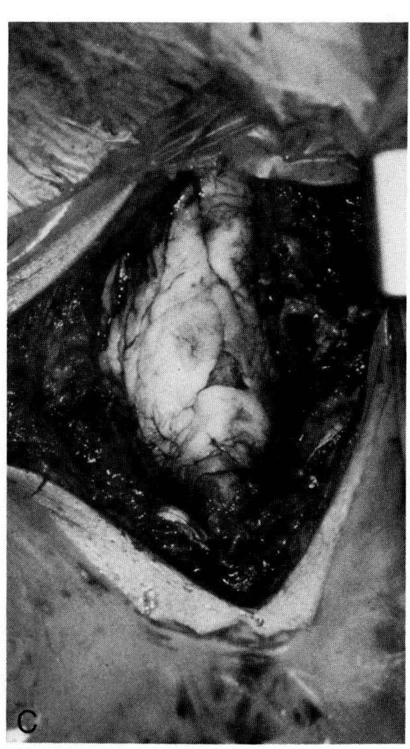

Fig. 10-14. (*A*) Operative view of posterior cervical spine of a 32-year-old spondylitic male suffering a fracture–dislocation of C6–C7 following automobile injury. The spinous processes of C5 and C6 are noted above the fracture line, the spinous processes of C7 and T1 below. The patient suffered partial quadriplegia with some initial improvement and subsequent worsening due to malposition and instability at the shear fracture site. The instability problem is magnified by the solid column of bone above and below. The patient was placed in a halo vest, and halo suspended along the normal line of his neck and the operation performed under local anesthesia in the sitting position. The fracture–dislocation was reduced under direct vision. (*B*) Posterior operative view of reduced shear fracture–dislocation with threaded Compere wires in position through the posterior arches of C5, C6, C7 and T1. The threaded wires were inserted percutaneously through the left lateral aspect of the neck, transfixing the bases of the spinous processes, the wires then being cut lateral to the spine. Encircling stainless steel wires may be placed around the Compere wires to add to the methylmethacrylate fixation. (*C*) Posterior operative view showing methylmethacrylate incorporating Compere wires and spinous processes to maintain reduction and provide instant fixation of the unstable shear fracture site. This maintains normal alignment of the canal, prevents the deleterious effect of continuing motion on the neural elements, and allows spontaneous healing of the fracture to occur. If midline decompression is also required, bridges of methylmethacrylate may be placed laterally on each side, leaving the midline clear.

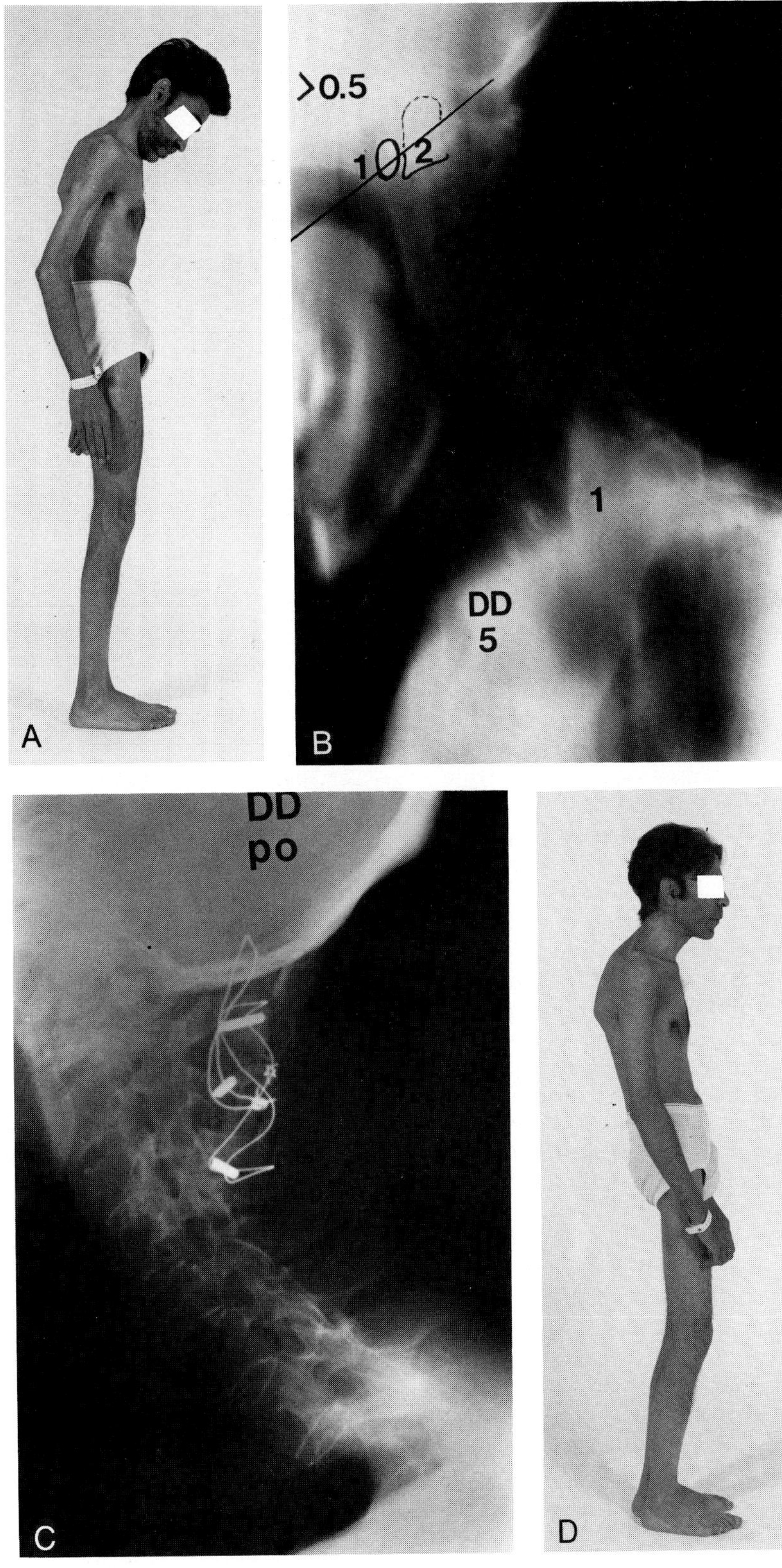

Fig. 10-15. (*A*) Lateral view of physicist with known ankylosing spondylitis and painful chin-on-chest deformity. The patient would hold his head with his hands when sitting to ease his discomfort. (*B*) Lateral tomogram of cervical spine showing normal cervical lordosis with normal alignment at cervicothoracic junction. The C1–C2 relationships are normal. The mandible approaches the cervical spine, indicating that the deformity is at the occipitoatlantal junction. Note the dense outline of the arch of C1 posteriorly, which was eroded and loose, likely causing dural irritation. A–P tomogram showed destructive changes at the occipitoatlantal joints, in keeping with his deformity. (*C*) Postoperative lateral radiograph following reduction of the patient's deformity with graduated halo traction, excision of the loose posterior arch of C1, and solid posterior occipitocervical fusion. Double onlay grafts were used, fixed to the skull and the upper cervical spine augmented by cancellous bone. (*D*) Postoperative lateral view of patient showing correction of chin-on-chest deformity with restoration of normal chin-brow to vertical angle. The patient's pain was relieved by solid fusion.

ture, had the fracture been diagnosed previously. This experience stresses the fact that early recognition of the fracture and adequate immobilization are essential, if the risk of increased deformity is to be avoided.

TECHNIQUE OF CERVICAL OSTEOTOMY

As Urist recommended,[8] the operation is performed under local anesthesia with the patient in the sitting position. This avoids any major anesthetic hazards. It allows the most accurate of all forms of spinal cord monitoring and assessment of vital functions with the patient awake and the avoidance of any major neurologic complications. It allows the patient to assist with anatomic localization of the level during the decompression. The patient is able to indicate, at any time, any paresthesias or discomfort along the distribution of his cervical nerve root, which is of real value in confirming the C8 nerve root canal and the level of the root. The level between C7 and T1 vertebrae is selected for correction of the deformity. As Mason and coworkers[1] and Urist[8] indicated, this interspace is more receptive to surgical treatment than any other level of the cervical region. The spinal canal is relatively wide. The cervical cord and eighth cervical nerve roots have reasonable mobility in this area. Any weakness caused by compromise of the eighth cervical nerve roots will cause less disability than compromise of other roots. The vertebral artery and veins usually pass in front of the transverse process of the C7 vertebra and enter the transverse foramen at the C6 vertebra. The position of these vessels above the level of the T1 vertebra protects them from injury during osteotomy at the C7–T1 level (Fig. 10-16). An adequate excision is carried out posteriorly with subsequent fracturing and extension of the spine at the cervicothoracic junction. One to two days preoperatively the patient is fitted with a rigid plaster or fiberglass body jacket incorporating the supports for the halo unit. It is important to recognize that this is a most important and essential part of the procedure. The jacket must be rigid and of a material that does not soften with body heat. It must be very skillfully contoured to the patient's trunk so that it can slide neither upward nor downward. This involves molding under the rib cage and the sides of the chest to prevent it from going upward, as well as being well molded over the pelvis and iliac crest to prevent it from moving distally. It should be understood that a commercial plastic halo jacket is totally inadequate

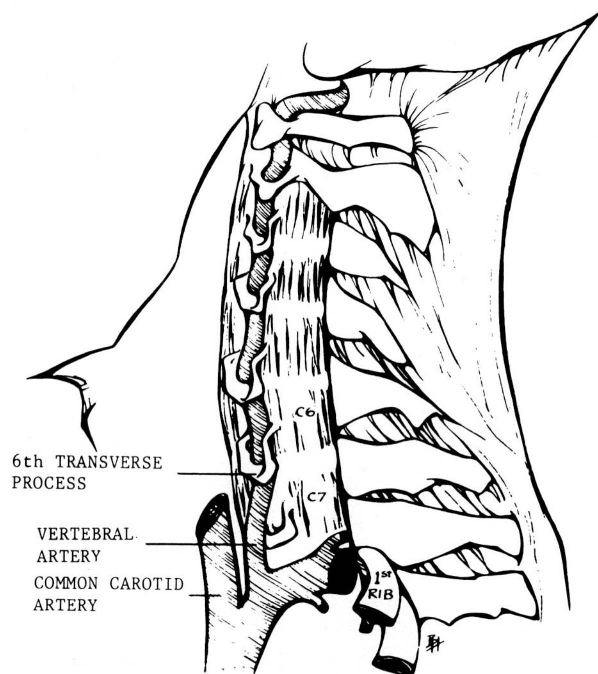

Fig. 10-16. Anatomic diagram showing lateral aspect of the cervical spine with the normal passage of the vertebral arteries and veins in front of the transverse process of the C7 vertebra, entering the transverse foramen at the C6 vertebra.

for the immobilization that is required for these patients postoperatively. In most instances, the spine is completely solid above and below the area of osteotomy. This creates excessive forces, tending to cause movement at the osteotomy site with almost any activity. If patients are not rigidly immobilized, they will have extreme distress in attempting to get in or out of bed or move about, and excessive mobility can result in neurologic compromise with irritation of the eighth cervical nerve roots. It is therefore wise to apply the jacket and test it carefully with the patient up and about to be certain that it is well contoured and secure. It should be applied early enough that it can be changed, if necessary, before the operation. A halo is fitted to the skull under local anesthesia in a stable position, below the maximum circumference of the skull.

The operation is performed with the patient in the sitting position (Fig. 10-17). A dental-type chair is used to allow the patient to be placed in a recumbent position, if necessary (Fig. 10-18). Valium is used for preoperative sedation, with the expo-

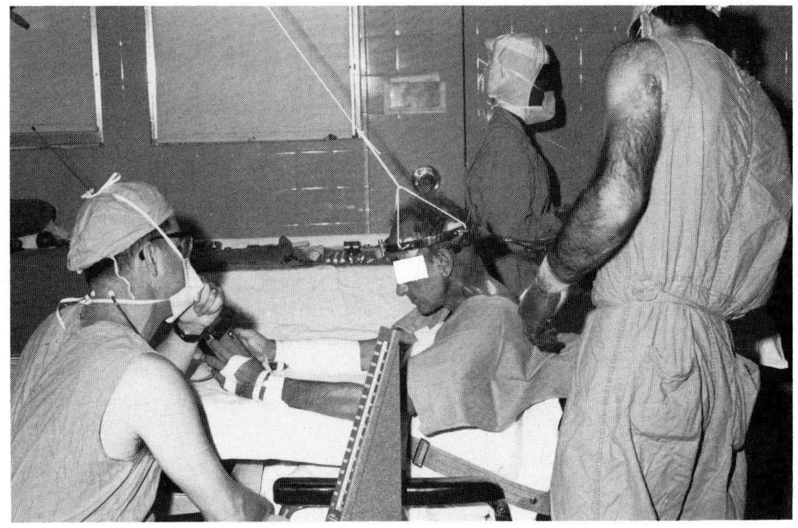

Fig. 10-17. Photograph showing operative position of patient awake, sitting in a dental-type chair with 9 lbs halo traction along the line of his neck. The halo and a plaster jacket containing the supports for the halo have been fitted preoperatively. The patient is able to enjoy the music of a transistor radio with continuing cheerful conversation between the anesthetist and himself.

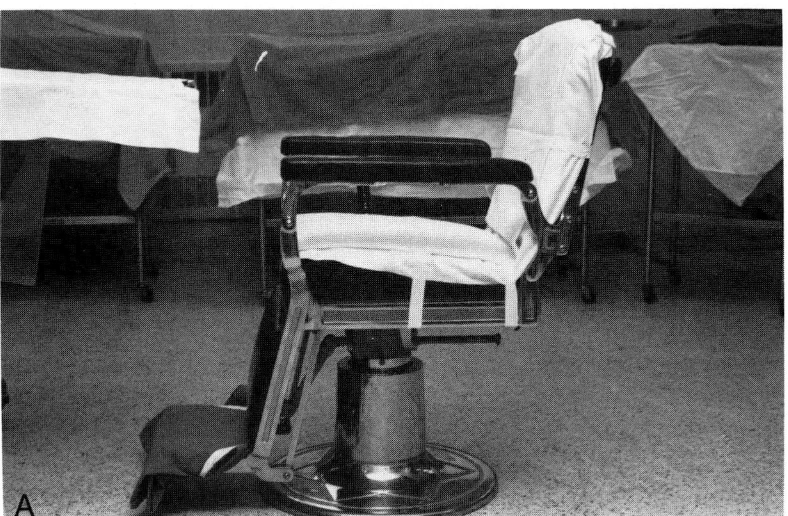

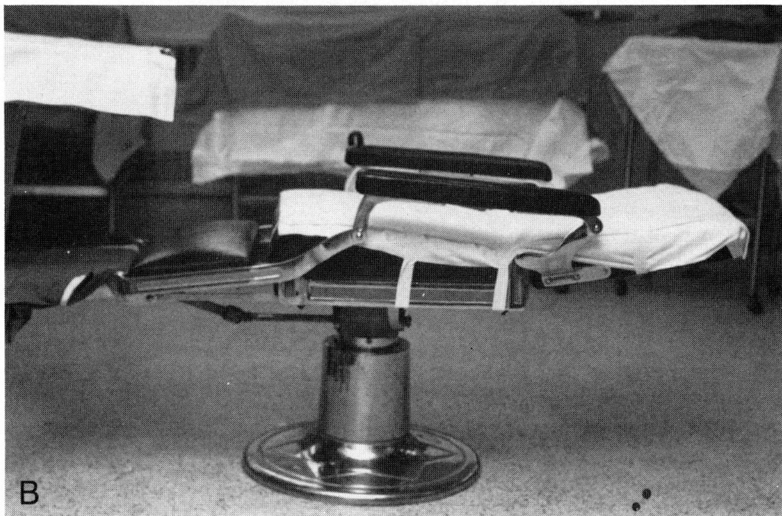

Fig. 10-18. (*A*) Dental-type chair in the erect position as used for the patient during the procedure. Its height may be adjusted. (*B*) Side view of the chair showing ability to extend it to the horizontal position, if necessary.

sure carried out posteriorly under local infiltration (1% lodocaine [Xylocaine] and epinephrine 1:200,000). Fentanyl is used as supplementary analgesia during the procedure. The last bifid spinous process of C6 is usually easily identified. The architecture of the lower cervical spinous processes, following exposure, are compared with a lateral radiograph of the cervical spine. If any difficulty is encountered in anatomic localization, radiographic confirmation of the level is obtained. This is rarely necessary.

The C7 spinous process, the inferior spine of C6, and the superior spine of T1 are removed in strips and preserved for grafting. The entire posterior arch of C7 is removed along with the inferior half of the arch of C6 and the superior half of the arch of T1. The spinal canal is opened. The dura and spinal cord are protected with cottonoid patties. Decompression is extended laterally on each side beyond the lateral margin of the spinal cord to the level of the pedicles. The laminae are undercut above and below the decompression to avoid impingement following extension correction. The eighth cervical nerve root is identified, and a curved probe is passed into its canal. The patient may be able to assist in confirmation of the level by indicating the distribution of any paresthesias associated with displacement of the root. The resection is extended through the fused area of the posterior joints of C7–T1, decompressing the C8 nerve roots completely (Fig. 10-19). The amount of bone requiring resection is indicated by the angle of correction that is desired, as determined from preoperative studies. The chin-brow to vertical angle is determined, and this angle is transposed to a lateral radiograph of the cervical spine with the apex of the angle at the posterior margin of the C7–T1 disc space. A lateral tomogram will likely be necessary to show this clearly. The angle is centered over the posterior arch of C7. The amount of bone that must be resected is determined from the radiograph with the superimposed angle, at the level of the spinous processes, the laminae, the posterior margin of the posterior joints, and at the posterior margin of the spinal canal at the level of the pedicles (Figs. 10-20, 10-21*D*, 10-21*E*). The lines of resection are beveled upward at the superior margin and downward at the inferior margin. Following correction, the two surfaces are parallel and in apposition. The inferior aspect of the pedicles of C7 and the superior aspect of the pedicles of T1 are exposed. The pedicles are cut through in a curved fashion, away from the eighth cervical nerve root, leaving

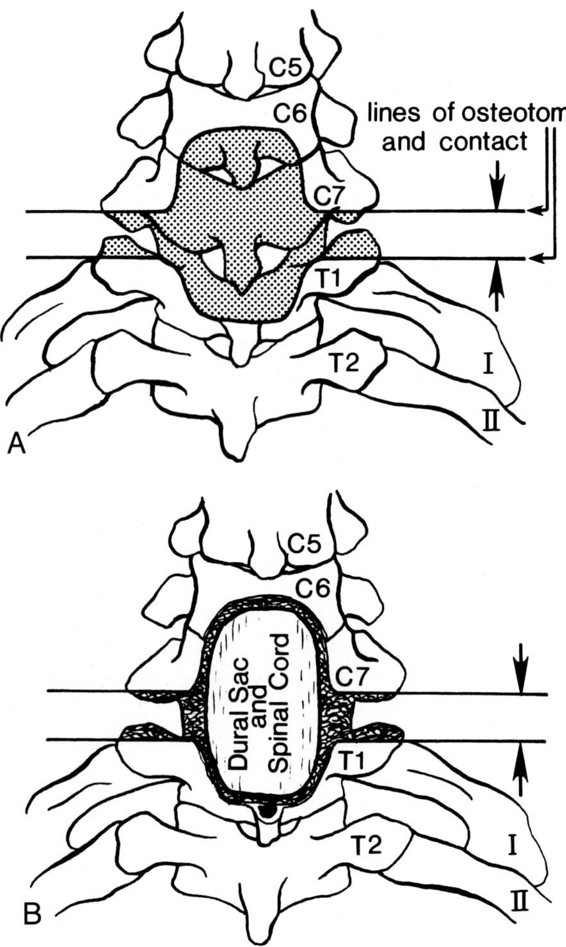

Fig. 10-19. (*A*) Posterior diagrammatic view of cervicothoracic spine showing level of resection and the area of bone removed. The entire posterior arch of C7 is resected along with the inferior half of the arch of C6 and the superior half of the arch of T1. The eighth cervical nerve root canal is identified and the overlying bone resected symmetrically on each side. The resections are planned so that following extension the lateral masses will come together posteriorly. (*B*) Diagram of posterior aspect of cervicothoracic spine showing completed resection with exposure of dural sac and spinal cord. The superior and inferior margins are undercut to avoid impingement following extension. The lateral resections are made symmetrical, converging toward each other posteriorly, so that following extension the lateral masses will come together posteriorly.

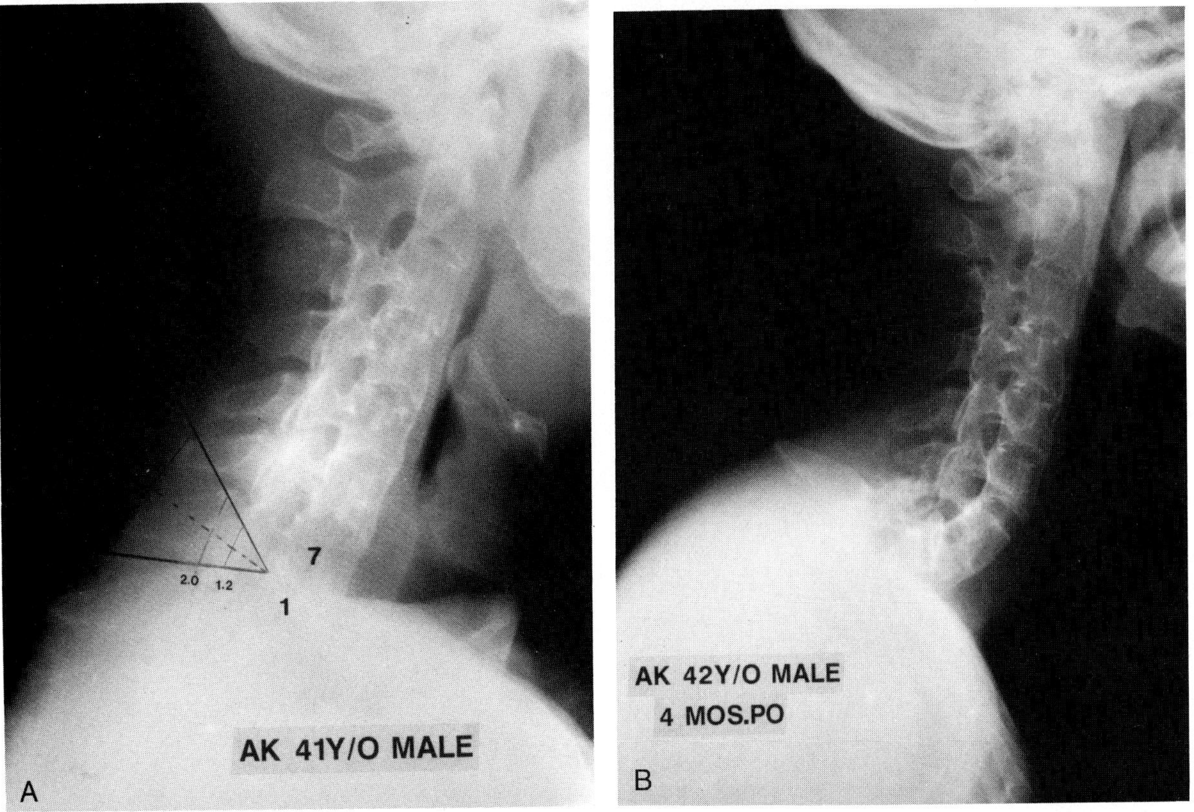

Fig. 10-20. (*A*) Lateral radiograph of the cervical spine of a 41-year-old male who has had known ankylosing spondylitis since the age of 19. He had a flexion deformity of the cervical spine with his chin-brow to vertical angle measuring 50 degrees. It was planned to carry out a 55-degree wedge resection–extension osteotomy. This angle has been transposed to the radiograph with the apex at the posterior margin of the C7–T1 disc space. The amounts to be resected at each level are indicated. (*B*) Postoperative lateral radiograph showing extension correction and solid fusion at 4 months. His deformity was completely corrected with his chin-brow to vertical angle 0.

a shell to protect the nerve root as the main bone is removed; the shell is finally removed at the completion of the nerve decompression. This is done to undercut the pedicles above and below adequately, so that following the extension correction there will be a bony recess for the eighth cervical nerve root, which will avoid impingement or a pincher effect on it (Fig. 10-22). The nerve root is followed laterally, and all the bone that could impinge upon it is removed. The lateral resections must be made evenly throughout their length, and they should be symmetrical on both sides. The lateral masses must be resected completely through, from medial to lateral, so that there is no remaining bridge of bone laterally, which could interfere with extension correction (Fig. 10-19).

Supplemental oxygen may be administered by the anesthetist during the procedure, either by nasal catheter or face mask. The patient is allowed to enjoy the music of a radio or tape recorder. This is an important part of the anesthetic management, along with a continuing cheerful conduct of conversation between the anesthetist and the patient or an attendant, concerning areas of interest to the patient. When this is done well, the amount of discomfort or concern expressed by the patient is minimal.

When the decompression is complete, the patient is given a small dose of short-acting barbituate (thiopental sodium), usually in a dose of 75 to 100 mg. When the anesthetist indicates that this is effective, the neck is extended by grasping the halo

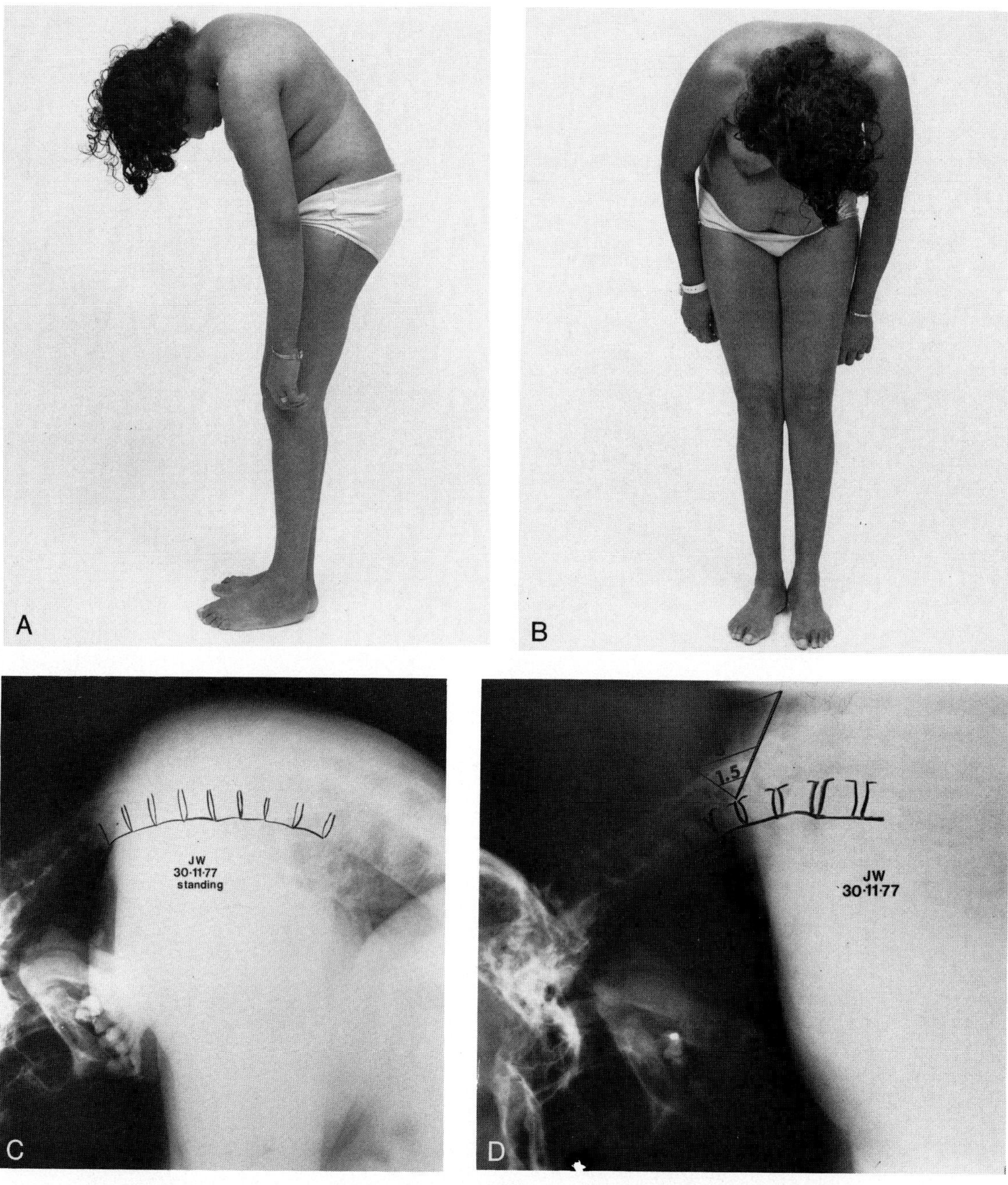

Fig. 10-21. (*A*) Lateral view of a 43-year-old female with combined severe flexion deformity of the cervical spine and flexion deformity of the lumbar spine. Bilateral total hip replacement arthroplasties had been performed with some residual hip flexion deformity. (*B*) Anterior view showing severe restriction of field of vision. Her arthritic disease had commenced in her teens. (*C*) Standing lateral radiograph of spine showing flexion deformity of the cervical spine with chin on her chest and lumbar flexion deformity. (*D*) Lateral radiograph of cervicothoracic spine showing plan of extension osteotomy.

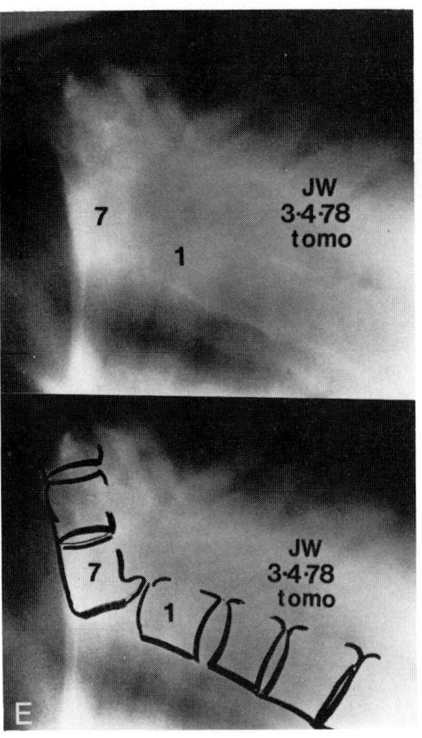

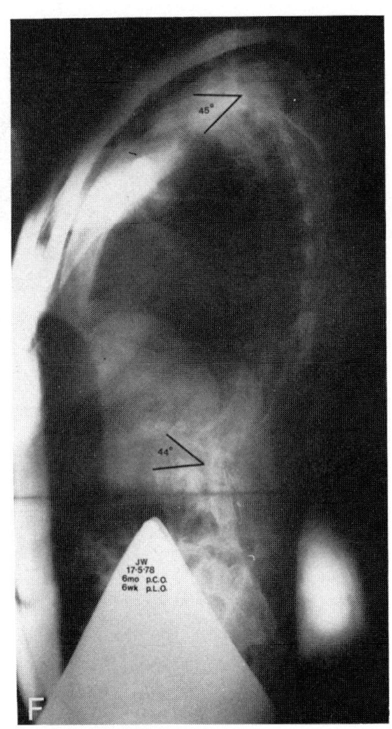

Fig. 10-21, *cont'd.*
(*E*) Postoperative lateral tomogram showing resection–extension osteotomy at C7–T1 (*above*) with vertebra outlined (*below*). (*F*) Postoperative standing lateral 3-foot radiograph of spine following resection–extension osteotomy of midlumbar spine. The weight-bearing line has been shifted posterior to the lumbar osteotomy site. (*G*) Postoperative lateral view of patient following union of her osteotomies, showing complete correction of spinal deformities with restoration of normal chin-brow to vertical angle. The patient was able to manage her family and return to work. (*H*) Postoperative anterior view of patient demonstrating normal field of vision, which is in marked contrast to preoperative state (*B*).

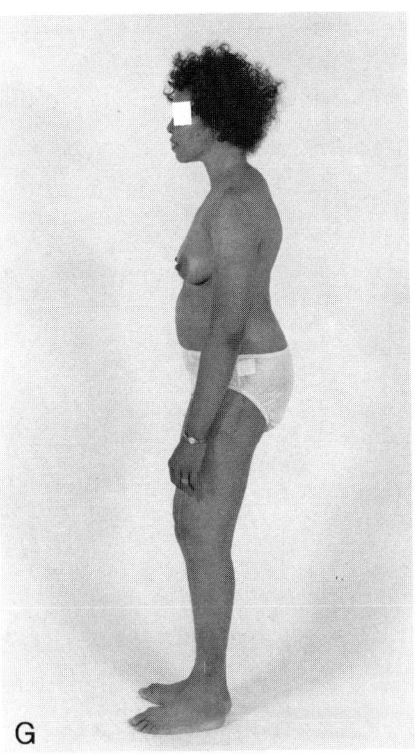

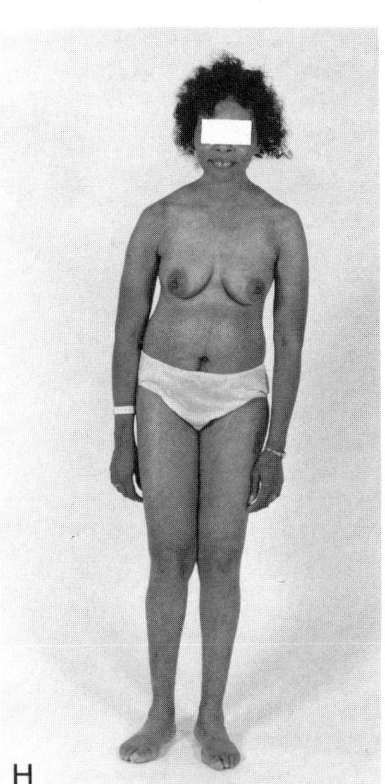

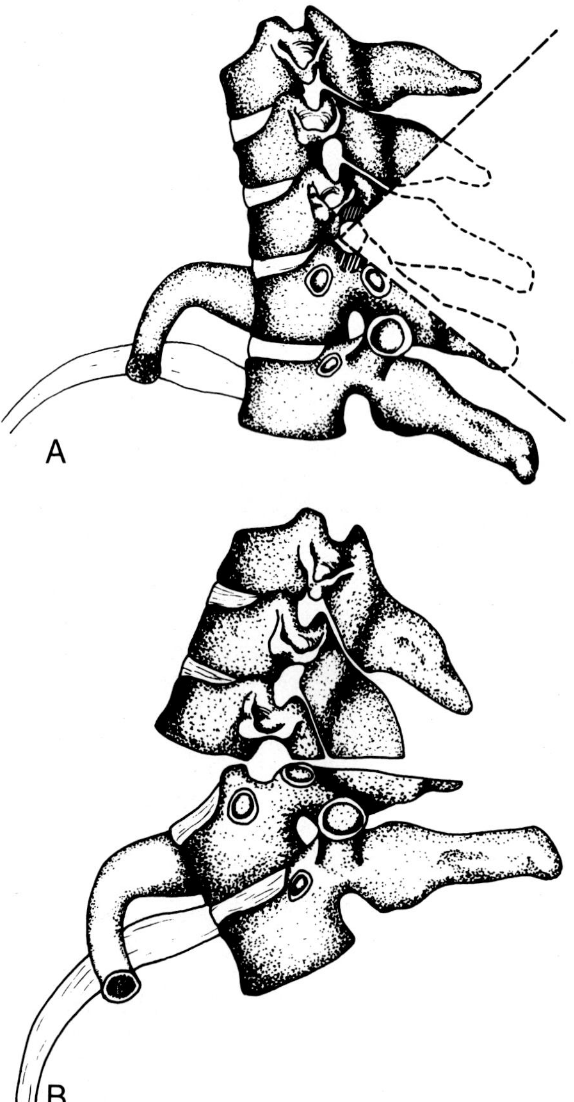

Fig. 10-22. (*A*) Lateral diagram of cervicothoracic spine showing area to be resected. The shaded areas show where the inferior aspect of the pedicles of C7 and the superior aspect of the pedicles of T1 are removed to prepare a recess for the eighth cervical nerve roots. (*B*) Lateral diagram of cervicothoracic spine after extension osteotomy, showing the lateral masses coming together posteriorly with the ossified disc space fracturing and opening up anteriorly. The area where the pedicles have been undercut leaves space for the eighth cervical nerve roots.

firmly and tilting the neck backward. An audible snap may be heard and a physical sense of fracture will be appreciated. The neck is extended until resistance occurs. The lateral masses can be palpated coming together posteriorly on each side (Fig. 10-22*B*). The patient is awake almost instantly and is able to confirm normal neurologic function of his extremities with the ability to move his upper and lower limbs, without sensory complaint. With the head held firmly in the corrected position, an assistant then stabilizes the head by connecting the anterior supports for the halo unit to the cast. The bone, which has been removed during the course of the decompression, is placed posterolaterally on both sides over the apposed lateral masses. It is not placed in the midline over the exposed dura. The deep closing sutures and a suction drain are inserted before the osteoclasis is carried out. The deep sutures are tied after extension correction, and the wound closure is completed. The skin is usually closed with interrupted silk or nylon sutures, which allow more accurate approximation that is necessary, owing to the redundancy of tissue that occurs following correction of the flexion deformity (Fig. 10-23). In all instances, at the end of the procedure the patient has been able to stand and walk to a circoelectric bed, which is turned vertically to allow the patient to back into it. The bed is then tilted horizontally with the patient supine. It may be partly flexed for comfort. Overcorrection should be avoided, particularly in individuals with a rigid cervical spine and no compensatory movement at the occipitocervical junction. The final position should represent a compromise between being able to look ahead for walking, and being able to work at a desk (Figs. 10-11, 10-21, 10-24, and 10-25).

Excessive force is not required to straighten the neck, providing there has been an adequate and complete decompression posteriorly. If the spine does not fracture readily, the surgeon should check to be sure there is not a bridge of bone remaining laterally and that the correct level has been operated upon and not a level below. Although full correction is usually obtained at the time of the procedure, on occasion with severe deformity, full correction is limited by tightness of the musculature anteriorly, or by the patient's apprehension that overcorrection will occur. The main correction can be established at the time of surgery with further correction added 7 to 10 days postoperatively. At this time, the soft tissues have had an opportunity to stretch, and the patient has had an opportunity to assess the amount of correction that

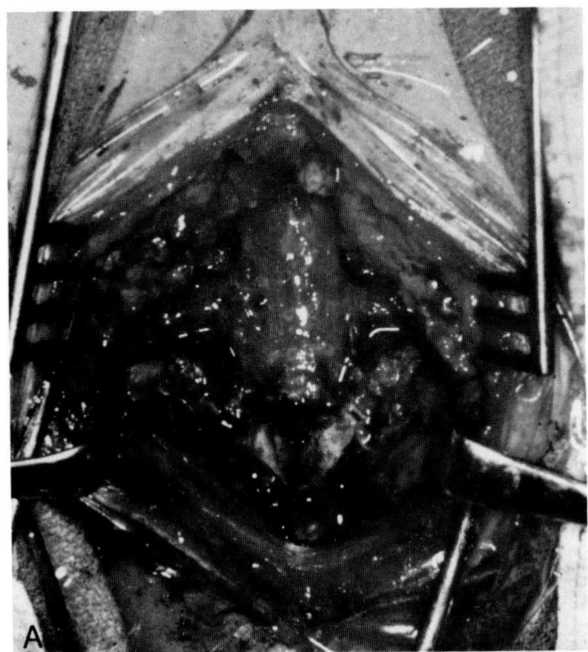

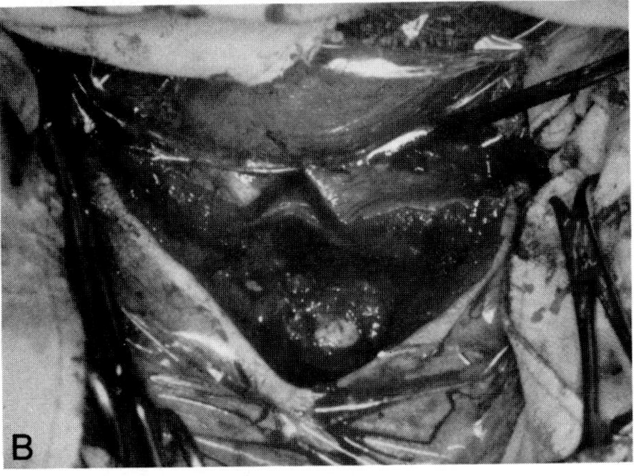

Fig. 10-23. (*A*) Posterior operative view showing decompression of spinal cord and eighth cervical nerve roots bilaterally. The pedicles have been undercut above and below. The wound is linear in configuration. (*B*) Posterior view of operative site after extension correction. The lateral masses have come together on each side. The wound is now transverse in configuration with redundancy of soft tissue on each side. This illustrates the advisability of placing the deep closing sutures and suction drain before the osteoclasis is carried out, to facilitate wound closure.

has been achieved and his or her adjustment to it. At that stage, with the patient supine under diazepam (Valium) and fentanyl sedation, the head may be supported by the surgeon, the attachments for the halo released, and the neck allowed to extend within the range of comfort obtaining full correction. The patients are nursed in the immediate postoperative period on a circoelectric frame. This allows them to be brought to the vertical fairly easily, to stand and walk about, and the return to the recumbent position without difficulty. When sufficiently mobile to get in and out of a regular bed, the patient is transferred to a hospital bed with or without trapeze attachment. The patient is immobilized in a halo cast for 4 months, at the end of which time it is removed and careful radiographic studies are performed, including lateral tomography centered at C7–T1. Clinical assessment of union with lack of pain is noted. Further splinting is then carried out, using a Somi brace for an additional 2 months or until it is certain that there is solid clinical and radiographic union.

The same technique has been followed in a consistent fashion without any major deviation, over the past 21 years in a total of 101 patients.[3–6] The results have been exceedingly satisfactory with a relative minimum of complications, considering the nature of the deformity and associated disease process. Union following osteotomy occurred fairly readily in most instances. However, in four patients nonunion occurred, an incidence of 4%. Three of these responded to anterior cervical fusion at the C7–T1 level with a keystone iliac strut graft,[7] one of these being performed under local anesthesia (Fig. 10-24). The fourth patient required not only anterior cervical fusion, but also posterior segmental instrumentation and fusion to obtain solid union. Transient neurologic complaints occurred, including a Horner's syndrome and mild symptoms of a central cord syndrome beginning 2 weeks postoperatively; 13 patients had transient C8 paresthesias or signs, and one transient ninth and tenth cranial nerve lesion, believed to be on a traction basis. All of these cleared spontaneously without any definitive treatment. Five patients had more sustained eighth cervical nerve root deficit, and one of these required further decompression with improvement. All improved with minimal residual signs and no gross functional handicap. There has been no major permanent injury to the spinal cord. One dramatic intraoperative experience demonstrates the necessity for surgery performed under local anesthesia. This involved a 70-year-old man with severe flexion de-

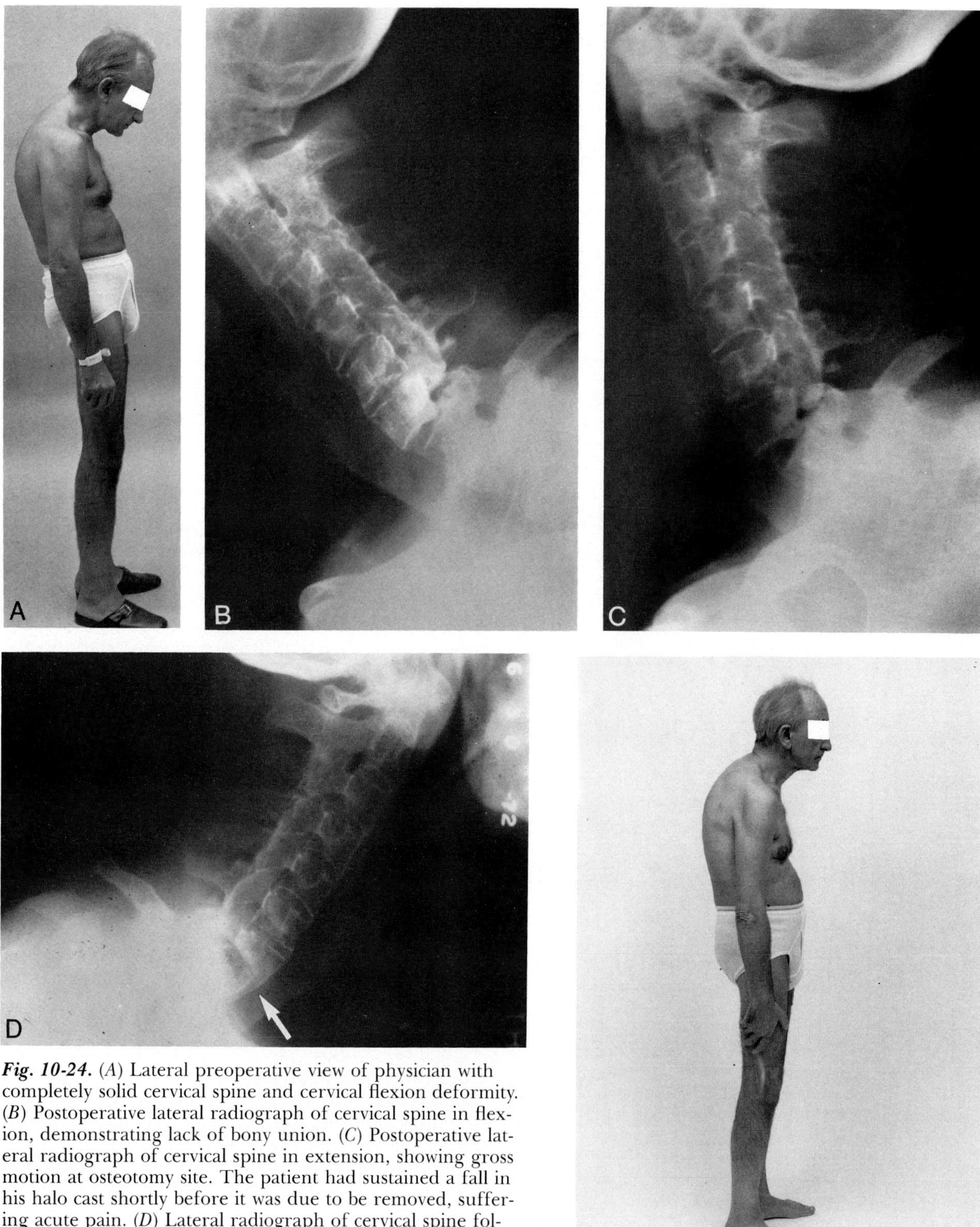

Fig. 10-24. (*A*) Lateral preoperative view of physician with completely solid cervical spine and cervical flexion deformity. (*B*) Postoperative lateral radiograph of cervical spine in flexion, demonstrating lack of bony union. (*C*) Postoperative lateral radiograph of cervical spine in extension, showing gross motion at osteotomy site. The patient had sustained a fall in his halo cast shortly before it was due to be removed, suffering acute pain. (*D*) Lateral radiograph of cervical spine following successful anterior fusion of the osteotomy site, using a keystone graft at C7–T1, under local anesthesia. (*E*) Final lateral view of patient showing correction of deformity with restoration of normal alignment.

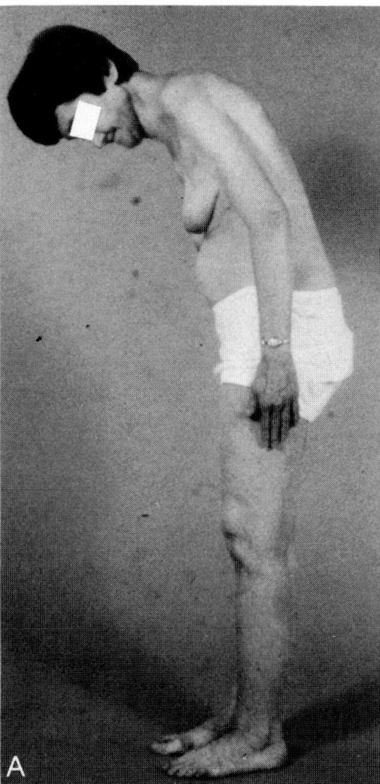

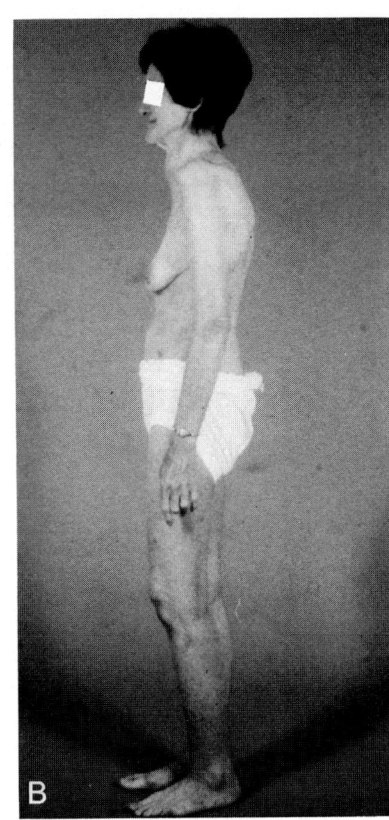

Fig. 10-25. (*A*) Preoperative lateral view of female patient with combined cervical and lumbar flexion deformities, with chin-brow to vertical angle of 87 degrees. Note loss of lumbar lordosis with lumbar flexion deformity, as well as flexion deformity of cervical spine. (*B*) Postoperative lateral view of patient following combined cervical and lumbar resection–extension osteotomies. A normal lordosis has been established with a normal chin-brow to vertical angle of 0.

formity accentuated by an unrecognized fracture that had healed with his chin on his chest. On decompression posteriorly, dense scarring was noted about the dura related to the previous trauma. As the spine was decompressed in the midline, the patient suffered increasing weakness of his lower limbs and subsequent difficulty with speech. The dura was exceedingly tense with dense scarring about it. In view of this, the dura was split longitudinally down to the arachnoid, which was not violated. As this was done there was an immediate dramatic return of neurologic function in the lower extremities, and his speech returned to normal. The operation was continued and, as the decompression was being completed on the last side, he again developed weakness of his lower extremities. The remaining exposed dura was split further distally, again with immediate recovery of neurologic function. The operation was completed without any further difficulty and the patient went on to a satisfactory result without neurologic deficit (Fig. 10-26). This observation is in keeping with the report of McKenzie and Dewar[2] describing the results of laminectomy for cord compression associated with kyphoscoliosis. Their review of the reported literature and their own cases indicated that the only patients who did not become worse following laminectomy or who had any benefit were those in whom there was an extensive splitting of the dura. They related the compression effect of the dura to the kyphosis, and they recommended that the dura be split not only longitudinally but transversely. Surgeons undertaking this type of surgery should be familiar with this recommendation. If this problem occurs during surgery, adequate splitting of the dura should be performed, not only longitudinally, but likely transversely as well.

No major intraoperative problems were noted immediately following the osteoclasis. However, in one patient, toward the end of the decompression, a sudden cardiac arrest occurred. The chair was flattened, and the patient responded quite well to resuscitation without late sequelae. Air embolism was considered as a possibility, but aspiration of the heart revealed no air. The cause of the cardiac arrest is unknown. To detect the possibility of air embolism, routine monitoring is now carried out

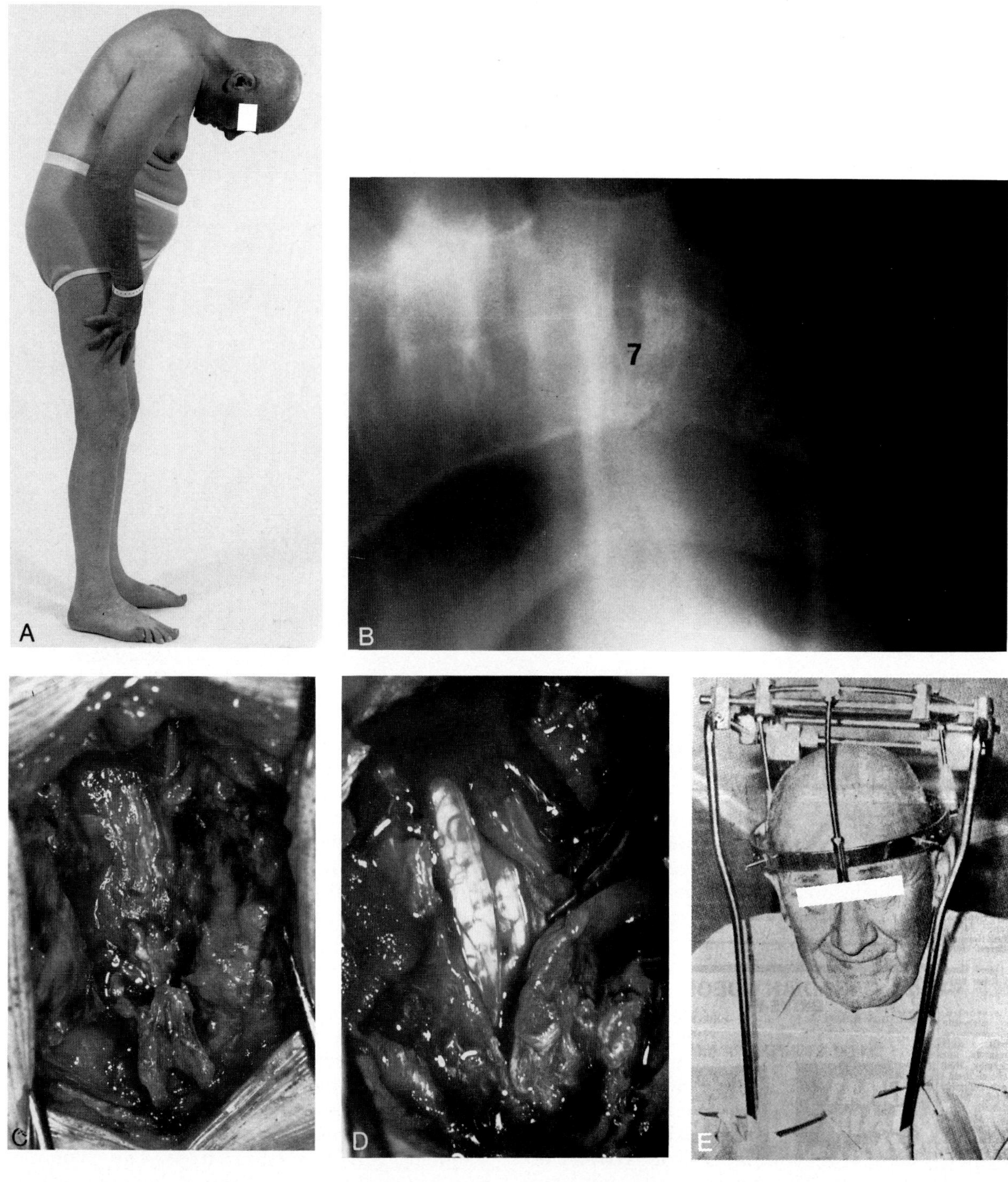
A
B
7
C
D
E

Fig. 10-26. (*A*) Lateral view of 70-year-old male with severe flexion deformity of the cervical spine. The patient's main concern was difficulty with a tendency to choke when swallowing. His deformity had been accentuated by an unrecognized fracture that had healed in flexion. (*B*) Lateral radiograph of cervicothoracic junction showing healed unrecognized previous fracture and fracture flexion deformity. (*C*) Posterior operative view of midline decompression showing extensively scarred dura. Following midline decompression, he suffered increasing weakness of his lower limbs and difficulty with speech. The dura was exceedingly tense. (*D*) Posterior operative view of patient showing vertical incision of the scarred dura down to the arachnoid, which was not violated. The cervical spinal cord was exposed. There was immediate return of neurologic function and speech. As the lateral decompressions were being completed, he developed further neurologic symptoms, which were again relieved by extending the dural incision distally. The operation then proceeded uneventfully. (*E*) A–P view of patient on discharge from hospital to his home region. He had no neurologic deficit. The use of local anesthesia to perform the operation allowed precision monitoring with instant recognition of the difficulty, allowing immediate corrective measures.

using a Doppler apparatus fixed to the patient's chest or by using an esophageal stethoscope. One 79-year-old female patient died suddenly 21 days postoperatively of fatal pulmonary embolism, her lungs showing multiple previous areas of embolism that had not been recognized clinically. Despite the procedure being performed under local anesthesia, pulmonary embolism must still be recognized as a hazard. One recent patient suffered a fatal pulmonary embolism before the osteotomy was done. Autopsy revealed multiple thrombi in his leg veins with evidence of previous pulmonary infarctions.

Other complications have been related to the age of the patients and associated disease processes, including one nonfatal pulmonary embolism, a perforated peptic ulcer, a perforated abdominal viscus, and a myocardial infarction. Considering the age and medical risk factors of these patients, the results and complication rate compare favorably to any other type of joint reconstructive procedure in a similar group of patients with the same disease process. These patients have an increased tendency for peptic ulceration. Considering the lethal nature of any intraabdominal catastrophe in these patients, who breathe entirely with the diaphragm, we now place all patients routinely on cimetidine or ranitidine (Zantac).

The average desired angle of correction that was achieved in these patients was 60 degrees. In 15 patients, cervical osteotomy was combined with lumbar osteotomy for major deformity in both areas, the procedures being performed either on separate admissions or during the same hospitalization. When planned during the same admission for severe combined deformity, the cervical osteotomy is done first, followed by the lumbar osteotomy 2 to 3 weeks later. Both procedures are done under local anesthesia. The patient is placed on the side, and the posterior portion of the plaster is removed in the lumbar area to allow the lumbar osteotomy to be performed; the remaining plaster immobilizes the cervical spine. Following correction, the lower portion of the cast is completed in the new position (Figs. 10-21 and 10-25).

The concept of resection–extension osteotomy of the cervical spine for severe fixed flexion deformity, when performed under local anesthesia and in the sitting position, is a valid technique with a high success rate and acceptable risks. It is to be emphasized that the essential safety factor in the technique is performing the surgery under local anesthesia with the patient awake. This allows accurate and continual monitoring of the patient's neurologic functions, so that the surgeon is able to react instantly if any major dysfunction should occur.

ACKNOWLEDGMENTS

The author acknowledges with sincere appreciation the excellent assistance of the Departments of Medical Photography of the Buffalo General Hospital, and the Toronto East General and Orthopaedic Hospital.

REFERENCES

1. MASON C, COZEN L, ADELSTEIN L: Surgical correction of flexion deformity of the cervical spine. Calif Med 79:244, 1953

2. *McKENZIE KG, DEWAR FP:* Scoliosis with paraplegia. J Bone Joint Surg 31B:162–174, 1949
3. *SIMMONS EH:* Surgery of rheumatoid arthritis. In Cruess RL, Mitchell N (eds): Surgery of the Spine in Rheumatoid Arthritis and Ankylosing Spondylitis, pp 93–110. Philadelphia, JB Lippincott, 1971
4. *SIMMONS EH:* The surgical correction of flexion deformity of the cervical spine in ankylosing spondylitis. Clin Orthop 86:132, 1972
5. *SIMMONS EH:* Kyphotic deformity of the spine in ankylosing spondylitis. Clin Orthop 128:65, 1977
6. *SIMMONS EH:* Surgery of the spine in rheumatoid arthritis and ankylosing spondylitis. In Evarts CM (ed): Surgery of the Musculoskeletal System, Vol II, p 85. New York, Churchill Livingstone, 1983
7. *SIMMONS EH, BHALLA SK:* Anterior cervical discectomy and fusion (keystone technique). J Bone Joint Surg 51B:225, 1969
8. *URIST MR:* Osteotomy of the cervical spine: Report of case of ankylosing rheumatoid spondylitis. J Bone Surg 40A:833, 1958

CHAPTER 11

Degenerative Disorders

Symptoms in Cervical Disc Degeneration

IAN MACNAB

ANATOMIC CONSIDERATIONS

The morphology of the articulations between the cervical vertebrae is of great clinical significance. The lumbar vertebral segments are connected together by three joints: the intervertebral disc anteriorly and the two zygapophyseal joints posteriorly. The lower five cervical vertebrae are connected together by five joints: the intervertebral disc anteriorly, the two zygapophyseal joints posteriorly, and, in addition to these, the neurocentral joints (Fig. 11-1).

The neurocentral joints consist of a projection of bone arising from the posterolateral portion of the vertebral body articulating with the vertebra above. They lie between the disc and the nerve root canal (Fig. 11-2). Versalius illustrated these joints very accurately in his book *De Corporo Humanica,* and they were subsequently described in detail by Luschka, whose name they commonly bear.[2,3]

PATHOGENESIS

Cervical spondylosis and all its manifestations are a product of cervical disc degeneration; it is therefore necessary to clarify from the outset the meaning of the term *disc degeneration.*

As in the lumbar spine, some clinicians fail to differentiate between disc degeneration and disc rupture or prolapse; these are two entirely different pathologic entities. Although every patient with a cervical disc rupture has a preceding cervical disc degeneration, the symptoms are produced by entirely different mechanisms.

In disc rupture, there is an anular protrusion, with or without extrusion of nuclear material, producing symptoms by means of tension on the dura or root, or by means of cord compression (Fig. 11-3*A*). Disc degeneration, on the other hand, implies a mechanical breakdown of the integrity of a cervical disc productive of symptoms initially because of mechanical instability, and only in the later stages productive of root or cord compression owing to the development of osteophytic outgrowths. In the first stage of cervical disc degeneration, the

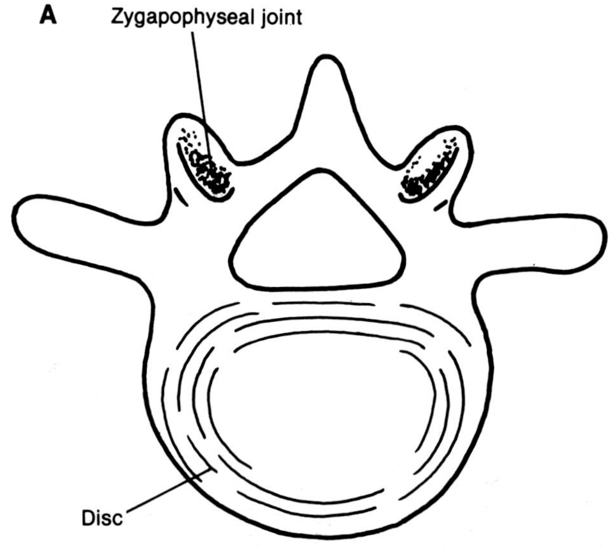

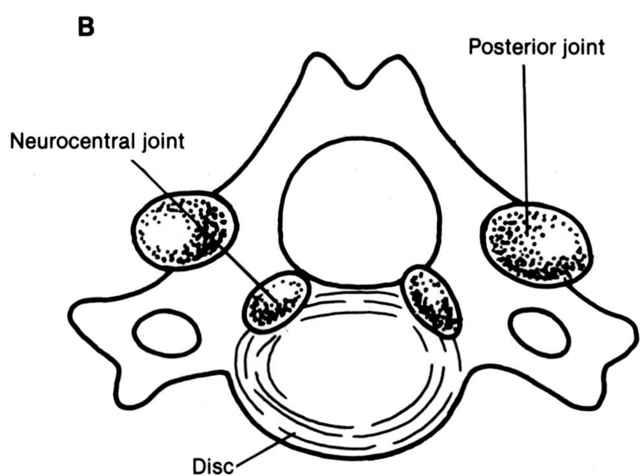

Fig. 11-1. (*A*) The lumbar vertebrae are connected together by three joints: the intervertebral discs anteriorly and the two zygapophyseal joints posteriorly. (*B*) In the cervical spine, the vertebrae are connected together by five joints: the two zygapophyseal joints, the two neurocentral joints, and the intervertebral discs.

involved segment becomes unstable and the movement of the related vertebrae becomes uneven, excessive, and irregular (Fig. 11-3*B*). As a result of this instability, the segment becomes very vulnerable to trauma, and symptoms arise from injured ligaments or damaged joints. Once instability develops, the patient has a "wobbly" segment that is easily strained and, once strained, is very difficult to rest.

Strangely enough, the presenting symptom is rarely just a pain in the neck. The patient usually also presents with pain referred to a distance: shoulder pain, suboccipital pain, occipital headaches, interscapular pain, or pain down the arm or into the chest. In addition, the patient may have vague symptoms such as blurring of vision, tinnitus, or dysphagia.

In the early stages of disc degeneration these symptoms are not due to nerve root irritation. They can be reproduced by the injection of hypertonic saline into the supraspinous ligament or by discography. Following the experimental injec-

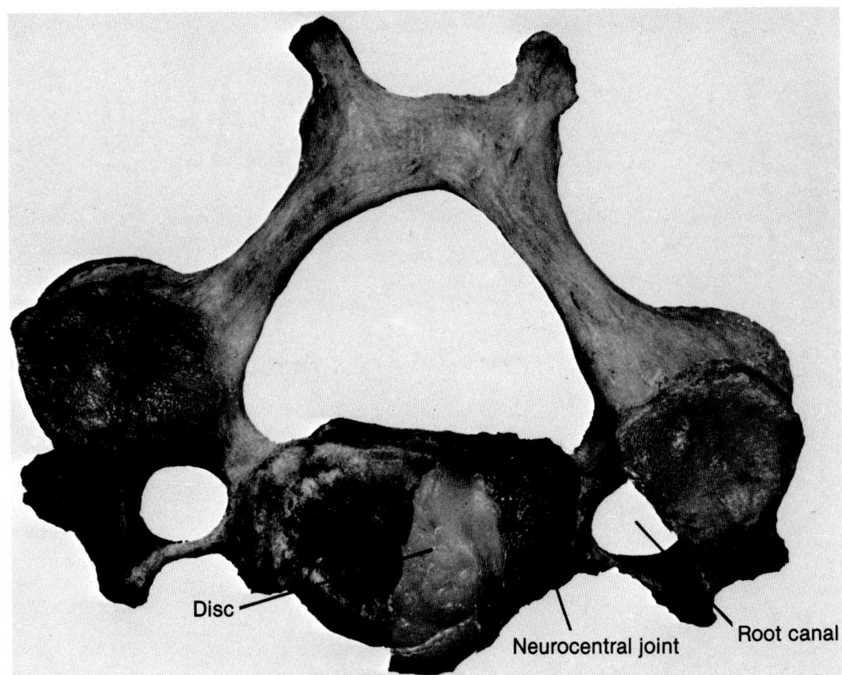

Fig. 11-2. Cervical vertebral segments as seen from the superior surface. Note that the neurocentral joints lie between the disc and the root canal.

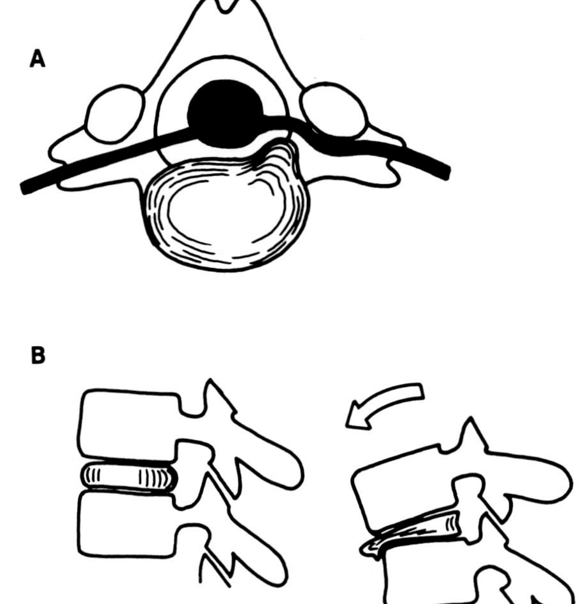

Fig. 11-3. (*A*) A ruptured disc compromising a cervical root as it enters the root canal. (*B*) Segmental instability associated with disc degeneration, giving rise to posterior joint strains.

tion of hypertonic saline into the supraspinous ligament, not only is pain referred to a distance but there are also areas of "referred" tenderness.

In the later stages of degenerative disc disease, however, because of bony outgrowths forming in relation to the neurocentral joints, the symptoms complained of are frequently due to nerve root compromise.

With the onset of disc degeneration, the intervertebral disc loses height. As it does so, the bony prominences formed by the neurocentral joints approach one another and eventually touch. With further disc degeneration these processes are firmly pressed together and osteophytic excrescences form (Fig. 11-4).

Further loss of height can only take place anteriorly, resulting, therefore, in a loss of the normal cervical lordosis and the typical posture of cervical disc degeneration, namely, the patient carrying his chin thrust well forward.

The osteophytic outgrowths that develop around the neurocentral joints may encroach upon the nerve root canal (Fig. 11-5). The emerging nerve root may therefore be compressed by an osteophyte derived from the neurocentral joint, by an osteophyte derived from the posterior joint, or

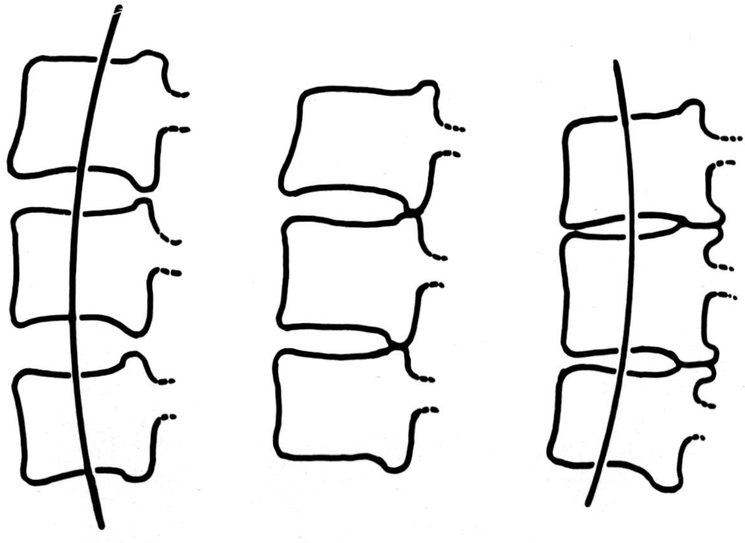

Fig. 11-4. With disc narrowing, the neurocentral facets are brought into firm contact. Further narrowing of the discs can only take place anteriorly, resulting in reversal of the normal cervical lordosis.

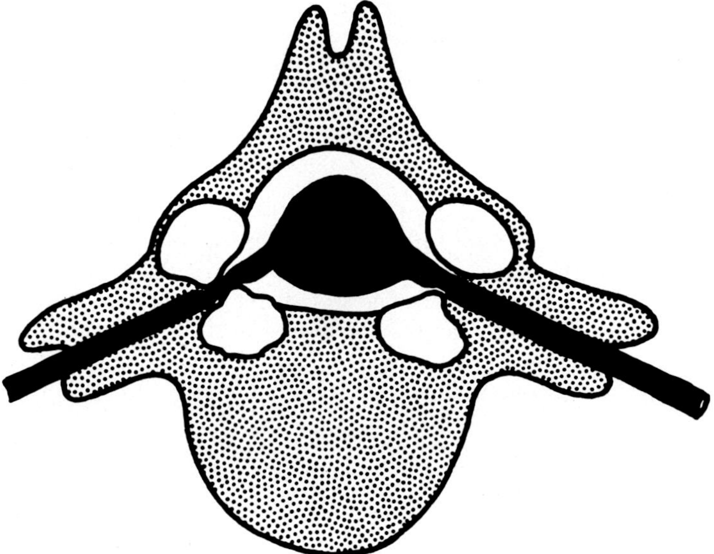

Fig. 11-5. Osteophytes derived from the neurocentral joints and the posterior joints intruding into the root canal, producing root compression.

by osteophytes derived both from the neurocentral joints and from the posterior joint.

On clinical x-ray examination, though the lateral view of the spine may show encroachment of the intervertebral foramen by osteophytes associated with a neurocentral joint, these osteophytes are more clearly shown in the anteroposterior view (Fig. 11-6). The encroachment of the foramen is readily demonstrated on oblique views of the cervical spine. On the lateral view, it is possible to demonstrate encroachment of the intervertebral foramen by osteophytes derived from the posterior joints (Fig. 11-7).

The neurocentral joints play an important role in modifying the effects of disc rupture in the cervical spine. Prolapse of nuclear material from the disc must pass medial to the neurocentral facet and therefore cannot produce a pure nerve root lesion unless the extruded disc material runs into the nerve root canal (Fig. 11-8). On careful clinical examination, it is possible in many instances of true disc ruptures to find evidence of long tract involve-

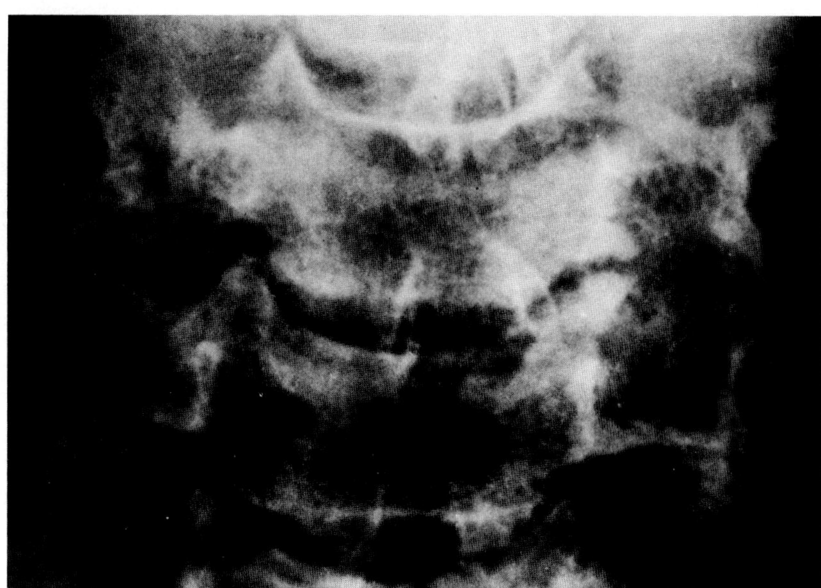

Fig. 11-6. A–P radiograph of a cervical spine demonstrating large neurocentral osteophytes at C5–C6 on the left.

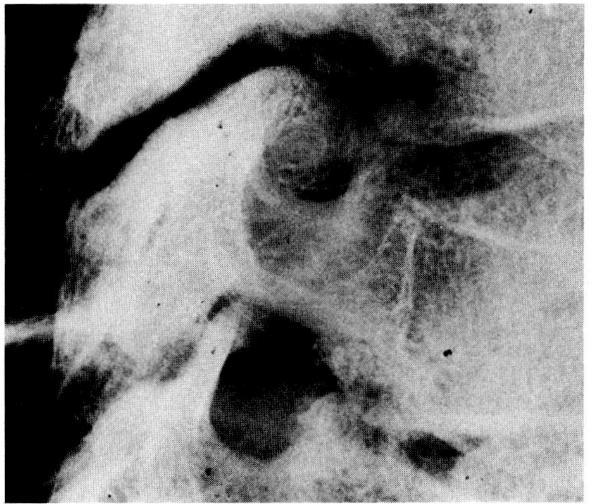

Fig. 11-7. Large osteophyte derived from the posterior joint intruding into the C5–C6 foramen.

ment in addition to the signs of impairment of peripheral nerve root conduction.

A diffusely bulging disc will eventually produce a transverse bar of bone at the discal edge of the vertebral body. When this protrudes posteriorly, the anteroposterior diameter of the cervical spinal canal is narrowed (Fig. 11-9). Compression of the cervical spinal cord in this manner, combined with minor vascular impairment produced by compression of the radicular arteries, may lead to the development of a progressive myelopathy.

If an osteophyte developing on the neurocentral joint extends laterally, the vertebral artery foramen may be encroached upon and the vertebral artery may be compressed to a significant degree (Fig. 11-10). Minor degrees of vertebral artery compromise may be responsible for the so-called vertebral artery syndrome, consisting of dizziness, tinnitus, intermittent blurring of vision, and occasional episodes of retroocular pain. Occasionally, a neurocentral osteophyte may produce severe kinking of the artery, resulting eventually in a vertebral artery thrombosis that may extend superiorly and involve the posteroinferior cerebellar artery. Occlusion of this artery leads to the development of the Wallenberg's syndrome, which is associated with the following symptom complex:

1. Dysphagia, ipsilateral palatal weakness, and vocal cord paralysis from involvement of the nucleus ambiguous of the vagus
2. Impairment of sensation to pain and temperature on the same side of the face from involvement of the descending root and nucleus of the fifth nerve
3. Horner's syndrome in the homolateral eye from the involvement of the descending sympathetic fibers
4. Nystagmus due to the involvement of the vestibular nuclei

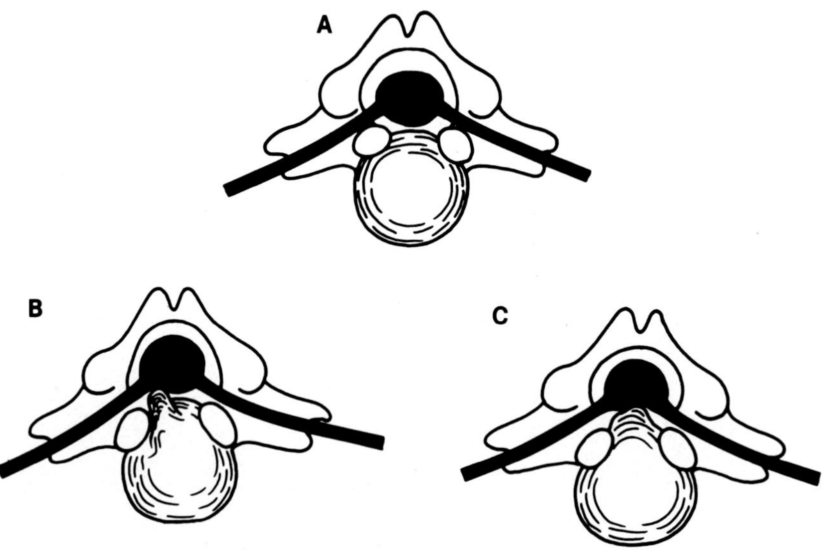

Fig. 11-8. (*A*) The neurocentral joint "protects" the nerve root against pressure from a prolapsed disc. (*B* and *C*) A central disc protrusion will cause cord compression.

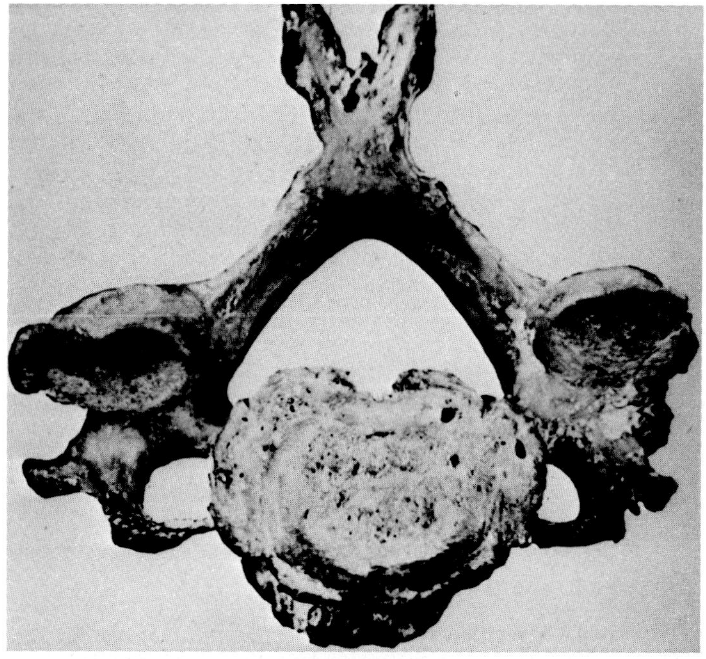

Fig. 11-9. A specimen showing a transverse posterior bar, giving rise to insidiously progressive myelopathy.

5. Cerebellar dysfunction in the ipsilateral arm and leg from interference of the function of the midbrain and cerebellum
6. Impairment of sensation to pain and temperature on the side of the body opposite from the involvement of the spinothalamic tract.

Obstruction of the vertebral arteries can lead to sudden death, as in the man described by Ford and Clark in 1956 who died 10 hours after his wife manipulated his neck.[1] Immediately following the well-intended manipulation, the unfortunate husband experienced tinnitus, vertigo, and right hemianopia, followed by a posteroinferior cerebellar syndrome. At autopsy, a thrombus was seen to extend from one vertebral artery into the basilar and posterior cerebellar arteries.

The midcervical region is the most common site

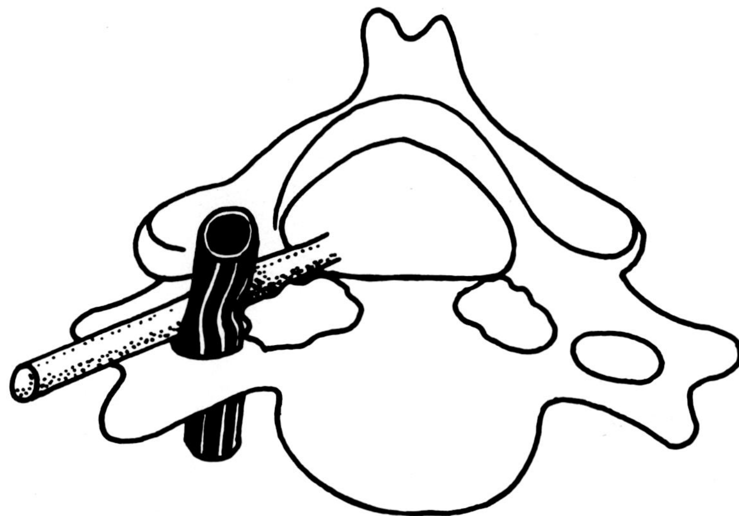

Fig. 11-10. A lateral neurocentral osteophyte compressing the vertebral artery.

for cervical disc degeneration. With the onset of disc degeneration this portion of the spine falls into flexion, and practically all movement at the involved segment is lost. The cervical spine above this level must hyperextend to keep the head erect. If patients with this condition are subjected to an extension injury of the neck, occasioned either by a direct blow or, in the elderly, by the extension strain occasionally associated with the introduction of an endotracheal tube for anesthesia, the vertebral artery may be seriously stretched and damaged as it runs from C2 to C1 or as it passes from the atlas to the foramen magnum, because this is the only region of the cervical spine capable of significant extension in such patients.

Anteriorly, osteophytic outgrowths may give rise to trouble, although this is rare. Severe dysphagia may, however, be produced by an anterior osteophyte and the osteophyte may indeed require surgical removal (Fig. 11-11).

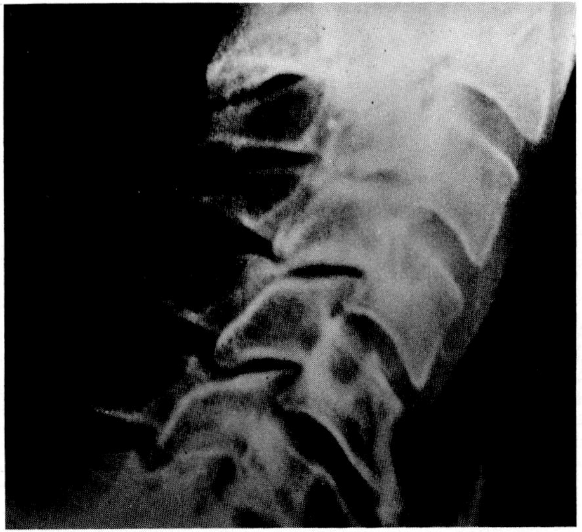

Fig. 11-11. Severe dysphagia produced by an anterior osteophyte.

In summary, then, cervical disc degeneration may occur and may remain asymptomatic. It may give rise to local pain or it may give rise to local and referred pain from posterior joint strains, resulting from spinal instability. It may lead to the production of a neurocentral osteophyte, giving rise to root irritation or impairment of root conduction. Bizarre symptoms may arise from irritation of the sympathetic plexus around the vertebral artery, and, on occasion, symptoms may be related to obstruction of the vertebral artery itself by a neurocentral osteophyte.

A diffuse posterior osteophyte, sometimes referred to as a posterior bar, may give rise to insidiously progressive myelopathy, especially if it is associated with some impairment of vascularity of the cervical cord.

A large anterior osteophyte may give rise to mechanical dysphagia.

REFERENCES

1. *Ford FR, Clark D:* Thrombosis of the basilar artery. Bull Johns Hopkins Hosp 98:37, 1956

2. *Luschka H:* Entwickelungsgeschichte der Formbestandheile des Eiters und der Granulationen, Vol 7, 54 pp, 1 l., 3 pl. 8°. A Emmerling, Freiburg im Breisgau, 1845

3. *Versalius A:* De corporus fabrica libri septem cum indice rerum & verborum memorabilium lucupletissimo. Venetiis, Apud F Franciscium, Seniensem J Creigher Germanum, 1568

Differential Diagnosis of Neck and Arm Pain Relative to Symptoms Caused by Degenerative Disorders of the Cervical Spine

Joseph F. Cusick

Although cervical nerve root compression resulting from lateral disc or osteophyte formation usually has a well-defined clinical presentation, other less common conditions, either singularly or in combination, may mimic or coexist with these entities. The first important diagnostic step is to determine whether the offending process is intraspinal (i.e., in spinal cord or nerve roots) or extraspinal (i.e., in nerve roots, brachial plexus, or peripheral nerves). The intraspinal lesions may exhibit varying patterns of pain, motor, and sensory loss relative to the relationship of the lesion to the spinal cord or nerve roots. Intramedullary spinal cord processes such as tumors or hydromyelia usually have a pattern of diffuse deep pain involving that specific cervical paraspinal area, a dissociated sensory loss, and relatively normal motor examination until the later stages of the disease.

Extramedullary tumors, such as nerve sheath tumors, frequently cause radicular pain at the site of the lesion, which is exacerbated by the Valsalva maneuver. These neoplasms, including the solitary schwannoma or neurofibroma, may have a selective root presentation with progressive sensory loss that closely replicates the effects of a lateral disc; however, the sensory loss is usually more profound, for these tumors generally arise from the sensory roots. Additionally, plain radiographs of the cervical spine show foraminal widening, and the patients may manifest stigmata of the neurocutaneous phakomatosis on physical examination. The radiologic identification of foraminal widening on oblique views of the cervical spine is further defined by computed tomography (CT). The trumpet-like erosion created by the dumbbell extension of these tumors usually results in a widened intraspinal component, whereas rarely occurring vertebral artery vascular lesions may demonstrate a greater element of extraspinal foraminal erosion, requiring vertebral angiography to fully define the process. Anterior horn cell disease with paralytic effects on the proximal musculature of the shoulder, or rarely occurring radicular pain resulting from meningeal involvement during the early stages of acute poliomyelitis, may result in upper extremity pain. However, the predominant motor weakness, fasciculations, widespread evidence of denervation on electromyography, or debilitating prodromal symptoms usually confirm the presence of these gray matter abnormalities of the spinal cord. Demyelinating processes may present with painful dysesthesias of the upper extremities, which may occasionally be initiated by forceful flexion of the cervical spine causing the dysesthesias to radiate into the upper limbs and down the axis of the spinal column (Lhermitte's sign). Diagnostic differentiation of a demyelinating process is assisted by neurologic and electrophysiologic (visual, auditory, and somatosensory-evoked potentials) examinations that show evidence of disseminated white matter abnormalities, alterations of cerebrospinal fluid cell counts, and biochemical analysis (myelin basic protein, oligoclonal bands, IgG, and IgG index). The diagnosis is also aided by magnetic resonance imaging (MRI) that demonstrates demyelinating white matter plaques.

The occurrence of foraminal narrowing during combined extension and ipsilateral rotation of the cervical spine may be accentuated during certain athletic pursuits, especially football. During such activities, forceful hyperextension and rotation of the cervical spine may cause painful paresthesias in the ipsilateral extremity. This process, termed "stinger" or "burner," is usually a self-resolving entity, but its course may be recurrent or partially resolving. Radiologic studies in these healthy young individuals are usually normal without any evidence of segmental instability.

As the nerve roots exit from the cervical foramen, the anterior primary rami of segments C5 through T1 continue on to form the initial portions of the brachial plexus, whereas the posterior primary rami of these nerve roots proceed to supply the paraspinal musculature (Fig. 11-12). This pattern of neural supply shows that electrophysiologic abnormalities in the cervical paraspinal muscles, especially if segmental, greatly help to identify the presence of a foraminal or juxtaforaminal lesion; evidence of paraspinal denervation in that location indicates an intraspinal lesion proximal to the origin of the posterior primary rami. Alterations of sensory action potentials also assist in defining the location of nerve root lesions, because lesions of the nerve root distal to the posterior root ganglion result in Wallerian degeneration

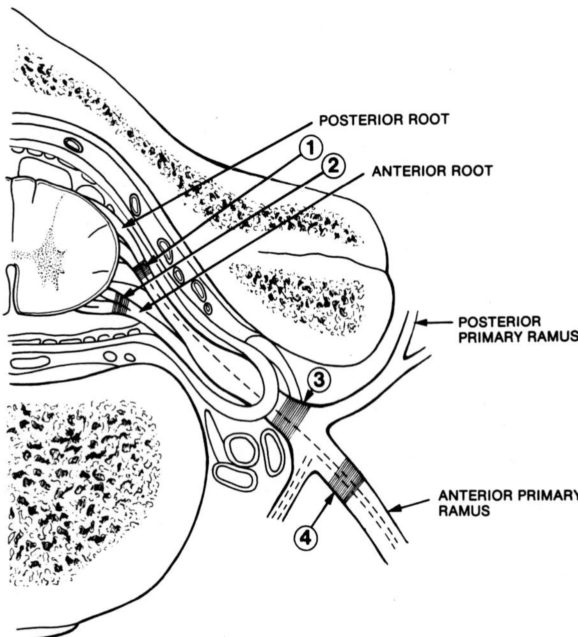

Fig. 11-12. Transverse segmental projection demonstrating the pattern of neural interruption associated with intraspinal and extraspinal lesions. Demyelination in the sensory pathways (*broken lines*) will be present only in lesions distal to the posterior root ganglion (*3, 4*), but absent in lesions proximal to the ganglion (*1*). Electromyographic abnormalities in the paraspinal musculature will be evident with intraspinal involvement (*2*) including the lateral aspects of the foramen (*3*), but absent in isolated involvement of the anterior primary ramus (*4*).

of the axon, whereas nerve root lesions proximal to the posterior root ganglion do not result in degeneration (Fig. 11-12). Therefore, sensory action potentials will be abnormal or unobtainable in lesions of the brachial plexus and peripheral nerves, but normal in lesions of the intraspinal nerve roots.

The anterior primary rami of C5 through T1 continue downward in a moderately oblique direction to form the trunks of the brachial plexus. Proximal to the source of the trunks of the brachial plexus, the dorsal scapular nerves originate from the anterior primary rami of the fifth and sixth cervical roots. These nerves supply the rhomboid muscles, the levator scapulae muscles, and the long thoracic nerves that innervate the serratus anterior muscles (Fig. 11-13). Clinical weakness of these specific muscles, therefore, indicates involvement of the fifth and sixth cervical roots in their extraspinal postganglionic location adjacent to the vertebral column. Disease processes that directly affect the brachial plexus may result in a variety of abnormalities of the upper extremities. Trauma is the process most commonly resulting in brachial plexus injury, and careful attention to the patient's history would implicate this cause. If possible traction injury to the cervical nerve roots in conjunction with the brachial plexus injury is a diagnostic problem, myelography or contrast-enhanced CT will be of assistance in documenting diverticulum or disruption of the nerve roots.

Other forms of brachial plexus neuropathy may result from compression by vascular and skeletal structures, fibrous bands, or tumors. The relationship of these structures is depicted in Figure 11-13, which illustrates the close approximation of the brachial plexus to the subclavian artery and vein as these elements pass through a triangle formed by the scalenus anticus muscle, scalenus medius muscle, and the first rib. This space may be compromised by a cervical rib, elongated transverse process of the seventh cervical vertebra, abnormalities of the scalenus anticus muscle, or narrowing of the space between the first rib and the clavicle resulting from hyperabduction of the upper extremity. One of the more popular syndromes of neurovascular compression proposed to occur at this level has been termed the *scalenus anticus syndrome,* in which vague shoulder and upper-extremity pain associated with positional exacerbation results from neural compression of the plexus by the scalenus anticus muscle. There is controversy regarding the validity of considering this a syndrome. Nevertheless, the absence of focal neurologic abnormalities associated with it permits easy differentiation from nerve root lesions, which have specific motor, reflex, and sensory alterations. Additionally, it must be emphasized that the scalenus musculature can participate in the diffuse muscle spasm associated with cervical radiculopathy. Consequently, local alterations in the area of the scalenus musculature must be interpreted relative to this general involvement.

A more defined but rare form of neurovascular compression has been reported to occur with rudimentary cervical ribs or fibrous bands, resulting in compression of the lower portion of the brachial plexus (Fig. 11-13). The clinical presentation is usually an ill-defined pain in the medial aspect of the arm and forearm associated with weakness and atrophy of the intrinsic musculature of the hand that results from compression of the lower segments of the brachial plexus. Compromise of this portion of the brachial plexus affects structures constituted mainly by the C8 and T1 nerve roots

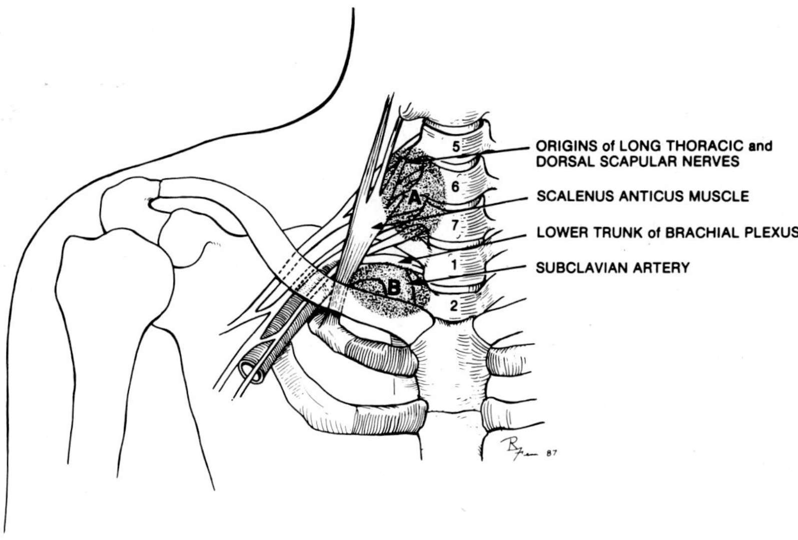

Fig. 11-13. Anterior primary rami of C5 through T1 proceeding to form the brachial plexus and peripheral nerves. Extraspinal lesions may result in certain patterns of neural involvement, as shown, by segmenting into two zones. In Zone A, involvement of the dorsal scapular and long thoracic nerve will cause abnormalities in the rhomboid, levator scapulae and serratus anterior muscles, but brachial plexus involvement distal will result in preservation of function. In Zone B, which is the area usually implicated in the thoracic outlet syndrome, the involvement of the lower trunk will result in abnormalities of the structures supplied by the ulnar nerve and partially by the portion of the median nerve derived from the C8 and T1 roots.

as they form the ulnar nerve and portions of the median nerve (Fig. 11-13). Involvement may be documented by electromyographic evidence of a conduction delay in the proximal ulnar distribution and neurogenic changes in the intrinsic musculature of the hands served by both the C8 and T1 nerve roots. Although thenar eminence atrophy may be prominent, the pattern of neural supply permits differentiation from the carpal tunnel syndrome, because the patient will demonstrate muscle involvement more extensive than would be expected with isolated median nerve involvement. Furthermore, the patient will have relatively normal sensory conductions at the wrist because of preservation of the C6 and C7 nerve root contributions to the median nerve. Positive vascular responses to the Adson, costoclavicular, or hyperabduction maneuvers have been proposed to confirm a probable thoracic outlet syndrome, but these findings have limited diagnostic value because of their frequent positive occurrence in asymptomatic individuals.

The so-called cryptogenetic brachial plexus neuropathy, which has also been termed paralytic brachial neuritis, neuralgic amyotrophy, and localized neuritis of the shoulder girdle, may prove difficult to distinguish in its initial stages from a cervical root lesion, especially that of the fifth cervical nerve root. This process, which is more common in middle-aged males, is characteristically initiated with severe pain of a sharp or aching character that is exacerbated by movement of the upper extremity, but relatively unaffected by neck motion or the Valsalva maneuver. These latter negative mechanical findings, in association with the diffuse and progressive character of the motor weakness in a pattern suggesting peripheral nerve involvement, reduced amplitude of sensory nerve action potentials, and absence of paraspinal muscle denervation, help to differentiate this form a brachial plexus neuropathy from C5 or C6 radiculopathy originating from a lateral cervical disc or osteophyte.

Apical carcinomas of the lung may encroach upon the brachial plexus, subclavian artery, or vein, resulting in irritation or compromise of these structures. In the early stages of involvement, the absence of a palpable supraclavicular mass and the poor definition of this region on routine chest radiographs may cause difficulties in detecting the tumors. Apical lordotic views of the chest help to clarify this entity, and the infiltrating character of these lesions usually results in a progressive lower brachial plexus involvement that ultimately proceeds to a profound neurologic loss accompanied by deafferentation-type pain. The presence of Horner's syndrome associated with intense and diffuse pain of the upper limb significantly raises the index of suspicion of an apical carcinoma of the lung.

Angina pectoris may cause varying patterns of left-shoulder or upper-extremity pain, but this process usually is easily defined by its deep aching or crushing pain, exacerbation by exertion, associated precordial pain component, absence of aggravation by cervical spine movement or by the

Valsalva maneuver, and a positive response to coronary artery vasodilators—especially nitroglycerin. Angina pectoris can occasionally be misinterpreted as a cervical radiculopathic process. However, far more commonly a patient with a quite clearly defined clinical presentation of left cervical radiculopathy will first be vigorously evaluated for the presence of coronary artery insufficiency.

Although primary disorders of the shoulder may occasionally implicate cervical radiculopathy, physical examination generally shows clinical signs localized to the shoulder. Patients with frozen shoulder or adhesive capsulitis have limited passive glenohumeral abduction and rotation of the shoulder with pain symptoms reproduced by stretching them to the extremes of their available motion. Patients with subachromial bursitis, when presenting with a sudden onset of pain, have an acutely tender shoulder on palpation, and marked aggravation of shoulder motion that is most prominent in the middle arc of motion. Shoulder radiographs may often demonstrate calcium deposits in the subachromial area. Shoulder pain resulting from a tear of the rotator cuff is usually subachromial and associated with weakness in initiating and sustaining shoulder abduction. In this situation, an arthrogram will verify the diagnosis of a rotator cuff tear. Patients with elbow problems may also occasionally have a pain pattern resembling that seen in a cervical nerve root compression. It has been previously noted that conditions resulting in weakness of the girdle muscles of the upper extremity are frequently associated with pain as a result of the instability of the shoulder joint. Such a consideration can be extended to the initial manifestations of the myasthenic syndrome or to any of the polyneuritis affecting the peripheral nerves innervating the muscles of this region. This group of somewhat vague pain complaints, sometimes referred to as the pseudoradicular syndromes, and those primary structural abnormalities of the shoulder or elbow joints are not associated with the typical motor, sensory or reflex changes that occur with cervical nerve root involvement. These processes also do not have the corresponding electromyographic alterations indicative of an intraspinal preganglionic lesion and do not manifest pain in the paracervical musculature or aggravation by motion of the cervical spine, which is frequently found with the cervical nerve root compression syndromes.

Peripheral nerve involvement, especially compressive neuropathy, occasionally manifests patterns of upper-extremity pain that exceeds the expected regional involvement of the specific peripheral nerve. Radial, median, or ulnar nerve entrapment neuropathy can usually be differentiated by their pattern of motor and sensory loss as well as topographical evidence of conduction abnormalities on electromyographic studies. These peripheral nerve entrapment lesions, however, may coexist with cervical root compression in a process that has been termed the double-crush nerve entrapment syndrome. It has been hypothesized that axons compressed in one region become more susceptible to impairment at a distant site and, therefore, that subclinical cervical nerve root compression may be a contributing factor in the development of compressive ulnar or medial neuropathy. The failure of a patient to respond to an uncomplicated decompression of a peripheral nerve should alert the investigator to the possibility of a coexisting cervical root compression that was obscured by the clinical and electromyographic findings of entrapment neuropathy.

In summary, it may be difficult, especially in the early stages, to distinguish some of these entities from the usual cervical radiculopathy originating from cervical nerve root compromise by a lateral disc or osteophyte. However, careful attention to clinical presentation, electromyographic abnormalities, and radiographic findings generally permit both differentiation of these various disorders and localization of the process to the appopriate region of neural compromise.

REFERENCES

1. *Adson AW, Coffey JR:* Cervical rib: A method of anterior approach for relief of symptoms by division of scalenus anticus. Ann Surg 85:839–857, 1927
2. *Dyck PJ, Law PA, Stevens JC:* Diseases of peripheral nerves. In Baker AB, Baker LH (eds): Clinical Neurology, Vol 3, pp 52–58. Philadelphia, Harper & Row, 1981
3. *Gilliatt RW:* The classical neurological syndrome associated with a cervical rib and band. In Greep JM, Lemmens HAJ, Roos DB, Urschel HC (eds): Pain in Shoulder and Arm: An Integrated View, pp 173–183. The Hague, Martinus Nijhoff, 1979
4. *Hardy RW Jr, Wilbourn A, Hanson M:* Surgical treatment of compressive cervical band. Neurosurgery 7:10–13, 1980
5. *Upton ARM, McComas AJ:* The double crush in nerve entrapment syndromes. Lancet 7825:359–362, 1973
6. *Urschel HC Jr, Razzuk MA:* Management of thoracic outlet syndrome. N Engl J Med 286:1140–1143, 1972

An Algorithm for the Diagnosis of Neck Pain

WILLIAM A. ROBERTS, STEVEN R. GARFIN, AND AUGUSTUS A. WHITE III

SUGGESTED PATIENT EVALUATION PLAN

If the patient's symptoms and signs are clear and relatively classic for one of the disorders described in the preceding section of this chapter, the treatment can be appropriately directed. However, often the source of the pain is unclear, and the diagnosis and treatment cannot be rapidly and efficiently localized. These latter conditions, which lead to confusion, are the focus of this section.

In order to summarize the information presented, a suggested patient flow plan is provided (Figs. 11-14 to 11-16). Although certainly this plan cannot be useful for every patient, the concept of an organized approach should be considered in the work-up and treatment of these individuals. Appended to this section is a detailed algorithm that includes almost all the diagnoses that can affect the neck, shoulder, and arm.

INITIAL PRESENTATION

Most patients, because of intense pain, present to the physician within 1 to 2 weeks of the onset of their symptoms. At that time a detailed history and physical examination should be performed. This should include evaluation of the neck and shoulder as well as of the neurologic function of the upper and lower extremities. For localized symptoms, radiographs of the appropriate area(s) can be obtained. If a systemic disorder is suggested, one should consider obtaining a radiograph of the chest and should order hematologic and chemistry studies to include CBC with a differential sedimentation rate (SED), chemistry panel (including a creatine phosphokinase [CPK]), and a serum protein electrophoresis. These latter studies do not routinely have to be obtained on the first visit, unless there is a suggestion of systemic disorder, myelopathy, tumor, or infection. If, however, concern is raised about the possibility of a serious underlying disorder, in addition to the laboratory studies listed, a medical evaluation, bone scan, CT scan, MR scan, or myelogram should also be considered with relative urgency. Most patients with degenerative disc disease will improve in the first few weeks if they have rest, some degree of immobilization (collar or sling), antiinflammatory medications, and analgesics. If the pain does not completely resolve or decrease to an acceptable level, then a physical therapy evaluation and treatment can be added in the early phase.

If the pain persists for 2 to 3 weeks without relief, the patient should be reevaluated with a detailed history and physical examination. In most patients, the generalized pain complaint will have subsided, and it will be possible to localize the pain and the nature of the discomfort at this time. If the pain is migratory, one could consider a diagnosis of fibrositis or polymyalgia rheumatica. However, at this stage these are diagnoses of exclusion, rather than primary diagnoses, and they are not easily confirmed during the second or third week of pain. If the pain is localized and there are focal neurologic findings or limited range of motion of the shoulder, then x-ray studies of the appropriate areas and specific treatment can be ordered. Antiinflammatory medications and physical therapy are the type of treatment required for most pain-related complaints in the neck, shoulder, and upper extremity.

When the pain appears to be localized in the shoulder, subacromial bursa injections with lidocaine (Xylocaine) or bupivacaine hydrochloride (Marcaine) and/or a long-acting glucocorticosteroid may prove useful not only in treating but also in helping to diagnose the anatomic location of the discomfort. Physical therapy and antiinflammatory medications are extremely useful in the treatment of shoulder disorders. If the pain persists despite this regimen, arthrography, CT or MRI of the shoulder, or possibly arthroscopy, should be considered.

If the pain localizes to the neck, further evaluation may delineate trigger points that can be treated with injections. If there is radiating pain, EMG/NCV studies may be helpful (after at least 2 to 3 weeks of pain). If these are positive or if there are appropriate neurologic deficits, and the patient has failed normal conservative care, MR scans or enhanced or unenhanced CT scans of the cervical spine can be performed to better evaluate the possibility of cervical disc disease as the cause of pain. With this diagnosis there is no urgency in performing these studies, as nonoperative means will most likely succeed in controlling the patient's symptoms. At this point, if the pain remains nonfocal and the work-up (including electrophysiologic and

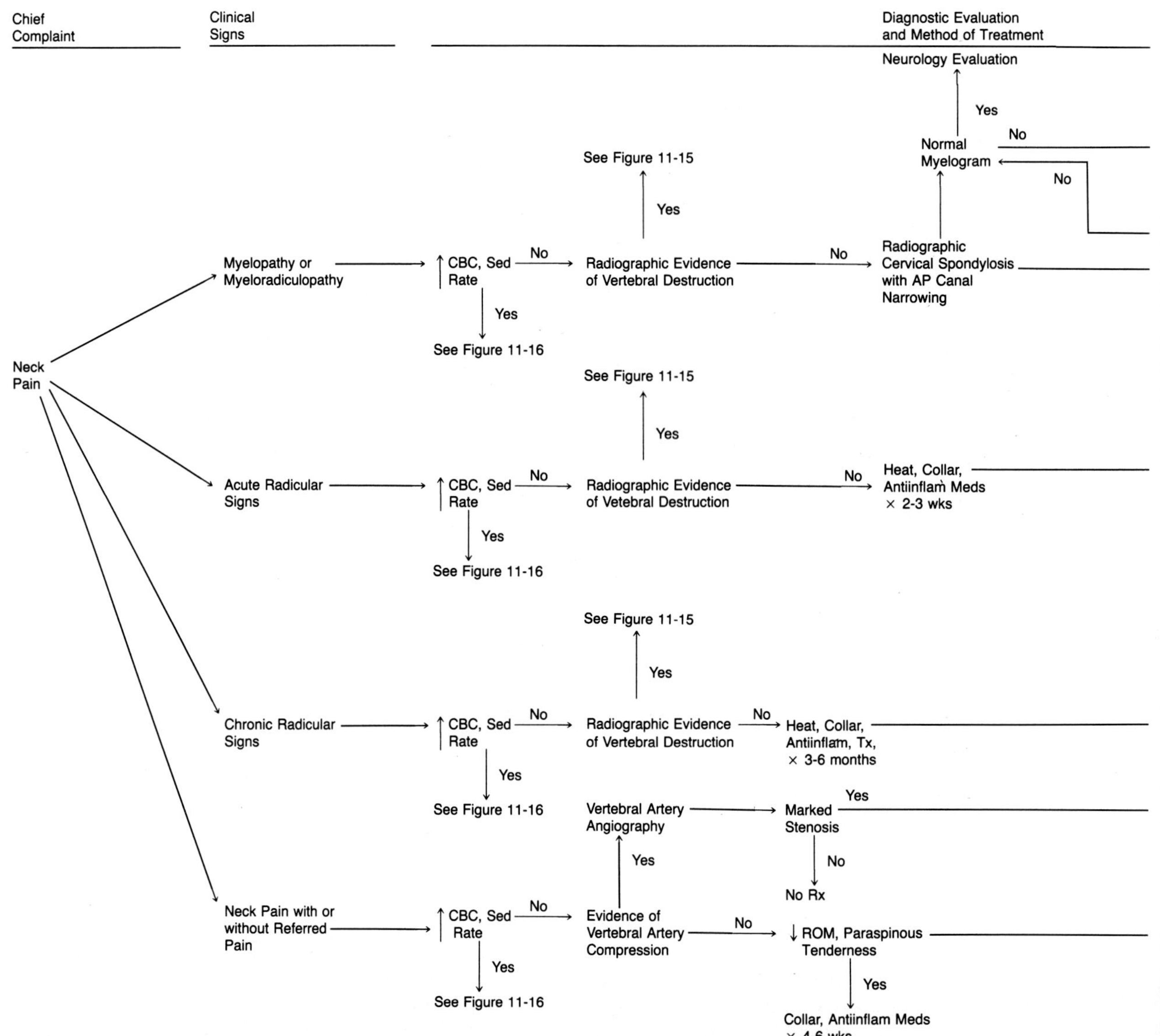

Fig. 11-14. Neck pain algorithm.

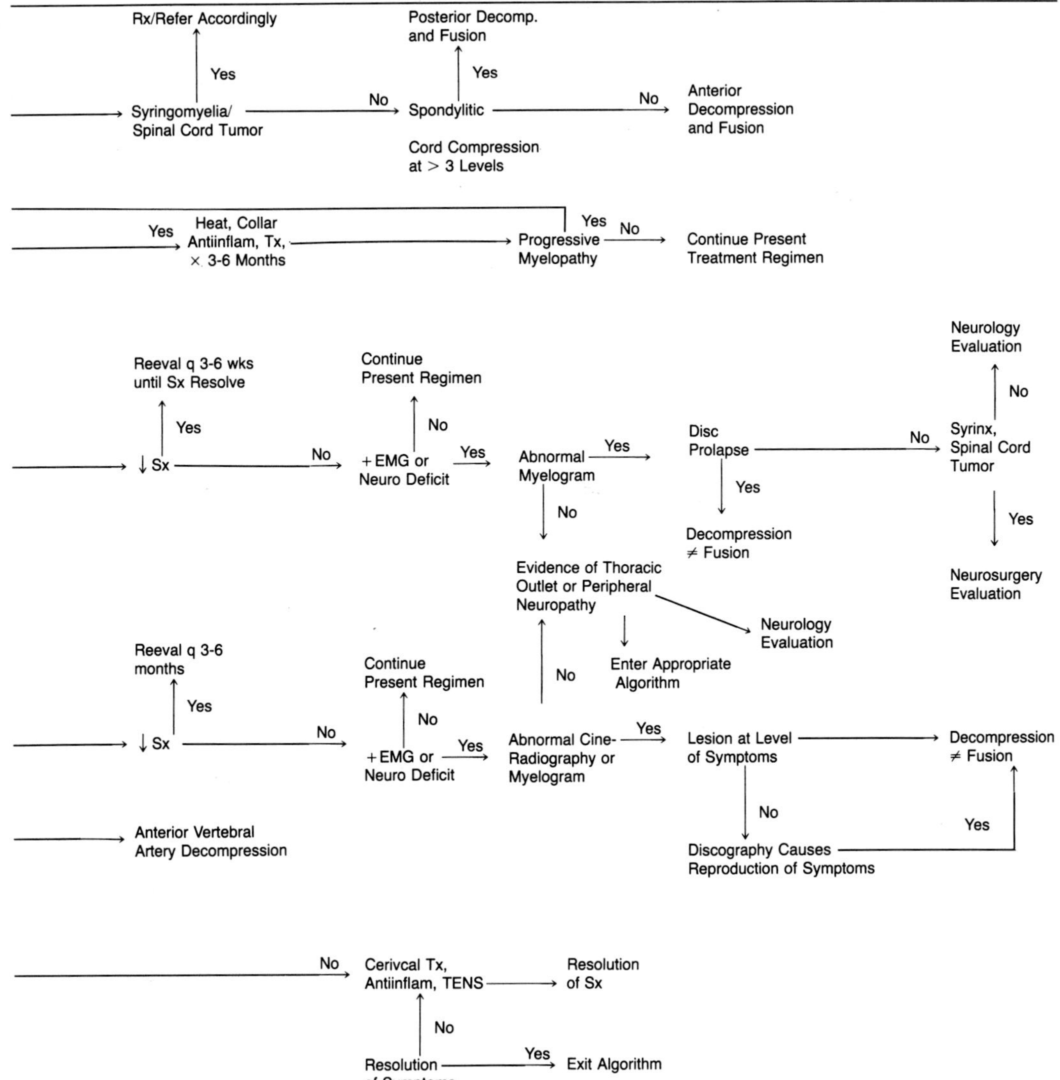

Rx/Refer Accordingly
Yes
Syringomyelia/ Spinal Cord Tumor
No
Posterior Decomp. and Fusion
Yes
Spondylitic
Cord Compression at > 3 Levels
No
Anterior Decompression and Fusion
Yes
Heat, Collar Antiinflam, Tx, × 3-6 Months
Yes
No
Progressive Myelopathy
Continue Present Treatment Regimen
Reeval q 3-6 wks until Sx Resolve
Yes
↓ Sx
No
Continue Present Regimen
No
+EMG or Neuro Deficit
Yes
Abnormal Myelogram
Yes
Disc Prolapse
No
Syrinx, Spinal Cord Tumor
Neurology Evaluation
No
Yes
Neurosurgery Evaluation
Yes
Decompression ≠ Fusion
No
Evidence of Thoracic Outlet or Peripheral Neuropathy
Neurology Evaluation
Enter Appropriate Algorithm
Reeval q 3-6 months
Yes
↓ Sx
No
Continue Present Regimen
No
+EMG or Neuro Deficit
Yes
No
Abnormal Cine-Radiography or Myelogram
Yes
Lesion at Level of Symptoms
Decompression ≠ Fusion
No
Yes
Discography Causes Reproduction of Symptoms
Anterior Vertebral Artery Decompression
No
Cerivcal Tx, Antiinflam, TENS
Resolution of Sx
No
Resolution of Symptoms
Yes
Exit Algorithm

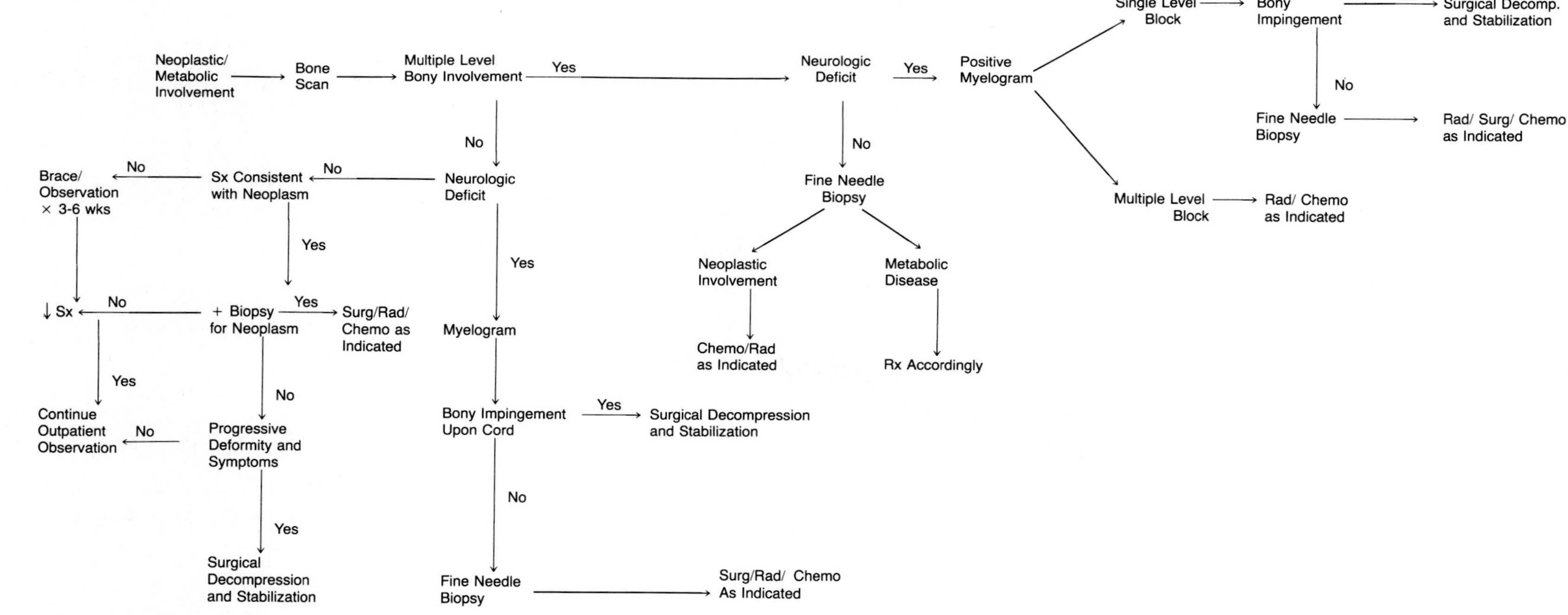

Fig. 11-15. Neoplastic/metabolic disease algorithm.

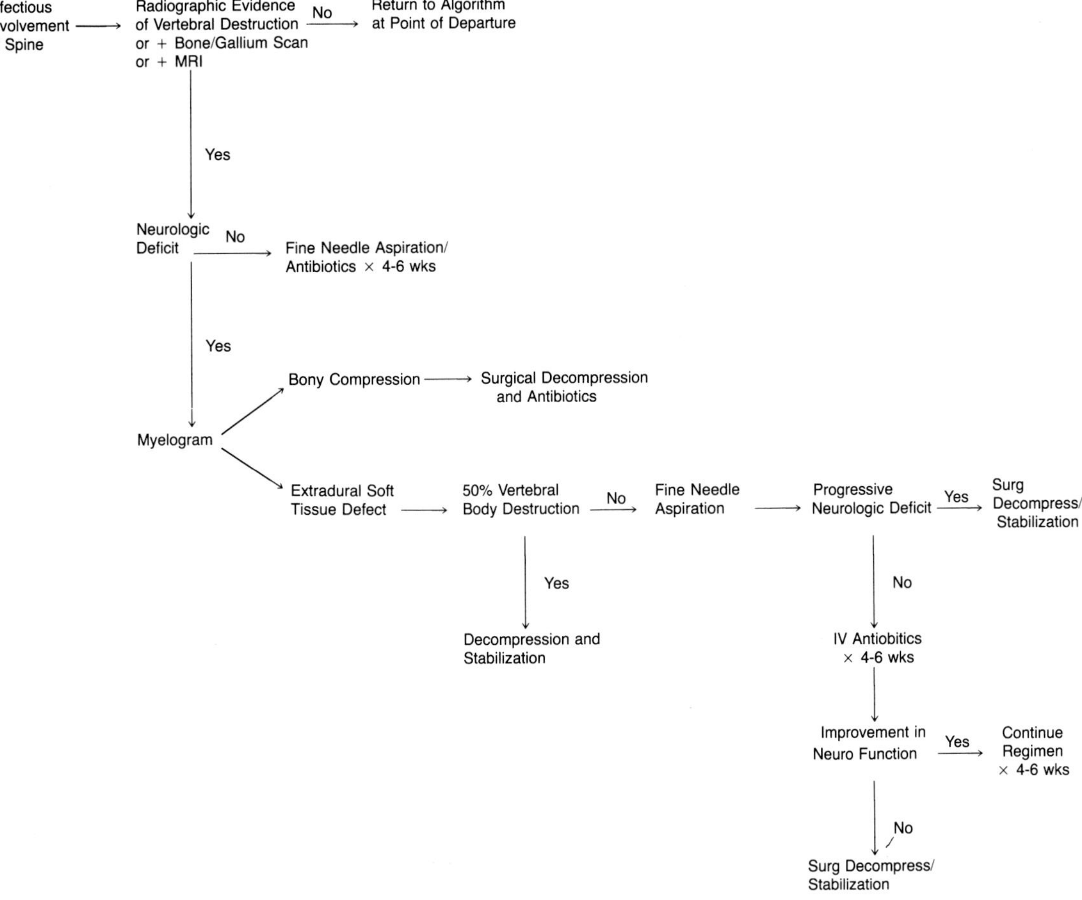

Fig. 11-16. Infectious process algorithm.

radiologic studies) is negative, the possibility of a systemic disease should be considered. Consultation with the appropriate specialist (internist, pulmonologist, rheumatologist, or gastroenterologist) might be necessary to establish the nature of the systemic disorder.

SPECIFIC LABORATORY TESTS

Certain tests should be emphasized because of their usefulness in making relatively specific diagnoses. An increased *white blood count* (WBC) is usually suggestive of an infection, leukemia, or lymphoma. Although nonspecific, an increased *sedimentation rate* can be seen with infections, tumors, rheumatoid arthritis, polymyalgia rheumatica, or collagen vascular diseases. An elevated *creatinine phosphokinase (CPK)* is seen with polymyalgia rheumatica, collagen vascular disorders, dermatomyositis or polymyositis, and occasionally in a myofascitis (fibrositis) syndrome following muscle massage. *Bone scans* are extremely useful in diagnosing infections and tumors. The *MR scan* is becoming increasingly useful and specific in the evaluation of (1) cervical disc disease (herniated discs and stenosis), (2) soft-tissue tumors, (3) infections (bone and soft tissue), (4) the sternoclavicular joint, (5) spinal cord syrinx, (6) spinal cord tumors, and (7) rotator cuff abnormalities of the shoulder. The *CT scan,* an extremely important tool in the cervical spine and shoulder, frequently requires enhancement (*enhanced CT scans*). It remains the most effective study for evaluating bony shoulder abnormalities (Hill-Sachs and Bankart lesions), cervical stenosis, sternoclavicular joint abnormalities (particularly hyperostoses), infections, and tumors, particularly in bone. Although the CT scan does not, and enhanced CT scans may, require hospitalization, the latter is the preferred study for the definitive diagnosis of herniated discs or stenosis as well as spinal cord tumors in the cervical spine. Enhanced CT scans (*arthro-CT*) should also be considered to evaluate shoulder pathology. *EMGs* are diagnostic of many neuromuscular disease disorders, peripheral nerve entrapment syndromes and useful in cervical nerve root lesions. *Nerve conduction velocities* should routinely be ordered to evaluate peripheral nerve entrapment syndromes.

Management of Radiculopathy Secondary to Acute Cervical Disc Degeneration and Spondylosis by the Posterior Approach

ALEXANDER E. BRODSKY

The choice of the posterior approach for cervical nerve root decompression over the anterior route rests on the personal preference of the surgeon. Most neurologic surgeons prefer the posterior approach because this was the traditional approach to such problems for many years before the popularization of the anterior approach by Smith and Robinson and Cloward in the early 1950s.[2,3,18] It is also the approach most neurosurgeons use for other conditions such as tumors, spinal cord injuries, syringomyelia, and so forth.

Orthopedic surgeons and younger neurosurgeons often favor the anterior method because of the excellent results achieved as well as the comparative safety in not exposing the spinal cord and nerve roots.

There are many of us who use both approaches, employing that which is most suited to the individual case with the realization that either method is equally suitable for the majority of cases. In those cases in which there is a coexistence of cervical spinal stenosis and monoradiculopathy, one can decompress the cervical spinal cord posteriorly with a complete laminectomy and then decompress the individual nerve root by partial facetectomy with or without removal of the underlying spur or disc.

Extruded fragments in cervical disc ruptures do not usually migrate as they do in lumbar lesions. However, many surgeons feel more secure visualizing fragments posteriorly and exploring above and below with a blunt nerve hook for additional fragments of the disc material. Furthermore, advocates of the posterior approach, such as Simmons, point out that there is a higher potential for complication anteriorly, and mention such things as injuries to the esophagus, carotid arteries, sympathetic chain, larynx, recurrent laryngeal nerve, vertebral arteries, spinal cord, and nerve roots, as well as displacement of bone grafts, pseudoarthrosis of fusion, and degeneration of discs above or below the fusion, which occurs in 2% to 3% of cases.[17] Of course, the posterior approach carries with it the potential for serious complications such as spinal cord or nerve root injury as well as the potential for destabilization of one or more segments. Obviously it is necessary to be aware of these potential complications and minimize them by careful technique in either approach.

The anterior approach is preferable in the following situations:

1. For midline lesions, either soft or hard
2. When one opts for the stability of a fusion
3. When ease of positioning is a consideration

The posterior approach would be preferred as follows:

1. For lesions above C2–C3 or below C7–T1
2. When the presence of spinal cord neoplasm is suspected
3. To enable the decompression of multiple nerve roots, preferably unilaterally, without the need to consider fusing multiple segments
4. When spinal stenosis requires posterior decompression

TECHNIQUE

The posterior approach to cervical nerve roots and discs or spurs can be accomplished through a hemilaminectomy with removal of the medial third or half of the facet joint to decompress the affected nerve root, or through a smaller "keyhole" foraminotomy as described by Scoville.[15,16] The choice depends upon the extent and severity of the compressive lesion and the preference and training of the surgeon.

In general, the "keyhole" foraminotomy is adequate for dealing with a sharply localized soft disc herniation or rupture, whereas the wider decompression afforded by hemilaminectomy is preferable for a hard disc or spur and narrowed foramen of the spondylotic spine. Obviously, surgery by whatever approach in such cases is employed only if adequate conservative treatment has failed. However, surgery should not be unduly delayed when there is significant motor weakness, signs of spinal cord compression, or clinical indications of an extruded fragment. Failure of symptoms to significantly diminish in less than 1 week on intensive conservative treatment would tend to indicate an irreversible herniation or extruded fragment. Extruded fragments are often associated with symptoms of constant deep burning pain in the scapular region with an associated tilt of the head and the usual absence of trauma in the his-

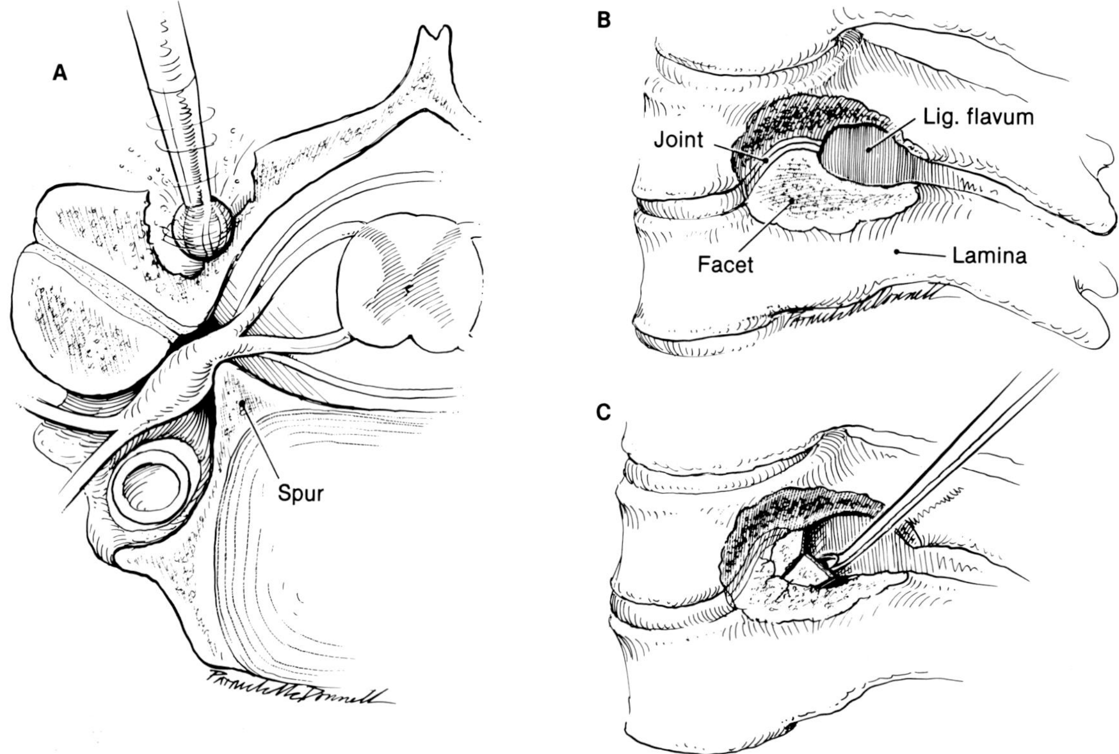

Fig. 11-17. (*A*) A high-speed diamond bur is used to thin out the bone over the outer part of the lamina and the medial part of the inferior articular facet. The ventral spur compressing the root is graphically demonstrated. The thinned-out bone (*B*) can then be removed easily with a curette (*C*). (After Frykholm R: Cervical nerve root compression resulting from disc degeneration and root-sleeve fibrosis: A clinical investigation. Acta Chir Scand (Suppl) 160:v, 1951; and Brain WR, Wilkinson JL: Cervical Spondylosis and Other Disorders of the Spine. Philadelphia, WB Saunders, 1967)

tory. Some advocates of posterior root decompression recommend only posterior decompression of the nerve root by removing the medial third or half of the facet (posterior wall of the foramen); they further advise against retracting a nerve root or attempting to remove spurs or discs beneath the root (Fig. 11-17). Others, led by Epstein, advocate removal of the underlying hard spurs with special reverse-curve curettes and rasps, and removal of soft, herniated, or ruptured discs that lie beneath the nerve root.[5]

The first group claimed good results without incurring the added risk of nerve root deficit from retraction, but this viewpoint is not fully accepted. Epstein has presented a series of cases in which two almost equal groups were treated in the above manner.[5] Ninety percent of those who had spur removal had good results as opposed to the 50% in whom simple posterior root decompression was carried out (Fig. 11-18).

POSITIONING

For the posterior approach the patient may be either prone or sitting up (Figs. 11-19, 11-20, and 11-21).

In the more traditional prone position, the neck is flexed and the forehead rests upon the cerebellar headrest. The upright position is achieved either by taping of the head to the Mayfield headrest or by using the special Gardner tongs, preferably in a slightly flexed or neutral position (Figs. 11-20 and 11-21). In cases of cervical spondylosis, flexion is to be avoided because of the danger of compressing the cord against the ventral spurs.

The upright position carries the added risk of

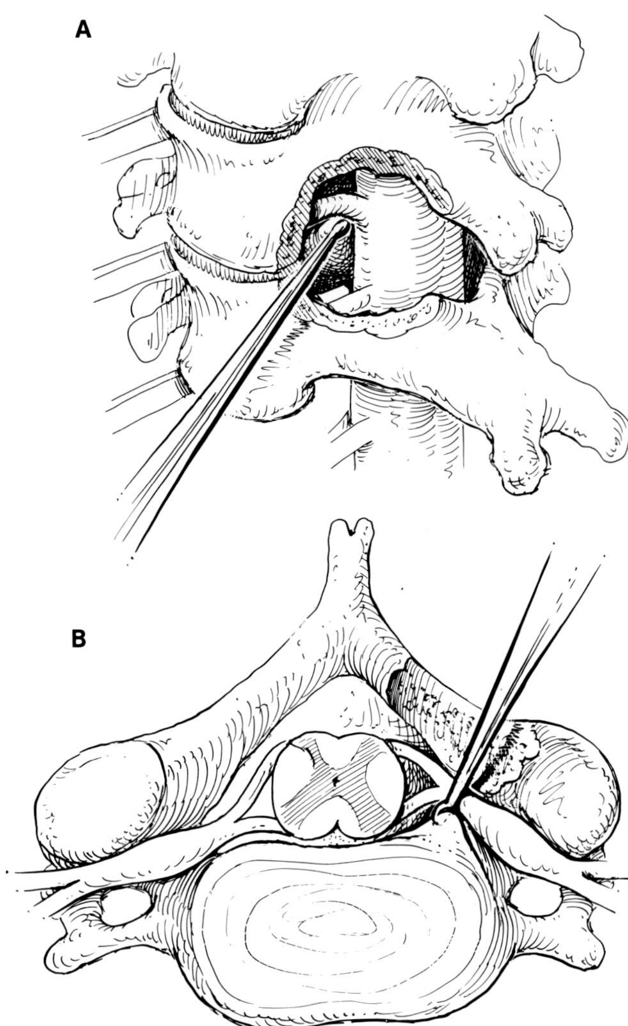

Fig. 11-18. Removal of spurs ventral to the root using small straight or reverse bent curettes of Epstein. (*A*) Posterior view. (*B*) Coronal section.

air embolism through veins that might be opened, as well as the risk of cerebral hypoxia should there be a severe and prolonged drop of blood pressure. However, this position carries the advantage of a drier field owing to a diminished venous distention and bleeding. Our own preference is for the sitting position with a sensing catheter in the right atrium to detect and evacuate an air embolus promptly, should one develop. The patient's legs are wrapped with elastic bandages from the toes to the upper thighs to reduce postural hypotension, and the eyes are protected assiduously in both upright and prone positions. One should avoid excessive flexion in cases of spondylotic spinal cord compression to avoid pressing the cord against the ventral spurs lest there be postoperative signs of cord compression on awakening.

Almost all ruptured cervical discs present in the posterolateral corner since the posterior longitudinal ligament is thicker in its central portion and becomes extremely thin as it approaches the lateral corner. Thus, most extruded fragments lie in the posterolateral corner and can usually be found and removed both anteriorly as well as posteriorly. Cloward advocates removing the posterior longitudinal ligament in selected cases and exploring the anterior extradural space for fragments.[3] However, this carries a risk of extradural bleeding with hematoma and acute cord compression, as reported by Hoi Song and Wilson.[9] For this reason,

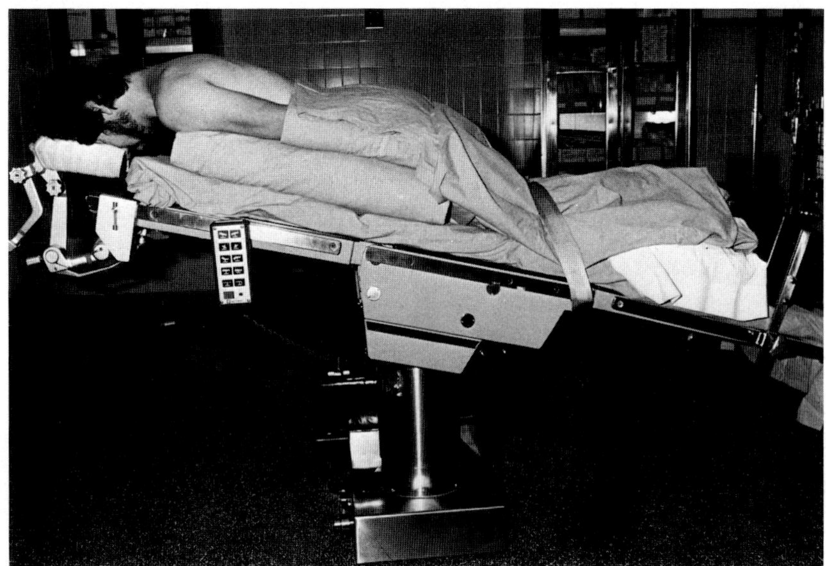

Fig. 11-19. The patient is in the prone position on the cerebellar headrest, reverse Trendelenburg 20°, with the neck in flexion for posterior cervical surgery.

we do not advocate that this procedure be carried out routinely and advise against blindly running a nerve hook up and down in the extradural space, especially if the patient is in the upright position in which bleeding might go unnoticed. Through a midline incision with or without infiltration of dilute adrenalin, the laminae of the cervical vertebrae is exposed either unilaterally or bilaterally and self-retaining retractors inserted. Excessive stripping of the erector spinae muscles posterolaterally off the laminae should be avoided since it may contribute to denervation of the posterior muscles and thereby create a permanent kyphotic curve of the cervical spine.*

A lateral roentgenogram should be taken with a metallic marker on a spinous process for localization. One or more laminae are removed unilaterally (hemilaminectomy) with Leksel or Fulton rongeurs. The posterior wall of the medial third or half of the facet joint is removed with curettes or with a high-speed diamond bur. The compressed nerve root is thus exposed; it is gently retracted upward, and the extruded disc fragments are removed with a small blunt hook, pituitary forceps, or suction. If the soft disc protrusion is as yet unruptured, it is carefully opened with a number 11 blade, and several small fragments are removed with a pituitary forceps. One should not attempt to evacuate much of the disc or curette it, as would be done in the lumbar region.

* Epstein JA: Personal communication

If the case is one of spondylotic radiculopathy, there will be spurs projecting into the ventral portion of the foramen from the margins of the vertebral bodies. There are often perineural fibrous adhesions binding the root to the surrounding bony canal. The technique for such lesions is similar to that described above with removal of the medial half of the facet joint—careful lysis of the perineural adhesions with a small, blunt hook under magnification. The underlying spur is then removed with Epstein's small reverse-angle curettes and rasps introduced beneath the nerve root from below, with the curette or rasp always pulled toward the surgeon and not toward the cord or neural structures.[5] Again, in such cases of spondylosis the head should be positioned in neutral or slight extension to prevent compression of the cord against the ventral spurs. Epstein also recommends abduction of the shoulders with the arms on armrests to relax the nerve roots, placing them at a right angle or an upward angle.[5] This facilitates the introduction of curettes and rasps and diminishes the amount of tension exerted on a nerve root during such a procedure.

"KEYHOLE" FORAMINOTOMY OF SCOVILLE

Scoville has popularized a more limited decompression of the root by creating a hole over the nerve root and removing the medial half of the facet and a small portion of the adjacent lam-

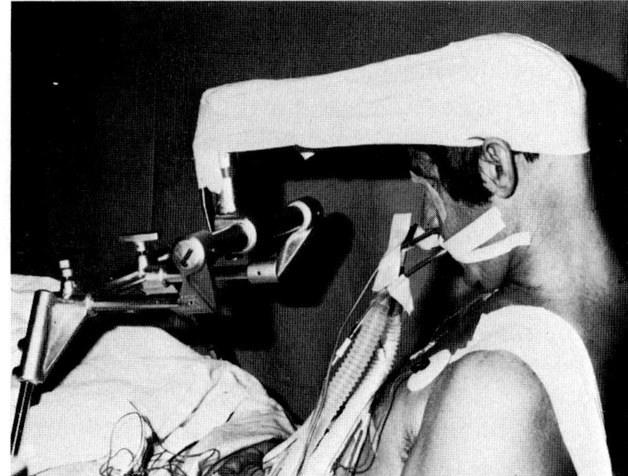

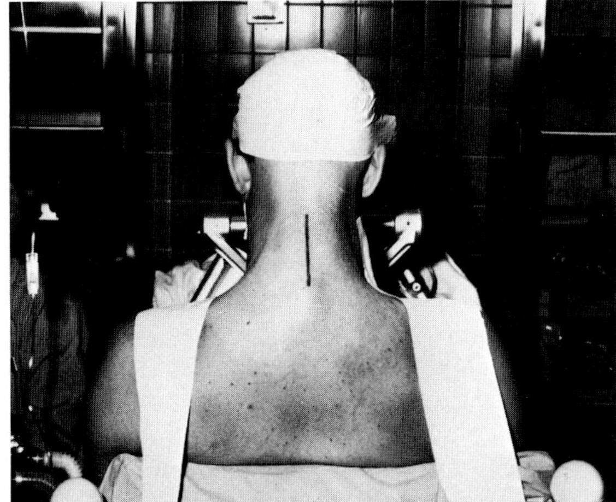

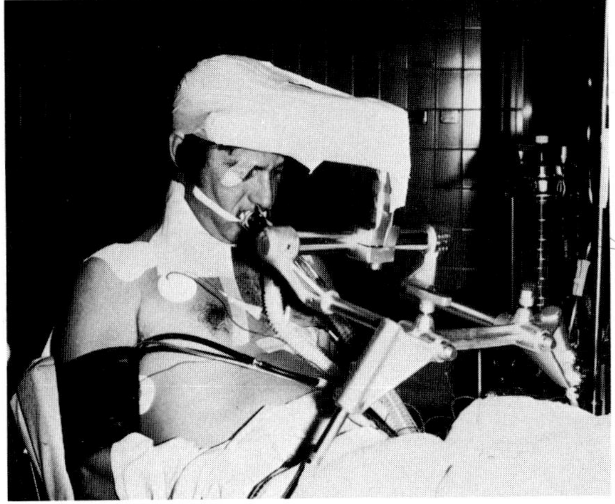

Fig. 11-20. The patient is in the sitting position for posterior cervical surgery, with Mayfield headrest and adhesive tape. The eyes are protected, the left atrial line is in place, the hips and knees are flexed, and the arms are placed in abduction.

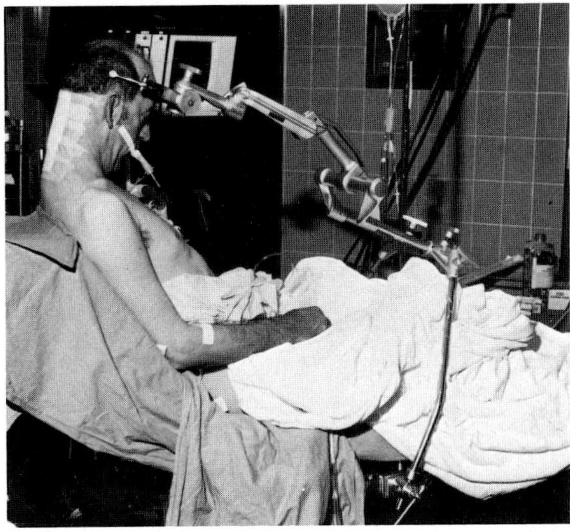

Fig. 11-21. The patient is positioned in the upright position with the Garner headrest and tongs.

inae, either with a diamond bur or small, sharp curettes (Figs. 11-17 and 11-22).[15] The laminae is exposed as for the hemilaminectomy but usually with a smaller incision. The foraminal opening is then created with a curette or burr, avoiding the introduction of the Kerrison or Schlesinger punch because this might further compress the underlying root. When dealing with an unusual degree of compression, one can enlarge the opening by removing a larger amount of lamina above and below, depending on the amount of compression that is disclosed by use of nerve hooks or dural elevators. Similarly, when it is necessary to introduce curettes or small pituitary forceps for removal of the spurs or extruded fragments, respectively, the opening may have to be enlarged inferiorly by removing more of the superior laminae of the vertebrae below (Figs. 11-18 and 11-23).

MULTIPLE LESIONS

The best results using the posterior approach are secured in patients who present a single-level disc extrusion or soft disc herniation as opposed to those who present with multiple root compression defects as visualized on the myelogram. Decompression of multiple levels increases the risk of neurologic deficit (usually temporarily), even with the gentlest of techniques. Epstein and colleagues report no such problem in a series of 57 cases with decompression of three or four levels in 70% of the patients.[5] Spinal fusion is rarely indicated in

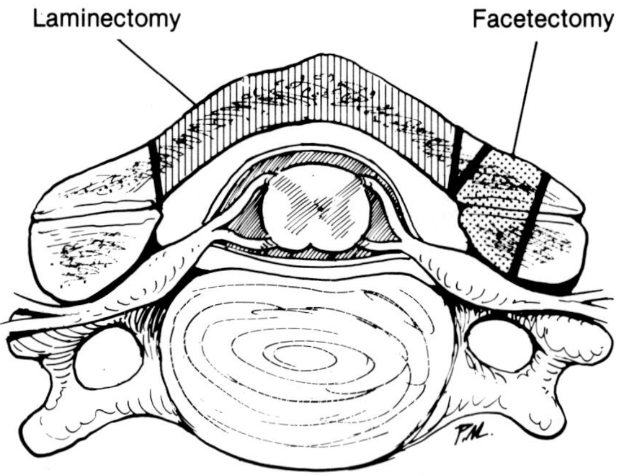

Fig. 11-22. Cross section graphically illustrating the areas of removal for central laminectomy and those for a partial facetectomy. (After Brain WR, Wilkinson JL: Cervical Spondylosis and Other Disorders of the Spine. Philadelphia, WB Saunders, 1967)

such cases but can be carried out either posteriorly or anteriorly in those cases in which it is desirable or necessary to stabilize one or more interspaces. When it is desirable to combine an anterior fusion with posterior decompression, we prefer that the anterior fusion be staged electively at a later date, although we have in the past done both at the same time.

Occasionally one encounters small extruded disc fragments associated with intraluminal spurs in cases of spondylotic radiculopathy, and one must, therefore, be on the lookout for such lesions at the time of spur removal. Meticulous hemostasis must be secured with adequate exposure, with bipolar coagulation and the use of small pledgets of gel foam and gentle packing with small cottonoids.

As pointed out by Ruge and Wiltse, gentleness and restraint are essential in retracting neural structures when searching for extruded disc fragments or attempting to expose spurs (Fig. 11-24). The desire to produce a specimen should be suppressed.[14] If such lesions are not readily visualized, one should be content with adequate posterior decompression and hemostasis. Medial retraction of the spinal cord is contraindicated.

The use of a head lamp and magnification with an operating microscope or loupe greatly enhances the safety and accuracy of the procedures described herein.

STABILITY

In performing posterior decompression it is important to avoid destabilization caused by remov-

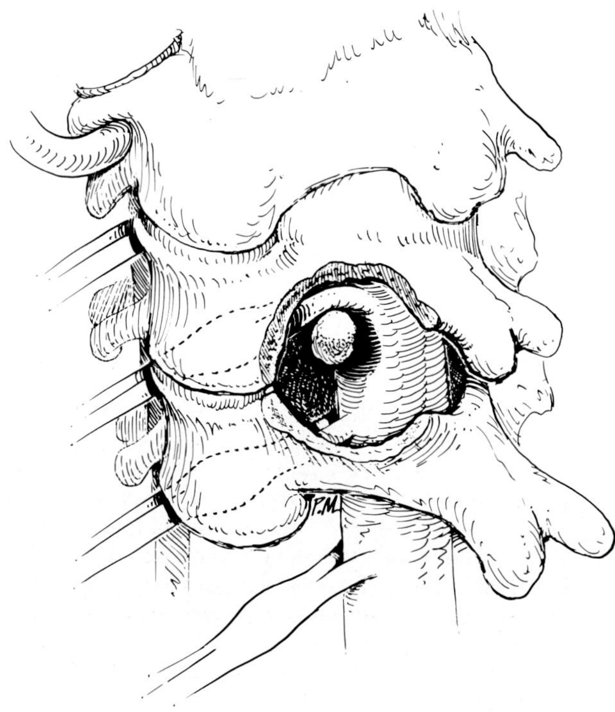

Fig. 11-23. Extruded disc fragment presenting ventral and inferior to the nerve root. (After Ruge D, Wiltse LL: Spinal Disorders. Philadelphia, Lea & Febiger, 1977)

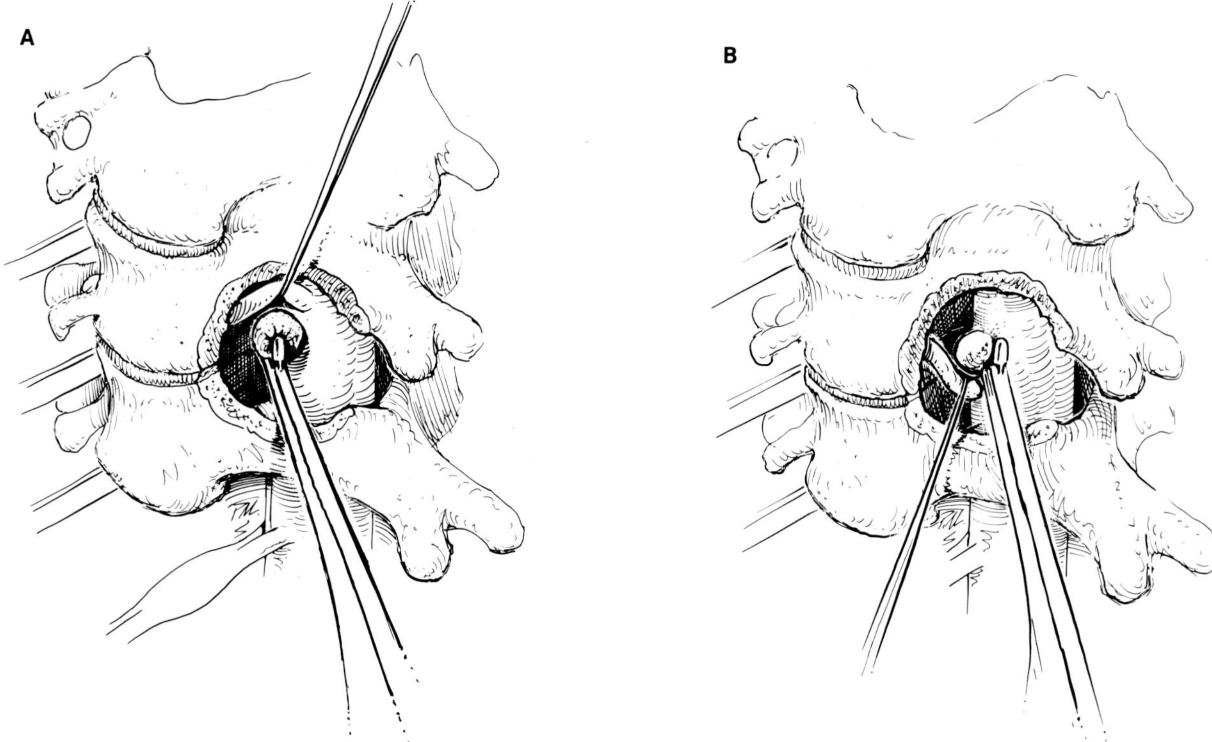

Fig. 11-24. Removal of the disc. (*A*) Removal distal to the root with a gentle retraction of the nerve root. (*B*) Removal cephalad to the root. Fragments present inferiorly much more commonly. (After Ruge D, Wiltse LL: Spinal Disorders. Philadelphia, Lea & Febiger, 1977)

ing too much of the facet, especially if the procedure is done bilaterally. There have been instances of anterior subluxation occurring at a given interspace because the central laminectomy has been extended too widely on either side. Removing the stabilizing effects of the spinous processes, the interspinous and superspinous ligaments, and ligamentum flavum, and then removing too much of the facets, may permit the development of a spondylolisthesis. This may endanger the spinal cord, which would then have to be corrected by spinal fusion.

In other patients, taking away too much of a facet, even unilaterally, can destabilize an interspace, from a mechanical standpoint. This may lead to mechanical neck pain, which requires stabilization.

In patients for whom there has been an extensive central laminectomy requiring spinal fusion, the preferred method is that of Robinson and Southwick,[12,13] using multiple wires through the inferior articular processes into laterally placed iliac grafts. On the other hand, when the instability is confined to one or two interspaces, an anterior fusion is my preference.

REFERENCES

1. *BRAIN WR, WILKINSON JL:* Cervical Spondylosis and Other Disorders of the Spine. Philadelphia, WB Saunders, 1967
2. *CLOWARD RB:* Treatment of ruptured intervertebral discs; observations on their formation and treatment. Am J Surg 84:151, 1952
3. *CLOWARD RB:* The anterior approach for removal of ruptured discs. J Neurosurg 15:602, 1958
4. *EPSTEIN JA, CARRAS R, HYMAN RA, ET AL:* Cervical myelopathy caused by developmental stenosis of the spine canal. J Neurosurg 51:362, 1979
5. *EPSTEIN JA, CARRAS R, LAVINE LS, ET AL:* The importance of removing osteophytes as part of the surgical treatment of myeloradiculopathy in cervical spondylosis. J Neurosurg 30:219, 1969
6. *EPSTEIN JA, EPSTEIN BS, LAVINE LS, ET AL:* Clinical

monoradiculopathy caused by arthrotic hypertrophy. J Neurosurg 49:387, 1978

7. *Epstein JA, Lavine LS, Aronson HA, et al:* Cervical spondylotic radiculopathy. Clin Orthop 40:113, 1965
8. *Frykholm R:* Cervical nerve root compression resulting from disc degeneration and root-sleeve fibrosis: A clinical investigation. Acta Chir Scand (Suppl) 160:v, 1951
9. *Hoi Song U, Wilson CB:* Postoperative epidural hematoma as a complication of anterior cervical discotomy: Report of 3 cases. J Neurosurg 49:288, 1978
10. *Holt S, Yates PO:* Cervical spondylosis and nerve root lesions: Incidence and routine necropsy. J Bone Joint Surg 48B:407, 1966
11. *Murphey R, Semmes J:* Ruptured cervical discs. Am J Surg 32:83, 1966
12. *Robinson RA, Southwick WO:* Indications and techniques for early stabilization of neck in some fracture dislocations of the cervical spine. So Med J 23:565, 1960
13. *Robinson RA, Southwick WO:* Surgical approaches to the cervical spine. Instruct Course Lecture, AAOS 17:299, 1960
14. *Ruge D, Wiltse LL:* Spinal Disorders. Philadelphia, Lea & Febiger, 1977
15. *Scoville WB:* Cervical spondylosis treated by bilateral facetectomy and laminectomy. J Neurosurg 18:423, 1961
16. *Scoville WB, Whitcomb BB, McLaurin R:* The cervical ruptured disc: Report of 115 operative cases. Trans Am Neurol Assoc 76:222, 1951
17. *Simmons JCH:* In Edmonson AS, Crenshaw AA (eds): Campbell's Operative Orthopaedics, 6th ed, Vol 2, p 2126. St. Louis, CV Mosby, 1980
18. *Smith GW, Robinson RA:* Anterior lateral cervical disc removal and interbody fusion for cervical disc syndrome. Bull Johns Hopkins Hosp 96:223, 1955
19. *Smith GW, Robinson RA:* The treatment of cervical spine disorders by anterior removal of the intervertebral disc and interbody fusion. J Bone Joint Surg 40A:607, 1958
20. *Spurling RG, Scoville WB:* Lateral rupture of the cervical intervertebral discs: A common cause of shoulder and arm pain. Surg Gynecol Obstet 78:350, 1944
21. *Spurling RB, Segerberg LH:* Lateral intervertebral disc lesions in the lower cervical region. JAMA 151:354, 1953
22. *Teng P:* Spondylosis of the cervical spine with compression of the spinal cord and the nerve roots. J Bone Joint Surg 42A:392, 1960

The Surgical Management of Cervical Spinal Stenosis, Spondylosis, and Myeloradiculopathy by Means of the Posterior Approach

JOSEPH A. EPSTEIN AND NANCY E. EPSTEIN

The management of cervical spinal stenosis and spondylotic myeloradiculopathy has passed through many phases. Initial results of the various approaches justified optimism that has since been tempered by experience and technical innovations, with larger groups of patients over extended periods of time. The number of surgical procedures now used provides ample evidence that no single technique can solve all the anatomic and pathologic problems presented by this disorder; each patient must be evaluated based on the particular characteristics of the set of clinical findings. Methods presently used include anterior and anterolateral approaches, as well as decompression by means of laminectomy, foraminotomy, and neurolysis, with and without the excision of osteophytes. In addition, newer procedures initiated by our Japanese colleagues and referred to as "open-door expansive laminoplasty" have been used to enlarge the spinal canal over multiple segments by preserving a laminar roof over the intact dura. Conservative treatment, however, still has a role in the management of this disorder.

The most common cause of failure, as for all operative procedures, is the improper selection of the patient. At times, it is extremely difficult to separate individuals with evidence of early motor neuron disease and demyelinizing disorders from those who have myeloradiculopathy caused by cervical stenosis and spondylosis. Indeed, the conditions may coexist. The decision to operate must be based on meticulous neurologic evaluation supplemented by appropriate x-rays, including CT scanning after myelography. Magnetic resonance imaging (MRI) is now used as a supplementary diagnostic aid. Valuable information is also derived from electromyography and from the study of sensory-evoked potentials in the search for nuchal delay. CT scanning of the brain is also helpful in elderly individuals suspected of having normal-pressure hydrocephalus or cerebellar dysfunction on a degenerative or vascular basis.

Cervical spondylosis without coexisting stenosis can be productive of myelopathy. However, individuals with preexisting congenital stenosis become early candidates for myeloradiculopathy associated with the development of degenerative arthropathy that further intrudes into available space. Patients with normal or large canals may develop evidence of advanced spondylosis with little or no relevant spinal cord or nerve root dysfunction until the spondylotic intrusions increase in size and the canal becomes significantly compromised. Other factors causing the cervical canal to narrow are found in patients with hyperlordosis and shingling, with thickening of the yellow ligaments and arthrotic deformities that involve both the posterior facets and the lamina.[13,15,17]

DIAGNOSTIC EVALUATION: CLINICAL FINDINGS

Patients spontaneously develop symptoms of myelopathy over an extended time interval. This includes an unsteady gait with long-tract signs, such as spasticity, hyperreflexia, and extensor plantar responses. Minor trauma can accentuate or precipitate symptoms. Motor abnormalities dominate. Weakness and atrophy of the upper extremities occurs, with a loss of dexterity that progresses, at times, to complete uselessness of the hands. Here atrophy and motor alterations are compounded by sensory deficits approaching stereoanesthesia. This usually occurs in the higher cervical lesions. Lhermitte's sign with flexion or extension of the neck is an important indication of spinal compression. A neurologic level determined principally by reflex changes has diagnostic value. For instance, when the biceps reflex is diminished or absent, and is associated with hyperreflexia of the triceps and finger flexor responses, the anatomic level of the major pathology is usually at C5–C6.

Long-tract signs may precede or follow the alterations in hand function, but they usually occur earlier in patients with congenital spinal stenosis. Sensory changes initially are poorly localized and may ascend from the lower extremities to the mid-level areas of the trunk, and rarely to a cervical level. If the hands are involved, the fingertips lose sensation to light touch, number writing, and other forms of superficial sensation, although position sense is preserved. Weakness of the shoulder girdle, hyperactive biceps, and pectoralis reflexes usually indicates a lesion higher in the cervical canal. In older individuals, a positive snout or palmar mental reflex may be elicited. These findings, especially in the presence of gross fasciculations, may be the earliest manifestations of motor neuron disease. We prefer to maintain a conservative attitude under such circumstances. Multiple small strokes and/or normal-pressure hydrocephalus make surgery rarely rewarding. MRI preoperatively helps to exclude demyelinizing diseases, cerebral vascular disease and neoplastic or cystic lesions of the cervical cord and brain stem. Sphincter disturbances occur, but they are not an outstanding finding. They indicate a less favorable prognosis, especially in association with posterior column dysfunction.[16,18,19]

Pain is not a dominant complaint. The various cervicobrachial disorders with nerve root pathology only are not discussed in this report.[50]

Approximately 10% will have associated lumbar stenosis, which may or may not have clinical manifestations.[17] In such patients, if myelopathy is present, it is mandatory to perform the more critical cervical decompression first, and then to consider a secondary lumbar laminar decompression as conditions permit. Total myelography is indicated for this reason.

NEURORADIOLOGIC EVALUATION

A complete radiologic examination is essential for confirming the clinical impression of cervical spinal stenosis in its various manifestations. The ventrodorsal diameter of the stenotic canal usually measures less than 1.2 cm.[14,18,68] Stenosis is further confirmed by tomograms, CT myelography, and MRI studies, the latter being supplemented by both flexion and extension views. In the congenitally narrowed canal (Fig. 11-25), almost the entire length of the spinal canal is narrowed to critical levels.[12,14] The uppermost levels at C1 and C2 must also be carefully evaluated, since stenosis may be overlooked in this region. Here it is often associated with congenital anomalies, most often block vertebrae.[19,47] Failure to recognize high levels of stenosis will compromise the results of the laminar decompression, which may not be adequately extensive.

Iohexol is the best tolerated water-soluble contrast agent currently used for myelography. Unfortunately, the need for the patient to remain in the upright position for at least 8 hours after the procedure usually results in the loss of spinal fluid through the needle opening in the dura, resulting in a flaccid dural envelope at surgery. This loss of the "dural tampon" can lead to excessive bleeding from the epidural veins. Waiting several days for the opening to seal itself, and for the restored fullness of the dural envelope, can be helpful. The patient should be properly hydrated and medicated before myelography. Deterioration after myelography can occur, especially if the patient's head and neck are maintained for long intervals in a position of hyperextension during the procedure.

Myelography usually reveals multiple levels of block with the cord splayed out in its transverse diameter (Fig. 11-26). In most patients with spondylostenosis limited to only one or two levels, the changes are apparent in a restricted segmental pattern.[12] If neither finding is present, it is doubtful that the disorder is a spondylotic-stenotic myelopathy. The most common trap set for the unsuspecting clinician is the appearance of myelographic ladder-like defects without compressive changes in the spinal cord or nerve roots in patients with large canals.[13,14,17–19]

CT and CT myelography of the cervical spine provide valuable information, especially the A–P diameter of the spinal canal at any given level. This study can define the shape of the spinal cord, the presence of osteophytes, and foraminal changes caused by arthrotic posterior facets and associated disc protrusions. Changes in the angle of the gantry may result in artifacts that simulate narrowing. Delayed studies using CT myelography have shown multiple cystic changes, which may be of prognostic value, within the spinal cord.[34]

MRI has proved to be an important diagnostic tool in evaluating both intrinsic and extrinsic spinal cord changes including atrophy, cystic degeneration, and the effects of posture on the spinal cord itself. The use of surface coils in MRI is extremely helpful for obtaining sharper images. Such studies are also important postoperatively in the presence of complications or as a means of following adequate displacement of the spinal cord posteriorly into an expanded dural sac (Fig. 11-27*A*,*B*).

PATHOLOGY

Ono and colleagues described the clinical and pathologic findings at the postmortem examination in five patients who were never treated surgically for spondylotic myelopathy.[51] In these patients with typical stenosis, spinal cord atrophy occurred over multiple segments and was not confined to a single level. Pyramidal tract involvement was particularly profound, with ascending and descending demyelinization. There was severe gray matter destruction, with obliteration of the intrinsic vessels. Infarction extended over both gray and

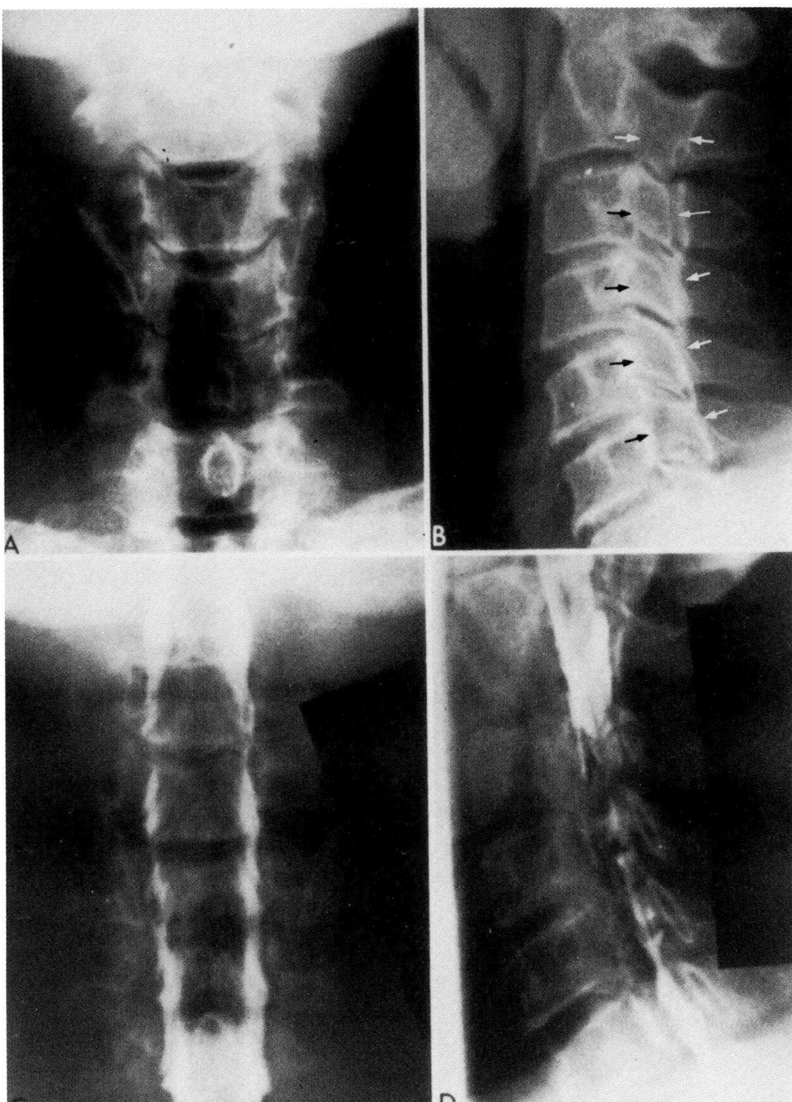

Fig. 11-25. These films are of a 24-year-old man with weakness of his upper extremities and a spastic gait following a hyperextension neck injury. There are no significant degenerative changes on plain films (*A*). The canal in the lateral view (*B*), is narrowed ventrodorsally averaging 1.2 cm from C2 through C7, with a shallow neural arch indicated by the base of the spinous processes and lamina approximating the tips of the facets (*white arrows*). The myelogram (Iophendylate) shows splaying of the spinal cord over multiple segments (*C* and *D*).[17]

white matter, although the former was more seriously compromise. A variable and inconstant pattern was observed among the patients. In all patients the anterior white columns were spared. Aberrant proliferation of Schwann cells was noted in the posterior white column. The levels of maximal cord compression corresponded to the most severely infarcted areas of the cord.

Holt and Yates studied 120 cervical spines removed at autopsy from elderly patients.[30] Osteoarthritis of the apophyseal joints was found in 78, and was most common in the middle and upper cervical regions. Degeneration and scarring of the nerve roots was frequently found with diseased discs. These changes were accentuated in the presence of apophyseal arthrosis. No root changes could be attributed to ischemia from narrowing or distortion of the vertebral arteries. Cysts with arachnoidal diverticula excavating the posterior root ganglia were found in 36 cases. The main histologic changes were essentially limited to the dorsal nerve root and ganglion. There was a diffuse increase in the fibrous tissue of the endoneurium in the ganglia, with degeneration of axis cylinders and myelin sheaths. Such changes are closely related to the clinical findings in advanced cases and

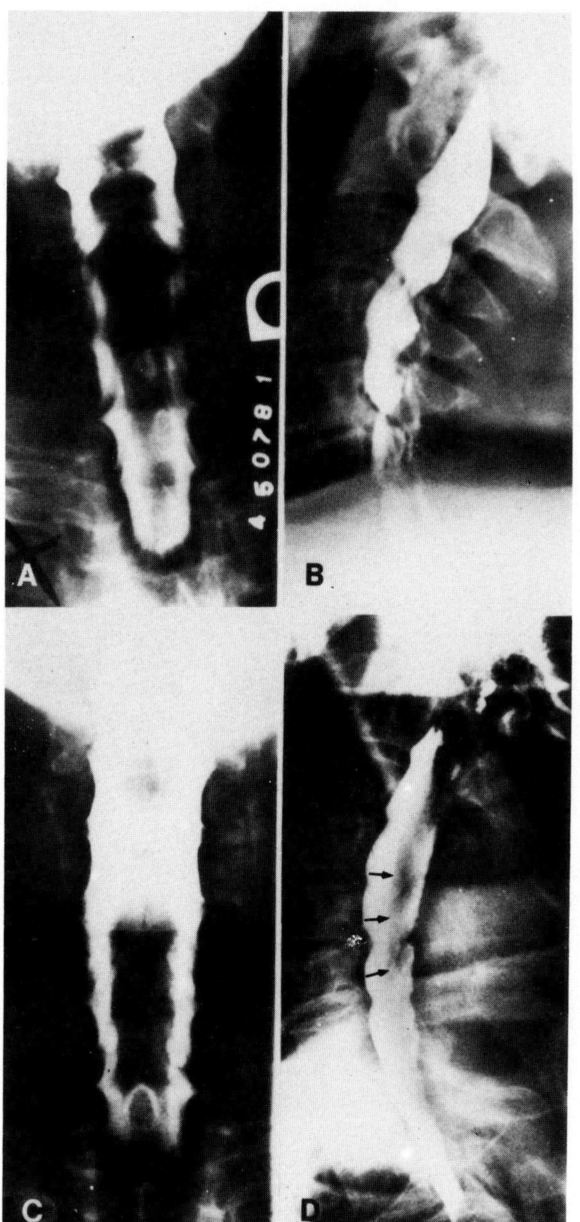

Fig. 11-26. A 54-year-old man with myelopathy caused by cervical stenosis and complicated by spondylosis. The preoperative myelogram (Iophendylate) (*A* and *B*) shows flattening of the cord in the A–P projection at both C4–C5 and C5–C6 caused by dorsal and ventral intrusions into the spinal canal. Spur formation is most evident at C5–C6, with prominent dorsal intrusions extending from C3–C4 to C6–C7 and a "pincer" effect at C5–C6. Shingling of the lamina is seen at C3–C4 and C4–C5, the latter complicated by infolding of the yellow ligaments and dura extending into the lower cervical segments. The postoperative myelogram (*C* and *D*), following laminectomy from C3 to C7, foraminotomy and excision of the ventral spurs at C5–C6, shows a resumption of the normal spinal cord pattern in the A–P projection (C) and a dorsal migration of the cord in the lateral exposure (D) into a new, expanded canal. The lordotic curve is well preserved, the minor intrusions in the floor of the canal are well away from the ventral surface of the negative cord shadow that is clearly evident in this extraordinary film (*arrows*). (From Epstein JA, Epstein BS: Handbook of Clinical Neurology, Vol 32, pp 342–343, 1978)

account for the lack of improvement after operation.

INDICATIONS FOR SURGERY

Surgical decompression is indicated in patients with progressive impairment of function without sustained remission. Irreversible changes may well occur within the spinal cord and nerve roots, including the ganglia; therefore, the time factor is critical. The best results are obtained in patients whose symptoms are less than 6-months duration, with evidence of only mild myelopathic alterations and few sensory changes.

Nonoperative care has a definite role in management, especially in patients who are poor operative risks, who have dense neurologic deficits, or who for any reason are reluctant to undergo

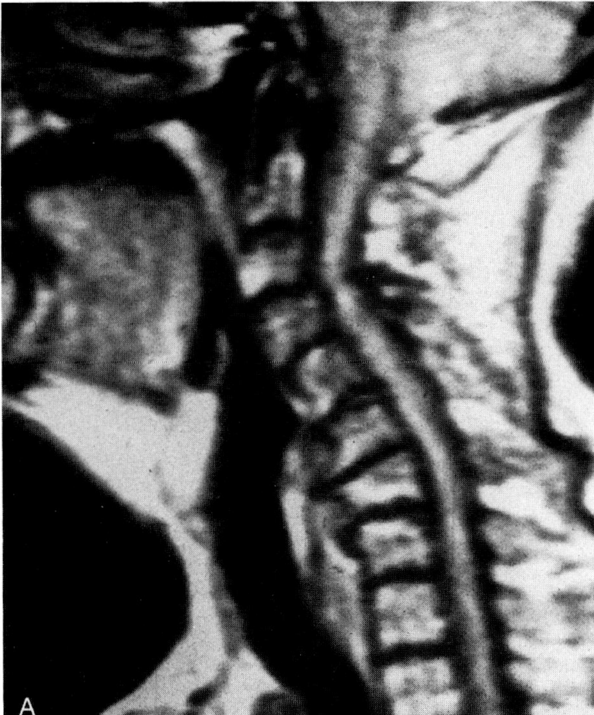

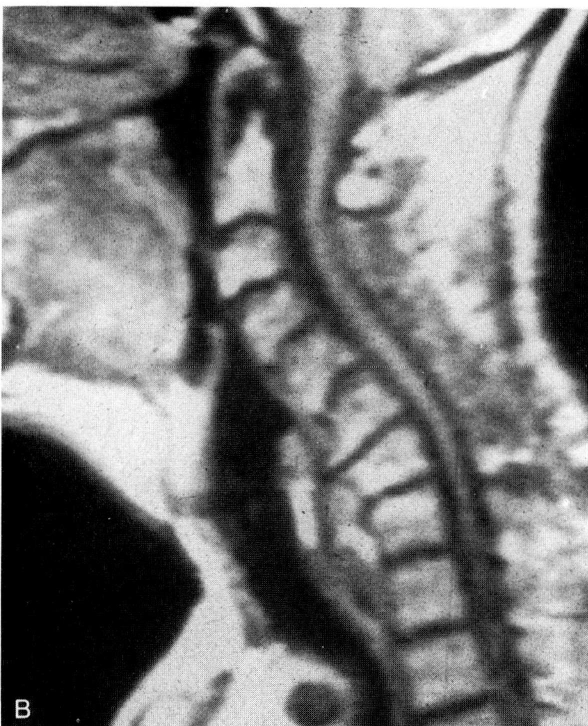

Fig. 11-27. Preoperative and postoperative MRI studies in a 76-year-old man with hyperlordosis and shingling, and severe myeloradiculopathy with extreme functional loss of both hands. The preoperative study (T1-weighted image) (*A*) shows marked impingement on the cord both ventrally and dorsally at C3–C4 and C4–C5. The postoperative scan (7 days) (*B*) shows dorsal migration of the cord into an expanded canal with resolution of the previous effects of the spurs and infolded yellow ligaments.

surgery.[6,42,49,56] Supportive care includes the use of a cervical collar to restrict cervical motion, physical therapy, and nonsteroidal antiinflammatory drugs, especially if pain complicates the clinical picture.

Poor surgical candidates are individuals with advanced neurologic changes and essentially fixed lesions in the spinal cord, nerve roots, and ganglia.[30,51] This most often occurs in older patients whose diagnosis has been delayed because of obscure findings and avoidance of medical care. The best result that could be anticipated under such circumstances would be the prevention of further deterioration and perhaps some slight improvement in gait and hand function. Diabetic patients and patients who are chronic alcoholics have associated neuropathy and myelopathy, cerebellar dysfunction, cerebral disorders, and a higher incidence of complications such as infection and poor wound healing. Cerebrovascular disease is a negative factor, as previously indicated. Although age is apparently no contraindication to surgery, the patient who elects to be operated on should be well motivated and robust, with significant family support. Depressed individuals and those using disability for secondary gain must be avoided. Patients who have fluctuating signs, a rapidly changing clinical picture, and a history of multiple trauma, rarely do well with surgery performed on an urgent basis. In fact, such rapidly advancing and changing patterns contraindicate surgery until the patient's status has stabilized.[65] This is especially true in patients with central cord injuries.[5]

Laminectomy is not indicated in patients who have a kyphotic deformity of the cervical spine. Those with flexion abnormalities are best treated by anterior vertebrectomy and strut fusion, although decompression through the foramen magnum has been suggested by Aboulker and Alsharif.[1,3] With reversal of cervical curve and swan-neck deformities, any procedure permitting further kyphosis, such as laminectomy and facetectomy, is contraindicated.

In patients born with congenitally narrowed spinal canals (Fig. 11-25), hyperextension injury without fracture or dislocation may result in devastating trauma to the spinal cord, usually in association with a central cord injury, including hematomyelia.[16] Laminectomy should be considered only after the neurologic status has stabilized, and it may result in further improvement.[5]

PREOPERATIVE PREPARATION

The patient's entire head, cervical, and shoulder areas should be shampooed with Betadine soap the night before surgery and once again the morning of the procedure. The neck and occipital areas are shaved after the head is placed in a neutral position using the three-pin head holder. The seated position has proved to be invaluable for the performance of this procedure. A relatively dry field is obtainable so that precise identification of the nerve roots is possible, while unusual trauma in the foramenal areas is avoided. Air embolism has not been a significant factor in our large series of patients if the proper precautions are taken.[44,46] These include elevating the flexed lower extremities, wrapping the extremities securely in ace bandages, or more recently using alternate compression stockings. A central venous line is inserted as a precautionary measure; this procedure has recently been questioned, because the possible complications from using the central venous line far exceed the benefits. However, its presence is reassuring to the operating physician should embolism occur despite the usual preventive measures. Only the lowest levels of Post Expiratory End Pressure should be employed, if it is used at all. It must not be used in patients with suspected septal defects.[44,46] The monitoring of arterial pressure is mandatory. Any drop in pressure with impaired perfusion to a critically stressed spinal cord may result in quadriparesis or plegia. End tidal CO_2 values and the Doppler apparatus provide the means of early detection of air embolism, both quantitatively and qualitatively. If possible, adequate fluids (1 L Ringer's lactate) should be given to fully hydrate the patient before sitting him up to maintain blood volume. The neutral position of the head and neck avoids stretching the spinal cord against a ventral ridge. Hyperextension is also contradindicated because of dorsal intrusion into the spinal canal of hypertrophied, infolded yellow ligaments coincident with thickening of the cord.[8,52,55]

The patient is given 10 mg of dexamethasone intravenously, prior to the induction of anesthesia. It is continued for 4 to 7 days postoperatively, in decreasing doses, beginning with 4 mg q6h, with the supplementary use of antacids and/or cimetidine. Local infiltration of the paraspinal muscles with a long-acting local anesthetic supplemented with epinephrine is used prior to making the incision. This relieves local pain considerably, limits blood loss, and less anesthesia is needed.

Patients with pulmonary fibrosis, emphysema, or similar disorders have elevated thoracic venous pressure and can bleed excessively from engorged epidural veins. This should be treated before surgery to minimize complications. All nonsteroidal antiinflammatory drugs should be stopped for an adequate period before surgery.

OPERATION

Intubation is best achieved with the patient awake, avoiding hyperextension of the neck. Fiberoptic assistance may be helpful.

Laminectomy is performed using an en face technique (Fig. 11-28). This technique may be facilitated by cutting longitudinal channels in the extreme lateral portions of the lamina using a high-speed air drill and/or a small Kerrison punch and by lifting the free lamina away from the underlying cord.[20] This avoids inserting any instrument beneath the lamina. Removal of the lamina is begun inferiorly and extended toward the more cranial segments with the decompression extending at least two segments above and below the major areas of stenosis. If stenosis is multisegmental, as in the developmental type, the laminae from C3 through C7 should be removed. If the canal is also narrowed at the C1–C2 level, the arch of C2 may be undercut or removed entirely. It rarely is necessary to remove the arch of C1. The spinous process at C2 provides the major attachment for the erector spinae muscles, and its preservation is a major factor preventing subsequent flexion deformity. The erector spinae muscles should not be dissected laterally beyond the facets in order to avoid denervation, another factor disposing to flexion deformity postoperatively. Self-retaining retractors should be relaxed periodically to avoid compromising circulation with subsequent tissue necrosis.

The cervical lordosis must be maintained. With removal of the lamina, the dura bulges posteriorly into the area of decompression. The spinal cord moves away from the floor of the canal and away from ventral intrusions, assuming a shorter course with less axial tension (Figs. 11-26 and 11-29). This also facilitates manipulation beneath the nerve roots and dura. The dura is not opened, and its tamponade effect is preserved. The lateral recesses are unroofed, and foraminal decompression is then performed, primarily by means of a medial facetectomy that removes, at most, one quarter to one third of the medial margins. Undercutting is done if further decompression is necessary (Fig. 11-28*A* to *C*).[54] A small diamond bur may be helpful. Under most circumstances, however, small micropunches of 2 to 3 mm, with the tips angled at 30 degrees and filed to a thin point, should be adequate to remove the portions of the superior and inferior articular facets that cover the nerve root. Small, but extremely sharp, up-biting curettes also aid in this portion of the procedure (Fig. 11-28*A* to *C*). It should be noted that with the patient in the seated position, the nerve roots are usually oriented horizontally or are directed upward; this is especially evident at the levels of C4–C5 and C5–C6, where the nerve roots closely approximate the pedicles and are cradled in the hook formed by the superior articular facets (Fig. 11-28*A* to *C*). Since the foramen is essentially funnel-shaped with its narrowest portion situated medially, only limited portions of the facets need to be sacrificed, and stability is preserved. Root sleeve adhesions are separated using small micro hooks and dissectors (Fig. 11-28*A* to *C*).

In at least one third of these patients, the motor and sensory nerve roots are often separate structures.[30] The sensory root usually covers the upper portion of the smaller motor root. The latter has only a thin cover of dura, and therefore, it is unusually vulnerable to trauma (Fig. 11-28*A*,*B*). It also has a slightly reddish color compared with the more yellow-white color of the more prominent and protected sensory root, where the covering of dura is of greater thickness. Once the nerve root is released from the tethering effect of root sleeve adhesions, the insertion of small down-biting sharp curettes beneath and medial to the nerve root makes it possible to scrape out the underlying spurs. These spurs usually rest on the cortical bone surface of the vertebral body and can be removed down to this level (Fig. 11-28*C*). When the spinal cord has moved posteriorly away from the floor of the canal after the laminar decompression (the "bow string" position), we have found it unnecessary to vigorously attempt to remove any medially lying spurs, although this can be accomplished (Fig. 11-29). In poor-risk individuals, where the difficulty of the procedure has been further compromised by bleeding or other untoward reactions, a simple foraminal decompression may be adequate to provide essential relief of neural entrapment.[35,59] Concern for spurs in the midventral quadrants has decreased, since the spinal cord can tolerate plastic deformity if the canal is expanded and dorsal migration occurs. Removal of spurs is almost impossible with the patient in the prone position, because of poor visibility and a wet field.

In individuals with myelopathy caused primarily by congenital spinal stenosis extending over multiple levels, it is only necessary to perform extensive laminectomy and limited foraminal decompression (Fig. 11-25). Such individuals are usually younger, and they present primarily with long-tract signs. Degenerative changes are absent or minimal, and the foramina are rarely compromised.[14,28]

When bleeding does occur from epidural veins despite precautions, the use of bipolar coagulation and strips of gelfoam soaked in thrombin and peroxide can be extremely helpful in controlling oozing in the lateral gutters. Small pledgets of Oxycel cotton* or Surgicel,† if used in a similar manner, must be removed. These substances swell and if placed in the immediate proximity of a nerve root or the spinal cord itself can cause further compression. The use of Avitene‡ has also been helpful and has not caused any specific problems. Hydrogen peroxide appears to aid in achieving hemostasis, either by raising the local temperature or by contributing to coagulation by aggregation of platelets on the foamy surface. Although nonabsorbable sutures were used previously, we now use absorbable coated Vicryl§ with satisfactory results, reducing the amount of foreign material left in the wound. Suction drainage, even if remotely indicated, should be used for the first 12 to 24 hours if oozing persists or if the dura remains flaccid after myelography.

Transfusion is rarely required in the seated position. Every effort is made to maintain perfusion pressures and oxygenation during and after the operative procedure, followed by close monitoring for the first 24 to 48 hours. Patients are allowed to stand and void the day of surgery if vital signs

* Oxidized cellulose

† Oxidized regenerated cellulose

‡ Microfibrillar collagen hemostat

§ Polyglactin-910

are stable, caution being taken to avoid any abrupt change of posture. Ambulation is gradually resumed the following day. The patient wears long elastic stockings and, if needed, an abdominal support. A Philadelphia collar is worn for the first 7 to 14 days postoperatively, after which a moderately firm foam collar may be used for an additional 1 to 2 weeks.

The majority of these patients are in the sixth and seventh decades of life and if significant intraoperative problems develop, the surgeon should not hesitate to abort the procedure. Unusual blood loss with hypotension, electrocardiographic changes, and other alterations in the vital signs, especially those suggesting impaired perfusion, are examples of the major problems that can occur.

Braughler and Hall demonstrated that methylprednisolone sodium succinate (MPSS) in experi-

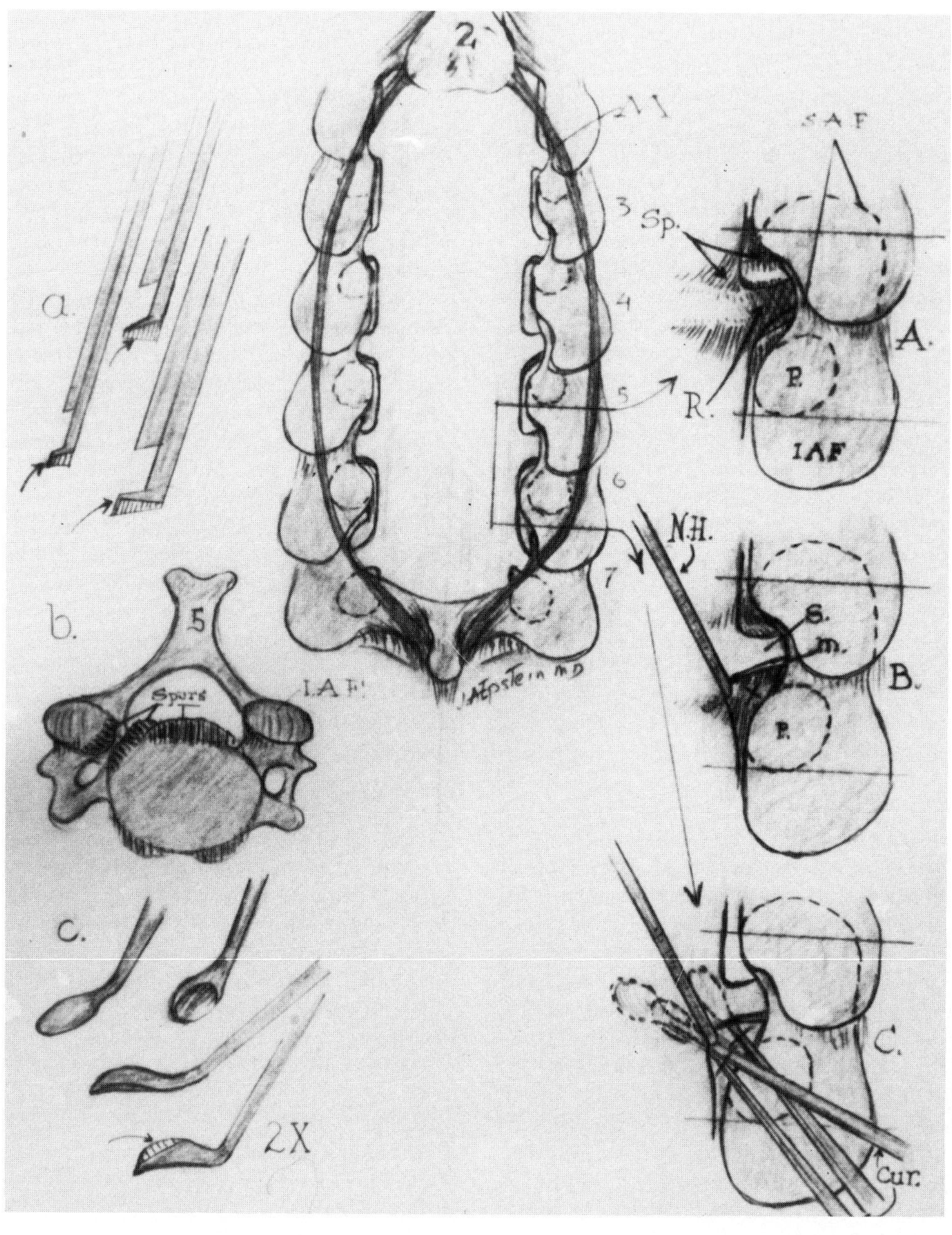

mental animals can prevent posttraumatic spinal cord ischemia.[7,27] Once ischemia has developed, however, its effect is limited and is probably lost within a few hours of onset, which underscores the need for early treatment. The use of dexamethasone or MPSS intraoperatively may have definite advantages in this regard in the presence of inadvertent or unrecognized injury to the cord or impaired perfusion. The advantages appear to outweigh the disadvantages of this drug.[7,27,32]

Dexamethasone also reduces postoperative pain significantly and permits early ambulation. Older individuals have depleted adrenal reserves and tolerate stress poorly; specifically in this type of person it has proven essential in postoperative management. Vital signs are more readily stabilized. The patient becomes more alert and responsive to a program of early ambulation and self care. Patients with diabetes require more restricted use of dexamethasone which is usually discontinued sooner. Blood sugar values are followed closely and controlled with the judicious use of insulin and diet. A peptic ulcer or a history of gastrointestinal bleeding requires the supplementary use of Cimetidine and antacids under careful supervision. Prophylactic antibiotics are used for 2 days.

The average postoperative stay in the hospital is approximately 7 days. Isometric exercises are started as soon as the incisional pain has subsided and are followed by supplementary physical therapy and a program of rehabilitation. Exercises are mandatory to strengthen the cervical musculature and to maintain the normal lordotic curve of the cervical spine.

The advantage of this technique is that circumferential decompression of the cervical spinal canal and foramina can be obtained by a single operative procedure. Only rarely is additional anterior decompression and fusion required, because of abnormal mobility or subluxation. An anticipated satisfactory result with improvement or stabilization can be achieved in 80 to 85% of such patients.

The charts outline and summarize the factors affecting prognosis (Table 11-1, 11-2) as well as deterrents (Table 11-3), operative precautions (Table 11-4), and complications (Table 11-5).

Fig. 11-28. The central illustration indicates the dorsal decompression required by laminectomy with unroofing of the lateral recesses and foraminotomy. This, at most, includes the innermost one quarter to one third of the foramina, which can be enlarged by an undercutting technique using the filed-down Kerrison punches indicated in *A*. In *A*, the root sleeve adhesions (*R*) are removed by use of microdissection if necessary, with care taken to preserve both motor and sensory roots. The sensory root (*S*), for the most part, covers the underlying motor root (*M*), with the latter often being obscured by scar formation that binds it to the underlying osteophyte. After freeing the root, a nerve hook (*NH*) is used to elevate the root upward and slightly medially; various downbiting curettes (c) can then be used to remove the underlying spurs down to the cortical bone surface both at the level of the foramen and medially as in *C*. The deltoid is uniquely innervated by a single root (C5), in which the motor fibers are the dominant constituent. This may result in paralysis following manipulation. The motor changes usually resolve in time. Elevation of the arms at surgery reduces axial tension on all roots and is recommended to help avoid this complication. In *B*, the spurs are shown not only arising from the vertebral margins in the midline and laterally into the foramen, but also involving the facet. The oval area (*M*) in the central illustration indicates the extent of muscle retraction. The attachments of the muscles to the spinous process of C2, and to the spinous processes below, should be preserved. Note that in *A*, various sized Kerrison punches are filed down at the tips (*arrows*), as in the dome of the curette in *C*. This increases the safety of manipulation in confined spaces, avoiding undue pressure on neural elements. Note that excision of osteophytes should be performed only with clear visualization of the critical anatomy of the nerve roots. In our experience, this can best be achieved during the sitting position (see text). Since foraminal decompression can often be adequate to relieve most symptoms, one should be judicious in the selection of proper candidates for the more extensive procedure. (From Epstein JA: Contemporary Neurosurgery, Vol 7, No 18, p 4. Baltimore, Williams & Wilkins, 1985)

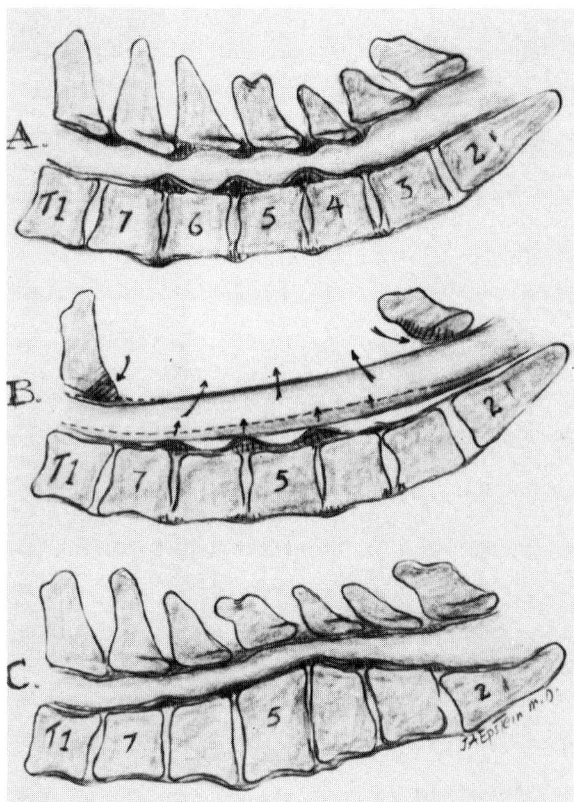

Fig. 11-29. (*A*) The narrowing of the spinal canal is further compromised by the ventral spurs at the three levels indicated, supplemented by intrusion of the ligamentum flavum dorsally. As a result of decompression (*B*), the dura expands and the cord migrates dorsally into the operative defect away from the ventral osteophytes (bow-string effect). This results in shortening of the cord, lessening of axial tension, and improved perfusion. (Epstein JA: Contemporary Neurosurgery, Vol 7, No 18, p 3. Baltimore, Williams & Wilkins, 1985)

BIODYNAMICS

The significance of osteophytes contributing to the development of radiculopathy and myelopathy has been investigated by Brieg and coworkers and by Reed, using a biomechanical approach.[8,55] These authors emphasize the need to avoid sustained contact of the spinal cord ventrally against spondylotic bars. In flexion, axial tension on the spinal cord increases. The anteroposterior diameter of the spinal cord decreases, deforming the lateral columns and the anterior horns while compromising circulation. Hyperextension results in relaxation of the spinal cord with thickening, as axial

Table 11-1. Factors Affecting Prognosis in Spondylostenosis Neurologic Disorders

1. Severity
2. Duration
3. Sensory motor
4. Myelopathy
5. Radiculopathy
6. Myeloradiculopathy
7. Entrapment syndromes: carpal tunnel
8. Peripheral neuropathy
9. Myopathy: steroid, thyroid, toxic, metabolic
10. Spincter disturbance
11. Duration of preoperative changes: fixed lesions
12. Age
13. Associated neurologic disorders: coexisting or latent, motor neuropathy (ALS), posterior lateral sclerosis, demyelinizing, central cord injury, vascular disease of spinal cord

Table 11-2. Factors Affecting Prognosis in Spondylostenosis Age-related Factors

1. Attitude, personality
2. Psychological disorders: depression
3. Socioeconomic factors
4. Cerebrovascular: stroke
5. Cardiovascular
6. Cerebral disorders: degenerative, normal pressure hydrocephalus
7. Peripheral vascular disease
8. Pulmonary obstructive disease
9. Anemia
10. Degenerative arthritis: knee, hip
11. Osteoporosis
12. Toxic-metabolic disorders: alcoholism, diabetes, myopathy, radiculopathy, myelopathy, polyneuropathy
13. Nutritional problems
14. Obesity

Table 11-3. Deterrents

1. Motor neuron disease
2. Long history in older individuals with fixed neurologic deficit (rare exceptions)
3. Alcoholic, diabetic
4. Pulmonary hypertension, heart disease, cerebrovascular disease
5. Cervical kyphosis
6. Depression, no motivation, no family support
7. Acute onset of symptoms with rapid progression

Table 11-4. Operative Precautions

1. Head-neck, neutral position
2. Infiltrate muscle, skin, fascia with Marcaine-Epinephrine
3. Keep PEEP to reasonable low levels or avoid
4. Avoid long periods of retraction of muscle: let up retractors (necrosis, denervation)
5. Preserve C2: anchor
6. Dura intact: wait several days after myelography—for turgid dural sac
7. Decadron 5 to 7 days (may start 24 hours preoperatively
8. Avoid hypotension—perfusion maintained

Table 11-5. Complications

1. Air embolism: rare and overrated as a primary concern; monitor, doppler, end tidal CO_2
2. Hematoma/blood loss: postoperative—avoid preoperative nonsteroidal antiinflammatory drugs; seated position used
3. Infection: prophylactic antibiotics—2 days
4. Quadriplegia: paresis, traumatic, vascular perfusion, hematoma
5. Monoplegia: Motor root vulnerable; adherent to osteophytes, especially C5
6. Postoperative subluxation: preserve facets; avoid muscle necrosis secondary to prolonged retraction and denervation; preserve attachments to C2 spinous process

tension is reduced and circulation is improved.[52] Infolded yellow ligaments, however, have intruded dorsally into the canal, especially in patients with hyperlordosis and shingling. These findings dictate the importance of the cervical spine being in a neutral position during cervical spine surgery in order to avoid undue iatrogenic trauma to the spinal cord through either an anterior or a posterior approach. Reed noted increased tension of the nerve roots over spurs with flexion of the neck, resulting in root sleeve fibrosis and interference with radicular blood flow.[55] He found that the normal function of the dentate ligaments is to transmit cephalocaudal axial stresses between the spinal cord and dura rather than to provide a mechanism to hold the cord in a particular dorsal or ventral position. Therefore, sectioning of the dentate ligaments has been discontinued. Leaving the dura intact avoids complications such as meningocele and spinal fluid leakage. A postoperative wound hematoma in the presence of an open dura can have catastrophic results.

The functional pathology of the cervical spine, including dynamic factors, has been well described by Penning.[52]

EVALUATION OF SURGICAL AND NONSURGICAL RESULTS: A REVIEW OF THE LITERATURE

In any evaluation of the results of treatment, patients who are operated on must be compared with those who are managed conservatively. Table 11-6 reviews the management of cervical myelopathy in 1355 patients gathered in 1982 and compares the results of conservative treatment with the results obtained by surgical procedures performed anteriorly, posteriorly, and anterolaterally.[19] In a combined group of 114 conservatively treated patients, 36% improved and 64% did not improve. However, of the latter group, 38% remained the same, whereas only 26% continued to deteriorate. Since only 26% failed to maintain their neurologic status (the others becoming either stable or improving) nonoperative care certainly deserves consideration for poor-risk patients or for individuals who refuse surgical intervention.[6,42,49,56]

Among the 1241 remaining patients that were operated on, 353 procedures were performed by an anterior approach, 444 by extensive laminectomy and 116 by extensive laminectomy with foraminotomy and removal of osteophytes. The remaining 328 procedures were performed in the various manners indicated in the table. Because of the numerous variables, such statistics are not significant. At best, however, they do provide a gross means of comparison. Seventy-three percent of patients treated by an anterior approach improved, whereas 68% to 85% of patients treated by a posterior approach improved. Patients with limited laminectomy and patients in whom dentate section was performed showed similar results. Of the patients operated on by means of extensive laminectomy, foramenotomy, and removal of osteophytes, 85% improved.[15,19,45] Only a limited number of surgeons performed the procedures, which reflects the importance of experience and mastery of the technique for the excision of osteophytes through a posterior approach. Nevertheless, even without removing osteophytes, a satisfactory result can often be obtained in the majority of patients by means of laminectomy and foraminotomy.[2,19,59] With the present use of magnification and proper instrumentation, these techniques can be facilitated. This applies both to the removal of osteo-

Table 11-6. Results of Management of Cervical Spondylotic Myelopathy in 1355 Patients[19]

Type of Management	Total No. of Patients	Improved	Nonimproved
Conservative[6,42,49,56]	114	36%	64%
Anterior cervical surgery[8,21,24,25,37,43,45,58,60,64–66]	353	73%	27%
Extensive laminectomy[9,10,15,22–25,44,52,59,67]	444	68%	32%
Extensive laminectomy, foraminotomy, excision of osteophytes[15,19,45]	116	85%	15%
Limited laminectomy, foraminotomy, excision of osteophytes[2]	30	70%	30%
Extensive laminectomy and dentate section[2,45]	46	57%	43%
Extensive laminectomy, dentate section, dural graft[10,53,61]	82	60%	40%
Limited laminectomy, variable foraminotomy, dentate section[23,25,26,50]	116	66%	33%
Limited laminectomy, dentate section[25,26]	54	63%	37%

phytes from an anterior as well as a posterior approach.

Motor function was the most challenging index of operative success in a study by Allen. He operated on 30 patients by means of limited laminectomy, foraminotomy, and the excision of osteophytes.[2] Thirty percent of the patients failed to respond or deteriorated further, and four patients died of motor neuron disease. Seventy percent improved objectively. Eighty percent improved on performance, and 60% were able to return to work or to equivalent physical activity. Allen presented two patients who, after simple laminectomy and dentate ligament section, had a relapse of the neurologic deficit after 15 months. Removal of osteophytes at a second procedure resulted in significant and sustained improvement. This report stimulated the addition of osteophyte excision to the technique.

Of the 27 patients operated on by Mayfield by means of laminectomy, foraminotomy, and removal of osteophytes, improvement was observed in 21 (78%); operations in six patients were regarded as failures.[45] Concern over subluxation and the problem of a painful and prolonged rehabilitation led him to prefer a subsequent anterior approach. The former can be prevented by limiting the facetectomy, and the latter has not been of specific concern since the introduction of steroids and the newer methods of pain inhibition.

Epstein and colleagues, in reviewing 50 patients operated on during a 10-year period, noted that beyond 70 years of age fixed lesions became more frequent.[19] No patient over 70 had an excellent result. Satisfactory responses were noted in six, and one patient remained the same (Table 11-7).

In 1965, Aboulker and associates, described complete laminar decompression of the cervical canal from the foramen magnum through the second thoracic vertebra. Subluxation was not observed. The dura expanded and the cord migrated dorsally. Every effort was made to preserve the cervical lordosis by allowing a dense scar to form in the midline of the incision, which provided a bolstering effect.[1]

In 1976, Jung reviewed Aboulker's experiences with 345 patients. Of these, six died and two had a postoperative increase in myelopathy. The cause of myelopathy was stenosis of the foramen magnum in two patients, and cervical stenosis with or without arthrosis in 112; the remaining 106 patients had cervical spondylosis.[1,38]

Table 11-7. Results of Surgery Relating to Age[19]

AGE	EXCELLENT	GOOD	SAME	POOR	TOTAL
37–50	3	6	0	0	9(18%)
51–60	2	12	2	3	19(38%)
61–70	5	9	0	1	15(30%)
71–84	0	6	1	0	7(14%)
Total	10(20%)	33(66%)	3(6%)	4(8%)	50(100%)

Gorter compared the results of limited laminectomy at one or two levels and division of the dentate ligaments with results achieved by means of laminectomy by the Aboulker technique.[23] He discovered an improvement rate of 51.4% in 26 patients with limited laminectomy, whereas the rate was 66.6% in 37 patients with total laminectomy. Younger patients showed more improvement than older patients, and the shorter the duration of illness, the better the result.

The 1979 report of Alsharif and coworkers on the use of the Aboulker technique in spondylotic myelopathy indicated that one benefit was relief of the cranial anchoring of the spinal cord by decompression of the C1 segment and the foramen magnum.[3] By this means, the cord moved dorsally in a wide arch that protected it, even in flexion positions. This may be of advantage when the cervical curve is reversed, and it is the only posterior approach suggested for deformity of this nature.

Galera and Tovi, in one of the rare negative reports on the results on anterior disc excision with interbody fusion, noted progression of the neurologic signs in 41% of 51 patients with spondylotic myelopathy.[21] Only 17% showed a satisfactory response and 83% showed a poor response. Lunsford and coworkers reviewed their results of anterior cervical surgery for the treatment of cervical spondylotic myelopathy 1 to 7 years postoperatively in 32 patients.[43] In an excellent statistical review, 55% improved and the remainder were failures. The results could not be linked to the patient's age, duration of symptoms, severity of myelopathy, cervical canal size, or the performance of single- or multiple-level operations. None of the anterior surgical techniques showed superior results. Notably, they failed to surpass those obtained by Lees and Turner and Nurick who employed conservative, nonoperative measures alone.[42,49]

Cervical laminectomy in which the facets are not disturbed is well tolerated. Deformity occurs more frequently in children than in adults, especially in those with spinal cord tumors where the anterior horn cell innervation of supportive muscles is destroyed. Raynor and associates, employing biomechanical studies of the cervical spine motion segments in human cadavers, has clearly demonstrated that shear strength is not compromised until more than 50% of the facets have been removed bilaterally.[54] This is avoided with the current techniques that remove, at most, one quarter or one third of the medial facet and augment the foraminal decompression by undercutting, if necessary.

Albouker, Alsharif and coworkers, Bishara, Epstein and coworkers, Jenkins, Rogers, and Stoops and King have not encountered postoperative instability or subluxation as a problem inimical to the performance of cervical laminectomy and limited foraminotomy (Fig. 11-30).[1,3,4,19,36,57,59]

Rogers, reporting the results of extensive laminectomy on 33 patients, noticed no weakness of the cervical spine from the surgery, if care was taken not to damage the posterior vertebral muscles by heavy retraction.[57] Jenkins was able to follow five of the patients operated on by Rogers after an interval of 12 to 17 years. Using repeated x-ray studies, he found no evidence of instability.[36] These patients had achieved lasting improvement. He thought the intervertebral joints were primarily responsible for spinal stability and that the lamina and spinous processes were redundant structural factors after maturity.

Stoops and King noted that of 42 patients operated on for spondylostenosis, seven were found to have a congenital anomaly of the cervical spine.[59] Six had congenital fusion of two vertebral bodies, five at C2–C3 and one at C4–C5. One patient had two pairs of congenitally fused vertebral bodies at C3–C4 and C6–C7. Spondylotic changes were most marked at the adjacent interspace. These authors were among the first to specifically refer to the dorsal migration of the dural tube following laminectomy, whereby the spinal cord was transposed into a new position of shorter length, less subject to stress incident to flexion and extension. In their series, the high incidence of congenital interbody fusion associated with spondylosis and myelopathy made them hesitant to consider employing anterior interbody fusion. Of their 42 patients, 35 (83.3%) showed definite improvement after laminectomy and foraminotomy with neurolysis, whereas the conditions of seven (16.7%) remained stable.

Alsharif and coworkers, whose decompression included the posterior rim of the foramen magnum, found no evidence of instability in any of their 26 patients.[3] Alsharif believed, as did Galera and associates,[21] that the anterior operation mod-

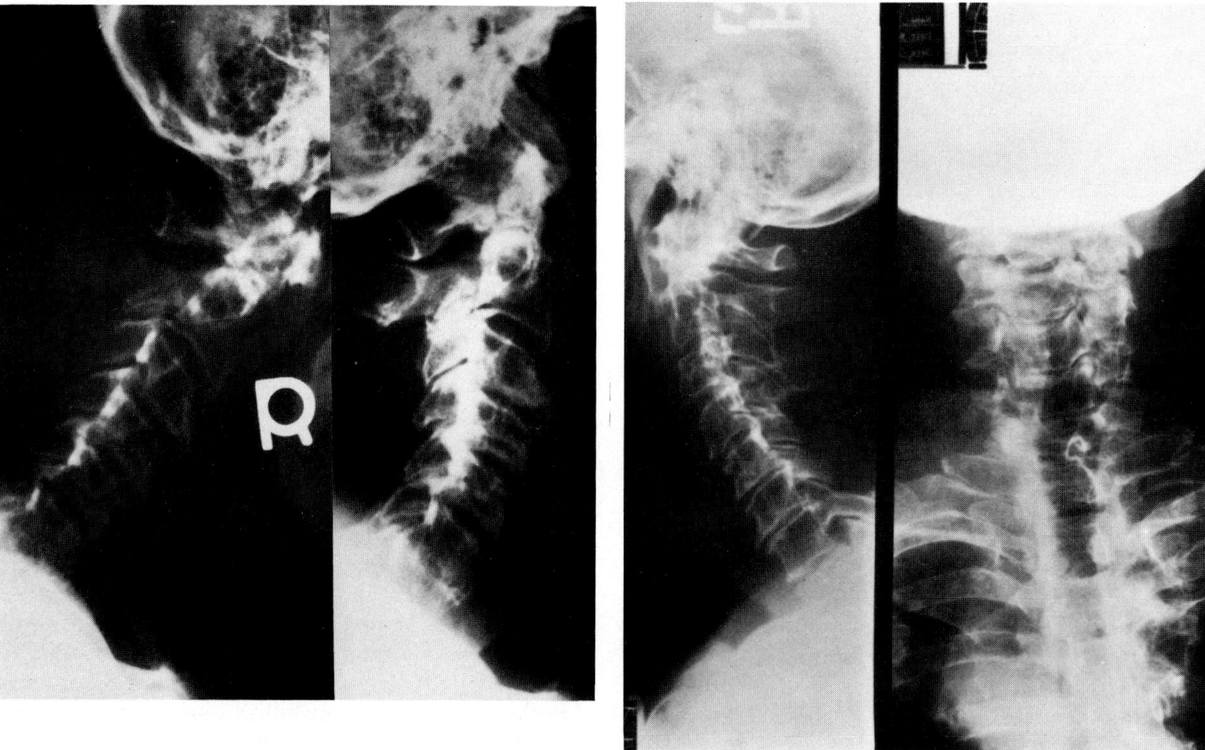

Fig. 11-30. Postoperative x-ray studies of two patients taken 26 years (*left*) and 32 years (*right*) after laminectomy for spondylostenosis. Both are essentially asymptomatic with no neurologic deficit. The lordotic curves are adequately maintained, with no evidence of subluxation.

Both patients are now 72 years old, one is a practicing anesthesiologist, the second an extremely active retiree. The patient on the left required a second, more extensive laminar decompression with excision of osteophytes before an adequate result was obtained.

ified only one aspect of the pathogenesis of spondylotic myelopathy, namely, the excision of ventral osteophytes. He believed that it resulted in bony fusion of the vertebrae akin to the Klippel-Feil deformity, which eventually was always associated with marked osteoarthritic changes.

Crandall and Gregorius, in a study of the surgical treatment of cervical spondylotic myelopathy by means of both an anterior or posterior approach noted dramatic recoveries in patients who had undergone either operation.[11] These patients were followed for an average of 85 months; and for as long as 20 years. In patients who underwent anterior interbody fusion, disability tended to decrease; following laminectomy, disability generally increased. Symptoms became more severe for as long as 8 to 12 years after improvement and plateau had been reached. It was difficult to explain the reason for deterioration. The presence of sphincter disturbances and excessive lower-extremity weakness was associated with a poor surgical result. In two patients, pseudomeningocele had occurred after laminectomy, and a retained laminar arch of C3 was present in three patients who were inadequately decompressed. Both complications are avoidable and could significantly change the prognosis.

A long-term study of the results of laminectomy in the treatment of cervical spondylosis and myelopathy was provided by Bishara.[4] The postoperative period of observation ranged from 5 to 20 years with an average of 10 years. Initially, 36 patients improved following surgery, 24 considerably. In 15, further deterioration was prevented. Five years after operation, 33 patients were still improved and in 5 patients, coexistent disease had become apparent. Ten years after operation 30 patients had maintained their initial improvement, and disease progression accounted for a drop of only 10% in the initial success rate. No patient in this series developed postoperative instability, including those in whom foraminotomy was performed.

Vaquero and coworkers, in 1982, in a retrospective study of the results of laminectomy in 34 patients after a minimum follow-up period of 5 years, noted that amelioration of the myelopathic symptoms occurred in only 8 of the 20 patients subjected to anterior fusion by the Cloward technique.[63] In contrast, 10 of the 14 patients who had laminectomy improved. Of patients with radiculopathy as well as myelopathy, 6 of 11 patients with anterior fusion improved, whereas 4 of 5 patients subjected to laminectomy improved. It was suggested that laminectomy offered the best results in the treatment of myelopathy with or without radiculopathy, when two or more intervertebral spaces were affected.

Jeffries in 1986 reported his results in the surgical treatment by both an anterior and posterior approach of 137 patients with cervical myelopathy due to spondylosis.[35] Of these, 108 underwent the Cloward procedure and 29 had laminectomies. Ten patients, following the initial Cloward operation, required second operations, five of which were laminectomies. The result of the anterior decompression was a 90% satisfactory rate, 54.6% of whom were in the excellent category. After the posterior approach was used, 62% improved, of whom only 20.7% were in the exceilent category. An unusually high percentage of patients (24%) in the anterior group had disc herniations. It should be noted that only 55% of the patients in the anterior group were severely neurologically impaired, as compared with 76% in the posterior group. Such factors seriously influence the statistical results.

The most recent papers on the advantages of expansive "open-door" laminoplasty in the treatment of ossification of the posterior longitudinal ligament (OPLL) and spondylostenosis emphasize the safety of the procedure and the absence of significant postoperative complications.[29,31,33,39,41,48,62] There was no evidence of postoperative malalignment of the vertebral segments. The ankylosis that occurred on the side where the hinge was placed apparently reduced the movement of the spine by at least 50%, thereby limiting kinetic, dynamic-related injury to the spinal cord caused by excessive mobility. The open-door segment filled with fibrous tissue, as did the space beneath the lamina. No thickened laminectomy membrane was encountered. Foraminotomy was possible on one side, a disadvantage since foraminal decompression could only be used on the side where the open door was placed. It was possible, however, to consider the use of a keyhole type of foraminotomy on the hinged side, as suggested by Koyama and Handa.[41]

All of these patients were operated on in the prone position with the head elevated approximately 30 degrees. However, blood loss was considerable, varying from 190 cc to as much as 580 cc. The average blood loss was 350 cc. The time factor varied from as little as 1 hour and 15 minutes to approximately 2 to 3 hours. Patients wore a brace for 3 to 6 months, required bed rest for 1 to 2 weeks, and were hospitalized for approximately 6 weeks. Tsuji[62] noted bone union across the open door after 6 months. Of the 30 cases reported by Itoh and Tsuji, 16 patients had excellent results, 11 had good results, and three had fair results. None had poor results.[33] Tsuji reported on twelve patients, with two excellent, five good, and five fair results, and one death caused by pulmonary embolus.[62] In Hirabayashi's 40 cases, good results were obtained in 66% of his patients. There were two failed cases, one patient having a Brown-Séquard syndrome. Postoperatively, three patients had transient weakness in the C5–C6 motor elements (Table 11-8).[29]

As in other reports, the Japanese surgeons noted that the more severe the symptoms and the older the patient, the poorer was the end result. The "open-door" technique is best applied to patients with multiple-level disease and is quickly replacing the anterior approach for both OPLL and spondylostenosis. Fusion of the laminae can be further achieved by placing bone chips along the hinged sides if instability is present, adding to the usefulness of the procedure. The progression of OPLL is not affected, and it may present future problems.

One of the most common complications in the early cases was the "sinking" of the lamina into the open door. Correction was achieved by using bone grafts in the open door, regardless of whether it was laterally or dorsally situated. Only a 4-mm expansion of the canal was needed to provide adequate decompression of the spinal cord. More recently, Nakano has observed no need to perform foraminotomy, because the relief of radiculopathy occurs without decompression in this area.[48] He also preserves the spinous processes and places a

Table 11-8. Results—Laminoplasty for Cervical Spondylostenosis (OPLL)

	No. Patients	Average Age	Average Follow-up (Months)	OPLL	Spondylo-stenosis	Results			
						Excellent	Good	Fair	Fail
Tsuji (1982)	12	47–70	6–24	8	4	2 (16%)	5 (42%)	5 (42%)	0
Hirabayshi (1983)	40		54(maximal)	29	11	"Most good results" (66% recovery rate)			2 (5%)
Kimura (1984)	24	58(47–67)	29	15	9	OPLL—2 (13%)	12 (80%)	1 (7%)	0
						SP ST—2 (20%)	6 (60%)	1 (10%)	0
Itoh (1985)	30	63(35–77)	17.6	13	17	16 (53%)	11 (37%)	3 (10%)	0
Hukuda (1985)	13	48(20–79)	31		13	"Improved from 8.0 ± 3.1 to 12.0 ± 3.5" (Grade—Japanese Orthopaedic Assoc)			
Koyama (1985)	31	53(24–72)	19.8		31	14 (45%)	10 (32%)	4 + 1 (16%)	2 (6%)
						(33% required anterior operations)			
Nakano (1986)	78		48	47	31	"75–90% improved"			

fat graft into the gap of the open door. This deserves confirmation since it could further simplify the procedure (Table 11-8).

Hukuda and coworkers in 1985 reported that over the past 19 years they had operated on 269 patients with spondylostenosis who were followed for an average of 31 months.[31] A posterior decompression provided results superior to those from an anterior approach for patients with more advanced myelopathy, especially when three or more disc levels were involved and the canal was stenotic. Patients with spondylotic lesions at one or two segmental disc levels without narrowing of the spinal canal were treated by means of an anterior approach. Their results showed no definite superiority of any individual anterior or posterior operation. In the anterior approach, they preferred the Robinson-Smith to the Cloward procedure, because it provided greater stability and mechanical support. Of the posterior operations, laminoplasty of the "French-window" type was used in their last 13 patients. Only one patient developed an unstable spine. The severity and the duration of the clinical symptoms influenced the surgical outcome in a negative manner, although the age of the patient was not significant. When there was stenosis of the spinal canal, the resection of posterior vertebral osteophytes through an anterior approach at multiple levels was hazardous to the spinal cord. However, single-level disease with radicular symptoms was treated most successfully by an anterior procedure.

It should be noted that the ossification of the posterior longitudinal ligament is being recognized with increasing frequency in Caucasians.[40]

Matjasko and coworkers reviewed the results of anesthesia in surgery in the seated position in 554 cases.[46] They regarded the seated position as safe in experienced hands, if appropriate surgical and anesthetic skills were exercised. Caution was advised in patients with atherosclerotic cardiovascular disease, severe hypertension, cervical stenosis, and right-to-left intracardiac shunts. Young and coworkers more recently compared the surgical and anesthetic complications in neurosurgical patients using the seated position.[69] Most of the complications were related to the operative procedure, not to the position or to venous air embolism. The episodes of embolism that were encountered were not significant factors in the perioperative morbidity and mortality. The patients included those operated on for both posterior fossa disorders and cervical decompression. The authors caution against the use of cervical flexion in the performance of laminectomy. They also indicate that the alternative prone or lateral positions do not guarantee the avoidance of such complications. In their series of 255 patients, a total of only three were found to have morbidity resulting from either venous air embolism or operation in the seated position. In their opinion, this position offers the advantages of optimal surgical exposure and anatomical orientation, a drier surgical field with relative ease in obtaining hemostasis, a good diaphragmatic excursion during ventilation, and access to the airway with lower airway pressure when compared with alternative positions. By improving operative conditions, the surgeon is afforded advantages that actually reduce the incidence of surgical complications, improve outcome, and permit the safe excision of osteophytes.

SUMMARY

No conclusive statistical evidence establishes the superiority of the anterior or the posterior approach in the management of spondylostenosis, although some order is developing. The consensus is that in spondylostenosis, the anterior approach may be preferred for disc or osteophyte protrusion limited to one or two levels. This will correct segmental stenotic changes and will create an adequate spinal canal at the critical areas of narrowing. Laminectomy is the procedure of choice in patients with a narrowed canal and multiple-level protrusions. Patients with congenital stenosis involving all the major segments, with or without superimposed developmental changes, require more extensive laminar decompression. Proper attention must be given to the craniocervical junction where anomalies may occur. By means of extended laminectomy and foraminotomy, the spinal canal can be enlarged in patients with developmental narrowing. This can be performed expeditiously with acceptable risk, and without the problems associated with multiple-level interbody fusion and vertebrectomy with strut fusion. The success of laminar decompression is dictated by the preservation of cervical lordosis. In patients with major dorsally located abnormalities, such as seen in hyperlordosis, shingling, and arthrosis with hypertrophy of the yellow ligaments, dorsal decompression is essential. Such patients usually have little or no ventral intrusions from vertebral margins. Subsequent stabilization is rarely required, if proper surgical and postoperative rehabilitation is maintained. This option, however, is still available as a secondary procedure. Indeed, both an anterior and posterior approach may be indicated in unique circumstances of segmental spondylosis complicated by subluxation and instability.

The development of laminoplasty, which again enlarges the dorsal quadrants of the spinal canal but preserves the laminar roof, has led to a generalized reversal of the former commitment to the anterior approach for the treatment of OPLL. Posterior decompression is now used as a safer, shorter operative procedure with better sustained results. Supplementary fusion is readily achieved.

Ultimately, the success of either approach depends on the selection of the proper surgical candidate and the skill and judgment of the surgeon and his associates.

ACKNOWLEDGMENTS

The authors wish to thank Dominic Nardi, M.D., for his invaluable suggestions regarding anesthetic management.

Our gratitude to Ms. Sherry Lynn Grimm cannot be fully expressed—her care in the preparation of this manuscript exceeds definition.

REFERENCES

1. *Aboulker J, Metzger J, David M, Engel P, Ballivet J:* Les myelopathies cervicales d'origine rachidienne. Neurochirurgie 11:88, 1965
2. *Allen KL:* Cervical spondylosis with accompanying myelopathy: Its alleviation by removal of the bony spur. S Afr J Surg 6:5, 1968
3. *Alsharif H, Ezzat SH, Hay A, Motty NA, Malek SA:* The results of surgical treatment of spondylotic radiculomyelopathy with complete cervical laminectomy and posterior foramen magnum decompression. Acta Neurochir (Wien) 48:83, 1979
4. *Bishara SN:* The posterior operation in treatment of cervical spondylosis with myelopathy: A long term follow-up study. J Neurol Neurosurg Psychiatr 13:393–398, 1971
5. *Bose B, Northrup BE, Osterholm JL, Cotler JM, DiTunno JF:* Reanalysis of central cervical cord injury management. Neurosurgery 15:367, 1984
6. *Bradshaw P:* Some aspects of cervical spondylosis. Q J Med 26:177, 1957
7. *Braughler JM, Hall ED:* Current application of "high-dose" steroid therapy for CNS injury. J Neurosurg 62:806, 1985
8. *Brieg A, Turnbull I, Hassler O:* Effects of mechanical stresses on the spinal cord in cervical spondylosis: A study of fresh cadaver material. J Neurosurg 25:45, 1966

9. *COMBALERT A, PELLET W:* Indications therapeutiques et resultats operatoires obtenus dans une serie de 80 myelopathies par cervicoarthrose. Therapeutique 48:498, 1972
10. *CRANDALL PH, BATZDORF I:* Cervical spondylotic myelopathy. J Neurosurg 25:57, 1966
11. *CRANDALL PH, GREGORIUS FK:* Long-term followup of surgical treatment of cervical spondylotic myelopathy. Spine 2:139–146, 1977
12. *EHNI G:* Developmental variations, including shallowness of the cervical spinal canal. In Post JD: Radiographic Evaluation of the Spine. New York, Masson Publishing, 1980
13. *EPSTEIN JA, CARRAS R, EPSTEIN BS, LAVINE LS:* Myelopathy in cervical spondylosis with vertebral subluxation and hyperlordosis. J Neurosurg 32:421, 1970
14. *EPSTEIN JA, CARRAS R, HYMAN RA, COSTA S:* Cervical myelopathy caused by developmental stenosis of the spinal canal. J Neurosurg 51:362, 1979
15. *EPSTEIN JE, CARRAS R, LAVINE LS, EPSTEIN BS:* The importance of removing osteophytes as part of the surgical treatment of myeloradiculopathy in cervical spondylosis. J Neurosurg 30:219, 1969
16. *EPSTEIN JA, DAVIDOFF IM:* Chronic hypertrophic spondylosis of the cervical spine with compression of the spinal cord and nerve roots. Surg Gynecol Obstet 35:27, 1951
17. *EPSTEIN JA, EPSTEIN BS:* Lumbar and cervical spinal stenosis with related cauda equina radiculopathy and myelopathy. In Post JD: Radiographic Evaluation of the Spine. New York, Masson Publishing, 1980
18. *EPSTEIN JA, EPSTEIN BS, LAVINE LS:* Cervical spondylotic myelopathy: The syndrome of the narrowed canal treated by laminectomy, foraminotomy, and the removal of osteophytes. Arch Neurol 8:307, 1963
19. *EPSTEIN JA, JANIN Y, CARRAS R, LAVINE LS:* A comparative study of the treatment of cervical spondylotic myeloradiculopathy: Experience with 50 cases treated by means of extensive laminectomy, foraminotomy and excision of osteophytes during the past 10 years. Acta Neurochir (Wien) 61:89, 1982
20. *FAGER CAL:* Results of adequate posterior decompression in the relief of spondylotic cervical myelopathy. J Neurosurg 38:684, 1973
21. *GALERA RG, TOVI D:* Anterior disc excision with interbody fusion in cervical spondylotic myelopathy and rhizopathy. J Neurosurg 28:305, 1968
22. *GODLEWSKI D:* Les myelopathies par stenose cervicale et par cervicoarthrose (A propos de cinquante cas operes et revises avec un recul de 2 a 10 ans). Cah Sociol Demogr Med 13:1069, 1972
23. *GORTER K:* Influence of laminectomy on the course of cervical myelopathy. Acta Neurochir (Wien) 33:265, 1976
24. *GREGORIUS FK, ESTRIN T, CRANDALL PH:* Cervical spondylotic radiculopathy and myelopathy: A long term follow-up study. Arch Neurol 33:618, 1976
25. *GUIDETTI B, FORTUNA A:* Long terms results of surgical treatment of myelopathy due to cervical spondylosis. J Neurosurg 30:714, 1969
26. *HAFT H, SHENKIN HA:* Surgical end results of cervical ridge and disc problems. JAMA 186:312, 1963
27. *HALL ED, WOLF MS, BRAUGHLER MJ:* Effects of a single large dose of methylprednisolone sodium succinate on experimental post-traumatic spinal cord ischemia. J Neurosurg 61:124, 1984
28. *HINCK VC, SACHDEV NS:* Developmental stenosis of the cervical spinal canal. Brain 89:27, 1966
29. *HIRABAYSHI K, WATANABE K, WAKANO K, ET AL:* Expansive open-door laminoplasty for cervical spinal stenotic myelopathy. Spine 8:693–699, 1983
30. *HOLT S, YATES PO:* Cervical spondylosis and nerve root lesions—Incidence at routine necropsy. J Bone Joint Surg 48B:407, 1966
31. *HUKUDA S, MOCHIZUKI T, OGATA M, ET AL:* Operation for cervical spondylotic myelopathy. A comparison of the results of anterior and posterior operations. J Bone Joint Surg 67B:609–615, 1985
32. *IIZUKA H, IWASAKI Y, YAMANOTO T, KADOYA S:* Morphometric assessment of drug effects in experimental spinal cord injury. J Neurosurg 65:92, 1986
33. *ITOH T, TSUJI H:* Technical improvements and results of laminoplasty for compressive myelopathy in the cervical spine. Spine 10:729–736, 1985
34. *IWASAKI Y, ABE H, ISU T, MIGASAKA K:* CT myelography with intramedullary enhancement. J Neurosurg 63:363, 1985
35. *JEFFRIES RV:* The surgical treatment of cervical myelopathy due to spondylosis and disc degeneration. J Neurol Neurosurg Psychiatr. 49:353–361, 1986
36. *JENKINS DHR:* Extensive cervical laminectomy. Br J Surg 60:852–854, 1973
37. *JOMIN M, BOUSQUET C, DELANDSHEER J-M, LAINE E:* Traitment des complications radiculomedullaires de la cervicoarthrose par la methode de Cloward-Resultats a propos de 370 malades operes. Neurochirurgie 21:21, 1975
38. *JUNG A:* La chirurgie des syndromes cervicaux. Rev Chir Orthop (Suppl II)62:63, 1976
39. *KIMURA I, OH-HAMA M, SHINGU H, ET AL:* Cervical myelopathy treated by canal expansive laminoplasty. J Bone Joint Surg 66A:914, 1984
40. *KLARA PM, MCDONNELL DE:* Ossification of the posterior longitudinal ligament in Caucasians: Di-

agnosis and surgical intervention. Neurosurgery 19:212, 1986

41. *Koyama T, Handa J:* Cervical laminoplasty using apatite beads as implants. Surg Neurol 24:663, 1985
42. *Lees F, Aldren Turner JS:* Natural history and prognosis of cervical spondylosis. Br Med J 2:1607, 1963
43. *Lunsford LD, Bissonette DJ, Zorub DS:* Anterior surgery for cervical disc disease. Part 2: Treatment of cervical spondylotic myelopathy in 32 cases. J Neurosurg 53:12, 1980
44. *Magnaes B, Hauge T:* Surgery for myelopathy in cervical spondylosis: Safety measures and preoperative factors related to outcome. Spine 5:211, 1980
45. *Mayfield FH:* Cervical spondylosis: A comparison of the anterior and posterior approaches. Clin Neurosurg 13:181, 1965
46. *Matjasko J, Petrozza P, Cohen M, Steinberg P:* Anesthesia and surgery in the seated position: Analysis of 554 cases. Neurosurgery 17:695, 1985
47. *Michie RH, Clark M:* Neurological syndrome associated with cervical and craniocervical anomalies. Arch Neurol 18:241, 1968
48. *Nakano N:* Cervical laminoplasty for OPLL—spondylosis and stenosis. Bessatsu Seikei Oteka, Orthopaed Surg 9:23–26, 1986 (Nauko-do Japan).
49. *Nurick S:* The natural history and the results of surgical treatment of the spinal cord disorder associated with cervical spondylosis. Brain 9S:101, 1972
50. *Odom GL, Finney W, Woodhall B:* Cervical disk lesions. JAMA 166:23, 1958
51. *Ono K, Ota H, Tada K, Yamamoto T:* Cervical myelopathy secondary to multiple spondylotic protrusions. Spine 2:218, 1977
52. *Penning L:* Functional pathology of the cervical spine. Baltimore, Williams & Wilkins, 1968
53. *Piepgras DG:* Posterior decompression for myelopathy due to cervical spondylosis: Laminectomy alone vs laminectomy with dentate ligament section. Clin Neurosurg 24:508, 1977
54. *Raynor RB, Pugh J, Shapiro I:* Cervical facetectomy and its effect on spine strength. J Neurosurg 63:278, 1985
55. *Reed JD:* Effects of flexion-extension movements of the head and spine upon the spinal cord and nerve roots. J Neurol Neurosurg Psychiatr 23:214, 1960
56. *Roberts AH:* Myelopathy due to cervical spondylosis treated by collar immobilization. Neurology 16:951, 1966
57. *Rogers L:* The surgical treatment of cervical spondylotic myelopathy. Mobilization of the complete cervical cord into an enlarged canal. J Bone Joint Surg 43B:3, 1961
58. *Rosomoff HL, Rossman F:* Treatment of cervical spondylosis by anterior cervical diskectomy and fusion. Arch Neurol 14:392, 1966
59. *Stoops WL, King RB:* Chronic myelopathy associated with cervical spondylosis. JAMA 192:281, 1965
60. *Tezuka A, Yamada K, Ikata T:* Surgical results of cervical spondylotic radiculomyelopathy observed for more than five years. Tokushima J Exp Med 23:9, 1976
61. *Thomalske G, Wild von K, Lammert E:* Zur chirurgischen behandlung der cervicales myelopathie. Nervenarzt 43:520, 1972
62. *Tsuji H:* Laminoplasty for patients with compressive myelopathy due to so-called spinal canal stenosis in cervical and thoracic regions. Spine 7:28, 1982
63. *Vaquero J, Cabezudo JM, Leunda G, Bravo G:* Subjective postoperative results in cervical spondylotic myelopathy. Acta Neurochir 62:95, 1982
64. *Verbiest H:* Les operations anterieures dans la cervicoarthrose et les hernies discales cervicales. Neurochirurgie (Suppl)16:91, 1970
65. *Verbiest H:* The management of cervical spondylosis. Clin Neurosurg 20:262, 1973
66. *Verbiest H, Paz Y, Geuse HD:* Anterolateral surgery for cervical spondylosis in cases of myelopathy or nerve root compression. J Neurosurg 25:611, 1966
67. *Vignon G, Colcombet P, Bochu M, et al:* Les myelopathies des cervicoarthroses: A propose de 14 observations personelles dont 12 operees. Rev Rhum 44:239, 1977
68. *Wolf BS, Khilnani M, Malis LI:* The sagittal diameter of the bony cervical spinal canal and its significance in cervical spondylosis. J Mount Sinai Hosp 23:283, 1956
69. *Young ML, Smith DS, Murtagh F, Vasquez A, Levitt J:* Comparison of surgical and anesthetic complications in neurosurgical patients experiencing venous air embolism in the sitting position. Neurosurgery 18:157, 1986

Management of Radiculopathy and Myelopathy by the Anterior Approach

THOMAS S. WHITECLOUD III

Clinical manifestations of cervical disc disease are highly variable. Patients present with a variety of complaints and physical findings. Signs and symptoms can broadly be categorized as neurogenic or discogenic in nature.[16] Neurogenic symptoms result from pressure on the cervical nerve roots or the spinal cord by disc material or by posterior or posterolateral osteophytes. Patients may manifest radicular symptoms alone, or may present with simultaneous signs and symptoms of nerve root and spinal cord compression.

Patients with discogenic symptoms have no objective neurologic findings. They complain of intermittent, chronic pain in the posterior cervical region, shoulder, chest wall, and scapular regions. Occipital headaches are frequent. It is postulated that the pain experienced by patients with discogenic symptoms results from the stimulation of the sensory receptors of the sinovertebral nerve that is located in the anulus fibrosus and in the posterior and anterior longitudinal ligaments.[15]

Regardless of the presenting symptoms, it may become necessary at some point to consider surgery as a method of alleviating the symptom complex. In almost all instances, a trial of nonoperative treatment is mandatory prior to considering operative intervention.

The surgical procedure first used for the treatment of symptomatic cervical spondylosis was the posterior route. The primary problem with this approach is the difficulty in exposing and removing compressive structures that lie anterior to the spinal cord and nerve roots. As early as 1928, Stooky noted that difficulty was encountered in removing "chondromas" by the posterior transdural route.[68] Although posterior surgery for degenerative disease of the cervical spine is satisfactory in certain pathologic conditions, it became apparent that an alternative surgical approach was needed that would reliably produce better clinical results.

The anterior approach to the cervical spine was developed and popularized in the early 1950s. Bailey and Badgley pioneered anterior cervical surgery for the treatment of traumatic and postsurgical dislocations and destructive vertebral lesions.[3] This procedure was first performed in 1952 for stabilization of the cervical spine of a woman with a lytic lesion involving the fourth and fifth cervical vertebrae. In 1955, Robinson and Smith described a surgical technique for spinal fusion via the anterior approach for cervical disc disease.[60] Cloward first reported his technique for interbody fusion in 1958.[14] The generally excellent results of the anterior approach for cervical disc disease for neurogenic or discogenic symptoms led to a rapid switch to that approach during the 1960s (Fig. 11-31).

During the past 30 years, numerous refinements in the anterior approach for the treatment of cervical radiculopathy and myelopathy have been developed. These include the use of operative magnification and modification of graft materials and their configurations. A number of authors have also reported techniques of anterior disc excision alone producing results comparable to those of series in which bone grafting is used.[6,21,26,37–39,47,50,51,55,58,62,64,79]

SURGICAL APPROACH

Regardless of whether the surgeon elects to fuse the cervical spine by any number of the techniques that have been described or simply removes the offending disc or discs, Southwick and Robinson report that the surgical approach is essentially the same.[67]

The patient is supine on the operating table with either head-halter traction or skeletal traction in place. Traction helps to stabilize the cervical spine in a slightly extended position on the operative headrest. If a graft is to be inserted, additional weight can be added to distract the disc space at the appropriate time. The anterior aspect of the cervical spine is prepared, as well as the donor site. Towels are then sutured to the anterior neck, which facilitates visualization for operative roentgenograms.

The surgical approach can be made from either the left or right side. Although the recurrent laryngeal nerve is in greater jeopardy on the right, a right-handed surgeon generally finds the approach from that side technically easier. The location of the skin incision is determined by the location of the cricoid cartilage, which is generally opposite the body of C6, and from palpation of the carotid tubercle (Chassaignac's tubercle), located on the anterior aspect of the transverse process of C6. Once these landmarks have been identified, the skin incision may be placed higher or

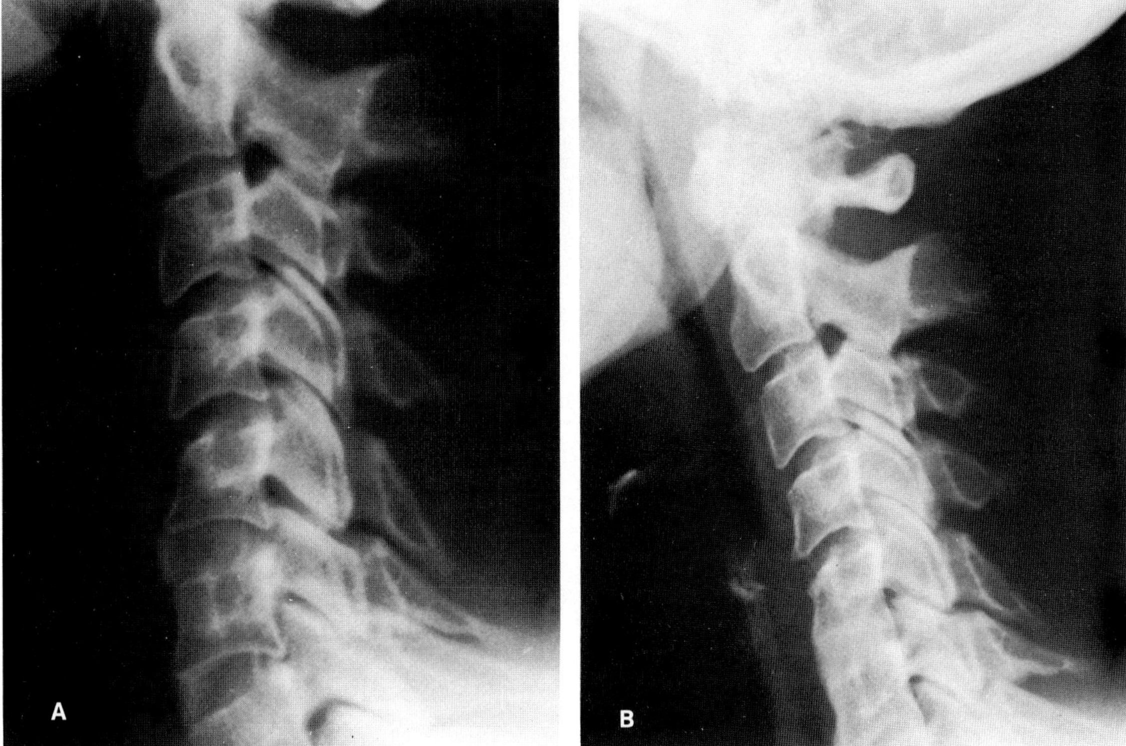

Fig. 11-31. (*A*) Lateral roentgenogram in the immediate postsurgical period showing Smith-Robinson grafts inserted in the C5–C6 and C6–C7 interspaces. (*B*) Two years after surgery, solid arthrodesis has occurred.

lower than C6, depending on the level that is to be approached. If one or two discs are to be exposed, a transverse skin incision is placed in a skin crease, extending from the midline well over the body of the sternocleidomastoid muscle. If three or more discs are to be approached, an incision vertically along the medial border of the sternocleidomastoid is recommended. The platysma is sectioned in line with the skin incision. After the platysma is sectioned, the pretracheal fascia is incised longitudinally. The interval between the medial border of the sternocleidomastoid muscle and the strap muscles is developed using blunt dissection. The carotid sheath is palpated and retracted laterally. The trachea, esophagus, and thyroid are retracted medially. The prevertebral fascia is then exposed and sectioned longitudinally. Care must be taken to remain in the midline. The longus colli muscle fibers lie laterally, and the anterior longitudinal ligament overlies the disc and vertebral bodies in the midline. Once the discs have been exposed, a spinal needle is inserted, and a roentgenogram is obtained to verify the disc level. Visualization of the disc and posterior structures after removal of the disc is greatly enhanced by the use of operative loupes or the operative microscope. The fiberoptic light source also facilitates visualization. All discs from C2–C3 downward to C7–T1 can be adequately exposed by this approach. It is relatively simple, makes use of natural anatomic planes, and is relatively bloodless. Furthermore, it allows adequate visualization of the cervical disc and has a low morbidity. Complications are rare and can be minimized by thorough anatomic knowledge of the region.

TYPES OF GRAFTS FOR ANTERIOR CERVICAL FUSION

Bailey and Badgley first reported their technique for fusing the cervical spine anteriorly in 1960.[3] They reported on 20 patients with cervical instability from trauma, tumor, or infection. Two patients had persistent symptoms due to cervical disc disease that was previously treated by posterior surgery. The authors did not recommend treatment of herniated cervical discs by anterior surgery in their initial report.

The technique of Bailey and Badgley consists of identifying the vertebra to be fused and cutting a trough in the anterior aspect of the vertebral bodies about ½ inch in width and 3⁄16 inch in depth. The trough is cut into the full vertical height of the vertebra. The discs are cleaned with a rongeur to a depth of 3⁄16 inch, and the cartilaginous plates on the inferior and superior aspects of the vertebral bodies to be fused are removed. A cortical cancellous iliac graft is obtained that corresponds in shape to the trough that was fashioned in the anterior aspect of the vertebrae. Chips of cancellous iliac bone are packed into the cleaned disc spaces, and the cortical cancellous graft is mortised into the trough. Sutures that have been previously placed in the prevertebral fascia are tied; this helps to maintain the graft in its bed (Fig. 11-32).

In the initial series of Bailey and Badgley, patients were maintained in traction for 6 weeks, then allowed up in a cervical thoracic orthosis. The brace was worn until fusion occurred, usually from 4 to 6 months. Fusion occurred in all 18 of the patients who were followed for at least 6 months.

The first report of anterior cervical fusion performed for symptoms of cervical spondylosis appeared in 1955.[60] Robinson and Smith postulated that disc degeneration led to osteophyte formation, disc narrowing, subluxation, instability of one cervical vertebra on another, or disc protrusion, which were the pathologic changes producing neck, arm, hand, and chest pains stemming from the cervical spine. They developed a technique of interbody fusion that would restore disc height and, by stopping motion, allow resorption of posterior and posterolateral osteophytes. Their first report presented eight patients, only one of whom had follow-up at 1 year. They were encouraged by the initial clinical results.

A more detailed report on operative technique by the same authors appeared in 1958.[66] This technique is as follows. After appropriate preoperative evaluation, the pathologic disc or discs are approached anteriorly. Using sharp dissection, the disc space is entered and the intervertebral disc material removed entirely. The cartilaginous endplates and subchondral bone at the top and bottom of the intervertebral disc spaces to be fused are also removed. (Subsequently, the authors modified this technique and did not remove the subchondral bone.) No attempt is made to remove posterior or posterolateral osteophytes. The empty disc space is then measured; it usually accepts a block of bone 10 to 15 mm high, 10 to 15 mm wide, and 10 to 15 mm deep. The disc space is widened as much as possible prior to insertion of the graft by either instrumentation or traction. The bone graft is then countersunk into the disc space.

If one level is fused the patient uses no brace postoperatively, unless neck pain persists, in which case a neck brace is used for 1 to 3 months. When multiple levels are fused, bracing is used for 3 to 6 months.

Robinson and associates reported on the clinical results of their technique on a series of 55 patients in 1962.[61] Generally, preoperative symptoms consisted of what was termed a chronic neck syndrome; in the treatment of patients with definitive and obvious cervical root or spinal cord compression, anterior spine fusion was not usually a primary procedure. Nineteen patients, however, did have previous posterior surgery. Postoperative results were excellent in 45.5% of the patients, good

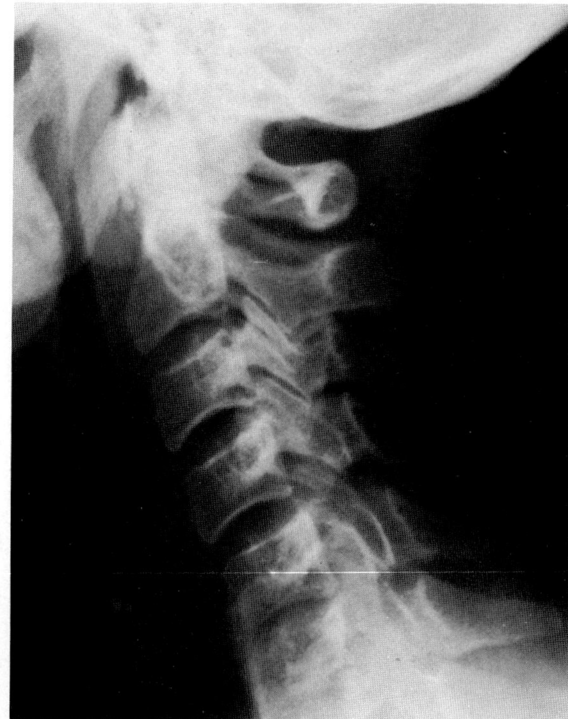

Fig. 11-32. Cortical cancellous grafts of the Bailey-Badgley type spanning C5–C6 and C6–C7 interspaces. The roentgenogram was taken in the immediate postoperative period.

in 27.2%, and fair in 21.8%. The results were poor in 5.5%. One-level fusions were found to produce better clinical results. Ninety-four percent of the patients with one-level fusions had good or excellent results, 73% with two-level fusions had good or excellent results, but only 50% of the patients with three-level fusions had good or excellent results. The overall fusion rate was 88%. The authors' postulation that a solid fusion would result in absorption of bony spurs was not proven. Only 50% of the spines evaluated postoperatively by roentgenogram showed evidence of remodeling of posterior or posterolateral osteophytes. This, however, did not seem to affect the clinical result. A higher instance of resorption of posterior and posterolateral osteophytes has been reported by Gore and Sepic.[30] Eighty patients of 119 undergoing anterior cervical arthrodesis had osteophytes present on their preoperative evaluations. Solid arthrodesis occurred in all these cases. The osteophytes decreased in size in 67 and remained the same in 13. In no case did they increase in size.

Cloward's first report on his technique of interbody fusion appeared in 1958.[14] He modified instruments designed for posterior interbody fusion of the lumbar spine. His instrumentation allows drilling of a round hole in the intervertebral disc space, into which is inserted a prefit dowel of bone. A drill is used with a guard that permits the intervertebral disc space and adjacent vertebrae to be drilled to any desired depth. The drill and guard are removed two or three times during the procedure in order to check the depth and direction of the hole and adjust the length of the guard accordingly, and to remove soft tissue of the disc. Drilling is continued downward until the bone at the bottom of the hole is entirely cortical in nature. This remaining cortical bone is then removed with curettes and rongeurs to expose the posterior longitudinal ligament. Care is taken to remove all posterior and posterolateral osteophytes. The posterior longitudinal ligament is not opened. Once removal of all bone and disc is completed, a precut dowel of bone is tapped into place; it should be slightly shorter than the depth of the drill hole. The dowel of bone is cancellous in its midportion, with cortical bone on both ends. Bone was obtained from cadaveric sources in all but one of Cloward's first reported cases.

Cloward's initial report consisted of 47 cases, 27 with evidence of neural compromise and 20 with neck-shoulder and interscapular pain. Four patients had evidence of myelopathy. The results reported were excellent in 42 of 47 cases. Three patients demonstrated graft resorption and did not achieve fusion. One patient sustained spinal cord injury at the time of surgery. Subsequent series reported by Cloward continued to show a high percentage of good to excellent results with a high rate of fusion.

Bailey and Badgley, Robinson and Smith, and Cloward are considered to be the pioneers of the anterior approach to the cervical spine for the treatment of a variety of pathologic conditions.[3,14,60] They use graft materials of different configurations, but all believe that stabilization following disc excision is necessary for achievement of the best possible clinical result. Cloward emphasizes the removal of posterior and posterolateral osteophytes at the time of surgery.[14] It is also possible to remove these compressive structures with the exposure offered by the Smith-Robinson technique,[66] although that exposure is somewhat less than with the Cloward technique. Whether the direct removal of compressive structures enhances the overall clinical result is impossible to ascertain and remains the choice of the individual surgeon. However, it appears that the risk of spinal cord injury increases if there is an attempt to remove compressive structures.[5,44,70] The type of graft to be inserted also remains the surgeon's choice.

Experimental data on the load-bearing capabilities of the previously described graft configurations are available. The horseshoe-shaped graft developed by Robinson-Smith is much more resistive to compressive forces.[74]

Numerous series appeared in the literature reporting the clinical results and rate of fusion in patients undergoing anterior surgery for degenerative disease of the cervical spine.[2,3,16,18,30,31,43,57,61,65,69,78] The pseudarthrosis rate varied from 26% in the series of White and coworkers to 3% in that of Gore and Sepic.[30,75] Table 11-9 tabulates the pseudarthrosis rate in selected series from the literature.[2,10,18,23,30,57,61,69,75,78] Several series reflect an increasing pseudarthrosis rate as fusion is attempted at more than one level.[10,18,61,75] Only Riley noted poorer clinical results in patients with a pseudarthrosis.[57] These patients had clinical improvement following subsequent posterior fusion.

Difficulty in obtaining stabilization on multiple levels has led to various modifications in graft materials. Simmons reported on a modification of the Smith-Robinson graft in 1969.[65] Sixty-eight patients were treated by a keystone type of graft. A 100% fusion rate was obtained. There were 4 three-level, 36 two-level, and 28 one-level fusions. In this technique, a keystone square of rectangular

Table 11-9. Incidence of Pseudarthrosis

Author	Incidence (%)
White	26
Connolly	21
Riley	18
Robinson	12
DePalma	12
Williams	10
Stuck	5
Aronson	4
Gore	3

tissue is removed and beveled upward into the vertebra above and downward into the vertebra below. Disc material is removed completely. A rectangular graft is obtained from the iliac crest and prepared to fit the shape of the prepared trough. The ends are beveled upward and downward to lock into place. With the neck extended and traction applied, the graft is driven into place and the traction released, locking the graft firmly into position and maintaining fixed distraction and immobilization of the disc space. When two levels are fused, the trough and graft are extended across the intervening vertebra into the one above and the one below. Gore's high rate of arthrodesis was achieved utilizing a modification of this keystone technique.[30]

Whitecloud and LaRocca reported on the use of cortical bone obtained from the fibula to achieve multilevel stabilization in 1976.[77] Verbiest and coworkers also used cortical bone for multilevel stabilization.[73]

The fibula strut graft consists of a full segment of fibula. It is roughly triangular, and the apical aspect of the graft is inserted into a trough cut in the anterior aspect of the vertebral bodies to be fused. After all the disc material has been removed from the cervical segments to be fused, a trough is begun in the anterior aspect of the vertebral column with a rongeur and completed with a dental bur on an air drill. Partial vertebrectomies are performed, if indicated; this allows decompression of the spinal cord and nerve roots under direct visualization. Notches are cut on both ends of the graft; those on the end to be inserted superiorly are of equal length, but the posterior extension of the inferior notch is slightly shorter than the anterior one. This allows easier insertion. The endplates of the superior and inferior receptor vertebrae are prepared to accept the graft with the dental bur. A hole is undercut to preserve the anterior portion of the vertebral body so that the posterior extension of the notched fibula can lock into place. The anterior preserved portion of the vertebral bodies serves as a barrier against dislodgment. The graft is inserted after applying more traction to the patient's head. The superior portion is inserted first, and an impactor is used to sink the inferior portion of the graft into the trough. Once this is accomplished, the graft is grasped by an instrument and pulled distally. This locks the graft into place, with both posterior extensions inserted into the prepared holes in the vertebral endplates. Thus two thirds of the graft is deep in the anterior aspect of the vertebral column (Fig. 11-33).

This graft technique has a fusion rate of 99% and requires that at least two disc spaces be fused. There have been no incidences of graft fracture, but extrusion in the immediate postoperative period is a complication that has occurred on occasion. Although graft incorporation takes 8 months to 1 year, postoperative immobilization is now utilized for only a 3-month period following surgery (Fig. 11-34). Bone-bank fibula has a similar rate of fusion and eliminates donor-site complications.[45]

COMPLICATIONS OF ANTERIOR CERVICAL FUSION

It is true that the anterior approach to the cervical spine is relatively simple and has a low morbidity rate. However, numerous complications can occur with this procedure. If forewarned, the prudent surgeon will prevent them from occurring when possible.

Complications relating to failure of graft incorporation were discussed previously. Grafts may also collapse or extrude; such complications are discussed in the series reviewed.[2,23,28,57,65,69,75] A higher rate of arthrodesis is obtained, if only an attempt is made to fuse one disc level.[10,18,23,30,57,61,69,75,78] Multilevel arthrodesis is perhaps best accomplished by utilizing a graft configuration that spans multiple segments.[30,65,77] Failure of incorporation does not necessarily compromise a clinical result. Reports in the literature indicate that anterior disc excision without fusion can also obtain a satisfactory clinical result.[6,21,47,55,62]

Major complications can occur at the time of the surgical approach itself. The carotid and vertebral vessels are susceptible to perforation, as are the esophagus and trachea. Temporary or permanent

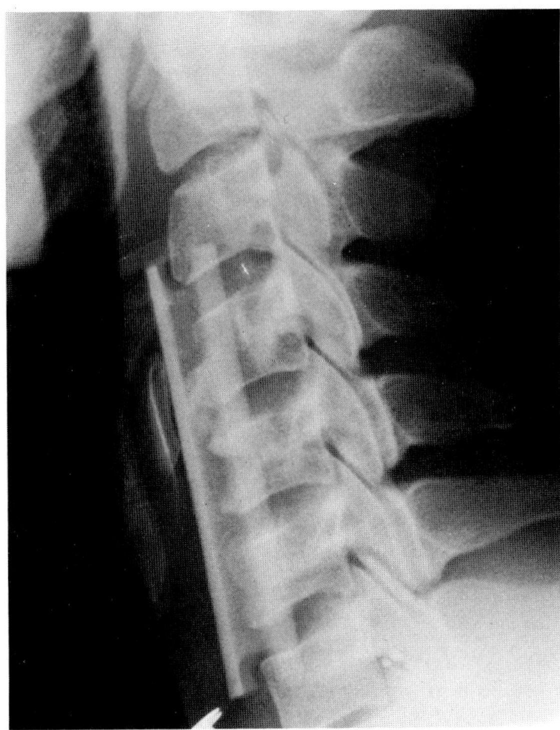

Fig. 11-33. Lateral roentgenogram takes in the immediate postsurgical period of a fibular strut graft extending from C3 to C7. The patient has congenital spinal stenosis, and anterior spinal cord decompression was accomplished by disc removal and partial vertebrectomy from C3 to C7.

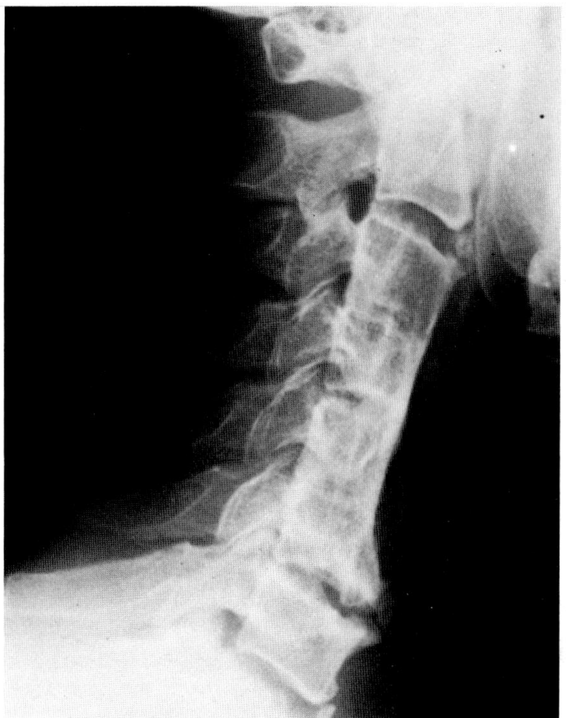

Fig. 11-34. Solid arthrodesis achieved between C3 and C6 using the fibular strut graft technique. Eight years have elapsed since surgery.

damage can occur to nerve root, cervical sympathetic chain, spinal cord, or recurrent laryngeal nerve. With osteophyte removal, dural tears can occur and are quite difficult to repair. Osteomyelitis, either of the cervical spine or donor site, can complicate postoperative management, and pneumothorax can result from surgery on the lower cervical levels.[71,76]

Perforating injuries may be minimized by using retractors without sharp points. Cloward or Richardson retractors provide adequate exposure. No instrument should be inserted into the disc space without both the carotid sheath and the esophagus protected by retractors. Thorough anatomic knowledge of the anterior and anterolateral neck will help to eliminate other serious complications. The recurrent laryngeal nerve, on the right, enters a groove between the esophagus and trachea, accompanied by the inferior thyroid artery; it should be located when operating from C6 downward. By staying in the midline and only stripping the longus colli muscles laterally at each disc level, possible injury to the cervical sympathetic chain can be avoided. The superior thyroid artery, accompanied by the superior laryngeal nerve, must be avoided when approaching the C4 level or above.

Permanent spinal cord injury is the most serious operative complication of the anterior approach. Kraus and Stauffer reported six cases of permanent cord damage in patients undergoing anterior interbody fusion.[44] Bohlman reported six cases with quadriparesis secondary to anterior spinal surgery.[5,70] Sugar carefully analyzed six cases of myelopathy following anterior cervical surgery. In none of these patients did intraoperative trauma cause the neurologic deficit; nor was there evidence that the bone graft had been inserted improperly. The risk of spinal cord injury has been calculated to be less than 2 per 1000.[27] It is obviously a devastating complication, and must be considered whenever anterior spinal surgery is recommended.

Fortunately, most complications are minor. The

most common postoperative complaints are transient hoarseness and dysphagia; their incidence can be decreased by the routine use of dexamethasone during and after the surgical procedure.

Wound complications are frequent at the donor site. The donor site is by far the most painful of the two incisions. Persistent drainage, hematoma formation, superficial or deep wound infections with osteomyelitis, or injury to the lateral femoral cutaneous nerve have been reported. In 1244 cases reviewed in a 1978 report, the incidence of donor-site complications was 20%, as compared with a 0.2% incidence of complications from neck incision.[76] Lunsford and coworkers reported a 23% complication rate in patients undergoing disc excision and fusion, but this included graft extrusion, infection, or nonunion.[47] Routine postoperative drainage decreases donor site complications.

The use of cadaveric allografts eliminates the numerous difficulties occurring when the patient's bone is used. Brown and coworkers reported on a comparable series of patients undergoing anterior cervical fusions with autogenous graft material or cadaveric allografts obtained under aseptic conditions and stored at −20°C.[11] A total of 76 allografts were inserted in 53 patients. In 45 patients, 63 levels were fused with autogenous iliac bone. In this series, 94% of the allografts and 97% of the autografts were united. However, a 28% incidence of graft collapse was seen in patients receiving allografts, as compared with 16% in those receiving autografts. Cloward reported on a "simplified bone bank" for interbody fusion in 1980.[17] Cadaveric graft material is harvested under nonsterile conditions and is thoroughly cleansed of soft tissue. The graft is sterilized with ethylene oxide gas and aerated for 72 hours. The allografts are stored in an unfrozen state. Fifty cervical interbody fusions were performed on 28 patients. The fusion rate was 100%, although three cases of graft collapse were noted.

A lack of ready availability has prevented the use of allografts by most surgeons. If, and when, allografts become available, prospective clinical studies will be needed to determine whether their use results in a different rate of fusion than that achieved by autogenous bone. Experimental research is being conducted on the use of bone graft substitutes in the cervical spine.[19] Recently, concerns have arisen regarding transmission of the AIDS virus by bone allografts. These concerns may limit the use of allografts in the future.

RESULTS OF ANTERIOR DISC EXCISION FOR RADICULOPATHY AND DISCOGENIC CERVICAL PAIN

Numerous reports have appeared in the literature tabulating the clinical results of anterior disc excision and interbody fusion. A critical comparison of these series is not possible because of different preoperative criteria and modes of follow-up. Most series include patients with and without objective evidence for neurologic compromise, although the series of Riley and coworkers and Robinson and associates included only patients with no obvious neural deficit.[57,61] Table 11-10 presents results from selected series in the literature.[12,18,,22,25,57,61,65,69,75,78] All these series used Odom's crite-

Table 11-10. Results of Anterior Disc Excision and Fusion

AUTHOR		NO. CASES		EXCELLENT TO GOOD(%)	FAIR (%)	POOR (%)
Robinson	(1962)	55		73	22	5
Stuck	(1963)	151		73	21	6
Connolly	(1965)	63		54	24	22
Dohn	(1966)	210		51	29	20
Williams	(1968)	60		63	15	22
Riley	(1969)	93		72	18	10
Simmons	(1969)	68		81	15	4
Jacobs	(1970)	62		82	13	5
DePalma	(1972)	229		63	29	8
White	(1973)	65		67	22	11
Chirls	(1978)	467		92	6	2
Gore	(1984)	133		96	2	2
Total		1656	Mean	72.25%	18%	9.75%

ria, or a similar modification, for their postoperative clinical evaluation; these criteria are as follows:

Excellent: All preoperative symptoms relieved; abnormal findings improved
Good: Minimal persistence of preoperative symptoms; abnormal findings unchanged or improved
Fair: Definite relief of some preoperative symptoms; other symptoms unchanged or slightly improved
Poor: Symptoms and signs unchanged or exacerbated[37]

It is important to note that patients in the fair category have been improved by surgery.

In the series presented, the Cloward technique was used by Stuck, Dohn, and Chirls.[12,25,69] The remaining authors used the Smith-Robinson technique, except Simmons and Gore, who reported on the keystone technique of arthrodesis.[30,65]

In contrast to results of surgery on the lumbar spine, several reports note that the results of patients involving litigation are not statistically different from those in nonlitigation patients.[18,23,61,75] Furthermore, White found no difference in the results in patients who had a Cornell Index indicating a neuropsychiatric or psychosomatic disturbance.[75]

Williams and coworkers and White and colleagues present data indicating that the best results are obtained when surgery is performed on patients with radicular symptoms.[75,78] Seventy-five percent of the patients in Williams' series had radicular symptoms, and 73% had a good or excellent result, as compared with 27% without radicular symptoms.[78] In White's series, 57% of the patients had radicular symptoms, with 75% good or excellent results.[75] Without radicular symptoms, 57% had results that were good or excellent. In Dohn's series, however, 137 patients had radiculopathy, and 72 (53%) had good to excellent results.[25] In his much smaller group of 34 patients with discogenic symptoms, 62% were in the good or excellent category. Robinson and coworkers and Riley and coworkers had no patients with radicular findings, and both series had 73% of patients in the good or excellent category.[57,61]

Another series not presented in Table 11-10 is that of Aronson, who analyzed the results of 88 patients with soft disc protrusions or extrusions in over 500 patients treated by the Smith-Robinson technique.[1] All had neurologic deficits, and all but one were rated in the good or excellent category following surgery. Aronson postulates that the diseased disc acts as a hydraulic wedge, and believes that anterior removal and fusion will decompress the nerve root sufficiently to provide complete relief of nerve root pressure symptoms, even if a small amount remains intraspinally. It is recommended, however, to attempt removal of all extradural material by the anterior approach.

The problem of cervical myelopathy is not directly addressed in the series presented here. Dohn had 39 patients in this diagnostic category, and his results were the poorest in this group of patients.[25] White and coworkers make a similar observation.[75] However, Connolly and coworkers did have good or excellent results in two thirds of their patients with this diagnosis.[18] Aronson had three patients with massive midline disc protrusions producing a myelopathy; all were treated successfully by the anterior approach.[1] He noted, however, that the duration of symptoms was short, and believed that the disease process was different in patients who present with longstanding deficits due to multilevel spondylitic involvement.

The literature certainly supports using the anterior approach for the treatment of cervical disc disease that produces a radiculopathy or discogenic-type symptom complex. Approximately 90% of patients undergoing this procedure benefit from it, 70% dramatically so. Generally, better results are obtained if surgery is required at only one interspace.

RESULTS OF ANTERIOR SURGERY FOR CERVICAL SPONDYLOTIC MYELOPATHY

The etiology of degenerative cervical disc disease producing nerve root irritation directly by disc herniation or a posterolateral osteophyte formation is fairly well understood. This is also true of the painful disc, or discogenic syndrome, in which no objective neurologic findings are present in patients with chronic neck, occipital, chest, and shoulder pain. As has been well documented, these conditions are quite readily treated by anterior surgery.[1–3,13,14–17,18,22,25,57,61,66,69,75,78]

The most serious consequence of cervical disc degeneration is cervical spondylotic myelopathy. It is known that cervical spondylotic myelopathy is invariably associated with a narrowed neural canal, although a narrow canal does not always lead to myelopathy.[53] This diminution in the circumferential diameter of the canal may be congenital or secondary to disc degeneration with subsequent osteophyte formation. Patients with this disease process often begin with a congenitally narrowed canal and develop associated spondylotic changes.

Further reduction in the functional diameter of the osseous canal occurs with motion. Flexion stretches the cord across the ventral spurs, and extension may cause retrolisthesis of a vertebral body or inbuckling of the ligamentum flavum.

The narrowed canal produces direct mechanical pressure on the spinal cord at one or more levels. This pressure may directly produce neural damage or may cause ischemic changes secondary to vascular compromise.

Experimental studies have shown that the ischemia and compression can separately cause cord lesions resembling those found in human cervical spondylotic myelopathy. The effects of compression and ischemia are additive; separately, each has less profound effects on neurologic function than when combined.[29]

Initial presenting complaints of patients with this disease process vary, from those with minimal spinal cord involvement and normal gait to those with profound neural involvement and inability to walk. Symptoms may be intermittent, progressing slowly in a steplike fashion, and may be associated with multiple remissions. Other patients may present with a progressive unrelenting neural deterioration. Generally, these patients have difficulty with gait and upper-extremity weakness. There is no prognostic indicator of what course a particular patient's disease will follow. Consequently, it is not surprising that there is no standard mode of treatment for this condition.

Lees and Turner document quite well the clinical findings in a series of 44 patients with cervical spondylotic myelopathy followed for as long as 40 years.[46] Most patients were followed for at least 10 years and demonstrated that with this condition, long periods occur without new or worsening symptoms. The authors recommended most conservative treatment of this condition because the overall clinical results of such treatment were as good as the series in the literature at that time tabulating the results of cervical laminectomy. They also noted the danger of neurologic deterioration occurring in the immediate postoperative period.

Nurick's excellent studies of cervical myelopathy confirmed the findings of Lees and Turner. In the majority of cases, initial phase of neural deterioration is followed by a static state lasting several years.[52,53] Nurick's classification of the disability associated with cervical spondylotic myelopathy is generally used today in evaluating patients with this condition.

The prognosis for patients presenting in Grades I to III was thought by Nurick to be good, that is, few progressed to a higher classification of disability. Patients presenting in Grades IV or V, however, had a poor prognosis.

A comparison was made between a larger number of patients who had undergone surgery for this condition and another series who had undergone no surgery.[53] It was concluded that laminectomy and anterior cervical fusion produced results slightly superior to those of nonoperative management, but the overall results were not statistically significant. Another conclusion was that in view of the benign nature of the disease, surgery should be considered only for patients whose disability is progressive, particularly in patients 60 years or older.

If surgery is to be considered in patients with cervical spondylotic myelopathy, either the anterior or posterior approach may be used. Posterior decompression had been used exclusively, before the development of the anterior approach. The results have generally been less than satisfactory. Improvement is noted in approximately 50% of patients undergoing posterior decompression, and the hazards of postoperative loss of neural function have been well documented.[8,9,13,20,32,34,56,72]

Numerous reports in the literature now indicate a 60% to 70% improvement in symptoms in patients undergoing anterior surgery for cervical spondylotic myelopathy.[5,7,20,24,33,35,36,41,43,49,63,80,81] Most series recommend anterior decompression with removal of disc material and all posterolateral osteophytes producing pressure on neural structures. Dereymaeker and coworkers noted a 64% improvement rate after anterior spinal stabilization; his series consisted of 31 patients.[24] Guidetti and Fortuna had 45 patients who underwent anterior surgery, with 82% in the very good, good, or fair category.[33] The condition of two patients was made worse by the surgery, and one continued to deteriorate. Crandall and Batzdorf noted a 71% improvement rate in 21 cases.[20] Philips reported on 65 patients who underwent Cloward procedures, with a 74% improvement rate following surgery.[56] He emphasized the removal of all compromising structures at the time of surgery, and stated that the results of anterior surgery are markedly superior to those of laminectomy or conservative management. Zhang and coworkers reported on 121 cases of cervical spondylotic myelopathy treated by anterior disc excision and fusion.[81] The average number of segments fused per patient was 2.9. Ninety-one percent of patients were believed to be improved by the procedure, and 73% were able to resume their full normal activities.

Bohlman presented a series of 17 patients who underwent anterior stabilization by the Smith-Robinson technique, with no attempt having been made to remove posterior or posterolateral osteophytes.[5] He expressed concern that attempted removal of posterior osteophytes may produce an increased neural deficit through the manipulation of an already diseased spinal cord. All but one patient showed improvement.

Satisfactory results utilizing radical anterior decompression, with partial vertebrectomies over multiple segments followed by fusion, have been reported.[4,7,36,80] Boni reported on 29 cases of spondylotic myelopathy treated by resection of the central portion of three or more vertebral bodies followed by stabilization with a cortical cancellous iliac graft. Good results were reported in 53% with moderate improvement in 39%. Bernard and Whitecloud performed a similar procedure on 21 patients in whom all compressive structures were removed anteriorly over multiple segments, followed by stabilization with autogenous fibular strut graft. Three segments were decompressed in 13 cases, four levels in four cases, and two levels in the remaining four patients. Nineteen of the 21 patients were improved by operative intervention. Hanai's series consisted of 30 patients undergoing subtotal vertebrectomy and fusion. Follow-up evaluation is based on the Japanese Orthopaedic Association's score for myelopathy, 17 points being normal. In the patients reported, the postoperative score ranged from 9 to 16 points. All patients thought that surgery was beneficial. Yonenobu and coworkers compared three surgical procedures for multisegmental cervical spondylotic meylopathy in 95 patients.[80] Twenty-four patients had undergone extensive laminectomies, 50 anterior interbody fusion alone, and 21 a subtotal vertebrectomy and fusion. The results of the subtotal vertebrectomy were significantly better than those of the other two procedures. However, they did recommend that if involvement was over four segments or more, a posterior procedure should be carried out.

Another method of performing multilevel decompression has been presented by Mann and coworkers.[49] They reported on a prospective study of 50 patients undergoing anterior decompression. They removed all disc protrusions, or bony osteophytes measuring 1.5 mm or larger based on myelography. If protrusions were between 2 and 4 mm, no fusion was carried out. If they were larger than 4 mm, fusion was performed at the same time of removal. Therefore, these patients underwent disc excision with and without fusion. Sixty-four percent of the patients undergoing this type of procedure improved two or more preoperative grades. Thirty-six percent improved one grade.

Anterior decompression without fusion has been reported by Hankinson and Wilson and Hoff and Wilson for the treatment of cervical spondylotic myelopathy.[37,40] Their results are similar to those of series reporting on the use of interbody fusion techniques for the treatment of this disease process.

Not all reports of anterior surgery have been optimistic. Galera noted only a 39% improvement rate in 33 patients with cord compromise who underwent Cloward procedures, with a definite tendency toward deterioration as the follow-up period was lengthened.[28]

Lunsford and coworkers reported only a 50% improvement rate in patients who had undergone anterior cervical surgery and were followed 1 to 7 years later.[48] Fifty percent of the patients did not improve or deteriorated despite surgery. In his series, various types of anterior procedures were performed, none showing results better than another. Results could not be statistically linked to the patient's age, duration of symptoms, severity of myelopathy, cervical canal size, or the performance of a single or multilevel operation. Surgical results in this series were no better than results of nonoperative management.

There are still no clear-cut criteria for determining when surgery is to be recommended for patients with cervical spondylotic myelopathy. Hukuda's large retrospective analysis of 269 patients undergoing operative procedures for cervical spondylotic myelopathy showed no technique had overall superiority.[41] Three different types of anterior procedures and three different techniques of posterior procedures were utilized. As others have shown, a short duration of symptoms before the operation is associated with more favorable results.[4,43,63]

RESULTS OF ANTERIOR DISC EXCISION WITHOUT FUSION FOR CERVICAL DISC DISEASE

In 1960, Hirsch reported on the anterior removal of cervical discs without interbody fusion.[38] Surgery was performed on patients with radicular symptoms, and initial clinical results were satisfactory. Hirsch's first series consisted of 18 patients, 7 of whom underwent surgery. All patients undergoing surgery had positive myelography, and five of the seven underwent disc excision at two levels. The operative technique consisted of a routine anterior approach to the cervical spine. After the correct disc level was identified, disc fenestration was performed by opening the disc space through an incision measuring approximately 3 × 5 mm. No attempt was made to completely remove the disc or cartilaginous end-plates. The posterior anulus and the posterior longitudinal ligament were not disturbed.

A subsequent report in 1964 detailed further experience with anterior disc excision without fusion in a group of 35 patients who had positive myelograms. Forty-three percent made a complete recovery, 40% were improved, and 17% had no improvement.[39] Follow-up roentgenograms of 28 patients obtained 1 year after surgery showed osseous union in half the cases. The remaining patients had achieved intervertebral stability by fibrous union. Some of his patients experienced transient postoperative cervical pain following disc excision without fusion. Kadoya and coworkers performed microsurgical anterior osteophytectomy for cervical spondylotic myelopathy and abandoned his "without fusion" procedure because of a similar problem of postoperative neck discomfort.[43]

Murphy and Gado performed a similar operation on a group of 26 patients and reported their results in 1972.[51] Ninety-two percent of the patients undergoing simple anterior disc excision had a good result. One patient who had two discs removed showed no initial improvement and was reexplored anteriorly, only to develop an acute kyphotic angulation measuring 25 degrees. Mann and coworkers also had one patient who had multilevel anterior decompression followed by a rather alarming subluxation that required bony stabilization.[49] Excessive anterior angulation would seem to be a potential complication of disc excision without fusion, especially over multiple levels. Follow-up roentgenograms were available from 20 patients. Seventy-two percent had achieved bony union; the remaining patients had a fibrous union and a stable joint complex. It was noted that a kyphotic angulation at the level of disc removal between 5 degrees and 15 degrees generally occurred.

The use of the operating microscope for anterior disc excision was reported by Robertson and others.[6,21,37,58,59] His operative technique removed all the anulus, the entire disc, and the cartilaginous end-plates, but he did not recommend removal of the posterior longitudinal ligament. All interspaces undergoing disc removal achieved bony or fibrous union. He reported excellent results in 16 patients with lateral disc herniation, and marked improvement in 80% of patients with painful disc syndromes. The clinical series consisted of 40 patients.

Martins presented a series of 51 patients with neural compromise, who randomly underwent either a Cloward interbody fusion or anterior disc excision alone.[50] There were 25 patients in the Cloward group, and 26 in the disc excision group. Ninety-two percent of both groups were in the good or excellent category at the time of follow-up. The operative technique presented by Martins is described as a radical discectomy with foraminotomy. The disc is removed entirely along with the cartilaginous end-plates. The posterior aspects of the superior and inferior vertebral bodies are removed to facilitate the exposure of the posterior

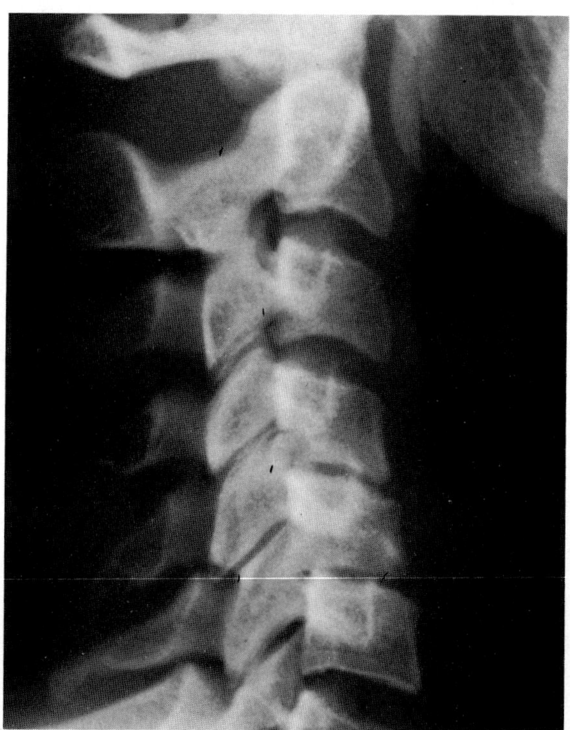

Fig. 11-35. Lateral roentgenogram of the cervical spine 18 months after disc excision at C4–C5 and C5–C6. Note the posterior settling of the C4 and C5 vertebral bodies. The patient still experiences symptoms.

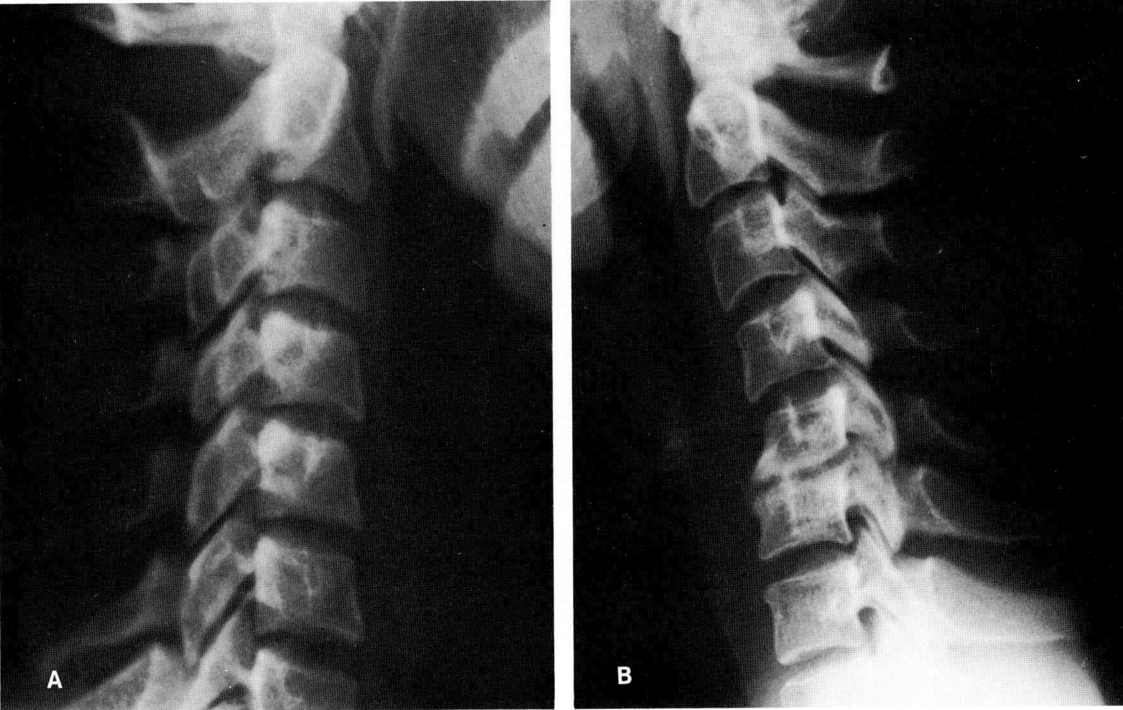

Fig. 11-36. (*A*) Preoperative roentgenogram prior to C5–C6 disc excision without fusion. (*B*) Roentgenogram taken 18 months postoperatively showing fibrous ankylosis. The patient is without symptoms.

longitudinal ligament. The ligament is incised and removed along with any posterior or posterolateral osteophytes. The dura and nerve roots are seen to be free of any encroachment at the termination of the procedure. Anterior bone and soft tissues on the anterior aspect of the vertebrae are not removed, with hope of preventing excessive anterior angulation as the disc narrows. It was concluded from this series that discectomy without fusion is as effective as interbody fusion, and the complications of interbody fusion are eliminated. It was believed, however, that in cases of advanced spondylosis, the exposure offered by the dowel fusion technique was needed for adequate decompression (Figs. 11-35 and 11-36).

Dunsker performed the same type of radical excision of intervertebral disc contents, and thought that removal of the posterior longitudinal ligament was indicated to prevent it from buckling and causing root compression as the disc narrowed.[26]

Hankinson and Wilson reported on 51 patients undergoing anterior disc removal using the operating microscope in 1975.[37] Their series included patients with and without neural deficits, 12 with myelopathy. They highly recommended the operating microscope in performing anterior discectomy. Besides use of the microscope, the operative technique emphasizes preservation of lateral columns of disc material with an opening no more than 10 mm wide in the anterior anulus. Vertical exposure is gained through this opening by drilling away 5 mm to 6 mm of the superior and inferior vertebrae. Drilling is directed more laterally as the posterior aspect of the body is approached. Posterior and posterolateral osteophytes are removed under direct vision. The posterior longitudinal ligament is generally open. In this series, 26 patients underwent disc removal at multiple levels; three had four discs removed at the time of surgery. Instability did not develop in any of these patients, possibly owing to preservation of lateral columns of disc material and minimal removal of anterior bone. Results in this series were comparable to the others, with 84% of the patients showing adequate follow-up in the good or excellent category.

Wilson and Campbell reported on 71 cases of

anterior disc excision in 1977.[79] The surgical technique evolved as the series progressed, but most patients only had disc removal down to the posterior longitudinal ligament and laterally to the uncinate process. The cartilaginous end-plates were not removed, the posterior longitudinal ligament was not incised, and osteophytes were not removed. Only one patient had two discs removed at one time; the remainder had only one level excised. In 68 patients, the results were good or excellent. The three patients who were not improved by surgery had no localizing neurologic signs. O'Laoire and Thomas reported on 26 patients presenting with spinal cord compression due to a soft cervical disc prolapse.[55] This condition is to be differentiated from cervical spondylotic myelopathy secondary to chronic degenerative changes. Utilizing operating microscope and simple disc excision, they report good or excellent results in 25 of the 26 patients.

The elimination of the donor site from the operative procedure certainly decreases the operative morbidity. Lunsford reported that, of the 334 patients undergoing anterior surgery for hard or soft disc herniations with or without fusion, the postoperative complications were more frequent and hospitalizations longer in patients undergoing fusion.[47]

A critical evaluation of the series presented in the literature indicates that the overall results of anterior disc excision without fusion compares quite favorably with the series of excisions followed by interbody fusion. It is interesting that the proponents of the anterior approach without fusion are also divided on whether or not radical decompression with removal of posterior and posterolateral osteophytes is necessary for a satisfactory clinical result. Results of the series using radical excision (Martins, Dunsker, Hankinson) are essentially the same as those with only simple disc excision (Hirsch, Murphy, Robertson, Wilson).[26,37,39,51,58,79]

REFERENCES

1. *Aronson NI:* The management of soft disc protrusions using the Smith-Robinson approach. Clin Neurosurg 20:253, 1973
2. *Aronson N, Filtzer DK, Bagan M:* Anterior cervical fusion by the Smith-Robinson approach. J Neurosurg 29:397, 1968
3. *Bailey RW, Badgley CE:* Stabilization of the cervical spine by anterior fusion. J Bone Joint Surg 42A:565, 1960
4. *Bernard TN Jr, Whitecloud TS III:* Cervical Spondylotic Myelopathy and Myeloradiculopathy. Clin Orthop Rel Res 221:149–160, August, 1987
5. *Bohlman HH:* Cervical spondylosis with moderate to severe myelopathy: A report of seventeen cases treated by Robinson anterior cervical discectomy and fusion. Spine 2:151, 1977
6. *Bollati A, Galli G, Gandolfini M, Marini G, Gatta G:* Microsurgical anterior cervical disk removal without interbody infusion. Surg Neurol 19:329, 1983
7. *Boni M, Cherubino P, Benazzo F:* Multiple subtotal somatectomy: Technique and evaluation of a series of thirty-nine cases. Spine 9:358, 1984
8. *Brain WR, Northfield D, Wilkerson M:* The neurological manifestations of cervical spondylosis. Brain 75:187, 1952
9. *Brain WR, Wilkerson M:* Cervical Spondylosis and Other Disorders of the Cervical Spine, 1st ed, p 226. Philadelphia, WB Saunders, 1967
10. *Brodsky AE, Summer JM, Khalil MA:* Fusion or no? Better imaging criteria needed. Presented at 50th Annual Meeting of the Western Orthopaedic Association, San Francisco, Jan 1987
11. *Brown MD, Malinin TI, Davis PB:* A roentgenographic evaluation of frozen allografts versus autografts in anterior cervical spine fusions. Clin Orthop 119:231, 1976
12. *Chirls M:* Retrospective study of cervical spondylosis treated by anterior interbody fusion (in 505 patients performed by the Cloward technique). Bull Hosp Joint Dis 39:74, 1978
13. *Clark E, Robinson PK:* Cervical myelopathy: A complication of cervical spondylosis. Brain 79:483, 1956
14. *Cloward RB:* The anterior approach for removal of ruptured cervical disks. J Neurosurg 15:602, 1958
15. *Cloward RB:* Cervical discography contribution to the etiology and mechanism of neck, shoulder and arm pain. Ann Surg 150:1052, 1959
16. *Cloward RB:* Lesions of the intervertebral disks and their treatment by interbody fusion methods. Clin Orthop 27:51, 1963
17. *Cloward RB:* Gas-sterilized cadaver bone grafts for spinal fusion operations: A simplified bone bank. Spine 5:4, 1980
18. *Connolly ES, Seymore RJ, Adams JE:* Clinical evaluation of anterior cervical fusion for degenerative cervical disc. J Neurosurg 23:431, 1965
19. *Cook SD, Whitecloud TS, Reynolds MC, Harding AF, Routman AS, Kay JF, Jarcho M:* Hydroxylapatite graft materials for cervical spine fusions. In Kehr P, Weidner A (eds): Cervical Spine I—Strasbourg 1985, p 257. Wien, New York, Springer-Verlag,

20. *Crandall PH, Batzdorf U:* Cervical spondylotic myelopathy. J Neurosurg 25:57, 1966
21. *Cuatico W:* Anterior cervical discectomy without interbody fusion: An analysis of 81 Cases. Acta Neurochir 57:269, 1981
22. *DePalma AF, Rothman RH:* The intervertebral disc in operative treatment of cervical disk disease, pp 429. Philadelphia, WB Saunders, 1970
23. *DePalma AF, Rothman RH, Lewinneck RE, et al:* Anterior interbody fusion for severe cervical disc degeneration. Surg Gynecol Obstet 134:755, 1972
24. *Dereymaeker A, Ghosez JP, Henkes R:* Le Traitment Chirurgical de la Discopathie Cervacle. Resultats compares de l'abord posterieur (laminectomie) et de l'abord ventral (fusion corporeale) dans une cinquantaine de cas personalles. Neurochirurgie 9:13, 1963
25. *Dohn DF:* Anterior interbody fusion for treatment of cervical disk condition. JAMA 197:897, 1966
26. *Dunsker SB:* Anterior cervical discectomy with and without fusion. Clin Neurosurg 24:516, 1977
27. *Flynn T:* Neurologic complications of anterior cervical fusion. Spine 7:536, 1982
28. *Galera GR, Tovi D:* Anterior disc excision with interbody fusion in cervical spondylotic myelopathy and rhizopathy. J Neurosurg 28:305, 1968
29. *Gooding MR, Wilson CB, Hoff JT:* Experimental cervical myelopathy: Effects of ischemia and compression of the canine cervical spinal cord. J Neurosurg 43:9, 1975
30. *Gore DR, Sepic SB:* Anterior cervical fusion for degenerated or protruded discs: A review of one hundred forty-six patients. Spine, 9:667, 1984
31. *Green PWB:* Anterior cervical fusion: A review of thirty-three patients with cervical disc degeneration. J Bone Joint Surg 59B:236, 1977
32. *Gregorius F, Estrin T, Crandall P:* Cervical spondylotic radiculopathy and myelopathy. Arch Neurol 33:618, 1976
33. *Guidetti B, Fortuna A:* Long-term results of surgical treatment of myelopathy due to cervical spondylosis. J Neurosurg 30:714, 1969
34. *Haft H, Shenkin HA:* Surgical end results of cervical ridge and disk problems. JAMA 186:312, 1963
35. *Hanai K, Inouye Y, Kawai K, Tago K, Itoh Y:* Anterior decompression for myelopathy resulting from ossification of the posterior longitudinal ligament. J Bone Joint Surg 64B:561, 1982
36. *Hanai K, Fujiyoshi F, Kamei K:* Subtotal vertebrectomy and spinal fusion for cervical spondylotic myelopathy. Spine 11:310, 1986
37. *Hankinson HL, Wilson CB:* Use of the operating microscope in anterior cervical discectomy with fusion. J Neurosurg 43:452, 1975
38. *Hirsch C:* Cervical disc rupture: Diagnosis and therapy. Acta Orthop Scand 30:172, 1960
39. *Hirsch C, Wickbon I, Lidstrom A, et al:* Cervical disc resection. A follow-up of myelographic and surgical procedure. J Bone Joint Surg 46A:1811, 1964
40. *Hoff JT, Wilson CB:* Microsurgical approach to the anterior cervical spine and spinal cord. Clin Neurosurg 26:513, 1979
41. *Hukuda S, Mochizuki T, Ogata M, Shichikawa K, Shimomura Y:* Operations for cervical spondylotic myelopathy. J Bone Joint Surg 67B:609, 1985
42. *Jacobs B, Krueger EG, Leivy DM:* Cervical spondylosis with radiculopathy: Results of anterior diskectomy and interbody fusion. JAMA 211:2135, 1970
43. *Kadoya S, Nakamura T, Kwak R:* A microsurgical anterior osteophytectomy for cervical spondylotic myelopathy. Spine 9:437, 1984
44. *Kraus FR, Stauffer ES:* Spinal cord injury as a complication of elective anterior cervical fusion. Clin Orthop 112:130, 1975
45. *LaRocca SH:* Personal communication, 1984
46. *Lees F, Turner JWA:* Natural history and prognosis of cervical spondylosis. Br Med J 2:1607, 1963
47. *Lunsford LD, Bissonette DJ, Jannetta PJ, Sheptak PE, Zorub DS:* Anterior surgery for cervical disc disease. Part 1: Treatment of lateral cervical disc herniation in 253 cases. J Neurosurg 53:1, 1980
48. *Lunsford LD, Bissonette DJ, Zorub DS:* Anterior surgery for cervical disk disease: Treatment of cervical spondylotic myelopathy in thirty-two cases. J Neurosurg 53:12, 1980
49. *Mann KS, Khosla VK, Gulati DR:* Cervical spondylotic myelopathy treated by single-stage multilevel anterior decompression: A prospective study. J Neurosurg 60:81, 1984
50. *Martins AN:* Anterior cervical discectomy with and without interbody bone graft. J Neurosurg 44:290, 1976
51. *Murphy MG, Gado M:* Anterior cervical discectomy without interbody bone graft. J Neurosurg 37:71, 1972
52. *Nurick S:* The pathogenesis of the spinal cord disorder associated with cervical spondylosis. Brain 95:87, 1972
53. *Nurick S:* The natural history and the results of surgical treatment of the spinal cord disorder associated with cervical spondylosis. Brain 95:101, 1972
54. *Odom GL, Finney W, Woodhall B:* Cervical disk lesions. JAMA 166:23, 1958
55. *O'Laoire SA, Thomas DGT:* Spinal cord com-

pression due to prolapse of cervical intervertebral disc (herniation of nucleus pulposus): Treatment in 26 cases of discectomy without interbody bone graft. J Neurosurg 59:847, 1983

56. *Philips DG:* Surgical treatment of myelopathy with cervical spondylosis. J Neurol Neurosurg Psychiatr 36:879, 1973
57. *Riley LH Jr, Robinson RA, Johnson KA, et al:* The results of anterior interbody fusion of the cervical spine: Review of ninety-three consecutive cases. J Neurosurg 30:127, 1969
58. *Robertson JT:* Anterior removal of cervical disc without fusion. Clin Neurosurg 20:259, 1973
59. *Robertson JT:* Anterior operations for herniated cervical disc and for myelopathy. Clin Neurosurg 25:245, 1978
60. *Robinson RA, Smith GW:* Anterolateral cervical disc removal and interbody fusion for cervical disc syndrome. Bull John Hopkins Hosp 96:223, 1955
61. *Robinson RA, Walker AE, Ferlic DC, et al:* The results of an anterior interbody fusion of the cervical spine. J Bone Joint Surg 44A:1569, 1962
62. *Rosenorn J, Hansen EB, Rosenorn MA:* Anterior cervical discectomy with and without fusion: A prospective study. J Neurosurg 59:252, 1983
63. *Sakou T, Miyazaki A, Tomimura K, Maehara T, Frost HM:* Ossification of the posterior longitudinal ligament of the cervical spine: Subtotal vertebrectomy as a treatment. Clin Orthop 140:58, 1979
64. *Sandre RL, Wilson DH:* The surgery of cervical disc disease: New perspectives. Clin Orthop 146:119, 1980
65. *Simmons EH, Bhallia SK:* Anterior cervical discectomy and fusion: A clinical and biomechanical study with eight year follow-up. J Bone Joint Surg 51B:225, 1969
66. *Smith GW, Robinson RA:* The treatment of certain cervical spine disorders by the anterior removal of the intervertebral disc and interbody fusion. J Bone Joint Surg 40A:607, 1958
67. *Southwick WO, Robinson RA:* Surgical approaches to the vertebral bodies in the cervical and lumbar regions. J Bone Joint Surg 39A:631, 1957
68. *Stooky G:* Compression of the spinal cord due to ventral extradural cervical chondromas: Diagnosis and surgical treatment. Arch Neurol Psychiatr 20:275, 1928
69. *Stuck RM:* Anterior cervical disc excision and fusion: Report of two hundred consecutive cases. Rocky M Med J 60:25, 1963
70. *Sugar O:* Spinal Cord Malfunction after Anterior Cervical Discectomy. Surg. Neurology 15:4, 1981
71. *Tew JM Jr, Mayfield FH:* Complications of Surgery of the Anterior Cervical Spine. Clin Neurosurg 23:424, 1975
72. *Tezuka A, Yamada K, Ikata T:* Surgical results of cervical spondylotic radiculo-myelopathy observed more than five years. Tokushima J Exp Med 23:9, 1976
73. *Verbiest H, Paz Y, Geuse HD:* Anterolateral surgery for cervical spondylosis in cases of myelopathy or nerve root compression. J Neurosurg 25:611, 1966
74. *White AA III, Hirsch C:* An experimental study of the immediate load bearing capacity of some commonly used iliac grafts. Acta Orthop Scand 42:482, 1971
75. *White AA III, Southwick WO, DePonte RJ, et al:* Relief of pain by anterior cervical spine fusion for spondylosis: A report of sixty-five cases. J Bone Joint Surg 55A:525, 1973
76. *Whitecloud TS III:* Complication of anterior cervical fusion. In the American Academy of Orthopaedic Surgeons: Instructional Course Lectures, p 223. St. Louis, CV Mosby, 1978
77. *Whitecloud TS III, LaRocca SH:* Fibular struct graft in reconstructive surgery of the cervical spine. Spine 1:33, 1976
78. *Williams JL, Allen MD Jr, Harkess JW:* Late results of cervical discectomy and interbody fusion: Some factors influencing the results. J Bone Joint Surg 50A:277, 1968
79. *Wilson DH, Campbell DD:* Anterior cervical discectomy without bone graft: Report of seventy-one cases. J Neurosurg 47:551, 1977
80. *Yonenobu K, Fuji T, Ono K, Okada K, Yamamoto T, Harada N:* Choice of surgical treatment for multisegmental cervical spondylotic myelopathy. Spine 10:710, 1985
81. *Zhang, AH, Yin H, Yang K, Zhang T, Dong F, Dang G, Lou SQ, Cai Q:* Anterior intervertebral disc excision and bone grafting in cervical spondylotic myelopathy. Spine 8:16, 1983

Anterior and Posterior Approaches to the Cervical Spinal Cord, Discs, and Roots: A Comparison of Exposures and Decompressions

RICHARD B. RAYNOR

Two operations are routinely used for cervical radiculopathy and/or spondylosis. The diseased area may be approached anteriorly by removing the intervertebral disc and, usually, parts of the adjacent vertebral bodies. The operation is extended laterally to achieve root decompression by removing more disc and bone.

Osteophytes on the posterior border of the vertebral bodies at the interspace are easily accessible. The uncovertebral joints, which are at the lateral margins of the interspace, should also be within the operative field. The lateral bony walls of this joint form part of the anteromedial wall of the neural foramen and canal through which the nerve root exits.

The root may be visualized directly by approaching it posteriorly. This requires resection of the facet joint along its medial side to expose the root axilla and its lateral extension into the neural foramen. For spondylosis and cord compression, a laminectomy extending over multiple levels is required. This can be combined with facetectomy if root problems coexist.

Few objective criteria are available to evaluate the merits and shortcomings of either an anterior or a posterior approach. Our purpose is to establish objective criteria, where possible, and to evaluate the potential advantages and disadvantages of each approach in light of these criteria.

BACKGROUND

To accurately evaluate what could be accomplished by each operation, isolated cervical spine segments were studied.[13] These consisted of the C4–C5 or C6–C7 vertebrae with all their interconnecting ligaments and discs intact but stripped of their muscular attachments.

For an anterior decompression, the standard Cloward technique was used. This provides good visualization of the area, allowing an assessment of what was thought to have been done at the time of surgery. Later, the joint was disarticulated for a more accurate evaluation of what was actually done. The largest Cloward drill compatible with leaving a lateral rim of vertebral body was used. In a group of specimens, x-rays were taken at each stage of the dissection to evaluate their usefulness in determining what had actually been accomplished surgically. These x-rays were later evaluated in comparison with the disarticulated specimen.

To evaluate root decompression via the posterior approach, a facetectomy was performed and appropriate measurements and x-rays were made. The same specimen was used for both an anterior and posterior decompression, allowing a careful comparison of the procedures. The initial procedure was changed from posterior to anterior on alternate specimens to obtain a more random appraisal.

ANTERIOR APPROACH

Orientation and Landmarks

The cervical spine is approached anteriorly in the plane between the great vessels laterally and the tracheoesophageal complex medially. The initial dissection is from a somewhat lateral position toward the midline. When the anterior aspect of the vertebral bodies is reached, the midline must be identified. The longus colli muscles, which are attached to the anterolateral aspect of the vertebral bodies, are the best landmark since there is a bare space between the right and left muscles.[10] Frequently there is also a small bony ridge in the middle of this bare space. However, in the degenerative spine the longus colli muscles can be asymmetrical in size and location. An anterior osteophyte can be present on either side of the midline to further distort the surgeon's orientation. The anatomic midline may be difficult to determine, causing the surgical approach through the vertebral bodies to be placed more to one side. The consequences of this difficulty are significant when the posterior longitudinal ligament is reached and the decompression part of the operation is performed.

Surgical Exposure

The lateral extent of the exposure can be overestimated since the full width of vertebral body to its attachment to the lateral mass is not normally exposed. The medial borders of both longus colli muscles are dissected from the vertebral body, especially if they are used to anchor self-retaining retractors. However, this dissection is generally limited, because the sympathetic chain lies near the lateral border of the muscle (as do the recurrent laryngeal nerves in the lower part of the cervical spine). A sufficiently lateral dissection can also bring the roots into the operative field. Thus, the body-lateral mass junction is usually not exposed, again making uncertain the true midline orientation and precise lateral extent of the vertebral body.

Root Decompression

The midline orientation problem becomes compounded with the approach to the posterior aspect of the vertebral body, regardless of whether this is accomplished by removing disc only, or both disc and bone. Many surgeons do not remove the posterior longitudinal ligament. The most reliable landmark, the edges of the dural tube, is not seen. Even when the posterior longitudinal ligament is removed, the dural tube borders may not be visualized, especially if an osteophyte has flattened the dura and caused it to extend laterally to fill the transverse diameter of the canal. The lateral extension of the bony exposure tends to be narrower than the central part, at least ventrally near the posterior longitudinal ligament, creating the illusion that one is viewing the roots in these lateral extensions. Figure 11-37 illustrates the problems of visualization and exposure.

Root decompression can be minimal if the lateral extension of disc and bone removal is not carried beyond the line of direct vision. Note in Figure 11-37 that neither the dural edge nor the root can be seen on the right, even though the drill hole through the vertebral body is relatively large. On the left, the edge of the dural tube can just be seen if the posterior longitudinal ligament is opened.

The most effective means of extending the decompression laterally is by the use of 30 to 0 upbiting currettes. These are gradually worked laterally sweeping upward and toward the midline, first from the superior edge of the lower vertebral body and then from the inferior edge of the upper vertebral body bordering the interspace. No more than the posterior one quarter of the body, measured by depth, should be removed. If the vertebral body is divided into quarters, proceeding in an anterior-to-posterior direction, the vertebral artery lies approximately opposite the second or third quarter of the body, as shown in Figure 11-37.[13] Using the full lateral reach of the curettes, beyond the surgeon's field of vision, 3 to 5 mm of nerve can be decompressed. This assumes that the initial approach is relatively close to the lateral margin of the spinal canal.[13]

Although magnification enhances anatomic detail,[9] it in no way increases the extent of the visual field.[13]

Maximum visualization for lateral decompression is obtained by standing on the side opposite the root being worked on. The up-angled currettes are then used with the distal end reaching beyond the visual field of the operator.

OSTEOPHYTE RESECTION

In their early descriptions of the anterior approach, Smith and Robinson noted that it was not necessary to remove an osteophyte projecting into the spinal canal.[17] The immobilization provided by fusion would alleviate symptoms in two ways. First, the osteophyte would tend to resorb if the irritative focus due to motion was removed. Second, immobilization of the joint would decrease the irritative focus due to motion of neural structures over the bony protuberance. Although some osteophytes do eventually resorb after immobilization, some do not.[4] If the osteophyte persists and is large, it will continue to compress neural structures, regardless of whether they move over it. On balance, it is desirable to remove large osteophytes.

MIDLINE OSTEOPHYTES

In spondylosis the cephalad-caudad extent of an osteophyte along the posterior margin of the vertebral body must be considered. In most instances this is only a matter of a few millimeters on each body, and the standard methods of doing the operation will result in an adequate removal, especially if up-angled currettes or the air drill is used on the posterior margin of the vertebral body just anterior to the posterior longitudinal ligament. Again, this is basically a blind procedure since the posterior body margin must be undercut to remove the osteophyte.

With the Cloward technique, the midline osteophytes are rarely a problem, provided the drill hole is properly placed. However, the lateral extensions of the bony ridges can be missed, unless the lateral edges of the drill hole are curetted. Using the Smith-Robinson technique, some of the

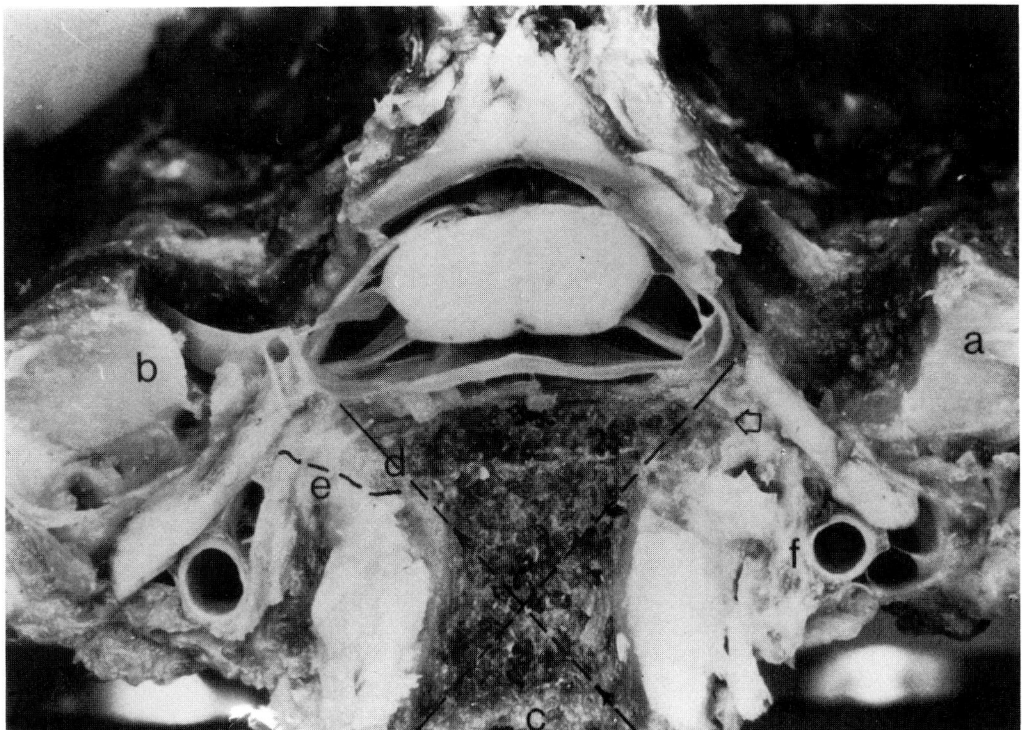

Fig. 11-37. The C4–C5 interspace has been disarticulated and the viewer is looking superiorly at the undersurface of C4. A bilateral facetectomy has been done, with one half of the facet removed on the right (*a*) to expose 4 mm of root. On the left (*b*), one quarter of the facet has been resected and 5 mm of root has been exposed. A Cloward procedure (*c*) has been performed. The line of vision from the right side of the specimen to the left root has been drawn (*d*). Note that neither the dural edge nor the root can be seen. On the opposite side, the line of maximal lateral visualization is also drawn. The bone of the uncovertebral joint has been resected for several millimeters laterally (*open arrow*), beyond the limits of visualization. The dural edge and the roots would be seen if the posterior longitudinal ligament and its lateral expansion were removed. On the left, the resection of the uncovertebral joint has been retouched (*e*). X-ray films with markers verified that the extent of lateral root exposure achieved was the same anteriorly and posteriorly. Note the vertebral artery position (*f*) in relation to the depth of the vertebral body. (Raynor RB: Anterior or posterior approach to the cervical spine: An anatomical and radiographic evaluation and comparison. Neurosurgery 12:7, 1983)

midline bars can be left, unless enough of the posterior body under the posterior longitudinal ligament is resected cephalad and caudad as indicated by the location of the osteophyte.

At times, the osteophytic ridge can extend a considerable distance in a cephalad-caudad direction. It then becomes difficult to determine whether bone removal has been adequate. The operator sees only the posterior edge of the vertebral body but cannot see around the corner to accurately evaluate the vertebral body–dura interface. Attempts to translate preoperative measurements to the intraoperative situation are difficult because of the lack of direct vision (Fig. 11-38).

Long-Term Considerations

The number of levels that should or can be operated on anteriorly has not been determined by

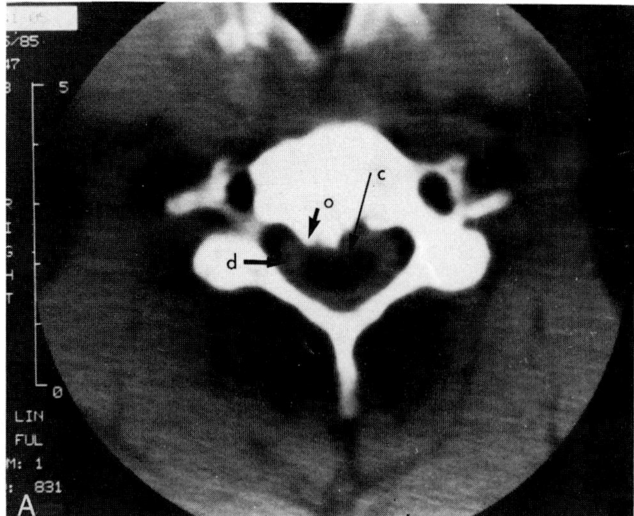

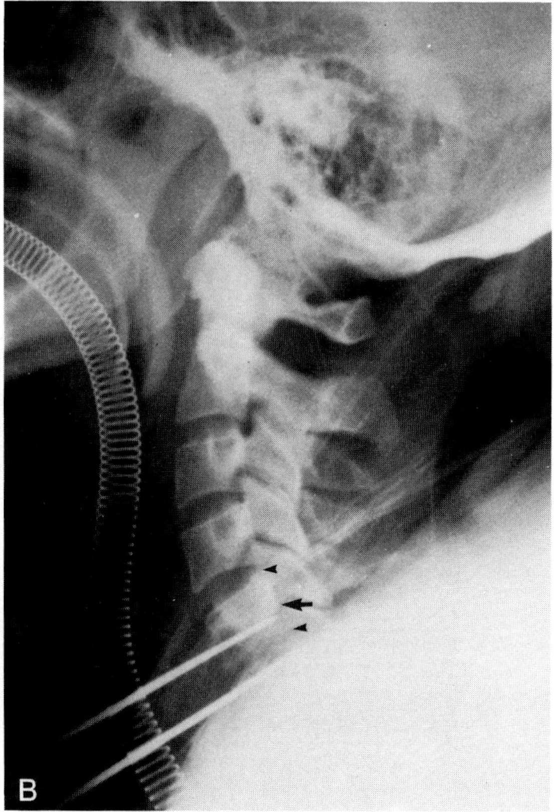

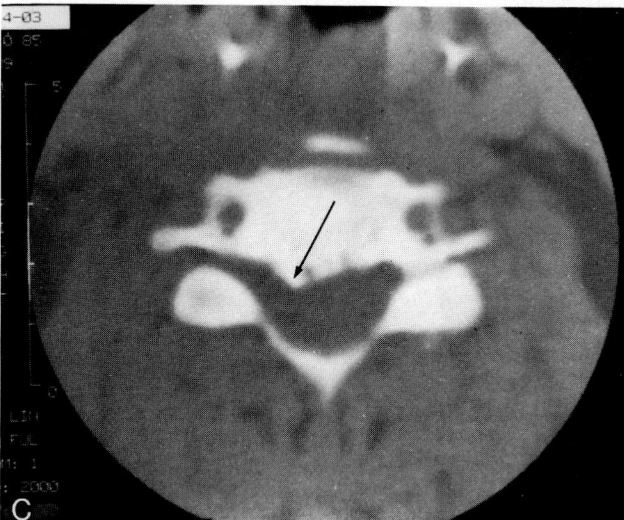

Fig. 11-38. (*A*) Preoperative CT myelogram showing a large osteophyte (*o*) impinging on the spinal cord (*c*) and right root. The dural tube (*d*) contains contrast material. Measurements indicated that the osteophyte extended about one third up the body of the vertebra. (*B*) An attempt was made in the operating room to measure the length of the vertebral body resection. A forceps has been placed in the resected area. The arrowheads indicate the upper and lower limits of the vertebral body. The arrow indicates the upper limit of vertebral body resection achieved by undercutting the posterior rim of the body next to the posterior longitudinal ligament. (*C*) Postoperative CT scan. The arrow indicates remaining osteophyte, in spite of what was believed to be an adequate length of bone resection.

hard and fast data. When making this decision, several factors should be considered. Each interspace fused decreases overall spine motion. The adjacent interspaces attempt to compensate and are placed under increased stress. In a number of patients examined 2 to 5 years after a one- or two-space anterior fusion, an increase in degenerative changes has been noted at the adjacent interspaces immediately above or below (Fig. 11-39).[2] In the younger patient, especially, the possible long-term consequences of this effect must be considered. If three, or perhaps even four, spaces have been

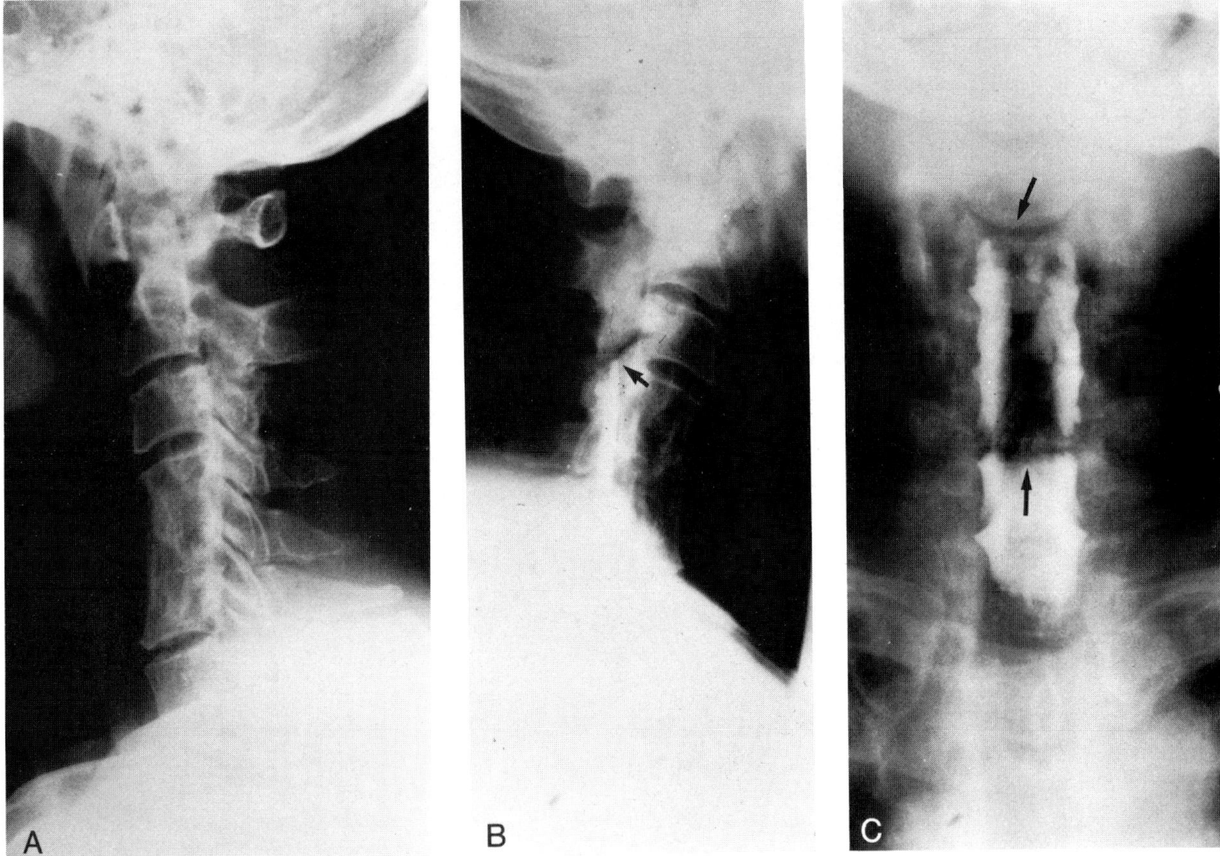

Fig. 11-39. (*A*) Anterior fusion performed 5 years ago at C4–C5 and C5–C6. Myelogram at the time was normal at C3–C4 and C6–C7. (*B*) Myelogram shows high-grade block to the flow of contrast material at C3–C4 (*arrow*). (*C*) Posteroanterior projection showing large defect in contrast at C6–C7 and block at C3–C4 (*arrows*).

done initially, the prognosis regarding functional capacity and complications must be weighed.

Lateral Osteophytes

Lesions in the uncovertebral joint can best be approached anteriorly (Fig. 11-37). The ventral part of the joint is easily removed, affording good decompression into the root axilla region. This area is important because in its normal course the root curves anteriorly as it exits laterally. Degenerative changes here can tether the root and prevent the normal cephalad-caudad motion of the cord that occurs with movement of the cervical spine.[3] The lateral wall of the joint also forms the anteromedial wall of the neural foramen. An osteophyte here may cause local root compression. Opening the uncovertebral joint therefore decompresses the neural foramen.[7,13]

THE POSTERIOR APPROACH

Technical Considerations

Decompression of a nerve root by a posterior approach requires a facetectomy. Less than half of the facet joint should be removed so that the possibility of instability is kept to a minimum. Resecting more than 50% of the joint significantly decreases its strength.[14]

The facetectomies on isolated motion segments were performed with the high speed air drill using standard operative technique. The estimate of the amount of facet resection was reasonably accurate,

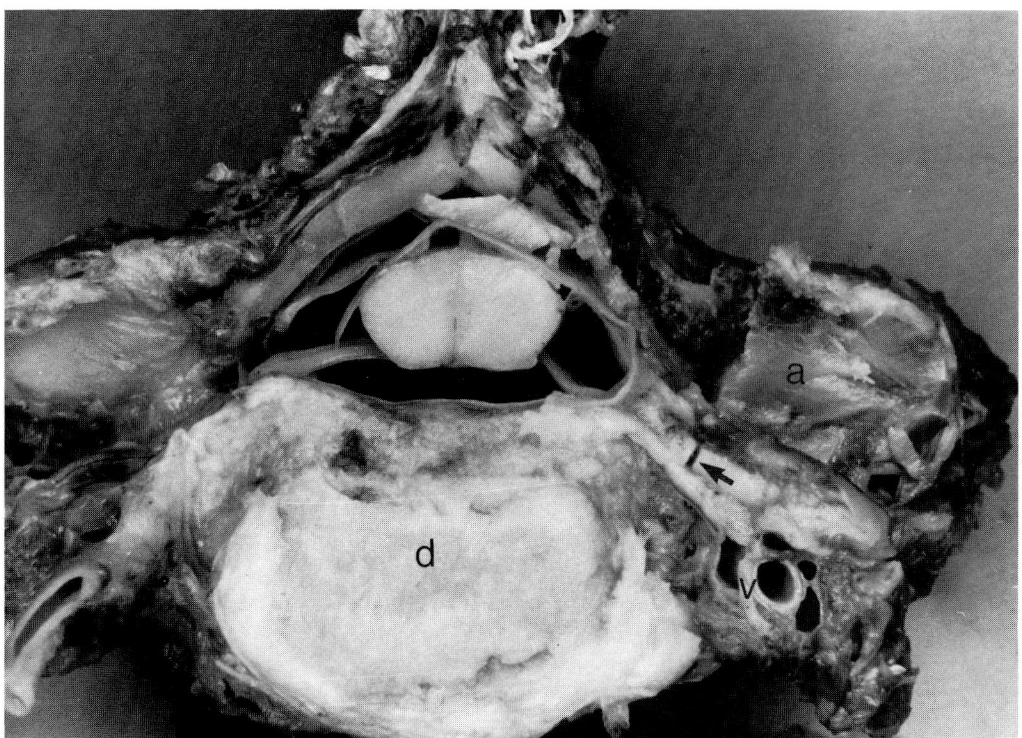

Fig. 11-40. The observer is looking upward at the inferior surface of C6. One quarter of the facet (*a*) has been resected on the right. The arrow points to an incision made in the root at its lateral limit of visualization after facetectomy, but before the joint was disarticulated. By measurement, 3 mm of root could be seen after facetectomy. Note the position of the vertebral artery (*v*) and its venous plexus with regard to the anteroposterior diameter of the disc (*c*). (Raynor RB: Anterior or posterior approach to the cervical spine: An anatomical and radiographic evaluation and comparison. Neurosurgery 12:7, 1983)

as verified later in the disarticulated joint. In no instances did the actual resection exceed the estimate.

The amount of nerve root actually exposed by the facetectomy was measured. The distance from the dural tube to the posterolateral margin of exposed root was 3 to 5 mm when less than 50% of the facet was removed (Fig. 11-40).[13]

The position of the nerve root relative to the interspace was somewhat surprising. Of six specimens examined, three roots left the dural tube horizontally, directly overlying the intervertebral disc. Two roots were angled caudad at fifteen degrees. One root exited at an angle of 38 degrees from the horizontal in a markedly oblique, caudad course (Fig. 11-41). Its point of egress was opposite the vertebral body above the intervertebral disc, and remained so in its exposed length.[7,13] Roots can also angle cephalad in the spondylytic patient, although this rarely happens.

Uncovertebral Joint Decompression

The posterior longitudinal ligament is opened just above and below the root in two specimens. The air drill is passed ventral to the ligament, and bone is resected under the root in the area of the uncovertebral joint. Using this method, clinically smaller lateral spurs have been removed. A 3- or 4-mm bur is passed behind the ligament and under the root, then medially and/or laterally for about 4 to 5 mm. This is the distance that the exposure and configuration of the drill allows (Fig. 11-42).

Multiple Level Spondylosis

For spondylosis involving multiple levels, laminectomy is a very effective treatment, providing a lor-

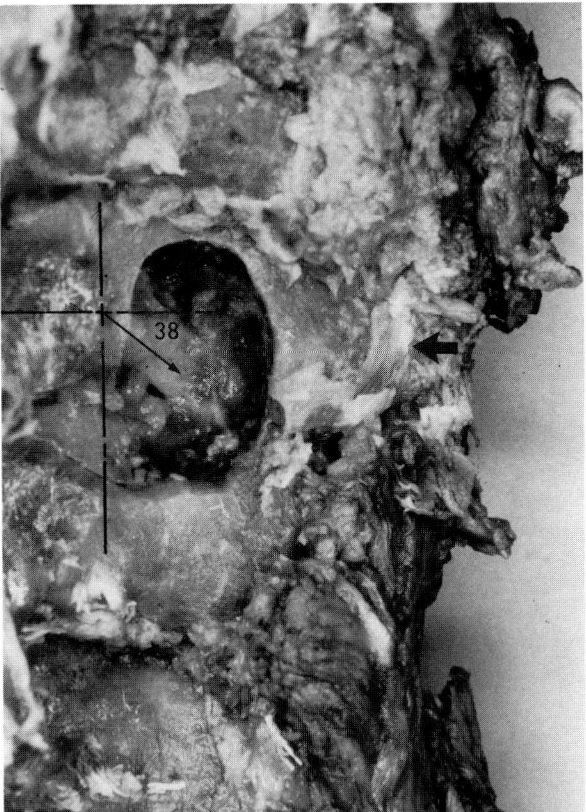

Fig. 11-41. Exposure of the C5 root after facetectomy. Slightly less than half of the inferior facet and about one third of the superior facet has been removed. Five millimeters of root are exposed. The root (*long arrow*) forms an angle of 38 degrees with the horizontal. Heavy arrow marks the lateral edge of the facet joint. (Raynor RB: Anterior or posterior approach to the cervical spine: An anatomical and radiographic evaluation and comparison. Neurosurgery 12:7, 1983)

dotic curve is present in the cervical region.[1,2] Removing the lamina allows the cord to float backward away from the vertebral ridges.[1,15] The decompression must extend above and below the area of compression to provide the necessary cord mobility. C3 to C6 laminectomy is usually the minimum decompression necessary. C7 and T1 are done frequently, and C2 rarely.[6] In severe cases with large ventral ridges, bilateral facetectomies are performed at two or three levels.[15] Approximately 25% to 30% of the joint is taken. This relieves the tethering effect of the root caught in a narrow foramen and further facilitates the ability of the cord to migrate posteriorly away from the ventral ridges (Fig. 11-43).

There is a group of patients in whom the posterior elements contribute to the cord compression of spondylosis.[18] Mechanically, this may result in the same compressive pattern as anterior pressure.[12] Hypertrophy or accordian-like infolding of the ligamentum flavum is almost always the problem. Laminectomy corrects this by removing these structures.

For spinal stenosis with a narrow canal, a posterior approach with decompression is obviously the procedure of choice.

DISCUSSION

Exposure of a cervical root from a posterior approach offers certain advantages. The principal one consists of direct visualization of the nerve roots and cord, thus evaluating the effectiveness of decompression. If soft-disc herniation is the problem, it is unlikely that fragments will be missed, especially if the root is above the interspace and fragments have migrated between the posterior longitudinal ligament and the vertebral body or laterally into the foramen. Three to 5 mm of root can be exposed if half of the facet joint is removed.[13] The joint remains mobile since only a small amount of disc or bone has been removed.

When root compression is caused by a hard disc or osteophyte ventrally in the area of the uncovertebral joint, an anterior approach offers better access and more effective decompression. However, the lateral extent of the decompression can be easily overestimated, especially if the posterior longitudinal ligament is kept intact and the dura is not visualized. If the lateral limits of the operative field are still under direct vision, at most a few millimeters of root are exposed. More usually, only the edge of the dural sac has been reached. It is even possible that no root decompression has been achieved, if the root does not leave the dural sac at the interspace, but leaves above it. To achieve the 3 to 5 mm of root decompression possible anteriorly, the full length of the up-angled curettes must be used with the end beyond the direct vision of the operator. The initial side-to-side extent of disc removal is the limiting factor, and it is doubtful that the lateral anatomic limit of disc is reached using any of the standard approaches.

Other anterolateral approaches to the area can expose most of the root. Verbiest has described one in which the anterior ramus is exposed behind the anterior tubercle of the transverse process.[19] The anterior wall of the neural canal is then resected. Hakuba sections the longus colli and ex-

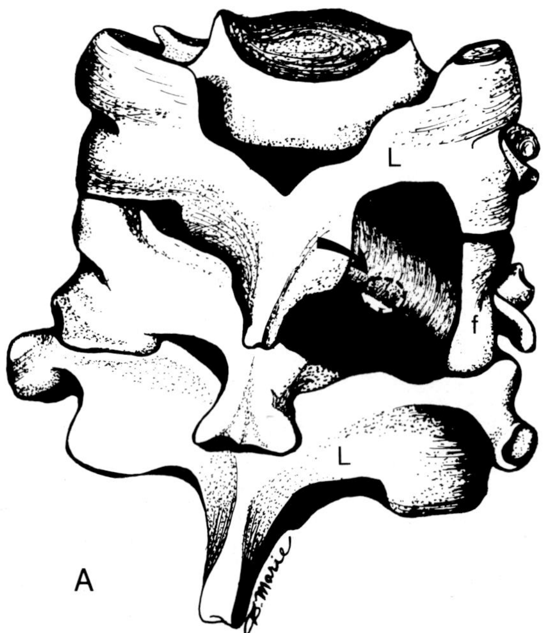

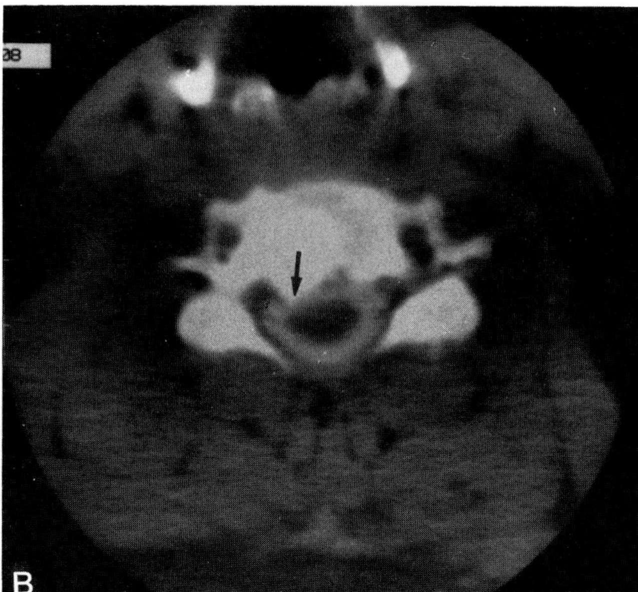

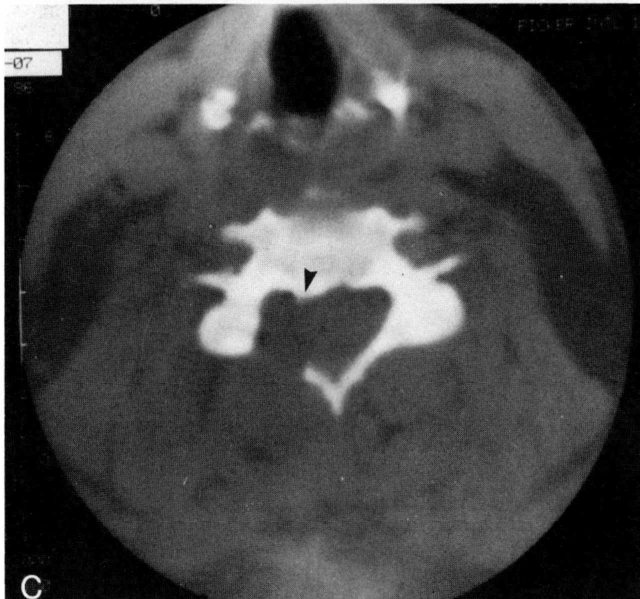

Fig. 11-42. (*A*) Drawing showing resected facet joint with root exposure. Arrow points to area of root undercutting (*f* = facet, *L* = lamina). This can also be accomplished superior to the root, if indicated. (*B*) CT myelogram showing osteophyte (*arrow*) impinging on root. (*C*) CT following hemilaminectomy with facetectomy. The posterior longitudinal ligament was opened below the root as shown in *A*. A 4-mm bur was passed through the opening, and the osteophyte was resected (*arrowhead*).

poses the vertebral artery after resecting the uncovertebral joint.[8] Neither of these operative techniques is in common use.

Care must be taken not to resect more than the posterior quarter of the lateral vertebral body since the vertebral artery lies in the middle third of the body.

A greater length of root can be easily exposed from a posterior approach in most cases, because the medial edge of the facet joint is easily identified and at least half of it can be removed without significantly affecting its strength. The length of decompressed root is under direct vision and can be confirmed. However, as much root can be exposed anteriorly if the dissection is vigorously pursued beyond the line of direct vision. Occasionally, epidural bleeding can be a problem.

Osteophytes arising from or near the uncover-

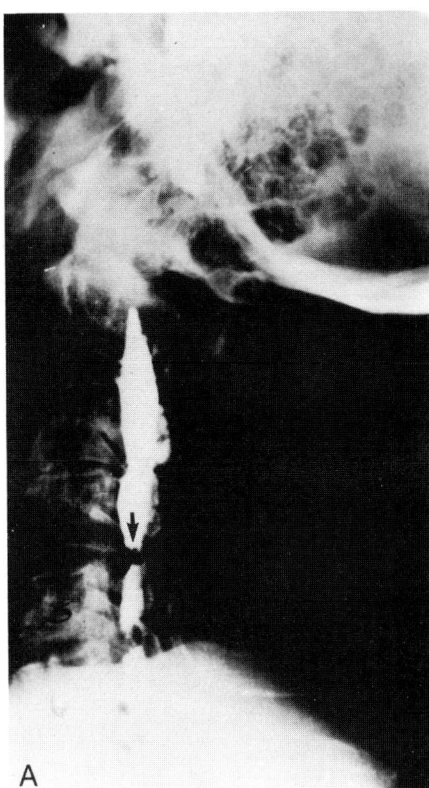

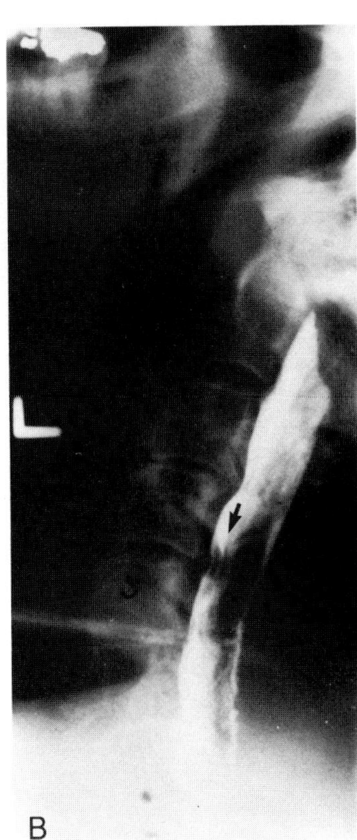

Fig. 11-43. (*A*) Myelogram showing defects in the contrast material at multiple levels both anteriorly and posteriorly. Note the particularly large ventral defect at C4–C5 (*arrow*) and the smaller defect at C5–C6. (*B*) Myelogram obtained 9 months after laminectomy of C3 through upper half of C7, with small facetectomies at C4–C5 and C5–C6. Contrast is present dorsal to the cord. At C5–C6 there is good filling of the subarachnoid space. At C4–C5 filling is still poor (*arrow*). Following the laminectomy, the patient had marked improvement in long tract signs and hands but continued to have proximal arm weakness. An anterior excision of the osteophyte at C4–C5 with particular attention to the lateral osteophytes for root decompression was done with marked improvement.

tebral joints are usually the cause of root compression in spondylosis. Anteriorly, this region is relatively easy to reach. However, even anteriorly the actual area of compression may be missed if the dissection is not carried far enough laterally to obtain part of the anteromedial wall of the neural foramen.

Posteriorly, it is difficult to decompress the area of the uncovertebral joint. However, if a bony excresence is large enough, it will cause atrophy of the intervening soft tissues between it and the ventromedial surface of the root. Only the posterior longitudinal ligament would then separate bone and dura. The posterior ligament can be opened above and below the root and the air drill can be used to resect bone under the root, using the posterior longitudinal ligament to protect the root.

A cervical root may leave the dural tube above the interspace.[4,7] If soft-disc herniation is the cause of root compression, the disc fragment may migrate behind the vertebral body out of the actual interspace.[4] When the root is clearly visualized from a posterior approach, the point of root compression can be seen and felt, and the disc fragment can be removed.[6] If an anterior approach is elected, the interspace-disc relationship should be carefully evaluated. When the root sleeve lies above the interspace, careful attention must be paid to the inferior edge of the superior vertebra.[4] This should be removed to provide the exposure necessary to facilitate mobilization of a high disc fragment.

The most effective way to remove a midline osteophyte is by the anterior approach, because no neural structures impede access to the lesion. A careful evaluation should be made preoperatively to determine the length of the bony bar in order to ensure an adequate cephalad-caudad decompression. It can be difficult to determine whether the cord is decompressed when viewing the area from an anterior approach, especially if the posterior longitudinal ligament remains intact.

When one or two levels are involved, an anterior decompression is indicated for midline osteophytes. If more than two levels are involved, a laminectomy with or without facetectomies may offer some advantages. Neck motion is not reduced by multiple fusions. Minimal stress is placed

Table 11-11. Anterior and Posterior Approaches to the Cervical Spine: Advantages and Disadvantages

Anterior Approach
- Advantages
  1. Removal of midline ridge
  2. Access to uncovertebral joint underlying root
  3. Immobilization of joint by fusion
- Disadvantages
  1. Orientation difficulty
  2. Restricted visualization, possibly resulting in inadequate superior-inferior decompression or inadequate root exposure and decompression
  3. Loss of joint mobility (even with simple disc excision, 60 to 70% of joints will fuse)

Posterior Approach
- Advantages
  1. Direct visualization of structures
  2. Multiple-level decompression
  3. Posterior soft-tissue decompression
  4. Functioning joint maintained
- Disadvantages
  1. Large ventral mass possibly continuing to cause pressure
  2. Risk in approaching midline area ventral to the dura
  3. Difficulty in decompressing uncovertebral joint ventral to root
  4. Possible instability

on the adjacent unfused levels reducing the possibility, especially in the younger patient, that these levels will become pathologic and require later treatment. Soft-tissue pathologic conditions, such as infolding or hypertrophy of the ligamentum flavum, are relieved.

The question of stability after a multiple-level laminectomy with some facetectomy has been raised.[5,11,16] In my experience, with patients in whom most of the facet joint is kept intact, the problem has occurred only once in a patient with spondylosis. Other authors have verified this result.[6] In the patient with intrinsic cord disease such as a tumor, different conditions exist and instability does occur. This is especially true in children.

There is a group of spondylytic patients in whom both an anterior and posterior operation may be indicated. They have multiple levels of anterior osteophytes, but the most severe compression occurs at one or two levels. The cord is frequently compressed from behind by ligamentum flavum. A long laminectomy relieves many but not all of the symptoms (Fig. 11-43). Although the cord may migrate posteriorly, it may not be sufficient to relieve pressure from a particularly large ventral ridge. Anterior excision at this level provides the necessary decompression, while maintaining mobility at the other involved levels that have been decompressed by laminectomy. The advantages and disadvantages of anterior and posterior approaches to the cervical spine in the treatment of cervical spondylosis are summarized in Table 11-11.

REFERENCES

1. *ABOULKER J, METZER I, DAVID M, ENGEL P, BAILLERET J:* Les Myelopaties cervicales d'origini rachidienne. Neurochirurgie 11:87, 1965
2. *BATZDORF U, BATZDORF A:* Analysis of cervical spine curvature in the surgical management of cervical spondylotic myelopathy: A pilot study. Presented at American Association of Neurological Surgeons, Denver, April 13–17, 1986
3. *BRIEG A:* Biomechanics of the Central Nervous System, pp 62–95. Chicago, Yearbook Publishers, 1960
4. *DUNSKER SB:* Anterior cervical discectomy with and without fusion. Clin Neurosurg 24:516, 1976
5. *DUNSKER SB:* Summary of panel on management of myelopathy and radiculopathy of cervical spondylosis. Clin Neurosurg 24:522, 1976
6. *FAGER CA:* Management of cervical disc lesions and spondylosis by posterior approaches. Clin Neurosurg 24:488, 1976

7. *Frykholm R:* Cervical nerve root compression resulting from disc degeneration and root sleeve fibrosis. Acta Chirurg Scand (Suppl)160, 1951
8. *Hakuba A:* Trans-unco-discal approach: A combined anterior and lateral approach to cervical discs. J Neurosurg 45:284, 1976
9. *Hankenson HH, Wilson CB:* Use of the operating microscope in anterior cervical discectomy without fusion. J Neurosurg 43:452, 1975
10. *Henry AK:* Extensile exposure, 2nd ed, p 69. Edinburgh, London, E & S Livingstone Ltd, 1959
11. *Mayfield F:* Cervical spondylosis: A comparison of the anterior and posterior approaches. Clin Neurosurg 13:181, 1965
12. *Raynor RB, Koplik B:* Cervical cord trauma: The relationship between clinical syndromes and force of injury. Spine 10:193, 1983
13. *Raynor RB:* Anterior or posterior approach to the cervical spine: An anatomical and radiographic evaluation and comparison. Neurosurgery 12:7, 1983
14. *Raynor RB, Pugh J, Shapiro I:* Cervical facetectomy and its effect on spine strength. J Neurosurg 63:278, 1985
15. *Scoville WB:* Cervical spondylosis treated by bilateral facetectomy and laminectomy. J Neurosurg 18:423, 1961
16. *Sim FH, Svien HJ, Bickel WH, Jones JM:* Swan-neck deformity following extensive cervical laminectomy. JBJS 56A:564, 1970
17. *Smith GW, Robinson RA:* The treatment of certain cervical spine disorders by the anterior removal of the intervertebral disc and interbody fusion. JBJS 40A:607, 1958
18. *Taylor AR:* The mechanism of injury to the spinal cord in the neck with damage to the vertebral column. JBJS 33B:543, 1951
19. *Verbiest H:* A lateral approach to the cervical spine: Technique and indications. J Neurosurg 28:191, 1968

Nonoperative Treatment of Cervical Spine Pain

MICHAEL J. MURPHY AND JONAS V. LIEPONIS

Pain of cervical origin has long been a challenge to physicians and a plague to mankind. The timeless phrase "pain in the neck" has characterized the human condition for centuries. The incidence of neck pain is largely unknown. Some attempts have been made to identify the incidence of degenerative changes in the cervical spine. Brain quoted an English series by Kellgren and Lawrence who found some degree of degenerative disc disease in 80% of all persons over the age of 55.[1] Although it is tempting to conclude that these degenerative changes are directly responsible for cervical pain syndromes, this may not necessarily be the case. Friedenberg and Miller compared series of symptomatic and asymptomatic patients and found that 75% of the asymptomatic group had degenerative changes comparable to those in the symptomatic group.[6] They believed that roentgenographic changes were of questionable value in determining the clinical significance of degenerative changes in the cervical spine. Although nonoperative treatment of neck pain is firmly rooted in ancient medical texts, the topic remains a timely subject of current medical philosophy in an era during which access to medical attention makes it an increasingly prevalent complaint.

The patient with neck pain must be carefully evaluated. The time-honored process consisting of history, physical examination, and differential diagnosis based on the appropriate diagnostic studies is essential. These considerations are more appropriately covered in other chapters. It is essential, however, that these diagnostic steps be followed to ascertain the patients for whom nonoperative treatment is appropriate. Pain of cervical origin can be attributed to many causes, including soft-tissue injury, degenerative vertebral or disc disease, fracture, infection, or tumor. The primary criterion for conservatively treating any of these conditions is that it has a low probability of producing neurologic deficit. Under certain conditions, any of these causes is capable of producing devastating neurologic damage, and these situations must be determined by appropriate objective evaluation, including plain roentgenograms, computerized tomography (CT), myelography, and magnetic resonance imaging (MRI). The nonoperative treatment of infection, tumors, and fractures is fully covered in other chapters. Therefore, the focus of this chapter is the nonoperative treatment of soft-tissue injuries of the cervical spine as well as of degenerative disease of the vertebral column and cervical discs.

Much of the confusion surrounding the treatment of the various types of neck pain arises from a cumbersome body of terminology. Such terms as whiplash, cervical strain, soft-tissue injury, hard disc, soft disc, cervical bar, spondylosis, facet arthrosis, foraminal spurring, uncodiscarthrosis, and spondylytic myelopathy may have different connotations for different observers. For the sake of simplicity, it is convenient to think of all these as points within a single disease spectrum that has resulted in abnormal or excessive biomechanical stress. This can occur acutely, as in traumatic lesions in which soft tissue (muscle, ligament, or disc) is more likely to be involved. It can also occur as the result of chronic biomechanical stress in which soft tissues are first altered but in which the major effect is seen in bony architecture (degenerative joints and osteophyte formation). The pain derived from this spectrum is first characterized as mechanical, with hypermobility resulting from soft-tissue laxity or trauma, or from degeneration of the disc itself. The pain may finally become neurogenic as subluxation or narrowing of the neural canal or foramina resulting from osteophyte formation begins to exert direct pressure on neural structures. Between these two points is a broad zone where the two overlap and the pain is both mechanical and neurogenic in nature. We will use this concept of a disease spectrum in formulating a rational approach to the nonoperative treatment of neck pain.

GENERAL PRINCIPLES OF NONOPERATIVE TREATMENT

Regardless of etiology, certain general principles of nonoperative management apply to all conditions resulting in pain that originates in the cervical spine, when there is no apparent ongoing risk to the neural elements.

Immobilization

One of the primary principles of managing any painful musculoskeletal problem is immobilization. In the cervical spine this is most easily accomplished by the use of an orthotic device. A great number of appliances are available, but the two most popular are (1) the soft collar—a band of contoured foam rubber that provides moderate restriction of flexion and extension, as well as rotation and side bending, and (2) the Philadelphia collar, which is more rigid and provides somewhat more immobilization.[8] The purpose of immobilization is the reduction of intervertebral motion that may lead to compression, mechanical irritation, or stretching of the affected nerve roots. The position of the cervical spine is of great importance. In general, mild flexion is more beneficial than extension because of the tendency to open the neuroforamina and, thus, to mechanically decompress the nerve roots. Ultimately, however, stabilization of the vertebral motion segments is best accomplished by increasing the resting tone of the muscular cuff surrounding the spine. Prolonged usage of a collar or brace eliminates paracervical muscle stimulation and therefore is counterproductive after the initial period of pain, inflammation, and muscle spasm has resolved. It is important to begin weaning patients from the collar or brace as soon as the initial "crisis" has passed. This can be accomplished over a period of time to allow the paracervical muscles to regain their tone without the spasm that accompanies the overloading of atrophic muscles. This process can also be facilitated by the performance of simple isometric neck exercises. These can be accomplished simply by placing the palm of a hand sequentially on all four quadrants of the skull with the neck in neutral position and exerting pressure without allowing either the skull or neck to move.

Bed Rest

Bed rest is actually another form of immobilization, but it has the advantage of eliminating the axial compression forces of gravity. Another benefit of bed rest is the activity modification it imposes. It is imperative that the position assumed in bed rest allow the cervical spine to be flexed slightly or held in the neutral position. Generally, standard pillows must be somewhat modified. Many commercially available "cervical" pillows accomplish this function reasonably well. We generally tell patients to arrange two standard pillows to create a V with the apex located cranially. A third pillow is then placed across the apex (Fig. 11-44). The advantage of this position is that it provides mild cervical flexion and also internally rotates the entire shoulder girdle, thus relieving some traction on the cervical nerve roots.

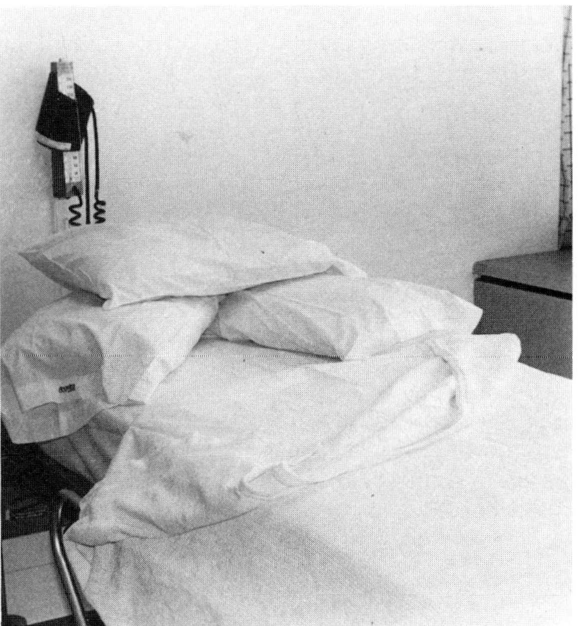

Fig. 11-44. A simple arrangement of three pillows—two forming an inverted V and the third across the apex—causes neck flexion and shoulder internal rotation. This position can offer significant relief to patients with cervical radiculopathy.

Traction

In a general sense, traction is another form of immobilization. Additionally, and probably most importantly, traction provides mechanical distraction of the cervical spine. Theoretically, this opens the neuroforamen and tends to flatten a bulging disc by placing the posterior longitudinal ligament under stretch. Furthermore, if accomplished with some flexion, it may relieve the pressure of osteophytes on the ventral floor of the neural canal. Some believe that it may increase blood flow, unload the facet joints, and, therefore, decrease ischemia in the synovial tissue of these joints. Whatever the mechanism, traction generally produces some relief of pain, particularly in the patients who exhibit a radicular component.

The presence of long tract signs or myelopathy is a relative contraindication to cervical traction in patients with severe spondylosis or disc disease. Patients with frank disc herniation may also complain of increased pain or radiculopathy, and, once traction has been initiated, this complaint should prompt further evaluation by means such as CT,

MRI, or myelography. Patients with massive paracervical muscle spasm may also complain of increased neck pain and spasm with the initiation of traction. Generally, it is advisable to control the spasm adequately before initiating traction.

The method of applying traction is very important. Although some physical therapy centers have special apparatus for applying cervical traction in the supine position, we have found this impractical to reproduce at bed rest. The standard home cervical traction is usually accomplished in the sitting position with a commercially available apparatus obtainable from most large pharmacies and surgical supply houses. This apparatus affixes to the back of an interior door and consists of a cervical halter, a length of cord over a pulley attached to the door frame, and a weight, most commonly, a plastic bag, that can be filled with water to a specific level corresponding to a certain number of pounds. We have found that the optimum position, imparting mild cervical flexion, is achieved with the patient facing the door (Fig. 11-45). As a general rule of thumb, 8 to 12 pounds of traction are applied for 15 to 20 minutes per session. These parameters can be adjusted according to patient tolerance, and several sessions per day may be optimum. Traction is continued as long as it appears to contribute to clinical improvement.

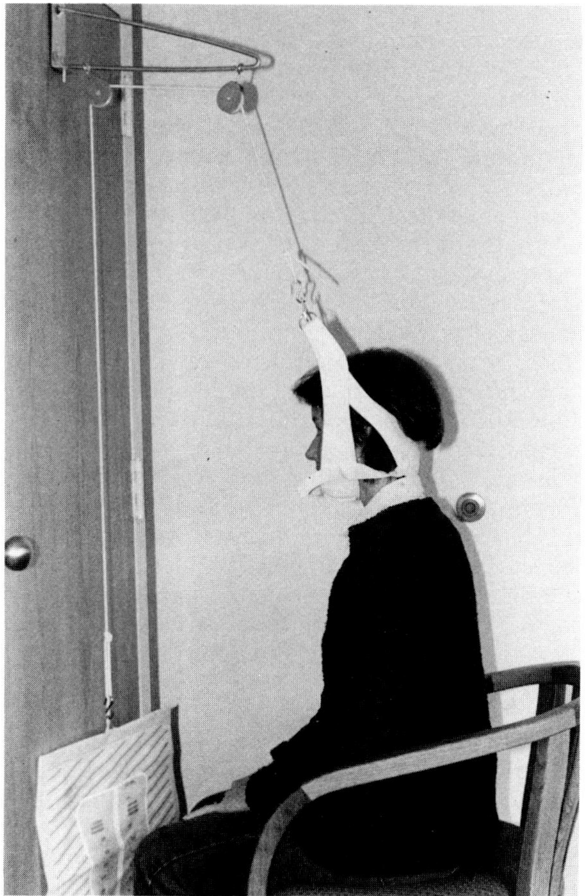

Fig. 11-45. Home cervical traction can be performed easily using a simple overhead frame, available at most pharmacies. The patient should be instructed to face the door, thus changing the angle of traction to gentle flexion.

Medication

Medication can play an important role in the management of cervical pain, particularly in the initial phase of treatment. Three broad categories of medication are commonly utilized: analgesics, muscle relaxants, and antiinflammatories. In our experience, no specific medication has universal application, and often patient tolerance dictates the choice of one drug over another.

Analgesics certainly play a major role in the initial treatment of acute cervical pain. Codeine in combination with aspirin or acetaminophen generally provides adequate analgesia. Synthetic opiates may occasionally be required, but the potential for addiction should always be kept in mind, especially if its use is anticipated to be greater than several weeks.[15]

Muscle spasm frequently accompanies acute cervical pain syndromes and can often be the source of a large component of the overall pain problem. This probably occurs by increasing the tension on the insertion of muscles into the periosteum and by creating a relative state of ischemia within the muscle allowing the build-up of products of anaerobic metabolism, thus setting up a "cycle" of repetitive spasm. Breaking this cycle can contribute greatly to patient comfort. Several authors have noted good results with carisoprodol (Soma), and we commonly use this medication. Effective alternatives are methocarbamol (Robaxin) or diazepam (Valium). A common side effect of these medications is drowsiness, although at times this may prove to be an advantage, initially, by restricting activity.

Currently, many excellent nonsteroidal anti-inflammatories are on the market. This group of drugs is particularly beneficial when a large portion of the cervical pain is believed to derive from degenerative joint disease. It has been our experience that this group of drugs has the highest potential for individual patient intolerance, and it is not uncommon to try two or three before a beneficial result without side effects is obtained. Ibuprofen (Motrin) at maximum dosage is often effective, in our experience. Oral steroids have an extremely limited application because of their undesirable systemic complications.

A number of other types of drugs may have analgesic activity or may enhance the efficacy of other analgesics in patients with chronic pain. Tricyclic antidepressants such as amitriptyline, imipramine, desipramine, and doxepin may provide direct analgesia for chronic pain and may potentiate other analgesic actions. Amitriptyline has gained a certain preeminent position among this group of drugs, but it is sometimes poorly tolerated because of its anticholinergic side effects. Because of their sedative effects these drugs may be given at bedtime with double benefit.

MANAGEMENT OF CERVICAL PAIN BY REGIONAL BLOCK TECHNIQUES

Persistent cervical pain may result in both physical and psychological chronic dysfunction. Once surgically correctable lesions are ruled out, it is often necessary to provide symptomatic pain relief, not only for patient comfort, but also to prevent the development of a chronic pain syndrome. Surgical or chemical denervation of sensory pain fibers frequently produces disorders such as dysesthesias, which may cause greater discomfort than the original pain. For these reasons, destructive procedures should be reserved for patients who do not respond to conservative therapy, or for those with a short life expectancy.

Often, in order to achieve the best possible outcome, it is beneficial to combine regional block techniques with other modalities such as relaxation exercises, physical therapy, and oral medication.

Myofascial pain syndrome involving the trapezius muscle is a common cause of cervical pain. If trigger points can be identified, infiltration using a local anesthetic (3 ml of 1% lidocaine or 0.25% bupivacaine) combined with 10 mg of depot steroid (triamcinolone diacetate or methylprednisolone) can be quite effective and may often break the pain cycle. In chronic resistant myofacial pain syndromes, trigger-point injections with 2 ml of 2.5% phenol in water may provide pain relief for prolonged periods of time.

Severe headaches are a common sequela of cervical pain as a result of paracervical muscle spasm. This may partly result from the fact that the greater and lesser occipital nerves travel through the trapezius muscle at the base of the skull, and the resulting muscle spasm may cause severe neurologic pain. An occipital nerve block with 3 ml of 0.25% bupivacaine and 10 to 20 mg of depot steroid often alleviates the neck pain and accompanying headache.

On rare occasions, degenerative facet joint disease may cause chronic persistent pain aggravated by movement of the neck. Facet joint blocks using the previously mentioned combination of 0.25% bupivacaine and depot steroid may offer prolonged pain relief. This procedure must be performed under fluoroscopy by an experienced operator to ensure a good result. The procedure may also be an effective diagnostic test.

Cervical radiculopathy resulting from cervical spondylosis or disc protrusion is in part due to the inflammatory process of the affected nerve roots with secondary edema. Therefore, reduction of edema and inflammatory response should significantly reduce symptoms. It has been our experience that cervical epidural injection of a local anesthetic (4 ml of 0.5% lidocaine) and steroid (40 to 60 mg of triamcinolone diacetate) often achieves this goal. Repeated injections may be necessary to produce a longer period of pain relief. Again, it is imperative that this procedure be performed by an experienced operator to avoid serious complications.

Tumors of the cervical spine or adjacent tissue may produce severe pain of bone destruction or mass effect on cervical nerve roots or cord. If the tumor is judged to be inoperable, or if life expectancy is so short that surgery is unwarranted, palliative regional blocks may be effective in controlling the pain. Epidural blocks, as described above, can offer significant relief in these situations. Neurolytic agents (absolute alcohol or phenol) are indicated in instances of tumor invasion of extravertebral cervical root invasion or involvement with the brachial plexus. Similarly, in inoperable vertebral body involvement with intractable pain, the use of subarachnoid block with neurolytic agents is indicated. Because of the potential disastrous complications of these procedures, they should only be performed by an experienced operator.

Recently, intractable and uncontrollable neck pain of nonmalignant or postoperative origin has been managed by the administration of opiates, (morphine or fentanyl) into the spinal canal (epidural or intrathecal). This procedure is still in the developmental stage, and further experience is needed to establish its efficacy and risk factors.[10]

TRANSCUTANEOUS ELECTRICAL NERVE STIMULATION

Transcutaneous electrical nerve stimulation (TENS) has been widely applied to a variety of pain management problems ranging from postoperative pain to the various chronic pain syndromes. The exact mechanism by which TENS reduces pain perception is still not clearly understood. Initially, many investigators used the spinal gate theory of Melzack and Wall developed in 1965 to explain the mechanism of action.[14] This theory proposed the existence of interneurons between large-diameter afferent fibers (touch and pressure) and small-diameter afferent fibers (pain), which could be activated to presynaptically inhibit transmission of one or the other tract, depending on which had the greater stimulus. This theory was not universally accepted and has since been modified to incorporate the discovery of endogenous opiate receptors, which are thought to play a modulatory role in the transmission of noxious stimuli to pain receptor regions of the thalamus.[7] Although the exact mechanism of action, remains to be fully explained, the technique can be beneficial in both acute and chronic cervical spine pain. Dougherty studied a group of 750 patients with chronic pain of various etiologies in which 55% obtained good pain relief, 17% obtained fair relief, and 29% achieved poor or no relief.[4] Generally our clinical experience has yielded similar results, and TENS continues to be an occasionally very effective, although not spectacular, technique in the management of chronic neck pain. Two major types of TENS are commonly used; high frequency (40 to 150 H_z, 50 to 100 μsec pulse width), low frequency (1 to 4 H_z, 100 to 400 μsec pulse width) with several variations.[7,5,12] Commonly, these various parameters are empirically altered using the patient's response as a guideline. The literature does not supply strict guidelines in regard to application of various modalities, although Mannheimer and Carlsson[12] suggest that high frequency is more effective in arthritic (rheumatoid) pain. Furthermore, Eriksson and coworkers[5] demonstrated that in a series of 123 chronic pain sufferers, 70% of the patients chose high-frequency treatment.

We use TENS as an adjunct to other forms of nonoperative therapy in an attempt to reduce symptoms, particularly, chronic pain. In this setting, TENS can be a very effective technique.

MANIPULATION

Manipulation is an ancient technique to alleviate spinal pain. Hippocrates is said to have first descrived spinal manipulation in 400 BC in the "Corpus Hippocrateum."[2] Though used more frequently for lumbar spine pain syndromes, some advocate its use in the cervical spine. Despite positive experience by Cyriax and others, there are also a number of disastrous results reported. We feel that the potential benefits of manipulation do not outweigh the potential risks involved and do not use this technique in the cervical spine.

PHYSICAL THERAPY

The physical therapist can be an invaluable assest in the nonoperative management of cervical pain. A good physical therapist has several techniques which can benefit a patient with neck pain both in terms of symptomatic relief during the treatment and in possibly shortening the overall length of treatment.

Heat is one of the basic techniques used by a physical therapist. The underlying theory is the theoretical increase in blood flow to the involved area. This should theoretically decrease muscle ischemia, help in the removal of products of anaerobic metabolism and aid in soft tissue repair. Heat may be applied in the form of moist heat packs—a technique the patient can be taught for home use—or via the use of diathermy. Paradoxically, some patients with severe acute muscle spasm respond better to ice packs applied to the area of involvement.

Direct electrical stimulation of the muscle groups that are in spasm can offer dramatic relief of pain. This effect is probably the result of increasing blood flow and its attendant benefits, as well as its interference with abnormal electrophysiologic activity in the muscle groups, which break the "spasm cycle." The use of ultrasound is a variant of this principle, and it probably acts in a similar fashion. In addition, it theoretically provides deep heat to the muscle groups.

The physical therapist may oversee the program of traction, and may exercise and educate the patient in proper body mechanics. It is our philosophy that both the physician and physical therapist should not only provide passive treatment to the patient, but should also educate and motivate the patient to take an active role in rehabilitation and accept a healthy share of the responsibility for recovery.

IMPLEMENTING A TREATMENT PLAN

With a knowledge of the various modalities and techniques available for the nonoperative treatment of cervical spine pain, the physician can determine which one is appropriate for the individual patient. The key to the success of such a plan is a solid physician–patient relationship, in which all the options and the probability of the success of each has been discussed. The patient then becomes an active partner in the plan and assumes much of the responsibility for its success. We believe that this is a very important point, and, in our experience, patients who prefer to assume a passive role in their treatment fare much worse.

Previously, we discussed the concept that the majority of nonneoplastic and noninfectious causes of cervical pain fell within a spectrum of pathophysiology, sharing a "common denominator" of altered biomechanics. This concept proposes that many of these pain syndromes begin as "mechanical pain" (e.g., muscle or ligament tear, degenerative joint disease) and that, if allowed to persist for long periods of time, result in anatomic lesions; these lesions initiate or compress neural elements, resulting in "neurogenic pain." Based on this concept, some modifications of the treatment plan must be made at different points along the spectrum.

Perhaps the most common cervical pain syndrome is the mechanical pain derived from minor injury. The classic flexion–extension injury or the whiplash (cervical strain) is a soft-tissue injury to the musculoligamentous support structures of the cervical spine. The injury sets up an inflammatory response accompanied by edema, decreased blood flow, and the tendency to paravertebral muscle spasticity. Initially, this is best treated with immobilization of the neck, mild analgesics, and muscle relaxants. Initially, ice (either packs or massage) will help to control edema and decrease muscle spasm. After the initial phase of acute pain has subsided, gentle range-of-motion exercises, isometric neck exercises, and applied heat (moist, hot packs, or diatheramy) will speed recovery. Persistent pain, especially related to "trigger-points," may respond very favorably to regional block techniques. Electrical muscle stimulation can also be effective in this phase. Generally speaking, rapid recovery is the rule and unless severe ligament injury has occurred, resulting in some degree of hypermobility, no long-term problems can be expected.

If the mechanical derangement has been more severe, resulting in vertebral hypermobility or early degenerative disc or joint disease, mechanical pain of a more chronic nature may ensue. Although immobilization may provide some symptomatic relief, the long-term solution to this problem is strengthening the internal support structures through a rigorous neck exercise program. This group will probably not benefit from pure analgesics and muscle relaxants but may significantly benefit from nonsteroidal antiinflammatories. Application of heat may provide some relief of symptoms, thus allowing the exercise program to continue unimpeded.

More severe degenerative disc or joint disease also responds to exercise, although to a lesser extent because exercise may be painful. Isometric exercises are the least irritating and should probably be the only ones used in this situation. Again, nonsteroidal antiinflammatory medication may offer significant benefit. Facet blocks and injections of steroid preparation may also help in these situations. Diathermy and ultrasound may provide temporary symptomatic relief, but the results are so short-lived that their use may not be warranted. In more severe degenerative disc disease, cervical traction may provide significant benefit.

As the disc herniates through acute trauma, or as the result of chronic degenerative changes, neurogenic pain ensues. Patients in this situation benefit greatly from immobilization in a cervical collar. Stronger analgesics are required in addition to muscle relaxants, if muscle spasm is present. Traction may be the most beneficial form of therapy in this group, but it should not be instituted until muscle spasm is controlled. Physical therapy probably has little to contribute in the initial phase of treatment, but as pain subsides an isometric neck exercise program can be of great value. We have had some promising results with epidural steroid injections; however, this technique should only be attempted by a physician experienced in these techniques.[10] TENS therapy may also provide significant relief.

Results of nonoperative therapy in this group of patients with cervical disc disease is generally good. DePalma and Subin reported a series of 225 patients treated in this manner for 3 months and cited complete pain resolution in 29%, partial relief in 49%, and no relief in 22%.[3] No surgical treatment was instituted prior to 1 year. Rothman and Subin reported on a series of 68 patients who were considered to be treatment failures after 1 year but who were followed for 5 years to determine their natural history.[16] At the 5-year point, 45% had achieved satisfactory pain relief and 55% reported unsatisfactory results, with 25% unable to return to their previous place of employment. Kumano and Umeyama reported a series of 20 athletes with acute cervical disc herniation.[9] With the exception of one who presented with myelopathy and underwent surgery, the remainder were treated nonoperatively. Seventeen of 20 athletes were able to return to full sports activity after an average of 17 weeks, and three never returned. Those who presented with neurologic deficits required up to 5 months to return to sports.

Once the pain has resolved from a cervical disc herniation, a program of isometric neck exercises and education in proper mechanics can be extremely valuable in preventing recurrence.

As the disc undergoes further degenerative change and becomes accompanied by peridiscal calcification, or if significant osteophyte formation results from altered biomechanics, a slightly different scenario unfolds. This group, in general, is more resistant to nonoperative treatment. Because of the chronic nature of this problem, immobilization with a collar is no longer practical, other than for short periods when symptoms flare. Traction also has less value, but warrants a trial. An isometric exercise program may be very beneficial in increasing the internal support of the cervical spine and relieving some of the mechanical stress at the site of involvement. Nonsteroidal antiinflammatories may provide significant benefit and may have to be augmented with analgesics. Because of the chronic nature of this problem, one of the tricyclic antidepressants may be very helpful. Furthermore, TENS therapy may provide significant benefit.

As degeneration progresses, often at multiple levels, osteophyte formation advances, and pressure on the spinal cord centrally or on nerve roots in the foramen produces an increasingly severe neurologic picture. This group is often referred to as having cervical spondylotic myelopathy. The changes may include hyperreflexia, clonus, gait disturbances, loss of sphincter control, and quadriparesis. This problem is often encountered in the sixth and seventh decades, and frequently these patients are not good surgical risks. Nonoperative treatment, although less successful, therefore assumes a more important role. Immobilization of the cervical spine can relieve some of the pain, and its long-term use may have to be accepted. Certainly, isometric exercises should cause no harm and may offer some benefit. Antiinflammatories and mild analgesics accompanied by tricyclic antidepressants may be of value. Experimental work has shown promising results from intrathecal opiate injection for controlling severe pain, but no significant benefit in regard to neurologic improvement. TENS therapy may also be helpful in the management of chronic pain. Certainly, surgical intervention should be considered for progressive neurologic deterioration.

In summary, nonoperative treatment of a great majority of the pain syndromes of the cervical spine can be expected to provide good results over a period of time. Time is, perhaps, the most important factor in considering this treatment. A thorough knowledge of the various modalities and techniques available to the treating physician, as well as an understanding of the limitations and appropriate application of each, may shorten the time involved and may certainly decrease symptoms during this period of recovery.

REFERENCES

1. *BRAIN R:* Some unsolved problems of cervical spondylosis. Br Med J 5333:771–77, 1963
2. *CYRIAX J, SCHIOTZ E:* Manipulation Past and Present, p 5. William Heinemann Books Ltd, 1975
3. *DEPALMA AF, SUBIN DK:* Study of the cervical syndrome. Clin Orthop 38:135–41, 1965
4. *DOUGHERTY RJ:* Transcutaneous electrical nerve stimulation: An alternative to drugs in the treatment of acute and chronic pain, p 10. Presented 34th Annual Scientific Assembly, American Academy of Family Physicians, 1982
5. *ERIKSSON M, SJOLUND B, NIELZEN S:* Long term results of peripheral conditioning stimulation as an analgesic measure of chronic pain. Pain 6:335–47, 1979
6. *FRIEDENBERG ZB, MILLER WT:* Degenerative disc disease of the cervical spine. J Bone Joint Surg 45A:1171–78, 1963
7. *GERSH MR, WOLF SL:* Applications of transcutaneous electrical nerve stimulation in the management of patients with pain. Phys Ther 65:3, 314–323, 1985
8. *JOHNSON RM, HART DL, ET AL:* Cervical orthosis: A study in normal subjects comparing their effectiveness in restricting cervical motion. J Bone Joint Surg 59A:323–39, 1977
9. *KUMANO K, UMEYAMA T:* Cervical disc injuries in

athletes. Arch Orthop Trauma Surg 105:223–226, 1986

10. *LILLEY JP, FROMME GA, WANG JK:* Management of acute pain. Adv Anesthesiol 4:347–364, 1987
11. *MACNAB I:* Cervical Spondylosis. Clin Orthop 109:69–77, 1975
12. *MANNHEIMER C, CARLSSON C:* The analgesic effect of transcutaneous electrical nerve stimulation in patients with rheumatoid arthritis. A comparative study of different pulse patterns. Pain 6:329–334, 1979
13. *MARVEL JP:* The clinical syndrome of cervical disc disease. Orthop Clin North Am 2:419–33, 1971
14. *MELZACK R, WALL PD:* Pain mechanisms: A new theory. Science 150:971–979, 1965
15. *PAYNE R, ET AL:* Principles of analgesic use in the treatment of acute pain and chronic cancer pain. American Pain Society. Syllabus.
16. *ROTHMAN AF, SUBIN DK:* Study of the cervical syndrome. Clin Orthop 38:135–41, 1965

Ossification of the Posterior Longitudinal Ligament in the Cervical Spine

K. HIRABAYASHI, K. SATOMI, AND T. SASAKI

Ossification of the posterior longitudinal ligament (OPLL) is noticeable as an abnormal radiopacity along the posterior margins of the vertebral bodies on lateral views of the roentgenogram. Although the pathogenesis of OPLL has not yet been clarified, it has come to be widely recognized that severe myelopathy or radiculopathy may be elicited by OPLL,[2–5,14,22,23] which is much more common among Japanese and other Oriental peoples than among Caucasians.[30,31]

It is said that the first report on the cervical compressive myelopathy due to OPLL was made by Key[13] in 1838. In Japan, Tsukimoto was the first to describe the pathologic condition of OPLL from autopsy findings in 1960,[29] and Onji and associates clinically reviewed 18 cases of OPLL in 1967.[23] Since then, many reports[28,33] of this disease have been made in Japan. The Investigation Committee[11,30] on Ossification of the Spinal Ligaments has been organized by the Ministry of Public Health and Welfare of Japan since 1974, which has been contributing to the clarification of epidemiology, etiology, and pathology of OPLL and to the treatment of myelopathy and radiculopathy due to OPLL.

OPLL of the cervical spine is reviewed here, because OPLL of the thoracic spine and lumbar spine is less frequent and shows different characteristics on a roentgenogram, and in regard to pathology and treatment.

INCIDENCE

In eastern Asiatic countries, including Japan, OPLL is observed in approximately 2% to 3% of the cervical roentgenograms of outpatients, as opposed to 0.2% at the Mayo Clinic and 0.6% in Hawaii.[30] In Italy 1.7% is reported.[11]

However, roentgenographic evidence of ossification is found much more frequently in the adult cervical spine for the reason that OPLL does not always cause clinical signs and symptoms. In fact, the incidence of asymptomatic ossification showed a roughly linear progression with advancing age; 11% of normal individuals in the sixth decade of life exhibited roentgenologic changes suggestive of ossification.[19]

ETIOLOGY

The etiology of OPLL remains obscure. Results of routine laboratory examination are all within normal range.

Studies of the family histories of patients with OPLL revealed the possibility of a hereditary dominant factor. It was suggested that the incidence of OPLL among family members of second-order kinship to the patient is about 30%, which is 15 times the general incidence.[31]

Concerning the general factors relevant to OPLL, it was suggested that patients with OPLL had a tendency toward generalized hyperostosis of the spinal ligaments,[21] such as diffuse idiopathic skeletal hyperostosis (DISH),[25] because ankylosing spinal hyperostosis (ASH) was observed in 23.9% to 30%[15] of the patients with OPLL and ankylosing spondylitis in 2.0%.[30]

Many authors[30] also maintained that a high incidence of diabetes mellitus was observed among patients with OPLL. Glucose tolerance tests in 535 patients resulted in 152 (28%) diabetics and 95 (18%) borderline diabetics, while the incidence of OPLL in diabetic patients was 16%.[11]

ROENTGENOGRAPHIC FINDINGS AND CLASSIFICATION

Early changes resulting from OPLL are inconspicuous on lateral films of the cervical spine.

Roentgenographically, cases of OPLL in the cervical spine are classified into the following types: the segmental type, in which OPLL is observed behind individual vertebral bodies; the continuous type, in which OPLL is observed through several vertebrae; the mixed type, which is a combination of the previous two types; and the "others" type in which OPLL is observed over intervertebral disc space (Fig. 11-46). The "other" type of OPLL are sometimes difficult to define on the lateral films of the cervical spine.

It is reported that the segmental type of OPLL occurred in 39.0%, the continuous type in 27.3%, the mixed type in 29.2% and the others type in 7.5% of patients.[30]

OPLL is most frequently observed at the C5, C4, and C6 levels on lateral films. The greatest thickness of OPLL is often seen at the same levels. The average number of vertebral bodies involved was 3.1, in the accumulated series.[30]

The narrowing of the spinal canal resulting

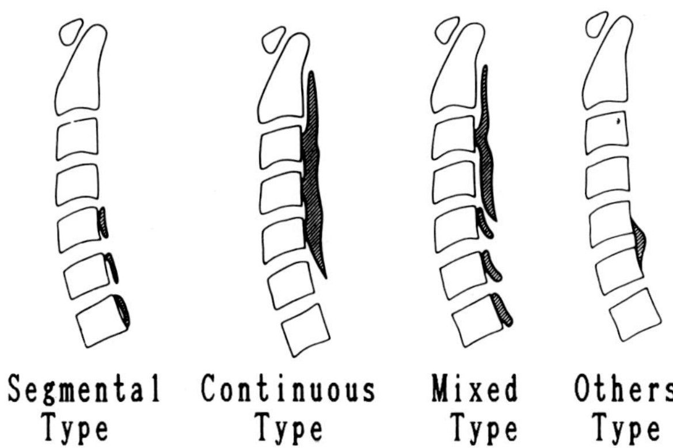

Fig. 11-46. Classification of OPLL as seen on lateral x-ray film.

from the ossified mass is calculated as a ratio of the maximal thickness of OPLL to the A–P diameter of the spinal canal on lateral views. The narrowing ratio is higher in the mixed and continuous types than in the segmental and "others" types of OPLL.

X-ray survey of the thoracic and lumbar spine and the pelvis is necessary for patients with OPLL, because various ligaments in these areas occasionally show ossification.[21] Yanagi and associates[33] reported that the incidence of ossification of the yellow ligament (OYL) in the thoracic spine, in patients with cervical OPLL, was 13%. OPLL and/or OYL in the thoracic spine combined with the cervical OPLL causes more severe disabilities than does cervical OPLL alone.

Computed tomography (CT) is particularly helpful in determining the existence of OPLL as well as its thickness, its lateral extension and the shape, and the extent of the narrowing of the spinal canal by OPLL. Authors classified OPLL on CT into three types: square, mushroom, and hill types, at the level of the most narrowed spinal canal (Fig. 11-47).

PATHOLOGIC CHANGES

The posterior longitudinal ligament (PLL) consists of deep and superficial layers and is connected continuously to the vertebral bodies and the intervertebral discs by fibrous tissue in the midline portion of the ligaments. On the other hand, the lateral portion of the PLL is connected only to the upper and lower margins of the vertebral bodies.

Pathohistologically, the ossification starts in the portion of the PLL connected by fibrous tissue to the vertebral body, at which point stress converges as a result of cervical motion. The ossified mass consists mainly of lamellar bone, with some irregular, woven bone surrounding the fibrocartilage and an area of calcified cartilage. Enchondral ossification plays a key role in the formation of OPLL. Ossification of the dura mater is occasionally observed in decompressive surgery, when the ossified mass is removed anteriorly.

In autopsy cases with OPLL,[7,17] the spinal cords were extremely compressed anteriorly as a result of the condition.[8,24] The total amount of neural tissue was remarkably decreased. Intensive damage was seen in the gray matter, as compared with the white matter. The most seriously damaged parts of the spinal cord showed tissue necrosis and cavity formation, which extended from the central parts of the gray matter to the ventral parts of the posterior columns (Fig. 11-48).[27] The horn cells were reduced in both number and size. Demyelinization was observed extensively in the white matter. It is suggested that these distributions of degeneration are caused by ischemia or venous stasis in the boundary areas of anterior and posterior spinal artery tributaries in the spinal cord.[17]

Relatively good spinal cord function, however, was preserved before death. From this fact, it can be understood that stability of the cervical spine provided by OPLL acts as a protective mechanism against damage to the spinal cord. In addition, the spinal cord has a high degree of tolerance to slowly increasing mechanical pressure from OPLL, until 50% to 60% of the A–P diameter of the spinal canal is occupied. On the other hand, in subclinical cases with severe OPLL in which the spinal cords are compressed to a critical degree, mild traumatic forces may readily cause complete tetraplegia.

CLINICAL SYMPTOMS AND NATURAL COURSE

It is widely recognized[20] that almost all patients with OPLL have only mild subjective complaints, such as neck pain and numbness in the hand, without disturbances in the activities of daily living

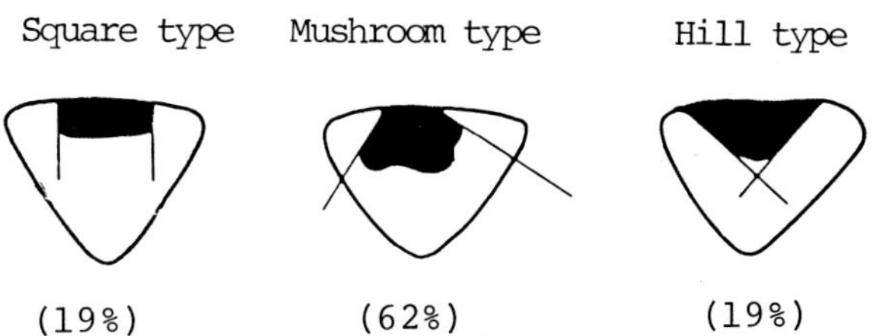

Fig. 11-47. Classification of OPLL as seen on CT scan.

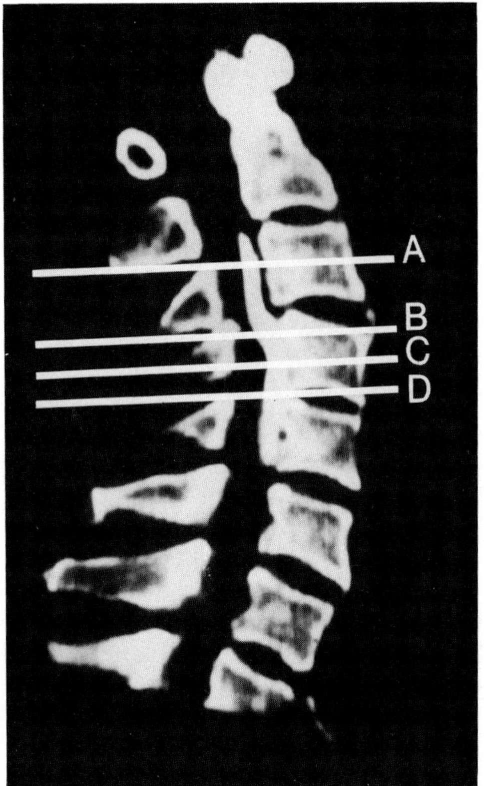

Fig. 11-48. Horizonal cross section showing the pathophysiology of a specimen (hematoxylin and eosin)[27] in a 74-year-old male.

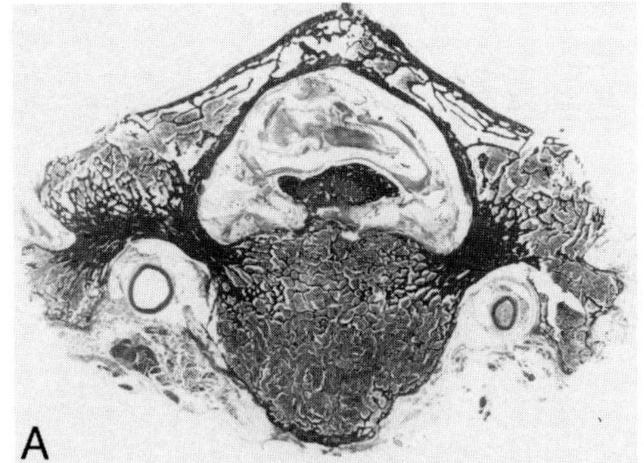

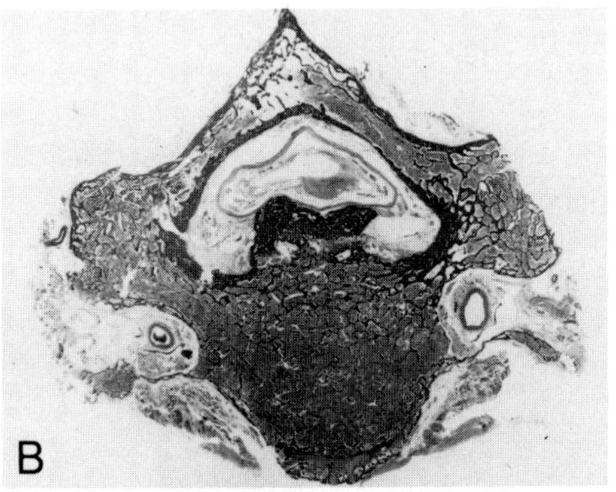

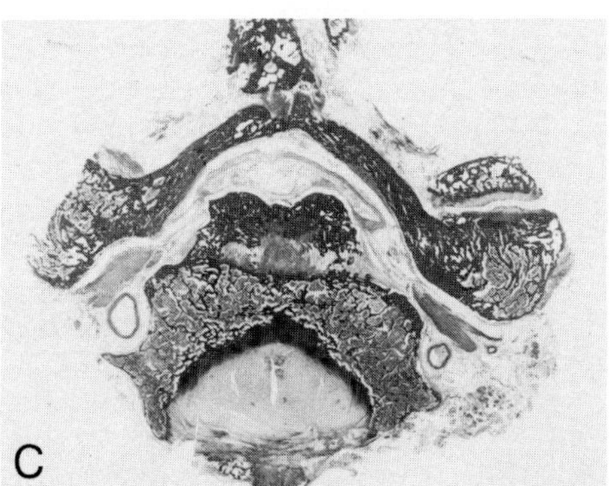

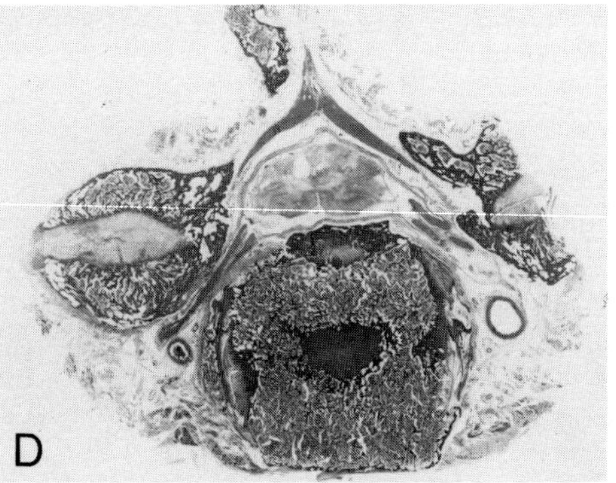

Table 11-12. Initial Symptoms of OPLL

Neck pain	41.9%
Pain or dysesthesia in upper extremities	47.7%
Motor dysfunction in upper extremities	10.4%
Dysesthesia in lower extremities	19.0%
Motor dysfunctions in lower extremities	15.4%
Bladder disturbance	1.0%

Percentage shows frequency of each symptom.
Total number of patients: 2162 (accumulated cases)[30]

(ADL). On the other hand, spastic gait disturbance and clumsiness of the fingers were recognized objectively in 15% and 10% of them, respectively (Table 11-12).[30]

An acute development or aggravation of tetraparesis after a minor trauma such as falling on the floor was noticed in 20.6% of the registered cases.[30] The average age of onset of the initial symptoms was at 51.2 years of age in males and 48.9 in females.[30]

In over 5 years follow-up, 54.8% of the patients with OPLL who were treated conservatively for mild disturbance of ADL showed no change, 26.7% of patients showed improvement, and 18.5% of patients showed aggravation of symptoms.[11]

DIAGNOSIS

OPLL can be diagnosed on plain lateral roentgenograms in the patients with myeloradiculopathy, but it can also be easily overlooked. Tomography is important for the demonstration of small foci of ossification and in most patients is indispensable for the visualization of the detailed outline of the ossified mass. The CT scan is most useful for determining the configuration of the ossification in

Table 11-13. Criteria for Evaluation of the Operative Results of Patients with Cervical Myelopathy by the Japanese Orthopaedic Association (JOA score)

I. Upper extremity function
  0. Impossible to eat with either chopsticks or spoon
  1. Possible to eat with spoon, but not with chopsticks
  2. Possible to eat with chopsticks, but inadequate
  3. Possible to eat with chopsticks, but awkward
  4. Normal

II. Lower extremity function
  0. Impossible to walk
  1. Need cane or aid on flat ground
  2. Need cane or aid only on stairs
  3. Possible to walk without cane or aid, but slow
  4. Normal

III. Sensory
  A. Upper extremity
    0. Apparent sensory loss
    1. Minimal sensory loss
    2. Normal
  B. Lower extremity, same as A
  C. Trunk, same as A

IV. Bladder function
  0. Complete retention
  1. Severe disturbance
    (1) Inadequate evacuation of the bladder
    (2) Straining
    (3) Dribbling of urine
  2. Mild disturbance
    (1) Urinary frequency
    (2) Urinary hesitancy
  3. Normal

Total 17 points

$$\text{Recovery rate} = \frac{\text{postoperative condition}^* - \text{preoperative condition}^*}{17 - \text{preoperative condition}^*} \times 100$$

(* signifies summated JOA score)

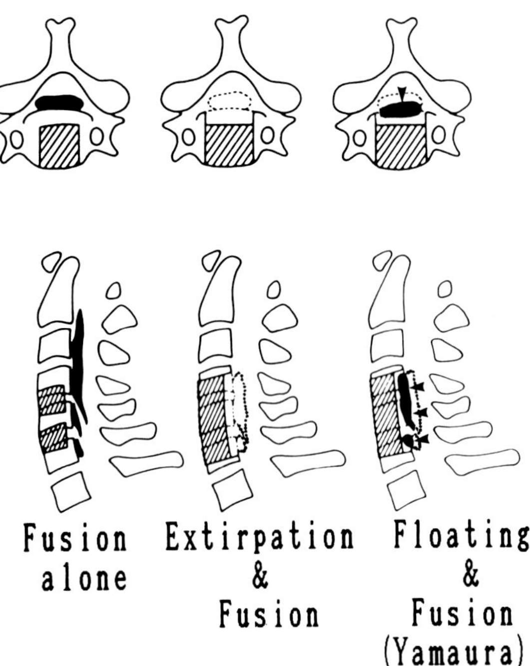

Fig. 11-49. Schema of anterior surgeries is shown.

the horizontal cross section of the spinal canal.[12,32] OPLL at the lower cervical levels, which otherwise may be masked by the massive shadows of the shoulder girdles, can be detected by CT scanning with ease.

However, clinical signs and symptoms do not always develop in OPLL, and many patients who have OPLL lead normal lives, as mentioned before. Thus, many patients with subclinical or latent OPLL may have no problems from the disease. Attention should be directed to the possibility of silent OPLL in any patient with myeloradiculopathy of unknown origin, and any patient in whom OPLL is suspected should be examined by tomography and preferably also by CT scanning.

TREATMENT

Conservative treatment for OPLL with myeloradiculopathy consists of continuous skull traction with halo brace, bed rest with halter traction, and application of a neck brace. With such conservative treatment, dynamic irritating factors would be eliminated; however, most of the patients with se-

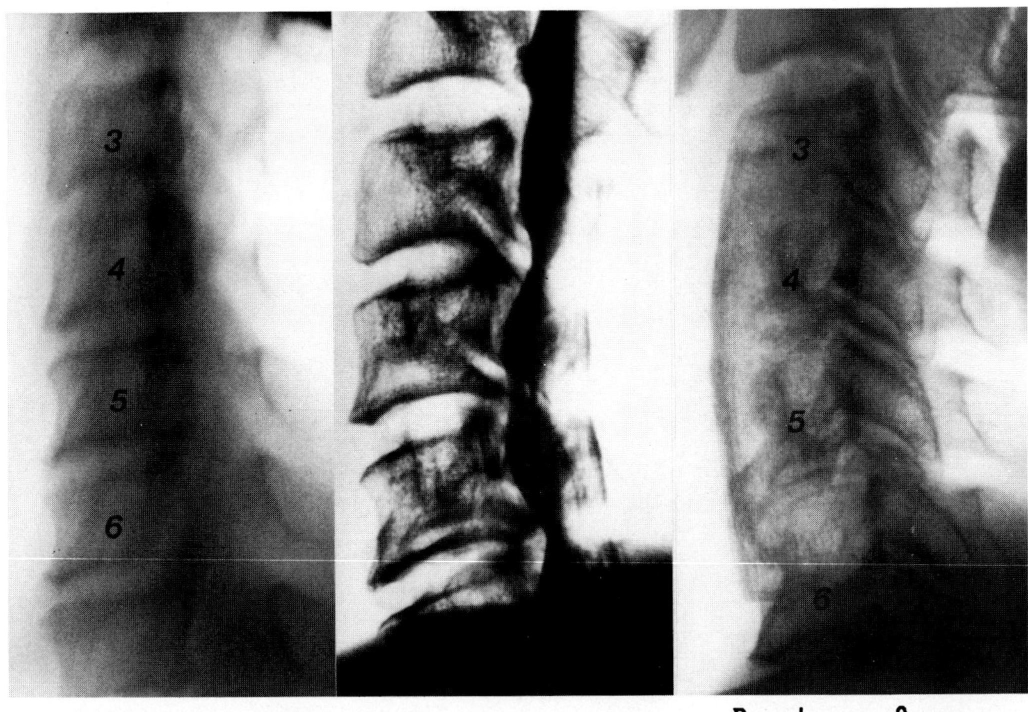

Fig. 11-50. (*A*) Lateral roentgenogram of a 57-year-old male who complained of muscle atrophy and weakness of the left arm showed segmental OPLL at C4 and C5 (left film). Myelogram showed the anterior indentation of the dural sac (middle film). Anterior extirpation of OPLL was performed with anterior spinal fusion between C3 and C6 (right film).

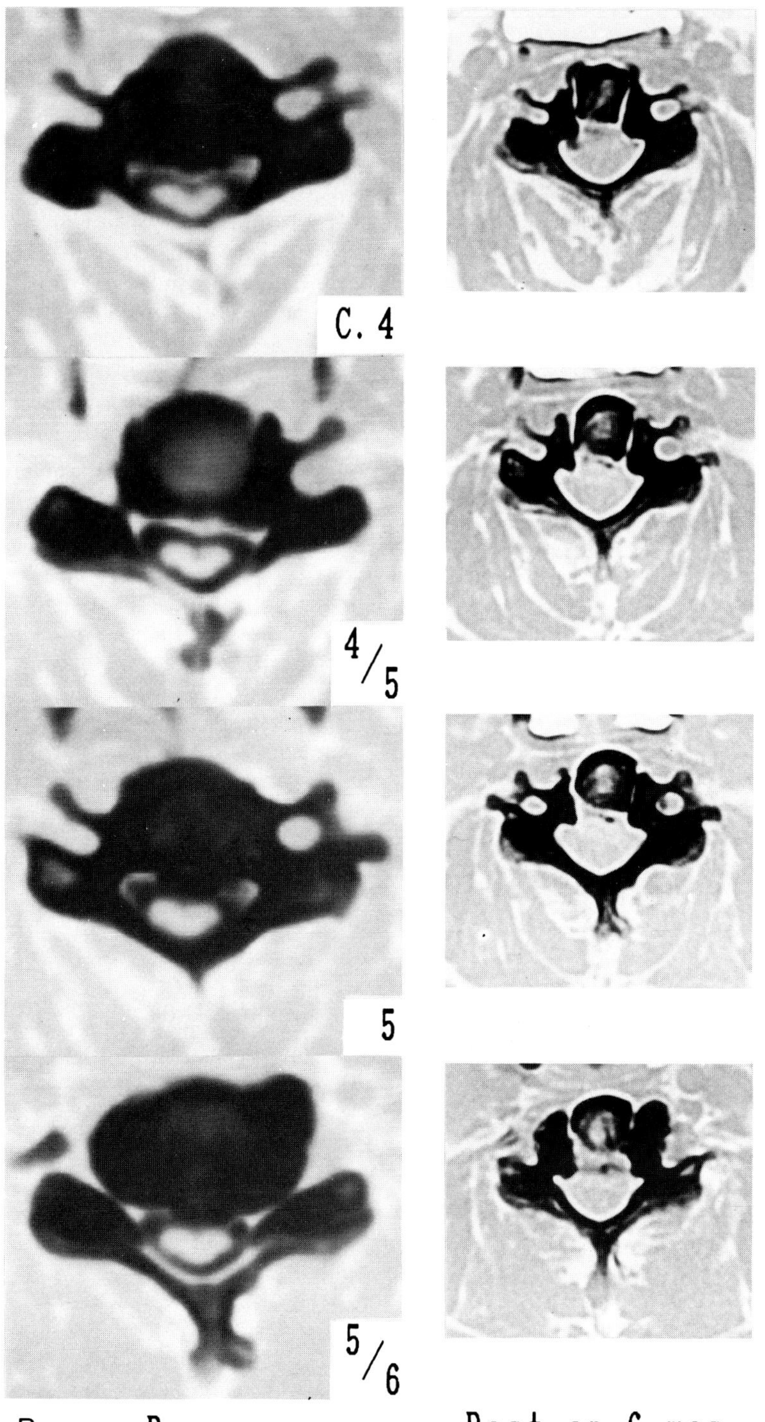

Fig. 11-50, *cont'd.*
(*B*) Preoperative CT-Myelography (CTM) showed that the spinal cord was compressed anteriorly by OPLL, and postoperative CT showed that OPLL was mostly removed by the anterior decompressive surgery.

vere myelopathy could not be treated sufficiently by the conservative therapy.

Surgery in patients with OPLL, taking their ages into consideration, is indicated for those who have been assigned six to twelve points according to the ADL criteria (JOA score), which have been established by the Japanese Orthopedic Association as standard for evaluation of the operative results of patients with cervical myelopathy (Table 11-13). Even if their myelopathy is not so severe, surgery may be indicated when patients are relatively young and have severe spinal stenosis. Patients with radiculopathy complaining of unendurable pain radiating to the upper arm are sometimes operated on as well, if conservative treatment is not effective.

CHOICE OF OPERATIVE METHODS

In the most radical type of operation, the ossified ligaments compressing the spinal cord and causing the neurologic symptoms are extirpated or floated[6] anteriorly to obtain anterior decompression (Fig. 11-49).

For the segmental and other types below the C3–C4 level, anterior decompression[1,26] followed by vertebral body fusion is routinely selected when fewer than three levels are involved (Fig. 11-50*A,B*). This operative procedure produces particularly good results for patients with clumsiness of the fingers and/or severe intrinsic muscle atrophy caused by lesions of the anterior horn cells, but sometimes causes neurologic complications to the vulnerable spinal cord.

On the other hand, the posterior decompressive operation[18] has only the effect of posterior shift of the spinal cord, but it is considered to be much safer to the severely deteriorated spinal cord (Fig. 11-51).[2,23]

For the continuous type, extensive laminectomy[16] and expansive laminoplasty for posterior decompression have been performed. Posterior decompression is performed as far as one level below and above the stenotic site and a medial third of the articular processes. In this fashion, nerve root decompression can be achieved.

Since 1977, the authors[9,10] have been applying open-door expansive laminoplasty according to Hirabayashi for posterior decompression, because he had observed dural tube pulsation before resection of the laminae as a whole. Using this method, the stenotic spinal canal can be widened without the structural loss caused by laminectomy, in which postoperative malalignment, instability, and fragility of the spine in response to neck trauma may occur.

For the special case of the mixed type, which has a locally prominent ossified mass, the authors have performed a two-stage combined operation, when necessary. The first operation, posterior decompression, is performed in order to provide space posteriorly for compressed spinal cord shifting. If necessary, anterior decompression is performed 3 to 6 weeks later (Fig. 11-52*A–E*). This posteroanterior combined operation is probably safer than the anteroposterior procedure.[1]

OPERATIVE PROCEDURES OF "EXPANSIVE OPEN-DOOR LAMINOPLASTY"

This operative procedures[10] proceed as follows (Fig. 11-53, parts 1 to 6): (1) After the spinal processes and laminae are exposed subperiosteally between one level below and above the lamina of the stenotic site, the spinous processes are partially resected to be shortened. (2) A bony gutter is drilled laterally and the thinned border of the laminae is excised. (3) Another bony gutter is drilled at the contralateral laminae, as well. (4) Sutures for preventing the laminar door from being closed are stitched around each facet of the hinge side. (5) The spinous processes and laminae are pushed laterally as in opening a door. (6) All the bases of the spinous processes are sutured to keep the laminar door open, using the threads already stitched in the fourth procedure.

Postoperatively, the patient is kept in bed for 2 days and then ambulates with a cervical brace for 3 months.

OPERATIVE RESULTS

Operative results were calculated using the recovery rates provided by JOA scores. A recovery rate over 75% is considered an excellent operative result, over 50% is good, over 25% is fair, and less than 25% is unchanged.

A group of 107 patients with OPLL have been operated on using various methods in our clinic since 1970. Relatively good operative results were obtained with all the operative methods, but better progress (63%) was achieved by expansive laminoplasty, as shown in Table 11-14.

Through observation of these patients, it was concluded that the operative results of surgery for OPLL were influenced by preoperative factors such as disability of activities of daily living (ADL), duration of the myelopathic symptoms, age, pres-

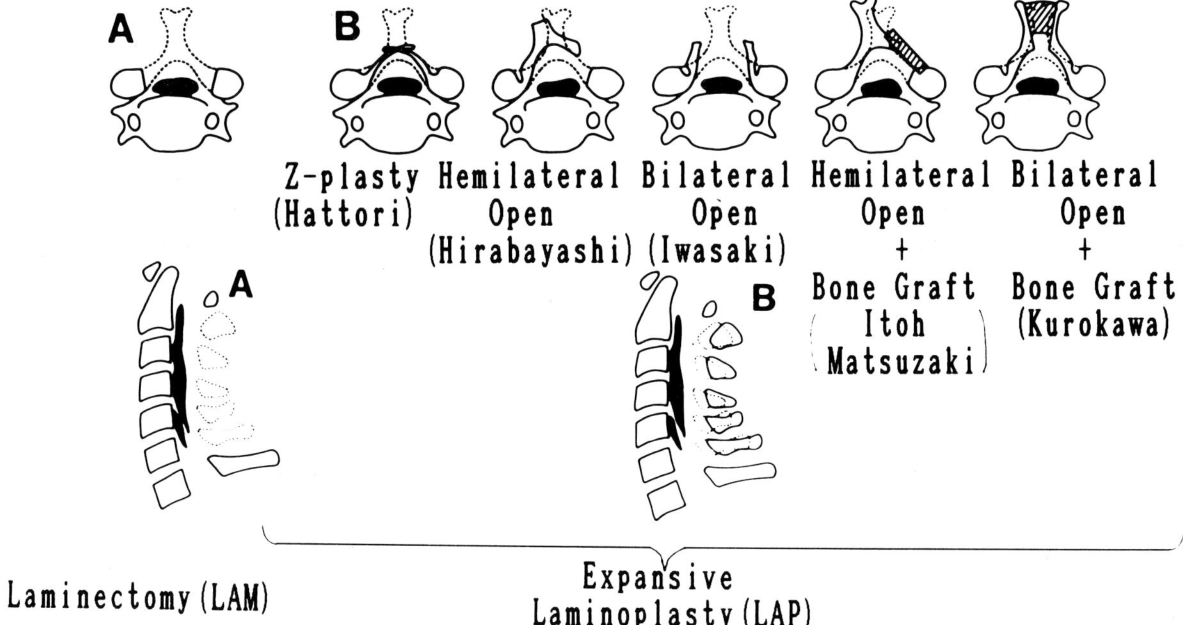

Fig. 11-51. Schema of posterior decompressive surgeries is shown.

ence of trauma at onset, stenotic condition of the spinal canal, and kyphotic curvative of the spine.

In fact, good operative results were not obtained in the following patients: those over 65 years old; those with severe disability of ADL (JOA score of less than 8 points); those with myelopathy for more than 2 years preoperatively; those with traumatic onset; those with severe stenosis of the spinal canal and kyphotic curvature of the spine.

In patients with every type of OPLL, the advancement of OPLL is sometimes found in either the longitudinal or transverse direction, although growth in the continuous and mixed types is much more frequent than in the segmental type, which also influences the long-term outcome. A 5-year follow-up showed the overall incidences of longitudinal and transverse growth of OPLL to be 24% and 11%, respectively, in the 338 nonoperative cases from the investigation committee, and to be 28% and 24%, respectively, in the 295 operative cases.[11] In our series, incidences of postoperative growth of continuous and mixed types of OPLL was 89% in the laminectomy group, 34% in the expansive laminoplasty group, and 20% in the anterior spinal fusion groups (Table 11-15). In comparing the laminectomy group and laminoplasty group, significant differences did not exist in longitudinal growth, but differences were seen in transverse growth. Thus, the frequency of "non-growth" cases of OPLL was three to four times higher in the laminoplasty patients than in those who underwent laminectomy, although the follow-up time of each group was different (Fig. 11-54). The progression to the final stage of ossification, such as from the mixed type to the continuous type of OPLL, was frequently observed in the laminoplasty patients showing growth of OPLL (Fig. 11-55).

COMPLICATIONS OF EXPANSIVE OPEN-DOOR LAMINOPLASTY

Enlargement of the spinal canal was not always maintained without supporting sutures. However, it is possible to keep the canal open successfully by adding the stay sutures, which are fastened between and around the bases of the spinous processes and the deep muscles and capsules around the facets in the position of an open door. Many modifications of laminoplasty have been devised in Japan, such as Itoh's with wiring, Matsuzaki's with iliac bone graft, and Kurokawa's with midlongitudinal bone graft, and so on (Fig. 11-51). All necessitate more operation time, with blood loss and a more difficult technique regarding safety of the patients than our method.

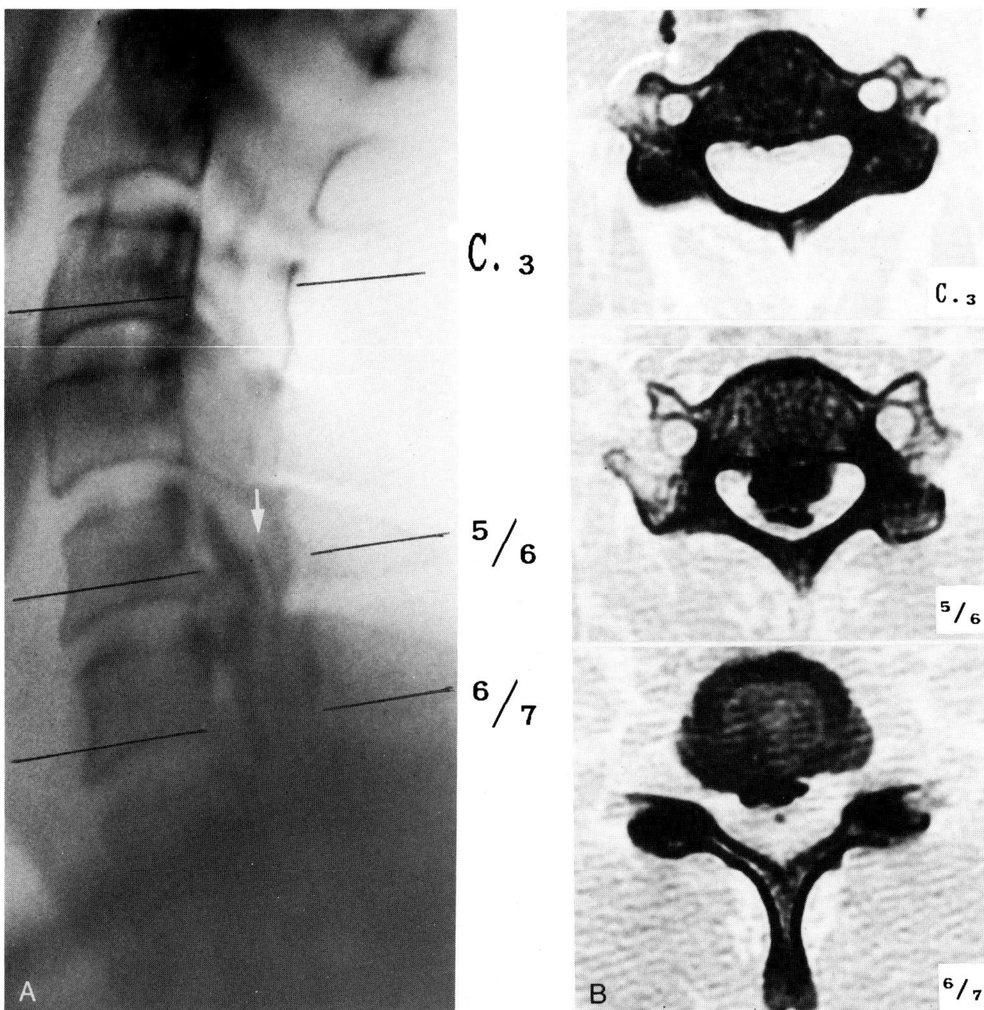

Fig. 11-52. (*A*) Lateral tomogram of a 57-year-old female, who complained of gait disturbance and muscle weakness of both hands, showed OPLL between C5 and C7. Ossification of the dura was also visible (*white arrow*). (*B*) OPLL was widely occupied in the spinal canal on CT. (*C*) The posterior shift of the spinal cord was observed on CTM after the expansive open-door laminoplasty, but the spinal cord was still compressed anteriorly by the OPLL. (*D*) Spinal canal was widened by the laminoplasty between C3 and C7 and the anterior spinal fusion between C4 and C7. (*E*) CTM after the combined operation showed that OPLL was mostly removed by the anterior decompression.

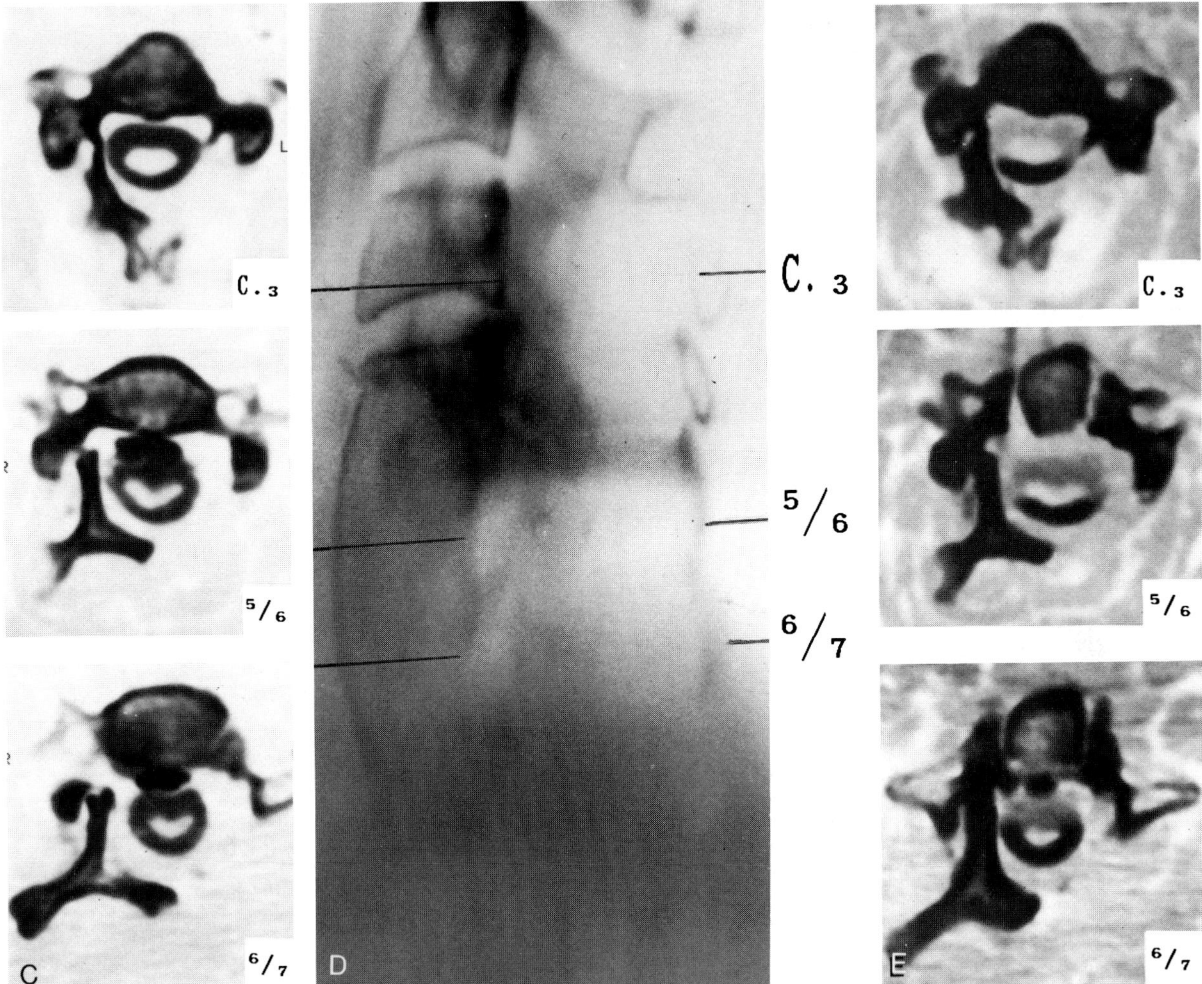

Fig. 11-52, *cont'd.*

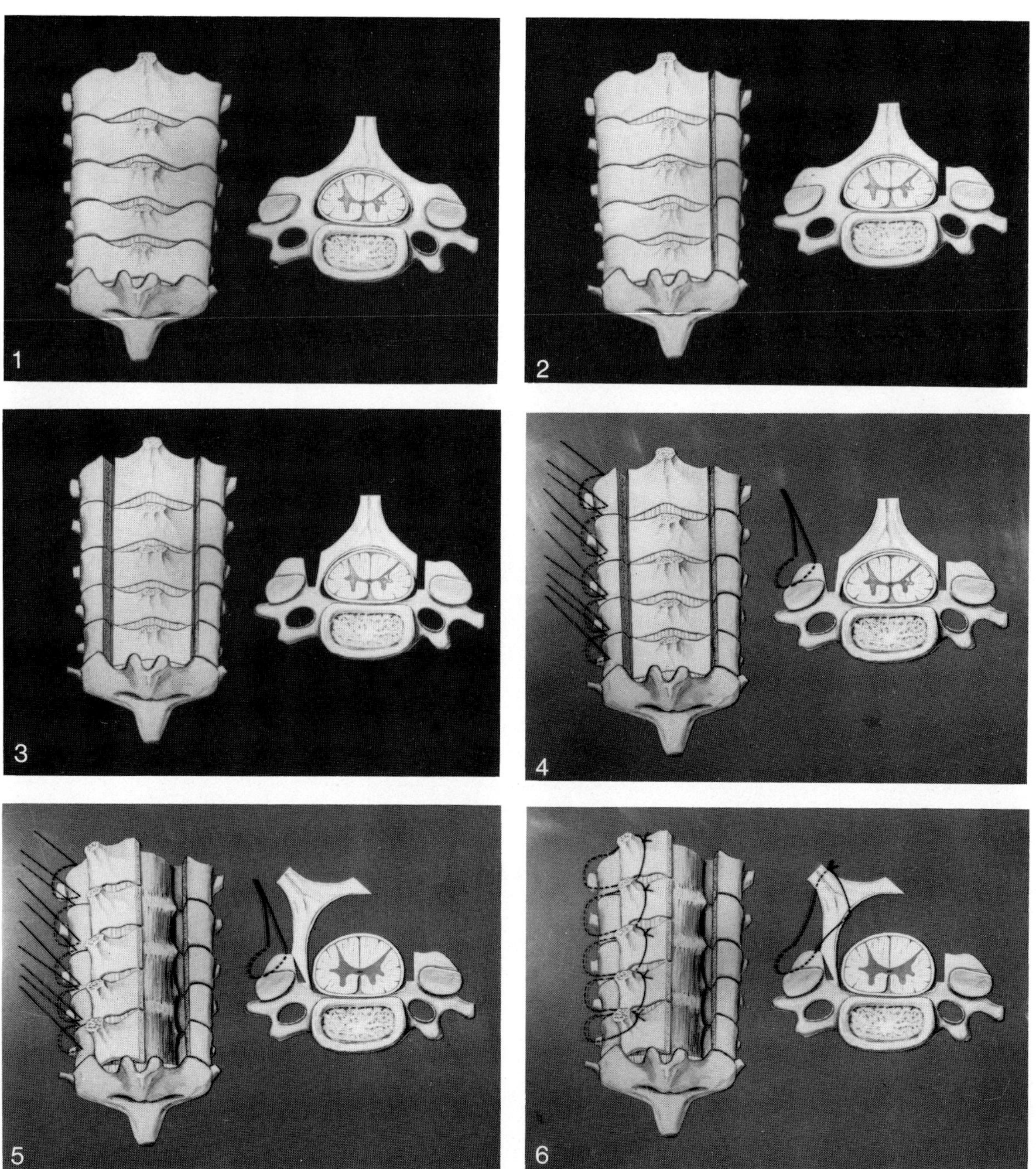

Fig. 11-53. Schema of expansive open-door laminoplasty (Hirabayashi) is shown.

Table 11-14. Operative Results for OPLL

	NO. OF CASES	RECOVERY RATE
Laminectomy (LAM)	28	53.4%
Expansive Laminoplasty (LAP)	54	62.8
Anterior Spinal Fusion (ASF)	16	57.7
LAM } + ASF LAP }	9	53.1

Table 11-15. Incidence of Postoperative Growth of OPLL (Continuous and Mixed Type)

Laminectomy (LAM)	16/18 cases	(89%)
Expansive Laminoplasty (LAP)	12/35	(34%)
Anterior Spinal Fusion (ASF)	1/5	(20%)
LAM + ASF	2/4	(50%
LAP + ASF	0/4	(0%)

One complication following expansive open-door laminoplasty is transient muscle paraparesis of the shoulder girdle and severe neck pain, resulting from tethering effect of the nerve roots of C5 and/or C6 and disjointing of the hinge. Disjointing of the hinge easily occurs in floating laminae and is followed by reclosure of the laminar door (Fig. 11-56). To prevent this complication, it is important that the hinge side of the bony gutter should be drilled, after completing resection of the medial side of the bony gutter at the open side (Fig. 11-53, *part 2*), and the stability of the hinge should be checked frequently by pushing the spinous processes. Although there is no way to prevent complications resulting from the tethering effect of the nerve roots, fortunately, spontaneous recovery can be expected in most cases.

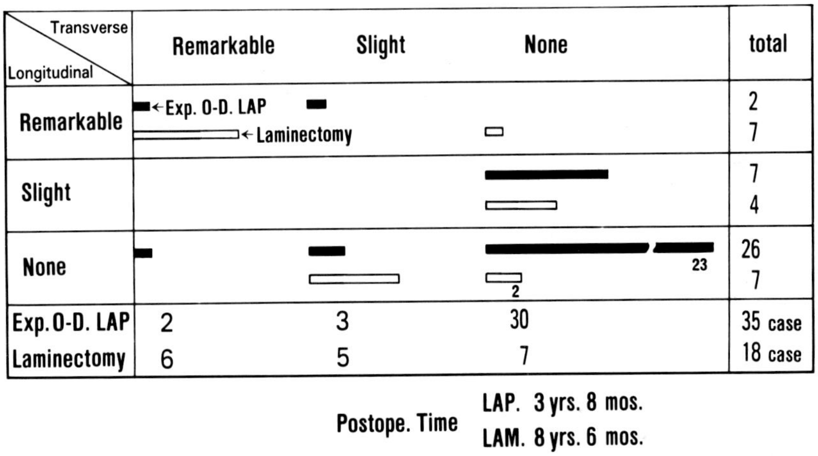

Transverse / Longitudinal	Remarkable	Slight	None	total
Remarkable	←Exp. O-D. LAP ←Laminectomy			2 7
Slight				7 4
None			23 2	26 7
Exp. O-D. LAP	2	3	30	35 case
Laminectomy	6	5	7	18 case

Postope. Time LAP. 3 yrs. 8 mos. LAM. 8 yrs. 6 mos.

Fig. 11-54. Postoperative growth of OPLL (continuous and mixed type) is represented.

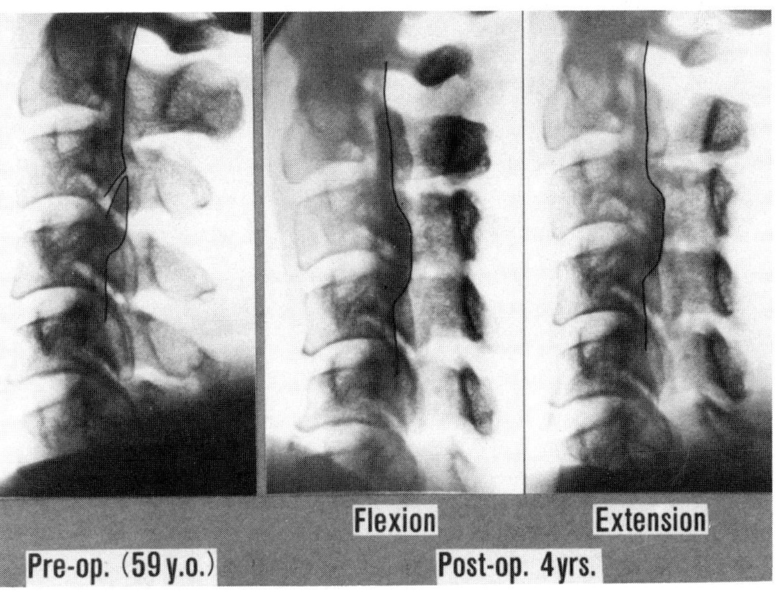

Fig. 11-55. End-stage growth of OPLL after expansive open-door laminoplasty is demonstrated.

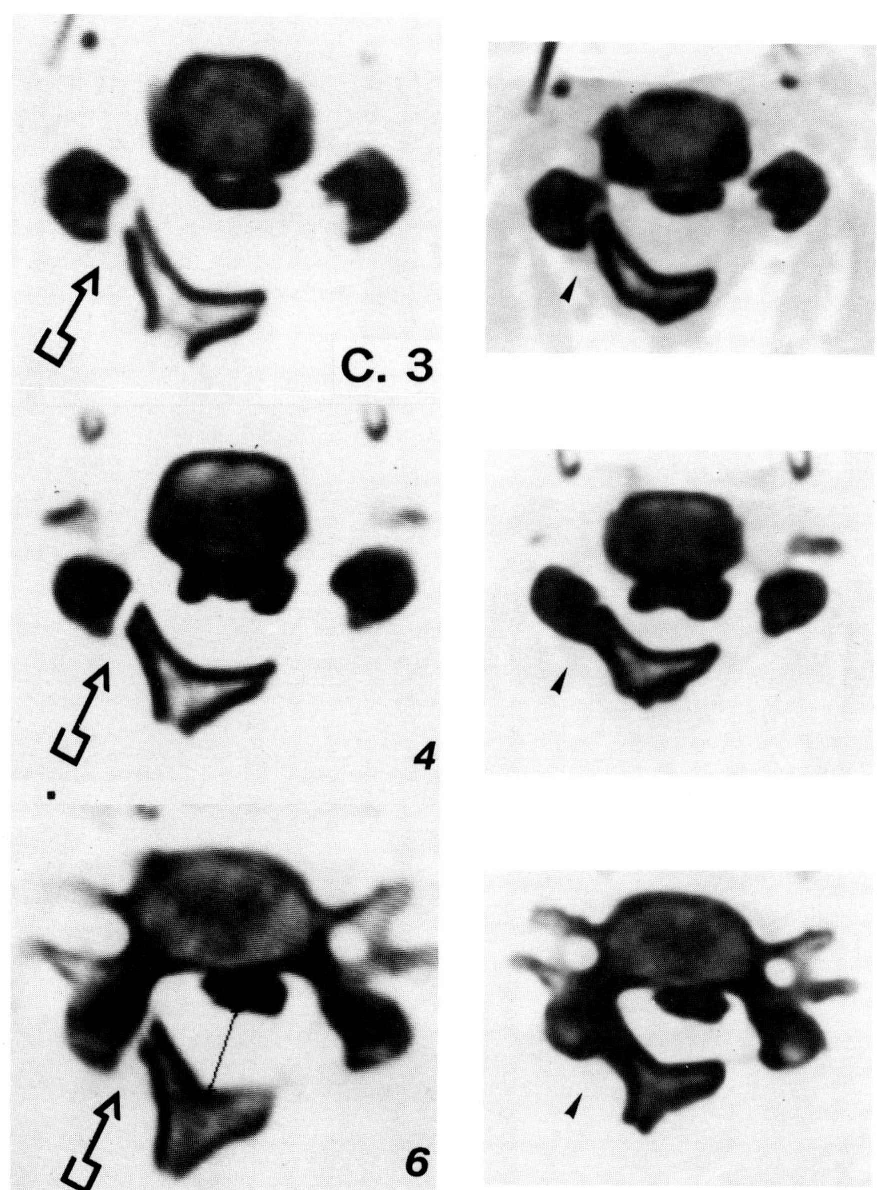

Fig. 11-56. Floating laminae causing reclosure.

SIGNIFICANCE OF EXPANSIVE OPEN-DOOR LAMINOPLASTY IN OPLL

The advantages of this operative method for posterior decompression of the spinal cord are as follows: (1) The operative technique is relatively easier and safer than others. (2) Postoperative supportability is better than with laminectomy. (3) Postoperative dynamic factor can be eliminated, because the range of motion of the preoperative cervical spine has been reduced to half by ankylosing of the bony gutter on the hinge side.

For the continuous and mixed types, the ossified ligaments may be biologically stimulated by the operative procedure, accelerating the postoperative growth of OPLL, as shown by the higher incidence of postoperative growth of OPLL, compared with nonoperative cases. The structural weakness caused by laminectomy may evoke postoperative growth of OPLL as a compensatory process. This is shown by the fact that the incidence in the laminectomy group was higher than in the laminoplasty group—especially the incidence of transverse growth. The mobility at the intervertebral space between OPLL may also evoke postoperative growth of OPLL, as shown by the fact that development from the mixed to the continuous type of OPLL was observed with elimination of the mobility at the involved disc space, while pseudarthrosis-like thickening is seen at the mobile disc space.

In conclusion, the expansive open-door laminoplasty as a decompressive procedure for the OPLL has several advantages. It prevents postoperative growth of OPLL, because loss of the posterior structural element is minimal. It also eliminates the range of motion in the cervical spine. Finally, it is an easy and safe operative technique.

REFERENCES

1. *Abe H, Tsuru M, et al:* Anterior decompression for ossification of the posterior longitudinal ligament of the cervical spine. J Neurosurg 55:108, 1981
2. *Bakay L, Cares HL, Smith RJ:* Ossification in the region of the posterior longitudinal ligament as a cause of cervical myelopathy. J Neurol Neurosurg Psychiatr 33:263, 1970
3. *Dietemann JL, Dirheimer Y, et al:* Ossification of the posterior longitudinal ligament (Japanese disease): A radiological study in 12 cases. J Neuroradiol 12:212, 1985
4. *Firooznia H, Rafii M, et al:* Computed tomography of calcification and ossification of posterior longitudinal ligament of the spine. J Comput Tomogr 8:317, 1984
5. *Gui L, Merlini L, Savini R, Davidovits P:* Cervical myelopathy due to ossification of the posterior longitudinal ligament. Ital J Orthop Traumatol 9:269, 1983
6. *Hanai K, Inouye Y, et al:* Anterior decompression for myelopathy resulting from ossification of the posterior longitudinal ligament. J Bone Joint Surg 64B:561, 1982
7. *Hashizume Y:* Pathological studies on the ossification of the posterior longitudinal ligament (OPLL). Acta Pathol Jpn 30:255, 1980
8. *Hashizume Y, Iijima S, et al:* Pathology of spinal cord lesions caused by ossification of the posterior longitudinal ligament. Acta Neuropathol 63:123, 1984
9. *Hirabayashi K, Miyakawa J, Satomi K, et al:* Operative results and postoperative progression of ossification among patients with cervical posterior longitudinal ligament. Spine 6:364, 1981
10. *Hirabayashi K, Watanabe K, Wakano K, et al:* Expansive open-door laminoplasty for cervical spinal stenotic myelopathy. Spine 8:693, 1983
11. *Japanese Ministry of Public Health and Welfare:* Investigation Committee Reports on OPLL (Jpn). Tokyo, 1981–1985
12. *Kadoya S, Nakamura T, Tada A:* Neuroradiology of ossification of the posterior longitudinal spinal ligament: Comparative studies with computer tomography. Neuroradiology 16:357, 1978
13. *Key CA:* Paraplegia depending on disease of the ligaments of the spine. Guy's Hops Rep 3:17, 1838
14. *Minagi H, Gronner AT:* Calcification of the posterior longitudinal ligament: A cause of cervical myelopathy. Amer J Radiol 105:365, 1969
15. *Mitsui H, Sonozaki H, et al:* Ankylosing spinal hyperostosis (ASH) and ossification of the posterior longitudinal ligament (OPLL). Arch Orthop Traumat Surg 94:21, 1979
16. *Miyazaki K, Kirita Y:* Extensive simultaneous multisegment laminectomy for myelopathy due to the ossification of the posterior longitudinal ligament in the cervical region. Spine 11:531, 1986
17. *Murakami N, Muroga T, Sobue I:* Cervical myelopathy due to ossification of the posterior longitudinal ligament, A clinico-pathologic study. Arch Neurol 35:33, 1978
18. *Nagashima C:* Cervical myelopathy due to ossification of the posterior longitudinal ligament. J Neurosurg 37:653, 1972
19. *Nakanishi T, Mannen T, Toyokura Y:* Asymptomatic ossification of the posterior longitudinal ligament of the cervical spine: Incidence and roentgenographic findings. J Neurol Sci 19:375, 1973

20. *NAKANISHI T, MANNEN T, TOYOKURA Y, ET AL:* Symptomatic ossification of the cervical spine. Neurology 24:1139, 1974
21. *OHTSUKA K, TERAYAMA K, ET AL:* An epidemiological survey on ossification of ligaments in the cervical and thoracic spine in individuals over 50 years of age. J Jpn Orthop Assoc 60:1087, 1986
22. *OKAMOTO Y, YASUMA T:* Ossification of the posterior longitudinal ligament of cervical spine with or without myelopathy. J Jpn Orthop Assoc 40:1349, 1967
23. *ONJI Y, AKIYAMA H, ET AL:* Posterior paravertebral ossification causing cervical myelopathy: A report of eighteen cases. J Bone Joint Surg 49A:1314, 1967
24. *ONO K, OTA H, TADA K, ET AL:* Ossified posterior longitudinal ligament: A clinicopathologic study. Spine 2:126, 1977
25. *RESNICK D, GUERRA J, ET AL:* Association of diffuse idiopathic skeletal hyperostosis (DISH) and calcification and ossification of the posterior longitudinal ligament. AJR 131:1049, 1978
26. *SAKOU T, MIYAZAKI A, TOMIMURA K, ET AL:* Ossification of the posterior longitudinal ligament of the cervical spine: Subtotal vertebrectomy as a treatment. Clin Orthop 140:58, 1979
27. *SASAKI T, ET AL:* An autopsy report of OPLL. Japanese Ministry of Public Health and Welfare: Investigation Committee Reports on OPLL (Jpn). Tokyo 127, 1980
28. *TERAYAMA K:* The ossification of the cervical posterior longitudinal ligament (Jpn). J Jpn Orthop Assoc 50:415, 1976
29. *TSUKIMOTO H:* A case report: Autopsy of syndrome of compression of spinal cord owing to ossification within spinal canal of cervical spine (Jpn). Arch Jpn Chir 29:1003, 1960
30. *TSUYAMA N, ET AL:* The ossification of the posterior longitudinal ligament of the spine (OPLL). J Jpn Orthop Assoc 55:425, 1981
31. *TSUYAMA N:* Ossification of the posterior longitudinal ligament of the spine. Clin Orthop 184:71, 1984
32. *YAMAMOTO I, KAGEYAMA N, ET AL:* Computed tomography in ossification of the posterior longitudinal ligament in the cervical spine. Surg Neurol 12:414, 1979
33. *YANAGI T, KATO H, ET AL:* Ossification of spinal ligaments (Jpn). Clin Neurol 12:571, 1972

CHAPTER 12

Tumors Involving the Cervical Spine

Diagnosis and Management of Tumors of the Cervical Spine

EDWARD J. DUNN, ROBIN I. DAVIDSON, AND SANJAY DESAI

Neoplastic disease of the cervical spine is a rare disorder. Because of the potential morbidity and mortality associated with cervical tumors, their significance to both patients and surgeon is much greater than their incidence. The improved longevity of patients with metastatic disease and increasingly sensitive techniques for demonstrating bone pathology have led to a greater recognition of cervical neoplasms.[4,7] These developments have occurred during a period of increasing knowledge about spinal cord pathophysiology and the development of surgical techniques emanating from the study of cervical trauma. Many of these surgical techniques and principles learned from the care of patients with cervical trauma have direct application to the treatment of cervical neoplasms.

The management of patients with cervical spine tumors involves the following four-part approach:

1. The establishment of a tissue diagnosis
2. The assessment and treatment of neurologic impairment
3. The correction of mechanical instability
4. Halting the progression of, or eradicating, the tumor when possible.

The general condition of the patient dictates the overall plan of care. The issue is not what can be done for a specific lesion, but what might optimally benefit the patient with such a lesion. A discussion of a general approach to patients with tumors of the cervical spine that considers both the diagnostic and the therapeutic issues is presented.

CLINICAL EVALUATION

Because neural tissues have limited tolerance of mechanical compression, tumors in the cervical spine may produce a wide variety of clinical syndromes, ranging from cervical or radicular pain to syncope, quadriparesis, and even death. Spinal cord and/or nerve root compression may result from the mass effect of an expanding vertebral tumor or the mechanical collapse and subluxation of the spine itself. In making treatment decisions, the distinction must often be made between these

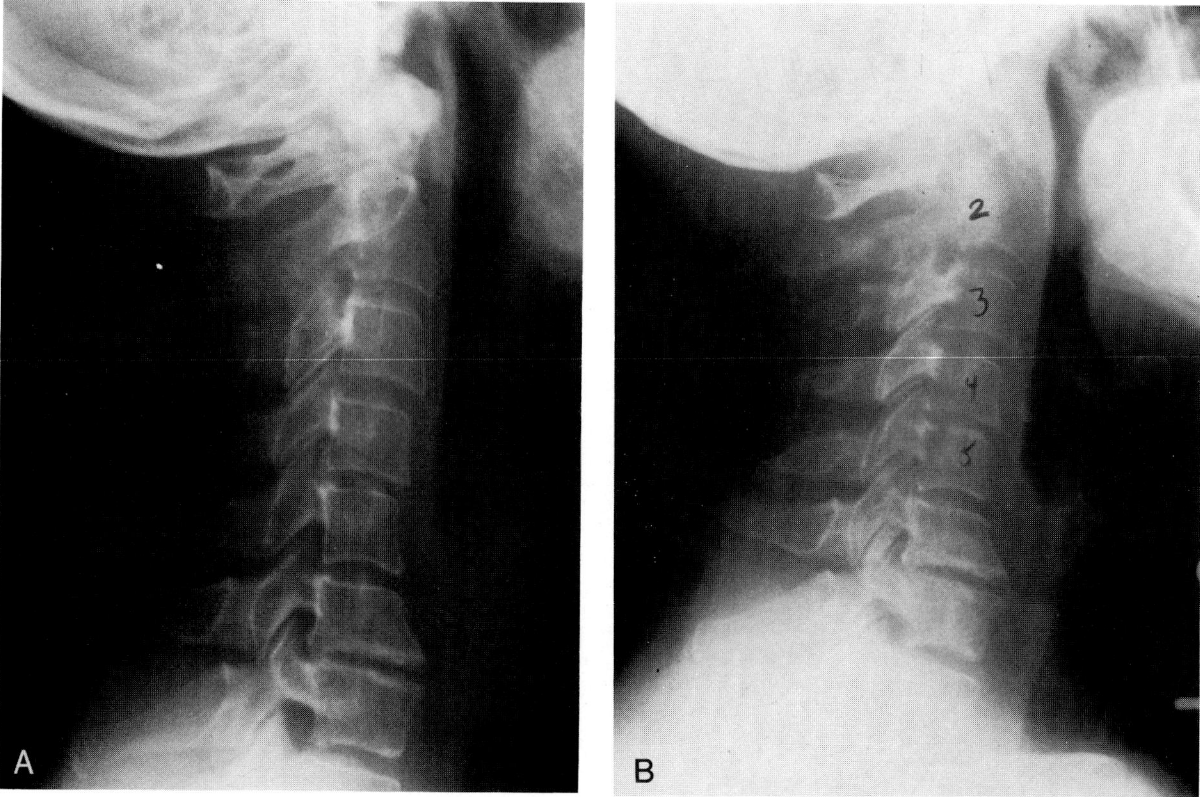

Fig. 12-1. A 50-year-old woman with metastatic carcinoma of the breast. She complained of neck pain and original x-ray films (*A*) failed to show evidence of metastases. It was believed that her pain may have been due to spondylosis at C6–C7. It is entirely possible that a bone scan and/or a CT scan performed at that time would have shown metastases. (*B*) Lateral x-ray films taken 4 months later showed lytic destruction of C2 and probable involvement of C4. Some posterior stabilization and grafting were being considered until a CT scan (*C*) showed marked involvement of the skull and upper posterior cervical area. It became obvious that the patient was losing the battle with her disease. She was given radiotherapy and a collar for support and died 2 months after the last x-ray study. It has been our experience that bone scanning is often the best means for detecting early metastases (*D*). Areas with positive uptake should be evaluated by plain x-ray films and CT scans when indicated.

pathologic processes. Localized pain is the most frequent symptom of cervical tumors. Generally, pain caused by neoplasm is persistent and not relieved by rest. Therefore, nocturnal and rest pain are particularly ominous. When a patient presents with neck pain, it is dangerous to accept the common diagnosis of spondylosis or intervertebral disc lesion without carrying out a full physical and radiologic evaluation (Fig. 12-1). Once the question of neoplasm has been raised, it must be fully evaluated. In addition to the clinical presentation of pain, radiographic abnormalities noted during the evaluation of incidental cervical trauma or asymptomatic lesions in the course of metastatic evaluation may also prompt patient referral. Clinical examination should include a careful assessment of local pain, range of motion, external deformity, and nerve root and spinal cord function. Hastings and McNab[45] reported that the earliest sign of tumors in the atlantoaxial region was a loss of rotatory motion. Pain noted on palpation of the spine is often the earliest localizing finding in posterior-element or lateral-mass involvement. A careful examination is necessary in order to elicit the

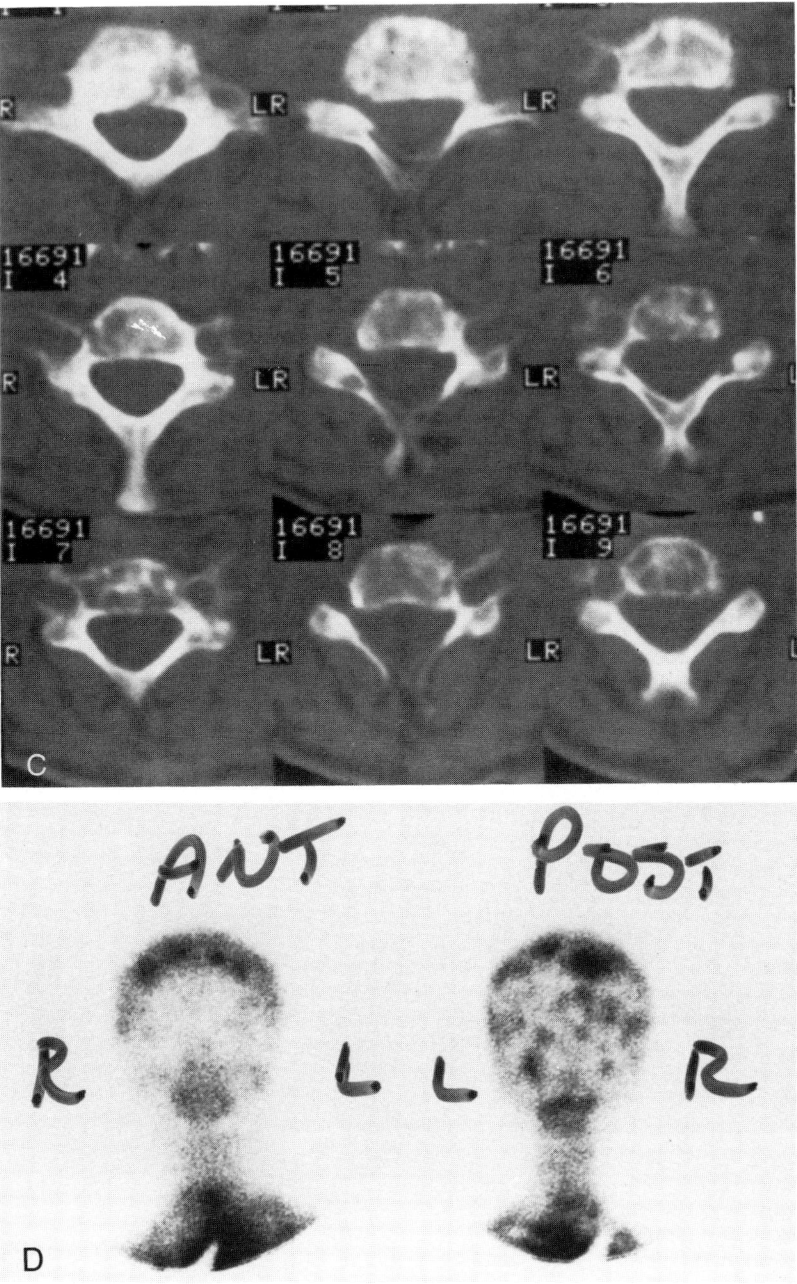

Fig. 12-1, *cont'd.*

earliest neurologic manifestations, since the ultimate goal of managing cervical tumors is obviously to prevent or correct neural deficit. Neurologic assessment at the time of the initial evaluation should include assessment of motor function proximally and distally in the upper and lower extremities, testing sensation to pinprick and light touch, testing position sense, and testing deep-tendon reflexes looking for hyperreflexia or asymmetric reflexes. A search for pathologic "long-tract" reflexes, including the Babinski and Hoffman signs and clonus, should also be carried out. Any of these signs, which indicate a progressing myelopathy, may require an accelerated course of action.

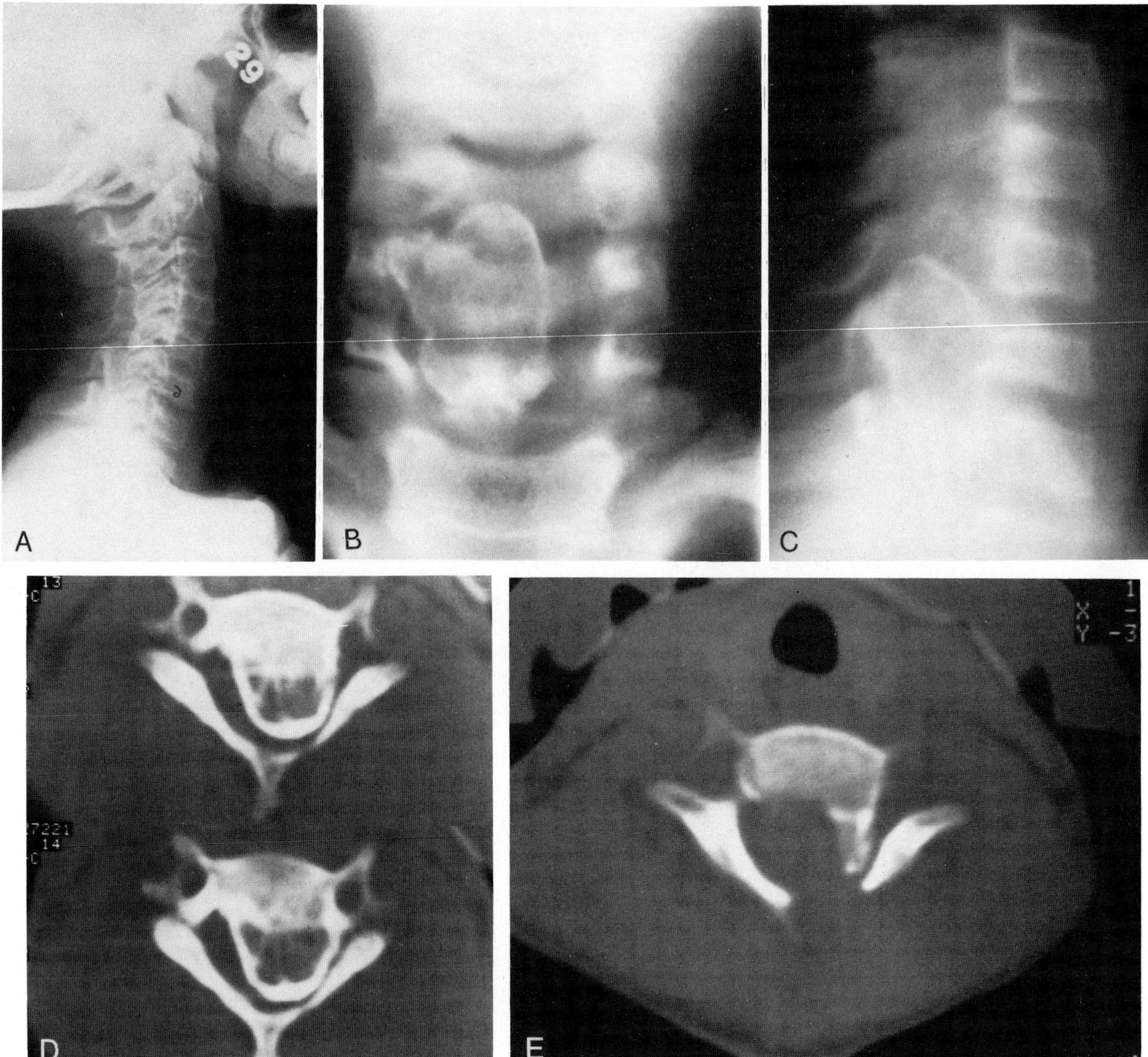

Fig. 12-2. An 11-year-old boy with progressive left upper-extremity weakness. He had a history of multiple osteochondromatosis noted since the age of 2. (*A*) Lateral x-ray shows bony mass in spinal canal at the C6 level along with irregularity of the posterior aspect of the vertebral body. (*B* and *C*) A–P and lateral tomograms show large well-defined mass extending posteriorly from the vertebral body of C6, superiorly to the spinal canal at C5, and inferiorly to the spinal canal at C7. (*D*) CT scan demonstrates well-delineated large bony lesion filling the spinal canal at C6. The preoperative diagnosis was osteochondroma. A left hemilaminectomy of C5–T1 was carried out, the main portion of the tumor was excised, and the nerve root decompressed. (*E*) When seen 21 months postoperatively, he had no neurologic deficit and no complaints referrable to his neck or arms. (In association with Dr. C. Atkins)

Although Dahlin[20] located 46 primary tumors of the cervical spine and Bohlman and coworkers[6] recently reviewed 23 similar neoplasms, no series exists that is large enough to allow a statistical approach to cervical spine tumors based on histologic diagnosis. Several broad generalizations can be offered to help guide the diagnosis, however. Metastatic involvement of the cervical spine is far more frequent than primary involvement. Multiple metastatic defects may coexist at different levels. With primary tumors, the incidence of benign tumors is greater than that of malignant neoplasms. In the cervical area, some tumors, although benign histologically, may produce severe consequences because of their location, the difficulty in excising them, and the resultant neurocompressive signs and symptoms caused by their expansile growth (Fig. 12-2).

A child with a tumor in the cervical spine is likely to have a benign process; an adult is likely to have metastatic spread from a malignancy elsewhere in the body. The primary cervical tumors of adults are likely to be malignant.

A lesion may often be diagnosed as metastatic when there is a recognized primary malignancy or multiple bony metastases elsewhere in the body. Not uncommonly, the first manifestation in malignant disease may be the appearance of a spinal metastasis. As in other regions of the skeleton, vertebral metastases are most frequently due to primary tumors of the breast, lung, prostate, and thyroid. It has been estimated that 50% to 70% of cancer patients have spinal metastases.[31] The vertebral bodies are involved seven times as often as the posterior elements.[51,107] The thoracic and lumbar spines are involved more frequently than is the cervical area. Metastatic lesions in children may arise from leukemia, neuroblastoma, retinoblastoma, or Ewing's sarcoma.

LABORATORY AND RADIOGRAPHIC EVALUATION

Laboratory evaluation may be helpful in the diagnosis of multiple myeloma (anemia, Bence-Jones protein in the urine, increased abnormal globulin on serum protein electrophoresis), mestastatic carcinoma of the prostate (acid phosphatase, prostatic fraction), and metastatic neuroblastoma (urinary vanillylmandelic acid). Depending on the patient's age and symptoms, other carefully directed laboratory studies may also be helpful in arriving at a final diagnosis of a primary or metastatic tumor.

Once the initial clinical and laboratory exams have been completed, the diagnostic process should progress to the evaluation of plain x-ray films. Because bone loss of 30% to 50% must occur in order to appreciate a radiographic change, the plain radiograph is not a highly sensitive method of detecting decreased bone density. The plain radiograph may, however, reveal a distinction between a lytic and blastic process, differentiation between slowly enlarging and rapidly expansile destructive processes, and a review of the mechanical integrity of the spinal support mechanism. Whereas benign tumors are generally demonstrable by the time that they produce symptoms, the same is not true of primary malignancy or metastatses. The exception to this general guideline is osteoid osteoma, which may be difficult to demonstrate by plain x-ray films. Despite negative plain films, a high degree of clinical suspicion should prompt further investigation (Fig. 12-3).

The most sensitive diagnostic procedure for demonstrating an occult cervical malignancy is the technetium bone scan. This modality is not very specific, however, and a high number of false positives are likely to occur in patients with previous surgery, trauma, or degenerative disease. Areas showing increased uptake on the bone scan should have plain x-ray films taken for further evaluation of the pathology. If these films fail to demonstrate pathologic findings, a CT scan of that area should also be obtained. Despite its high degree of sensitivity, care must be taken in interpreting isotope scans in patients undergoing chemotherapy because of occasional false-negative results.[109] This may be due in part to the toxic effects of chemotherapeutic agents on osteoblastic activity in bone formation.[34] A neoplasm such as multiple myeloma that often does not evoke significant reactive or lesional bone formation may also fail to produce a positive bone scan.

Tomograms and CT scans are useful in the evaluation of spinal integrity and the localization and delineation of compressive lesions. We found that CT scans often revealed metastatic involvement when plain films were negative. In addition, CT scanning of the spine in metastatic disease may demonstrate lesions not apparent on a radionuclide scan.[108] CT scanning is becoming the most important method of demonstrating the extent of bony tumor in the cervical spine (see Figs. 12-1, 12-2, 12-3, 12-10, 12-14, and 12-16).

Angiography may be of assistance in diagnosing tumor or planning an approach in the area of the vertebral arteries (Figs. 12-4 and 12-12). Malignant tumors may demonstrate bizarre tumor vessels, hy-

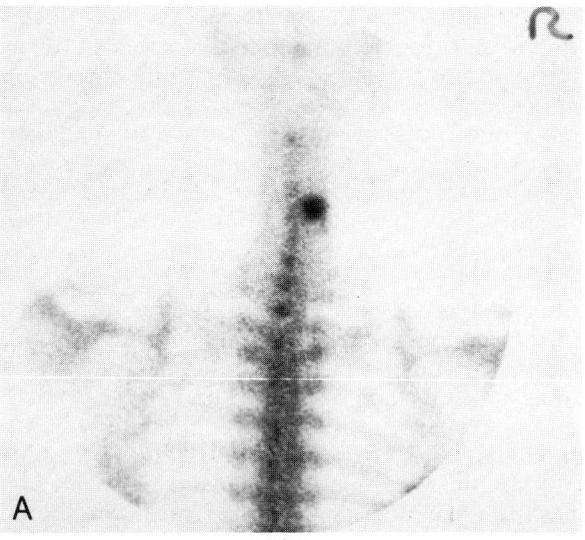

Fig. 12-3. A 21-year-old man who presented with increasing neck pain over a 2-year period. X-ray findings were within normal limits, but because of the persistence of pain and cervical spasm a bone scan was ordered. (*A*) Bone scan demonstrating increased uptake C5 on the right. (*B*) CT scan showing sclerotic lesion with possible nidus, pedicle of C5 on the right. (*C*) Using a posterior approach, a hemilaminectomy and partial resection of the articular facet allowed access to the spinal canal and excision of the lesion. Because of limited bone resection, no stabilization procedure was necessary. Pathology report confirmed the suspected diagnosis of osteoid osteoma. A positive bone scan may be the earliest clue to osteoid osteoma. CT scan often demonstrates pathology that is not seen on plain x-ray films. The patient is now 1.5 years postoperative and is asymptomatic.

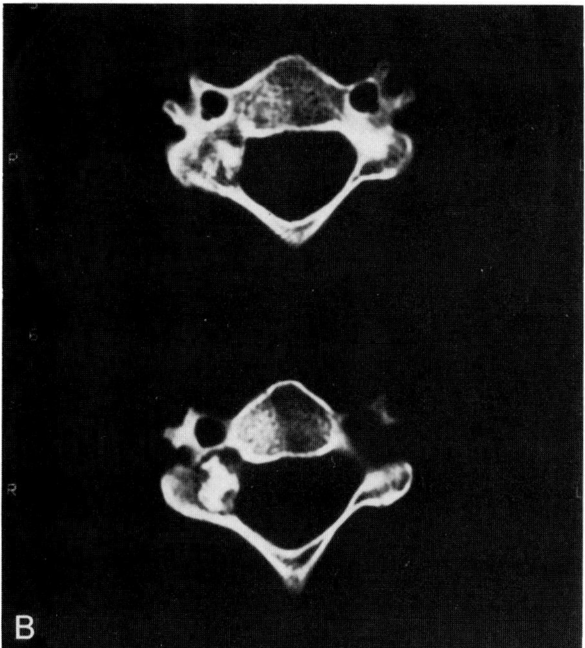

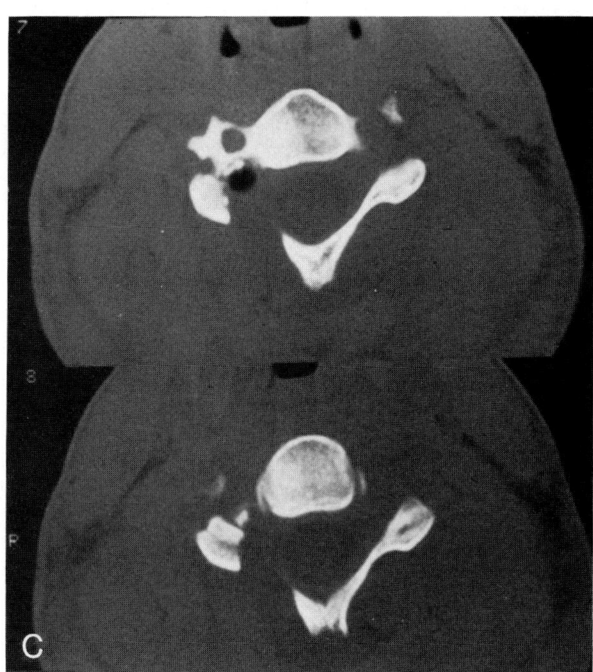

pervascularity, tumor staining, and dilatation. However, Ono and associates[76] noted that between 44% and 66.7% of benign primary tumors of the cervical spine also displayed these angiographic characteristics. Angiography demonstrates particularly hypervascular tumors, and selected embolization techniques may significantly decrease bleeding at the time of surgery. On angiography, one of the two vertebral arteries is generally larger and more dominant. Ligating the larger vertebral artery in the course of surgery may lead to significant vascular compromise. On the other hand, the lesser vertebral artery may often be ligated without difficulty, if necessary, in the course of surgery. In one series, 75% of primary malignant tumors, 86.8% of metastatic tumors, and 83.3% of benign tumors of the cervical spine were diagnosed prior to tissue confirmation, by means of a combination of plain films, isotope scanning and selected angiography.[76]

We also consider myelography to be an integral part of the evaluation of a patient with a cervical tumor. Myelography is helpful in differentiating an intradural lesion of the cord from a tumor of the bone that has extended into the spinal canal to compress the cord. Myelography is also used in assessing the presence of additional asymptomatic extradural lesions that have not yet produced plain film changes (the so-called skip metastases) (see Figs. 12-4, 12-5, 12-9, 12-10, and 12-14).

Magnetic resonance imaging (MRI) is a recently developed addition to the radiologic armanentarium that may assist in evaluating cervical spine tumors. McAfee and colleagues[72] used this imaging modality in diagnosing the causes of upper cervical cord compression. They found that one of the important advantages of MRI over CT consisted of the ability of the former to display an unreconstructed sagittal section of the cervical spine. Although MRI does not clearly delineate intraosseous details, it shows promise as the most effective method for demonstrating intrathecal structures such as the spinal cord itself and spinal cord tumors.

The combination of a thorough history, a careful clinical examination, and the outlined laboratory and diagnostic radiologic techniques should support an intelligent conjecture regarding the histologic characteristics of the tumor and will enable the physician to formulate a rational treatment plan that may include biopsy, surgery for tumor ablation, and the restoration of mechanical stability, if necessary.

TUMOR TYPES

Benign Tumors of the Cervical Spine[6,15,22,36,45]

Aneurysmal Bone Cyst.[8,57,80,104,110] Aneurysmal bone cyst is a destructive lesion of bone most often seen in children and young adults. Although it is most commonly located in the neural arch, the vertebral bodies may also be affected. It is characteristically an expansile lesion confined by a thin rim of new bone formation, and it may destroy adjacent vertebrae. Symptoms are usually related to pressure from the expanding mass. These lesions are best treated by excision and/or curettage and bone grafting (Fig. 12-4).

Eosinophilic Granuloma/Histiocytosis X.[21] Eosinophilic granuloma is a localized form of a group of related reticuloendothelial disorders called histiocytosis X. This entity can occur in the cervical spine of both children and adults and may be associated with neurologic signs and symptoms appropriate to the site and level of the lesion. Radiographic appearance may include a lytic lesion or the erosion and collapse of the centrum or the lateral supporting structures of the involved cervical vertebrae (Fig. 12-5).

Treatment of solitary eosinophilic granuloma is controversial. In some instances, biopsy is necessary in order to make the diagnosis. Traditional treatment methods have included biopsy, immobilization, and low-dose radiotherapy. Needle biopsy and local injection with methylprednisolone have been demonstrated to be efficacious in the treatment of eosinophilic granuloma in nonspinal locations.[12,16,97] Other authors have indicated that healing rates of lesions did not differ significantly among patients who received chemotherapy alone, chemotherapy plus radiotherapy, radiotherapy alone, or no treatment.[32,96] Furthermore, cases of untreated but resolved spinal eosinophilic granuloma exist in the literature.[11] We believe that, unless neurologic compromise occurs, therapeutic conservatism is warranted, including biopsy for diagnosis, steroid injection, and immobilization. Close clinical and radiologic follow-up should, of course, also be obtained.[50,65,90]

Osteochondroma.[29,37,53,54,59,73] These benign lesions consist of cortical and trabecular bone covered with a cartilaginous cap that may or may not be calcified. Although frequently asymptomatic elsewhere in the body, in the cervical spine this tumor may lead to spinal-cord or nerve-root compression. Osteochondromata may originate from the body or posterior elements of the vertebra and may undergo significant growth during adolescence, thereby leading to symptoms of neural compression in this age group. Incidences of malignant degeneration of this lesion to chondrosarcoma are less than 1%. Treatment of symptomatic lesions consists of surgical excision (Fig. 12-2).

Osteoid Osteoma.[27,58,60,82,122] Osteoid osteoma is generally seen in young people under 30 years of age. After the lumbar spine, the cervical spine is the second most common spinal location for this lesion.[60,120] In the cervical spine, osteoid osteoma is found almost exclusively in the pedicles and the posterior elements. Classic osteoid osteoma produces symptoms of night pain relieved by aspirin, and these symptoms may be present before the lesion is visible on plain radiographs. A typical radiographic appearance is a dense sclerotic reac-

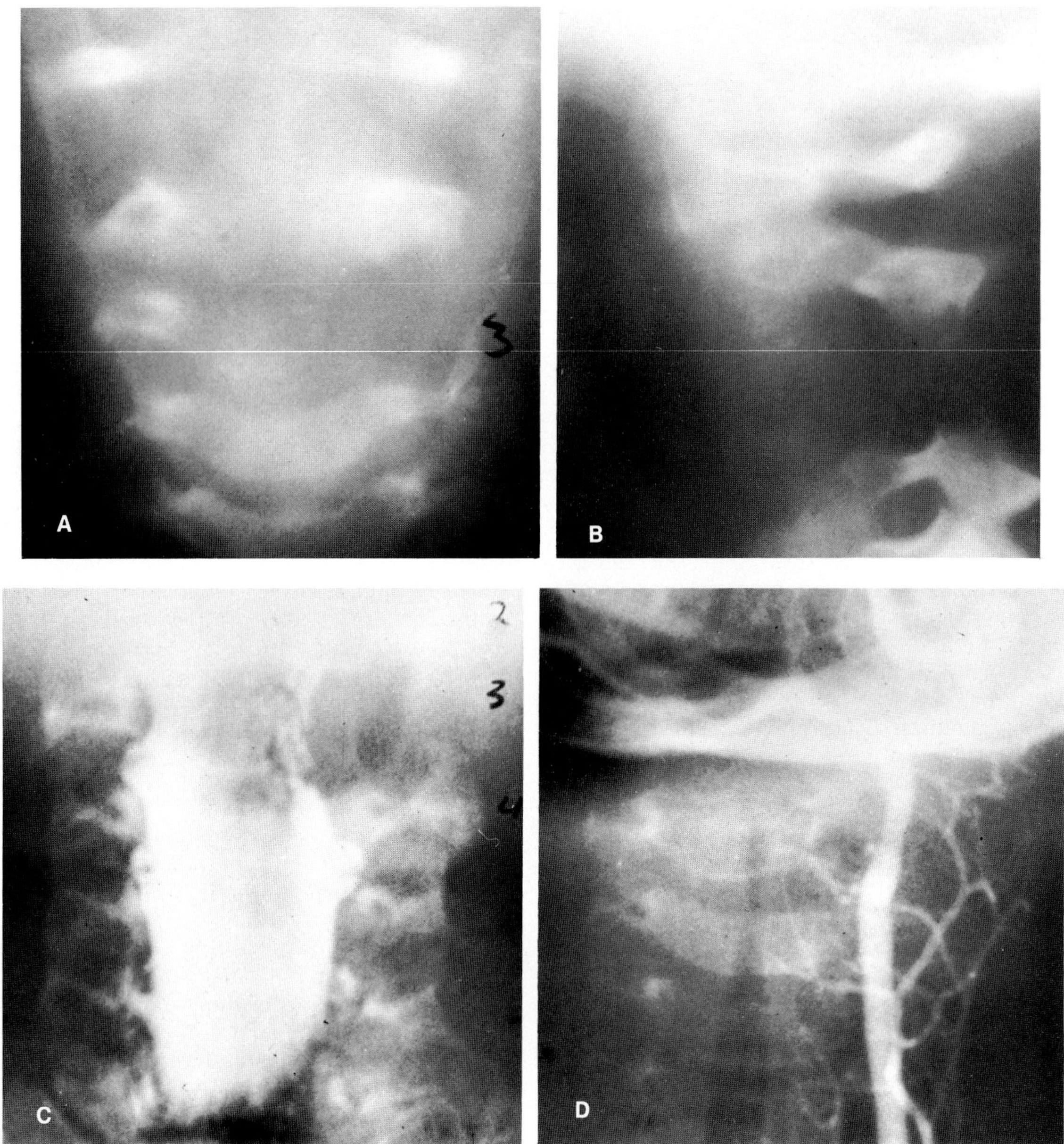

Fig. 12-4. Roentgenograms of a 5-year-old girl with aneurysmal bone cyst involving C3 primarily but extending into the pedicle and spinous process of C2. She was treated by halo cast, anterolateral and posterior resection, and bone grafting. (*A* and *B*) Tomograms showing involvement of the vertebral body, pedicle, and spinous process of C3 and the pedicle and spinous process of C2. (*C*) Myelogram. Note the defect in the dye column at C3. (*D*) Arteriogram. Note the displacement and compression of the vertebral artery at C3. (*E*) Intraoperative position in a halo cast. (*F*) One year postoperatively, there is solid fusion from C2 to C4 without recurrence. *Note:* This case was done before the availability of CT scanning. (Courtesy of Dr. S. Kopits and Dr. R. Robinson)

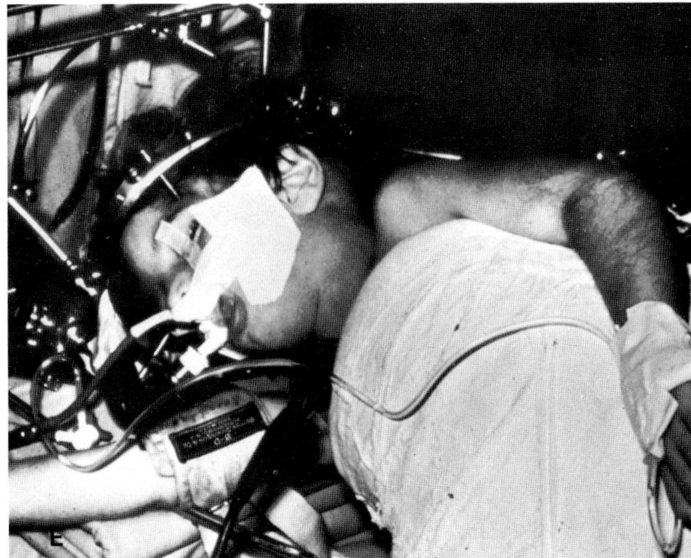

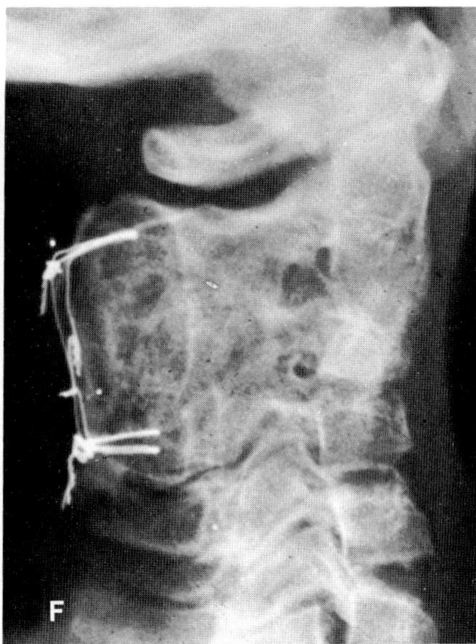

tion surrounding a small central nidus. A technetium bone scan may demonstrate the lesion before it becomes visible on plain radiographs, and a CT scan may assist in demonstrating the lesion in these instances. Treatment is excision of the central nidus (Fig. 12-3).

OSTEOBLASTOMA.[1,30,62,112] Osteoblastoma is often seen in children and teenagers. Pain appears to be the major presenting symptom with this lesion. However, this pain is neither consistently nocturnal nor necessarily relieved by salicylates, unlike osteoid osteoma. In one series consisting of 144 cases, 13% of osteoblastomas were located in the cervical spine.[67] The most frequent location within each vertebra appears to be in the posterior and lateral elements, with the vertebral body being an infrequent location. Osteoblastoma is generally larger than osteoid osteoma—hence the name giant osteoid osteoma—and may appear lytic or radiodense on x-ray films. The neoplasm is generally considered benign, but recent reports emphasize the locally aggressive nature of some osteoblastomata. One should also be conscious of the possibility that it may, in fact, represent primary osteogenic sarcoma, and a careful histologic evaluation of cell type is important in determining the exact nature of this growth.[63] The treatment is excision and bone grafting, when necessary.

HEMANGIOMA.[39,40] Hemangioma is a benign lesion that may be present in as many as 12% of spines at autopsies.[33] It produces a characteristic vertical striated lesion in the vertebral body on x-ray. In most instances, this neoplasm is asymptomatic and is an incidental radiologic finding. Hemangioma may also be seen posteriorly, and its appearance there may cause concern requiring biopsy. In general, no treatment is required for these tumors. Radiotherapy has been suggested as a satisfactory form of treatment for symptomatic hemangiomas (Fig. 12-6).

ANGIOMATOSIS. Although histologically similar to hemangioma, radiologic and clinical presentation of angiomatosis is strikingly different. Massive osteolysis has been reported to occur in the cervical spine as a result of two separate entities: angiomatosis and Gorham's disease. Both are thought to be angiomatous hamartomas and have the ability to relentlessly destroy the structural stability of the cervical spine. A few cases are reported in the literature,[13,24,49] and these suggest that attempts at surgical stabilization with bone graft are not always successful because of graft invasion and osteolysis by the pathologic process. Radiotherapy may be helpful, but no satisfactory method of treatment exists at this time.

GIANT CELL TUMOR.[17,19,48,87,97] In the cervical spine, these tumors can destroy the vertebral body and may even extend to the posterior elements. Signs of neural deficit can occur either from the lytic destruction of the vertebra or from the compressive effect from the growth of the giant cell tumor itself. Dahlin[19] believes that extrasacral

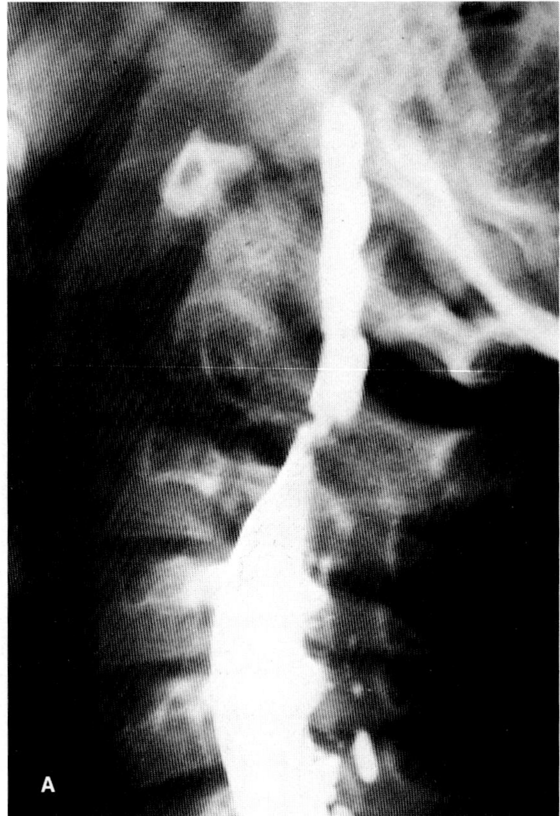

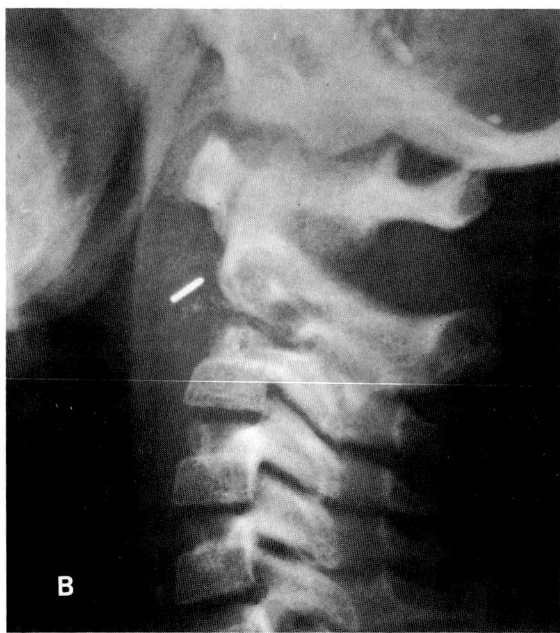

Fig. 12-5. (*A*) Roentgenogram of a 7-year-old boy with eosinophilic granuloma involving C2 and C3. Note the large anterior soft tissue mass. Biopsy and curettage followed by radiation led to pain relief. (*B*) Five months postoperatively there was good reconstitution of the lytic defect. (Davidson R, Shillito J: Eosinophilic granuloma of the cervical spine in children. Pediatrics 5:746, 1970)

spinal giant cell tumors might be basically different from such tumors elsewhere in the body. In his series, they occurred in a younger age group, had a female preponderance significantly higher than normal, and had a relatively benign course after excision. The potential for recurrent metastases does exist,[17,28] and treatment must take this fact into consideration. Excision with bone grafting is the treatment of choice. Routine radiotherapy after *en-bloc* excision is not recommended but may be appropriate after subtotal curettage or in inoperable cases (Fig. 12-7).

FIBROUS DYSPLASIA. The cervical spine may be affected by fibrous dysplasia in both the monostotic and polyostotic forms of this disease. Monostotic fibrous dysplasia of the cervical spine is extremely rare, and only a few cases exist in the English literature.[89,94] Vertebral involvement in polyostotic fibrous dysplasia is also reported as rare,[66] but various authors report an incidence of from 4% to 14%.[41,67,93] Radiographically, the lesions are often surrounded by sclerosis and may involve any part of the vertebra. The lesion can be lytic, or trabeculated, with or without a ground-glass appearance. Fibrous dysplasia in the spine has a poorer prognosis than its presence in the extremities, due to the much higher incidence of neural compression and the higher surgical morbidity and mortality associated with treating spinal fibrous dysplasia.[120] Treatment is generally directed toward preventing or correcting neurologic or structural compromise of the cervical spine by the use of orthoses or surgical fusion (Fig. 12-8).

OTHER BENIGN TUMORS. Reports have appeared in the literature describing chondromyxoid fibroma,[103] juxtacortical chondroma,[9] chondroma,[15,56] benign fibrous histiocytoma,[92] and intraosseous neurilemmoma[6,15,83] of the cervical spine. The treatment of choice in these benign lesions consists of complete excision when possible.

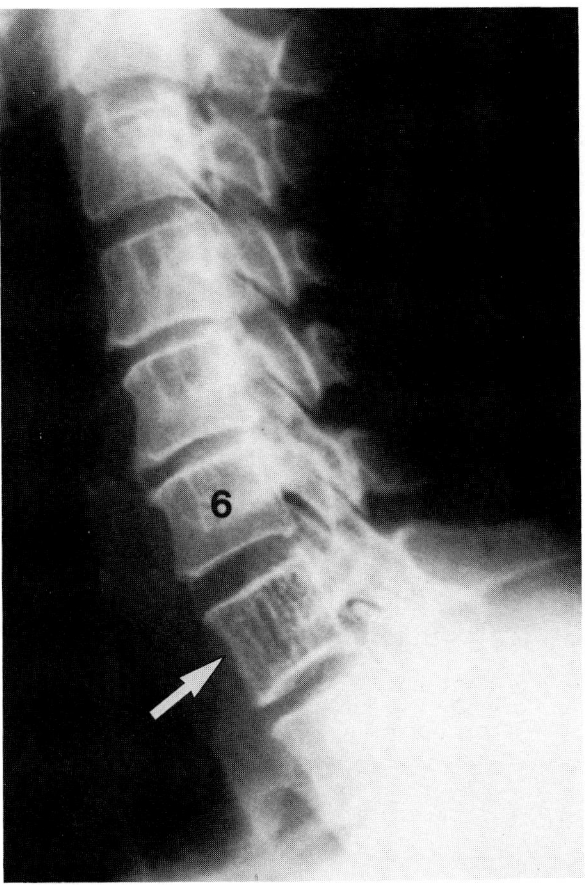

Fig. 12-6. Young man with hemangioma involving vertebral body of C7—note the vertical striated appearance. This patient was asymptomatic from this lesion discovered incidentally on x-ray film. No treatment was indicated in this case. (Courtesy of Dr. Henry Bohlman)

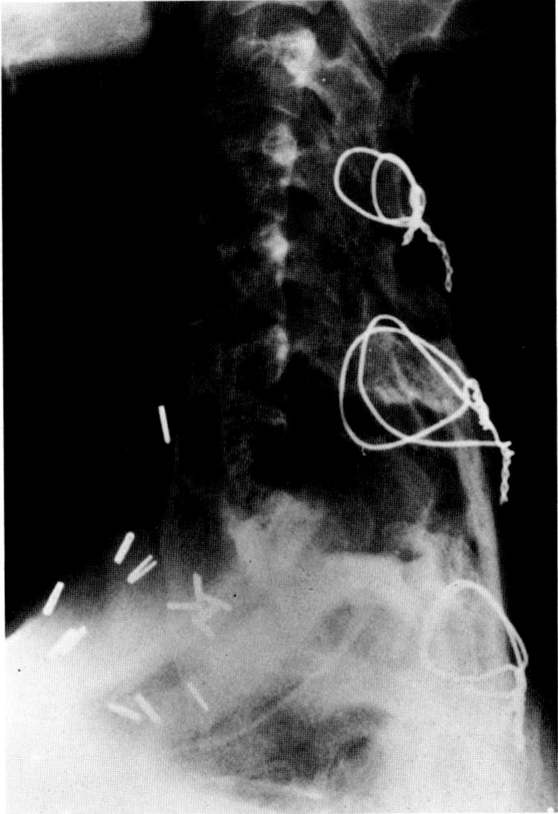

Fig. 12-7. Roentgenogram of a 28-year-old woman who underwent surgery for a giant cell tumor involving C7 and T1, with an associated thoracomediastinal mass. Her symptoms were pain and weakness of the left arm. Posterior exploration and excision of all tumor forward to the nerve roots, along with a posterior fusion, were followed 2 weeks later by a sternal splitting approach with bilateral claviculectomy for excision of the mediastinal mass and all tumor posterior toward the nerve roots. This resulted in essentially a two-level total vertebrectomy, with the exception of the pedicle of T1 on the right, which was not involved with tumor. The roentgenogram was taken 5 years after surgery and shows stable fusion without recurrence. The patient has no signs of neural compression.

Malignant Tumors of the Cervical Spine

MULTIPLE MYELOMA. The most common primary cervical tumor in the adult spine is multiple myeloma. Two thirds of myeloma patients have vertebral involvement and one third present with vertebral pain. Occasionally, patients appear to have some involvement of only a single vertebral body; this is called a solitary plasmacytoma. These patients generally have a more favorable prognosis and a much longer survival following a vertebral body resection and grafting. Myeloma is generally seen in patients over the age of 50 but may be seen in much younger people. Males are affected more often than females.

The x-ray appearance shows lytic defects in bones, generally without any significant new bone formation or sclerotic reaction. Bone scans may not show increased uptake. Laboratory abnormalities may include anemia, increased sedimentation rate, hypercalcemia, the appearance of an abnormal immunoglobulin specifically detectable by a serum protein electrophoresis, and the appearance of Bence-Jones protein in the urine. In the dissem-

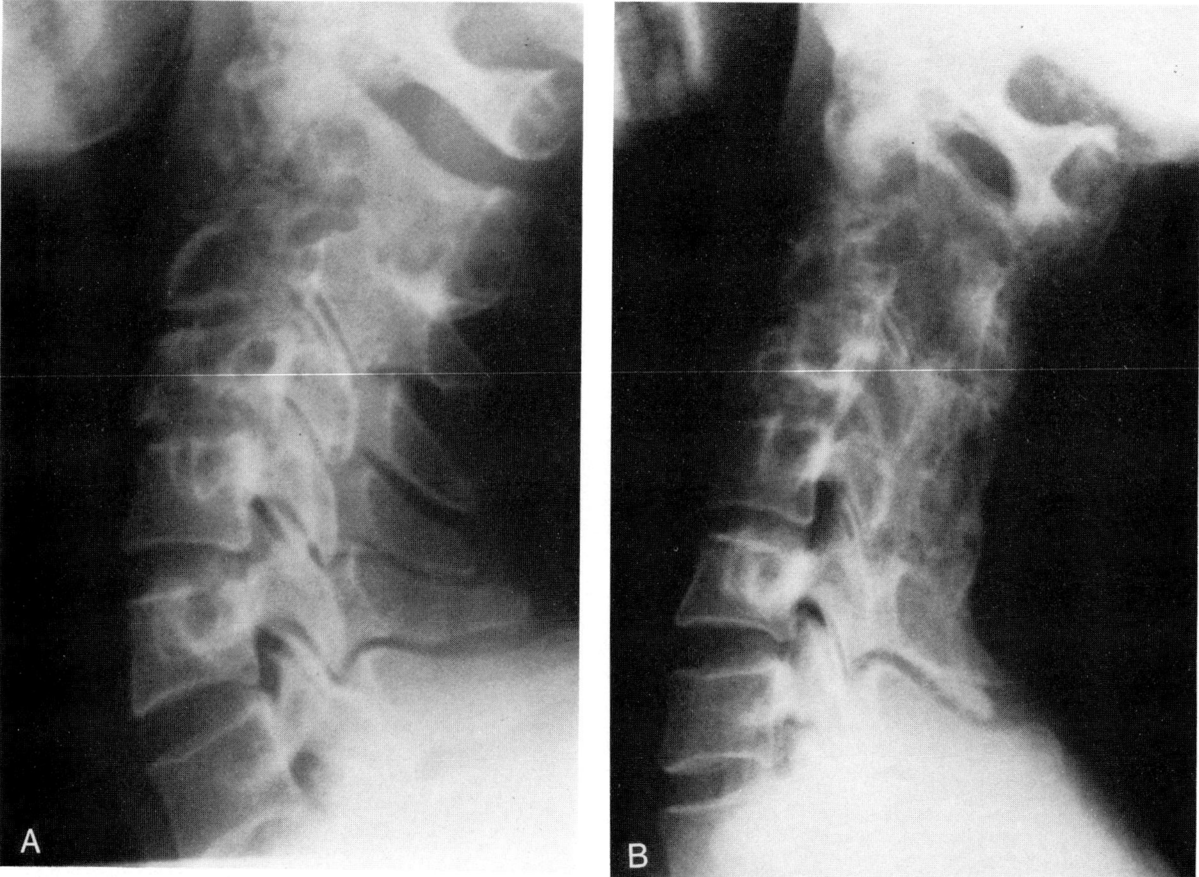

Fig. 12-8. A 27-year-old woman with fibrous dysplasia of the cervical spine and other areas. Because of increasing pain and the concern for vertebral collapse, a posterior fusion from C1 to C6 with autogenous iliac graft was carried out. Because of skull involvement, a halo was not used. Two and one half years later, the patient did not have any neural deficit and was working. (*A*) Lateral cervical spine x-ray at time of presentation showing extensive destruction of the vertebral body of C2 and C3, and involvement of C4. (*B*) Lateral x-ray films 2.5 years postoperatively demonstrating solid posterior cervical fusion and further destruction of C2, C3, and C4 vertebral bodies. Knowing the natural course of this disease allowed the surgeon to carry out an early stabilization procedure before vertebral collapse occurred. (Courtesy of Dr. David Fardon)

inated cases, diagnosis can often be made by bone-marrow biopsy. Treatment of this malignancy usually requires systemic chemotherapy and local irradiation of painful lesions. Often, an aggressive lesion compromises spinal stability and/or jeopardizes neurologic function to the point at which surgical stabilization or removal is required (Fig. 12-9, 12-15, and 12-16).

CHORDOMA.[42,69,84,99,105,106,121] Chordoma is a rare malignant neoplasm arising from the vertebral remnants of the embryonic notochord. In one series of 54 cases, only 9% of the vertebral chordomas were located in the cervical spine. Chordoma usually occurs in the second cervical vertebra, although any upper cervical vertebra may be involved. Although metastases are rare in cervical chordomas, they may extend locally within the central nervous system. The life-threatening potential of chordomas results from their critical location. Bony involvement generally occurs early in the course of chordoma, and the classic radiologic

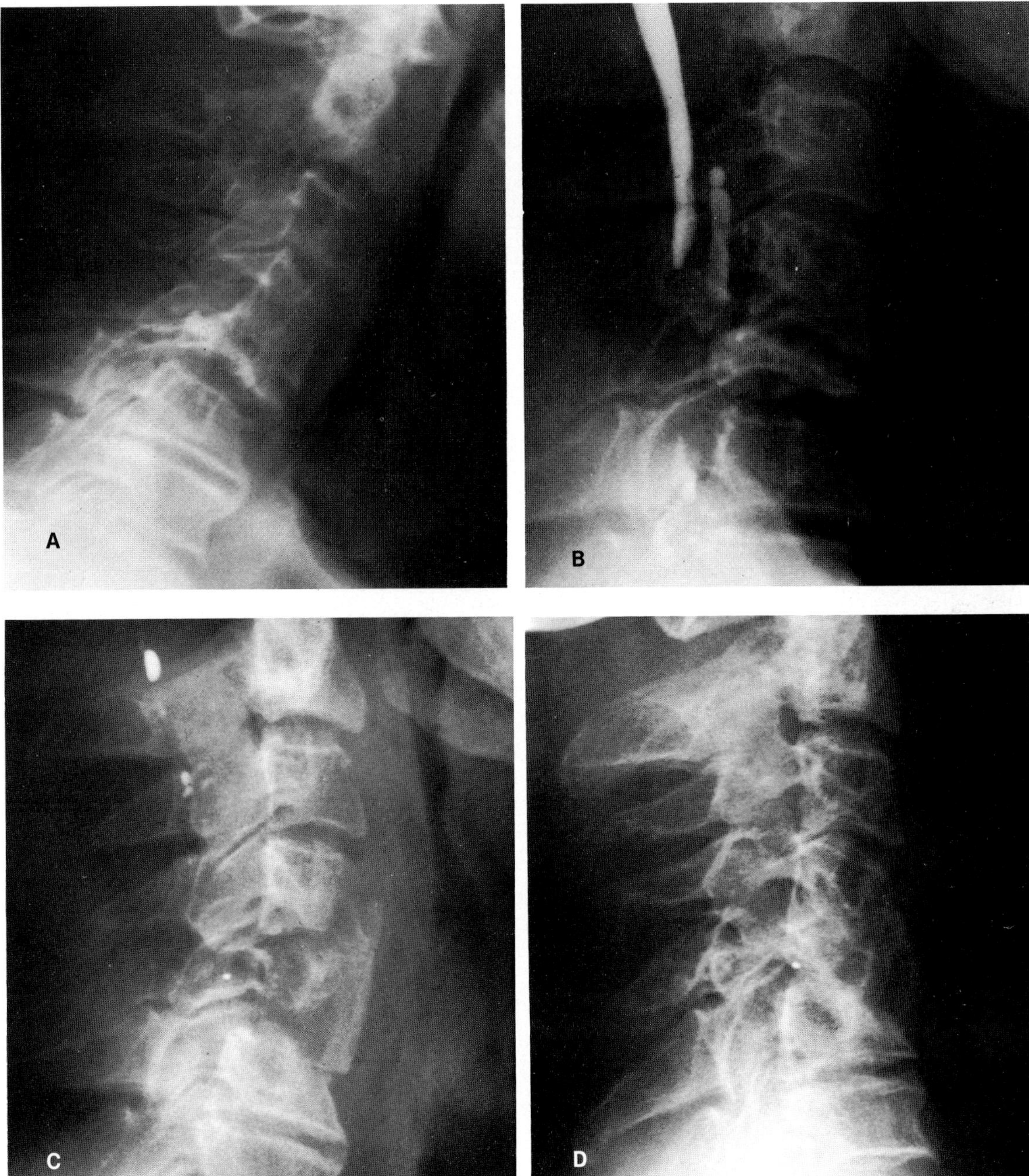

Fig. 12-9. Roentgenograms of a 55-year-old man with quadriparesis secondary to multiple myeloma. (*A*) Collapse of C5 with some posterior protrusion of bone. (*B*) Myelographic block at C5. (*C*) Excisional biopsy, decompression, and bone grafting. (*D*) Four years postoperatively, the patient was ambulatory and free of neurologic deficit. (In association with Dr. B. Northrup)

finding is an expansile osteolytic lesion. However, a combination of lysis and sclerosis may be encountered, making difficult the differentiation between chordoma and metastatic disease based on plains films. With the use of CT, a differentiation between these two entities is less difficult. Chordomas consistently have a significant soft-tissue mass, whereas bone metastases only rarely demonstrate soft-tissue extension (Fig. 12-10).

Treatment consists of radical removal and reconstruction. The use of radiotherapy postoperatively is not uniformly believed to be of any benefit. Recent reports seem to indicate that proton beam irradiation may have more benefit than previous types of radiation treatment.[105] The complete surgical removal is not generally possible but offers the greatest chance of cure. The use of the CT scan to improve delineation of the extent of the tumor may make complete surgical removal more feasible than it has been in the past. When total removal cannot be accomplished, the quality of life, and perhaps the length of survival, may be favorably affected by repeated local debulking procedures.

OTHER PRIMARY MALIGNANT TUMORS. Case reports have appeared in the literature describing chondrosarcoma,[5,47] osteosarcoma[26,63,68] Ewing's sarcoma,[81,118] malignant fibrous histiocytoma,[86] and fibrosarcoma[6] of the cervical spine. Chondrosarcoma may be slow growing and relatively well encapsulated, and because of this it may lend itself to a complete excision. If the history and radiologic studies suggest that this may be accomplished, then it should be attempted. The other tumors are considerably more invasive and more rapidly growing. In general, treatment would consist of biopsy, adjuvant chemotherapy, and/or radiotherapy.

METASTATIC TUMORS OF THE CERVICAL SPINE.[43,44,85,74] Metastatic lesions are the most common malignant tumors of the cervical spine. Frequent sites of primary involvement include the lung, breast, prostate, kidney, and thyroid, although any malignant tumor may metastasize to bone. As mentioned earlier, a careful history must be taken and should include questions concerning prior existence of a known malignancy. The appearance of metastatic disease is usually characterized by destructive and generally lytic but occasionally blastic features.

The vertebral body is usually the initial site of deposition; however, the pedicle may be the first area demonstrating involvement on x-ray film. This is because 30% to 50% of the cancellous bone in the vertebral body must be destroyed before any changes can be appreciated on plain x-ray films. Because cortical destruction of the pedicle is more easily appreciated on plain films, it is the type that is often first noted.[44] Metastatic lesions may cause symptoms prior to producing significant alterations in the x-ray appearance. The technetium-99 bone scans have provided an effective means of surveying the entire skeleton for metastatic disease and often demonstrate the location of metastatic disease before it is visible on x-ray film (Fig. 12-1). One must be aware that the round-cell type of tumors, such as multiple myeloma, may not show increased uptake on the bone scan. CT can demonstrate even small areas of vertebral destruction. CT is also helpful in the assessment of paravertebral soft-tissue masses and a clear visualization of the extent and direction of the tumor impingement on the spinal canal.[44] Major limitations of CT scanning for cervical spinal metastatic disease include potential failure to disclose a site of compression of the spinal cord.[3] In this regard, myelography may be helpful. Most metastatic foci remain relatively silent, but with an increase in the size of the lesion and destruction of the cortex, individuals may develop pain that is refractory to rest and mild analgesics, pathologic fractures, deformity, and often loss of function. Even a small mass in the spine may cause neurologic compromise and pain, if in a critical location. Treatment of metastatic disease is palliative. It is generally directed at reducing pain and improving or at least maintaining neurologic function. It often consists of irradiation and an immobilization device (Fig. 12-11). Occasionally, a surgical stabilization procedure is indicated. Some metastatic lesions are asymptomatic and therefore do not require any specific treatment.

TISSUE DIAGNOSIS

Guidelines for treatment of bone tumors elsewhere in the body also apply to the cervical spine.[18,61,77,78,101] An accurate diagnosis should be obtained and generally requires histologic confirmation. Possible exceptions include well-established metastatic disease with a previously determined tissue diagnosis or multiple myeloma proven by a bone marrow examination and serum protein electrophoresis.

All regions of the cervical spine are accessible by an open surgical technique or needle biopsy. With multiple metastases, bone lesions in the peripheral skeleton may be more amenable to open biopsy

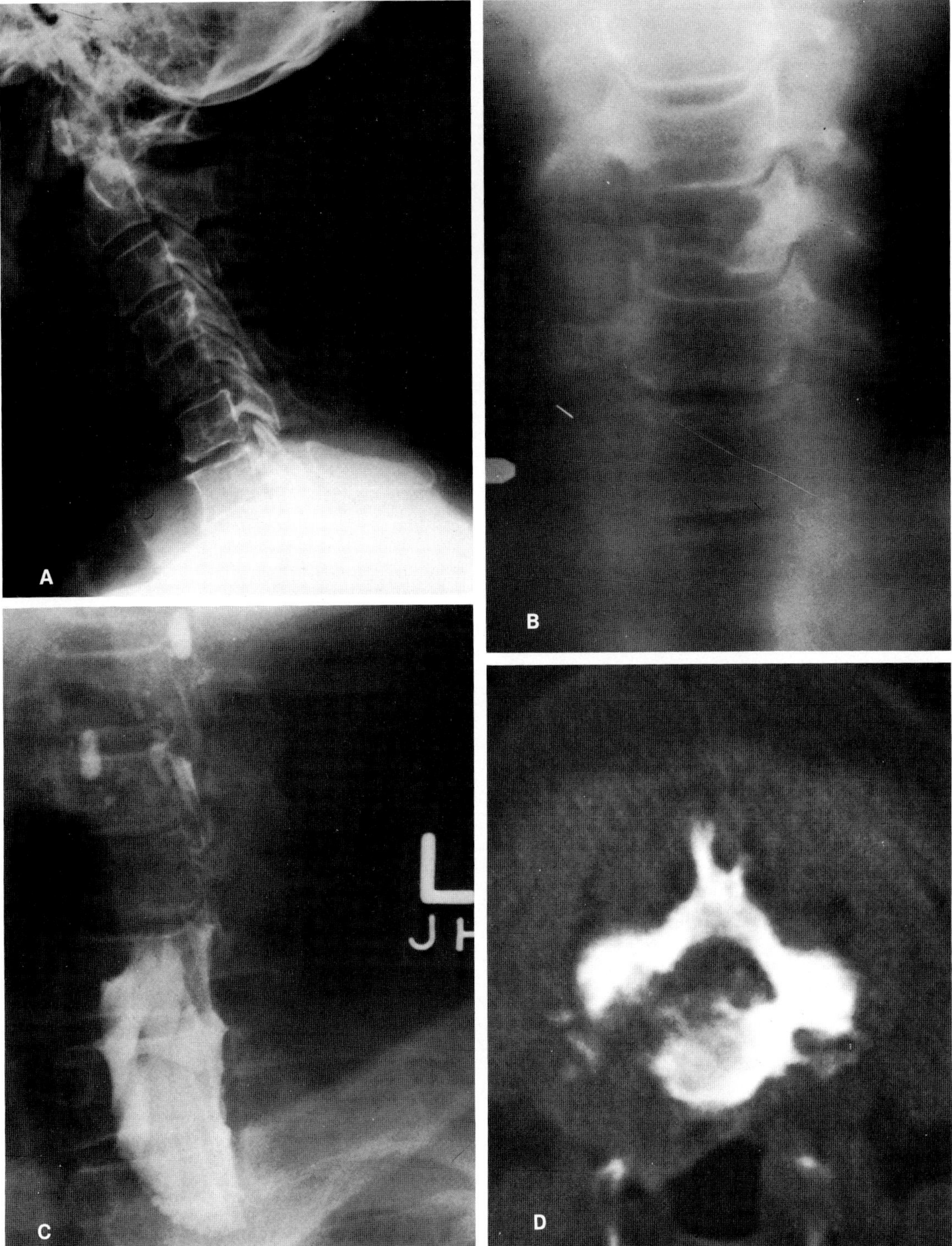

Fig. 12-10. Roentgenograms of a 57-year-old man with an 8-month history of neck pain radiating to the right shoulder and arm. (*A*) lateral view shows lytic changes of the C5 vertebral body. (*B*) Tomogram demonstrates a destructive lesion (*right*) of the pedicle and the body of C5. (*C*) Myelogram demonstrates a block at C4–C5. (*D*) CT scan shows an expanding soft tissue mass with impingement on the trachea and destruction of the vertebral body and the pedicle. A biopsy revealed chordoma. Treatment consisted of post fusion for stabilization followed by antero-lateral resection and bone grafting. (Courtesy of Dr. R. Thorne)

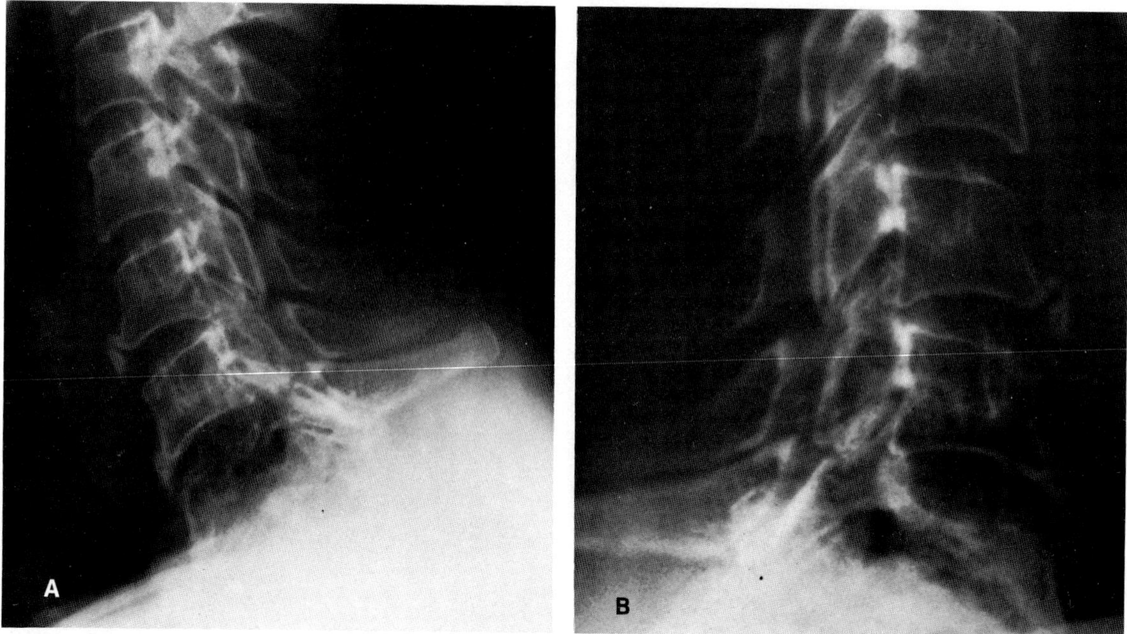

Fig. 12-11. (*A*) Roentgenogram of a 67-year-old woman with breast carcinoma metastatic to C7. (*B*) Two poster brace and radiation therapy provided pain relief and some reconstitution of vertebral body of C7.

than lesions in the spine itself. We prefer open biopsy and find that needle biopsy, when indicated, is most helpful anteriorly and in the upper cervical area. When carrying out an open biopsy, the incision must be planned with considerable forethought. It must allow access to a representative portion of the neoplasm but must not compromise the ability to make more extensive incisions and resections at a later date. When the type of tumor is strongly indicated by clinical and radiographic information, it is often possible and frequently preferable to combine open biopsy with a definitive surgical procedure. This has been our practice in recent years (Fig. 12-12).

MANAGEMENT CONCEPTS

Once the tissue diagnosis is established, the plan for management must consider (1) tumor ablation, (2) pain relief, (3) prevention or reversal of neurologic deficit, and (4) the reconstitution of mechanical stability. A multidisciplinary approach to therapy may include consultation with a radiotherapist, an oncologist, an orthopedist and a neurosurgeon. A patient's general condition and long-term prognosis dictate the necessary aggressiveness of management. An important concept in the management of tumors of the cervical spine is the prediction of the natural history or course of the tumor. Anticipation of future areas of instability and the need for obtaining spinal stability and solid fusion above and below the tumor are often a key to management. If the spine is stabilized early around an advancing tumor, a necessary decompression can be performed later without the need for external support (Fig. 12-8). Patients with limited prognosis for survival should not be made to suffer pain and neurologic deterioration, if surgery can be beneficial and carried out with little risk to the patient. Some patients who have metastatic disease will benefit from radiotherapy or chemotherapy and external support alone. When determining the type of orthosis to be used, we have been guided by principles established by Johnson and colleagues.[52]

SURGICAL CONSIDERATIONS

Benign Tumors

In a patient whose tumor appears benign, the lesion should be approached directly and completely removed, whenever possible. The anterior approach is used for those tumors located anteriorly, and the posterior approach is used for tumors

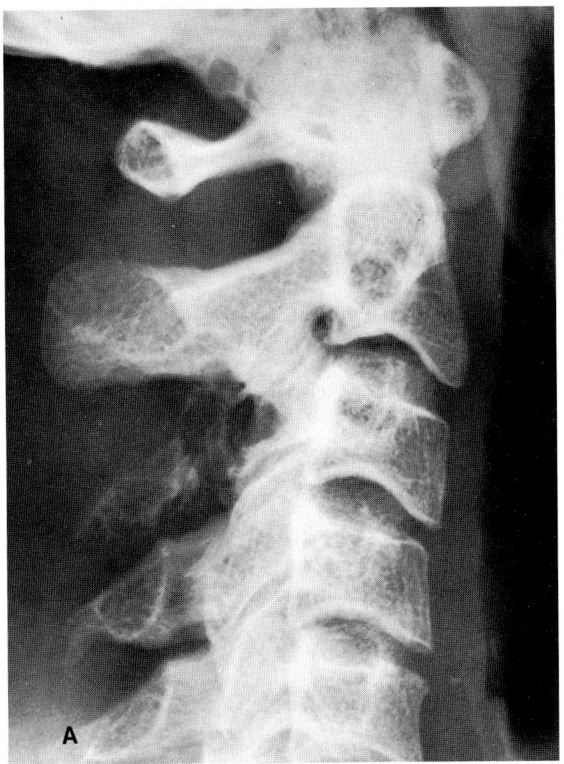

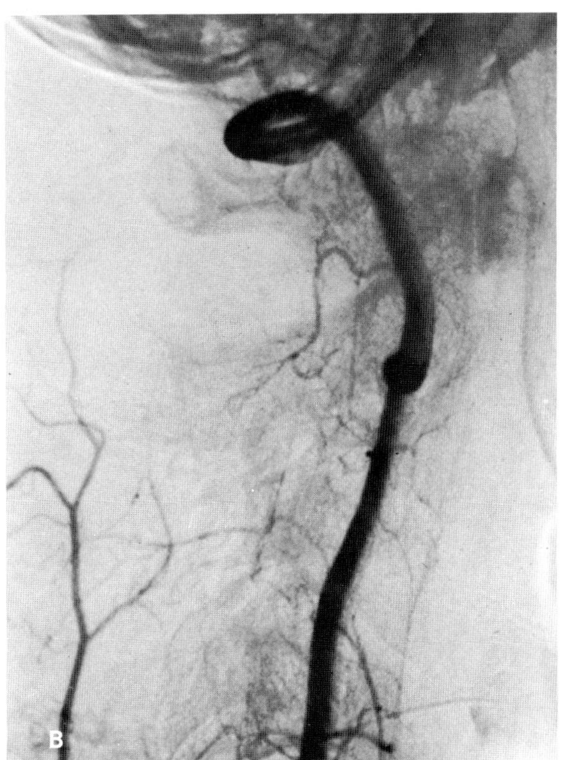

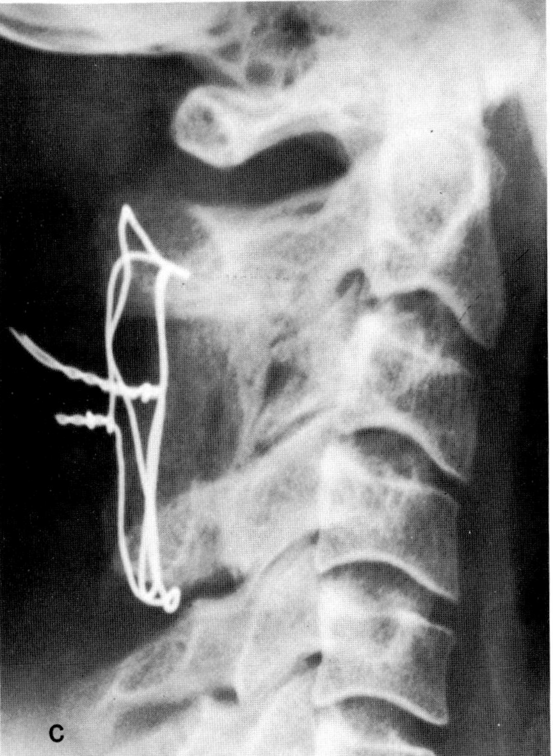

Fig. 12-12. (*A*) Roentgenogram of a 43-year-old man with an irregularly defined lytic lesion of the pedicle, lamina, and facet area of C3. (*B*) Minimal vascularity on arteriogram suggested a benign process. (*C*) Posterior excisional biopsy and fusion were carried out. The histologic diagnosis was hemangioma.

located posteriorly. When tumor surrounds or involves the vertebral artery, an anterolateral approach should be utilized.[110] If the tumor is extensive, a combined anterior and posterior approach will occasionally be necessary. In the slower growing tumors, it may be advantageous to first carry out a posterior stabilization and grafting, followed by an extensive resection at a later date. When benign tumors are removed, bone graft is the material more properly used for stabilization or reconstituting defects left behind.[28]

Primary Malignant Tumors

In many instances, surgery is confined to biopsy alone. If compression of the spinal cord or nerve roots is caused by tumor mass, radiotherapy and/or adjuvant chemotherapy may be indicated. In slow-growing malignant tumors, such as chondosarcoma or chordoma, initial attempts to completely extirpate the tumor may significantly prolong the patient's life and the period of freedom from neural deficit. If instability is seen secondary to bone destruction, some stabilizing surgery may be indicated.

Metastatic Tumors

It is in the treatment of metastatic tumors that our understanding of pathology and treatment concepts has changed most radically over the past few years. With the use of x-rays, myelography, bone scanning, and CT scanning, it is generally possible to know the location and extent of all spinal metastases in these patients. Furthermore, it is generally possible to localize the metastases in the cervical spine to intradural or epidural locations and also to note the exact degree and location of bony involvement.

In the past, the results of surgery for patients with metastatic disease of the cervical spine were not encouraging. This appears to have been largely the result of poor patient selection, a poor understanding of the pathophysiology of these tumors, and a poor application of surgical concepts.[22]

PATHOPHYSIOLOGY.[44] In a recent review, Harrington noted that vertebral metastases are often asymptomatic.[43] He also noted that when symptoms did develop they were a consequence of (1) an enlarging mass within the vertebral body that may break through the cortex and invade the paravertebral soft tissue, (2) compression or invasion of adjacent nerve root, (3) development of a pathologic fracture secondary to vertebral destruction, (4) development of spinal instability from such a fracture, and (5) compression of the spinal cord. He believed that the most common cause of compression of the spinal cord or a nerve root was the extrusion of tumor tissue and detritus of bone into the spinal canal, following partial collapse of the vertebral body that was infiltrated and weakened by a metastatic deposit. On occasion, tumor tissue may break into the canal and compress the cord, without causing significant destruction or collapse of the vertebral body. Rarely, compression of the cord or root results from a soft-tissue mass growing into the spinal canal through a neural foramen, from intradural metastases, or from carcinomatous meningitis. It is uncommon for the dura to be penetrated by metastatic tumor tissue. Patients who have one or more of these problems usually present with pain, neurologic involvement, radiologic signs of involvement of bone without collapse or instability, and radiologic signs of involvement of bone with collapse or instability, or a combination of all of these.

NONOPERATIVE TREATMENT. In patients who have bone scan and roentgenographic evidence of spinal metastases, but who have no pain, neurologic impairment, or vertebral collapse, no treatment may be necessary. Some physicians, however, believe that these people should undergo chemotherapy and in some instances radiotherapy, in order to stop what is usually a progressive metastatic involvement. Patients with pain but no neurologic impairment and involvement of bone but without collapse or instability will often obtain relief from chemotherapy or radiation.[44] Patients with major neurologic impairment without significant bone involvement usually respond to treatment with radiotherapy alone. Patients with epidural metastases are obviously included in this category. Occasionally, a patient with a rapid onset of neurologic symptoms of major proportions associated with epidural metastases may require surgical decompression in addition to radiotherapy.

OPERATIVE TREATMENT. Patients with vertebral collapse and pain due to mechanical causes or instability, but without significant neurologic compromise, and patients with vertebral collapse or instability combined with major neurologic impairment are often candidates for surgery. In patients who have a mechanical problem as the basis of their symptoms, it is unlikely that radiotherapy alone can relieve their symptoms. In the past, most of the surgery performed was posterior laminectomy, and little or no consideration was given to the location of the tumor. In our understanding of pathophysiology with newer biomechanical concepts, we are again indebted to Harrington[44] for the following summary of the indications for surgical intervention in these patients: (1) Patients with progressive impingement on the spinal canal and compression of the spinal cord by radio-resistant tumor, by recurrent tumor in an area that has already been subjected to maximum radiation, or by bone or soft-tissue detritus that has been extruded into the canal as a result of progressive spinal deformity, require direct decompression with spinal stabilization, when indicated. (2) Patients with progressive kyphotic spinal deformity with intact posterior structures, but with intractable pain due to mechanical causes, require anterior decompression and anterior stabilization. (3) Patients with progressive kyphotic deformity associated with disruption of the posterior elements and progressive shear deformity require anterior and posterior decompression and stabilization. (4) Patients who have had a decompression for epidural metastases may also require a stabilization procedure following that surgery.

We have been able to establish some patient selection criteria which have increased the ability to assist patients with metastatic involvement of the cervical spine. It should be stated, however, that the patients who meet the criteria for surgical stabilization of the cervical spine constitute an extremely small percentage of all patients with cervical spinal metastases. Patients with hormone-dependent primary tumors, such as those of breast, prostate, and thyroid, generally have a longer survival rate and therefore are more likely to benefit from surgery when indicated. Localized metastatic lesions from a well-differentiated primary tumor are often relatively slow growing, and these patients can also be expected to survive long enough to obtain significant benefit from surgery. Occasionally, patients present in an emergency situation with a rapidly evolving neural deficit associated with a collapsed vertebra secondary to an apparent malignancy, and in these instances surgery allows us to perform biopsy, to decompress and provide pain relief, and to restore stability, all in one procedure. We agree with Friedlander and Southwick[33] that a patient with metastatic tumor should not be denied the benefits of aggressive surgical stabilization when appropriate, but we believe that most patients with uncontrolled or unresectable primary cancer and/or lung metastases generally do not live long enough to benefit from this procedure. Multiple bone metastases may be a relative contraindication to surgical stabilization, but occasionally a nondisabled patient with one of the slower-growing tumors may benefit from surgery (Fig. 12-13). Retrospectively, we have realized that patients with metastases from the lungs or tumors of nasopharyngeal origin are not usually appropriate candidates for surgery, because their remaining life span is generally short. Active infection is generally a contraindication for stabilizing surgery, and when a longstanding tracheostomy has been present or the need for such can be anticipated, anterior surgery may be contraindicated because of the increased risk of infection. In patients with metastatic disease requiring anterior decompression and stabilization, we have been happy with the use of methylmethacrylate secured by anchor holes in the superior and inferior adjacent uninvolved vertebrae. Ono and coworkers have described the use of a ceramic prosthesis that is anchored by cement into anchor holes made in the superior and inferior adjacent normal vertebrae (Fig. 12-14). Another advantage of the prosthesis is that it serves as a mold to contain the cement and, to some extent, protect from extrusion of cement against the posterior longitudinal ligament and spinal cord. Harrington has described a combination of Knodt distraction rod and hooks in methylmethacrylate as an acrylic vertebral replacement.[44] According to several authors, acrylic cement used anteriorly for this purpose has excellent resistance to compressive loads, the normal load that would be placed on it. Those cases in which we have used posterior stabilization have been fewer. Following a midline laminectomy as long as the facet joints are intact some variation of the Robinson–Southwick method of posterolateral fusion may be utilized.[10] Under ordinary circumstances this is carried out by wiring bone grafts to the facet joint on either side. It is also possible to use Steinman pins encased in acrylic and wire them to the facet joints. Some surgeons use acrylic cement on one side and bone graft on the other side, hoping to ultimately achieve bony stability. It is possible to use acrylic cement, plates, and wires posteriorly in an attempt to prevent flexion deformity.[22] Recent studies by Penjabi, White, and Whitehill have demonstrated that posteriorly placed acrylic constructs are quite weak under this flexion force.[79,113,116] Good anchorage for acrylic or wires in sound bone is necessary to achieve an optimal result. Although still considered helpful these constructs should be restricted to those patients with limited longevity. Those with mechanical collapse anteriorly at the C2 level with or without neurologic deficit may be properly treated by posterior cervical stabilization and fusion. We have seen a number of patients with multiple myeloma

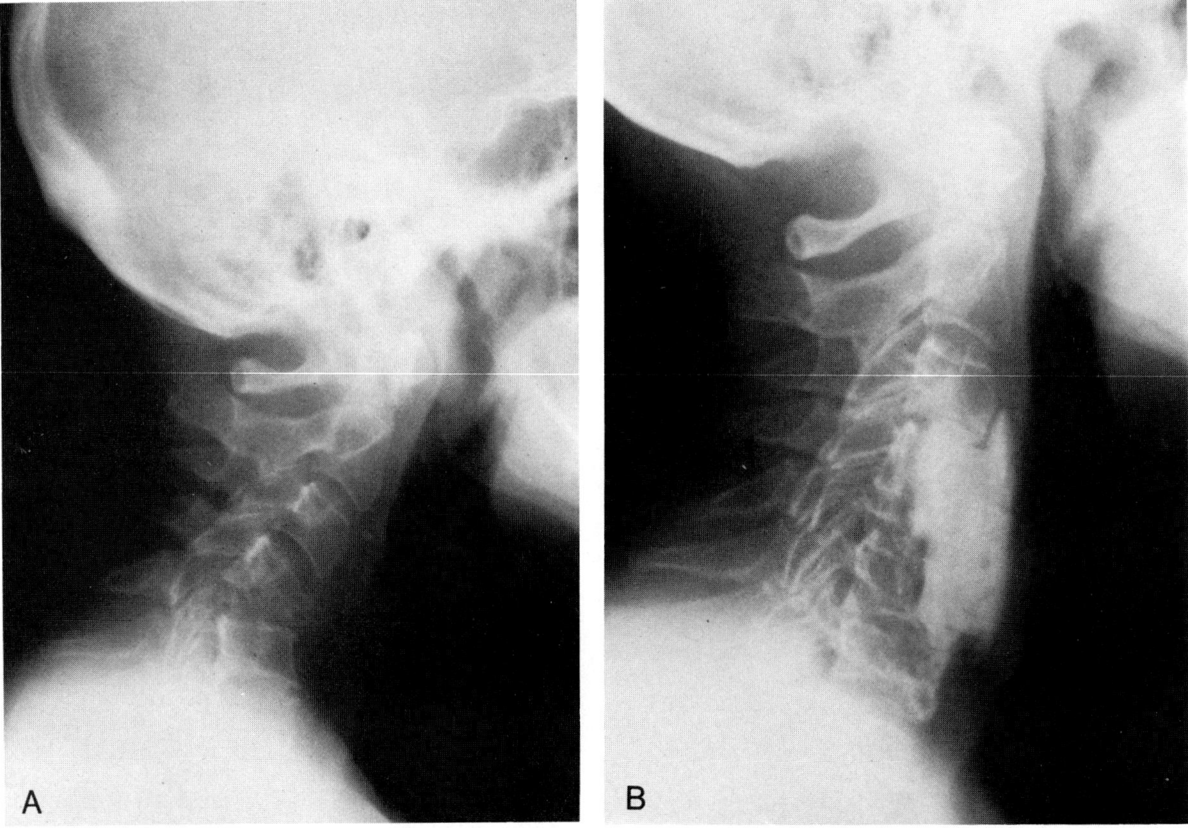

Fig. 12-13. A 55-year-old female with metastatic carcinoma of the breast. She presented with severe neck pain and weakness of the right arm. X-rays demonstrated (*A*) metastatic involvement of the body of C4 with partial collapse, extensive involvement of the body of C5 with marked collapse and angulation of C4 on C5. Gardner-Wells tongs were applied, and the patient was reduced on a Stryker frame. She obtained good pain relief and neural recovery in traction. She underwent an anterior decompression and stabilization using methylmethacrylate from C3 to C7 (*B*). (At the time of surgery C6 was also found to be involved with tumor.) Despite the presence of other metastases she lived a full life until her death 22 months later.

involving C2 and this presentation, who have been successfully treated with halo immobilization, occiput C2 arthrodesis and radiation (Fig. 12-16). The posterior occipital cervical plates described by Roy-Camille[95] or Steinman pins bent and wired to the occiput and facet joints are also an effective means of stabilization for these patients. Usually, patients with multiple areas of anterior vertebral collapse can be identified. In our experience significant difficulty in anchoring the prostheses or methylmethacrylate constructs in patients spanning three or more vertebral levels was encountered. We believe, therefore, that patients with vertebral body lesions spanning three or more levels should not undergo this type of surgical approach. When indicated radiation or some type of posterior instrumentation or bone grafting and possibly even the use of a halo combined with these measures would be preferable.

SURGICAL APPROACHES

Posterior Approach and Stabilization

The posterior elements from the occiput to the C7 vertebra are directly approachable through a posterior midline incision with subperiosteal dissection to the lateral facets. This approach is indicated for tumors involving the spinous processes, laminae, tumor extension from the lamina to the articular facets, and intraspinal tumor, and for posterior fusion and stabilization. If the spinous processes and laminae are to remain intact or are removed only to a limited degree, a standard Roger's type midline wiring and fusion with bone grafting would be the most appropriate stabilization procedure. Decompressive laminectomy performed for any reason may leave the patient with progressive instability and deformity in the post operative period. In this situation, appropriate measures to provide stability by means of the lateral facet fusion as described by Callahan and Southwick should be undertaken. Autogenous bone graft is the best material to secure long-term fixation. Stabilization with methylmethacrylate is possible, but generally we reserve this for patients with malignant or metastatic tumors. The possible options in dealing with posterior occipitocervical instability include the use of the halo jacket, while waiting for a bone graft to incorporate, and Roy-Camille plates, which stabilize the occiput to the lower cervical spine. We do not have any experience with the Roy-Camille technique but in theory at least it seems to offer stable fixation posteriorly without the use of cumbersome external fixation. This may be desirable in patients with a limited life span. (See also Fig. 12-17.)

Anterior Approach and Stabilization

Indications for an anterior approach to the cervical spine would include tumors that involve the vertebral body and compress the anterior cord and tumors that destroy the vertebral body to such an extent that mechanical stability is compromised. The third through the seventh vertebral body are readily accessible through a longitudinal incision anterior to the sternocleidomastoid muscle.[91] The anterior aspects of the atlas, axis, and C3 body require a more extensive exposure. The anterior lateral approach described by Riley offers exposure of this region, allowing tumor excision and fusion from the basiocciput to the first thoracic level.[89] This approach involves the proximal extension of the previous incision, angling the incision anteriorly at the mastoid process in a line paralleling the inferior border of the mandible. The exposure requires resection of the submandibular gland and dislocation of the mandible. The assistance of an otolaryngologist may be necessary for those unfamiliar with this route. The transoral approach of Fang[25] offers another alternative for exposure. This approach is simple and direct; however, several authors have reported a high incidence of infection with this technique. Our limited experience with the transoral approach to the anterior body of C2 has not been associated with infection. Our patients were prepared preoperatively with a program of dental hygiene, decongestants, and systemic and topical antibiotics. This approach does often limit the surgical field. In the anterior approach, once tumor ablation and cord compression have been completed, the final hurdle of providing reconstruction of the vertebral body remains. Full-thickness iliac crest or fibula provides suitable graft material. We prefer the iliac crest. The graft must be carefully countersunk within the cancellous portions of the contiguous vertebral bodies. Dislocation is a common postoperative problem and can be avoided only through care in fashioning and inserting the graft. Although not widely used in the United States, plate and screw stabilization of a bone graft, as suggested by Caspar and others in the European community, appears to be a reasonable alternative. The cervical surgery should be performed with a skeletal halo or tong traction device in place, with subsequent conversion to a halo jacket whenever necessary. One should not hesitate to maintain nasotracheal intubation in the immediate postoperative period. When malignancy is treated in the anterior cervical area, the use of methylmethacrylate or a ceramic prosthesis is often perferable to bone grafting.

Tumorous involvement of the lateral portion of the cervical vertebral bodies and extension into the lateral processes, pedicles, and posterior/lateral joints can be adequately treated by retraction of the longissimus capitis and colli muscles and resection of the anterior rims of the foramina transversaria and the anterior tubercles of the transverse processes. The resulting exposure of the primary rami of the spinal nerves and the vertebral artery allows for protection during surgical removal of lateral portions of the vertebral bodies, pedicles, posterior/lateral joints, or entire transverse processes, depending on the extent of tumor. A preoperative vertebral angiogram is indispensable for identification of possible displacement or other involvement of the vertebral artery. Verbiest popularized this exposure and used it extensively for resection of tumors in the locations described.[110] This exposure is more likely to be needed and used for the excision of benign tumors.

CONCLUSION

Although we do not have complete solutions to the problems of managing tumors of the cervical

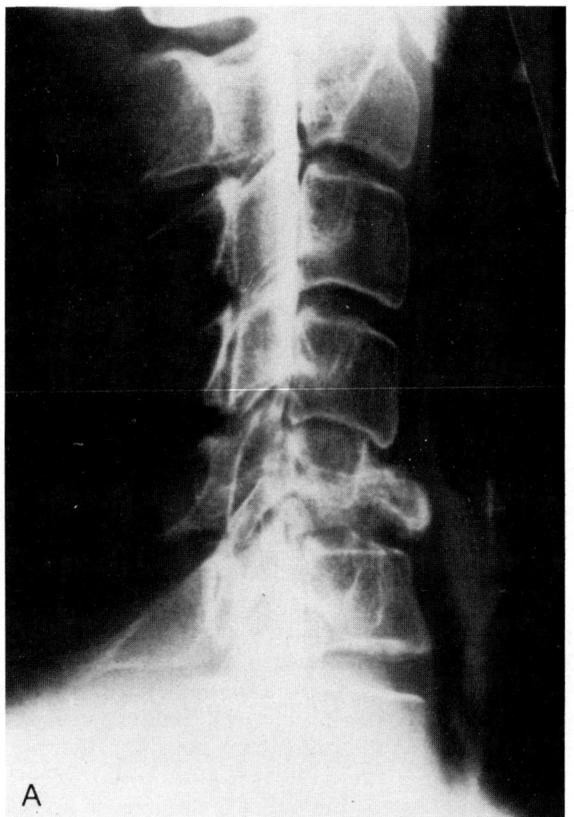

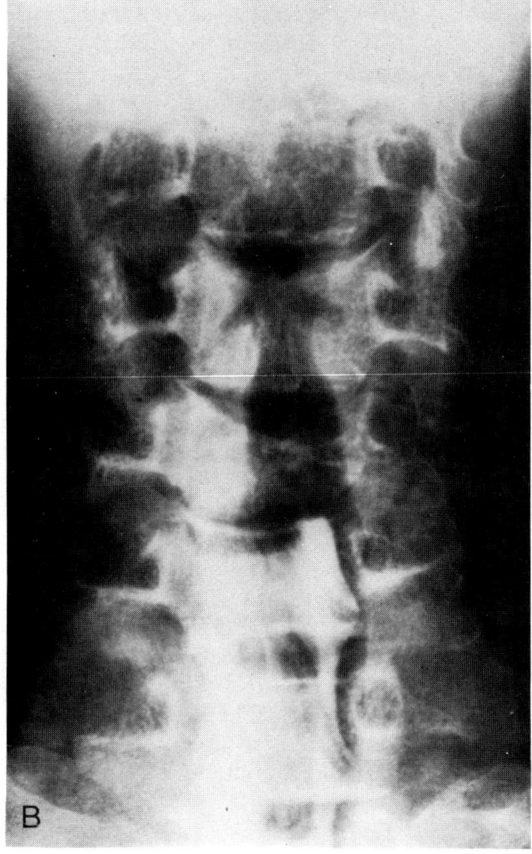

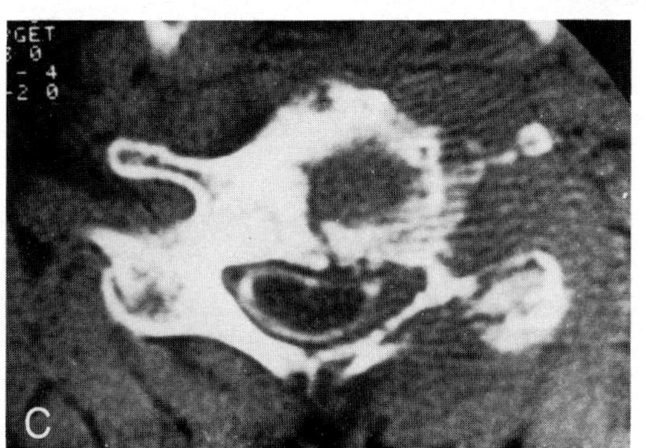

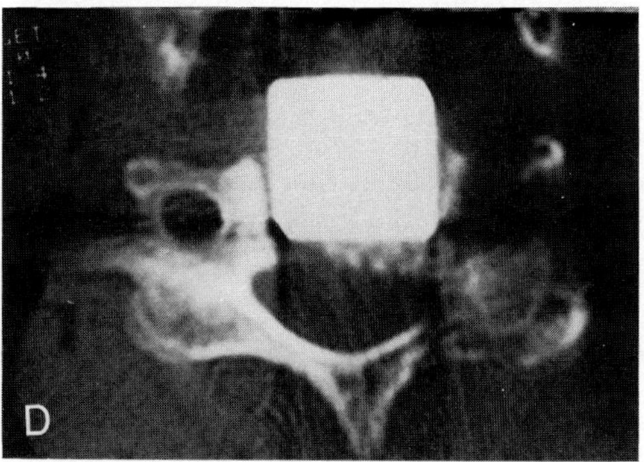

Fig. 12-14. A 36-year-old man with metastatic synovial sarcoma to C5. (*A*) Lateral myelogram shows collapse of vertebral body with pathologic fracture and protrusion into the spinal canal. (*B*) A–P film also demonstrates collapse of C5. (*C*) CT scan confirms extensive vertebral body involvement and extrusion of material into the spinal canal. (*D*) Postoperative CT scan demonstrates replacement of vertebral body by a ceramic prosthesis. (*E* and *F*) Lateral and A–P views of ceramic prosthesis. This patient was pain free, without external immobilizing devices until his death 7 months postoperatively. (Courtesy Dr. K. Ono)

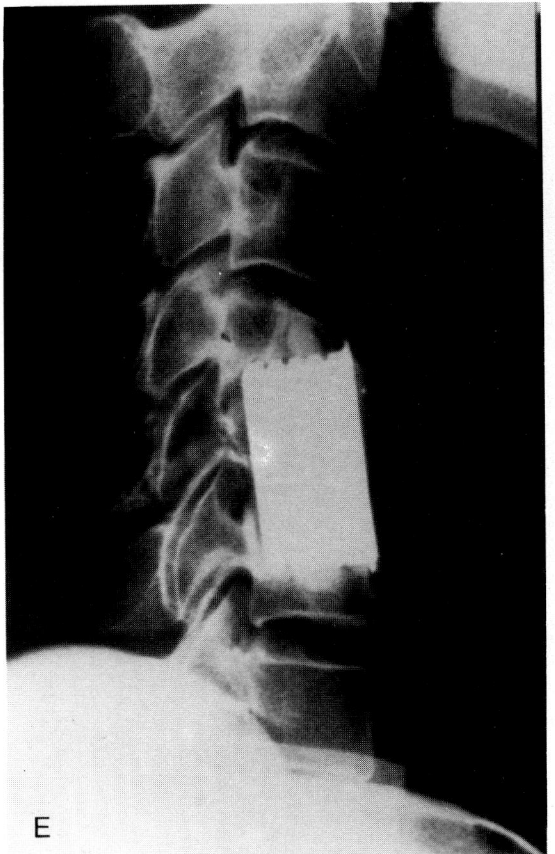

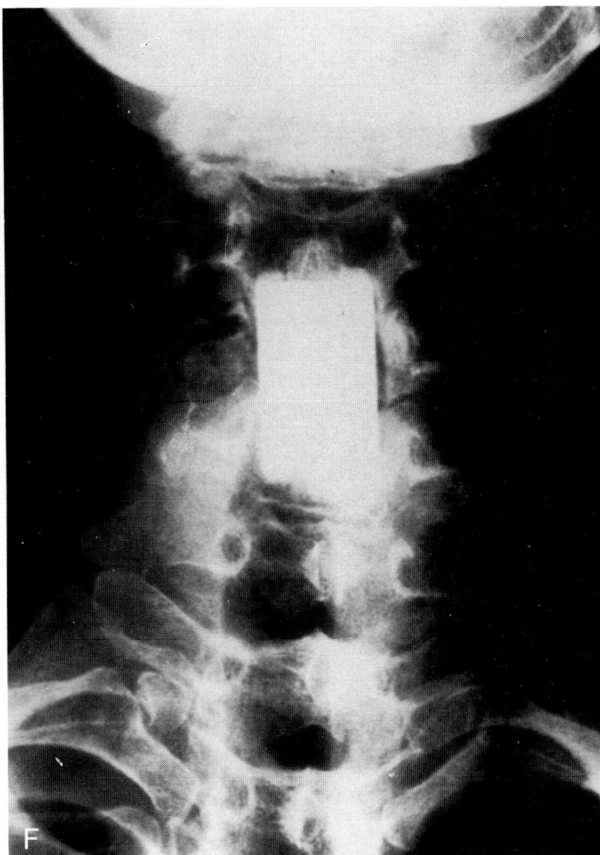

Fig. 12-14, *cont'd.*

spine, it should be obvious that great strides have been made in our ability to accurately diagnose the nature and extent of these tumors. Advances in chemotherapy, radiotherapy, and early detection of malignant disease have improved the life span of this group of patients. Careful application of the surgical indications and techniques that we have described should lead to a higher cure rate in patients with benign tumors, and it should contribute significantly to the dignity and general quality of life in patients with primary malignant and metastatic disease.

ACKNOWLEDGMENT

We have been assisted in the collection and preparation of this material by the teaching, discussion, clinical association, and case contributions of the following physicians:

Dr. Peter Anas, Boston, Massachusetts
Dr. Carlton Akins, Worcester, Massachusetts
Dr. Richard Bergland, New York, New York
Dr. Henry Bohlman, Cleveland, Ohio
Dr. Andrew Cederbaum, Worcester, Massachusetts
Dr. Alec Danylevich, Worcester, Massachusetts
Dr. David Fardon, Knoxville, Tennessee
Dr. James Hughes, Jackson, Mississippi
Dr. Stephen Kopits, Baltimore, Maryland
Dr. Bruce Northrup, Philadelphia, Pennsylvania
Dr. Keiro Ono, Osaka, Japan
Dr. Paul Riccardi, Worcester, Massachusetts
Dr. Lee Riley, Baltimore, Maryland
Dr. Robert Robinson, Baltimore, Maryland
Dr. Joseph Shillito, Boston, Massachusetts
Dr. Wayne Southwick, New Haven, Connecticut
Dr. Roger Thorne, La Jolla, California

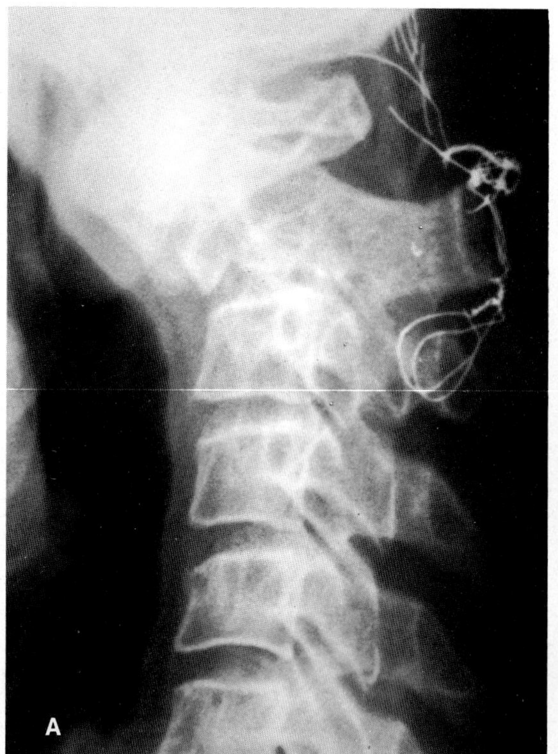

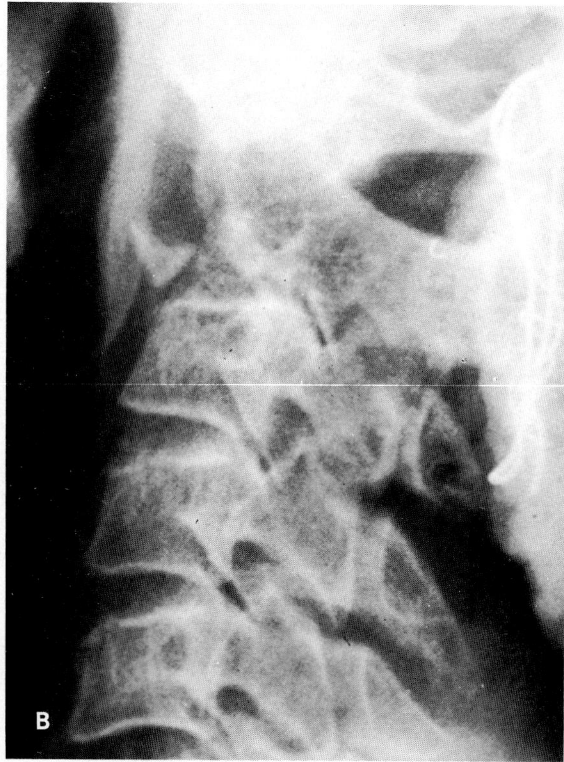

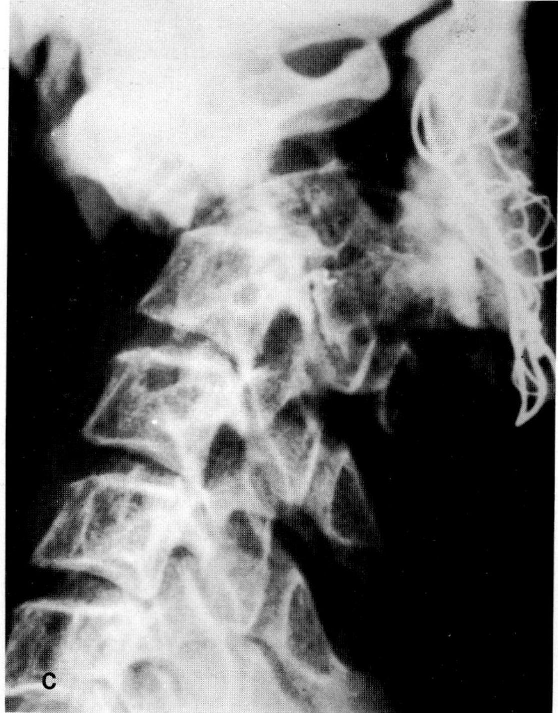

Fig. 12-15. Roentgenograms of a 50-year-old man with multiple myeloma and destruction of the body of C2. (*A*) Failed wire and bone graft. (*B*) Return of position following acrylic stabilization. (*C*) Loss of fixation following tearing fixation wire through spinous process of C3. Good anchorage for acrylic or wires in sound bone is necessary to achieve an optimal result. (Dunn E: The role of methylmethacrylate in the stabilization and replacement of tumors of the cervical spine. Spine 2:15, 1977)

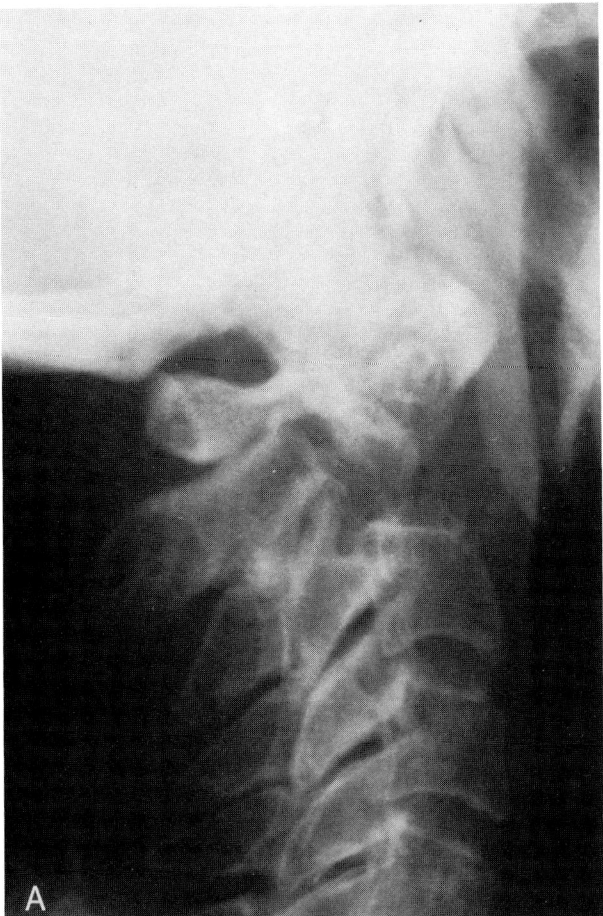

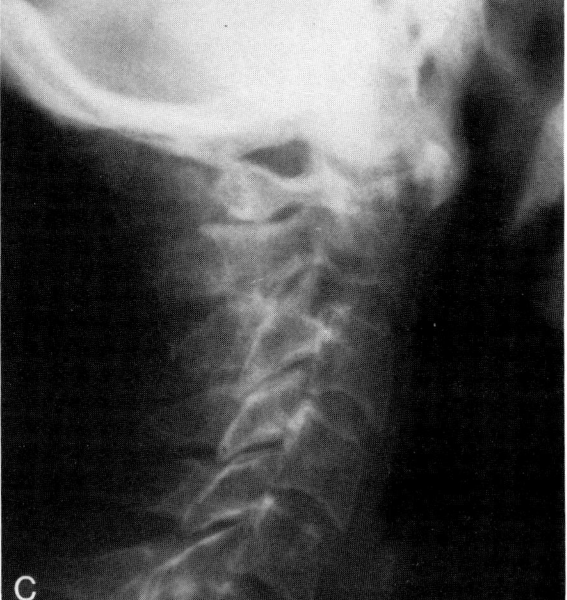

Fig. 12-16. A 77-year-old man who presented with sudden onset of pain in the neck and weakness preventing ambulation. (*A*) Lateral x-ray film in supine position showing destruction of the body of C2. (*B*) CT scan demonstrating bone loss in the body of C2. The diagnosis was multiple myeloma, suggested by serum protein electrophoresis and confirmed by bone marrow biopsy. He was placed in a halo and underwent a posterior occiput–C2 arthrodesis. (*C*) After satisfactory fusion had occurred (4 months), his halo jacket was removed and he was given radiotherapy. Note some reconstitution of the vertebral body of C2. The patient is still alive 2.5 years after surgery and without neural deficit or the need for external support. (In association with Dr. Alec Danylevich)

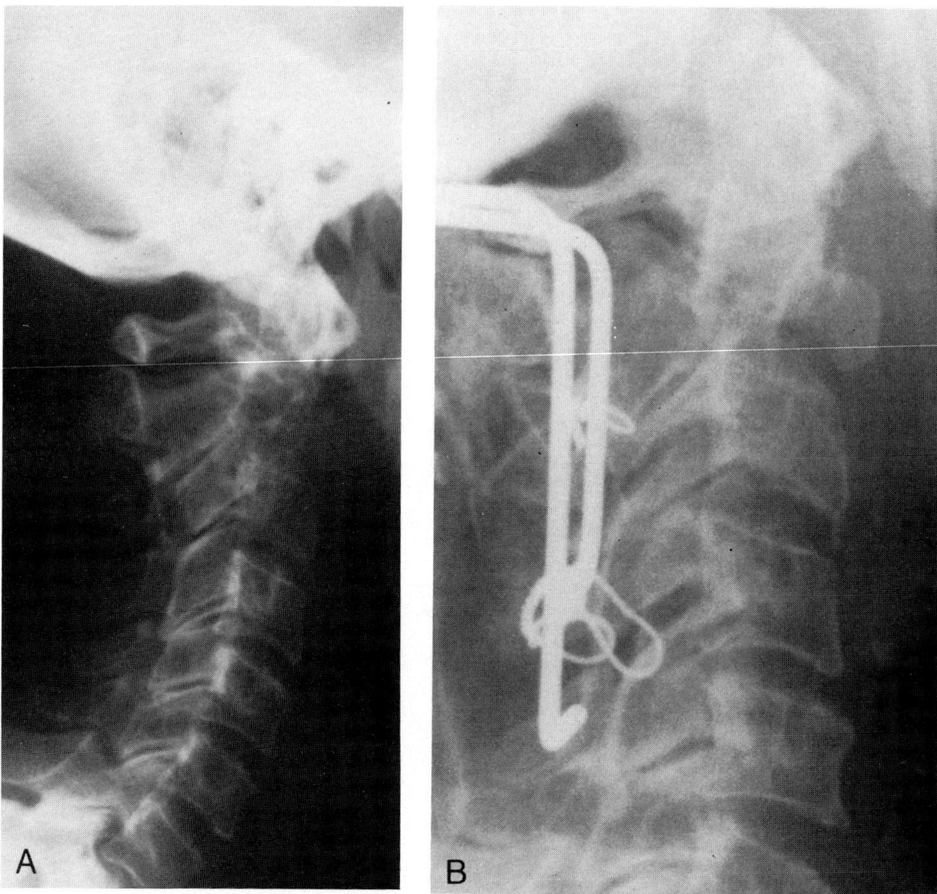

Fig. 12-17. A 64-year-old woman with carcinoma of the breast metastatic to C2. (*A*) lateral x-ray study demonstrates lytic destruction of C2 with a pathologic fracture. The patient had pain and instability but no neural deficit. She was frail and unlikely to be able to tolerate a halo jacket. Through a posterior approach, contoured Steinman pins were encased in methylmethacrylate and wired to the base of the skull and lateral facet joints of C2, C3 and C4. (*B*) Bone graft was placed between these struts over the lamina and spinous processes. Unfortunately, the patient died from disseminated disease 4 months postoperatively. Her neck was stable at that time. No autopsy was obtained. Although not optimal from the biomechanical point of view, some types of posterior internal stabilization may still be helpful in selected cases.

REFERENCES

1. *AMACHER AL, ELTOMERI A:* Spinal osteoblastoma in children and adolescents. Child Nerv Syst 1:29, 1985
2. *BARRON KD, HIRANO A, ARAKI S, ET AL:* Experiences with metastatic neoplasms involving the spinal cord. Neurology 9:91, 1959
3. *BERNAT JL, GREENBERG ER, BARRET J:* Suspected epidural compression of the spinal cord and cauda equina by metastatic carcinoma. Cancer 51:1953, 1983
4. *BLACK P:* Spinal metastasis: Current status and recommended guidelines for management. Neurosurgery 5:726, 1979
5. *BLAYLOCK RL, KEMPE LG:* Chondrosarcoma of the cervical spine. J Neurosurg 44:500, 1976
6. *BOHLMAN HH, SACHS BL, CARTER JR, ET AL:* Primary neoplasms of the cervical spine. J Bone Joint Surg 68A:483, 1986
7. *BOLAND P, LANE J, SUNDARESAN N:* Metastatic disease of the spine. Clin Orthop 169:95, 1982
8. *BUCK RE, BAILEY RW:* Replacement of a cervical

vertebral body for aneurysmal bone cyst. J Bone Joint Surg 51A:1656, 1969

9. *CALDERONE A, NAIMARK A, SCHILLER AL:* Case report 196. Skel Radiol 8:160, 1982
10. *CALLAHAN R, JOHNSON R, MARGOLIS R:* Cervical facet fusion for control of instability following laminectomy. J Bone Joint Surg 59A:991, 1977
11. *CANADELL J, VILLAS C, MARTINEZ-DENEGRI J, ET AL:* Vertebral eosinophilic granuloma. Spine II:767, 1986
12. *CAPANNA R, SPRINGFIELD DS, RUGGIERI P, ET AL:* Direct cortisone injection in eosinophilic granuloma of bone: A preliminary report on 11 patients. J Pediatr Orthop 5:339, 1985
13. *CASTLEMAN B, MCNEELY B:* Case records of the Massachusetts General Hospital. N Engl J Med 270:731, 1964
14. *COBB CA, LEAVENS ME, ECKLES N:* Indications for non-operative treatment of spinal cord compression due to breast cancer. J Neurosurg 47:653, 1977
15. *COHEN DM, DAHLIN DC, MACCARTY CS:* Apparently solitary tumors of the vertebral column. Mayo Clin Proc 39:509, 1964
16. *COHEN M, ZORNOZA J, CANGIR A, ET AL:* Direct injection of methylprednisolone sodium succinate in the treatment of solitary eosinophilic granuloma of bone. Diagnostic Radiology 136:289, 1980
17. *CHOW SP, LEONG JC, YAU AC:* Osteoclastoma of the axis. J Bone Joint Surg 59A:550, 1979
18. *CRAIG FS:* Vertebral-body biopsy. J Bone Joint Surg 38A:93, 1956
19. *DAHLIN DC:* Giant-cell tumor of vertebrae above the sacrum. Cancer 39:1350, 1977
20. *DAHLIN DC:* Bone tumors. General aspects and data on 3,987 cases. Springfield, Illinois, Charles C Thomas, 1967
21. *DAVIDSON RI, SHILLITO J:* Eosinophilic granuloma of the cervical spine in children. Pediatrics 45:746, 1970
22. *DUNN EJ:* The role of methacrylate in the stabilization and replacement of tumors of the cervical spine. Spine 2:15, 1977
23. *DUNN EJ, ANAS PP:* The management of tumors of the upper cervical spine. Orthop Clin North Am 9:1065, 1978
24. *EDWARDS WH, THOMPSON RC, VARSA W:* Lymphangiomatosis and massive osteolysis of the cervical spine. Clin Orthop 177:222, 1983
25. *FANG HS, ONG GB:* Direct anterior approach to the upper cervical spine. J Bone Joint Surg 44A:1588, 1962
26. *FIELDING JW, FIETTI VG, HUGHES JO, ET AL:* Primary osteogenic sarcoma of the cervical spine. J Bone Joint Surg 58A:892, 1976
27. *FIELDING JW, KEIM HA, HAWKINS RJ, ET AL:* Osteosid osteoma of the cervical spine. Clin Orthop 128:163, 1977
28. *FIELDING JW, PYLE RN, FIETTI VG:* Anterior cervical vertebral body resection and bone-grafting for benign and malignant tumors. J Bone Joint Surg 61A:251, 1979
29. *FIELDING JW, RATZAN S:* Osteochondroma of the cervical spine. J Bone Joint Surg 55A:640, 1975
30. *FLOMAN Y, MILEROM C, KENANA S, ET AL:* Spongious and cortical osteoblastoma of the axial skeleton. Orthopedics 8:1478, 1985
31. *FORNASIER VL, HORNE JG:* Metastases to the vertebral column. Cancer 36:590, 1975
32. *FOWLES JV, BOBECHKO WP:* Solitary eosinophilic granuloma in bone. J Bone Joint Surg 52B:238, 1970
33. *FRIEDLANDER GE, SOUTHWICK WO:* Tumors of the spine. In Rothman RH, Simeone F (eds): The Spine, 2nd Ed, pp 1022–1040. Philadelphia, WB Saunders, 1982
34. *FRIEDLANDER GE, TROSS RB, DOGANIS AC, ET AL:* Effects of chemotherapeutic agents on bone. J Bone Joint Surg 66A:602, 1984
35. *GILBERT RW, KIM JH, POSNER JB:* Epidural spinal cord compression from metastatic tumor: Diagnosis and treatment. Ann Neurol 3:40, 1978
36. *GLASAUER FE:* Benign lesions of the cervical spine. Acta Neur Chirurg 42:161, 1978
37. *GOLDBERG MJ, BELSKY MR, BRADER D, ET AL:* Solitary osteochondroma of the cervical spine. Orthopedics 3:759, 1980
38. *HALL AJ:* The results of laminectomy for compression of the cord or cauda equina by extradural malignant tumor. J Bone Joint Surg 55B:497, 1973
39. *HAMBACH R, PUJMAN J, MALY V:* Massive osteolysis due to hemangiomatosis. Radiology 71:43, 1958
40. *HARMON JD, BEVERIDGE W, EL GAMMAL T, ET AL:* Cervical spine hemangiomas: Report of a Case. Otol Head Neck Surg 90:501, 1982
41. *HARRIS WH, DUDLEY HR, BARRY RJ:* The natural history of fibrous dysplasia. J Bone Joint Surg 44A:207, 1962
42. *HARWICK RD, MILLER AS:* Craniocervical chordomas. Am J Surg 138:512, 1979
43. *HARRINGTON KD:* The use of methylmethacrylate for vertebral-body replacement and anterior stabilization of pathological fracture-dislocations of the spine due to metastatic malignant disease. J Bone Joint Surg 63A:36, 1981
44. *HARRINGTON KD:* Metastatic disease of the spine. J Bone Joint Surg 68A:1110, 1986
45. *HASTINGS DE, MCNAB I:* Neoplasms of the atlas and axis. Can J Surg 11:290, 1968

46. *HENRY AK:* Extensile Exposure, 2nd ed. Edinburgh, Churchill Livingstone, 1973
47. *HERMANN G, SACHER M, LANZIERI CF, ET AL:* Chondrosarcoma of the spine: An unusual radiographic presentation. Skel Radiol 14:178, 1985
48. *HESS WE:* Giant cell tumor of the cervical spine. J Bone Joint Surg 41A:480, 1960
49. *HEYDEN OD, KINDBLOOM LG, NIELSEN JM:* Disappearing bone disease. J Bone Joint Surg 59A:57, 1977
50. *HOCKING WG, SWANSON M:* Multifocal eosinophilic granuloma, response of a patient to etoposide. Cancer 58:840, 1986
51. *JAFFE WL:* Tumors and tumorous conditions of the bones and joints. Philadelphia, Lea & Febiger, 1958
52. *JOHNSON RM, HART DL, SIMMONS EF, ET AL:* Cervical orthoses. J Bone Joint Surg 59A:332, 1977
53. *JULIEN J, RIEMENS V, VITAL CL, ET AL:* Cervical cord compression by solitary osteochondroma of the atlas. Neurol Neurosurg Psychiatr 41:479, 1978
54. *LANZIERI CF, SOLODNIK P, SACHER M, ET AL:* Computed tomography of solitary spinal osteochondromas. J Comput Assist Tomogr 9:1042, 1985
55. *LIGHT TR, WAGNER FC, JOHNSON RM, ET AL:* Correction of spinal instability and recovery of neurologic loss following cervical vertebral body replacement. Spine 5:392, 1980
56. *LOZES G, FAWAZ A, PERPER H, ET AL:* Chondroma of the cervical spine. J Neurosurg 66:128, 1987
57. *MACCARTHY C, DAHLIN D, DOYLE J, ET AL:* Aneurysmal bone cysts of the neural axis. J Neurosurg 18:671, 1961
58. *MACLELLAN DI, WILSON FC:* Osteoid osteoma of the spine. J Bone Joint Surg 49A:111, 1967
59. *MADIGAN R, WORRALL T, MCCLAIN EJ:* Cervical cord compression from hereditary multiple exostosis. J Bone Joint Surg 56A:401, 1974
60. *MAIURI F, SIGNORELLI C, LAVANO A, ET AL:* Osteoid osteomas of the spine. Surg Neurol 25:375, 1986
61. *MANKIN HJ, LANGE TA, SPANIER SS:* The hazards of biopsy in patients with malignant primary bone and soft-tissue tumors. J Bone Joint Surg 64A:L1121, 1982
62. *MARSH BW, BONFIGLIO M, BRADY LP, ET AL:* Benign osteoblastoma: Range of manifestations. J Bone Joint Surg 57A:1, 1975
63. *MARSH HO, CHOI CB:* Primary osteogenic sarcoma of the cervical spine originally mistaken for benign osteoblastoma. J Bone Joint Surg 52A:1467, 1970
64. *MARSHALL LF, LANGFITTE TW:* Combined therapy for metastatic extradural tumors of the spine. Cancer 40:2067, 1977
65. *MARSHALL ME:* Chemotherapy for multifocal eosinophilic granuloma of bone. J Kentucky Med Assoc 617, 1983
66. *MATTHEW NT, BHAKTAVIZIAM A, ABRAHAM J:* Spinal cord compression in polyosteotic fibrous dysplasia. Can J Surg 14:228, 1971
67. *MIRRA J:* Bone Tumors. Philadelphia, JB Lippincott, 1980
68. *MNAYMNEH W, BROWN M, TEJADA F, ET AL:* Primary osteogenic sarcoma of the second cervical vertebra. J Bone Joint Surg 61A:460, 1979
69. *MURALI R, ROVIT R, BENJAMIN MV:* Chordoma of the cervical spine. Neurosurgery 9:253, 1981
70. *MURRAY JR, SEYMOUR RJ:* An anterior, extrapharyngeal, suprahyoid approach to the first, second and third cervical vertebrae. Acta Orthop Scand 45:43, 1974
71. *MURRAY J, HARRINGTON K:* Letter and reply. J Bone Joint Surg 69A:633, 1987
72. *MCAFEE PC, BOHLMAN HH, HAN JS, ET AL:* Comparison of nuclear magnetic resonance imaging and computer tomography in the diagnosis of upper cervical spinal cord compression. Spine 11:295, 1986
73. *NOVICK GS, PAVLOV H, BULLOUGH PG:* Osteochondroma of the cervical spine: Report of two cases in preadolescent mates. Skel Radiol 8:13, 1982
74. *ONIMUS M, SCHRAUB S, BERTIN D, ET AL:* Surgical treatment of vertebral metastasis. Spine 11:883, 1986
75. *ONO K, TADA K:* Metal prosthesis of the cervical vertebra. J Neurosurg 42:562, 1975
76. *ONO K, OKADA K, NAKAJIMA H:* Scintigraphy and selective angiography. In The Cervical Spine, edited by The Cervical Spine Research Society, pp 111–127. Philadelphia, JB Lippincott, 1983
77. *OTTOLENGHI CE:* Diagnosis of orthopaedic lesions by aspiration biopsy. J Bone Joint Surg 37A:443, 1955
78. *OTTOLENGHI CE:* Aspiration biopsy of the spine. J Bone Joint Surg 51A:1531, 1961
79. *PANJABI M, HOPPER W, WHITE AA, ET AL:* Posterior spine stabilization with methylmethacrylate. Spine 2:241, 1977
80. *PARRISH FF, PEVEY JK:* Surgical management of aneurysmal bone cyst of the vertebral column. J Bone Joint Surg 49A:1597, 1967
81. *PILEPICH MV, VIETTI TJ, NESBIT ME, ET AL:* Ewing's sarcoma of the vertebral column. Int J Radiol Oncol Biol Phys 7:27, 1981
82. *POLIVY KD, SLOTT RM, ZIMBLER S:* Osteoid osteoma of the cervical spine. Orthopedics 9:1101, 1986
83. *POLKEY CE:* Intraosseous neurilemmoma of the cervical spine causing paraparesis and treated by

resection and grafting. J Neurol Neurosurg Psychiatr 38:776, 1975

84. *Prete P, Thorne RP:* Low cervical chordoma: Report of two cases with documentation by computed tomography and review of the literature. Orthopedics 3:6433, 1980
85. *Raycroft JF, Hockman RP, Southwick WO:* Metastatic tumors involving the cervical vertebrae: Surgical palliation. J Bone Joint Surg 60A:763, 1978
86. *Rechtine GR, Hassan MO, Bohlman HH:* Malignant fibrous histocytoma of the cervical spine. Spine 9:824, 1984
87. *Regen EM, Haber A:* Giant cell tumor of cervical vertebra with unusual symptoms. J Bone Joint Surg 39A:196, 1957
88. *Resnik CS, Lininger JR:* Monostatic fibrous dysplasia of the cervical spine: Case report. Radiology 151:49, 1984
89. *Riley LH:* Surgical approaches to the anterior structures of the cervical spine. Clin Orthop 91:16, 1973
90. *Robert H, Dubousset J, Miladi L:* Histiocytosis X in the juvenile spine. Spine 12:167, 1987
91. *Robinson R, Smith G:* Anterolateral cervical disc removal and interbody fusion for cervical disc syndrome. Bull Johns Hopkins Hosp 96:223, 1955
92. *Roessner A, Immenkamp M, Weidner A, Hobik HP, et al:* Benign fibrous histiocytoma of bone. J Cancer Res Clin Oncol 101:191, 1981
93. *Rosencrantz M:* A case of fibrous dysplasia (Jaffe-Lichtenstein) with vertebral fracture and compression of the spinal cord. Acta Orthop Scand 36:435, 1965
94. *Rosendahl-Jensen SV:* Fibrous dysplasia of the vertebral column. Acta Chir Scand 111:490, 1956
95. *Roy-Camille R:* Personal communication
96. *Sartoris DJ, Parker BR:* Histiocytosis X: Rate and pattern of resolution of osseous lesions. Radiology 152:679, 1984
97. *Savini R, Ciherlinzoni F, Morandi M, et al:* Surgical treatment of giant-cell tumor of the spine. J Bone Joint Surg 65A:1283, 1983
98. *Scaglietti O, Marchetti PJ, Bartolozzi P:* Final results obtained in the treatment of bone cysts with methylprednisolone acetate (Depo-Medrol) and a discussion of results achieved in other bone lesions. Clin Orthop 165:33, 1982
99. *Shallat RF, Taekman MS, Nagle RC:* Unusual presentation of cervical chordoma with long-term survival. J Neurosurg 57:716, 1982
100. *Scoville WB, Palmer AH, Samra K, et al:* The use of acrylic plastic for vertebral replacement or fixation in metastatic disease of the spine. J Neurosurg 27:274, 1967
101. *Simon, MA:* Biopsy of musculoskeletal tumors. J Bone Joint Surg 64A:1253, 1982
102. *Southwick WO, Robinson RA:* Surgical approaches to the vertebral bodies in the cervical and lumbar regions. J Bone Joint Surg 39A:631, 1957
103. *Standefer M, Hardy RW, Marks K, et al:* Chondromyxoid fibroma of the cervical spine—a case report with a review of the literature and a description of an operative approach to the lower anterior cervical spine. Neurosurgery 11:288, 1982
104. *Stillwell WT, Fielding JW:* Aneurysmal bone cyst of the cervicodorsal spine. Clin Orthop Rel Res 187:144, 1984
105. *Suit HD, Goitein M, Munzenrider J, et al:* Definitive radiation therapy for chordoma and chondrosarcoma of base of skull and cervical spine. J Neurosurg 56:377, 1982
106. *Sundaresan N, Galidich JH, Chu FCH, et al:* Spinal chordomas. J Neurosurg 50:312, 1979
107. *Thompson JE, Keiller VH:* Multiple skeletal metastases from cancer of the breast. Surg Gynecol Obstet 38:367, 1924
108. *Tomita K:* Ceramic prosthesis of the cervical vertebra in metastatic tumor of the spine. Nippon Geka Hokkan 54:16, 1985
109. *Van Zantzen TG, Tevle GJ, Golding RP, et al:* CT and nuclear medicine imaging in vertebral metastases. Clin Nuc Med 11:334, 1986
110. *Verbiest H:* Giant-cell tumors and aneurysmal bone cysts of the spine. J Bone Joint Surg 47B:699, 1965
111. *Wang GJ, Reger SI, Shao ZH, et al:* Comparative strength of anterior spinal fixation with bone graft or polymethylmethacrylate. Clin Orthop 188:303, 1984
112. *Weatherley CR, Jaffray D, O'Brien JP:* Radical excision of an osteoblastoma of the cervical spine. J Bone Joint Surg 68B:325, 1986
113. *White AA, Panjabi MM:* Clinical biomechanics of the spine. Philadelphia, JB Lippincott, 1978
114. *Whitecloud TS, Larocca H:* Fibular strut graft in reconstructive surgery of the cervical spine. Spine 1:33, 1976
115. *Whitehill R, Reger SI, Fox E, et al:* The use of methylmethacrylate cement as an instantaneous fusion mass in posterior cervical fusions: A canine in vivo experimental model. Spine 9:246, 1984
116. *Whitehill R, Barry JC:* The evolution of stability in cervical spinal constructs with either autogenous bone graft or methylmethacrylate cement: A follow-up report on a canine in vivo model. Spine 10:32, 1985
117. *Whitehill R, Reger S, Weatherup N, et al:* A

biomechanical analysis of posterior cervical fusions using polymethylmethacrylate as an instantaneous fusion mass. Spine 8:368, 1983

118. *WHITEHOUSE GH, GRIFFITHS GJ:* Roentgenologic aspects of spinal involvement by primary and metastatic Ewing's tumor. J Can Assoc Radiol 27:290, 1976

119. *WHITESIDES TE, KELLY RP:* Lateral approach to the upper cervical spine for anterior fusion. South Med J 59:879, 1966

120. *WU KK:* Diagnosis and treatment of benign and malignant monostotic tumors of the spine. Detroit, National Reproductions Corporation, 1985

121. *WU KK, MITCHELL DC, GUISE ER:* Chordoma of the atlas: A case report. J Bone Joint Surg 59A:140, 1979

122. *ZWIMPFER TJ, TUCKER WS, FAULKNER JF:* Osteoid osteoma of the cervical spine: Case reports and literature review. Can J Surg 25:637, 1982

Benign Cervical Spine Tumors: Clinical Experience

HENK VERBIEST

Benign tumors of the cervical spine are rare, resulting in limited individual experiences of their treatment. Thus, further knowledge that might lead to more adequate treatment can only be gained by centralization of such cases in adequately distributed regional departments of spinal surgery, if such an endeavor could ever be realized. In this section no attempt is made to review the numerous reports of one or a small number of benign tumors of the cervical spine published so far. Nomenclature and pathology of these tumors are generally known and can be found in textbooks on bone tumors.[3,5,8,11,14] Therefore, this discussion is limited to particular features of their behavior in the cervical spine and is divided into four parts. The first part lists personal cases and presents some comparative data on benign and malignant tumors of the cervical spine. There are notes on particular features of some tumor types. The particular frequency distribution of tumor types may be due to the fact that they were referred to a neurosurgical department that had developed special interest in cervical spine lesions. The second part details diagnostic aids adapted to regional particularities of the cervical spine and the benign tumors in this area. The chronological order of these procedures is also outlined. The next part deals with the treatment of benign tumors, which is mainly surgical. Recent surgical techniques of operations on the lateral structures of the cervical spine, called lateral operations in this section, added to the more widespread anterior and posterior operations, allow one to approach the cervical spine at all sites without great technical problems and, if necessary, in one stage. The lateral operations were an essential part in the surgical procedure in 14 of the 32 cases. The fourth part in this section consists of short case histories and iconographies demonstrating problems and results of surgical treatment.

COMPARATIVE DATA ON BENIGN AND MALIGNANT TUMORS

Table 12-1 shows that in our experience the benign tumors were far more frequent than the primary unicentric malignant tumors and almost as frequent as the totals of groups B, C, and D. In groups A and B, about half of the patients were under 30 years of age and there was no difference between the average ages of these patients. The youngest patient in group B was 16 years old. In group A, 11 patients were between 9 and 16 years. The oldest patient in group A was 72, and the oldest in group B was 63. The average ages in groups C and D were definitely higher, and the limits in the ranges of ages were smaller.

The eosinophilic granulomas are listed among the benign tumors in the left column of Table 12-2 because of their tumorlike behavior, following the tradition of various textbooks on bone tumors. For the same reason, exceptionally expanding rheumatoid bursitis around the odontoid, compressing the spinal cord, was included (see Cases 31 and 32, Case Reports). Aneurysmal bone cysts are not universally accepted as tumors, but their behavior and treatment is the same as for benign tumors.

NEUROFIBROMATOSES. Abnormal curvature of the thoracic and lumbar spine in neurofibromatosis has been frequently reported. Its nature is still unclear. Deformities of the cervical spine have received less attention in the literature. There is a striking difference in the frequency of cervical spine involvement in neurofibromatosis as reported in recent publications of relatively large series of spinal deformities. Of 102 patients with spinal deformity and neurofibromatosis reported by Winter and associates, only 4 patients had predominant cervical deformity.[28] In contrast, Yong-Hing and coworkers found abnormalities of the cervical spine in 17 of 56 patients with neurofibromatosis.[29] Of 34 patients who had scoliosis or kyphoscoliosis, 15 (44%) had cervical lesions. Four of the 17 patients showed scalloping of vertebral bodies or foraminal enlargement. The other abnormalities were absent lordosis (3 cases), cervical kyphosis (8 cases), atlantoaxial rotatory subluxation (1 case), and fixed anterior slip of C2 on C3 (1 case). Seven patients were asymptomatic, four patients had some neural deficit, and the other patients had limited or painful neck motion. Curtis and associates found that in four of eight cases of neurofibromatosis and paraplegia due to alterations of the spine the lesion was situated in the cervical region.[2] None of these limited statistics is based on random sampling since the doctors do not choose the patients—the patients choose the doctors.[6]

The cases presented in Table 12-2 did not include scalloping or foraminal enlargement as the

Table 12-1. Age Distribution

	A BENIGN TUMORS: 32	B PRIMARY UNICENTRIC MALIGNANT TUMORS: 10	C SOLITARY PLASMOCYTOMA WITH CHARACTERISTIC BIOCHEMICAL AND BONE MARROW FINDINGS: 6	D SOLITARY METASTASES: 14
1st decade	3	—		
2nd decade	8	4		
3rd decade	6	1		
4th decade	4	1	Average age: 62 yr	Average age: 57 yr
5th decade	4	2	Range: 56 to 75 yr	Range: 46 to 68 yr
6th decade	4	—		
7th decade	2	2		
8th decade	1	—		
Arithmetic mean of ages	32.2 yr	32 yr		
Range	9 to 72 yr	16 to 63 yr		

Table 12-2. Notes on Some Particular Tumor Types

BENIGN TUMORS		PRIMARY UNICENTRIC MALIGNANT TUMORS (10 CASES)	
Tumor Type	*Sex and Age*	*Tumor Type*	*Sex and Age*
Neurofibromatosis (Cases 1–7)	Males: 15,15,21,44,55 yr Females: 9 and 37 yr	Chordoma (2 cases)	Females: 58 and 63 yr
Aneurysmal bone cyst (Cases 8–14)	Males: 9,40 and 65 yr Females: 11,15,27 and 32 yr	Mesenchymal chondrosarcoma (1 case)	Female: 21 yr
Benign giant cell tumor (Cases 15–17)	Males: 21 and 22 yr Female: 16 yr	Chondrosarcoma (1 case)	Female: 47 yr
Benign osteoblastoma (Cases 18, 19)	Male: 47 yr Female: 13 yr	Osteosarcoma (3 cases)	Male: 17 yr Females: 16 and 17 yr
Solitary eosinophilic granuloma (Cases 20, 21)	Males: 10 and 14 yr	Ewing's sarcoma (1 case)	Male: 26 yr
Solitary plasmocytoma (Cases 22)	Female: 30 yr	Aggressive Solitary plasmocytoma (1 case)	Female: 63 yr
Chondromyxoid fibroma (Case 23)	Male: 55 yr	Hemangiopericytoma (1 case)	Male: 39 yr
Desmoid tumor (Cases 24, 25)	Females: 11 and 61 yr		
Hemangioma (Case 26)	Male: 25 yr		
Osteomas, osteochondromas (Cases 27–30)	Males: 38,51 and 72 yr Female: 51 yr		
Tumor-size rheumatoid bursitis around the odontoid (Cases 31,32)	Male: 47 yr Female: 49 yr		

only lesion. All seven cases had considerable deformities of the anterior column of the cervical spine: kyphosis and atlantooccipital subluxation (1 case), tumor involvement and collapse of entire vertebral body with tumor outgrowth (1 case), considerable irreducible vertebral slip and kyphosis (2 cases), and kyphosis alone (3 cases). Five patients had neural deficit: tetraparesis (2 cases), hemiparesis (2 cases), and radicular symptoms (1 case). In two patients the deformity was discovered because of limited painful neck motion and abnormal head posture. In six patients anterior subligamentous neurofibromatosis or neurofibromatosis around other portions of the anterior bony structures with various degrees of bony involvement was noted. The seventh patient developed postlaminectomy kyphosis that recurred after each of two corrective anterior operations. Biopsy of a vertebral body showed areas of devitalized bone (see Case 7, Case Reports).

Desmoid Tumors. Desmoid tumors belong to the fibromatoses, a large variety of conditions that are built up by nonencapsulated fibroblastic tissue without nuclear atypism or mitoses.[10,18,19] The lesions may be mono- or multifocal, or generalized. They may infiltrate surrounding tissues but do not produce metastases. The nature of the fibromatoses is unknown, though there are reports on traumatic or endocrine influences. They are classified as congenital or juvenile in children and simply as fibromatoses in older age groups. In young patients the fibromatoses may be self-limiting and may vanish, or they may develop into benign fibromas, the latter being attributed to so-called maturation. They may, however, also progress, especially in older age groups. Incomplete excision of progressive lesions may be followed by recurrence.

Fibromatoses involving the spine are at present divided into two types, the so-called extraabdominal desmoids and the desmoplastic fibromas.[15,16] The extraabdominal desmoids were so named because they were first discovered in the muscles of the abdominal wall, and this area is still the most frequent site of localization.[13] The tumor is thought to arise from the muscular aponeurosis or other supportive tissues of muscle. Extraabdominal desmoids rarely affect the skeleton and still more rarely the vertebrae. They may have their onset from vertebral ligaments or periosteum and destroy the cortex of the vertebrae. The desmoplastic fibroma, first described by Jaffe, develops inside the bone from endostial structures, but it may secondarily extend to surrounding tissues.[4,8,15] The histologic pattern of desmoids and desmoplastic fibroma is the same. Hardy and Lehrer discussed problems of classification of these tumors as exemplified by a desmoplastic fibroma of the radius that had perforated its cortex and extended along the interosseous membrane into the periosteum of the ulna, where it behaved as a periosteal dermoid.[7]

So far only two cases of vertebral desmoplastic fibromas have been reported in the literature.[15,16] In addition, we have had experience with a desmoplastic fibroma localized in the laminae of T4 in a girl of 15. It had penetrated into the spinal canal through the bony cortex, producing paraparesis. The whole tumor mass was excised. At the time (1947), a diagnosis of fibrosarcoma was made and the patient had radiation therapy. Twenty-eight years later the patient had recurrent paraparesis because of kyphosis of T4–T5. Reoperation (1975) showed no recurrence. At repeated examination of the original tumor specimen, a diagnosis of desmoid tumor was made.

Of the other two tumors involving the cervical spine, one was certainly an extra abdominal desmoid. It was localized inside the cervical intertransverse spaces affecting the cortex of the body of C6 (see Case 24, Case Reports). The patient was a girl of 11. No recurrence has been observed so far, 4 years after operation. In the other patient, a woman of 61, the tumor had considerably destroyed the odontoid and its ligaments, and it compressed the cord (see Case 25). It was impossible to classify it as an extraabdominal desmoid or desmoplastic fibroma since the original site of growth was unknown. There were no metastases. A diagnosis of aggressive fibromatosis was made; this terminology is vague since the histologic picture showed dense fibrous tissue of low cellularity, as reported in similar cases of aggressive fibromatosis.[12] The diagnosis of aggressive fibromatosis is based upon the fact that the tumor recurs unless wide excision is performed. The possibility of wide excision depends, however, not on the nature of the tumor but upon its localization. Some authors classify aggressive fibromatosis as fibrosarcoma Grade I.

Solitary Plasmocytoma. Case 22 listed in Table 12-2 showed no biochemical or bone marrow changes. The tumor had invaded the entire vertebra of C5 with posterior epidural extension of tumor mass. The patient was quadriplegic. Complete vertebrectomy and removal of peridural growth resulted in complete recovery. The patient is well and alive 28 years after operation (see Case 22). The solitary plasmocytoma, listed in the right columns of Table 12-2, developed in a woman of 63 who had suffered for 33 years from rheumatoid arthritis. Osteolysis of C2 was noted 3 years before admission, followed by anterior atlantic subluxation a few months later. Two years before admission, destructive lesions of the atlas and the body of C3 were noted, and at admission the body of C4 was also destroyed. The patient had developed weakness of both arms and had bilateral Babinski responses. Biopsy revealed a plasmocytoma. No bone marrow or biochemical abnormalities were found. The patient died from respiratory insufficiency. Autopsy revealed no other localizations. In this respect this plasmocytoma differed from the solitary plasmocytomas of Group C of Table 12-1. It demonstrates the problems in prognosis of the real unicentric plasmocytomas of the spine.

DIAGNOSTIC AIDS

Clinical Examination

Cervical pains under various influences, pains radiating in various directions, tenderness, muscle spasm, and limited cervical spinal movement may be the only symptoms of benign tumor. Torticollis mainly occurs with tumors of the upper cervical spine. Concomitant signs of compression of spinal nerve roots or the spinal cord may be produced by bony displacement or outgrowth of tumor. There is no reason to repeat the well-known symptoms of these complications. It is important to identify the presence of primary ischemia of the spinal cord caused by constriction of arterial feeders by tumor growth. The evolution of its clinical picture is rapid and it does not improve after tumor removal. Power in the arms may be affected first. Among our patients this condition was only observed in a few cases of malignant tumors situated in the C2 to C5 region.

Radiologic Diagnosis

Roentgenographic findings of hyperdensity (increased density) or osteolytic lesions may occur with benign as well as with malignant tumors of the spine. Since the introduction of the CT body scan, its priority versus other radiologic methods of examination has been under discussion. In our opinion, *plain roentgenograms of the cervical spine* should precede all other radiologic examination.[26] So far, we have no experience with sagittal reconstruction of CT scans in cervical vertebral tumors. *Pluridirectional sagittal or frontal tomography* covering the entire cervical spine is of great value in identifying the extent of bony changes and resulting deformities of the vertebral canal and intervertebral foramina. In recent years, these findings in our patients formed the basis for determining the frequency of CT scanning. The advantage of CT is the demonstration of tumor extent outside the bone and densitometric examination of the tumor mass, which may, for instance, give strong support to a diagnosis of neurofibromatosis of the spine. *Myelography* may show tumor masses inside the vertebral canal beyond the level of bony destruction. Among the benign tumors of the cervical spine, this may be particularly observed in neurofibromatosis. In patients in whom myelography is indicated, using metrizamide as a contrast medium, the place of CT scanning in the chronological order of diagnostic procedure should be about 6 hours following myelography. At that time the metrizamide is sufficiently diluted not to produce artifacts. The density of the residual metrizamide is, however, sufficient in the scans to facilitate the localization and densitometry of extradural soft tissue masses. With the present tracers it remains impossible to make a differential diagnosis between benign and malignant tumors because there are no specific differences in uptake. *Total body scintigraphy* is of value in the presence of radiographically solitary tumors of the spine in order to detect or exclude other foci of abnormalities in uptake. Because the uptake of the radionuclide bears relation to the metabolic activity, increased uptake may occur in border areas of tumors or other lesions. Spondylotic osteophytes may also show increased uptake. *Vertebral arteriography* may show a tumor pattern of some benign tumors (see Cases 18 and 24, Case Reports). The vertebral arteries may be displaced (see Cases 3, 11, 12, and 23) or occluded (see Case 27) by tumor mass. They may be narrowed by severe kyphotic deformities (see Case 5). The visualization of position or condition of the vertebral arteries is of particular importance for the surgical technique of tumor removal (see Treatment). Experiences with *transosseous phlebography of the spine* in vertebral tumors is limited. Its most interesting indications are in hemangiomas, especially if combined with arteriography in order to evaluate the share of arterial feeders and capillary and venous constituents. Phlebography by means of puncture through the anterior border of the vertebral body is preferable since the lesion is reported to escape visualization by the transspinous route (see Case 26).

We have no experience with magnetic resonance imaging (MRI) of benign spinal tumors. It is expected that MRI will be superior to CT scanning in detecting bony medullary tumor involvement and tumor spread into adjacent soft tissue structures.

Spinal Biopsy

Needle Biopsy. For needle biopsy we use the Turkel needle, which consists of an outer splitting needle that, with stylet in place, is pushed through the tissues until the bone is reached.[20] The stylet is then removed and replaced by a trephining inner needle, which cuts through the cortical bone into the marrow. The plug of biopsy material found in the trephine needle is pushed out easily with a stylet. We have limited this procedure to tumors of the vertebral body because of the risk of penetrating too far when puncturing the laminae (additional risk of mechanical pressure upon the spinal cord) or lateral structures of the spine (risk of damaging the vertebral arteries or spinal nerves). The adult vertebral body instrument consists of an outer needle, 11 gauge, and an inner trephining needle, 13 gauge. With the children's instrument the sizes are 12 gauge and 14 gauge respectively. The procedure is performed under control of body image x-ray amplifier and TV monitor. Needle biopsy of the upper three vertebrae can be performed transorally.

For the lower cervical vertebral bodies, the cervical blood vessels are retracted laterally by finger pressure and the needle is introduced transcutaneously and medially to the blood vessels. The examination of the tissue obtained may be difficult because of crush effects. Needle biopsy may allow a reliable diagnosis with very cellular tumors such as metastatic cancer or myeloma. Among the benign tumors, neurofibromatoses are more readily diagnosed than, for instance, aneurysmal bone cysts or fibromatosis. Blood or other fluids aspirated through the trephine needle are also examined cytologically.

Open Biopsy. Open biopsy was performed in our patients if needle biopsy did not result in a reliable diagnosis. The access to the tumor should be made in a fashion that allows continuation of the operation for tumor removal during the same stage.

We must stress the importance of oncologic biochemical examination.

TREATMENT

Unfortunately, there are still protagonists of radiotherapeutic treatment without an exact diagnosis of the tumor type. In one of our patients, this had resulted in a radiation sarcoma, considerably differing from the original giant cell tumor (see Case 17, Case Reports). In addition, preoperative radiation may unfavorably influence the fusion of bone grafts. Radiotherapeutic treatment is only indicated if total removal of a radiosensitive benign tumor proves impossible.

Tumors of the cervical spine may impair one or both of its two principal functions: protection of the neuraxis, and postural and kinetic activities. Neurologic disturbances may be due to one of the following:

1. Tumor compression of the neuraxis or its vascular feeders (Tumor removal or, if impossible, decompressive laminectomy or foraminotomy may only be effective in the absence of ischemic cord lesion.)
2. Traction of the spinal cord and nerves caused by angulation of the spine
3. A combination of compression and traction (Traction of the spinal cord can be relieved by reduction of the angulation or, if impossible, by flattening the bony wall of the vertebral canal at the site of angulation.[24,25])

Impairment of postural and kinetic functions of the cervical spine is basically due to tumoral derangement of intrinsic spinal stability. The intrinsic or mechanical stability of the spine is ensured by the elasticity and resistance of the vertebral bones and ligaments to compressive torsion, shearing, and bending stresses under the eccentric load of the head and the action of muscles. Most of these muscles are directly anchored to the cervical spine, forming a connection with other vertebrae or other parts of the skeleton (skull, shoulder girdle, thoracic cage). Other muscles, such as the sternocleidomastoid and the suprahyoid and infrahyoid muscles, influence the cervical spine indirectly.

Reduced resistance and elasticity of bone and ligaments may result in various types of instability according to the extent of the tumor. The basic morphologic expressions of intrinsic instability are bony deformity, fracture, vertebral slip, and deviations from the normal curvature. Surgical removal of the tumor or other decompressive techniques may aggravate the intrinsic instability or be its principal cause. Iatrogenic instability is not always predictable.

Cervical laminectomy in cases of neurofibromatosis carries a high risk of secondary instability (see Case 7). In other cases it may occur unexpectedly many years later (see Case 15). This stresses the necessity of long follow-ups.

Because of the complicated biomechanics of the cervical spine and its various possible modes of derangement, one should aim, in stabilization of the spinal motor segments involved, to be all-inclusive. This may be achieved by external supports or braces, but with benign tumors surgical stabilization, even if the tumor cannot be completely removed, is preferable. Surgical all-inclusive stabilization requires the following:

1. Reduction of vertebral slip or deviations from the normal curvature of the cervical spine
2. The use of fixating material that is resistant to physiologic compressive bending, torsion, or shearing stresses
3. Immobilizing procedures including the vertebrae adjacent to the motor segment(s) involved

Surgical Techniques

In contrast to malignant tumors of the cervical spine, in which radiation and chemotherapy may interfere with surgical measures such as the use of bone grafts, the surgical treatment of benign tumors is not aggravated by these problems. The use of vertebral prostheses or other artificial devices should, in our opinion, be limited to instability following removal of malignant tumors in cases of relatively short life expectancy. Stabilizing measures following removal of benign tumors should be aimed at guaranteeing stability over long periods, since benign tumors of the spine are relatively frequent among the younger age groups (Table 12-1). For this purpose we have used autogenous bone grafts in all cases because homografts may elicit responses to their foreign proteins. For repair of abnormal curvature or replacement of vertebral bodies, we prefer the use of cortical grafts because of their weight-bearing properties and their resistance to other physiologic stresses upon the cervical spine. Our experience with cortical strut grafts for replacing fractured vertebral bodies covers a period of 26 years and indicates that they are capable of maintaining stability; the roentgenographic examination showed fusion and adaptive remodeling of the grafts. The problem of tumor spread to adjacent structures undermining the effects of stabilization, frequently occurring with malignant tumors, is rarely encountered following removal of benign tumors. It may occur after incomplete curettage of an aneurysmal bone cyst, but in our experience serious problems were encountered particularly in benign but extensive or progressive neurofibromatosis of the cervical spine. Although the occasions to operate upon cervical vertebral tumors are rare, the required surgical techniques are advanced owing to the more frequent surgical experiences with cervical fractures and spondylosis. At present, the cervical spine can be rapidly exposed at all sides with relatively low damage to surrounding structures, and, if necessary, in one stage (Fig. 12-18).

The posterior approach gives access to the laminae and the facets joints.

The anterolateral approach gives access to the anterior portion of the spine from C2 through C7, and, with more recently developed techniques, it allows simultaneous exposure of transverse processes and the vertebral artery at all levels, the altantoocipital joint and all posterolateral cervical joints, and the lateral aspects of the bodies and intervertebral foramina from C2 through C7. Although the anterior arch of the atlas and the odontoid may be exposed by an anterolateral approach, the transoral approach provides a better view of this field.

The transoral approach allows exposure of the anterior arch of the atlas, the odontoid, and the body of C2, but transoral surgery of the C1–C2 joints carries a higher risk of damage to the vertebral artery than the lateral access.

Surgical Indications

THE POSTERIOR APPROACH. The posterior approach is indicated for tumors involving spinous processes and laminae, tumor extension from the laminae into the articular facets included (see Cases 8, 11, 13, 14, 18, 21, and 29); associated intraspinal tumor (see Cases 4 and 7); or posterior fusion or wiring (see Cases 1, 5, 6, 8, 13, 22, 31, and 32).

THE TRANSORAL APPROACH. Tumors in the area of the odontoid or the anterior arch of the atlas, and central or cystic tumors of the body of C2 are most adequately exposed by a transoral approach. Our experience with benign tumors is limited to six cases: four cases of aneurysmal bone cysts (see Cases 8, 9, 10, and 11), one case of intraosseous

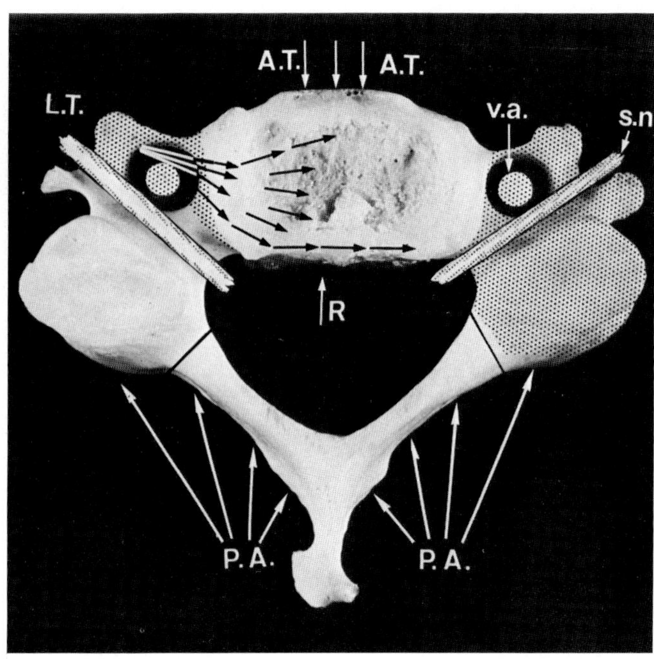

Fig. 12-18. The cervical vertebrae may be approached from all sides. Posterior operation allows exposure of laminae and facet joints (P.A. = posterior approach). Operations upon the anterior surface of the vertebral bodies and discs are accomplished by anterolateral approach (*A.T.* = anterior transvertebral). The anterolateral approach also allows exposure of the transverse processes, the articular processes, the lateral aspects of the vertebral body, and the vertebral artery. The dotted bony area on the left indicates bone to be removed for approaching lateral aspect of vertebral body (*L.T.* = lateral transvertebral). Proceeding in the direction of the arrows allows removal of the uncus and the intervertebral disc and, combined with the anterior approach, removal of the vertebral body. Removal of the most posterior portion of the disc or the body may be achieved in a plane parallel to the dural theca (*black arrows indicated by R*). The dotted bony area on the right shows bony structures that can be removed by lateral operation by way of anterolateral approach; *v.a.* = vertebral artery, *s.n.* = spinal nerve. The anterior and posterior primary rami are not drawn.

and extraosseous neurofibromatosis of the odontoid and the upper cervical spine (see Case 1), and two cases of rheumatoid expansive bursitis in the odontoid area (see Cases 31 and 32). In Cases 1, 8, 31, and 32 a combined posterior fusion was performed to prevent instability. Aneurysmal bone cysts in this area are curetted even as far as their extension into the pedicles. Filling the cavity with iliac bone is sufficient for repair. Extension into the medial portions of the laminae should not be neglected and must be treated by means of a posterior approach (see Case 8).

The Anterolateral Approach to the Anterior Surface of the Cervical Spine (Anterior Operations). Anterior operation is limited to central benign tumors of the vertebral body and their possible anterior subligamentous extension (see Cases 2, 17 and 21). In four patients, anterior operations were performed for correction of kyphosis or interbody fusion, following tumor removal by a posterior approach (see Cases 2, 4, 7, and 15).

The Anterolateral Approach for Exposure of the Lateral Structures of the Cervical Spine (Lateral Operation). Tumorous involvement of the lateral portions of the cervical vertebral bodies or tumorous extension into the lateral processes, pedicles, and posterolateral joints (see Cases 11, 12, 13, 19, 20, 23, 24, 27, 28, and 30) can be adequately treated by retraction of the longissimus capitis and colli muscles, and resection of the anterior rims of the foramina transversaria and the anterior tubercles of the transverse processes (Fig. 12-18). Resulting exposure of the primary rami of the spinal nerves and the vertebral artery allows for their protection during surgical removal of lateral portions of the vertebral bodies, pedicles, posterolateral joints, or entire transverse processes depending on tumor extent, possible extraosseous outgrowth included. Preoperative vertebral angiography is indispensable for identification of possible displacement or other derangements of the vertebral artery. Retraction of the vertebral artery, which could damage radicular arteries, should be avoided as much as possible. The use of the microscope is essential. Postoperative immobilization is usually not necessary following removal of tumors limited to the lateral portions of the cervical spine.

Combined Anterior and Lateral Operations Using the Anterolateral Approach. Complete corporectomy from C3 through C7 by means of an anterolateral approach is most safely performed by exposing both the anterior and lateral surfaces of the vertebral bodies to be removed.

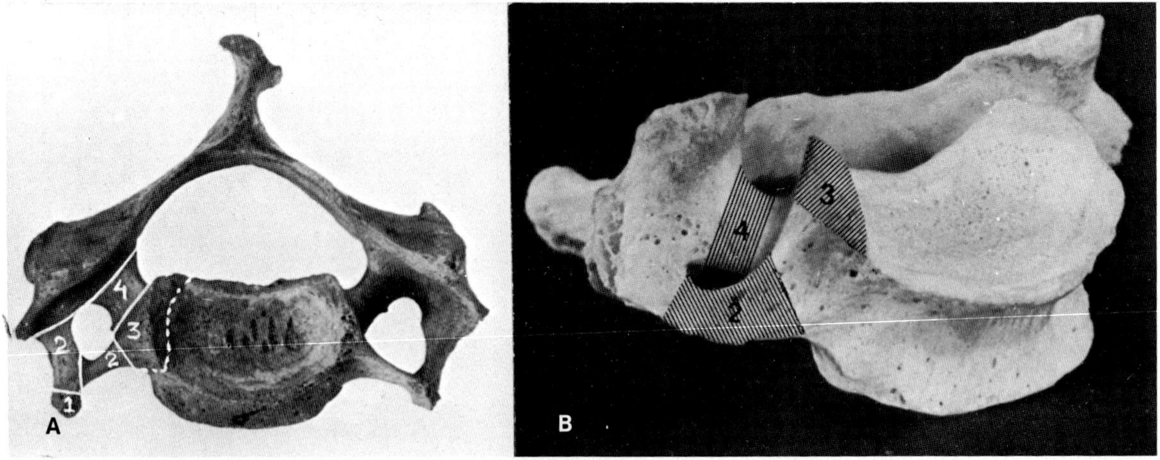

Fig. 12-19. (*A*) The numbers show the chronological order of removal of lateral bony structures preceding vertebral corporectomy. (*B*) Oblique view. Numbers of hatched areas correspond with those in *A*. (Reprinted by permission from Clinical Neurosurgery, Vol 20, © 1973, The Congress of Neurological Surgeons)

After exposure of the anterior surface of the body, the access to its lateral surface is obtained following the technique described in the paragraph above. This permits protection of the vertebral artery by means of thin-bladed spatulae applied under the control of direct eyesight during surgical removal of the vertebral body (Fig. 12-19). Again, the use of the microscope is essential.

In the early period we performed lateral operations on both sides for bilateral spondylotic foraminal narrowing during the same operation. In later years we observed three cases of temporary phrenic nerve paralysis following ipsilateral, unilateral operations on the middle cervical spine (about 3% of all cases operated on for spondylosis, disc protrusions, or disc extrusions). The phrenic nerve paralysis was noted immediately after operation in two patients and developed about 24 hours later in the third patient. The phrenic nerve may be particularly sensitive to minor mechanical or other noxious influences.[9] Although phrenic nerve function recovered in all three cases in a period of 6 weeks or less, it may present serious problems if occurring bilaterally after bilateral operations in one stage. Therefore, we have developed a method of *complete corporectomy* by means of exposure of one lateral aspect and the anterior surface of the vertebral body. The operation is started upon the lateral aspect of the body after resection of the anterior rim of its foramen transversarium and, according to the circumstances, of the foramina transversaria above and below. The uncus is separated from the vertebral body over its entire length by means of a mallet and small chisel directed toward the intervertebral disc (Fig. 12-19). The same procedure is performed with the uncus of the vertebral body below. This allows complete excision of the intervertebral discs above and below, and their posterior anulus and the adjacent portion of the posterior longitudinal ligament can be removed in a plane parallel to the anterior surface of the dural theca under eyesight (Fig. 12-18). Next, the vertebral body is removed piecemeal up to its contralateral cortical layer and uncus, followed by separation of the medial attachments of the contralateral longus capitis and colli muscles, which are retracted laterally. This allows careful removal of the medial portions of the anterior rims of the contralateral foramina transversaria. Using a fine rongeur, the remaining lateral cortex and uncus of the vertebral body are carefully removed while protecting the medial surface of the contralateral vertebral artery with a thin-bladed spatula. Next, if necessary, the pedicles can be removed on both sides of the dural theca.

REPLACEMENT OF ONE OR TWO COMPLETELY REMOVED VERTEBRAL BODIES BY MEANS OF CORTICAL STRUT GRAFTS. After complete corporectomy, the union of the bone grafts and ingrowth of the vessels and osteoblasts occur only at their extremities, bringing the end-plates of the adjacent ver-

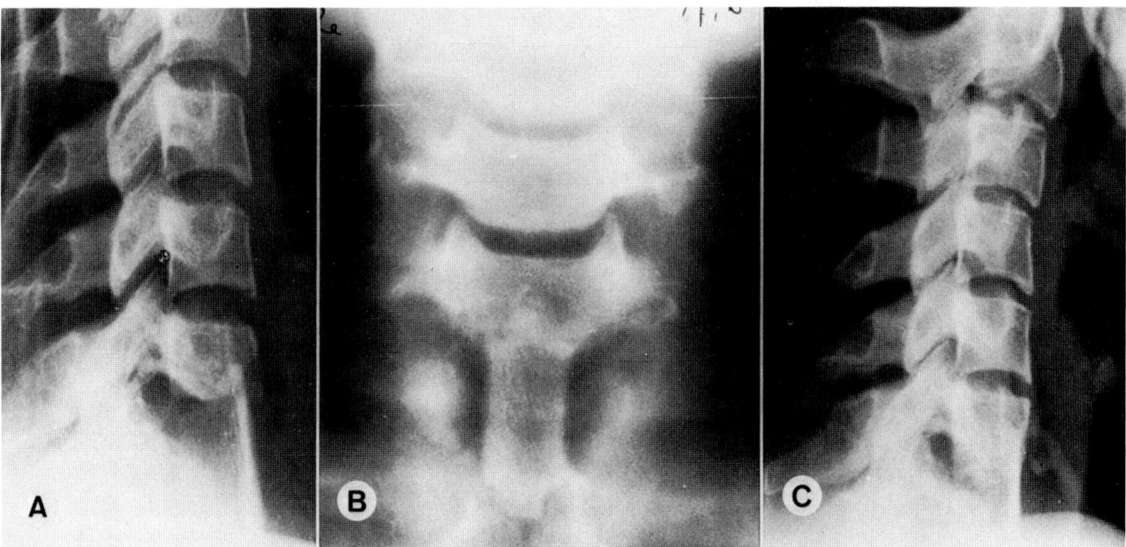

Fig. 12-20. Replacement of the vertebral body by a tibial strut graft inserted in end-plates of adjacent vertebral bodies. (*A*) Lateral view taken after operation. The cortical layer of the tibial strut graft is situated anteriorly, its spongious portion posteriorly. The cortical extremity is seen inserted into end-plate of the body above. (*B*) A–P view. The medial portions of the cortex of the strut graft are inserted into the end-plates of the vertebral bodies above and below. (*C*) Lateral view taken 2 years after operation shows increased density and remodeling of the spongious portion of the bone graft. Its cortical portion still shows higher density. This is a solid fusion.

tebral bodies into contact. Therefore, we have limited the use of cortical strut grafts to the replacement of one or two vertebral bodies. This is only possible in the cervical spine because of the relatively small size of its bodies. New bone formation occurs on the surfaces of the graft and by way of the haversian systems.[22,23] No significant loss of density was observed during the first year, and even in later years the original graft retained a somewhat higher density than the surrounding bone owing to its residual bulk of dead bone. The extremities of the struts are shaped as follows: One third of the diameter is removed laterally over a distance of about 6 mm to 8 mm so that the remaining central bar can be inserted to drill holes prepared in the end-plates of the adjacent vertebral bodies. The lateral portions of the extremities of the struts prevent further penetration (Fig. 12-20). Because the total length of these struts must exceed the length of the gap produced by the corporectomy, each strut is inserted first into the end-plate of the vertebral body below. Next, the gap is enlarged by skull traction and pressure against the lower surface of the chin, producing backward rotation of the spine. This latter movement is very important for allowing the introduction of the graft below the vertebral body above and insertion into its lower end-plate. The shaping of the extremities of the struts can be most adequately achieved with grafts taken from the proximal anterior surface of the tibia. Further fixation of the struts can be achieved by tying them to onlay grafts consisting of Kiel bone or bone bank material. The onlays are attached to the anterior aspects of the vertebral bodies above and below by mattress sutures passing through canals (made by special perforators in a dental drill) in the vertebral bodies behind the anterior inferior margin of the body above and the anterior superior margin of the body below. Initially, stainless steel wires were used. Although the extremities of the wire knots were carefully turned away from the esophagus and the carotid artery, postoperative rotation of these ends produced a perforation of the esophagus in one patient. Since then, strong silk sutures have been used instead without problems.

The use of metallic onlays attached by means of screws to the adjacent vertebral bodies carries a risk of loosening and outward displacement of the screws toward the esophagus. Surgical removal of those screws may be difficult because of surrounding scar tissue and resulting danger of tearing the wall of the esophagus. Immobilization of the head and neck for 3 months is the safest method of postoperative treatment. It may be achieved with bed rest and halo traction of the skull applying lateral pads to the head, or with mobilization using halo casts.[22] The latter not only helps the patient's general and psychological condition but also reduces hospitalization and the costs of health.

This method of vertebral body replacement has been performed in seven cases (one benign and six malignant tumors). In one other case, iliac crest grafts rather than tibial grafts were used (see Case 3). One patient with myelomatosis died a few days after operation. Roentgenographic checkups showed solid fusion in the other seven cases, though in four of the five malignant tumor cases, osteolysis in adjacent vertebral bodies was noted after 1 or more years. In the fifth case, solitary metastasis of prostata carcinoma, the patient is well 5 years after the vertebral body replacement. In young children the vertebral bodies are tiny and fragile, as are the autografts available. So far, however, we have not encountered the need for complete vertebral body replacement in such patients.

Replacement of More Than Two Vertebral Bodies by Means of Strut Grafts

Our experience includes two cases of extensive neurofibromatosis of the cervical spine (see Cases 5 and 6). Both patients presented considerable vertebral dislocation at the same time, constricting both vertebral arteries. Multiple corporectomies and bilateral decompression of the vertebral arteries had to be performed. Part of the iliac crest was used for their replacement and posterior wiring was performed for maintaining the cervical spine in extension. Postoperative immobilization in bed was preferred over mobilization in halo casts in these cases.

COMPLETE VERTEBRECTOMY. So far we have performed two complete vertebrectomies, in two stages: (1) corporectomy and removal of lateral structures and (2) removal of the residual neural arch and posterior fusion. In Case 22, benign solitary plasmocytoma operated on in 1952, the removed body of C5 was not replaced because of lack of experience in those days. This resulted in minor kyphotic deformity. In the second case, total vertebrectomy of C3 was performed because the vertebra was completely invaded by a hemangiopericytoma. The body of C3 was replaced by tibial grafts, and posterior fusion was performed after removal of the arch of C3. Good fusion and normal alignment of the cervical spine were noted in the year following the operation. The patient died from multiple metastases 1.5 years after operation without local recurrence of the tumor in the cervical spine.

REDUCTION OF KYPHOSIS. With the present techniques kyphosis in the area of C2 through T2 can be reduced or corrected by means of multiple-level interbody fusion with wedge-shaped cortical grafts or by using strut grafts. Angular kyphosis between C1 and C3 due to tumor involvement is difficult to correct in our experience.

In a number of cases, more than one type of the operations described above had to be performed (see Case Reports).

CASE REPORTS

Neurofibromatoses

CASE 1. A 37-year-old woman presented with subcutaneous neurofibromas and multiple *cafe au lait* pigmentations, thoracic kyphoscolioses, atlantic forward slip, kyphosis of C2–C4, neck-pains, and limited neck movements (Fig. 12-21*A*). Lateral tomograms showed too much blurring. Lateral stereograms showed half the odontoid and the anterior and posterior arch of the atlas. Pneumomyelograms showed interruption of air near the tip of the odontoid. There was no neural deficit.

March 21, 1969: Transoral removal of odontoid was performed, a difficult operation because of upper cervical kyphosis and the profound situation of the odontoid. A diffuse neurofibromatous mass was exposed, situated between the anterior arch of the atlas and the dural theca, surrounding the odontoid. This mass could be removed only incompletely. The operation was completed by posterior fusion (Fig. 12-21*B*). The patient died 5 years later from upper cervical cord compression.

CASE 2. A 9-year-old girl with a normal lumbar and thoracic spine presented with spastic tetraparesis because of sharp angular kyphosis of C2–C3, and left oculomotor and right facial nerve weakness. Myelography showed no intradural masses. Spastic quadriparesis was caused by kyphosis. There were cutaneous signs of neurofibromatosis, neck pains, and limited neck movements.

Right anterolateral approach revealed a large neurofibroma in front of the longissimus capitis and

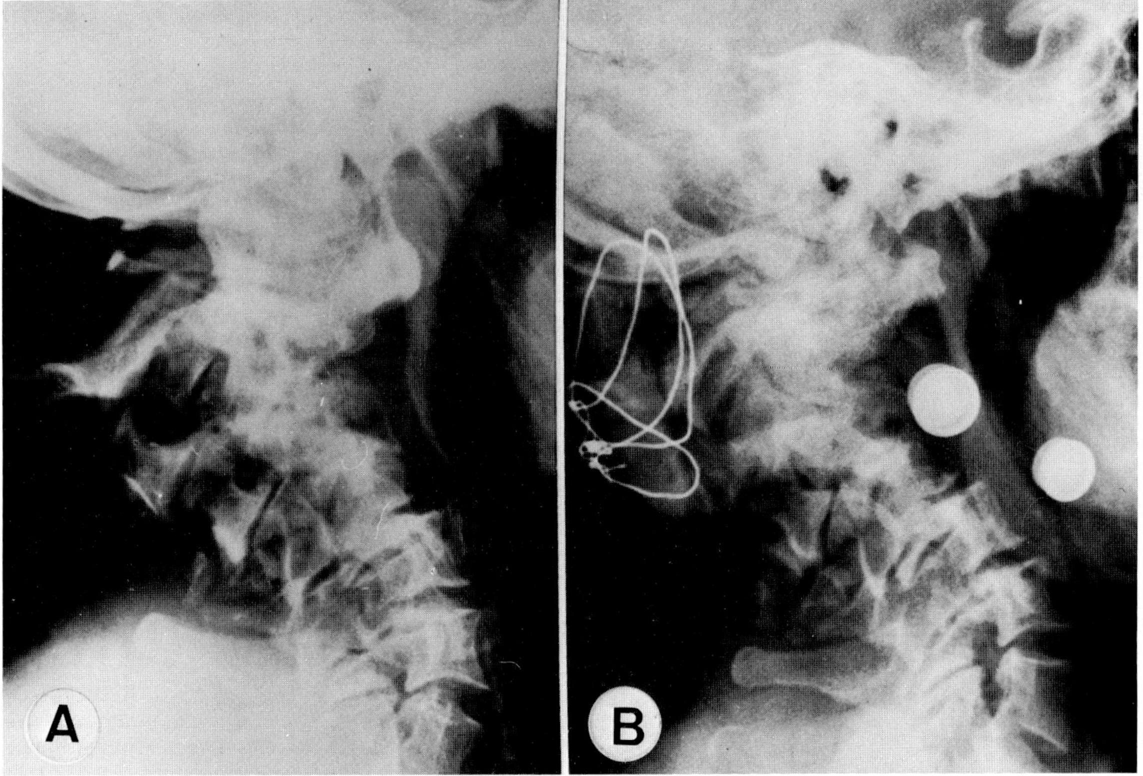

Fig. 12-21. Case 1. (*A*) Preoperative roentgenogram showing thoracic kyphoscoliosis, atlantal forward slip, and kyphosis of C2–C4. (*B*) Roentgenogram taken after incomplete removal of the diffuse neurofibromatous mass and posterior fusion.

colli muscles, connected with a small nonidentified nerve. There was diffuse neurofibromatosis below the anterior longitudinal ligament and the C2–C3 disc space was partly ossified.

Anterior columnotomy between C2–C3 and insertion of a wedge-shaped cortical graft, combined with skull traction, resulted in partial reduction of kyphosis. Microscopic examination showed neurofibromatosis infiltrating the anterior longitudinal ligament and fibromatosis of the intervertebral disc C2–C3. There was some improvement of quadriparesis. There was no follow-up because the patient returned to her home country.

CASE 3. A man of 52 had been operated on elsewhere (1956) because of a right dumbbell extradural neurofibroma at C3–C4; it had been removed by means of laminectomy. Eleven years later he experienced quadriparesis, collapse of the body of C3 with myelographic posterior displacement of contrast medium, and block at this level (Fig. 12-22*A*). Right vertebral angiography showed anterior displacement of the artery at the level of C3 (Fig. 12-22*B*). Turkel needle biopsy of the body of C3 revealed neurofibromatous tissue.

March 6, 1969: Right anterolateral approach was used, with decompression of the right vertebral artery and removal of a lateral vertebral neurofibroma the size of a goose egg. A complete corporectomy of C3 was performed by combined anterior and lateral operation, along with removal of anterior subligamentous and extradural spread in the areas of C2 and C4. The intervertebral foramen was cleaned. An iliac crest graft was used for replacement of the body of C3. The postoperative right vertebral angiogram, 5 months after operation, showed decompressed artery and overgrowth of bone in front of the graft (Fig. 12-22*C*). A plain lateral radiograph revealed a large mass of bone bridging the bone graft anteriorly from C2 to C4 (Fig. 12-22*D*). Neurologic disturbances had completely recovered within 3 months. At the last fol-

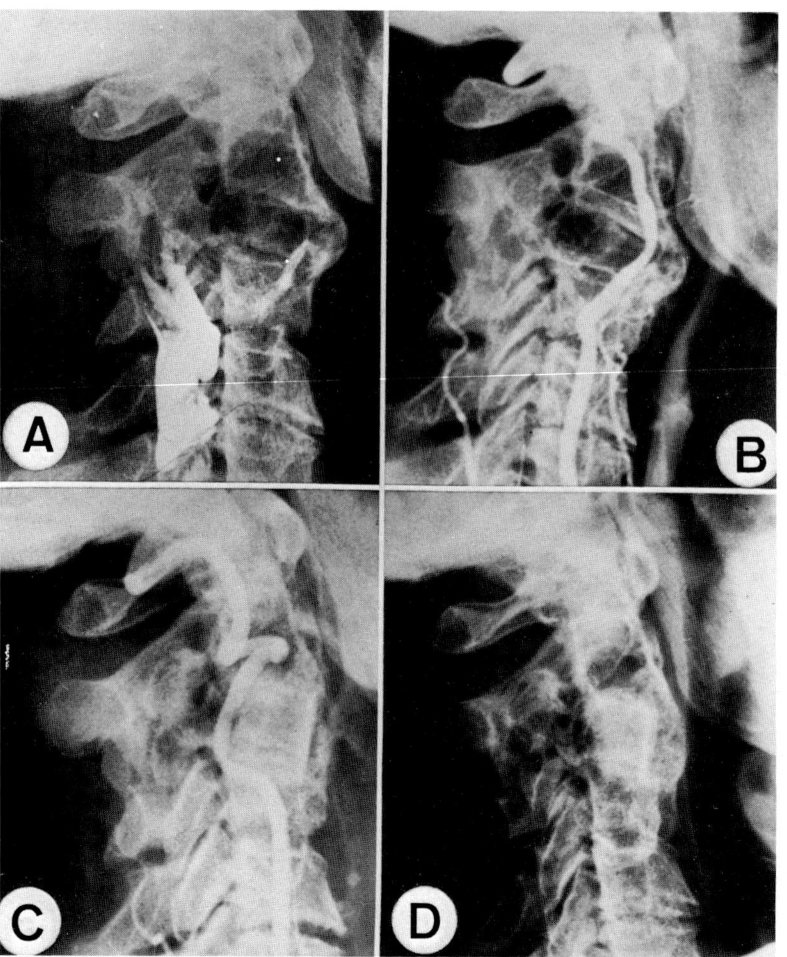

Fig. 12-22. Case 3. (*A*) Myelogram showing collapse of the body of C3, evidenced by the posterior displacement of the contrast medium and a block at this level. (*B*) Right vertebral angiogram showing anterior displacement of the artery at the level of C3. (*C*) Five-month-postoperative right vertebral angiogram showing decompressed artery and overgrowth of bone in front of the graft. (*D*) Lateral radiograph showing a large mass of bone bridging the bone graft anteriorly from C2–C4.

low-up, 11 years after operation, there were no signs of tumor recurrence.

CASE 4. A man of 44 had had an extensive cervical laminectomy, performed elsewhere (1969), for the intraspinal portion of a left dumbbell neurofibroma between C2 and C3. A postlaminectomy radiograph showed some anterior dislocation of C2 and kyphosis of C2–C3 (Fig. 12-23*A*). A 1970 radiograph revealed the development of cervical arcuate kyphosis (Fig. 12-23*B*) and a 1972 radiograph demonstrated calcification of the anterior longitudinal ligament in front of C3–C5 and ankylosis of the posterior joints (Fig. 12-23). This patient was admitted in May 1973 with quadriparesis, which had developed during the past months. Figure 12-23*D* shows enlargement of the left intervertebral foramen C2–C3 at the expense of the underlying foramina C3–C4. Myelography revealed recurrence of intraspinal neurofibroma.

First operation, June 5, 1973: A large intradural neurofibroma was sharply dissected from the cervical spinal cord using the posterior approach. At the same time an extraspinal mass was removed. For reduction of kyphosis, the posterolateral ankylosed joints C3–C4 and C4–C5 were resected and the other joint spaces were opened.

Second operation, June 27, 1973: An anterior columnotomy using the anterolateral approach was performed at the disc spaces between C2–C5 and wedge-shaped tibial cortical grafts were inserted. A biopsy of the body of C3 showed intraosseus neurofibromatous tissue.

A radiograph taken 6 months after second operation showed reduction of kyphosis (Fig. 12-23*E*). Power of the right arm, of the muscles of

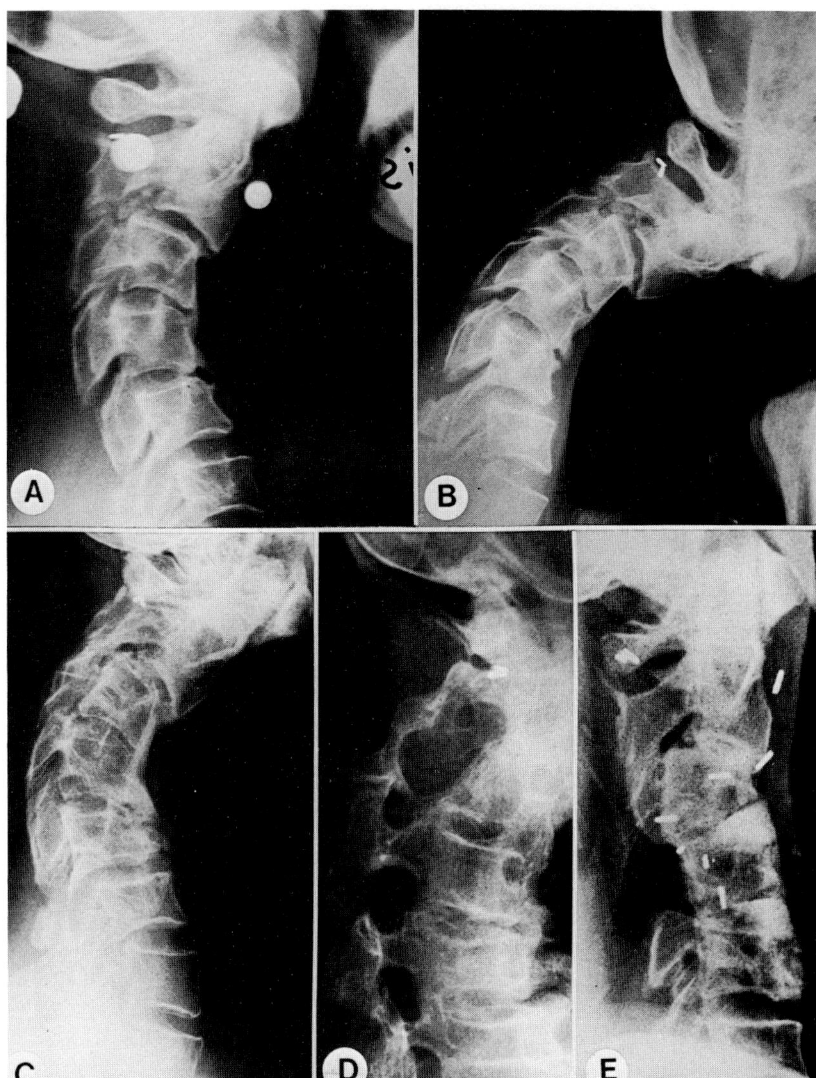

Fig. 12-23. Case 4. (*A*) Post-laminectomy radiograph showing some anterior dislocation of C2 and kyphosis of C2–C3. (*B*) Development of cervical arcuate kyphosis. (*C*) Calcification of the anterior longitudinal ligament in front of C3–C5 and ankylosis of the posterior joints. (*D*) Enlargement of the left intervertebral foramen C2–C3 at the expense of the underlying foramina C3–C4. (*E*) Reduction of kyphosis 6 months after operation.

the left forearm and hand, and of both legs had recovered. The patient was well until December 1980, when he developed a left-sided hemiplegia due to a chronic right-sided intracerebral hematoma. The patient is recovering from removal of the hematoma.

CASE 5. A young man of 15 presented with generalized neurofibromatosis (subcutaneous neurofibromas, *café au lait* spots, large fibroma pendulum of the right upper arm covered by pigmented hairy [animal] skin, torticollis, and thoracic kyphoscolioses). The patient's mother showed multiple neurocutaneous lesions. The patient was admitted in December 1974 because of rapidly progressive right-sided hemiparesis. X-ray films showed displacement of the bodies of C4 and C5 behind the superior aspect of the body of C6. Figures 12-24*A* and 12-24*B* show considerable narrowing of left and right vertebral arteries at the level of the posteriorly slipped C5 vertebral body. The inferior cervical spine was lordotic, and the anterior inferior border of the body of C3 contacted the anterior superior border of the body of C6 with resulting kyphosis (Fig. 12-24*C*).

First operation, January 29, 1975: The anterolateral approach was used. A large neurofibroma between the anterior aspect of the cervical spine and

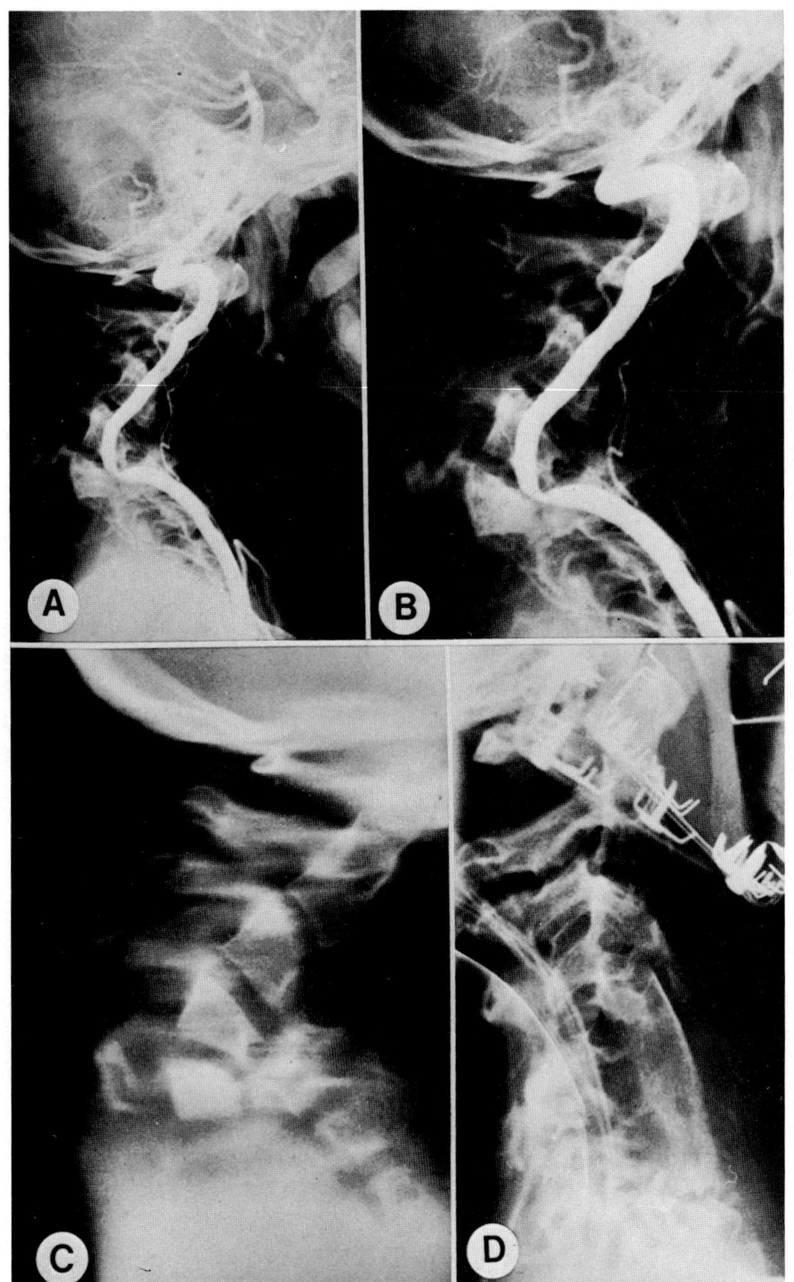

Fig. 12-24. Case 5. (*A* and *B*) Roentgenograms showing considerable narrowing of the left and right vertebral arteries at the level of the posteriorly slipped C5 vertebral body. (*C*) Lateral tomogram. (*D*) Roentgenogram following the final operation, showing the iliac crest graft replacing the bodies of C4, C5, and C6.

the visceral compartment had to be removed first. Anterior subligamentous neurofibromatosis was found at the level of kyphosis. The bodies of C4, C5, and C6 were removed by combined lateral and anterior operations. The body of C6 had to be removed first (for technique, see under Treatment). Figure 12-24*D* shows an iliac crest graft replacing the bodies of C4, C5, and C6. Figure 12-25*A* and 12-25*B* show decompressed right and left vertebral arteries.

Second operation, March 20, 1975: Posterior wiring was done for stabilization. A large neurofibroma covered the right laminae of C4 through C7. The arches C4-C6 and of the spinous processes

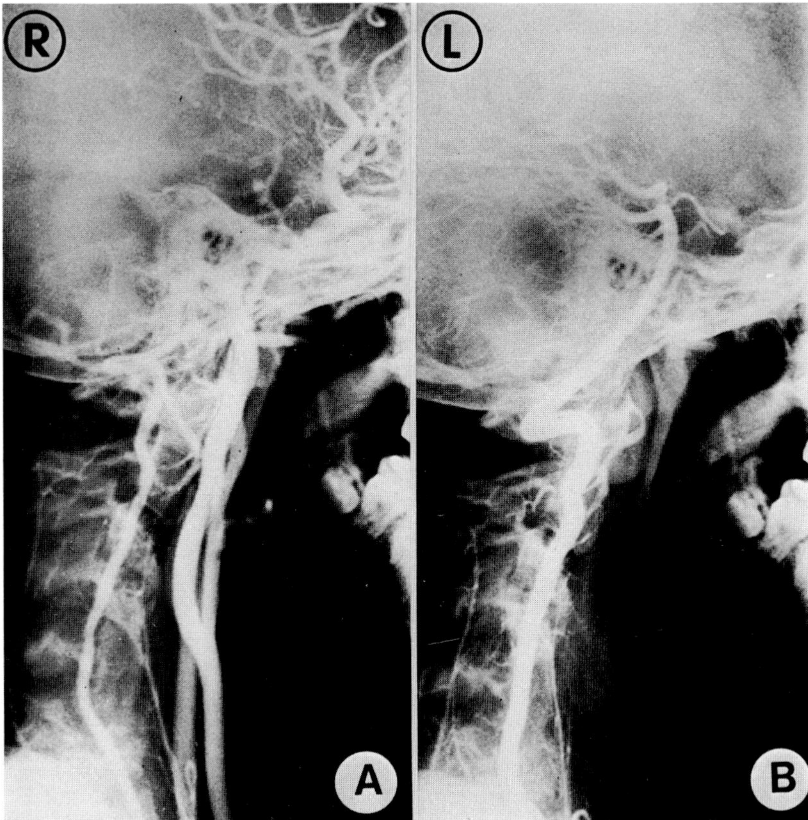

Fig. 12-25. Case 5. (*A* and *B*) Decompressed right and left vertebral arteries after iliac crest graft.

C4–C7 and C2–C7 were wired separately (Fig. 12-26*A*). The patient was mobile 2 weeks later. Hemiparesis completely disappeared 60 days after operation. The patient was readmitted on November 10, 1975 because of progressive wedge deformity of the body of C3 and resulting kyphosis of C2–C3. He had some weakness of the right arm.

Third operation, November 18, 1975: An anterolateral approach showed subligamentous neurofibromatosis eroding the body of C3. Interbody fusion of C2–C3 with a wedge-shaped cortical tibial graft and additional wiring of the spinous process of C2 to the laminae of C3 were done (Fig. 12-26*B*).

Four years after the last operation, the patient had no neural deficit. A lateral roentgenogram showed remodeling of the cervical spine; the bodies between C2 and C7 form a continuous column (Fig. 12-27). Kyphosis existed between C2–C3. There were no disturbances of spinal cord function.

CASE 6. A young man of 15, a quadriparetic patient in poor general condition referred from another country, presented with generalized neurofibromatosis. He had severe cervical kyphosis between C3 and C4 and anterior slip of C5 on the anterior surface of the body of C6 (Fig. 12-28*A*).

The vertebral bodies C4, C5, and C6 were replaced by iliac crest graft, and the arches of C2–C5, C5–C6, and C6–T1 were wired (Fig. 12-28*B*). The patient died 17 days after operation from pulmonary atelectasis and respiratory insufficiency.

CASE 7. A man of 21 presented with generalized neurofibromatosis, *café au lait* spots and subcutaneous neurofibromas, and lumbar-thoracic kyphoscoliosis.

First operation, July 7, 1973: Laminectomy of C2–T2 was performed because of cervical myelopathy caused by intradural multiple neurofibromas, which were larger at the right than at the left side.

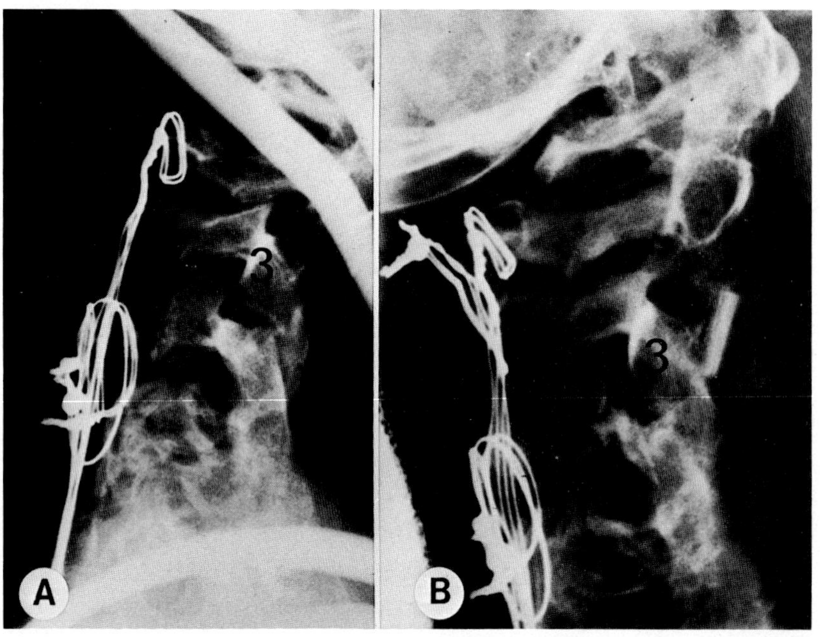

Fig. 12-26. Case 5. (*A*) Roentgenogram following a second operation shows separate wiring of arches C4–C6 and of spinous processes C4–C7 and C2–C7. (*B*) Roentgenogram following a third operation showing interbody fusion of C2–C3 with wedge-shaped cortical tibial graft and additional wiring of the spinous process of C2 to the laminae of C3.

The tumors spread dorsally and ventrally of the spinal cord. Many of them were attached to the posterior spinal nerve roots. The tumors also extended into the intervertebral foramina. Tumor removal was incomplete because small residual masses attached to nerve roots were not resected. Figure 12-29*B* shows enlarged intervertebral foramina. The operation was followed by complete recovery of neurologic disturbances. In 1975 the patient presented with kyphotic deformity in the cervical thoracic area and increased cervical lordosis (Fig. 12-29*C;* compare with preoperative radiograph 12-29*A*).

Second operation, July 11, 1975: Using the anterolateral approach, interbody fusion of C5–C6, C6–C7, and C7–T1 was done. This did not produce sufficient stability at the levels between C7 and T2.

Third operation, July 1, 1976: Using skull traction and the anterolateral approach, a tibial cortical strut graft was inserted in a trough prepared in the anterior surfaces of the bodies of C7 and T1; the extremities of the graft were inserted into the end-plates of the bodies of C6 and T2 behind their anterior rims. Biopsy of the bone removed from the C7 body showed devitalized areas of bone with disappearance of osteocytes. Figure 12-29*D* shows satisfactory correction of kyphosis and fusion of the graft. Figure 12-29*E* shows recurrent low cervical kyphosis and some separation of strut graft, better visualized in Figure 12-29*F*.

Aneurysmal Bone Cysts

The ages of two of the five patients treated for aneurysmal bone cysts were unusually high (Case 10, 40 years and Case 7, 65 years). Of the 104 patients collected by the Netherlands Committee of Bone Tumours, 97 patients were under 30 and only 7 patients were between 30 and 70.[14]

CASE 8. A young woman of 15 fell from a chair in April, 1972. She experienced neck pains 1 week later. A second fall in June of 1972 was followed by an increase of neck pains and limited head movements. Roentgenograms taken immediately after the second fall showed a lytic lesion in the upper portion of the body of C2 (Fig. 12-30*A*). X-ray films in June of 1972 showed "soap bubble" structures in the left lamina of C2 (Fig. 12-30*B*). A few weeks later the lytic lesion occupied the entire body of C2 (Fig. 12-30*C* and *D*), followed by anterior ballooning of the cyst (Fig. 12-30*E*) and lysis of the odontoid (*inset* Fig. 12-30*E* and *F*). There were no neurologic disturbances.

First operation, September 15, 1972: The transoral approach was used. After incision of the anterior longitudinal ligament, a large cyst was opened that contained a chocolate-colored fluid and crumbled

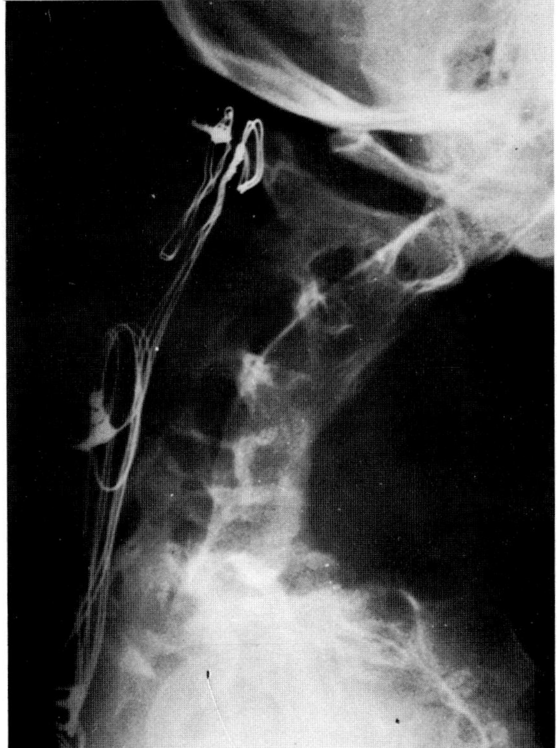

Fig. 12-27. Case 5. Lateral roentgenogram 4 years after the last operation shows remodeling of the cervical spine. The bodies between C2 and C7 form a continuous column. Note the kyphosis between C2–C3.

pieces of tumor and bone. The ballooned anterior bony wall of the cyst was excised. The residual cyst wall was removed by curettage. The cortical inferior end-plate and the lateral and posterior cortex of the body of C2 were still intact. The odontoid had disappeared with the exception of its tip. One graft of the iliac crest was inserted between the inferior end-plate of the body of C2 and the residual tip of the odontoid. A second graft was placed in the anterior opening of the cyst between the inferior end-plate of the body of C2 and the anterior arch of the atlas (Fig. 12-31*A* and *B*). The anterior ligament, the constrictor muscle, and the mucosa were sutured in layers.

Second operation, October 14, 1972: The posterior approach was used to remove the left lamina of C2, which was invaded by tumor. The right lamina was intact. Posterior bony fusion from the occiput through C5 combined with wiring was performed (Fig. 12-31*B*). Microscopic diagnosis of all tumor specimens indicated an aneurysmal bone cyst. X-ray films in March of 1973 showed perfect remodeling and fusion of the grafts (*inset* Fig. 12-31*B* and 12-31*C* and *D*). The anterior arch of the atlas was included in the fusion process.

Third operation, January 18, 1974: Posterior wiring and portions of the bone graft between the occiput and C1 and between C2 and C5 were removed. This resulted in improvement of mobility of the spine as shown in roentgenograms taken on May 9 and May 19, 1974 with the spine in extension (Fig. 12-32*C*) and flexion (Fig. 12-32*D*). Figure 12-32*A* and *B* were taken before the bone graft portions were removed.

Case 9. A man of 65 who had had a whiplash injury 2 years previously presented with neck pains and limitations of head movements of 1 year's duration. He was an inert, senescent patient with no neural deficit. X-ray films of the cervical spine showed collapse of the posterior portion of the body of C2 with some soap bell appearance and a ballooned-out area in front. Vertebral angiograms were normal. No lesions were found elsewhere.

May 29, 1975: Using the transoral approach, a large cyst was opened, which contained a brownish fluid. Removal of the cyst walls and smaller cavities posteriorly exposed the dura. Iliac grafts were introduced into the bony cavity. The microscopic diagnosis was aneurysmal bone cyst. The immediate postoperative course was uneventful. On July 15, 1975, pneumonia was observed, and by July 23, 1975, the patient had gram-negative sepsis, left-sided heart failure, and impaired renal function. He died from these complications on August 17, 1975.

Case 10. A 40-year-old man with no history of injury developed, in August 1980, a tender suboccipital area and local muscle spasms, although his head movements were painless and not limited. Figure 12-33*A* shows a large cystic lesion in the body of C2; the arrow at left points to undermining of the right superior articular process. A tomogram made more posteriorly shows lytic lesions inside the pedicles (Fig. 12-33*B*). Figure 12-33*C* and *D* show extension of the lytic lesion into the left and right pedicles and lateral portions of the laminae of C2.

November 15, 1980: Using the transoral approach, a large cystic cavity was opened that contained chocolate-colored fluid and crumbled solid masses. The large cavity, its extension into the pedicles and lateral lamina included, was cleaned of tumor masses by means of curettage and the cav-

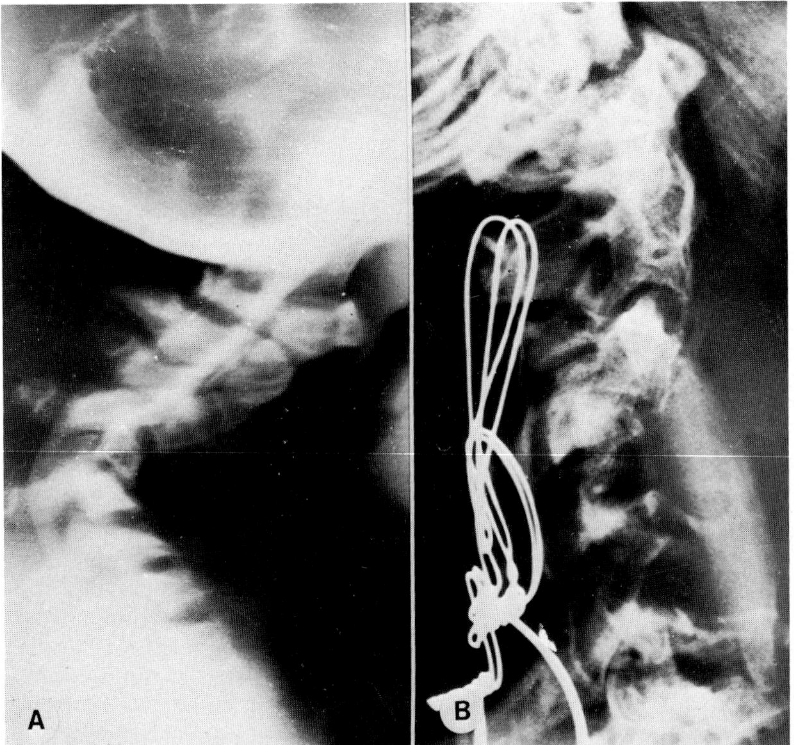

Fig. 12-28. Case 6. (*A*) Lateral tomogram showing generalized neurofibromatosis, severe cervical kyphosis, kyphosis between C3 and C4, and the anterior slip of C4 on the anterior surface of the body of C5. (*B*) Postoperative roentgenogram showing the replacement by iliac crest graft of the vertebral bodies C4, C5, and C6, and the wiring of the arches C2–C5, C5–C6, and C6–T1.

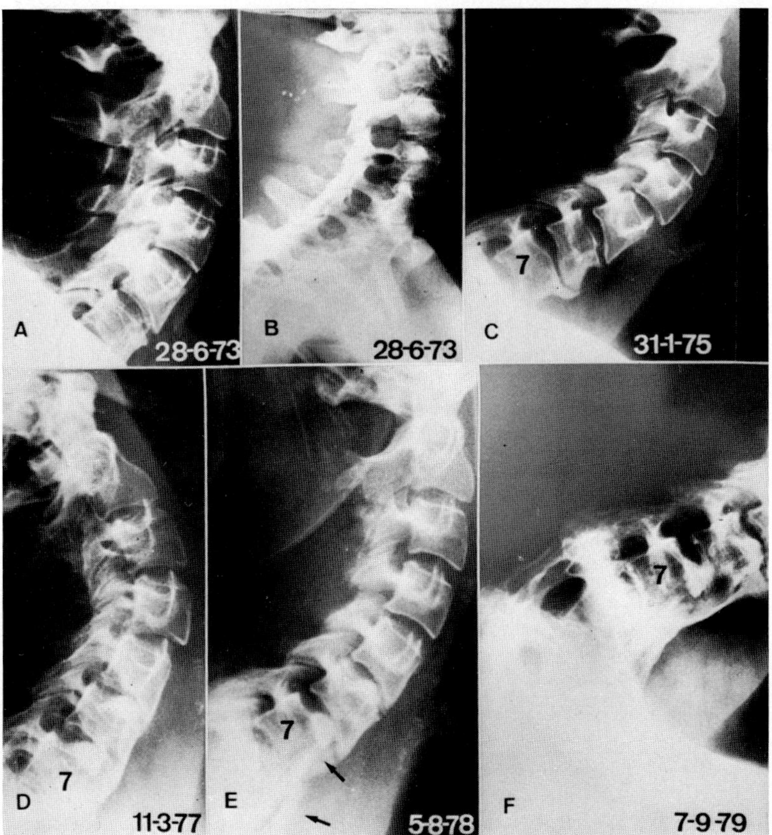

Fig. 12-29. Case 7. (*A* and *B*) Preoperative radiographs, with (*B*) showing the enlarged intervertebral foramina. (*C*) Postoperative radiograph. (*D*) Satisfactory correction of kyphosis and fusion of the graft. (*E* and *F*) Recurrent low cervical kyphosis and some separation of strut graft.

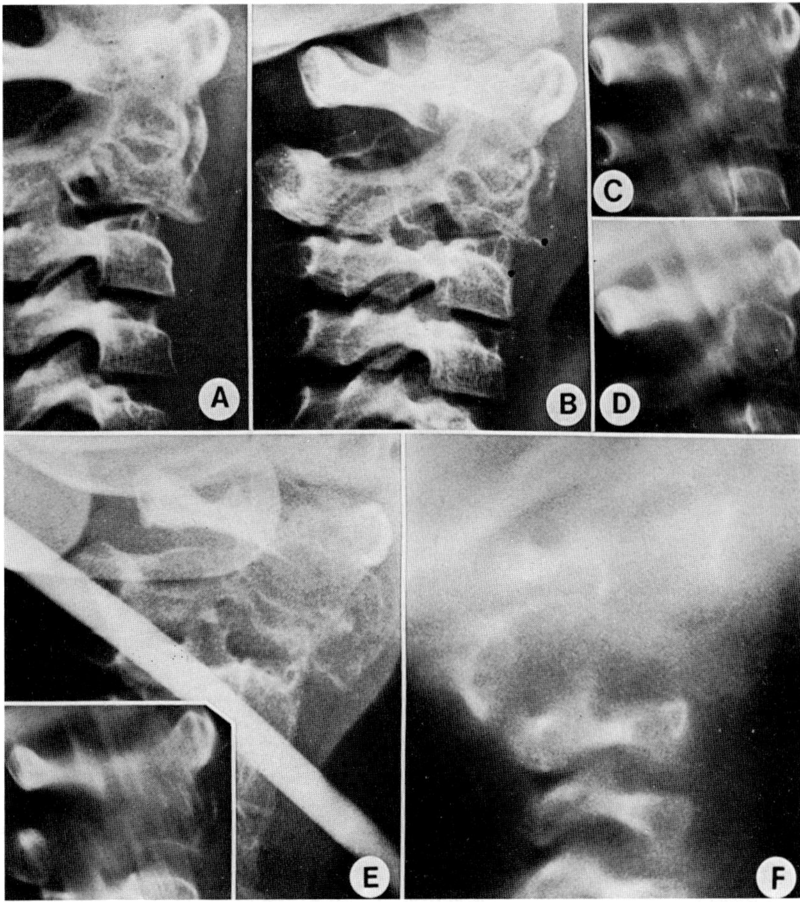

Fig. 12-30. Case 8. (*A*) Lytic lesion in the upper body of C2. (*B*) "Soap bell" structures in the left lamina of C2. (*C* and *D*) Lytic lesion occupies the entire body of C2. (*E* and *F*) Anterior ballooning of the cyst and lysis of the odontoid.

ities were filled with iliac bone grafts. Microscopic diagnosis indicated aneurysmal bone cyst. The operation was performed too recently for an evaluation of its results.

CASE 11. A woman of 32 received a head injury in a car accident on May 5, 1971, which resulted in right-sided neck pains. X-ray films taken after the accident showed no abnormalities of the cervical spine. Roentgenograms taken in July 1972 showed absence of the right portion of the posterior arch of the atlas. In December 1972, a fluctuating swelling was noted in the right suboccipital region.

The patient was admitted on January 29, 1973. She showed no neural deficit. X-ray films demonstrated disappearance of the right and medial portions of the atlas (Fig. 12-34*A*), suboccipital posterior displacement of the right vertebral artery (Fig. 12-34*B*), and no obstruction of the jugular foramen in the retrograde jugular venogram (Fig. 12-34*C* and *D*). Frontal tomograms showed destruction of the right atlantooccipital joint (Fig. 12-35*A*) and a defect in the right basal portion of the occipital bone (Fig. 12-35*B*).

First operation, February 20, 1973: The lateral approach was used; an incision was made from the right mastoid process along the inferior border of the mandibula and continued downward halfway to the anterior border of the sternocleidomastoid muscle. The mastoid process was sectioned for eversion of the sternocleidomastoid muscle. After anterior and medial retraction of the large cervical blood vessels, a grayish tumor capsule, situated between the transverse process of C1 and the occiput, was exposed. It contained a cystic cavity filled with a chocolate-colored fluid. The foramina transversaria of C2 and the atlas were opened for exposure of the vertebral artery, which allowed its separation from the tumor capsule more superi-

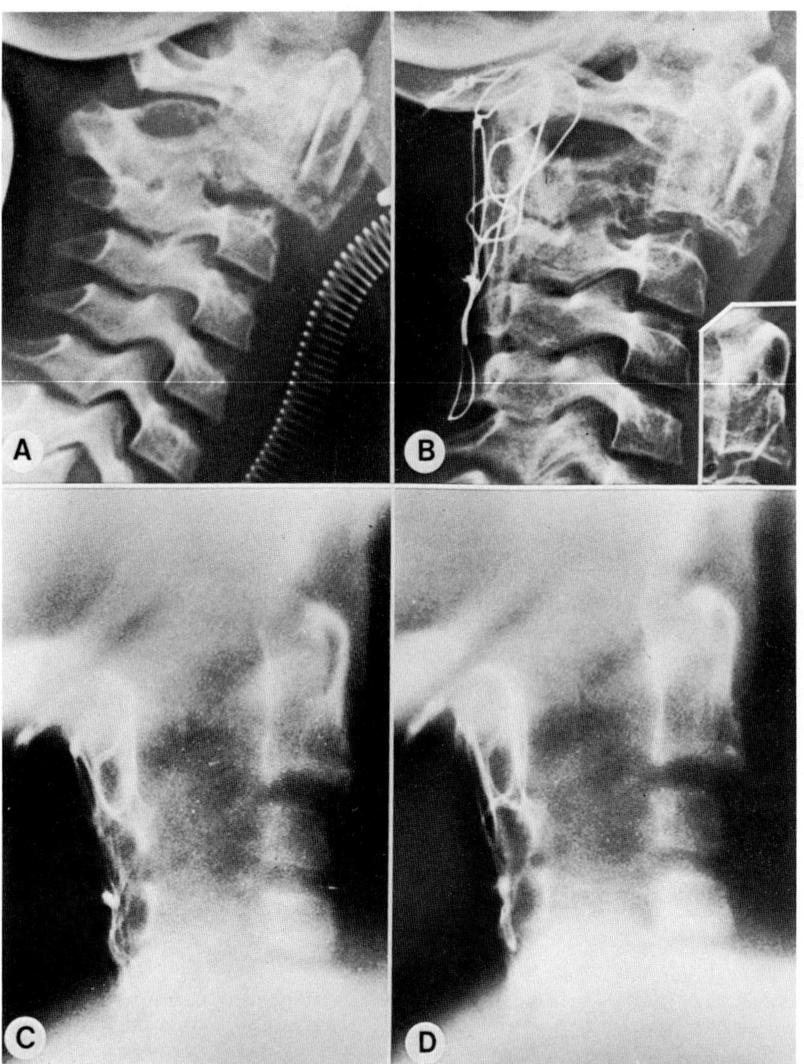

Fig. 12-31. Case 8. (*A*) Roentgenogram showing a graft placed in the anterior opening of the cyst between the inferior end-plate of the body of C2 and the anterior arch of the atlas. (*B*) Posterior body fusion from the occiput through C5 combined with wiring. (*B inset, C,* and *D*) Perfect remodeling and fusion of the grafts.

orly. The cyst extended into the right posterior cranial fossa and reached medially unto the odontoid. The cyst wall was carefully dissected. Iliac crest grafts were applied between the right occipital bone and the residual lateral mass of the atlas (Fig. 12-35*C*). The microscopic diagnosis was aneurysmal bone cyst. Figure 12-35*D* and *E* show good fusion of grafts in 1974 and 1975.

The patient did well until October 1978 when a left suboccipital swelling was noted. Tomography showed partial destruction of the right atlanto-suboccipital bone graft and destruction of the left atlantooccipital joint (Fig. 12-36*A*). The odontoid could not be visualized. The right sagittal tomogram showed blurring due to silver clips (Fig. 12-36*B, arrow*). Some remodeling of bone, difficult to identify, was noted between atlas and occiput. The left sagittal tomogram showed erosion of the atlantooccipital joint (Fig. 12-36*C*); the arrow points at a dense area possibly caused by the right-sided silver clips since one of these clips is also separately visible. The left suboccipital bone was also involved. The left vertebral artery was normal.

Second operation, January 17, 1979: The posterior midline approach was used and a cyst was found containing brownish fluid. It extended bilaterally into the neck muscles; posteriorly it had eroded the margin of the foramen magnum. Only the

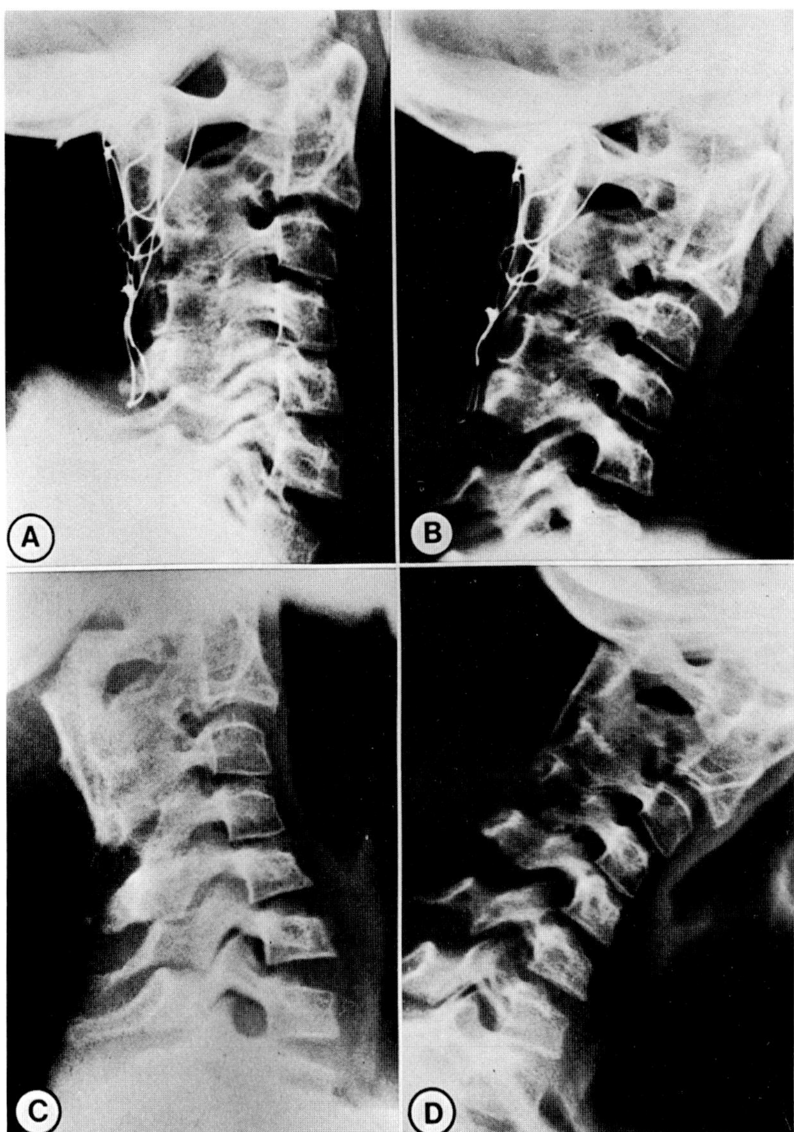

Fig. 12-32. Case 8. Limited extension (*A*) and flexion (*B*) of the spine before partial removal of the posterior grafts. (*C*) Extension and (*D*) flexion of the spine after partial removal of the posterior grafts.

right portion of the odontoid was preserved. The cyst encircled the odontoid completely. The cyst wall was excised as completely as possible, the cavity allowing the surgeon to proceed in front of the odontoid. Since the tumor was adherent to the posterior dural theca, it was excised and replaced by a fascia lata graft. The bleeding residual cavities were packed with muscle pieces taken from the upper leg. Microscopic examination indicated an aneurysmal bone cyst not differing in pattern from the one removed 6 years previously.

Third operation, February 2, 1979: Using the transoral approach, abrasion of the anterior rim of the foramen magnum was accomplished. An iliac crest graft was inserted by way of an opening of the anterior arch of the atlas, prepared by resection of its right half. The graft was placed against the residual right portion of the odontoid. The upper extremity of the graft contacted the anterior rim of the foramen magnum; its inferior extremity was inserted into the superior end-plate of the body of C2 behind its anterior superior margin. Empty spaces in front of and beside this main graft were filled with additional bone grafts. A roentgeno-

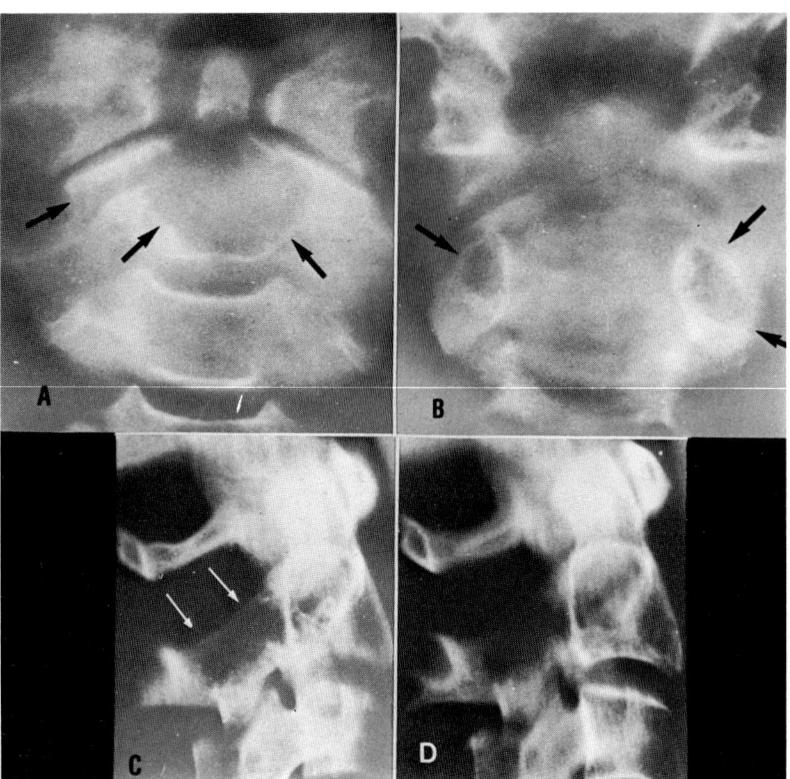

Fig. 12-33. Case 10. (*A*) Tomogram showing large cystic lesion in the body of C2. Arrow at left points to the undermining of the right superior articular process. (*B*) Posterior tomogram showing lytic lesions inside the pedicles. (*C* and *D*) Extension of the lytic lesion into the left and right pedicles and lateral portions of the laminae of C2.

gram taken 1 month after the third operation showed the position of the main graft and of additional smaller grafts, one of them projecting in front of the main graft (Fig. 12-37*A*). Lateral views taken 3 and 8 months later showed a calcified suboccipital mass (Fig. 12-37*B* and *C*), which does not reach to the midline (Fig. 12-37*D*). The tomogram also showed more density in the superior half of the odontoid. The grafts were demineralized but may be in the process of revitalization (Fig. 12-37*D*). As of January 15, 1981, the patient was doing well. Rotation and extension of the head were reduced but flexion was normal.

CASE 12. A woman of 27 had been operated on by Krayenbühl in 1972 because of an aneurysmal bone cyst involving the spinous process, the right lamina, and the right articular processes of C5 (Fig. 12-38*A* and *B*). The lesion was completely removed as seen in the postoperative radiographs (Fig. 12-38*C* and *D*). Some anterior angulation between C5 and C6 had developed (compare Fig. 12-38*B* with 12-38*D*). Progressive recurrence of the tumor was noted in 1973 and 1974.

Krayenbühl referred the patient to the Utrecht neurosurgical department; she was admitted on December 2, 1974 with right cervical and shoulder pains and radiating pains through the right arm into the hand and all fingers. She had some loss of power of all muscles of the right arm, but intact sensation. There was a palpable right-sided cervical tumor mass. X-ray films showed a large cyst of the right side of the spine bulging outward laterally and posteriorly; it presented a faint soap bubble pattern (Fig. 12-39*A*). Compared to 1972, there was additional destruction of the articular processes of C4 (Fig. 12-39*A*) and right lateral invasion of the body of C5 and the right inferior border of the body of C4 (Fig. 12-39*D* and *E*). The tumor had caused a slight lateral and considerable anterior displacement of the right vertebral artery at the level of C5 (Fig. 12-39*B* and *C*). The left vertebral artery was normal and of fair size (Fig. 12-39*B*).

December 11, 1974: Lateral operation was performed by means of a right anterolateral approach. After retraction of the right longissimus capitis and cervicis muscles the tumor was exposed. Tissue surrounded the vertebral artery and was firmly attached to its wall. The pathologic portion

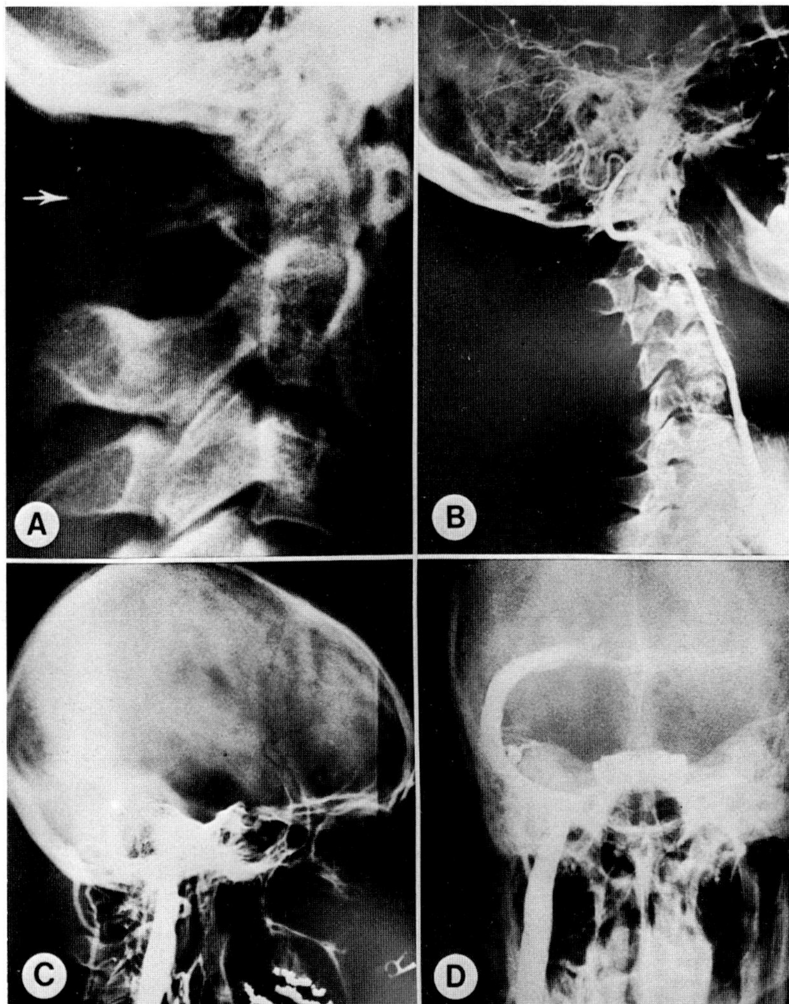

Fig. 12-34. Case 11. Preoperative roentgenograms demonstrating (*A*) disappearance of the right and medial portion of the atlas and (*B*) suboccipital posterior displacement of the right vertebral artery. (*C* and *D*) Retrograde jugular venograms show no obstruction of the jugular foramen.

of the artery was resected. The primary rami of the 5th and 6th spinal nerves were freed from surrounding tumor mass. Behind the spinal nerves was a large cyst whose wall was partly bony, partly tumorous. The cyst wall extending into the posterior cervical muscles and along the previous laminectomy defect was carefully removed. A spontaneously developed bony bridge between the spinous processes of C4 and C6 was left intact (Fig. 12-40*A*). Tumor growth into the interior lateral border of the body of C4 was removed. The cavity in the lateral half of the body of C5 was cleaned and filled with an iliac crest graft.

After the operation the patient had a temporary right recurrent nerve paralysis that recovered in March 1975. On February 14, 1976, x-ray films showed remodeling of the body of C5 (Fig. 12-40*B* and *C*). The patient, living in another country, was reported to be doing well (1979). No signs of tumor recurrence were noted. Power of the right arm had recovered. There were no complaints of pain.

Since the appearance of the first edition of this monograph we had experience with two other cases of aneurysmal bone cysts, which are interesting because the recovery process following operation could be checked in CT scans. Whereas in our first series of five aneurysmal bone cysts only one patient was younger than 20 years (patient was 15 years), now three of our seven patients are between 9 and 15 years of age.

Case 13. A 9-year-old boy for 1 year complained of neck pains and painful neck movements, with-

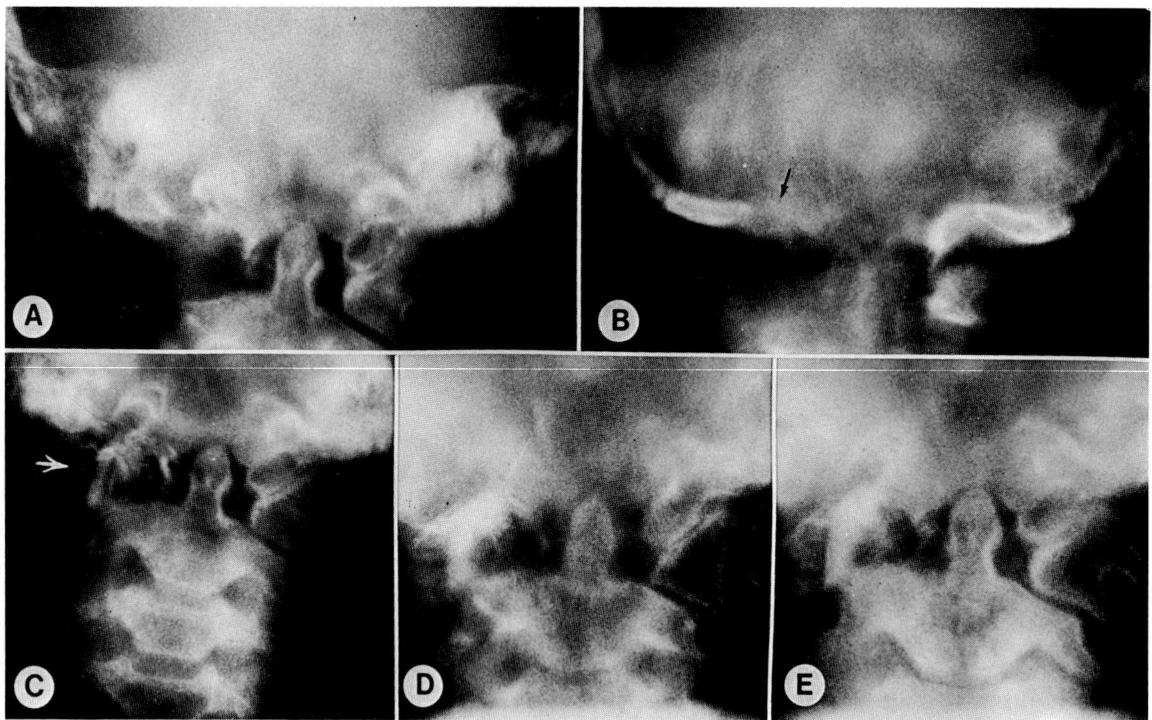

Fig. 12-35. Case 11. (*A* and *B*) Frontal tomograms show destruction of the right atlanto-occipital joint and of the lateral structures of the atlas. (*C*) Iliac crest grafts were applied between the right occipital bone and the residual lateral mass of the atlas. (*D* and *E*) Good fusion of grafts is evident.

out other disturbances. X-rays taken in February 1982 showed flattening of the disc space C3–C4, signs of anteroposterior enlargement of the body of L4 and of osteolysis in its upper half. Its spinous process was expanded, and its bone marrow cavity seemed to be cystic (Fig. 12-41*A*). A repeat X-ray in December 1982 showed a soap bubble appearance within the cortical surroundings of the spinous process of C4 (Fig. 12-41*B*). The patient was admitted in June 1983, and by a posterior approach the cavities within the spinous process and laminae of C4 were opened near the midline, excochleated, and occluded with cancellous bone chips. Because the extension of the tumor inside the vertebral bodies was to be treated during the same operation, the spinous processes C3–C5 were wired to ensure stability. Next, the lateral aspects of the vertebral bodies of C3 and C4 were exposed through a lateral approach. Lateral, transuncal excision of the disc C3–C4 was performed. The adjacent portions of the bodies of C3 and C4 showed cystic changes. The cavities were cleaned with a curette and occluded with cancellous bone chips.

Figure 12-41*C*, a profile view taken 1 year after the operation, shows a block of the vertebral bodies of C3 and C4. Figure 12-41*D*, taken 3 years after operation, shows ankylosis of the apophyseal joints between C3 and C5. The wires had been removed 1 year previously. The distance between the anterosuperior border of the body of C3 and the anteroinferior border of the body of C4 has increased in proportion to the anterior height of the body of C5, as compared with this proportion before the operation. It is a sign that the blocked bodies C3–C4 participate in skeletal growth. CT scans through the arch of C4, made 2 years after operation, show a residual paramedial cleft in the upper portion of the arch (Fig. 12-41*E*). The section through its lower portion shows some constriction of the thickness of the laminae in their central portions (Fig. 12-41*F*). Dense islands of graft material are seen in the spongious mass of the arch and the vertebral body. The boy shows free and painless cervical movements and has no complaints at all.

CASE 14. A girl, 11 years old, had been operated upon 7 years previously by means of a suboccipital

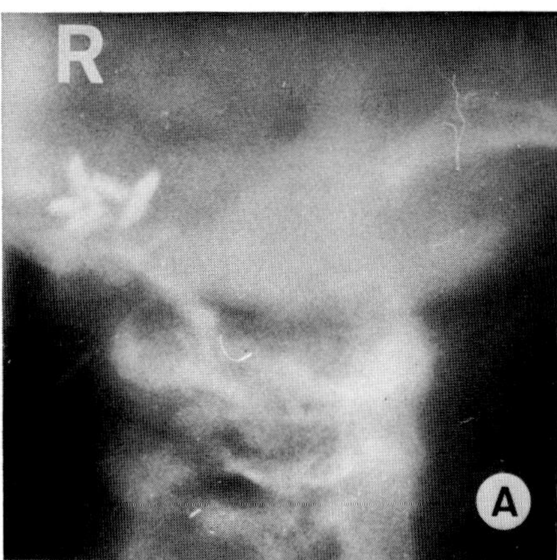

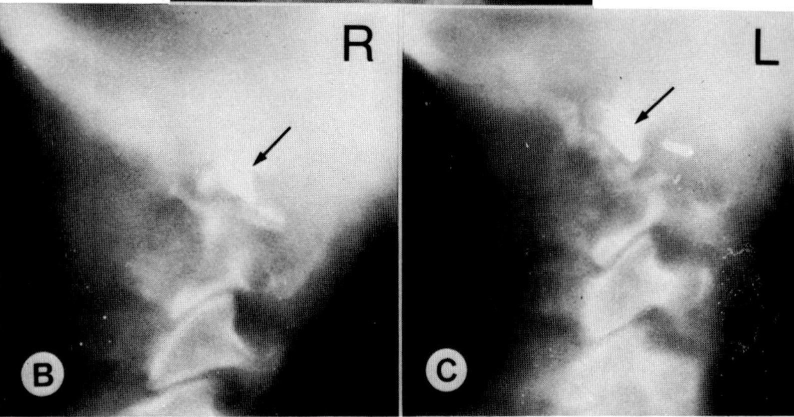

Fig. 12-36. Case 11. (*A*) Frontal tomogram showing partial destruction of the right altantosuboccipital bone graft and destruction of the left atlanto-occipital joint. (*B*) Right sagittal tomogram showing blurring due to silver clips (*arrow*). Some remodeling of bone, difficult to identify, was noted between the atlas and the occiput. (*C*) Left sagittal tomogram showing erosion of the atlantooccipital joint. Arrows point to dense areas possibly caused by the rightsided silver clips.

craniotomy with removal of a cerebellar ependymoma. She had received postoperative radiotherapy at a total dose of 5000 roentgens. At postoperative checkup 6 years later, x-rays of the skull revealed expansion of the spinous process of C2, which had a cystic appearance (Fig. 12-42*A*). The girl had no complaints at all, and her cervical movements were normal and painless. CT scans through the C2 vertebra showed osteolysis in the superior portion of its arch, reaching as far as the pedicles (Fig. 12-42*B*). The section through the inferior portion of the vertebral arch showed a vacuolated structure of the bone marrow cavity (Fig. 12-42*C*). The cortical layers of this vertebral arch were eggshell thin and showed discontinuities. The cavity was excochleated and occluded with cancellous bone chips by means of a posterior surgical approach (June 1983). Figure 12-42*D* shows a profile roentgenogram made in October 1984, 16 months after the operation. The arch of C2 shows a normal structure. CT scans through the upper and lower portions of the arch of C2 (Fig. 12-42*E* and *F*, respectively) show remodeling of the cortical bone and bone formation in the marrow cavity. The girl is free of signs and symptoms.

Giant Cell Tumors

Giant cell tumors are included among the benign tumors because the majority of cases show a benign course. Only in a few cases may they produce metastases. The case histories, roentgenograms, and microscopic illustrations of the histopathology of these cases have been published elsewhere, so that only a brief discussion is presented here.[21]

Case 15. A man of 21 had a spastic tetraparesis due to a giant cell tumor involving the left vertebral laminae of C4 and C5, occupying the left intervertebral foramina C4–C5 and C5–C6 and eroding the adjacent articular facets (see Case 1, Reference 21). Complete removal resulted in disappearance of neurologic disturbances in the year following operation. Ten years later the patient was found to be in good health. No signs of tumor recurrence were noted and the alignment of his cervical spine was normal. One year later, after a minor cranial injury, he developed neck pains.

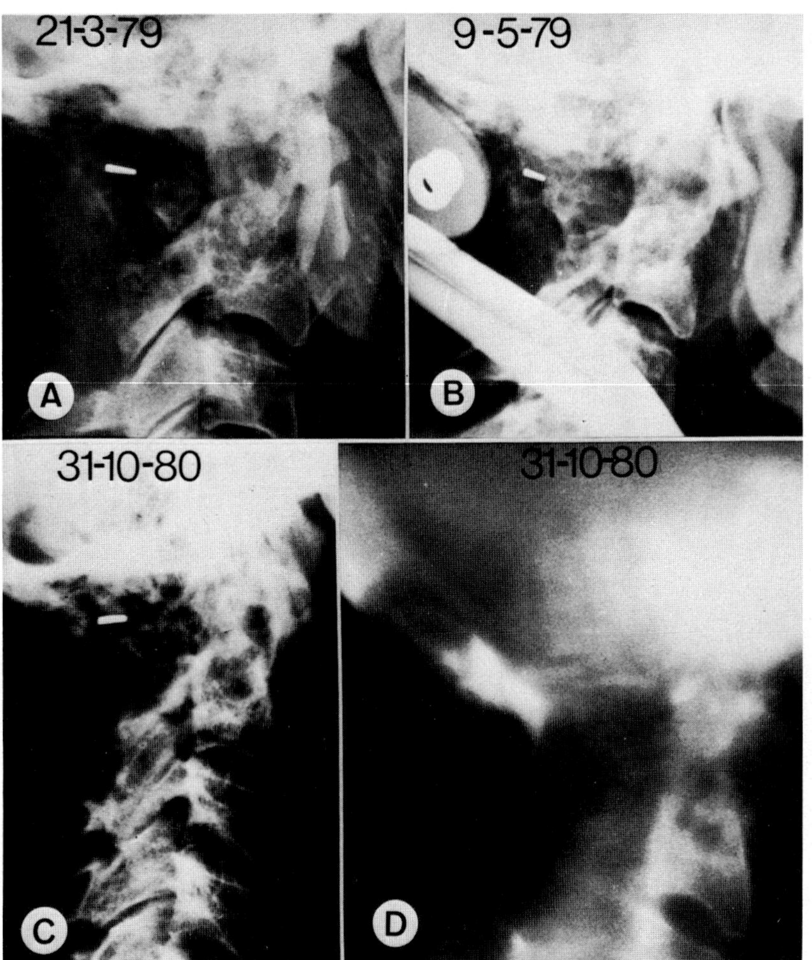

Fig. 12-37. Case 11. (*A*) Roentgenogram 1 month after the third operation showing the position of the main graft and of additional smaller grafts. (*B* and *C*) Lateral views taken 3 months and 8 months later show calcified suboccipital mass that does not reach to the midline. (*D*) Tomogram showing more density in the superior half of the odontoid.

Roentgenographic examination revealed instability and minor angular kyphosis between C5 and C6. There was no deformity of the vertebral bodies, instability being due to abnormal mobility between the right joint facets C5 and C6. As the left posterior joints C5 and C6 had been removed 11 years previously, overstress of the right joints during this period may have resulted in diminished resistance of its capsules and ligaments to minor cranial injury. The instability and disturbed curvature were corrected by means of an anterolateral approach and interbody fusion of C5 and C6 with a wedge-shaped tibial cortical graft.

Case 16. A young woman of 16 developed tetraplegia and loss of sensation below T4 (see Case 2, Reference 21). The tumor was found infiltrating the posterior muscles of the neck. It had destroyed the laminae and spinous processes of C5 and C6, and extended extradurally from C5 through C7. It also occupied the intervertebral foramina at these levels. Surgical removal by means of a posterior approach resulted in complete and rapid recovery of neurologic disturbances. Her last checkup 6 years after operation showed no signs of recurrence.

Case 17. A man of 22 had a giant cell tumor involving the entire seventh cervical vertebra and the extradural space from C6 through T1 (see Case 5, Reference 21). Microscopic diagnosis of tumor material removed in 1957 was giant cell tumor Grade II. After his first operation the patient received radiotherapy, a total dose of 4600 roentgens. At a repeat operation 3 years later because of instability, no evidence of tumor recurrence was found.

A third operation was performed in 1961 be-

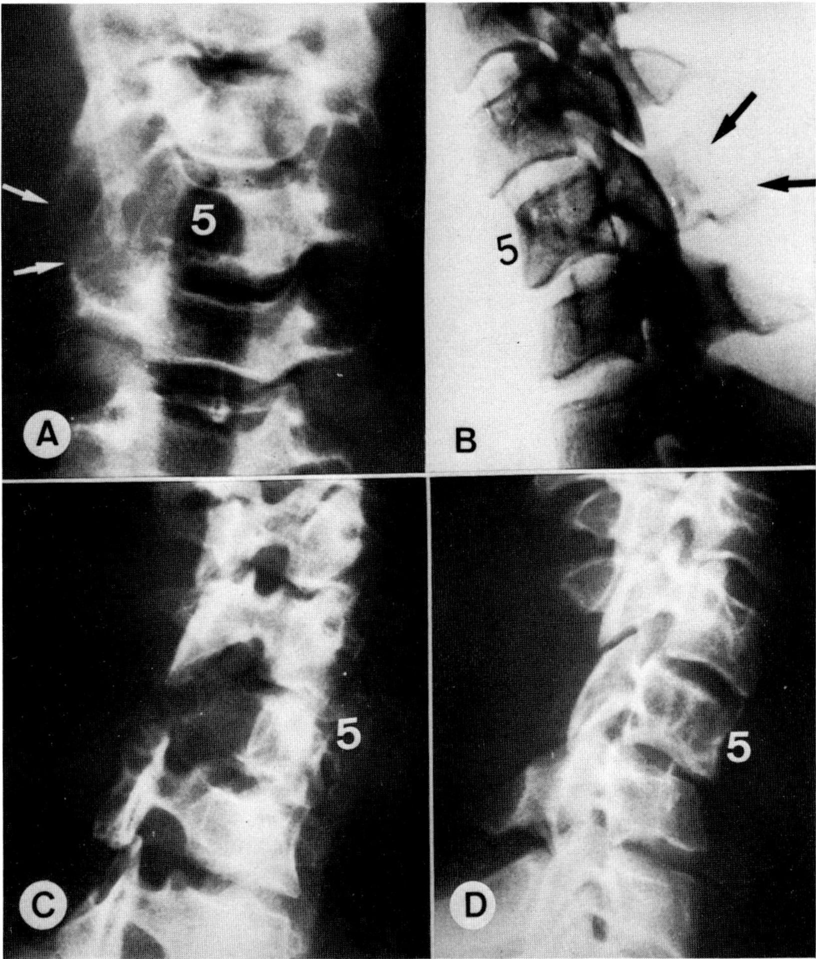

Fig. 12-38. Case 12. (*A* and *B*) Preoperative roentgenograms showing an aneurysmal bone cyst involving the spinous process, the right lamina, and the right articular processes of C5. (*C* and *D*) The lesion has been completely removed. Note the anterior angulation between C5 and C6.

cause of tumor recurrence. The microscopic diagnosis was again giant cell tumor showing no signs of malignancy. A fourth operation followed 3 months later because of rapidly occurring tumor growth. Histologic examination showed malignant transformation of the tumor.

Malignant transformation and metastatic spread of giant cell tumors may occur spontaneously. It is, however, equally possible that the malignant transformation in Case 17 was due to radiation therapy. Incomplete excision of a vertebral giant cell tumor harbors a possibility of malignant transformation, but radiation therapy of a vertebral giant cell tumor carries two risks. In the early phase it may produce exacerbation of the tumor, giving rise to increase or onset of serious neurologic disturbances, as seen in 2 of our 7 patients reported previously. The second risk of radiation therapy is the development of postirradiation sarcoma. Therefore, preoperative radiation therapy should not be practiced. Complete excision of the vertebral tumor appears to be preferable. With the present surgical techniques radical excision is possible, although it may require more than one operation. Even if a benign giant cell tumor cannot be completely excised, this does not indicate that radiotherapy should be used unless the residual tumor progresses rapidly and produces metastases.

Benign Osteoblastomas

Vertebral benign osteoblastomas occur most frequently in the posterior vertebral elements.

Case 18. A girl of 13 presented with posterior cervical pains and limited head movements that had had a sudden onset 1 month previously. Ten-

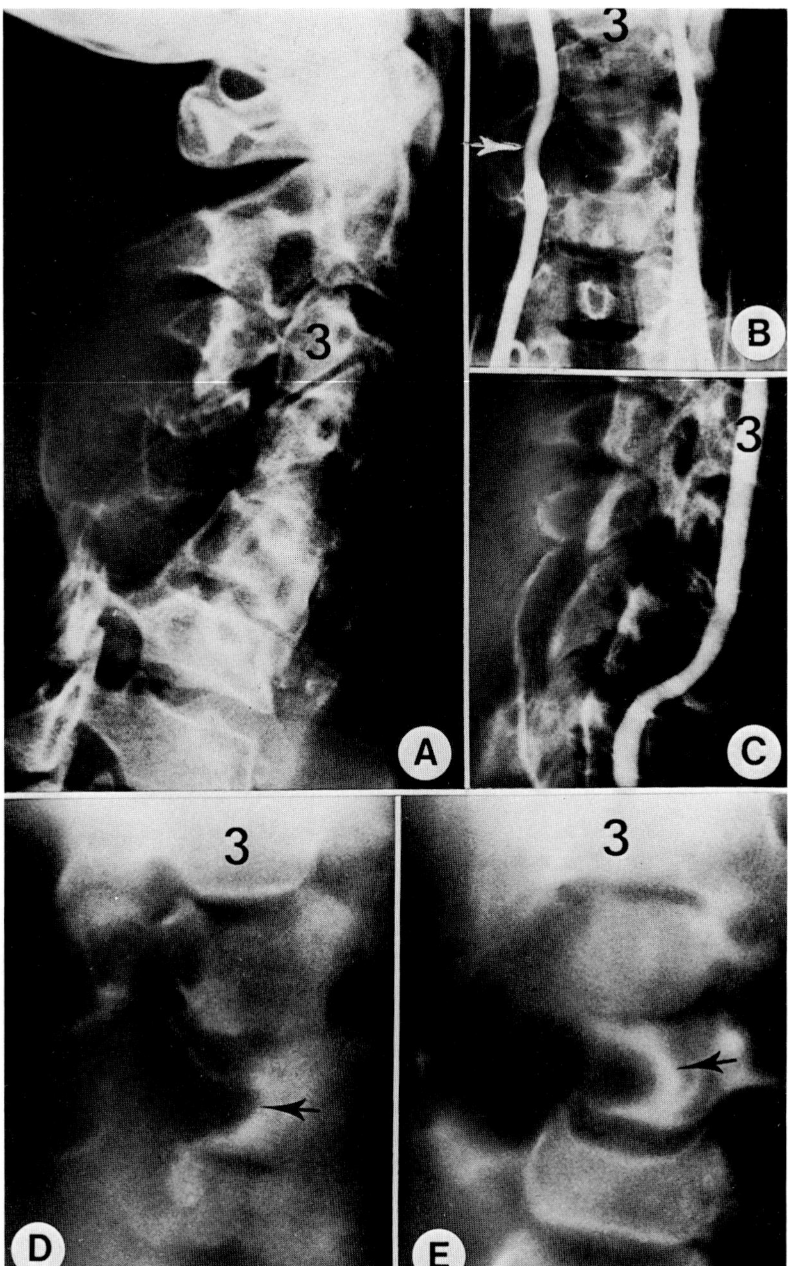

Fig. 12-39. Case 12. (*A*) Roentgenogram showing a large cyst bulging outward laterally and posteriorly from the right side of the spine. Note the faint soap bubble pattern and the additional destruction of the articular processes of C4 (compare with Fig. 12-38*C*). (*B* and *C*) Slight lateral and considerable anterior displacement of the right vertebral artery at the level of C5. (*D* and *E*) Frontal tomograms showing right lateral invasion of the body of C5 and the right inferior border of the body of C4.

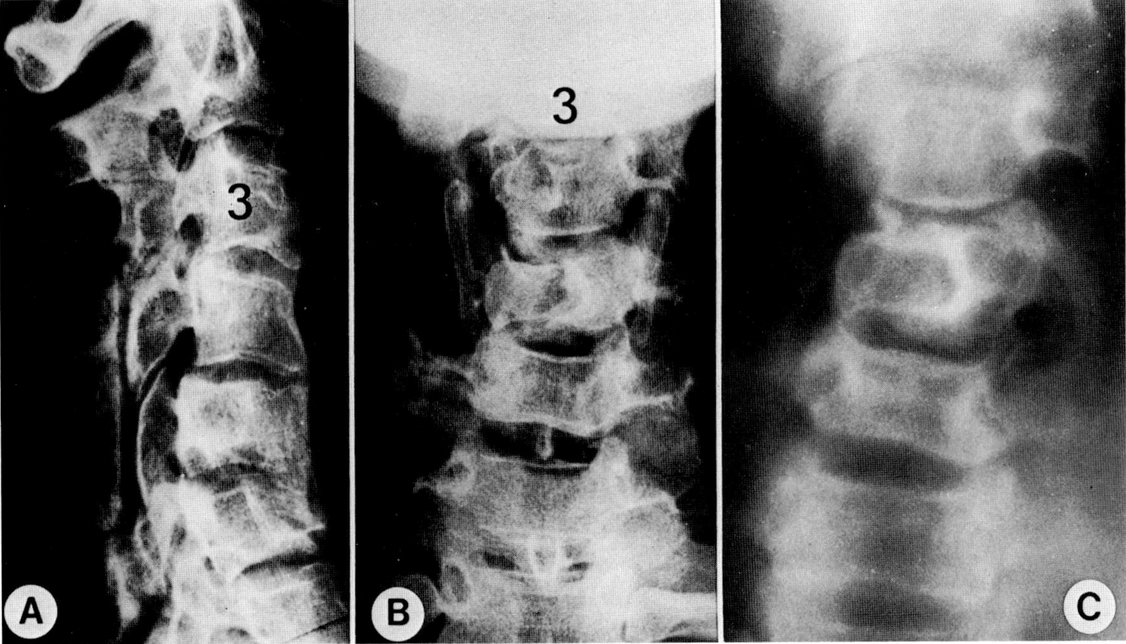

Fig. 12-40. Case 12. (*A*) The spontaneously developed bony bridge between the spinous processes of C4 and C6 was left intact. (*B*) Frontal view and (*C*) tomogram show remodeling of the body of C5.

derness was localized at the levels of the spinous processes of C5 and C7. The A–P roentgenogram showed an asymmetric enlargement of the basis of the spinous process of C6 (Fig. 12-43*A*, *arrows*). Its surrounding cortical layer was very thin. The profile roentgenogram (Fig. 12-43*C*) did not give much information, but the oblique view (Fig. 12-43*B*, *arrows*) showed the cystic lesion at the basis of the spinous process of C6. Its outline was denser inferiorly than superiorly. Vertebral angiography visualized a small tumor pattern supplied by a branch of the vertebral artery (Fig. 12-43*D* and *E*, *arrows*). Technetium phosphate scintigraphy showed increased uptake by the abnormality. There were no neurologic signs and symptoms.

November 1, 1977: Surgical exposure using the posterior approach revealed that the basis of the spinous process contained a soft grayish tumor extending in small adjacent portions of the laminae. The bony cortex was not perforated by the tumor. The spinous process and the laminae of C6 were removed. Diagnosis by the Netherlands Committee of Bone Tumours was "... tumor which bore a resemblance to a benign osteoblastoma as well as to an osteoid osteoma. Because of the presence of a great number of osteoblasts and the absence of sclerosing changes surrounding the nidus, the diagnosis of benign osteoblastoma was preferred." Since the operation the patient has been symptom free, and a roentgenogram taken 3 years after operation showed no signs of recurrence.

Case 19. A man of 47 suffered for 6 years from neck pains radiating to the head. Rotation of the head to the right became progressively limited. Physical examination revealed pronounced local tenderness of the superior lateral spine. A–P roentgenograms showed a translucent area in the region of the right transverse process and articular processes, bordered laterally by a bony shell (Fig. 12-44*A*). Medially there was intensive sclerosis. The oblique view showed an expanding bone lesion overlapping the intervertebral foramen of C3–C4 (Fig. 12-44*B*). There were no neural symptoms.

September 2, 1976: Using the right anterolateral approach, the transverse processes of C2 and C4 were exposed. The transverse process of C3 extended more laterally than the other transverse processes, thus producing kinking of the third spinal nerve at its exit from the neural groove. The lateral extremity of the transverse process, its

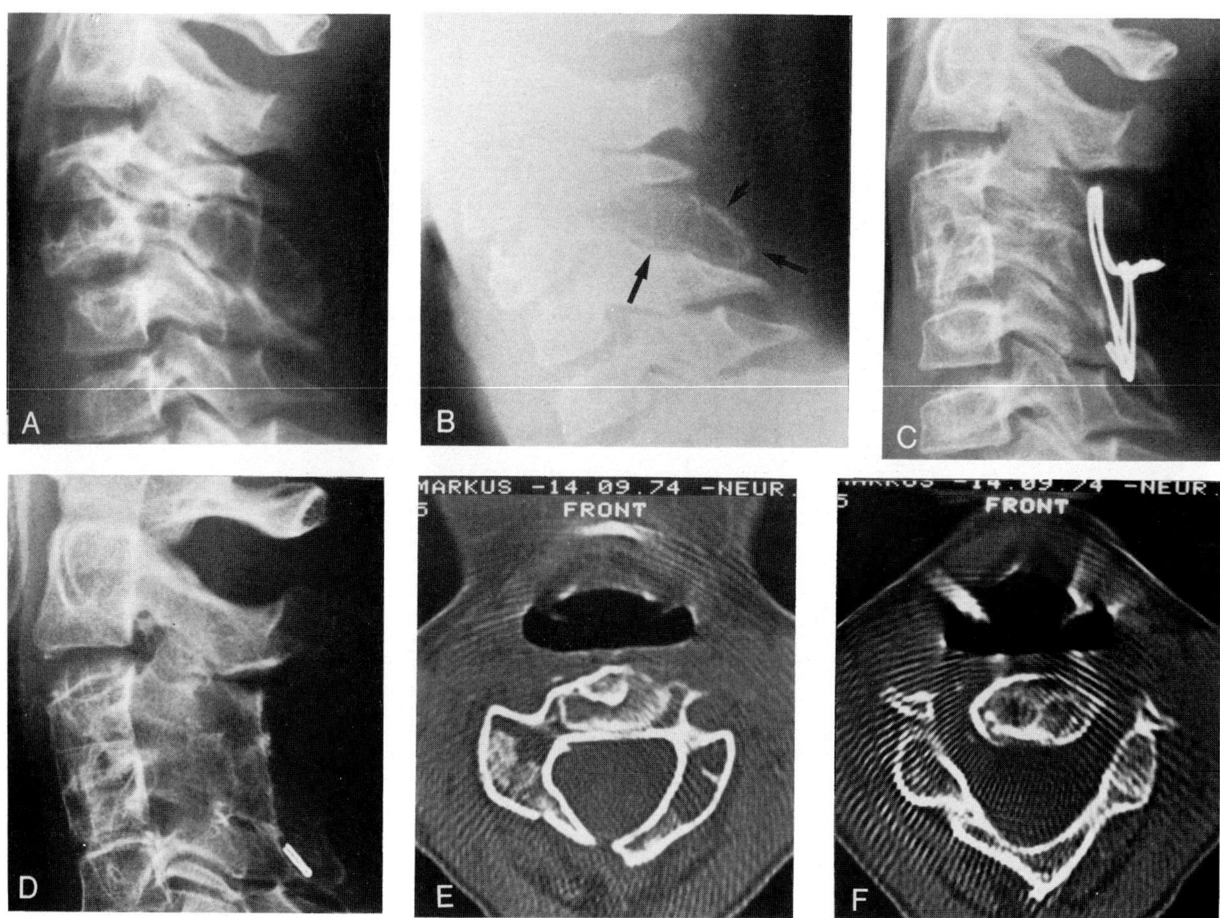

Fig. 12-41. Case 13. (*A*) Expansion of the spinous process of C4. Decreased density of its bony structure. The disc space C3–C4 is narrowed. Osteolysis in the upper position of the body of C4. (*B*) Arrows point to soap bubble structure of spinous process of C4. (*C*) One year after operation, block of bodies of C3 and C4 shows solid bony structure. (*D*) Three years after operation, wires have been removed. Ankylosis of apophyseal joints. (*E* and *F*) CT scans through upper and lower portions of the arch of C4 show a solid cortical surface and islands of transplanted bone chips.

cortical element, and the area of the uncus were thickened. Complete removal of these elements required uncusectomy. As the disc space was opened laterally, it was removed and replaced by a cortical interbody graft. The microscopic diagnosis was benign osteoblastoma.

Postoperative A–P roentgenograms showed disappearance of the bony abnormality, and the interbody graft between C3 and C4 (Fig. 12-44*C*). The oblique view no longer showed the abnormal shadow projecting over the intervertebral foramen of C3–C4 (Fig. 12-44*D*). The patient had no complaints.

Eosinophilic Granuloma

CASE 20. A 10-year-old boy presented with acute onset of neck pains accompanied by torticollis in December 1977. At admission on January 26, 1978, no neurologic disturbances were noted. The lateral roentgenogram showed a lytic lesion projecting in front of the spinous process of C3 (Fig. 12-45*A*). The oblique view showed a lytic lesion in

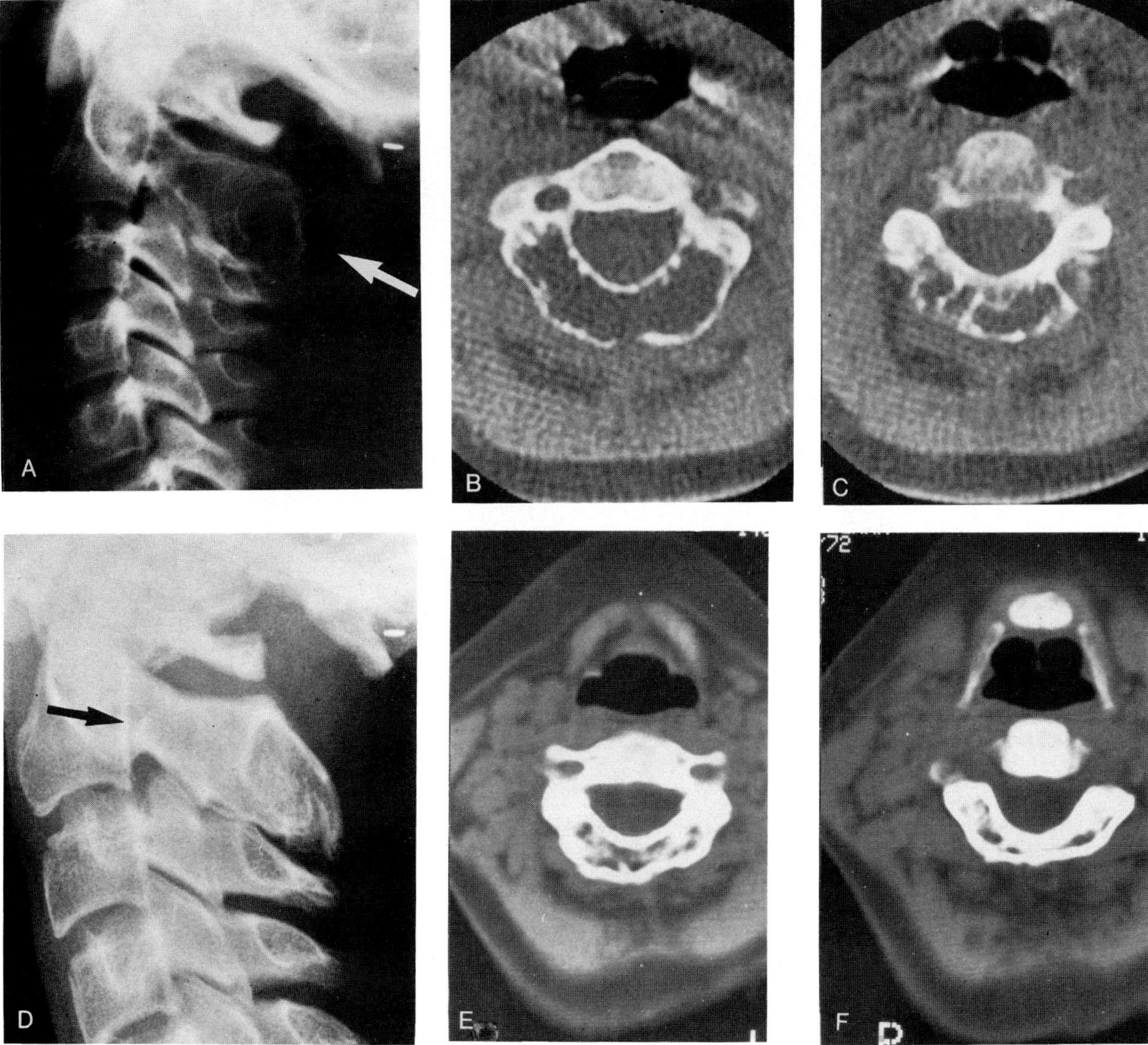

Fig. 12-42. Case 14. Expansion and marked osteolysis of the spinous process of C2 (*A*) confirmed in CT scans of upper (*B*) and lower (*C*) portions of the arch of C2. The cortex is eggshell thin and shows discontinuities (*B* and *C*). Complete osteolysis in the upper portion of the arch of C2 reaches as far as the pedicles (*B*), whereas residual bony trabeculae in lower portion of the arch produce a vacuolated appearance (*C*). One and one half years after operation the spinous process and laminae show normal structure (*D*), and CT scans show marked remodeling of cortical bony surfaces of the arch of C2 (*E* and *F*).

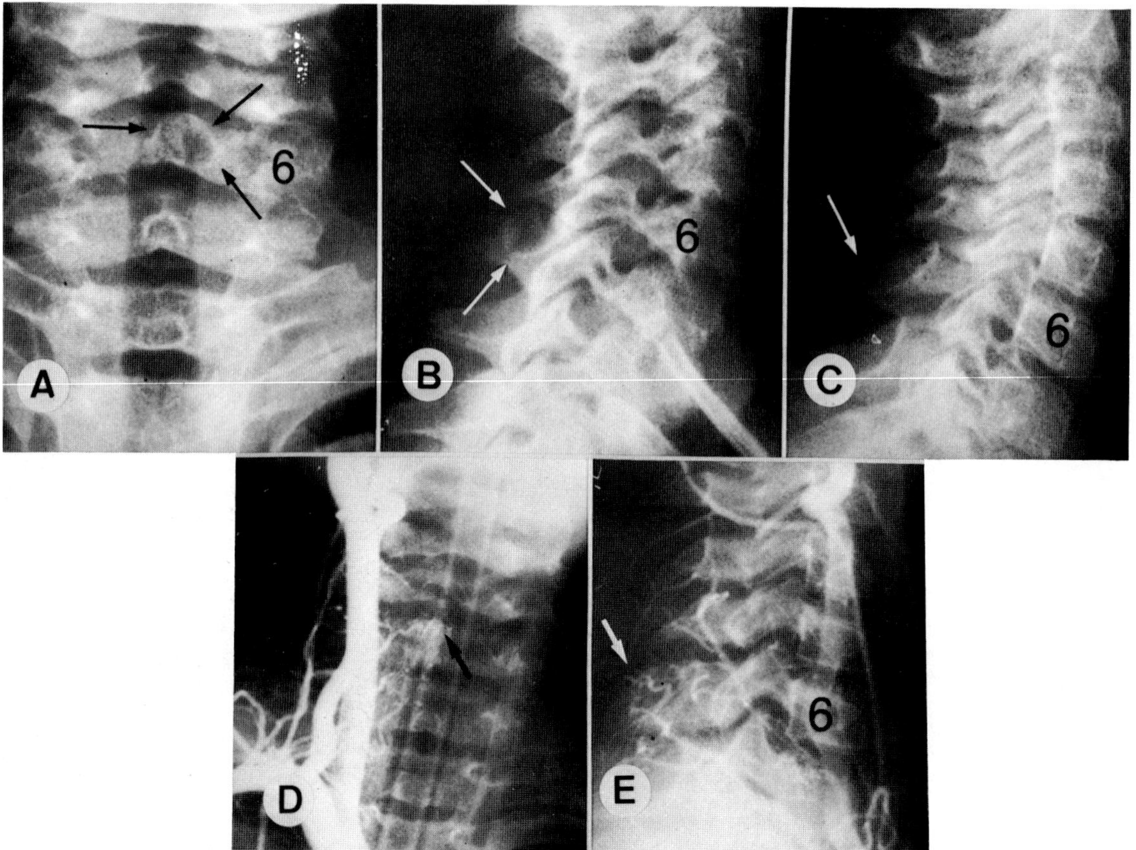

Fig. 12-43. Case 18. (*A*) A–P roentgenogram showing an asymmetric enlargement of the base of the spinous process of C6 (*arrows*). (*B*) Oblique view showing the cystic lesion at the base of the spinous process of C6. (*C*) Profile view. (*D* and *E*) Vertebral angiograms showing a small tumor pattern supplied by a branch of the vertebral artery (*arrows*).

the area of the right articular processes and the pedicle (Fig. 12-45*B*). CT scans showed hypodensic involvement of the right lamina, articular processes, and pedicle, and invasion of the lateral portion of the body of C3 (Fig. 12-46*A* through *F*). Vertebral angiography showed no abnormalities.

February 2, 1978: The transverse processes of C2 through C4 were exposed using the anterolateral approach. The foramina transversaria of C3 and C4 were opened. The lateral aspect of the body of C3 showed a cortical defect caused by a nonprotruding tumor mass. After removal of this tumor it appeared that it had been separated from the disc C3–C4 by the intact cortical end-plate only. The vertebral artery was encircled by a thin layer of tumor mass; this was removed. The articular processes were approached following upward retraction of the anterior primary ramus of the third spinal nerve. They were almost completely occupied by a cavity continuing into the right lamina of C3. All tumor mass was removed by curettage. The tumor had a grayish-red color. The cavity in the vertebral body was filled with iliac crest graft. The microscopic diagnosis was eosinophilic granuloma. The postoperative course was uneventful. Torticollis and pains disappeared. Control roentgenograms taken in August 1978 showed fusion of grafts inside the vertebral body. Cervical motion was normal.

CASE 21. In November 1968, a 14-year-old boy experienced the onset of neck pains radiating to the occipital region and left shoulder, followed in January 1969 by painful torticollis, with chin ro-

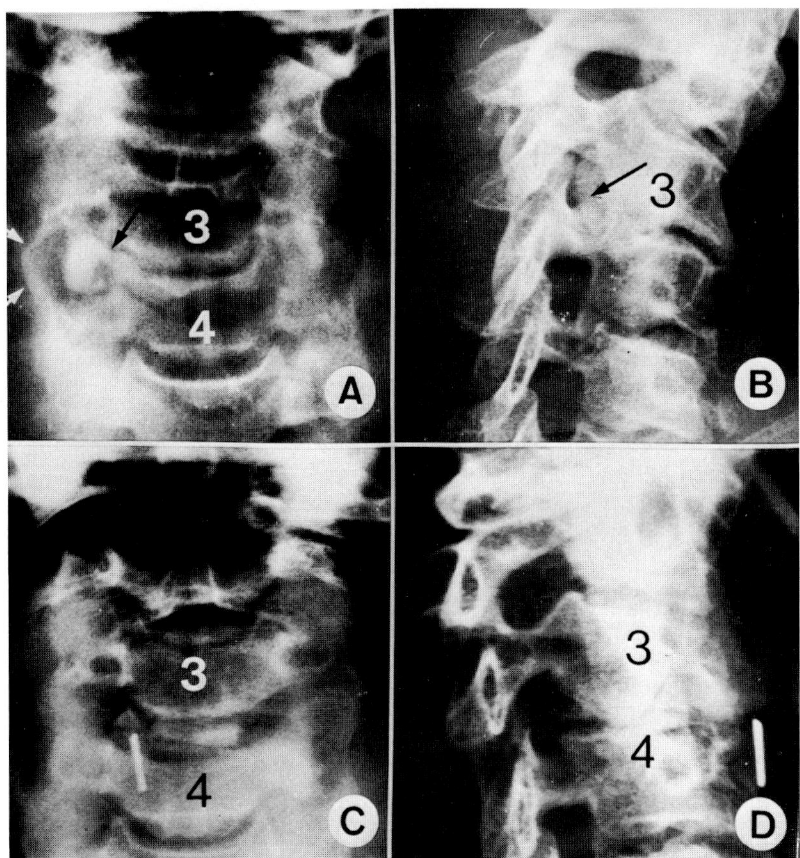

Fig. 12-44. Case 19. (*A*) A–P roentgenogram showing a translucent area in the region of the right transverse process and articular processes, bordered laterally by a bony shell. (*B*) Oblique view showing an expanding bone lesion overlapping the intervertebral foramen of C3–C4. (*C* and *D*) Complete removal of the lesion.

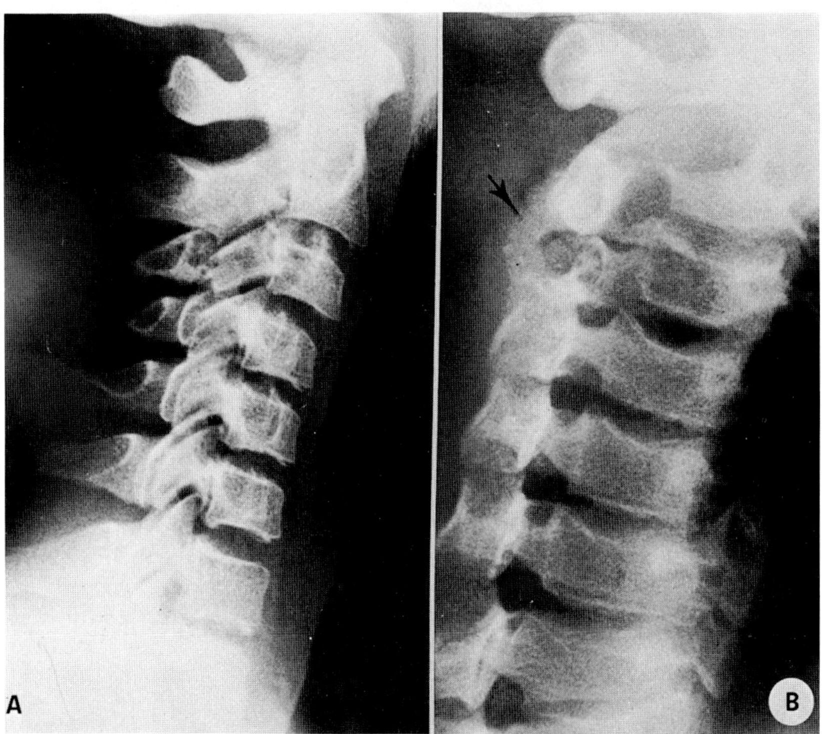

Fig. 12-45. Case 20. (*A*) Lateral roentgenogram showing a lytic lesion projecting in front of the spinous process of C3. (*B*) Oblique view showing a lytic lesion in the area of the right articular processes and the pedicle.

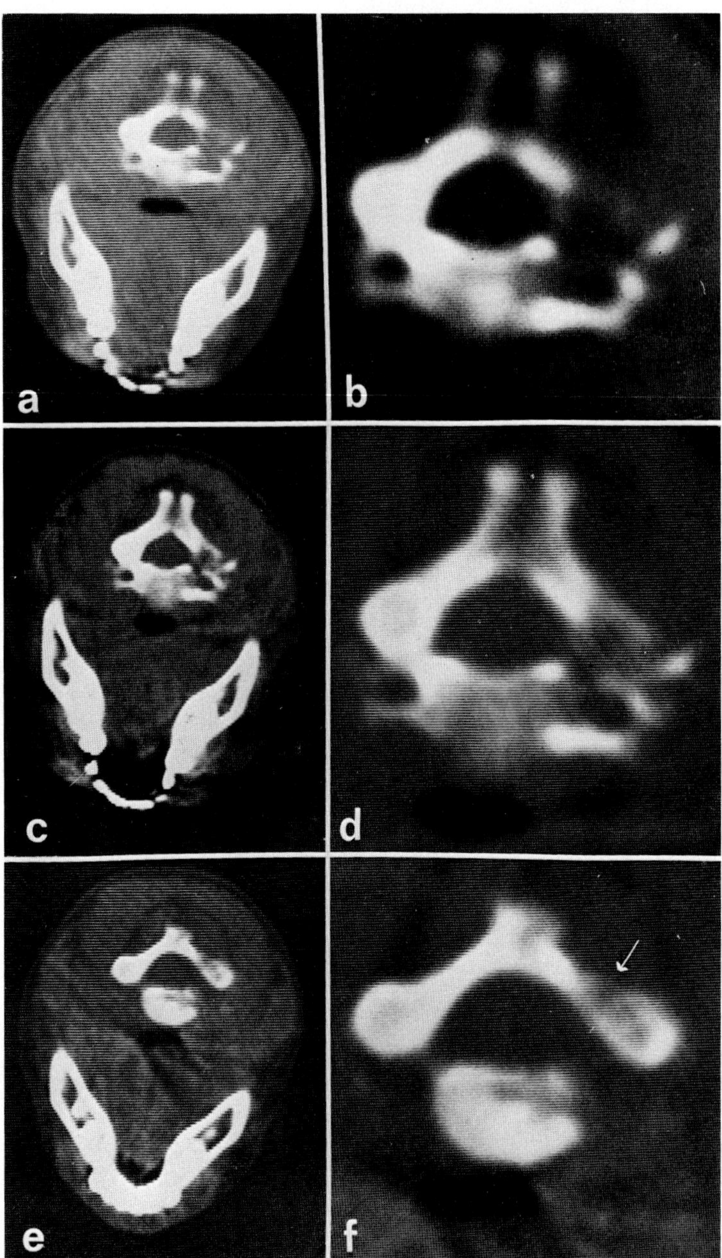

Fig. 12-46. Case 20. (*A* through *D*) CT scans showing hypodensic involvement of the right lamina (*B*), articular processes, and pedicle (*D*). (*E* and *F*) CT scans showing invasion of the lateral portion of the body of C3. The scans in the right column (*B, D,* and *F*) are magnifications of vertebrae in the left column scans (*A, C,* and *E*).

tated to the right. There were no neurologic disturbances. Roentgenograms showed collapse of the body of C3 and posterior dislocation of the C2 (Fig. 12-47*A*). Apart from signs of some interstitial pulmonary fibrosis and slightly reduced respiratory vital capacity, there were no other abnormalities. Needle biopsy (Turkel) from the C3 body yielded inconclusive findings. Vertebral angiograms were normal.

May 12, 1969: The right submandibular approach with skull traction was used. After division of the anterior longitudinal ligament, a cystic cavity inside the body of C3 was opened; its wall was formed by purple soft tissue. After removal of this tissue, the body of C3 appeared to have almost completely disappeared. Excision of the intervertebral discs C2–C3 and C3–C4 was performed. An iliac crest graft was inserted, replacing the body of

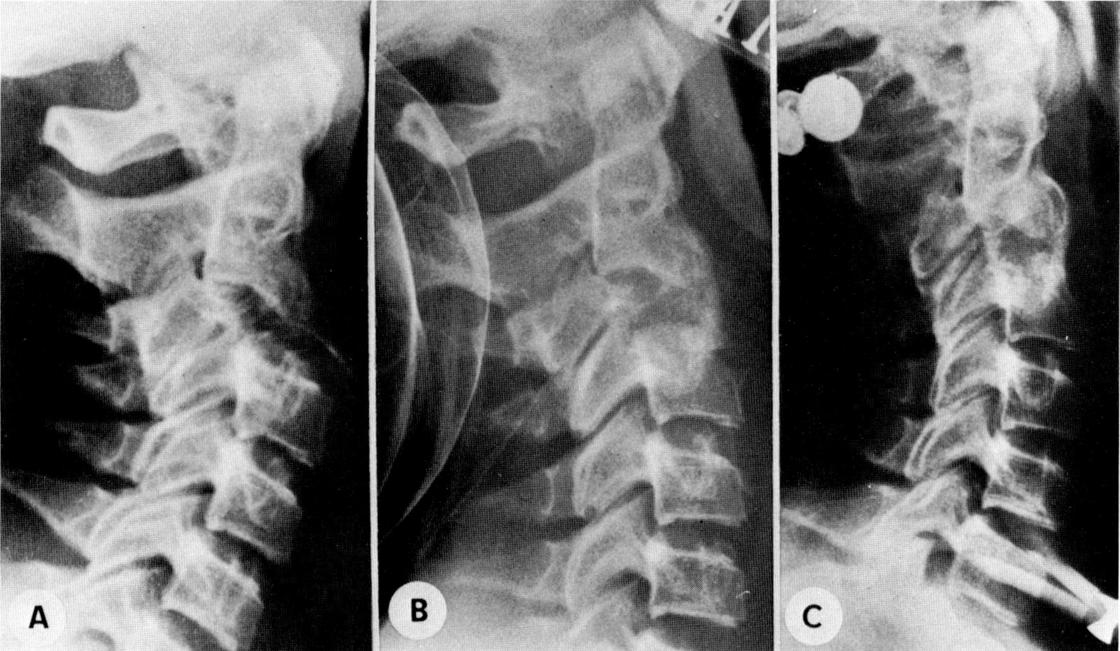

Fig. 12-47. Case 21. (*A*) Roentgenogram showing collapse of the body of C3 and posterior dislocation of C2. (*B*) An iliac crest graft was inserted, replacing the body of C3. (*C*) Roentgenogram 7 months after operation shows remodeling and fusion of the graft.

C3 (Fig. 12-47*B*). The microscopic diagnosis was eosinophilic granuloma.

Postoperative treatment consisted of skull traction for 3 weeks and 6 weeks of immobilization in bed, followed by mobilization with a cervical support for 3 months. Figure 12-47*C* shows remodeling and fusion of the graft 7 months after operation. No disturbances and no signs of recurrence in the radiographs were noted at the 5-year follow-up.

Benign Solitary Plasmocytoma

Case 22. A 30-year-old woman suffered from neck pains for 2 years before admission. She developed quadriplegia in the last 3 months. Figure 12-48*A* and *B* show collapse of the body of C5 and lytic lesion in its posterior element. Vertebral angiography was not performed at that time in tumor cases. (Some important data are discussed in the first section, Comparative Data on Benign and Malignant Tumors.)

First operation, October 13, 1952: Using the right anterolateral approach, the body of C5 was removed and the anterior portion of the transverse processes was resected, freeing the vertebral artery from surrounding bone. The microscopic diagnosis was plasmocytoma with no atypism of plasma cells and a rich framework of stroma.

Because of our lack of experience, the patient was immobilized in bed for 4 months. In this period, all neurologic disturbances disappeared. The anterior borders of the bodies of C4 and C6 had contacted each other with resulting kyphosis.

Second operation, April 2, 1953: Using the posterior approach, the laminae and articular processes of C5 and of the underlying epidural tumor mass were resected. Posterior fusion from C4 through C7 was accomplished with two tibial grafts. Roentgenograms were taken 1 year and 9 years after operation (Fig. 12-48*C* and *D*). The patient was doing well 27 years after operation, without neurologic or radiologic signs of recurrence. Figure 12-48*E* through *H* shows radiographs taken 17 years after the operation.

Chondromyxoid Fibroma

Chondromyxoid fibroma, a rare tumor that occurs most frequently in the lower limbs, has also been reported in the spine. It occurs mainly in the younger age groups. Of 24 cases of the Nether-

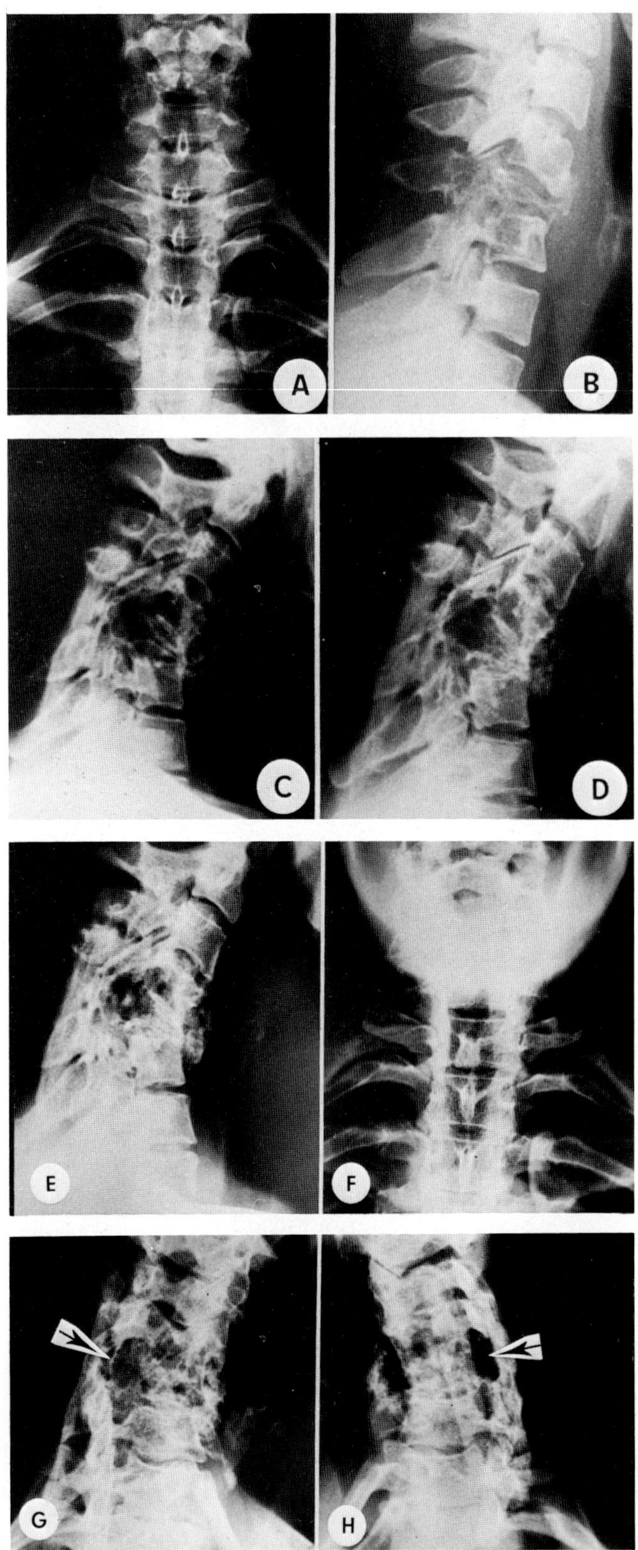

Fig. 12-48. Case 22. (*A* and *B*) Preoperative radiographs showing collapse of the body of C5 and lytic lesion in its posterior element. (*C*) Radiograph 1 year after operation. (*D*) Radiograph 9 years after operation (*E, F, G,* and *H*) Radiographs taken 17 years after operation.

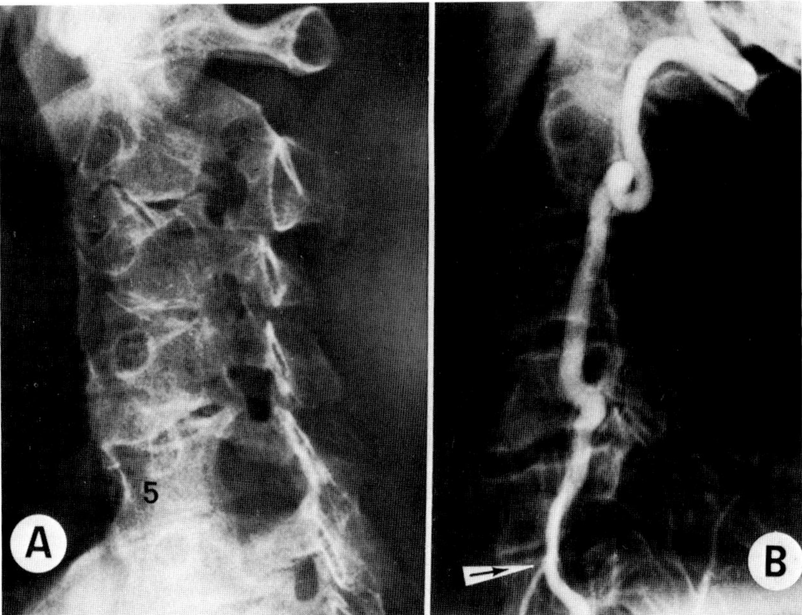

Fig. 12-49. Case 23. (*A*) Roentgenogram showing block vertebrae C5–C6 and enlargement of the left intervertebral foramen C5–C6. (*B*) Roentgenogram showing anterior displacement of the vertebral artery at C5–C6.

lands Committee of Bone Tumours, only three patients were older than 25 years (37, 40, and 54 years).[14] Case 23 is interesting because of the patient's advanced age and the tumor's localization in the cervical spine, its presentation as a dumbbell tumor, and its malignant degeneration 7 years after the first operation.[17]

CASE 23. A 59-year-old man developed loss of power in his legs and left arm of 1 year's duration before his admission on February 2, 1968. X-ray films showed block vertebrae C5–C6, enlargement of the left intervertebral foramen of C5–C6 (Fig. 12-49*A*), and anterior displacement of the vertebral artery at this level (Fig. 12-49*B*). Figure 12-50 shows a lytic lesion at the left side of the cervical spine with destruction of portions of the articular processes of C5 and C6 and erosion of the adjacent lateral borders of the bodies of C5 and C6.

First operation, March 4, 1968: Using the anterolateral approach, the vertebral artery was exposed followed resection of the anterior and lateral borders of the foramina transversaria of C5 and C6. A large encapsulated tumor was exposed. Incision of the capsule and evacuation of the crumbled grayish tumor mass allowed the collapse of the capsule and its separation from the vertebral artery. The primary rami of the C6 nerve had completely disappeared inside the tumor. The tumor was very adherent to the borders of the enlarged intervertebral foramen, necessitating sharp dissec-

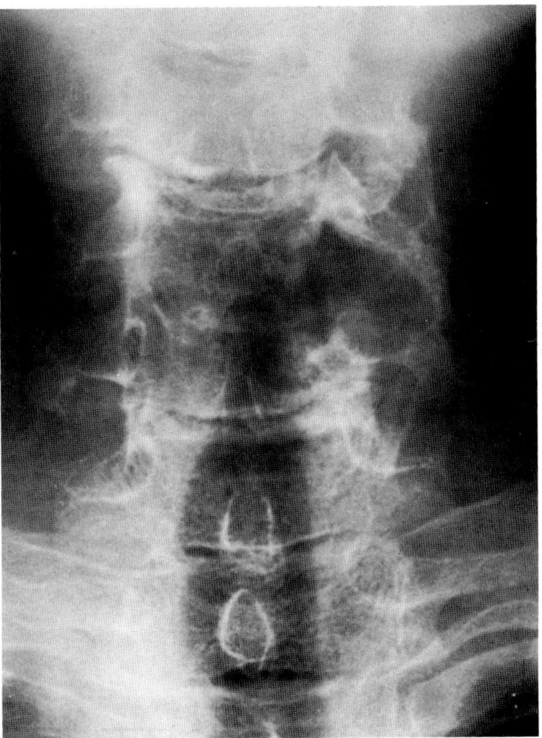

Fig. 12-50. Case 23. Roentgenogram of a lytic lesion of the left side of the cervical spine with destruction of portions of the articular processes of C5 and C6 and erosion of the adjacent lateral borders of the bodies of C5 and C6.

tion. Its intraspinal portion could be separated from the root pouch close to the dural theca. The microscopic diagnosis was chondromyxoid fibroma. There was rapid recovery of power in the legs and left arm with residual weakness of extension of the left arm and finger movements. The patient did well until August 1972, 4 years after the operation, when he developed a weakness of the entire left arm and hypaesthesia of the left hand. The roentgenograms showed more enlargement of the left intervertebral foramen than seen in 1968, but no other changes. Laminectomy was indicated in our opinion.

Second operation, October 10, 1972: The posterior approach was used. Tumor mass had invaded the posterior cervical muscles at C5–C6. The left laminae at this level were infiltrated by the tumor, which also extended at the left epidural space. The articular processes of C5 and C6 had been destroyed. The tumor was removed as far as it was visible. The microscopic diagnosis was chondromyxoid fibroma. The power of the left arm improved incompletely after the operation.

In January 1974, the patient experienced rapid loss of power in the left arm and some loss of power in the feet.

Third operation, February 2, 1974: The posterior approach was used again. There was recurrence of tumor in the posterior cervical muscles and epidural spread from C3 to C7, which was removed following laminectomy and resection of the left pedicles and articular processes, which were also involved by tumor. Removal of the tumor was decompressive but incomplete. The microscopic diagnosis was chondromyxosarcoma, Grade I. The power of the left arm did not improve, and the patient's gait was spastic. He resumed his work in June 1974.

February 1975: The patient experienced progressive loss of power in his arms and legs. X-ray examination showed a mottled appearance of the cervical vertebrae from C2 to C7. There was paralysis of the left diaphragm. The patient urgently requested surgery.

Fourth operation, February 26, 1975: Posterior approach was used. There was tumor recurrence in the left paraspinal region extending in front of the dural theca, which we removed by curettage. Microscopic examination revealed chondrosarcoma. In the first few days after the operation there was a rapid recovery of power in the right arm and both legs. Nine days after the operation, quadriplegia developed in 1.5 hours, accompanied by respiratory distress. Lumbar puncture showed manometric block. Because of the possibility of a late postoperative extradural hematoma, the wound was reopened. No hematoma was found, but the cavity left after the last operation was completely occupied by fresh tumor mass. The patient died the next day.

Desmoid Tumors

See the discussion in the first section, Comparative Data on Benign and Malignant Tumors.

CASE 24. A girl of 11 suffered from neck pains radiating to the right shoulder since November 1976. The patient developed torticollis (chin turned to the right). She elevated the shoulder for pain relief. There were no neurologic disturbances.

Radiographs showed progressive erosion of the posterior inferior portion of the body of C6 (Fig. 12-51*A*, Dec. 1976; Fig. 12-51*B*, Jan. 1977). A frontal tomogram through the bodies of C6 and C7 (Fig. 12-51*C*, Jan. 1977) showed a hypodensity in the lateral position of the body of C6 (*arrow*), a deformity in the lateral aspect of the body of C7 (*arrow*), and possibly osseous changes in the right transverse process of C6. Myelography showed a minor deformity of the right C7 root pouch. The right vertebral angiogram showed an abnormal vascular network in the right paraspinal region from about C5 to T1 (Fig. 12-52*A* and *B*).

February 1, 1977: Using the right anterolateral approach, the right transverse processes of C5 and C6 were exposed. After resection of the anterior rims of their foramina, the vertebral artery was found to be surrounded by a firm brownish membrane, which also covered the anterior sheath of the C7 spinal nerve. The abnormal tissue could be completely removed. The articular processes were not involved. The eroded lateral inferior border of the body of C6 was removed. The body of C7 was not invaded. As the disc space C6–C7 was opened laterally, its content was removed by way of the lateral surgical defect. No interbody graft was applied. The microscopic diagnosis was a desmoid tumor.

March 22, 1977: The patient had no pains, but a slight residual torticollis remained.

February 24, 1978: There was no torticollis, no pains, normal head movements, and remodeling of the body of C6 (Fig. 12-53*A* and *B*). Four years after operation there were no signs of recurrence.

CASE 25. A 61-year-old woman presented with neck pains and torticollis toward the right, of 6

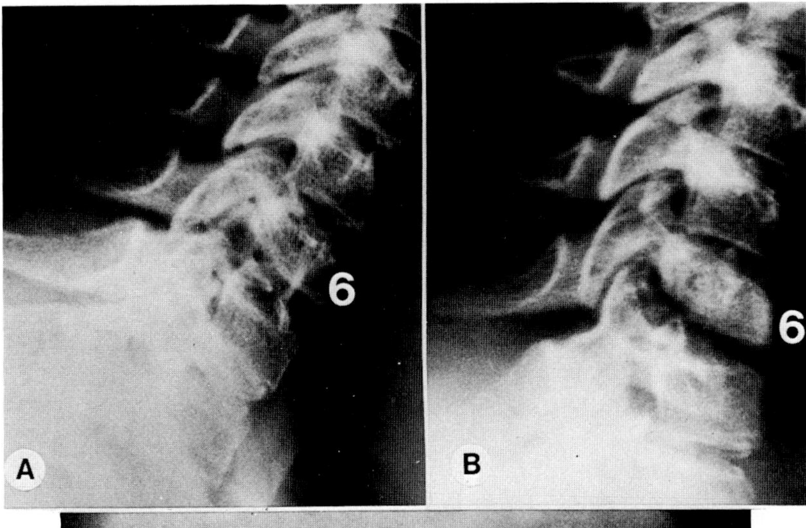

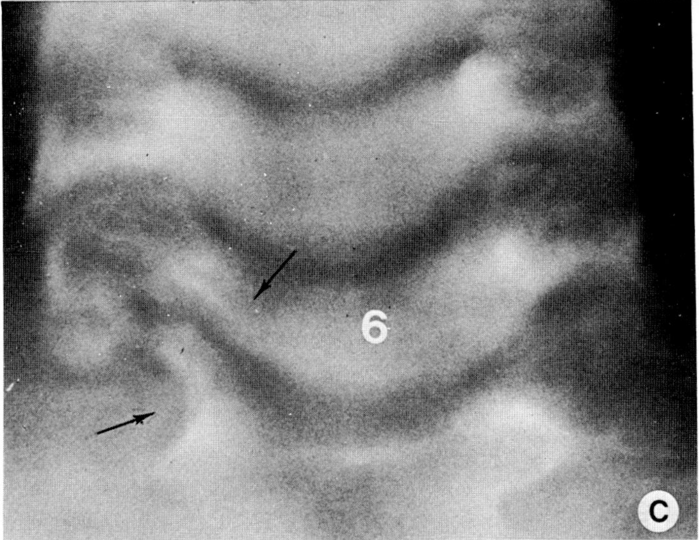

Fig. 12-51. Case 24. (*A* and *B*) Roentgenograms showing progressive erosion of the posteroinferior portion of the body of C6. (*C*) Frontal tomogram through the bodies of C6 and C7 showing a hypodensity in the lateral portion of the body of C6 (*arrow*), a deformity in the lateral aspect of the body of C7 (*arrow*), and the possible osseous changes in the right transverse process of C6.

weeks' duration. The day before admission she was temporarily unconscious with urinary incontinence. The patient also suffered from diabetes, urinary infection, and ventricular extrasystoles.

The patient was admitted on June 10, 1977. No neurologic disturbances were evident. The profile roentgenogram showed posterior dislocation of the anterior arch of the atlas (Fig. 12-54*A*, *upper arrow*) and erosion of the anterior surface of the odontoid. A frontal tomogram (Fig. 12-54*B*, *arrow*) showed erosion of the odontoid and irregular interruption of its attachment to C2. Carotid and vertebral angiograms were normal. Technetium phosphate scintigraphy showed slightly increased uptake in a transverse band-shaped area in the atlantooccipital region. Transoral needle biopsy was performed using a Turkel needle; the tissue removed did not allow a microscopic diagnosis.

July 11, 1977: A right submandibular incision was used, extending posteriorly to the mastoid process and inferiorly along the anterior border of the sternocleidomastoid muscle. We exposed the transverse processes of C1 and C2 and the vertebral artery up to the foramen magnum. After resection of the anterior arch of the atlas, we encountered a grayish nonencapsulated tissue mass. After removal of this mass the eroded odontoid was exposed. It was almost completely separated from the body of C2 by tumor mass. We removed the odontoid. The tumor reached to the dura. For complete decompression, the inferior portion of the clivus and a medial portion of the body of C2

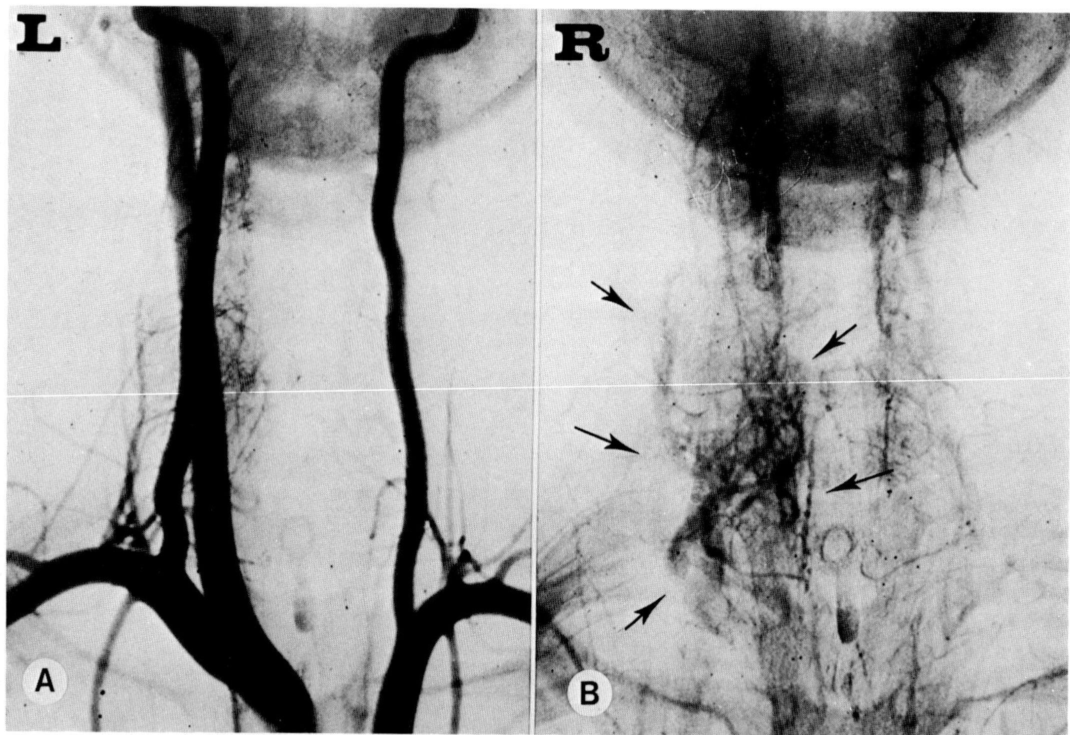

Fig. 12-52. Case 24. (*A* and *B*) Right vertebral angiograms showing an abnormal vascular network in the right paraspinal region from about C5 to T1.

had to be removed. The first 3 days after the operation were uneventful.

July 14, 1977: Tachycardia and oxygen undersaturation of the blood occurred. Artificial respiration was applied. The patient died the next day.

Autopsy findings included spontaneous pneumothorax and meningotheliomatous meningioma of the anterior cranial fossa. There were arteriosclerotic malacic areas in the brain stem. Coronary sclerosis and renal arteriosclerosis were observed. Residual abnormal tissue in the atlantooccipital region as well as the surgical specimens showed the microscopic picture of fibromatosis. No metastases were found. The desmoid tumor was labeled as aggressive fibromatosis (see the first section, Benign Tumors).

Vertebral Hemangioma

See also Diagnostic Aids: Transosseous Phlebography.

CASE 26. A 25-year-old man presented with a common type of mainly venous and cavernous hemangioma. Figure 12-55*A* shows typical vertical trabeculation of the body of C4; Figure 12-55*B* shows massive staining of the body of C4 with considerable venous outflow.

Figure 12-56*A*, a subtraction of a right vertebral angiogram, shows a vascular branch ascending beyond the fourth vertebral body. Vessels stained black in Figure 12-56*A* are white in Figure 12-56*B* because *B* is a subtraction of a later phase of the vertebral angiogram from *A*. The black-stained branch is filled in *B* but ends at the level of C5–C6. The hemangioma is not supplied by the right vertebral artery.

In Figure 12-56*C* and *D*, a branch of the left vertebral artery ramifies in front of the body of C4. It is white stained in Figure 12-56*D*, but a more recently black-stained vascular branch ends in a vascular nidus with a few ramifications at the level of the body of C4. A mainly cavernous and venous hemangioma with limited arterial supply from the left vertebral artery was the diagnosis.

Cartilaginous Exostoses

Cartilaginous exostoses are also known as osteochondrial exostoses or osteochondroma.[1,5,27]

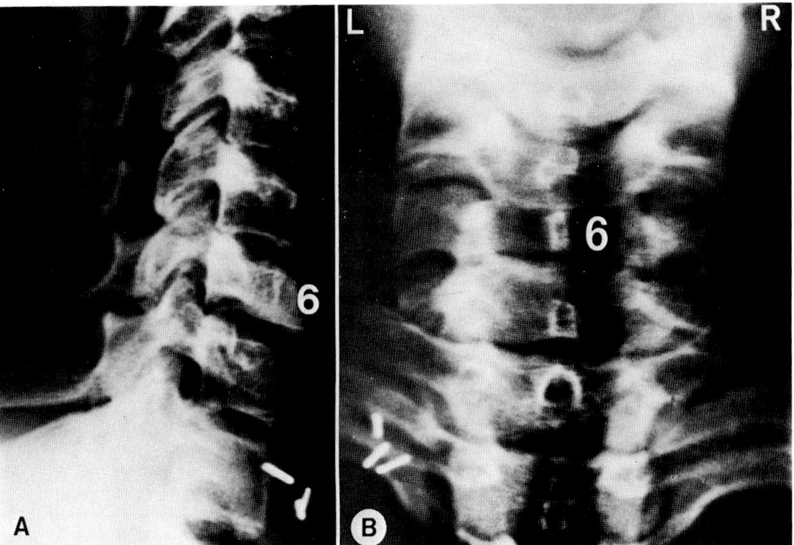

Fig. 12-53. Case 24. (*A* and *B*) Postoperative roentgenograms showing remodeling of body of C6.

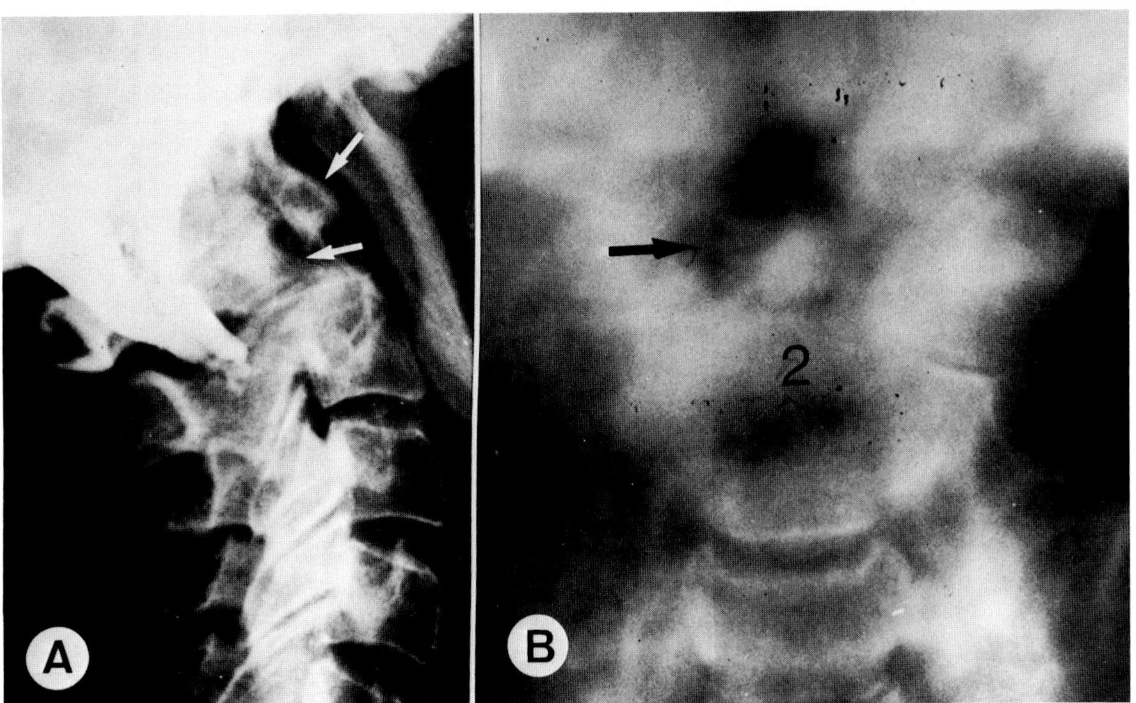

Fig. 12-54. Case 25. (*A*) Profile roentgenogram showing posterior dislocation of the anterior arch of the atlas (*upper arrow*) and erosion of the anterior surface of the odontoid (*lower arrow*). (*B*) Frontal tomogram showing erosion of the odontoid and irregular interruption of its attachment to C2 (*arrow*).

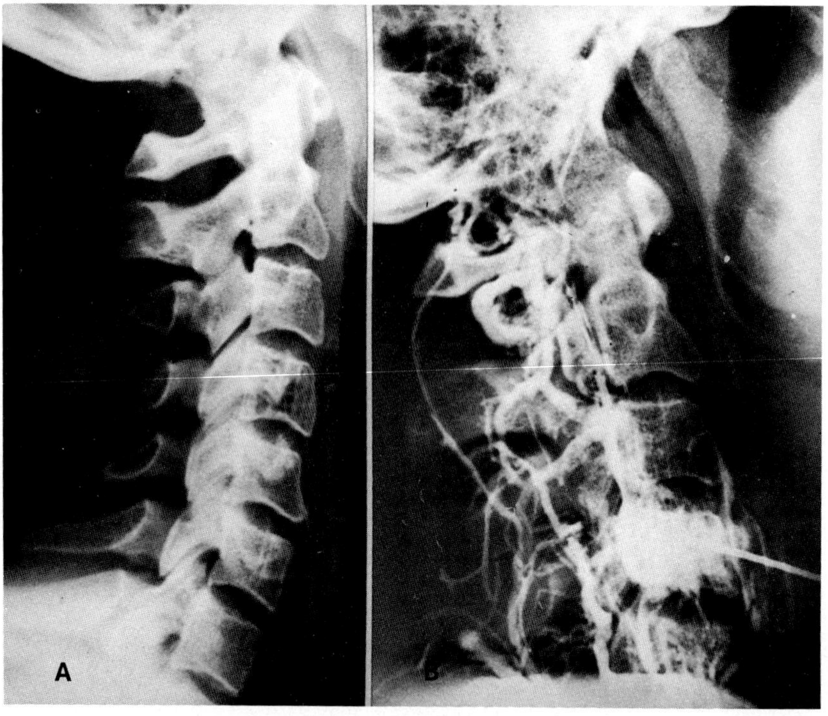

Fig. 12-55. Case 26. (*A*) Roentgenogram showing typical vertical trabeculation of the body of C4. (*B*) Percutaneous anterior transosseous phlebogram showing massive staining of the body of C4 with considerable venous outflow.

Case 27. A woman of 51 presented with multiple left-sided cartilaginous exostoses of the transverse processes of C4, C5, C6, and C7. The patient suffered for 25 years from paresthesias in the left little and ring fingers, and for 2 years from left-sided brachialgia. Two months before admission, she developed weakness of the left arm.

The patient was admitted on August 20, 1974, with painful flexion and extension of the head and weakness of all muscles of the left arm with depressed tendon reflexes. Hypoesthesia was evident in the area of C6 and C7. Figure 12-57*A* shows the exostoses of the left transverse processes of C4 through C7; view *B* shows narrowing of the left intervertebral foramina of C6–C7 and C7–T1. Figure 12-57*C*, shows complete occlusion of the vertebral artery from its onset to C3, where it is filled by collateral circulation through the deep and ascending cervical arteries. Figure 12-57*D* is a profile view of the left vertebral angiogram.

September 6, 1974: The left anterolateral approach was used. After retraction of the phrenic nerve the entire anterior scalenus muscle was resected. The anterior rami of the spinal nerves had been very compressed between the exostotic transverse processes posteriorly and the fibrous strands bridging the attachments of the anterior scalenus muscle anteriorly. The hyperostotic portions were removed (Fig. 12-57*E*). Cartilaginous masses were encountered at the junctions of the costal elements of the transverse processes with the vertebral bodies. The intervertebral foramina of C6–C7 and C7–T1 were narrowed. Anterior foraminal decompression was performed by means of a drill. Microscopic examination of the material removed showed normal structure of cartilage and bone. The postoperative course and rehabilitation were complicated by a pronounced left-sided shoulder-hand syndrome. One year later the patient had completely recovered power and mobility of the left arm.

Osteoma or Hyperostoses

In both conditions osteoblastic activity may be found at microscopic examination, but sometimes no such activity is found. Basically, no unanimously accepted definition exists to differentiate between conditions that should be classified as osteomas and those that should be classified as hyperostoses. Because of the increased bone volume in these conditions, both have a place in the discussion of benign tumors of the spine. Our experience covers three cases of hyperostosis or osteoma of the cervical spine. In two patients, hyperostosis resulted

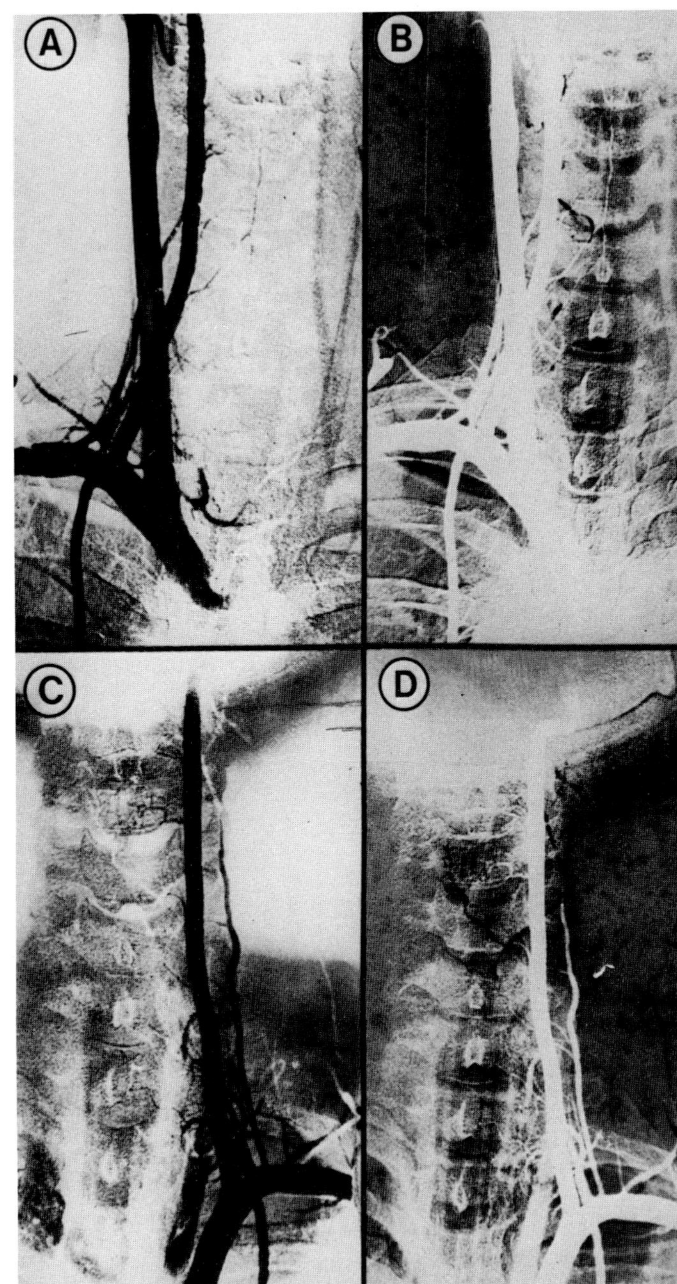

Fig. 12-56. Case 26. (*A*) Subtraction of early phase of right retrograde vertebral angiogram showing vascular branch ascending beyond the fourth vertebral body. (*B*) Subtraction from angiogram *A*, taken 1 second later, shows that the vascular branch ends at the level of C5–C6. (*C* and *D*) Subtractions from left vertebral angiograms showing the branch of the left vertebral artery ramifying in front of the body of C4.

in the increase of the volume of bony vertebral structures without loss of their characteristic shape. In Case 28, the pedicles were thickened, producing compression and a deficit of cervical nerve roots. The condition was combined with an exostosis, which may be classified as a tumorous outgrowth, an osteoma in the strict sense. In Case 30, the uncus was hyperostotic without loss of its original shape. In Case 29, the articular processes had increased in volume without loss of their original shape, but the fusion between the laminae was abnormal. Although this type of fusion may be attributed to abnormal bone formation, a congenital fusion of the laminae cannot be excluded with

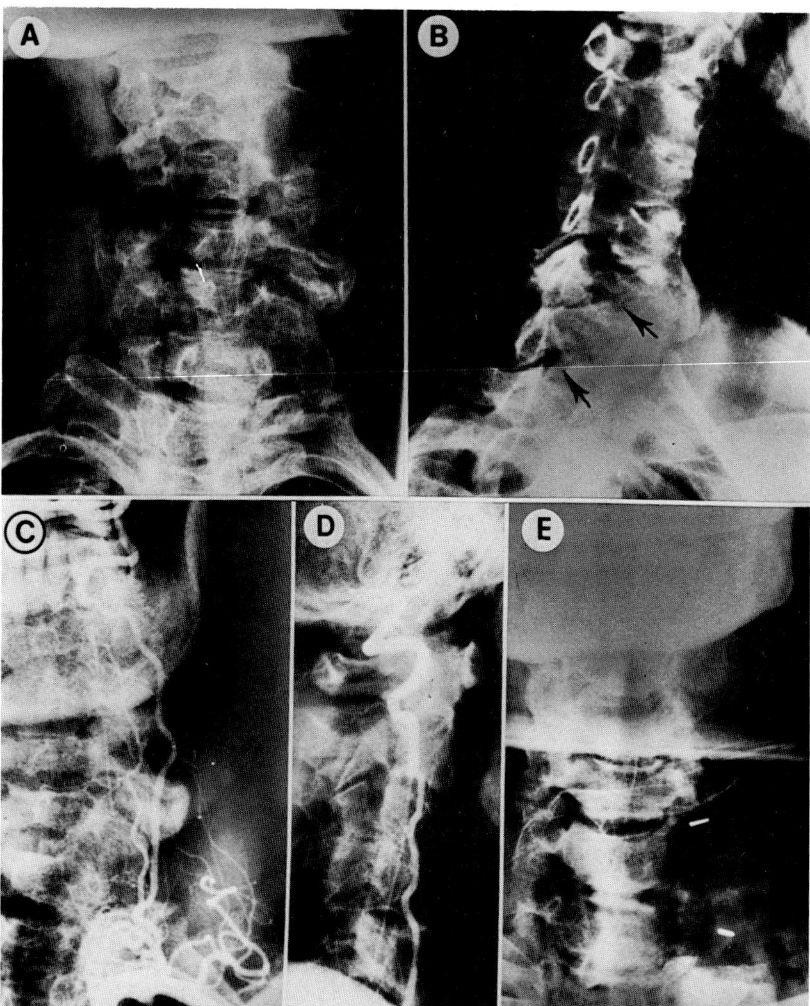

Fig. 12-57. Case 27. (*A*) Roentgenogram showing the exostoses of the left transverse processes of C4 through C7. (*B*) Oblique view showing narrowing of the left intervertebral foramina C6–C7 and C7–T1. (*C*) Left vertebral angiogram showing complete occlusion of the vertebral artery from its onset onto C3, where it is filled by collateral circulation through the deep and ascending cervical arteries. (*D*) left vertebral angiogram profile view. (*E*) Postoperative radiograph showing the removal of the transverse processes C4 through C7.

certainty. In none of the three patients did the microscopic examination of the abnormal bone reveal abnormal osteoblastic activity or other abnormal features.

CASE 28. A man of 72 suffered from periods of weakness of his right hand in the years 1975 and 1976 until his hands became permanently paralyzed in December 1976. He waited another 8 months before he visited his general practitioner.

The patient was admitted on August 31, 1977. All neck movements were very limited. There was pronounced atrophy of all hand muscles, thoracic scoliosis, and cervical spondylarthrosis. The bodies of C6 and C7 presented a large exostosis extending in front and right laterally. There was considerable thickening of the pedicles of C5 and C6 (Fig. 12-58*A*, *arrows*) and exostosis of the body (Fig. 12-58*B*).

September 7, 1977: Using the anterolateral approach, the lateral extension of the exostosis was removed; it had enclosed the anterior rims of the foramina transversaria and displaced the vertebral artery backward. The intervertebral foramina of C5–C6 and C6–C7 were decompressed by removal of thickened portions of the pedicles of C5 and C6 (Fig. 12-58*B*, *arrows*). Microscopic examination showed a normal structure of bone removed. No improvement of the hand muscles was noted in the year following the operation but when seen four years later they had considerably recovered.

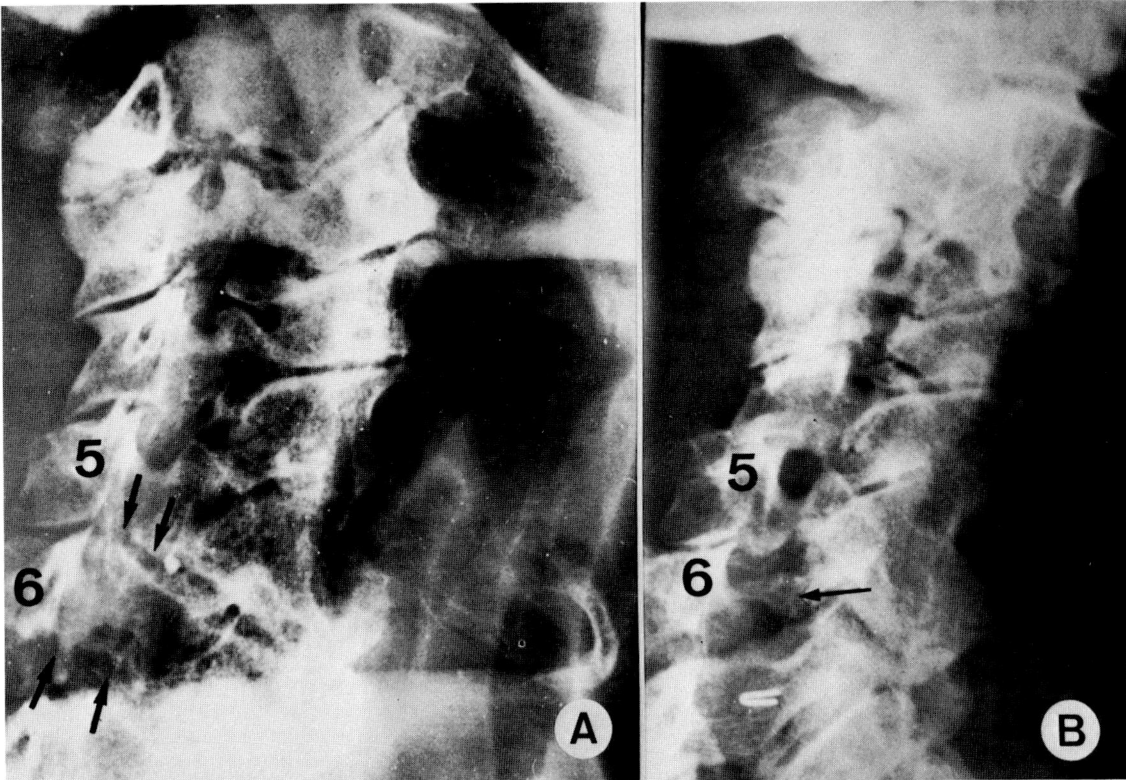

Fig. 12-58. Case 28. (*A*) Oblique roentgenogram showing considerable thickening of the pedicles of C5 and C6 completely occluding the intervertebral foramina C5–C6 and C6–C7 (*arrows*). (*B*) Roentgenogram showing exostosis of the body. The intervertebral foramina C5–C6 and C6–C7 are decompressed.

CASE 29. A 38-year-old man complained of neck pains of a few months' duration. Extension and rotation of the head to the right became limited. A hard swelling could be left in the right side of the nape of the neck. There were no neurologic disturbances. Vertebral angiograms were normal. The A–P roentgenogram showed only some right lateral protrusion of the posterior joints of C3 and C4 (Fig. 12-59*A*, *arrows*). The lateral tomogram showed considerable enlargement of the inferior articular process of C3 and the articular processes of C4 (Fig. 12-59*C*). Lateral tomograms taken more medially showed a bony bridge between the right laminae of C3 and C4 (Figs. 12-59*D* and *E*). The myelogram showed narrowing of the vertebral canal at C3–C4 (Fig. 12-59*B*); arrows point at tumor mass. The lesion had produced a slight kyphosis between the bodies of C3 and C4, with more flattening of the disc space anteriorly (Figs. 12-59*B*, *D*, and *E*).

April 4, 1975: Using a combined posterior and right anterolateral approach, laminectomy of C3 and C4 was performed, including the bony bridge between the right laminae and removal of the articular facets involved. No abnormality was found outside the abnormal bony structures, which were particularly soft. No cartilage lining was in the region of the posterolateral joints. Next, interbody fusion was performed between C3 and C4 by means of a wedge-shaped tibial cortical graft, because of the presence of kyphosis and possible instability following the removal of the right facet joints. Microscopic examination of the bone removed showed normal bone structure and osteoblast activity; the bone narrow showed no abnormalities. Figure 12-60*A* shows laminectomy defect and interbody graft 3 months after operation. Figure 12-60*B* is the same view taken 4 years after the operation; it shows solid fusion of the graft. There were no signs of recurrence of the exostosis.

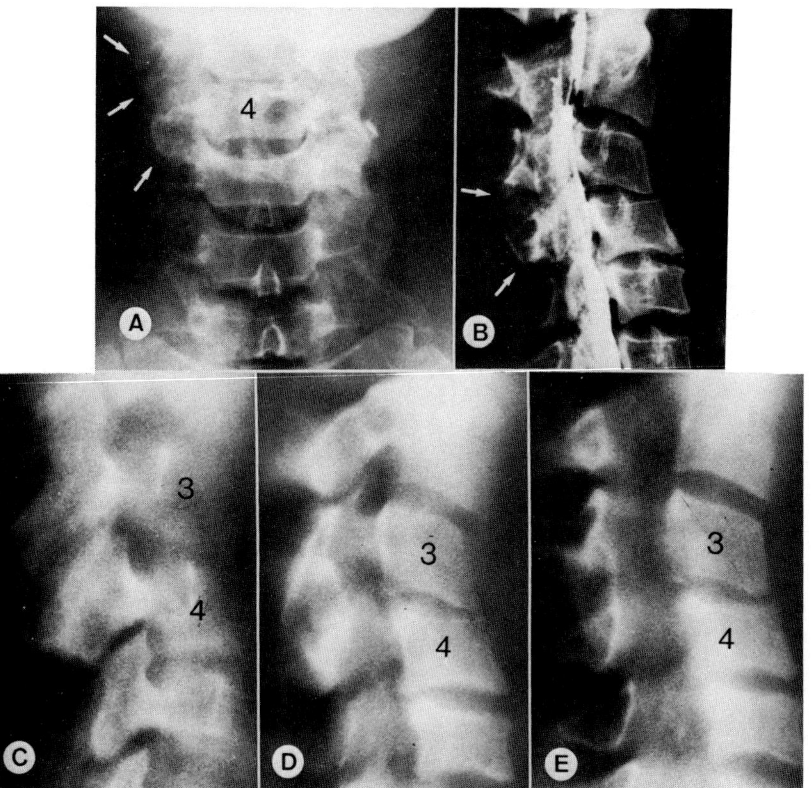

Fig. 12-59. Case 29. (*A*) A–P roentgenogram showing right lateral protrusion of the posterior joints of C3 and C4. (*B*) Myelogram showing narrowing of the vertebral canal at C3–C4. Arrows point to tumor mass. (*C*) Lateral tomogram showing considerable enlargement of the inferior articular processes of C4. (*D* and *E*) Lateral tomograms taken more medially showing a bony bridge between the right laminae of C3 and C4.

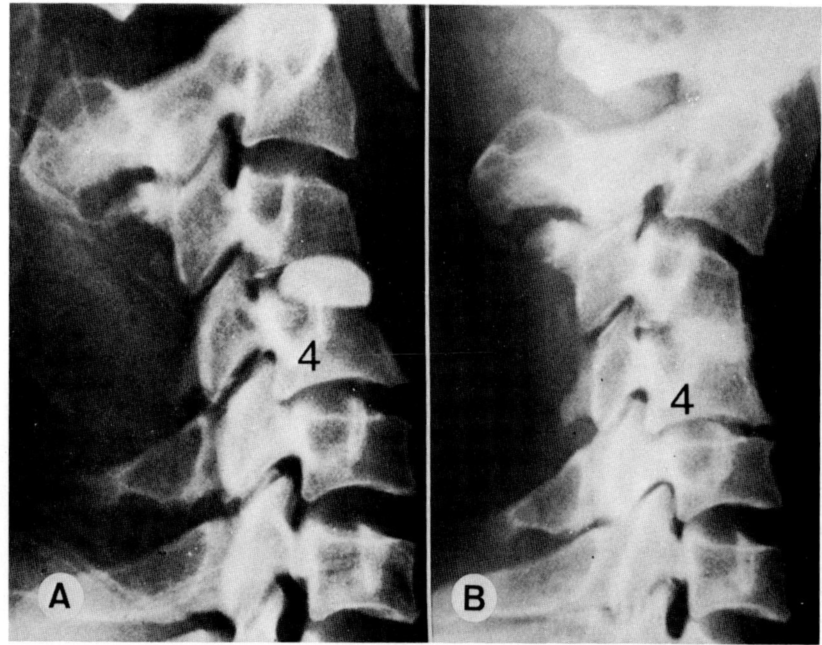

Fig. 12-60. Case 29. (*A*) Roentgenogram showing laminectomy defect and interbody graft 3 months after operation. (*B*) Same view 4 years after operation showing solid fusion of the graft.

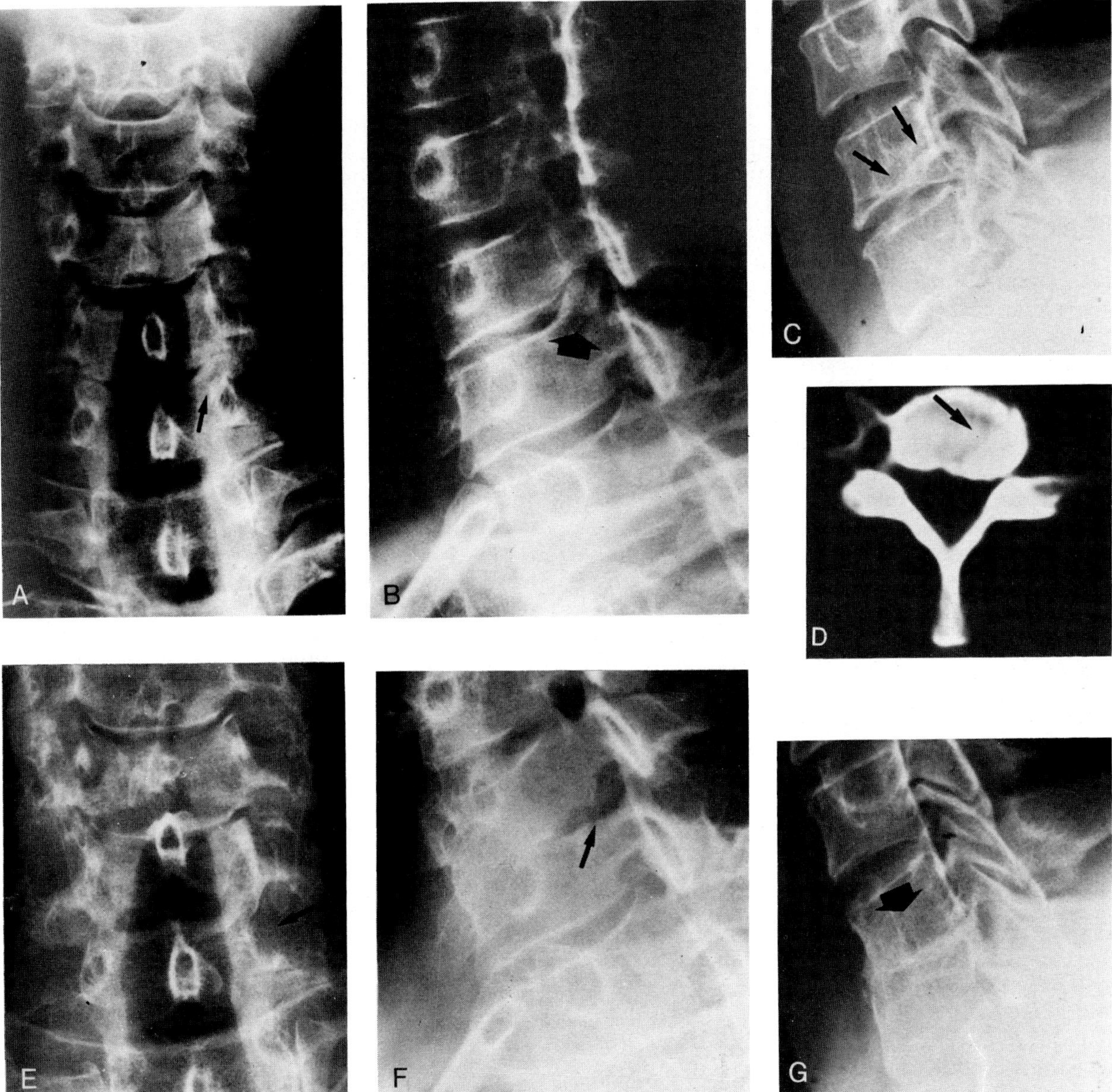

Fig. 12-61. Case 30. (*A*) Arrow points at hypertrophic left uncus of C7. The left intervertebral foramen is considerably narrowed by the hypertrophic uncus (*B*). Arrow points in profile view (*C*) to the projection of the upper border of the hypertrophic uncus. (*D*) CT scan shows greater extension of the left uncus of C7 than of the right one. The left anterior cortex of the vertebral body is also thickened. Arrow (*E*) points to defect in the body of C7 due to resection by means of a lateral approach. The left intervertebral foramen is completely decompressed following the removal of the left uncus (*F*). The bodies of C6 and C7 are fused (*arrow G*).

The patient had no complaints. Neck movements were normal. There was some anterior angulation between C2 and C3 (Fig. 12-60*B*).

CASE 30. A man, 51 years of age, complained for 2.5 years of pains in his left shoulder, radiating through the ulnar aspect of the left arm. The duration of these pains had increased in the past year, and the patient developed morning stiffness of cervical movements. In addition, he had periods of blocked movements of the cervical spine. Neurologic examination in June 1983 showed no abnormalities except slight hypalgesia in the ulnar aspect of the left arm. There was some limitation of rotation of the head to the right and to the left. X-ray examination of the cervical spine revealed marked hypertrophy of the left uncus of C7 (Fig. 12-61*A* through *D*). It narrowed the intervertebral foramen (Fig. 12-61*B*) and also showed lateral eversion. Left vertebral angiography showed only slight lateral displacement of the artery at this level. The disc space C6–C7 was flattened. Because CT scans showed enlargement of the left uncus of C7, as compared with the right uncus, and because the adjacent anterior cortex of the vertebral body was thickened (Fig. 12-61*D*), the diagnosis of hyperostosis was considered as the cause of enlargement of the left uncus. The uncus was removed by means of a lateral approach, which was the least mutilating and most adequate approach to this lesion. Since the nerve root of C7 was considerably compressed by the hypertrophic uncus, this structure was carefully removed by peeling layers with a small chisel. Because CT scanning had shown irregular thickening of the adjacent anterior bony cortex of the body of C7, this portion as well as the lateral superior portion of the body of C7, underlying the uncus, were removed (Fig.12-61*E*). Since the disc space C6–C7 was opened with this procedure, the disc was excised. After the operation, the left intervertebral foramen C6–C7 was completely decompressed (Fig. 12-61*F*). One year after the operation, x-ray examination showed a complete block of the bodies of C6 and C7, as a consequence of radical intervertebral disc excision (Fig. 12-61*G*). Microscopic examination of the removed uncus showed thickening of its cortex, but no signs of new bone formation. The surrounding portions of the vertebral body removed during operation revealed nothing abnormal. The diagnosis was hyperostosis of unknown origin. After the operation, the patient was considerably relieved from his pains; incidentally, however, he has some feelings of discomfort in his left arm and hand.

Tumor-Sized Rheumatoid Bursitis in the Odontoid Area

CASE 31. A man of 47 had suffered since about 1954 from rheumatoid arthritis. In 1966 and 1970 he had coronary infarctions. One year before operation he developed weakness of both legs, followed by loss of power in the arms and neck pains. He had bilateral Babinski responses.

The patient was admitted on July 7, 1971. The x-ray films showed no displacement of the odontoid or the atlas (Fig. 12-62*A*), but the lateral tomograms visualized considerable destruction of the odontoid (Fig. 12-62*C* and *D*). There was no obvious erosion of the atlantooccipital joints (Fig. 12-62*B*). A preoperative myelogram showed posterior displacement of the contrast medium at the level of the odontoid (Fig. 12-63*A*).

July 7, 1971: The transoral approach was used. After removal of the anterior arch of the atlas, the odontoid appeared to be surrounded by a grayish-yellow tissue mass. After freeing the odontoid from the abnormal tissue, it appeared to be eroded and diminished in size, whereas its bone had a mottled appearance. The odontoid was resected. The abnormal tissue had involved the transverse ligament and reached to the membrana tectoria, pushing it posteriorly. The abnormal tissue was removed as much as possible. The microscopic diagnosis was synovitis with much fibroblastic proliferation, fibrinoid degeneration, necrosis, and large numbers of inflammatory cells. In view of its situation, it originated from the synovial cavities between the front of the odontoid and the anterior arch of the atlas, between the posterior facet of the odontoid and the transverse ligament, and possibly also from a synovial cavity, which is often present between the transverse ligament and the membrana tectoria.

The postoperative myelogram showed the effect of the transoral decompression, which has resulted in an anterior dural recess as demonstrated by the contrast medium (Fig. 12-63*B*, *arrow*).

Because of the poor condition of this patient, posterior fusion by bone grafts and wiring from the occiput through C4 for stabilization was performed later on September 9, 1971 (Fig. 12-63*C*). There was some recovery of power in the arms and leg. One year later the patient walked small distances with the aid of a stick. His gait was spastic.

CASE 32. An Italian female, 49 years of age, had suffered for about the past 25 years from chronic rheumatoid arthritis. Since 10 years of age, she

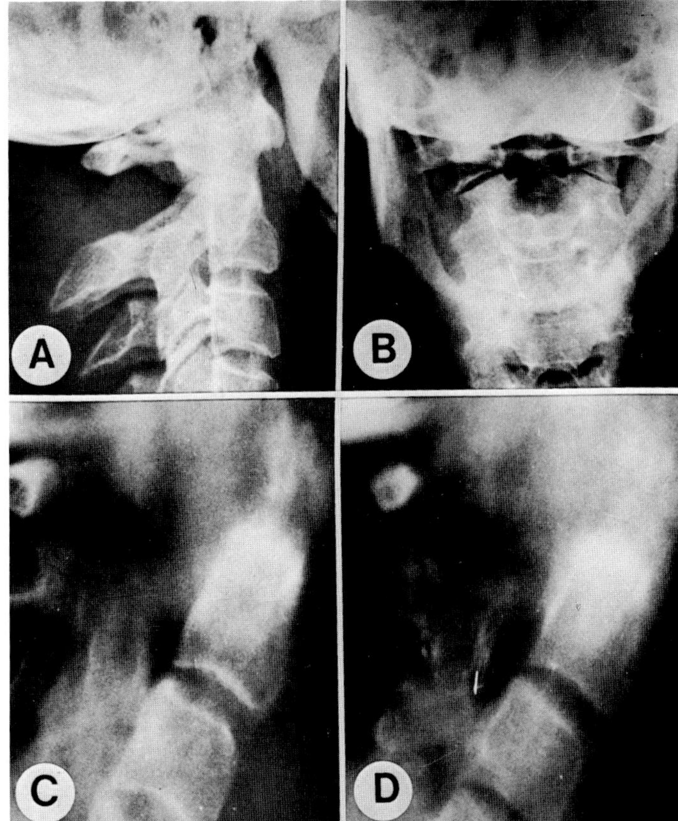

Fig. 12-62. Case 31. (*A*) Roentgenogram showing no displacement of the odontoid or the atlas. (*B*) Roentgenogram showing no obvious erosion of the atlantooccipital joints. (*C* and *D*) Lateral tomograms showing considerable destruction of the odontoid.

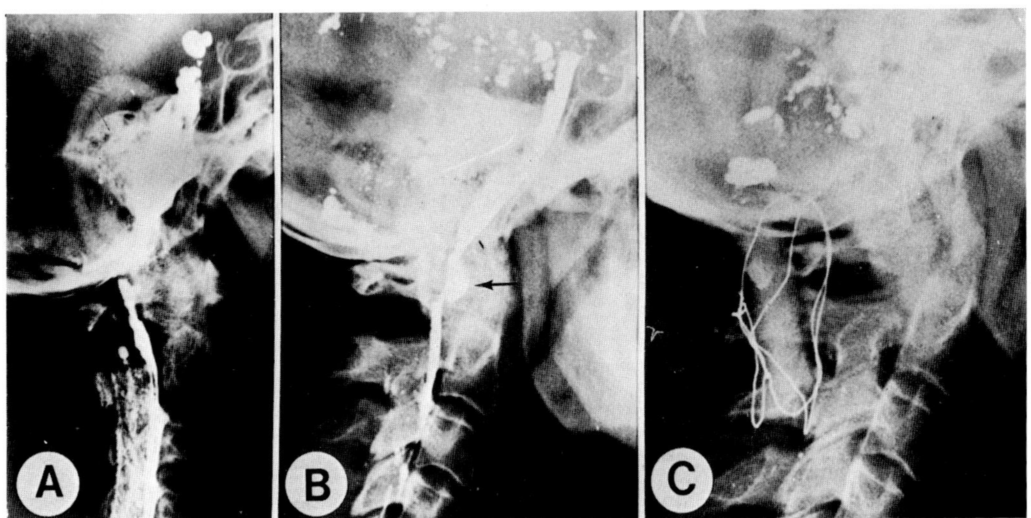

Fig. 12-63. Case 31. (*A*) Preoperative myelogram showing posterior displacement of the contrast medium at the level of the odontoid. (*B*) Postoperative myelogram showing an anterior dural recess. (*C*) Shows posterior fusion by bone grafts and wiring from the occiput through C4.

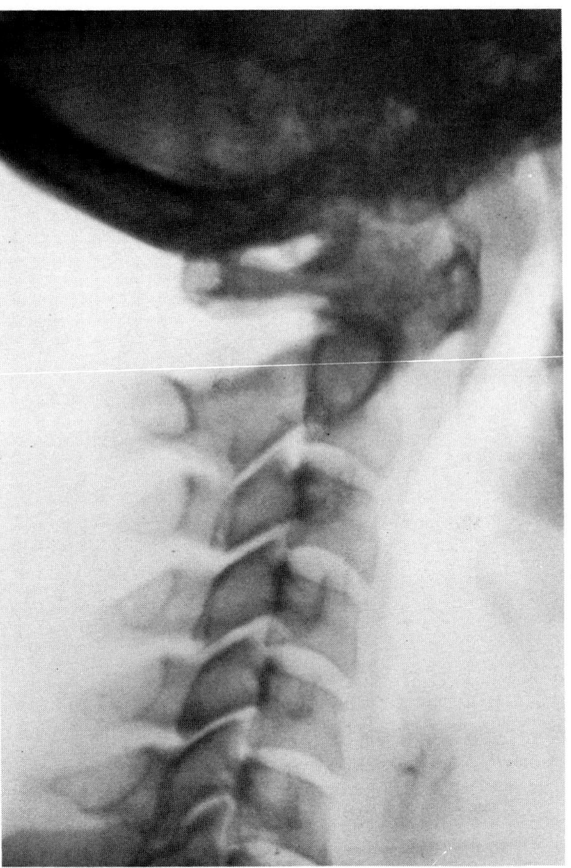

Fig. 12-64. Case 32. Anterior dislocation of the atlas. The odontoid process has completely disappeared.

had contractures in finger and wrist joints. Because of increasing neck pains and limited head movements, x-ray examination of the cervical spine was performed, revealing anterior dislocation of the atlas and disappearance of the odontoid process (Fig. 12-64). At neurologic examination, the only abnormality found was exaggerated tendon reflexes of arms and legs. On October 10, 1975, the atlantal dislocation was reduced by means of wiring between the arches of the atlas and axis. Additional bone grafts were applied to these arches. On February 26, 1976, the odontoid area was exposed via a transoral approach. The odontoid had completely disappeared, and the space between the anterior arch of the atlas and the dural theca was occupied by a massive granuloma. The granulomatous tissue was removed as much as possible. An iliac bone graft was inserted between the body of the axis and the anterior border of the clivus. The postoperative course was uneventful. The patient, who is living in Rome, reported recently that x-ray examination had shown stabilization of the reduced atlas. Neurologic examination revealed nothing abnormal. She still suffers from problems of rheumatoid arthritis.

Assessment of Results

In the presentation of the individual case histories, I have emphasized surgical indications, procedures, and results. They supply the basic material for the following facts and figures. They are presented not only for an assessment of results, problems and failures, but are also intended as some sort of contribution to efforts at standardization of surgical strategy in benign tumors of the cervical spine, which so far is wanting.

The practice of the four basic types of operations—posterior, anterior, lateral, and transoral—in 31 of the 32 patients is numerically presented in Table 12-3, which refers only to procedures during the first admission of the patients in our department. All operations performed in that period were aimed at being definitive; readmissions signified tumor recurrence or secondary spinal deformities. Three patients had been operated on elsewhere before the first admission by means of posterior operations (Cases 3, 4 and 12). The left column of Table 12-3 shows that in 22 of the 31 patients, two thirds of cases, the tumor could be removed by means of one of the four basic types of operations. The lateral and posterior operations were the most frequent. Fusion procedures, if performed in an area of tumor removal, are not mentioned in Table 12-3. In 10 patients (one third of total), fusion had to be performed by means of another operation outside the area of tumor removal. These procedures are mentioned in Table 12-3. Of the combined types of operations needed for tumor removal in nine of the 31 cases, the lateral approach was included in seven of them. One patient of the 32, Case 26 who had vertebral hemangioma, was not operated upon.

Three of 31 patients died owing to increase of neural deficit and respiratory failure (Case 6), consequences of pneumonia and gram-negative sepsis 1.5 months after operation (Case 9), or spontaneous pneumothorax and other complications not related to the operation (Case 25).

Preoperative principal roentgenographic abnormalities of the spine in 31 patients

Vertebral collapse :	5 cases
Osteolysis or erosion without collapse :	16 cases

Table 12-3. Types of Operations Performed

SINGLE TYPES OF OPERATIONS FOR REMOVAL OF TUMORS	COMBINED WITH OTHER TYPES OF OPERATIONS FOR CORRECTION OF KYPHOSIS OR FUSION
Posterior: 7 cases	Anterior Stabilization—interbody fusion: 2 cases Reduction of kyphosis: 2 cases
Anterior: 2 cases	None
Lateral: 7 cases	None
Transoral: 6 cases	Posterior fusion: 3 cases
MULTIPLE TYPES OF OPERATIONS FOR REMOVAL OF TUMOR	
Lateral + anterior: 4 cases	Posterior fusion: 3 cases
Posterior + anterior: 1 case	None
Lateral + posterior: 2 cases	None
Transoral + posterior: 1 case	None
Lateral + posterior + Transoral: 1 case	None

Kyphosis :	3 cases
Kyphosis and vertebral slip:	3 cases
Hyperostosis:	4 cases

Postoperative roentgenographic follow-up in 28 surviving patients

Good alignment and stability :	28 cases
Moderately reduced kyphosis :	2 cases
Kyphosis and atlantic dislocation unchanged :	1 case
Progressive kyphosis :	1 case

Fourteen of the 32 patients had preoperative neurologic disturbances due to the spinal deformities. After the operation one patient died; complete neurologic recovery was noted in eight patients, considerable improvement in two patients, some improvement in two patients, and no improvement in one patient. Only one patient had postoperative neck pains; 13 patients had more or less limited cervical movements and 11 patients had normal movements.

Late Results: The present condition is unknown in three cases. One patient had a second operation because of recurrence of an aneurysmal bone cyst (Case 11) and another patient needed two reoperations because of recurrent kyphosis (Case 7, neurofibromatosis).

Late Deaths: Three patients died. The causes of death were late malignant degeneration of a giant cell tumor 5 years later (Case 17) and malignant degeneration of a chondromyxoid fibroma 7 years later (Case 23). After the first operation both patients had been reoperated on three times. The third patient (Case 1) died 5 years after operation from diffuse progressive neurofibromatosis of the upper cervical spine.

According to information obtained during the past 3 years about the surviving patients, their condition has not shown untoward changes.

REFERENCES

1. *CHIURCO AA:* Multiple exostoses of bone with fatal cord compression. Neurology 20:275, 1970
2. *CURTIS BH, FISHER RL, BUTTERFIELD WL, ET AL:* Neurofibromatosis with paraplegia. J Bone Joint Surg 51A:843, 1969
3. *DAHLIN DC:* Bone Tumors. Springfield, IL, Charles C Thomas, 1957
4. *DAHLIN DC, HOOVER NW:* Desmoplastic fibroma of bone. JAMA 188:165, 1964
5. *EPSTEIN BS:* The Spine: A Radiological Text and Atlas, 4th ed. Philadelphia, Lea & Febiger, 1976
6. *FEINSTEIN AR:* Clinical Judgment. Baltimore, Williams & Wilkins, 1967
7. *HARDY R, LEHRER H:* Desmoplastic fibroma versus desmoid tumor of bone. Radiology 88:899, 1967
8. *JAFFE HL:* Tumors and Tumorous Conditions of the Bones and Joints. Philadelphia, Lea & Febiger, 1958
9. *KALENDA Z:* The prevention of irreversible lung changes following reversible phrenic nerve paralysis. Acta Anaesthesiol Belg (Suppl)27:305, 1976
10. *KEASBEY LE, FANSELAU, HA:* The aponeurotic fibroma. Clin Orthop 19:115, 1961
11. *LICHTENSTEIN L:* Bone Tumors, 3rd ed. St Louis, CV Mosby, 1965
12. *MANSEL RE, POWLEY PH:* Aggressive fibromatosis of the vertebral column. Clin Oncol 4:123, 1978
13. *MUSGROVE JE, MCDONALD JR:* Extra-abdominal desmoid tumors: Their differential diagnosis and treatment. Arch Pathol 45:513, 1948
14. *NETHERLANDS COMMITTEE ON BONE TUMOURS:*

Radiological Atlas of Bone Tumors, Vol 2. The Hague, Mouton & Co, 1973

15. *Rabhan WN, Rosae J:* Desmoplastic fibroma. J Bone Joint Surg 50A:487, 1968
16. *Scheer GE, Kuhlman RE:* Vertebral involvement by desmoplastic fibroma. JAMA 185:121, 1963
17. *Schutt PG, Frost HM:* Chondromyxoid fibroma. Clin Orthop 78:323, 1971
18. *Stout AP:* Juvenile fibromatoses. Cancer 7:953, 1954
19. *Stout AP:* The Fibromatoses. Clin Orthop 19:11, 1961
20. *Turkel H:* Trephine Technique of Bone Marrow Infusions and Tissue Biopsies. Detroit, Karl Schaltenbrand, 1961
21. *Verbiest H:* Giant cell tumours and aneurysmal bone cysts of the spine. J Bone Joint Surg 47*B*:699, 1965
22. *Verbiest H:* Anterolateral operations for fractures and dislocations in the middle and lower parts of the cervical spine. J Bone Joint Surg 51A:1489, 1969
23. *Verbiest H:* La Chirurgie antérieure et latérale du rachis cervical. Neurochirurgie (Suppl 2)16, 1970
24. *Verbiest H:* Lesions of the cervical spine: A critical review. In Carrea R (ed): Neurological Surgery, International Congress Series 433, pp 374–383. Amsterdam-Oxford Excerpta Medica, 1978
25. *Verbiest H:* From anterior to lateral operations on the cervical spine. Neurosurg Rev 1–2:47, 1978
26. *Verbiest H:* The value of CT of the spine to the neurosurgeon. In Donovan J (ed): Radiographic Evaluation of the Spine, pp 139–185. New York, Post. Masson Publishing, 1980
27. *Vinstein AL, Franken FA:* Hereditary multiple exostoses: Report of a case with spinal cord compression. AJR 112:405, 1971
28. *Winter RB, Moe JH, Bradford DS, et al:* Spinal deformity in neurofibromatosis. J Bone Joint Surg 61A:677, 1979
29. *Yong-Hing K, Kalamchi A, MacEwen G:* Cervical spine abnormalities in neurofibromatosis. J Bone Joint Surg 61A:695, 1979

CHAPTER 13

Surgical Approaches and Techniques

Posterior Approaches and Fusions

MICHAEL J. MURPHY AND WAYNE O. SOUTHWICK

The posterior approach to the spine seems the most natural one since the spinous processes of the neck vertebrae are easily palpable. Because of this seemingly easy accessibility, it is not surprising that posterior approaches were developed earlier than anterior approaches. However, even though the posterior elements of the vertebra seem superficial, the posterior approaches are more demanding than one would expect. A considerable amount of muscle detachment or separation from the posterior elements of the vertebrae is necessary, and attention to the natural anatomic planes is important to prevent unnecessary blood loss and to avoid damage to the spinal cord and nerve roots or to the articulations of the vertebra. In this chapter we attempt to give details of the most useful posterior approaches and fusion approaches as they are currently used from cephalad to caudad, along with some of their advantages and disadvantages. In general, the advantage of using posterior elements for fusion is that the lamina and spinous processes and facets are made up predominantly of cortical bone tissue and provide a large surface area for fusion. Obviously, if one can firmly attach bone grafts, wires, metal, and methylmethacrylate implants to these elements, a fusion becomes more stable immediately (providing an adequate fusion construct can be obtained). This approach obviously affords the best access to the posterior aspect of the spinal cord. A disadvantage of the posterior approach is the difficulty and tediousness of the dissection, including separation of the erector spinae muscle mass from its insertion. The other major disadvantage of the posterior cervical approach is that it is obviously a poor route to the anterior portions of the spinal canal, the anterior spinal cord, or the vertebral bodies.

INDICATIONS

There is much controversy over the indications for cervical fusion, particularly in any specific patient's situation, and over the definition of instability. The general categories of conditions that commonly produce clinical instability are trauma, neoplasia, rheumatoid arthritis, postlaminectomy, and so forth. In trauma, posterior cervical spine fusion is indicated when there is instability from posterior osteoligamentous disruption; when there is an anterior fracture with angulation or translation; when there is facet dislocation (the unstable type requiring open reduction); following laminectomy, particularly extensive laminectomies in young people; and for additional stability following excision and vertebral body replacement when there is an additional posterior ligamentous disruption. Neoplastic invasion of the anterior or posterior elements of the vertebrae often necessitate early extensive augmentation fusion posteriorly prior to or along with tumor resection. Severe spondylosis, particularly if there is posterior incursion of osteoarthritic material, may benefit from laminectomy; in these cases, facet fusion is an important adjunct to prevent further irritation of the cord and nerve roots.[2] Occasionally in rheumatoid arthritis or Marie-Strümpell arthritis, severe neurologic deficits require fusion posteriorly after laminectomy. There is some debate over the anterior *versus* the posterior approach for these latter two conditions.

Regardless of the indications, the surgeon must be certain that his skill and his facilities are adequate for this type of surgery to avoid aggravation or production of any neurologic deficit; that no other additional injury is produced; and that he will indeed achieve a stable construct. There are situations, such as deteriorating spinal cord injuries, where the condition is so desperate that reasonably high risk is justifiable. It is not possible to describe exact indications except in the most general terms in this introduction.

OCCIPITOCERVICAL FUSION

Since most of the flexion and rotation of the head, with respect of the thorax, occurs in the upper two cervical vertebrae, fusion of these elements should not be done without good reason. As stated in the previous section, some of the indications for such surgery include instability of these elements with impending neurologic damage, instability from trauma, intractable pain, or loss of bone substance from bone tumors. Occasionally, severe rheumatoid arthritis with neurologic damage is an indication for this procedure. Essentially, these procedures are carried out for types of instability that are more clearly defined elsewhere in this book (see Chap. 10).

The patient must be carefully prepared and positioned for this procedure, especially if there is gross instability. Usually such a patient will be in skull tong traction; if so, intubation and general endotracheal anesthesia may be somewhat difficult since the head position should not be changed. Prior to modern anesthesia techniques we used local anesthesia, but this has not been necessary for the past decade. Usually, with the patient asleep and intubated under continuous traction, he can be log-rolled into the face-down position using a Gardner head holder to maintain alignment (Fig. 13-1). If this maneuver is not considered safe enough, the patient may be maintained on a Stryker turning frame and operated upon in the frame. It is rather cumbersome to carry out the surgery on a Stryker frame, however; and if it is to be done on a frame, a reverse Trendelenburg tilt of 10° to 15° is needed. This frame can be elevated appropriately with various heights of shock blocks. In addition to all this, it is possible to use a wake-up technique, asking the patient to move his limbs or respond to stimuli to be certain that the maneuvers have not produced any injury to the neural elements.

After appropriate anesthesia, and once the patient's position is properly aligned, the skin is prepared with a sterilizing solution such as Betadine and draped so that one iliac crest donor site is available. The posterior occiput, neck, and shoulder should be widely prepped.

The posterior cervical incisions tend to ooze considerably, especially if the avascular midline is missed. We often use diluted epinephrine solution to reduce this bleeding to a minimum. A 1% solution of lidocaine (Xylocaine) with 1:100,000 epinephrine diluted with an equal volume of saline, injected 1 cc to 2 cc at a time into and just above the skin along the proposed incision site, is a very helpful method of reducing the bleeding. Small amounts along the muscle sheath will also improve identification of the fascial planes.

For the occipitoatlantal fusion, the skin incision and superficial dissection should extend to the midline of the back of the head at the external occipital protuberance to C4 or C5 (Fig. 13-2). The midpoint of the incision can be identified by palpation of C2 (about two finger breadths below the base of the occiput). Make a straight incision going down through the subcutaneous fat to the spinous processes. The C2 spinous process is large and bifid where the short external rotators to the head are attached. Once this landmark is identified, the midline dissection should be extended up and down from this point. The dissection is carried up

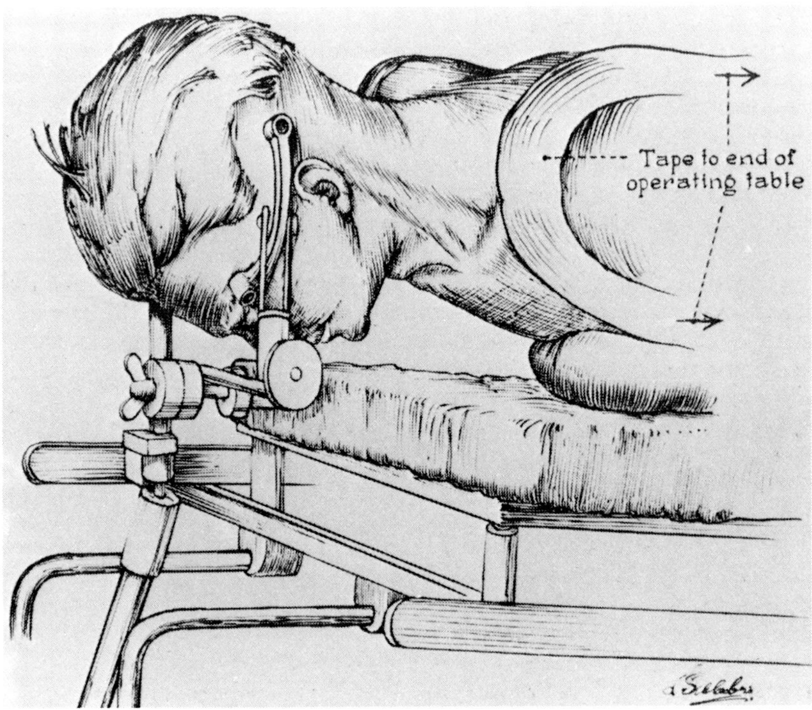

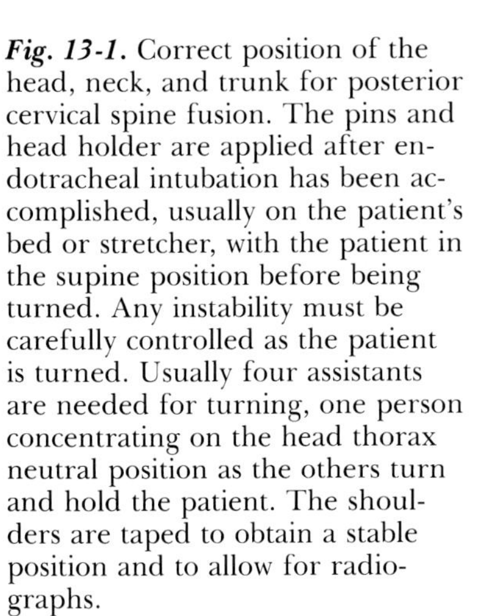

Fig. 13-1. Correct position of the head, neck, and trunk for posterior cervical spine fusion. The pins and head holder are applied after endotracheal intubation has been accomplished, usually on the patient's bed or stretcher, with the patient in the supine position before being turned. Any instability must be carefully controlled as the patient is turned. Usually four assistants are needed for turning, one person concentrating on the head thorax neutral position as the others turn and hold the patient. The shoulders are taped to obtain a stable position and to allow for radiographs.

to the base of the skull to about a finger breadth inferior to the external occipital protuberance. Careful dissection between the attachment of the erector spine muscles will allow adequate exposure of the lamina. The midline dissection should be carried down similarly to the spinous processes of C3, C4, or C5; there is no need to expose the spinous processes below this level. After the superficial midline structures have been exposed, a Weitlaner retractor is placed into the subcutaneous tissue (the superficial layer of fascia).

The dissection should then proceed throughout the length of the incision from the superficial fascia first down along the spinous processes of C2 and C3 and then down into the tubercle of C1 and the foramen magnum. Remove the small rotator attachments from the spinous process of C2 using a sharp scalpel and then a sharp curette. Proceed laterally exposing the lamina of C2 first on one side and then the other. Go then to the spinous process of C3 and the tubercle of C1, and then the midportion of the arch of the foramen magnum. Do not use large periosteal elevators since they may be more likely to result in excessive force. Use delicate strokes and delicate instruments. Remember that delicate subperiosteal dissection of the C1 arch is necessary to avoid the vertebral arteries and veins that pass cephalad from the vertebral foramen of C2 over the arch of C1, trailing medially or through the lateral portion of the arch of C1 to enter the foramen magnum. By using delicate dissection and care, the lateral superior edge of C2 and the arch of C1 can be exposed to the articulation of C1. Usually the exposure of the posterior two thirds of the arch of C1, the posterior two thirds of the arch of the posterior edge of the foramen magnum, about 3 cm of the posterior portion of the occiput, and two thirds of the lamina of C2 can be accomplished with minimal difficulty.

Although it is possible to fuse the occiput by merely abutting bone grafts to the sacrificed outer tables of skull, no early fixation is obtained and the chances of nonunion are high. It is much more preferable to create at least two holes, one on each side of the posterior midline of the foramen magnum. We described this column method 20 years ago.[6] After the foramen, lateral occiput, and cervical bones to be fused are well visualized, prepare two 1-cm holes in the occiput about 5 mm lateral to the midline and 5 mm away from the edge of the foramen magnum (Fig. 13-2). Make these rather large, shallow holes in the outer table either with a trephine drill or a round powered bur. If

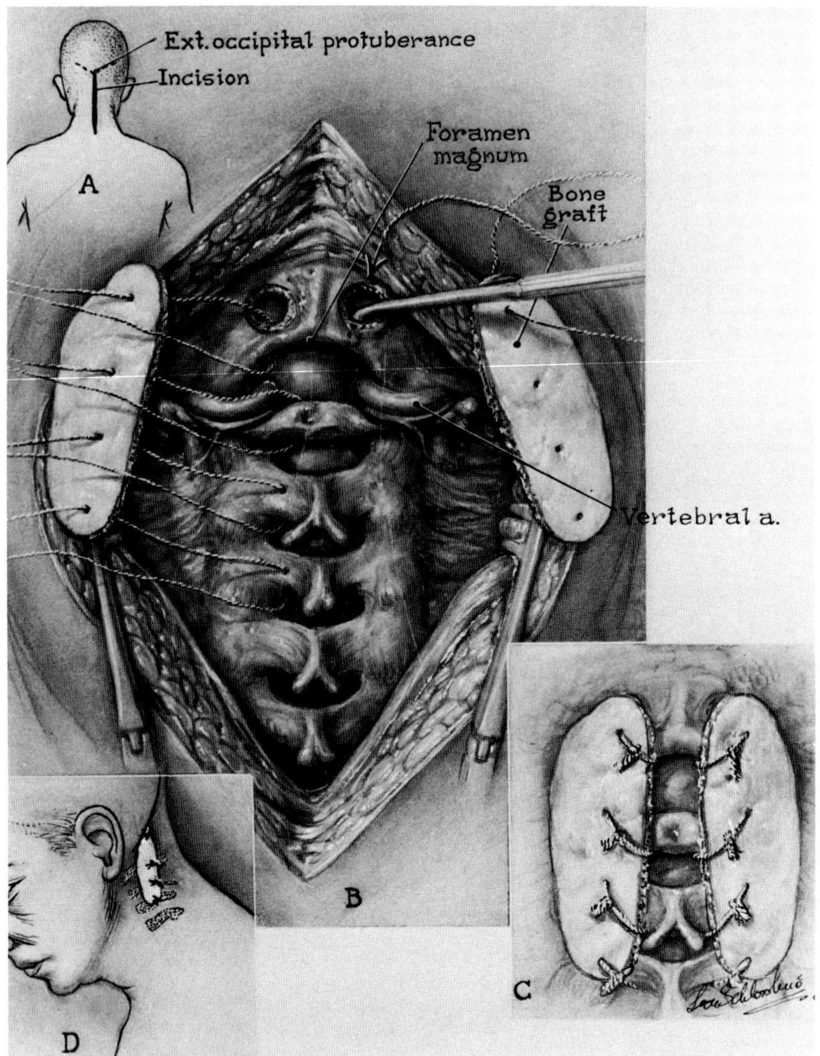

Fig. 13-2. The incision may not need to be as extensive as illustrated for exposure of the occipital C1, C2, and C3 segments. The donor grafts may be more "comma shaped," as described in the section on facet fusion, and the wires may also be passed around the grafts instead of through the grafts, especially if a laminectomy of C1 or C2 has been performed.

this is prepared with care, the inner table is very gradually perforated and no damage results to the dura. A large, shallow bed will be created for the onlay iliac graft, which can be wired into place.

At this point, the dura and periosteum stuck to the lamina of C2, the arch of C1, and the foramen magnum are carefully separated from the bone. Angle curettes and a Woodson dissector are used first in the midline to tease the soft tissue periosteum and dura away from the bone. These instruments must be delicately applied, their sharp edges scraping the bone constantly without making the slightest incursion into the spinal canal or cranial vault.

At this point, scrape away any remaining soft tissue from the bony surfaces to be fused. After the dura and periosteal tissues have been separated from the bones and the soft tissue free surfaces have been prepared, pass two 24-gauge twisted wires under each of these bony structures and loop them around an iliac bone graft.

The graft can be carefully measured and fashioned to fit snugly against the holes made in the occiput. Once these grafts and wires are placed satisfactorily, so that a strong piece of corticocancellous bone fits accurately to the host surfaces, the wires can be gently pulled upon the grafts and twisted to compress them. These wires should be uniformly twisted down to hold the grafts adjacent to the host recipient sites. Then, laterally placed cancellous grafts can be added to any gaps. This method prevents any bone graft material from falling into the central decompression area of the exposed dura.

Hemostasis should always be as complete as possible in these large oozing surfaces, especially at the time of closure. We use mostly cautery, pressure with Gelfoam and fibrin, and small ties to any aggressive bleeders. We apply pads of Gelfoam over the dura to protect it. We also prefer interrupted closure using 2-0 or single-0 chromic gut sutures primarily in the thick ligamentum nuchae or in the superficial layers of the deep fascia that enclose the erector spinae group. These sutures should be 1 cm apart; if oozing is not completely controlled, a small vaseline or rubber drain should be placed between these sutures to prevent pressure on the dura from the bleeding.

The subcutaneous tissue and the skin are then closed with interrupted sutures placed exactly over the same location as the deep sutures.

After Laminectomy. Occasionally following resection of a tumor or decompression laminectomy for other reasons, one is left with an unstable situation that requires fixation and fusion. If portions of the foramen magnum, the arch of C1, or the lamina of C2 has been removed, it may require considerable ingenuity to achieve immediate stability from the posterior aspect. In this situation it is usually possible to drill holes in the remaining bone above and below the laminectomy and attach grafts with wires. Wires are used to maintain grafts in the lateral position and to keep pressure off the midline. Rarely it is necessary to remove facet joints with the decompression, but if this is needed, facets above and below the lesion can be used for fixation.

One of us (Michael J. Murphy) has recently used compression rods from the Harrington set as an anchor for these wires. This will often achieve early stability and make it possible to avoid external support (Fig. 13-3).

Closure is performed as stated for occipitocervical fusion.

MODIFIED BROOKS ATLANTOAXIAL FUSION

Obviously, if the atlantoocipital joint can be spared, by all means it should be. This joint allows for a great deal of head flexion and extension. Years ago, Arthur Brooks of Vanderbilt University devised a fusion of C1 and C2 that was a considerable improvement over the midline wiring method originally described by Gallie.[1,3] Instead of simply passing the midline wire underneath the arch of the atlas and fixing it to the spinous process of C2,

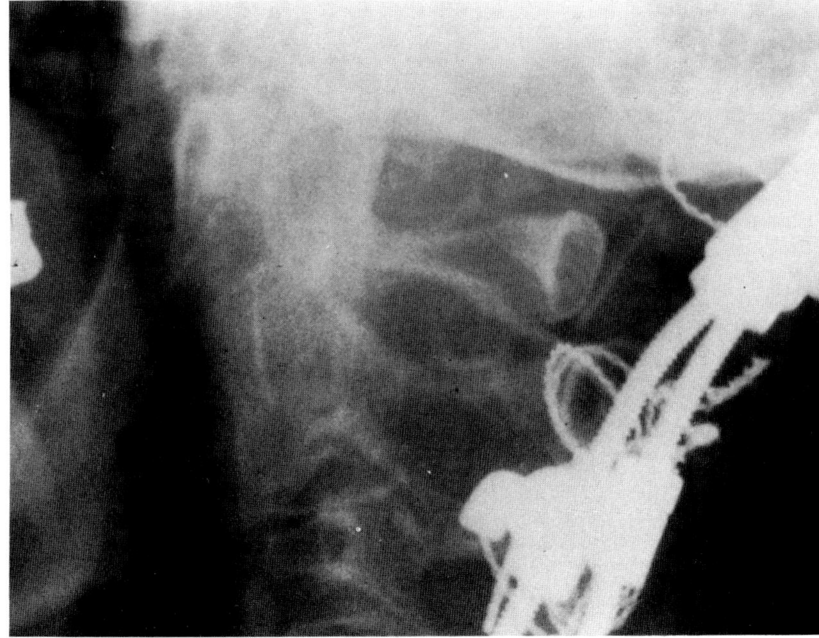

Fig. 13-3. Lateral view of a combined bone graft and rod and wire fixation of the occiput to C2–C3 in a 41-year-old woman with destruction of the C1–C2 facet joints from metastatic breast carcinoma. Since her survival time could easily be more than 2 years, the construct was augmented by a cortico-cancellous iliac bone graft. (The graft is visible between the arch of C1 and the Harrington rods. Half of the arch was removed because of tumor.) However, the threaded wires were bent to conform to the angles needed, and the hooks and wires fixed into the occipital trephine holes and the articulations of C2 and C3. The patient became comfortable in a brace in 8 days.

wires were passed under the lamina of C2 as well. These wires then could be moved somewhat laterally from the midline and could circumscribe fixed and compressed bone grafts of the lamina of C2 and the arch of C1. This gives a much more rigid construct that resists rotation. One must be extremely cautious, however, in passing the wires. We use a slightly modified version of his operation.[4]

The patient is routinely given endotracheal anesthesia, which is usually administered with the patient face up while the surgeons and the assistants maintain the position of the head by gentle traction. After the endotracheal tube has been placed in its proper position, the Gardner pin-vise head holder is applied to the patients' skull and the patient is turned onto the operating table. Make absolutely certain that the head–trunk relationships do not change. Attach the head-holding device to its base on the table, as shown in Fig. 13-1. If the neck is extremely unstable, simply operate with the head in traction on a Stryker frame, as described under Occipitocervical Fusion. When the patient is in the position considered desirable for operation, take a lateral roentgenogram to check the alignment. It is critical that the arch of C1 is properly aligned with the lamina of C2 and that there is sufficient head flexion to allow instrumentation between the foramen magnum, the arch of C1, and the lamina of C2 (Fig. 13-4*A*). This position is sometimes described as the "military tuck"; the cervical spine is in extension and the occipitoatlantal joint is maximally flexed.

Next, the midline skin incision is made from the occipital protuberance to the third and fourth spinous processes. If the ligamentum nuchae is carefully divided, the midline bleeding will be minimal. Small amounts of epinephrine solution can be used as described in the previous section. The bifid spinous process of C2 is identified with certainty and the small muscles removed with the curette of the scalpel. A sharpened Woodson dental instrument is used to separate the bone from the anterior soft tissues in the midline. A 60-cm piece of 24-gauge wire is bent over on itself and twisted three times per centimeter so as to make a smooth flexible cable. These wires are passed beneath the arch of C1 and the lamina of C2 at the midline (Fig. 13-4*C*, *D*, and *E*). Usually the wire can be passed through the undersurface of the lamina and the arch. An alternate method is to pass one aneurysm needle with a silk suture under the arch of C1 and the lamina of C2 and then tie the wire to the silk suture and pull the wire gently into position. The posterior arch of the atlas and the lamina of C2 are carefully denuded of all soft tissue with small sharp curettes. This is done very lightly and gently with special care not to disturb the dura or to move the lamina and arch with respect to other tissues. The arch and lamina should be held with a Kocher clamp to avoid motion.

Next, bone grafts are taken from the ilium. The posterior iliac spine is palpated and a transverse incision mark is made over this prominence directly down to bone. This ridge of bone is exposed for an area of about 4 square cm so that a piece of bone approximately 1.5 cm × 1.2 cm × 1.5 cm can be removed (Fig. 13-4*F*). Each graft should be slightly larger than the space to be grafted so it can be nibbled down to fit exactly. Small notches may be made in the edge of the graft to retain the wires. After the exact position of the graft is made, the wires are twisted together (Fig. 13-4*G* and *H*). A piece of Gelfoam is packed into the donor site and the wound is closed with figure-of-eight interrupted sutures to obtain a good bite to hold the gluteus muscle fascia to the bone and yet leave small gaps for oozing blood to escape from the wound site.

POSTERIOR FUSION FOR CERVICAL INSTABILITY

Cervical instability is a subject treated elsewhere in this volume and a careful study of this section is advised (see Chap. 10). White's definition of instability of the neck is as follows: "Clinical instability is defined as a loss of the ability of the spine under *physiologic loads* to maintain a relationship between vertebral segments in such a way that there is neither damage or *subsequent* irritation of the spinal cord or nerve roots, and, in addition, there is no development of *incapacitating deformity* or pain due to structural changes."[10] White has provided careful quantitative measures to determine this likelihood of the presence of cervical instability, which should be studied thoroughly to help decide on the indications for the operation described herein.

Although it is an oversimplification to describe fusion procedures for flexion, rotation, and extension injuries, it is of some value to think of the characteristic roentgenographic changes when deciding what type of fusion to perform with the various types of injury. Fortunately, with posterior fusions it is often possible to obtain stability that resists motion in all planes, at least with the help of minimal outside bracing. The most common causes of cervical instability arise from fractures or fracture-dislocations and from neoplastic invasion. Another relatively common cause of instability that we have seen is late cervical spine deformities (primarily kyphotic) following extensive laminectomy.

Obviously, in any of these situations in which there is instability, temporary safety measures, usually traction or brace immobilization, are mandatory to avoid spinal nerve root injury until the surgery herein described is performed. This matter is also handled in another section of the book (see Chap. 10).

MODIFIED ROGERS INTERSPINOUS WIRING AND FUSION

Dr. William A. Rogers, former editor of the Journal of Bone and Joint Surgery, was known throughout the orthopedic world for his careful, thoughtful, and conservative approach to orthopedic problems. His paper on operative management of cervical spine fractures changed markedly the ideas of treatment for neck injuries.[7] Prior to that time almost all these injuries were managed by long-term cast immobilization, a very uncomfortable method. Dr. Rogers noted the great problem with conservative treatment: that of not ever knowing if stability was achieved. He described an operative method that he found safe. His technique was very meticulous and cautious, and involved wiring bone grafts into place along the lamina of the injured segments. The Rogers method certainly helped immobilize the bone grafts and fixed the spine in place, but is was difficult to maintain exact position of the spine because of the rather circuitous route of the wires. Wires were somewhat more prone to slip through or fragment grafts with the resulting loss of internal fixation. It then became necessary to depend on additional external support. For these reasons we began wiring of intact lamina directly to each other and using onlay bone graft techniques on top of the wires. In the cervical spine, after careful curettage of the periosteum it is not necessary to remove curls of bone. The onlay of grafts, especially if some bone is supplied into the facet areas, results in a very satisfactory fusion.

A typical case for the illustration of our direct wire technique is one in which there is an anterior subluxation of a cervical vertebra above and an intact vertebral body or a slightly compressed vertebral body below. Often there will be an abnormal separation of these two spinous processes, which usually indicates that the interspinous ligament between these two segments is partially or completely torn and that the lesion is the result of a flexion force. In these cases, the anterior longitudinal ligament is intact; of course, the capsule and ligamenta flava are usually torn or the spinous process or lamina is cracked. The key to successful reduction and fusion in order to obtain immediate stability is to understand the exact extent of the injury and to fix together with tension only those segments that are unstable, making use of the soft tissue hinge. The prerequisite for interspinous wiring is obviously intact posterior osseous elements.

As anyone who has made a barbwire fence well knows, to achieve the most efficient tension the posts must be in a straight line and the wire must be in straight lines between the posts. Thus, in injuries in which the posterior elements have separated, the tension effect from this type of construct can be very useful. In situations in which extension and rotation are also factors, the construct must usually be different, usually that of lashing elements to a stable internal post. The original Rogers wiring technique did not provide control of specific forces, and the concept of affixing the vertebrae of unstable elements to a bone graft was essentially lacking. However, we now employ this modified wiring technique in most instances as a method of resisting increased flexion by wire tension bands.

With this concept in mind, we may proceed to the operating details. In these cases, the patient would have been in skull tong traction in the neutral position to maintain alignment. After the patient has been properly positioned on the operating table as described under Occipital Spinal Fusion, and after a lateral film demonstrates alignment position, an incision is scratched or marked into the skin over the area to be operated upon to ensure symmetry prior to full draping. After preparation and draping of the patient, the skin is opened down to the subcutaneous fascia. Since the skin is rather thick and since there are small bleeders under the skin not easily ligated, it is frequently possible to place Halsted or curved hemostats about one quarter inch apart from the subcutaneous layer just deep to the skin without particular regard to localizing the small bleeders. After skin towels are applied under the hemostats, the clamps are tied together in groups and help in the retraction. A small amount of epinephrine can be used as described previously in this section.

After the subcutaneous tissue has been separated in the midline over the spinous processes, the spinous processes are palpated. It is also wise at this point to make a lateral radiograph to be

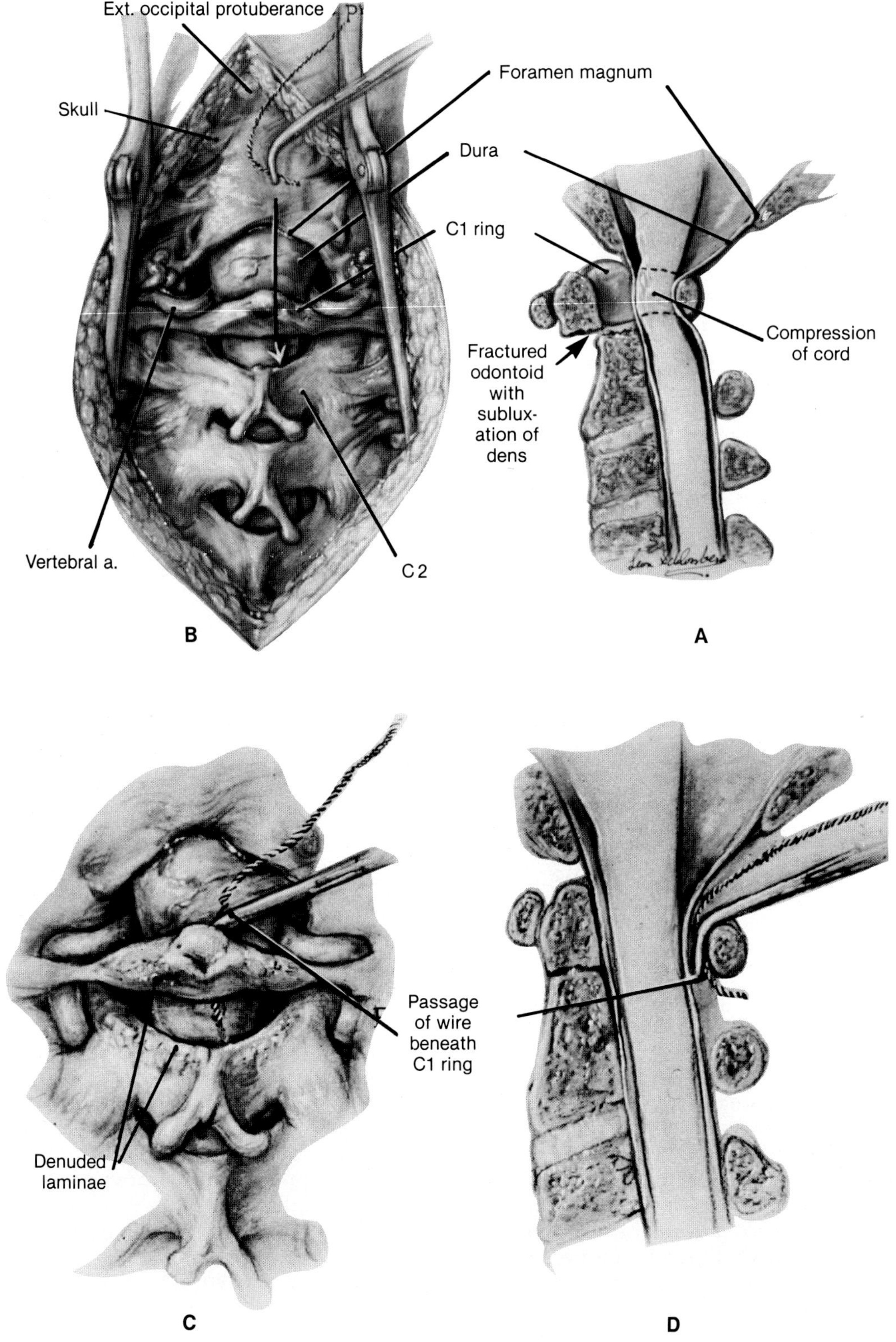
Ext. occipital protuberance
Skull
Foramen magnum
Dura
C1 ring
Vertebral a.
C2
B
Fractured odontoid with sublux- ation of dens
Compression of cord
A
Passage of wire beneath C1 ring
Denuded laminae
C
D

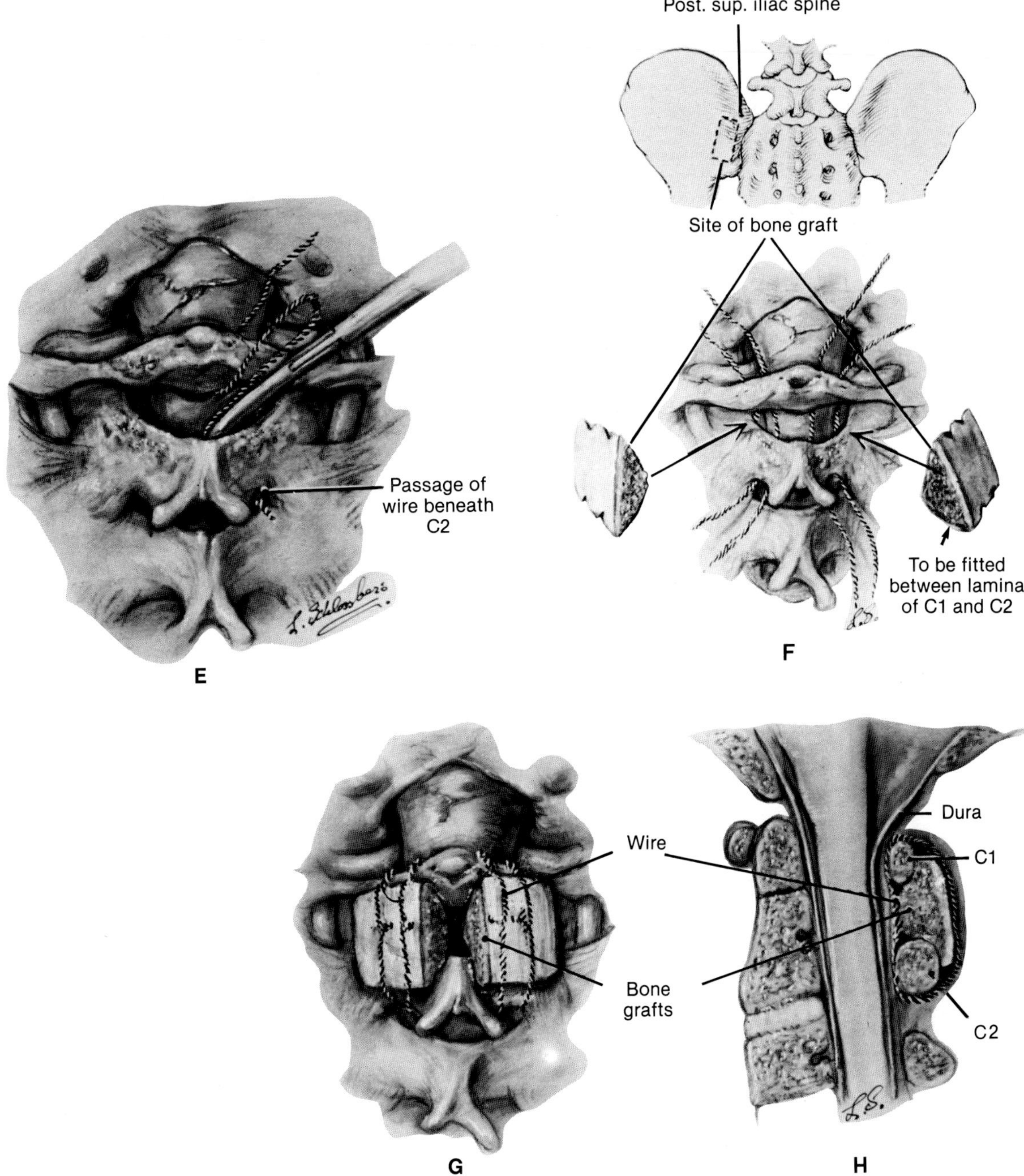

Fig. 13-4. Modified Brooks method of C1–C2 wiring.

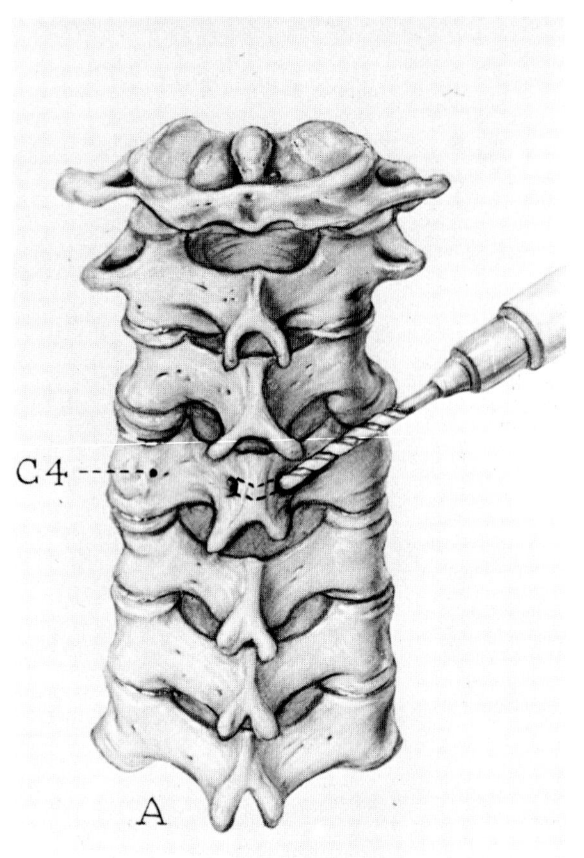
C4
A

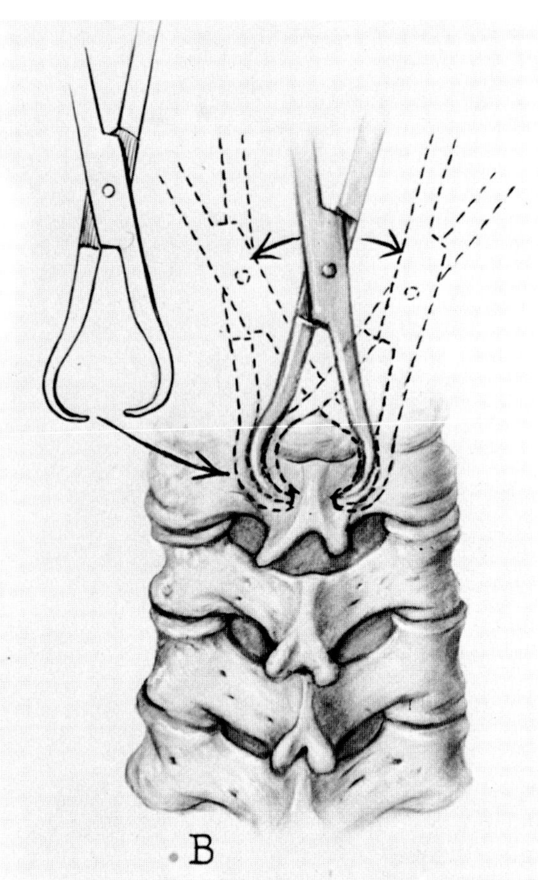
B

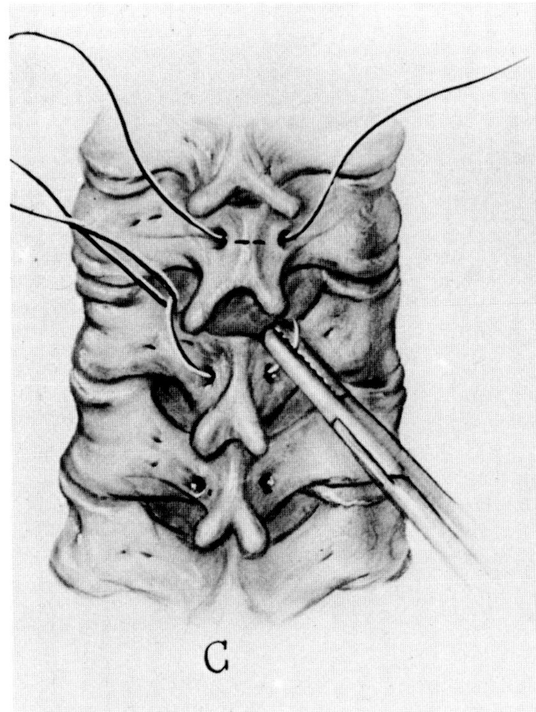
C

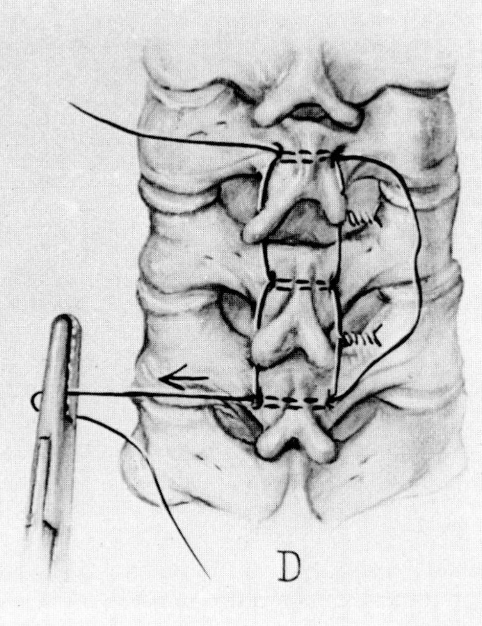
D

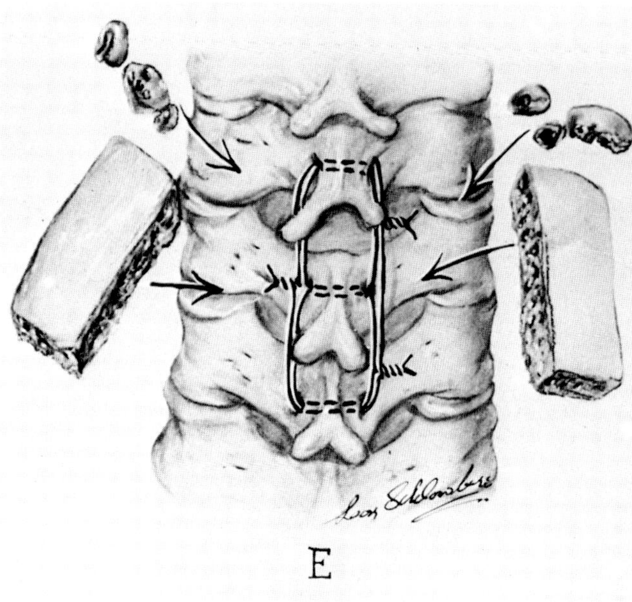

Fig. 13-5. Modified Rogers interspinous wiring and fusion.

certain of the level by attaching a hemostat to the spinous process in the middle of the incision and taking a lateral film for localization. It is also advisable to avoid dissecting periosteum from any of the laminae not to be fused because inadvertent extension of spine fusion does occur, especially in young people.

In a common situation, such as crush injury of the fifth cervical vertebra with separation of the interspinous ligament between C4 and C5, if there is a crack in the lamina of C5 as well, tension wiring will be required from C4 to C6. If, however, there is no evidence of a crack or defect in the lamina of C5, it may be quite sufficient to wire only one interspace. In order to join vertebral segments at the strongest possible location in the posterior bone for passing of wires, we usually choose the junction of the lamina to the spinous process, as seen in Figure 13-5*A*. In order to be absolutely certain of the exact location, meticulously scrape free of soft tissue the spinous process and lamina to be fused, using curettes and periosteal elevators, and visualize the edge of the vertebral foramina. Now, taking a new, sharp 7/64″ drill or a high-speed bur, make a 45° angle drill hole in each side of the base of the spinous process so that the drill holes meet without entering the spinal canal (Fig. 13-5*A*). If the hole is not widely open, passing a towel clip *gently* through the holes (always considering one's proximity to the spinal cord) will safely widen it (Fig. 13-5*B*). A loop of twisted 24-gauge wire or plain 18-gauge wire should then pass quite easily. Also, one can twist the wire around a Keith needle and then cut the needle off so that it has a blunt point. The wire or needle is passed through the hole and through a similar hole below or above. In this fashion a very strong tension band is constructed at the spinous process in the area of injury. Usually there are three wire loops, one through the spinous process of the level of injury (Fig. 13-5*C*), one through the injured vertebra to the intact spinous process below, and a third around both previous wire loops (Fig. 13-5*D*). Instead of making holes in the lower spinous process, one can pass the wire immediately inferior to the posterior spinous process.

As mentioned earlier, the wiring should extend only as far as needed to repair and stabilize the injured segment. Then, uniformly and gently tighten the wires by twisting them together, making certain each wire feeds into the twist so that one strand is not fatigued and broken. Also, be very careful that the loops are smooth and round, and that the segments are not overpulled (*i.e.*, into hyperextension). Excessive reduction resulted in diminishing of the vertebral canal in one case, with resultant injury. Alignment should be checked by a radiograph.

Next, take small iliac bone grafts from the posterior portion of the outer table of the iliac crest

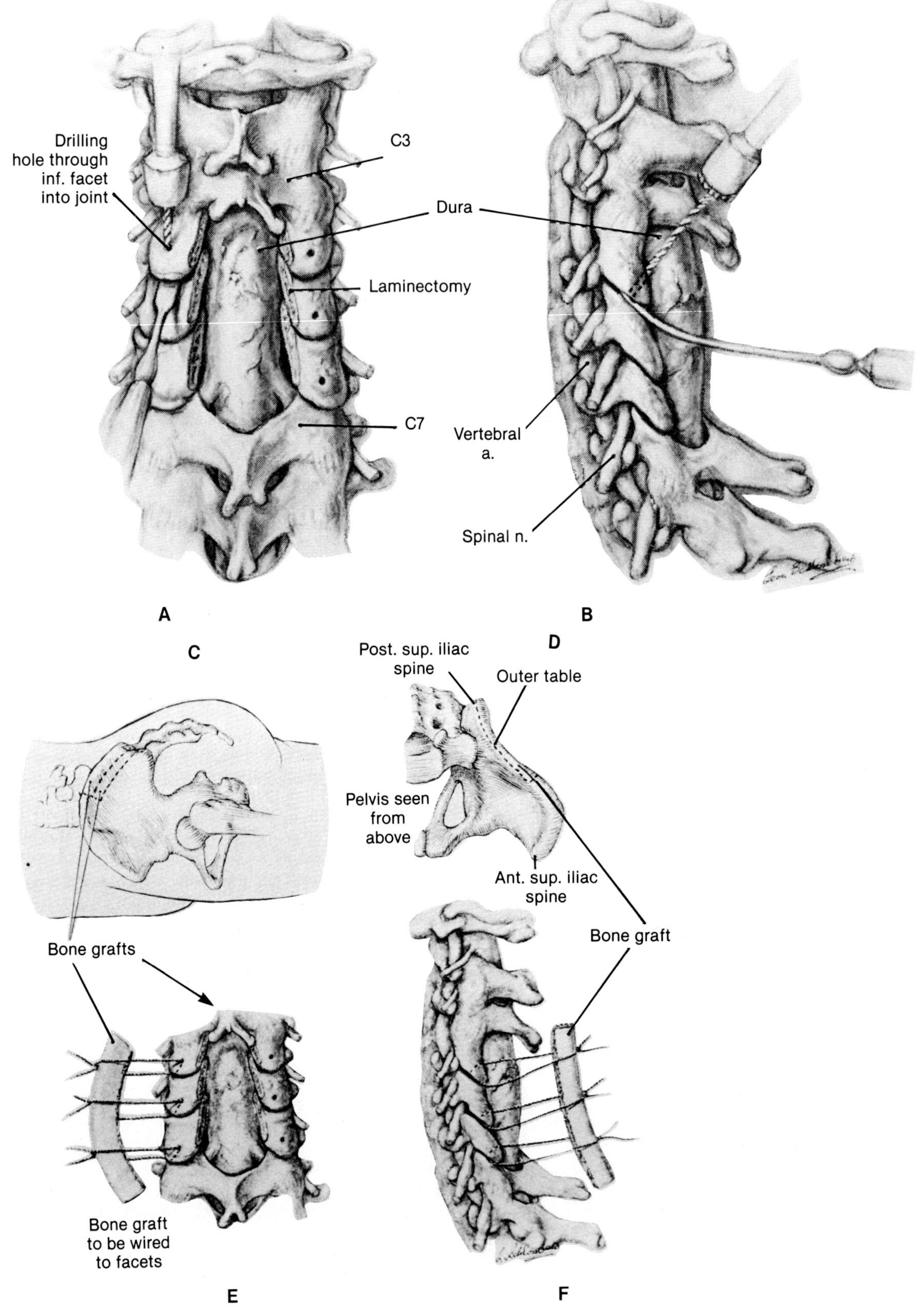
Drilling hole through inf. facet into joint
C3
Dura
Laminectomy
C7
Vertebral a.
Spinal n.
A
B
C
D
Post. sup. iliac spine
Outer table
Pelvis seen from above
Ant. sup. iliac spine
Bone graft
Bone grafts
Bone graft to be wired to facets
E
F

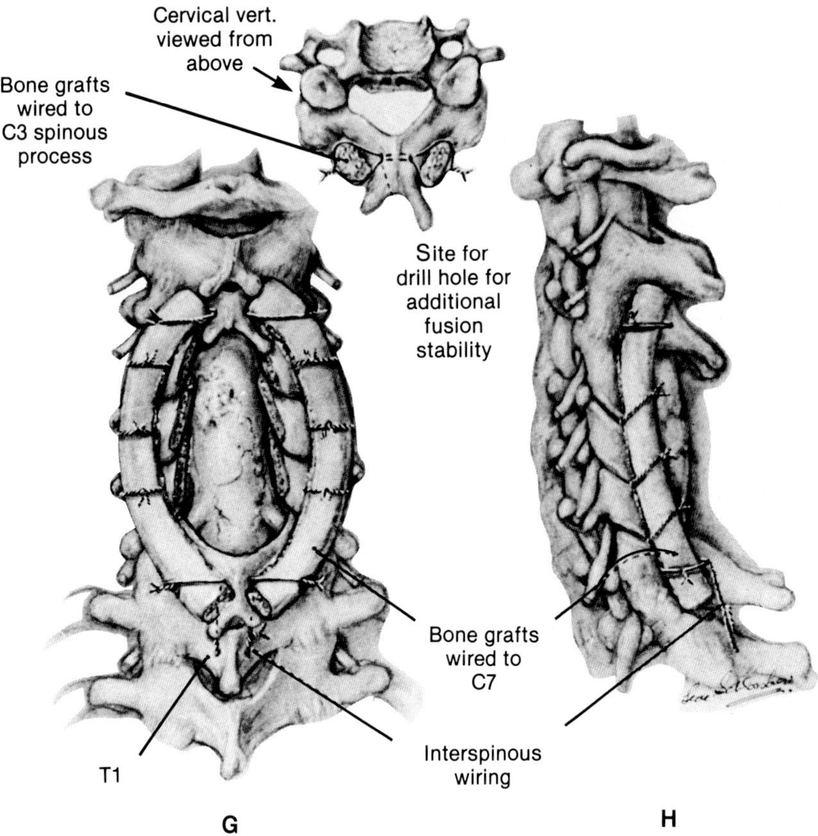

Fig. 13-6. Facet fusion used after laminectomy. After all of the soft tissues have been cleared away from the facet joints, they are pried open with a small curved osteotome, and the cartilage is removed with small curettes. (*A*) Cervical vertebrae, posterior view. (*B*) Cervical vertebrae, left lateral view. Drill holes are made into each articular process. (*C* and *D*) Note that the site of donor bone is important; one must obtain pieces of bone that fit the lordotic curve of the cervical spine. (*E*) A twisted 24-gauge wire is passed through each hole. (*F, G,* and *H*) The grafts are surrounded by wire and fit into place.

in a very small area and lay them in and around the wires (Fig. 13-5*E*). The grafts may not need to be as large as those illustrated. They should not extend beyond the fusion site. Since these grafts are simply laid on the denuded lamina, the posterior muscles must be sutured over the areas with 2-0 Dexon holding the grafts firmly in place. It is important to have a firm, solid suture line, especially for holding the superficial layer of the deep fascia since the trapezius and shoulder muscles tend to spread the wound open. The subcutaneous tissue is closed with 3-0 plain catgut and skin with interrupted 4-0 nylon sutures.

The patient is usually kept in a cervicothoracic orthosis for about 30 days to permit wound healing. Early after surgery the patient is encouraged to carry out general isometric neck muscle exercises. The responsible patient is also allowed to hold his neck in one position and remove the brace for showers. One great advantage of adequate internal fixation, of course, is early motion and prevention of cervical muscle atrophy along with the early removal of external supports.

POSTEROLATERAL FACET FUSION

When the posterior elements of the cervical spine are absent, either from laminectomy or tumor, there is danger of severe secondary deformity, primarily in flexion. This is an especially serious problem if the laminectomy was done at an early age, if the capsules of the facet joints have been damaged, if there has been an injury prior to laminectomy, or if multiple laminae have been re-

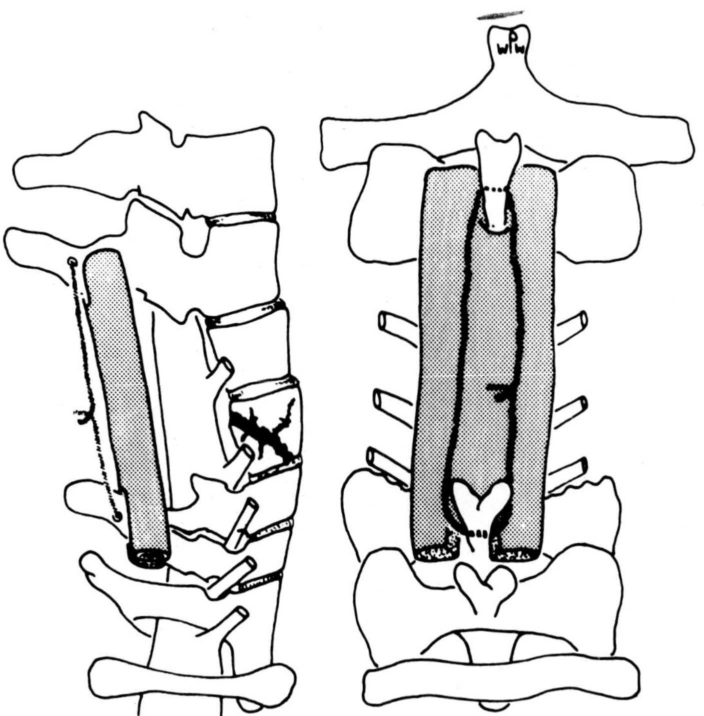

Fig. 13-7. Use of an H graft in instances of excessive posterior element trauma or surgical resection. The graft is fashioned from iliac crest in such a manner to accommodate the intact spinous processes above and below the deficient supporting structures. An interspinous wiring is then performed to lock these segments into the graft.

moved.[2,8,9] It has not been possible, apparently, to predict which cervical spines will develop a deformity, and there is controversy regarding the indications for posterolateral fusion. Generally it is better to perform the operation early in the above situations before the patient develops a significant deformity. On the other hand, it is desirable to avoid fusion of any more elements than necessary.

Position the patient for the posterior approach as described in the first section of this chapter, using the Gardner pin-vise head holder, endotracheal anesthesia, and so forth. It is always prudent to take a lateral radiograph during the procedure to check position. The skin preparation and draping should be simple; special drapes with an opening for the neck and the iliac graft make this less difficult. Take care to make the skin incision in the exact midline and the donor sites in the skin creases to obtain the least objectional cosmetic results.

In this dissection there are often no spinous processes to use as a guide, and there is often a previous incision scar. Using the same precautions described primarily to obtain hemostasis and a clean anatomic separation of tissues, begin the operation by finding the intact lamina above and below the posterior element defect. It is always wise to obtain exact normal anatomic landmarks and proceed from these. It is especially important to avoid midline scar tissue because it is very easy to inadvertently cut into the dura, making the procedure unnecessarily complicated. Of course, all of these problems are avoided if the procedure immediately follows the laminectomy.

In any event, carefully remove the soft tissues

→

Fig. 13-8. (*A*) Roentgenogram of a 35-year-old patient with cerebral palsy and marked cervical dystonia who developed progressive quadriparesis. His dystonia precluded the use of any external cervical support. (*B*) Myelogram shows the obliteration of the subarachnoid space at multiple levels. (*C* and *D*) The patient underwent multilevel laminectomy and lateral facet fusion. A contoured rod was used as an internal strut in addition to onlay bone graft, making external support unnecessary.

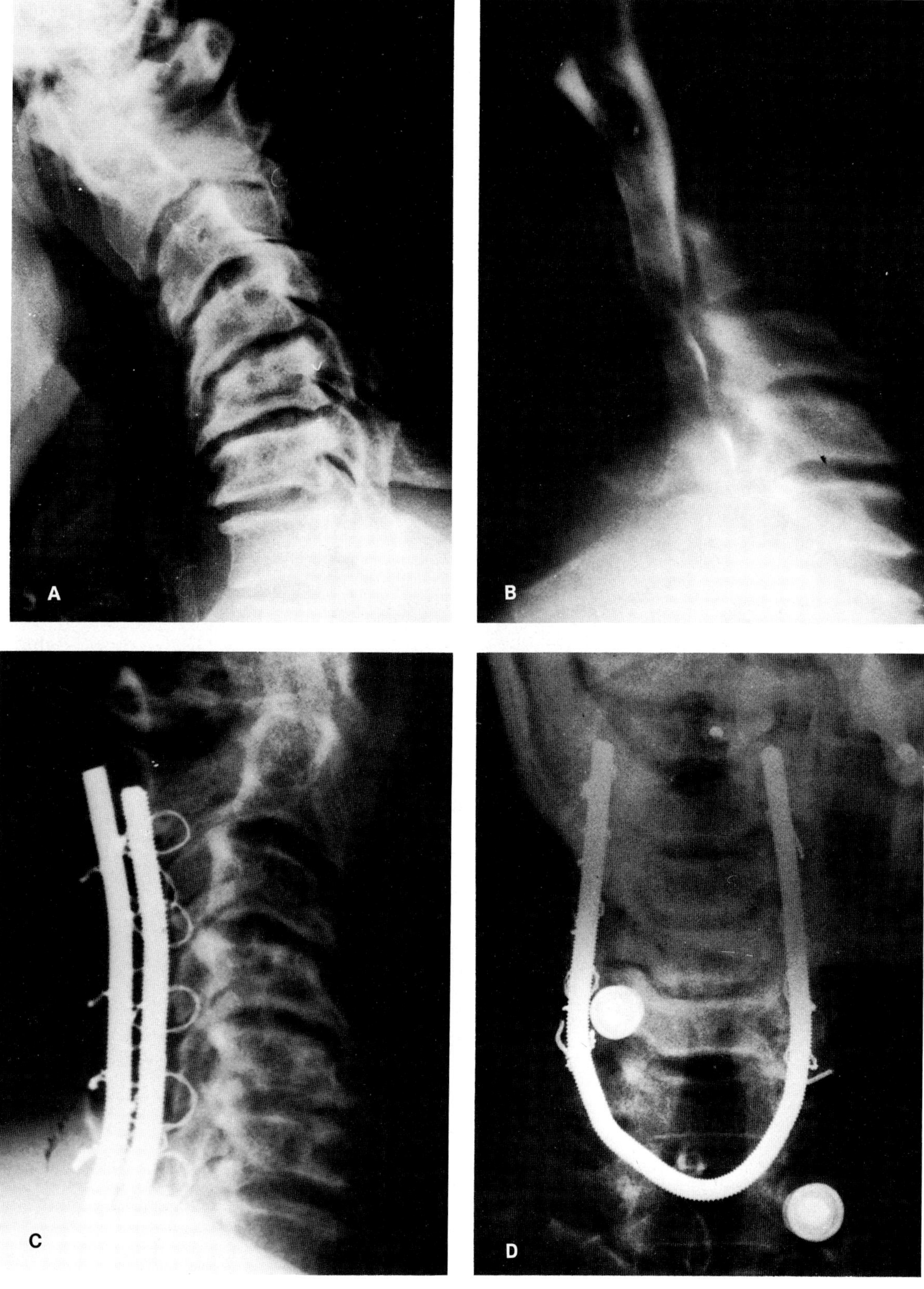
A
B
C
D

and ligaments from the superior and inferior lamina and from the facets (more properly termed the superior and inferior articular processes) and intervening posterior columns (where the laminae have been removed). After these bony elements are thoroughly cleaned and exposed, gently pry open the articular processes or facets with a thin curved osteotome. Then scrape away the articular surfaces with a fine twist drill or wire curettes to permit an opening in the joint about 2 mm wide. Next, make a new 7/64″ drill hole in the midportion of the superior facet at 90° to the articular surface of the joint (Fig. 13-6*A*).

Use this procedure of drilling a hole through each facet and cleaning out the joint at each level where spinous processes and laminae have been removed. In addition, make a drill hole in the spinous process of the first intact lamina below for anchoring the lower edge of the bone graft.

After all of the drill holes have been made and the joints cleaned between the facets to be fused, cut a 24-gauge stainless steel wire strand in 20-cm lengths; double each length and twist it about three turns per centimeter to form a strong flexible wire cable with a smooth end. Pass these wires through each drill hole down to a Halsted clamp that is placed in the joint. Each of these wires will circle the bone graft taken from the iliac crest (Fig. 13-6*C, D, E*, and *F*).

Proper removal of the combined cortical cancellous bone graft from the iliac crest is important. Because the superior bony surface of the iliac crest extending from the posterior iliac spine is curved in two planes (Fig. 13-6*C* and *D*), it is an ideal shape for a bone graft. Beginning at the iliac crest, remove a piece of cortical bone with its adjacent cancellous surface at least 2 cm wide and long enough to span the defect, using fine osteotomes

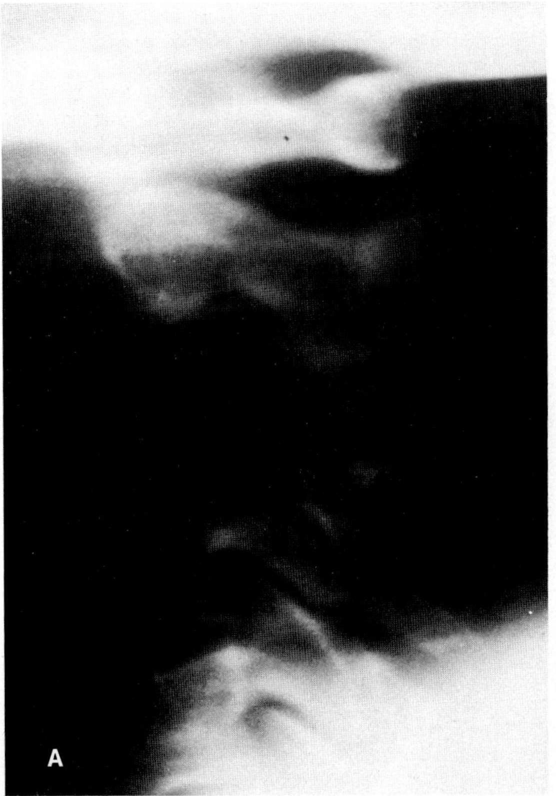

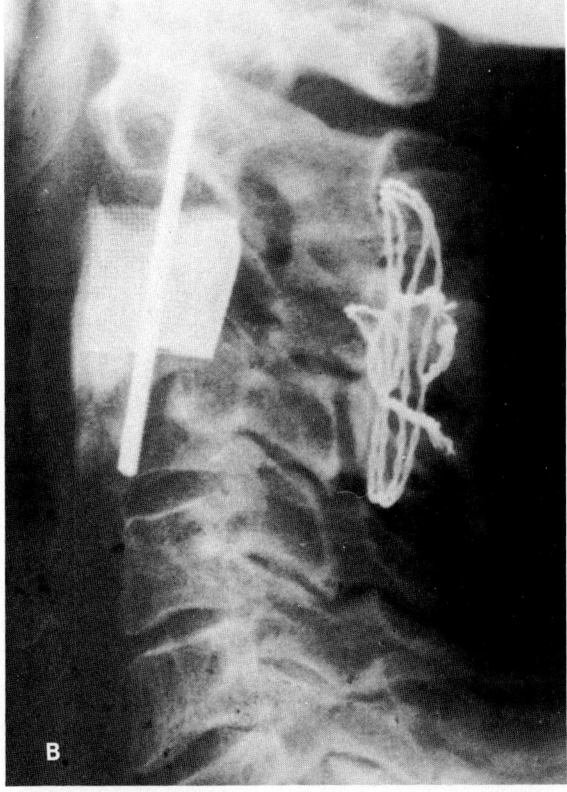

Fig. 13-9. (*A*) Lateral tomogram of a 56-year-old woman who presented with a myelopathy resulting from an undiagnosed metastatic breast carcinoma metastatic to the body of C3. (*B*) Posterior stabilization with a wire and methylmethacrylate construct was used to assure stability after anterior decompression. No bone graft was used because of the patient's anticipated aggressive chemotherapy and undetermined life expectancy.

and at times the alternating power saw. Split this piece of bone longitudinally into two 1.5-cm pieces and fit each into the lateral gutters that have been prepared. Then fit these grafts to the posterior column and twist the wires around the graft. The wires should be situated so that each wire coming from the drill hole passes medial to the graft (Fig. 13-6*E*). This fixes the graft into a lateral position and prevents pressure on the spinal cord. First twist the center wire into place so that the graft fits into the lordotic curve. Then tighten each other wire progressively. The lowermost portion of the graft should be made fast to the first intact spinous process as illustrated.

Recently Michael J. Murphy used threaded compression rods from the Harrington spinal instrumentation set as an anchor instead of the iliac bone grafts, thus obtaining immediate strength; this is especially useful with metastatic tumors and pathologic fractures (Fig. 13-3).

ALTERNATE MEANS OF FIXATION

From time to time, special circumstances will be encountered in which the standard posterior fusion techniques are inadequate, such as extensive trauma or surgical resection including both lamina and facet joints at multiple levels, metastatic tumor, exceptionally poor mechanical quality of bone graft, or conditions requiring maximum initial stabilization. These circumstances require a certain amount of ingenuity because no two cases are ever exactly the same. However, the principles defined for the standard fusions may be applied to these special circumstances, making their successful solution much easier.

For example, with extensive posterior element loss (*e.g.*, in multiple-level cervical laminectomy and facetectomy), we have used an H graft from the iliac crest with very satisfactory results.[5] This graft is placed from intact spinous process above to intact spinous process below (Fig. 13-7). In instances in which the mechanical strength of the bone graft is suspect or maximum initial stabilization is essential, such as severe cervical dystonia, we have substituted rigid metal rods for iliac struts and used only bone graft (Fig. 13-8*A*, *B*, *C*, and *D*). This has eliminated the need for postoperative cervical orthoses, which are very poorly tolerated in this group.

As Keggi and Clark from our department have recently demonstrated, debilitated patients who have a short life expectancy, such as those with metastatic tumors, may obtain adequate fixation with wire and methylmethacrylate constructs with or without bone grafts. The anterior and posterior combined approach is often advantageous in these cases. An example of such a patient is seen in Figure 13-9.

REFERENCES

1. *Brooks AL, Jenkins EW:* Atlantoaxial arthrodesis by the wedge compression method. J Bone Joint Surg 60A:279, 1978
2. *Callahan RA, Johnson RM, Margolis RN, et al:* Cervical facet fusion for control of instability following laminectomy. J Bone Joint Surg 59A:991, 1977
3. *Gallie WE:* Fractures and dislocations of the cervical spine. Am J Surg 46:495, 1939
4. *Griswold DM, Albright JA, Shiffman E, et al:* Atlanto-axial fusion for instability. J Bone Joint Surg 60A:285, 1978
5. *Murphy MJ, Ogden JA, Southwick WO:* Spinal stabilization in acute spinal injuries. Surg Clin North Am 60(5):1035, 1980
6. *Robinson RA, Southwick WO:* Surgical Approaches to the Cervical Spine. Instructional Course Lecture, American Academy of Orthopaedic Surgeons. St Louis, CV Mosby, 1960
7. *Rogers WA:* Fractures and dislocations of the cervical spine: An end-result study. J Bone Joint Surg 39A:341, 1957
8. *Sim FH, et al:* Swan neck deformity following extensive cervical laminectomy: A review of twenty-one cases. J Bone Joint Surg 56A(3):564, 1974
9. *Stauffer ES, Kelly EG:* Fracture dislocation of the cervical spine: Instability and recurrent deformity following treatment by anterior interbody fusion. J Bone Joint Surg 59A(1):45, 1977
10. *White III AA, Panjabi MM:* Clinical Biomechanics of the Spine, p 462. Philadelphia, JB Lippincott, 1978

Anterior Approaches to the Lower Cervical Spine

LEE H. RILEY, JR.

Anterior approaches to the lower cervical spine and the upper two thoracic segments are used to expose the vertebral bodies and the intervening intervertebral discs from the third cervical through the second thoracic level, the transverse processes and pedicles throughout that segment of the spine, the vertebral artery from the level of the seventh through the third cervical segment, and the emerging nerve roots in the lower cervical area. Exposure of these structures may be necessary for the treatment of cervical disc disease, tumors or infections of the anterior portion of the spine, and the sequelae of trauma involving the cervical region. This section describes two surgical approaches which permit exposure of these structures.

EXPOSURE OF THE VERTEBRAL BODIES AND INTERVERTEBRAL DISC SPACES FROM C3 THROUGH T2

The plane used to expose the anterior portion of the spine from the C3 through the T2 segment lies medial to the carotid sheath and lateral to the trachea, esophagus and thyroid gland. It is bounded superiorly by the hypoglossal and superior laryngeal nerves and by the stylohyoid and digastric muscles, and inferiorly by the rib cage and mediastinal structures. Although the stylohyoid and digastric muscles may be transected to permit superior extension of the exposure, the hypoglossal and superior laryngeal nerves may not, and therefore limit superior extension of the exposure unless the nerves are mobilized and retracted inferiorly, and the temporomandibular joint dislocated anteriorly to allow the clivus and the first two cervical segments to be visualized. The plane is crossed inferiorly by the omohyoid muscle and the superior thyroid vessels, which may be transected. This "highway to the cervical spine" allows excellent exposure of the anterior structures in the mid and lower cervical spine and the superior two thoracic segments.

The incision may be longitudinal or transverse (Fig. 13-10). A longitudinal incision is useful when three or more contiguous segments of the cervical spine are to be exposed; a transverse incision is used when three or fewer cervical segments are to be exposed. A transverse incision is preferred because of the superior cosmetic results. The key to placing either incision is the palpable anterior border of the sternomastoid muscle: the longitudinal incision is made along the palpable anterior border of the sternomastoid muscle, whereas the transverse incision is centered over the palpable anterior border of the sternomastoid muscle at the level of the cervical spine to be exposed. The level of the transverse incision is best determined by measuring the distance of the segment of the spine to be exposed superior to the clavicle on a lateral roentgenogram of the neck obtained in extension and marking that point on the skin of the neck to serve as a reference point for the incision. I prefer to expose the cervical structures through an incision based on the left side of the neck because of the more consistent position of the inferior laryngeal nerve on the left than on the right. The patient is placed in the supine position with the shoulders elevated, with a folded sheet placed transversely under the scapulae and a thyroid bag or rolled towel under the neck, and the neck is maintained in extension. Head-halter cervical traction of 5 pounds is useful in maintaining neck extension.

A transverse or longitudinal incision is made based upon the palpable anterior border of the sternomastoid muscle. The platysmal muscle fibers are easily identified deep to the subcutaneous fatty layer. The platysma is grasped between forceps and incised at the lateral corner of the incision (if a transverse incision is used) or at the inferior border of the incision (if a longitudinal incision is used). With Metzanbaum scissors or a dull clamp, the platysmal fibers are bluntly elevated from the underlying structures and incised in the line of the skin incision. Blunt elevation of the platysmal fibers before transection of the muscle prevents damage to the underlying muscle fibers and makes identification of the sternomastoid muscle easier (Fig. 13-11). The medial border of the sternomastoid is next mobilized throughout the extent of the incision to permit retraction of the medial border of the sternomastoid muscle laterally to allow identification of the underlying carotid sheath. The omohyoid muscle will be seen crossing the field in the midportion of the neck; it may be mobilized and retracted inferiorly or superiorly, or it may be divided. The carotid sheath is then identified and the middle layer or cervical fascia is sharply incised

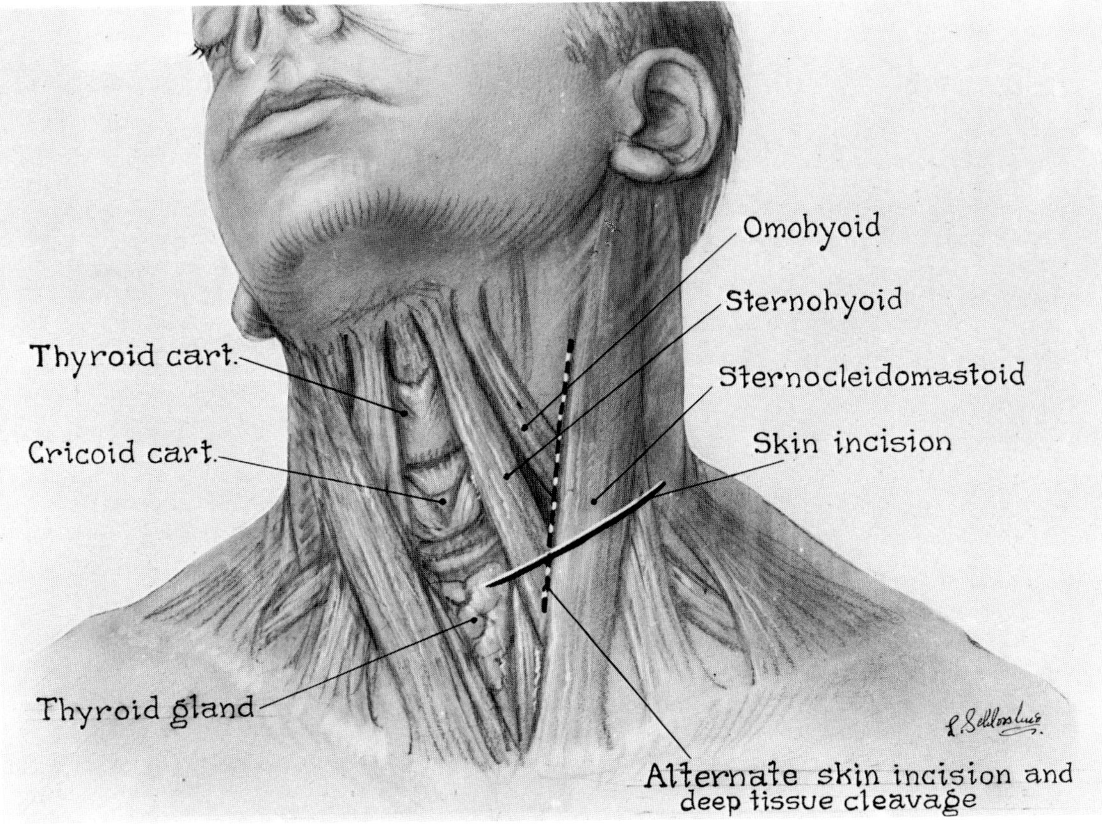

Fig. 13-10. The anterior cervical spine may be approached through a transverse or longitudinal skin incision. The key to either incision is the anterior border of the sternomastoid muscle. (Southwick WO, Robinson RA: Surgical approaches to the vertebral bodies in the cervical and lumbar regions. J Bone Joint Surg 39A:364, 1957)

just medial to and parallel with the carotid sheath throughout the extent of the exposure. This permits retraction of the carotid sheath and the sternomastoid muscle laterally, and retraction of the trachea, esophagus, and thyroid gland medially. The prevertebral fasciae are next incised longitudinally in the midline of the neck and retracted to either side. The prevertebral fasciae are swept from the anterior structures of the neck with a blunt Kidner dissector, exposing the anterior surface of the spine throughout the limits of the incision and the longus colli muscles on either side of the midline. The anterior tubercles of the transverse processes of the lower cervical vertebrae may be palpated within the substance of the longus colli muscles to either side of the midline. The superior thyroid artery and vein cross the plane of dissection at the sixth or seventh cervical segment and may be ligated and divided to permit extension of the exposure inferiorly to the second thoracic segment. The stylohyoid and digastric muscles, as well as the hypoglossal and superior laryngeal nerve, cross the plane of dissection superiorly at the level of the second cervical segment and prevent superior extension of the plane of dissection.

The longus colli muscles may be dissected from the anterior segments of the vertebral bodies and from the anterior portion of the transverse processes of the lower cervical segments, exposing the vertebral artery in the interval between the foramina transversarium of C3 through C6. The emerging nerve roots may be seen posterior to the vertebral artery as they descend to form the brachial plexus.

Closure of this incision is by reapproximation of the omohyoid muscle and the platysma muscle with fine nonabsorbable suture material, and the skin with fine sutures that may be removed on the

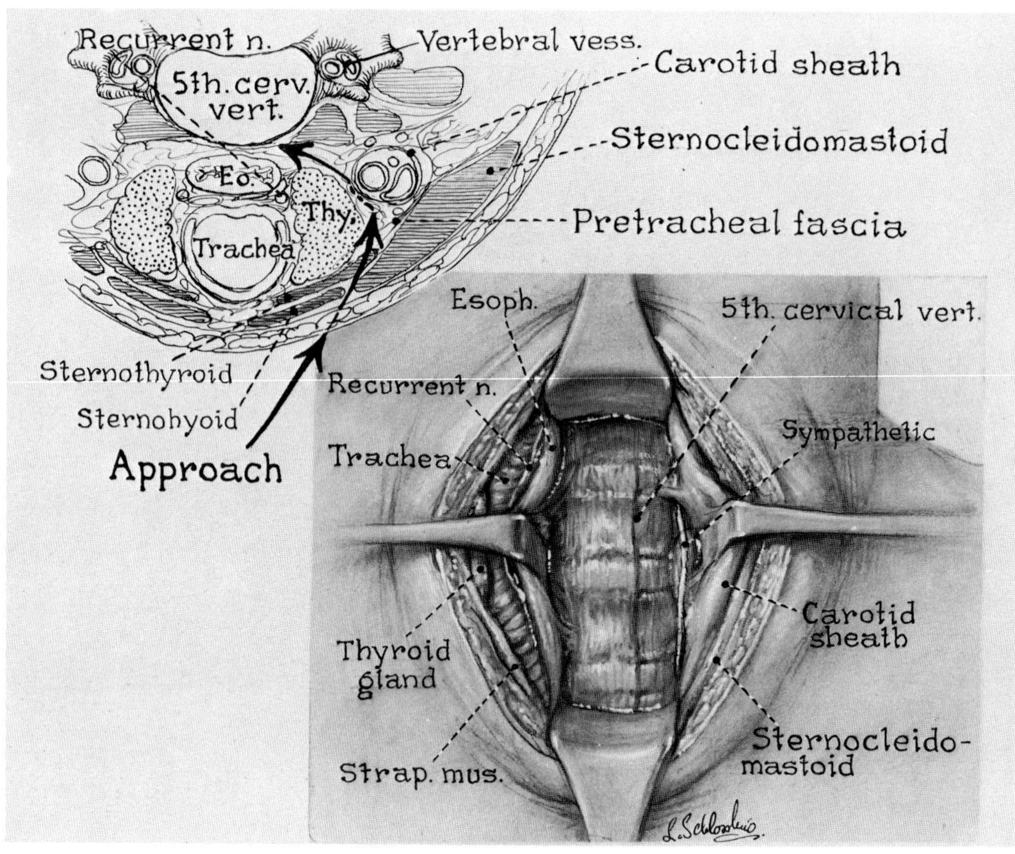

Fig. 13-11. The anterolateral approach to the cervical spine permits retraction of the sternomastoid muscle and carotid sheath laterally and the trachea, esophagus, and thyroid gland medially to permit visualization of the cervical spine. (Southwick WO, Robinson RA: Surgical approaches to the vertebral bodies in the cervical and lumbar regions. J Bone Joint Surg 39A:364, 1957)

third postoperative day to provide for an optimum cosmetic result.

EXPOSURE OF THE TRANSVERSE PROCESSES, VERTEBRAL ARTERY, AND PEDICLES FROM C3 THROUGH C7

Exposure of the transverse processes, pedicles, vertebral artery, and emerging nerve routes from the third through the seventh cervical vertebra is achieved through a transverse skin incision placed from the midline of the neck to a point several centimeters posterior to the posterior border of the sternomastoid muscle, with the patient supine on the operating room table and the chin rotated to the opposite side (Fig. 13-12). The platysma muscle is divided in line with the skin incision after bluntly elevating the platysma from the underlying structures to prevent inadvertent damage to underlying muscle structures. The flaps thus created (deep to the platysma muscle) are retracted superiorly and inferiorly, exposing the sternomastoid muscle. The anterior and posterior borders of the sternomastoid muscle are clearly identified throughout the length of the exposure. The sternomastoid muscle is bluntly elevated from the underlying structures and transected in the center of the wound, permitting superior and inferior retraction of the transected portions of the muscle. When this has been done, the phrenic nerve can be seen lying on the anterior border of the anterior scalene muscle, and the brachial plexis can be seen emerging from under the lateral border of the anterior scalene muscle. The phrenic nerve is

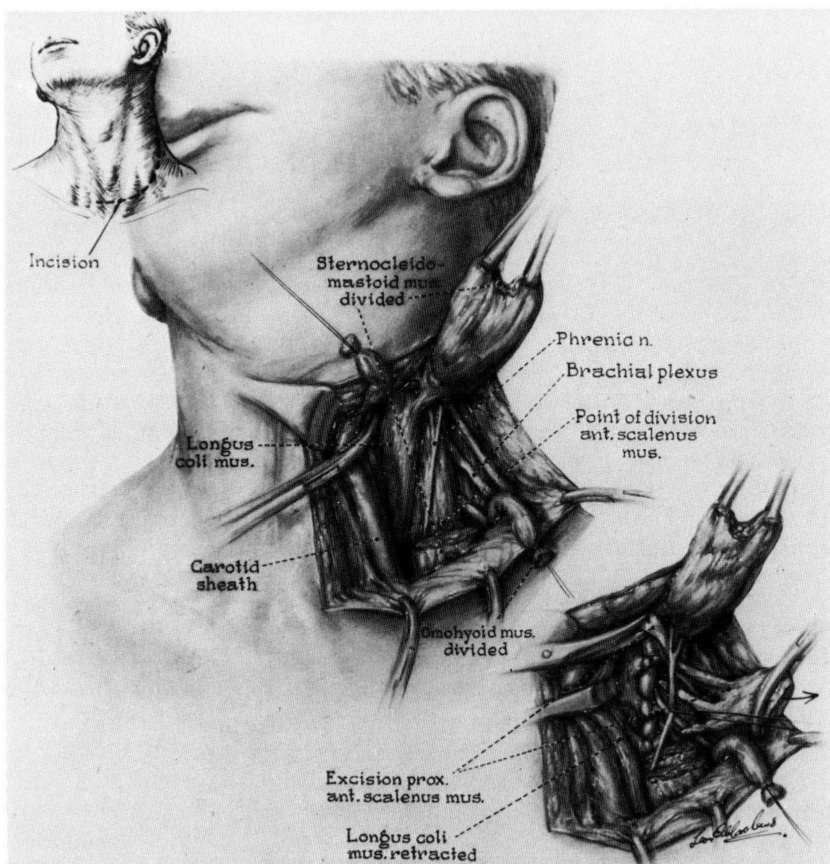

Fig. 13-12. The anterolateral structures of the neck are approached through a transverse incision, which will permit exposure of the anterior and posterior boundaries of the sternomastoid muscle. The transverse processes, the vertebral artery, and the nerve roots emerging at each level to form the brachial plexis are seen following excision of the superior portion of the anterior scalene muscle.

gently freed from the anterior border of the anterior scalene muscle and retracted anteriorly. The medial and lateral borders of the anterior scalene muscle are identified throughout the limits of the incision, and the anterior scalene muscle is transected just superior to its insertion into the first rib. The superior portion of the muscle is then dissected from its origin on the anterior tubercles of the transverse processes of C3 through C6. This exposes the anterior tubercles of C2 through C6, the vertebral artery passing through the foramen transversarium, and the intertransverse space between each segment, as well as the nerve root emerging at each level through the intervertebral foramen posterior to the vertebral artery. This exposure allows excellent visualization of the proximal portion of the vertebral artery, which may be mobilized and controlled; of the transverse processes and pedicles of the third through the seventh cervical segment; and of the emerging nerve roots and brachial plexis.

Closure is afforded by reapproximation of the sternomastoid muscle by interrupted sutures, closure of the platysma muscle by small interrupted sutures, and closure of the skin with fine suture material that may be removed on the third postoperative day to permit a pleasing cosmetic result. Drainage of the wound is recommended.

Lateral Retropharyngeal Approach to the Upper Cervical Spine

THOMAS E. WHITESIDES, JR.

Of the problems of the upper cervical spine presented to the orthopedist, the majority can best be taken care of either by nonsurgical means or by the more routine posterior surgical approach. On occasion, a direct anterior approach to the upper cervical spine may be required for either diagnosis or treatment. When occipitocervical extension and lateral rotation are possible, the classic approach medial to the carotid sheath as described by Southwick and Robinson can give exposure easily to C3.[1,2,12] The direct transoral approach as described by Fang and Ong gives exposure to C1 and C2 but not to the lower or middle aspects of the cervical spine in combination with it.[4] The major problem of postoperative infection associated with the transoral approach as reported by Fang and Ong and with the mandible and tongue-splitting transoral approach reported by Hall (50% in each report) makes them less attractive than the extrapharyngeal approach in the following circumstances: (1) when bony stability is not already present; (2) when bone graft to obtain fusion should be used; and (3) when penetration of the dura is a risk, because secondary meningitis may well be fatal.[4,5] Hodgson described another approach.[8]

Three extrapharyngeal anterior approaches to this area have been well established. Two of these are by routes medial to the carotid sheath. That described by deAndrade and McNab requires occipitocervical extension and dissection of the upper deck including the external carotid artery and the many neural structures surrounding it.[3] Another described by Riley requires anterior dislocation of the mandible on the side approached and resection of the submaxillary gland with an extensive dissection of the anatomic structures in this region.[10]

In 1963, I was directed by the late Robert P. Kelly to develop a lateral approach to this area to accomplish fusion of C1 and T2 anteriorly in a patient with cervical kyphosis secondary to laminectomy whose chin could neither be extended nor laterally rotated. Due to the problems with sepsis and lack of caudad extension associated with the transoral approach, and due to the complexities of the other approaches, we adopted Henry's approach to the vertebral artery, extending it just slightly further medially in the retropharyngeal space.[7] This approach is posterior to the carotid sheath. Our first three cases were reported in 1966, and a series of 31 procedures in 30 patients were reported in 1978.[13,14] Twenty-eight patients were followed until stable and satisfactory fusion occurred; these included 12 in whom anterior and posterior fusions were done, nine at the same operative procedure. The operation was performed for the following reasons: posttraumatic instability (ten patients including four with os odontoideum), rheumatoid arthritis or collagen disease (seven patients), primary tumor excision and fusion (three patients), biopsy of metastatic tumor (two patients), congenital malformations (two patients), postlaminectomy instability states (five patients), and infection (two patients, one with a purulent infection and a retained bullet and one with a tuberculous abscess).

Twenty-seven procedures were followed to a conclusive result, fusion having been attempted in all but four. These four included two for a metastatic tumor in which biopsy alone was performed, one for exploration of a complex fracture to determine the state of union, and one for drainage of an epidural abscess with removal of a retained bullet. All but three of the 27 patients achieved solid fusion with pain relief, arrest of neurologic deterioration, or reversal of neurologic deficits. All major complications occurred in this group and in one additional patient. In total, there was one failure of union, two early postoperative deaths, one infection in the anterior approach, and one infection in a distant wound associated with *Bacteroides* sepsis. Thus, of the 27 attempted fusions in 26 patients, there were one failure, two deaths, and one wound infection.

Since 1978, nine additional procedures have been done using the technique described below without complications. They have been of the same general distribution as the first group described above and shown in Tables 13-1 and 13-2, except that no fusions have been attempted in the mutilans form of rheumatoid arthritis. No nonunions of attempted fusions occurred, and there were no wound infections or other significant complications.

SURGICAL TECHNIQUE

The lateral retropharyngeal approach has remained essentially unchanged since it was originally reported. Because instability is usually a

*Table 13-1 Diagnostic Categories**

Instability			16
Os odontoideum		5	
Fracture nonunion or malunion		6	
Postlaminectomy deformity		5	
Collagen disease			8
Rheumatoid arthritis		4	
Ankylosing spondylitis		2	
Scleroderma		1	
Lupus erythematosus		1	
Tumor			5
Primary		3	
Myeloma	1		
Giant cell	1		
Fibroma	1		
Metastatic		2	
Breast	1		
Renal	1		
Infection			2
Tuberculosis		1	
Mixed purulent		1	
Retained foreign body (bullet)			1
Congenital deformity			2

* Four patients fell into more than one category, e.g., rheumatoid arthritis with postlaminectomy instability and ankylosing spondylitis with nonunion of odontoid fracture.

problem, the patients are generally operated upon with a halo ring in place and attached to a body cast through anteriorly placed uprights. A bone graft is usually obtained from the iliac crest through a window in the cast that is replaced at the end of the operative procedure. Nasotracheal intubation on the side opposite the approach is recommended; in order to maintain dental occlusion and keep the angle of the mandible from obstructing the area of dissection, neither this tube nor anything else should pass between the teeth. If it is not contraindicated, the neck is extended and rotated to the opposite side as much as is reasonable. The inside and outside of the ear area is prepared and the ear lobe is sewn anteriorly to the cheek to facilitate exposure of the operative incision.

A "hockey stick" incision is begun transversely across the tip of the mastoid process and carried distally along the anterior border of the sternocleidomastoid muscle. The greater auricular nerve is then identified and dissected in both directions to gain laxity, and retracted either cephalad or caudad as convenient; if it is in the way, it is often resected and a small acceptable sensory deficit results. In most cases the sternocleidomastoid muscle is detached from the mastoid process, but this is not necessary if only a limited exposure is needed and the patient is thin with small muscles. The spinal accessory nerve is then identified at its entrance into the sternocleidomastoid muscle approximately 3 cm from the mastoid tip. If only the C1–C2 area need be approached, the nerve is retracted anteriorly with the contents of the carotid sheath. If a more extensive approach is needed (extending distally into the mid and lower cervical or upper thoracic spine), the nerve is dissected from the jugular vein up to an area near the jugular foramen and then retracted laterally and posteriorly as the sternocleidomastoid muscle is everted.

Following eversion of the sternocleidomastoid muscle, the transverse processes of the cervical vertebrae, especially C1, are easily palpable. The transverse process of C1 extends more laterally than the rest. The dissection is then carried medially, often resecting the so-called jugular node or other large lymph nodes in the area. By proceeding transversely along the front border of the transverse processes and posterior to the carotid sheath, identifying the internal jugular vein and delineating it well, the vertebral artery can be avoided with safety. By extending the dissection further through the areolar plane, the fibers of Charpey (which moor the midline viscera to the prevertebral fascia and muscles) can be divided and the retropharyngeal space entered with ease.

Exposure of the appropriate vertebral bodies is now possible with subperiosteal stripping and, if needed, removal of the anterior cervical muscles (*e.g.,* the longus colli) that cover the lateral articulations of C1 and C2 and lateral reflection of these muscles more caudad. Localization is easy because of the prominent transversely oriented anterior arch of C1 and the prominent vertical midline ridge of the base of the odontoid and the body of C2. A fiberoptic headlight is essential for illumination. Malleable retractors bent to fit the differing needs that one may encounter are helpful also. This exposure has been useful for the simultaneous exposure of the right and left lateral C1 and C2 articulations through a unilateral approach for removal of vertebral bodies and the odontoid for various diseases; for biopsy of lesions of all areas of the anterior spine in this region; for fusion of C1 to T1; and to expose a small amount of the basiocciput for fusion to that area when needed. At the termination of the procedure, the sternomastoid muscle is sewn back into place after a small rigid suction drain has been installed. Only the platysma and skin layers are approximated there-

Table 13-2. Results of Treatment

Diagnosis	No. Patients with Diagnosis	Exploration or Incision and Drainage (No.)	Fusion Attempted (No.)	Fusion Successful (No.)	Fusion Failed (No.)	Died (No.)
Instability	16		16	16		
Os odontoideum	5		5	5		
Postfracture	6		6	6		
Postlaminectomy	5		5	5		
Collagen disease	8		9	7	1	1
Rheumatoid arthritis	4			3		
Ankylosing spondylitis	2			2		
Scleroderma	1			1		
Lupus erythematosus	1			1		
Tumor	5	2	3	2		1
Primary	3					
Myeloma	1		1			1
Giant cell tumor	1		1	1		
Nonossifying fibroma	1		1	1		
Metastatic	2					
Breast	1	1				
Renal	1	1				
Infection	2	1	1	1		
Tuberculosis	1		1	1		
Mixed purulent	1	1				
Retained foreign body		1				
(bullet)				2		
Congenital deformity	2		2			
Total		4	27 operations on 26 patients	24	1	2

after. Postoperative external immobilization is generally accomplished with a halo cast with special attention to windowing for abdominal breathing.

Due to difficulties with retropharyngeal edema in a few cases, tracheostomy is now done at the end of the surgical procedure in essentially all cases requiring significant retropharyngeal dissection. Resuscitation teams are now accustomed to performing intubation but are not familiar with the performance of emergency tracheostomy or difficult nasotracheal intubation techniques. It is better to carry out an elective tracheostomy than to risk the later need for an emergency procedure by inexperienced personnel. The presence of a halo cast makes the procedure more difficult, and there is a risk of serious injury if indiscriminate mobilization of the neck and head is carried out. Performance of this procedure at the termination of the operation and prior to extubation is more convenient than doing it at the beginning of the procedure.

If the procedure is done with the patient in halo cast immobilization, one has two options. If only the anterolateral procedure is planned, the halo uprights may be placed from the posterior aspect of the cast. They are then out of the way of the surgical procedure anteriorly. If a combined anterior and posterior surgical procedure is planned, it is probably better to use anterior uprights of the original design because this gives access to the posterior and lateral aspect of the neck. Tracheostomy postoperatively is a bit difficult but possible and safe; the major problem is retraction and draping. I prefer in this situation to prepare the ipsilateral anterior upright of the halo in the same manner as the skin and drape it into the operative field. This allows much greater facility in placing the retractors and so forth.

In the cephalad end of the wound superficially one may find the parotid gland. One should try to stay out of the gland because dissection into it might eventuate in a parotid fistula or facial nerve injury. Also, in the deep portion of the cephalad end of the wound lies the posterior belly of the digastric muscle. Sandwiched between this muscle and the base of the skull lies the facial nerve *en route* to the parotid gland. Owing to a complication noted below, care should be made not to retract against this area.

PATIENTS WITH MAJOR COMPLICATIONS

The occurrence of complications has to some degree affected how the procedure has developed. The most major complications were in patients with the mutilans form of rheumatoid arthritis with severe occipitocervical deformity. Fusions were attempted in three such patients. Two of these fusions were successful and in one the patient died. In another a severe complication occurred. I have had ten mutilans patients with severe difficulty in this region and have operated on three. Despite solid fusion in two of the three, all of these patients, including the seven I did not operate on, are now dead of other complications of their severe disease. I am now extremely cautious about recommending surgery in these patients.

An 86-year-old man became rapidly and progressively quadriplegic with a solitary destructive lesion of C3 but no other systemic disease. A resection of the lesion (myeloma) in conjunction with C2–C4 fusion was done using nasotracheal intubation. The patient died on the first postoperative day of massive epistaxis with aspiration of blood, cardiac arrhythmia, and cardiac arrest.

A 43-year-old woman with severe rheumatoid arthritis of only 3 years' duration had previously undergone an unsuccessful posterior C1–C2 fusion for anterior subluxation, quadriparesis, and pain. This had failed with dissolution of the graft and the posterior ring of C1. An anterior fusion from the basiocciput of C3 was performed with application of halo cast immobilization. She resumed ambulation with considerable pain relief. However, with progression of the disease the fusion mass was reabsorbed, and there was further destruction of C1–C2 articulations and migration of the body of C2 into the foramen magnum. Further neurologic deterioration including midbrain ganglion compression symptoms and inability to sit or walk because of pain necessitated a resection of C2 and another attempt at anterior fusion. After doing well in the immediate postoperative period, 5 hours following termination of the anesthetic she demonstrated signs of pontine stroke. She died 5 days later.

A 37-year-old woman was referred who had undergone a transoral biopsy of a giant cell tumor involving the odontoid, the body of C2, and the body of C3. There was severe pain and inability to sit but no neural deficits. A retropharyngeal approach was carried out with a resection of this lesion and bone grafting using an iliac crest graft from C1 to C4. On the second postoperative day retropharyngeal edema with apnea occurred. A tracheostomy had not been done at the time of surgery. Following orotracheal intubation, a breakdown of the pharyngeal wall at the site of previous biopsy occurred and a *Klebsiella* wound infection followed. With drainage of the wound and proper antibiotics, the wound healed and the graft solidified. However, the patient was left with intention tremors and mild ataxia due to anoxia. The fusion became solid but her status is unknown as she was lost to follow-up 6 months postoperatively. Thus her current status in regard to tumor recurrence is unknown.

A 51-year-old man with severe rheumatoid arthritis with only a 3-year history of the disease developed protrusion of the odontoid and body of C2 into the foramen magnum. An anterior and posterior fusion was done in sequence at the same operative procedure, followed by application of a halo hoop cast. A perforation of the cecum and retroperitoneal portion occurred on insertion of the right pelvic pin because of distortion of the pelvis. Generalized *Bacteroides* sepsis associated with infection in the subcutaneous portion of the posterior cervical wound occurred. These infections responded to appropriate antibiotics, drainage of the posterior cervical wound, and removal of the pelvic pins. The fusions became solid, relieving the neural deficit and severe upper cervical pain. However, the patient succumbed 2½ years later to the systemic ravages of severe rheumatoid arthritis.

A temporary facial palsy occurred in a patient described below (Case 1).

CASE REPORTS

Case 1

A 33-year-old woman with symptomatic os odontoideum had undergone two previous posterior fusions that had failed, the last being complicated by erosion and dissolution of the posterior arch of C1. Bilateral lateral approaches were made to the

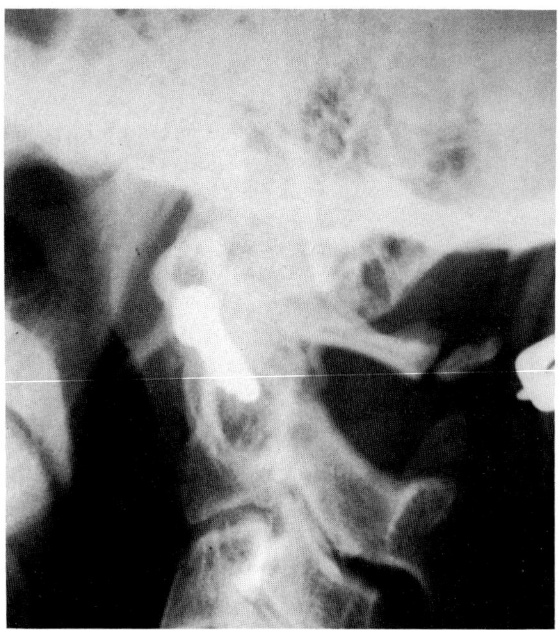

Fig. 13-13. Case 1. A–P roentgenogram of a 33-year-old woman who has undergone two previous unsuccessful posterior fusions with wiring, the last being complicated by erosion and dissolution of the posterior arch of C1. Bilateral lateral anterior C1–C2 screw fixation was carried out with curettage of lateral C1–C2 articulations and insertion of small amounts of autogenous iliac graft.

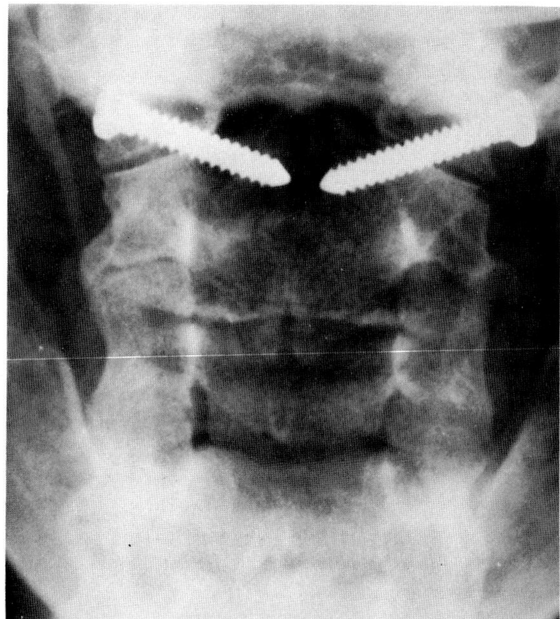

Fig. 13-14. Case 1. Postoperative A–P roentgenogram. Solid union was demonstrable within 3 months.

lateral articulations of C1 and C2 for screw fixation and fusion after the method of Barber. Temporary left facial palsy occurred, probably secondary to pressure of a retractor upon the digastric muscle under which runs the seventh cranial nerve. Four months postoperatively the patient had completely recovered from the facial palsy and had developed solid fusion of the lateral mass articulations, which were curetted at the time of surgery and packed with autogenous iliac graft (Figs. 13-13 and 13-14).

Case 2

A 27-year-old woman was seen with a 4-month history of progressive and severe upper cervical pain. An extensive destructive lesion of the entire vertebral body of C1 extending into the right pedicle and surrounding the right vertebral artery was identified. Though nulliparous, she had had a hysterectomy at age 24 for adenocarcinoma of the endometrium. An extensive search for other lesions (including bone scan and CT of chest and abdomen) and other possible primary sites revealed nothing. A right anterolateral approach was made extrapharyngeally and the majority of the lesion was removed by curettage. The lesion involved the body back to the posterior longitudinal ligament and down to the C2–C3 disc space. The superior articular surfaces and the odontoid were intact. A frozen section was examined and the lesion was felt to be malignant; a methylmethacrylate plug was then put in place. Halo cast fixation was used. After the original lesion was identified as a malignant histiocytic lymphoma, a posterior fusion was carried out, which relieved the local symptomatology. Irradiation of the primary site using a linear accelerator was carried out through lateral ports. The patient did quite well and began systemic chemotherapy 2 months later upon the identification of lesions in the pulmonary parenchyma and soft tissue of the right shoulder. She failed to respond and developed many other soft-tissue and bony tumor sites identified by bone scanning and other techniques. She succumbed despite her therapy 4 months from the time of her original operative procedure. During that time, the upper cervical area remained asymptomatic (Figs. 13-15, 13-16, and 13-17).

Case 3

A 30-year-old woman had, over the past several years, noted gradual inability to look up and dis-

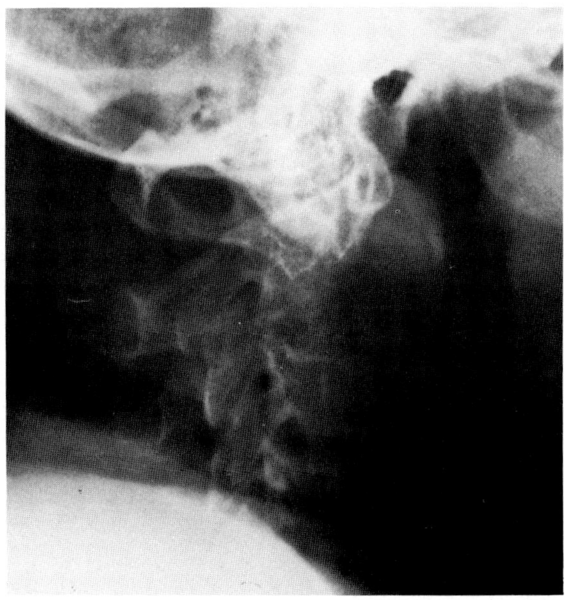

Fig. 13-15. Case 2. Lateral roentgenogram demonstrating destruction of the body of C2 in a 27-year-old woman. Biopsy revealed reticulum cell sarcoma.

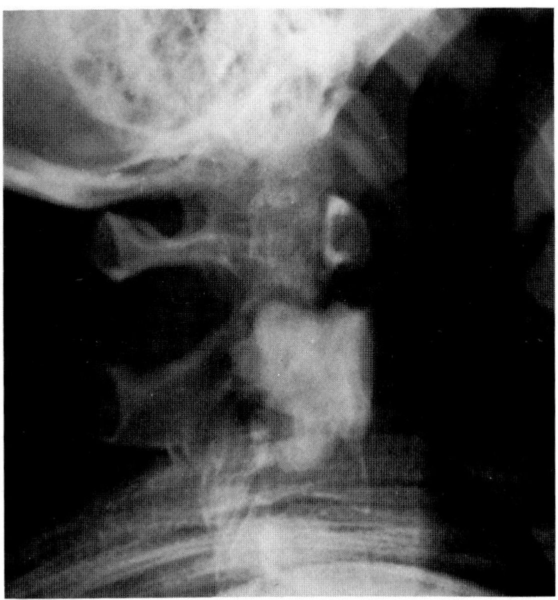

Fig. 13-16. Case 2. Postoperative anterior approach with methocrylate spacer. Lateral irradiation was carried out with a linear accelerator.

comfort on lateral rotation of the head. Over the previous months she had developed long-tract neurologic deficits while ambulating with resolution of the deficits on assuming the supine posture. X-ray films showed a fixed C1–C2 dislocation with an os odontoideum. Both she and her parents faintly recalled a fall from a bicycle in adolescence, following which she had a short period of neck pain but no disability. The patient was placed in a halo cast. Extensive traction and attempted posterior displacement failed to change the position; however, relief of all neurologic deficits occurred. Since posterior fusions alone in this area are subject to distraction forces (the center of gravity of the head is, as a result, anterior to its support column and the unsupported weight of the head causes flexion and distraction moments posteriorly), an anterior C1–C2 fusion and a posterior occiput-to-C2 fusion were carried out, one after the other during the same anesthetic, using autogenous iliac graft. The occiput was included in the posterior fusion because C1 was immobile in relation to the skull, suggesting no motion in the occipitocervical articulations. A tracheostomy was done at the end of the operative procedure and left in place until resolution of the retropharyngeal edema. The patient remained in her halo cast for a period of 3 months, at which time consolidation

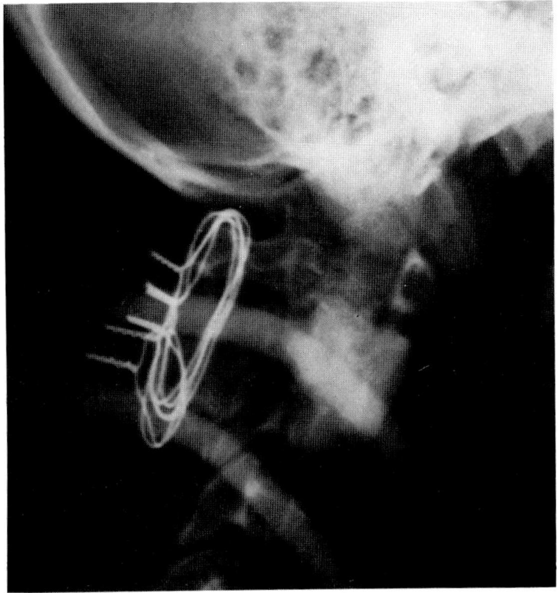

Fig. 13-17. Case 2. Lateral roentgenogram after posterior fusion to augment anterior fusion.

of the fusion masses appeared to be occurring. Three years postoperatively the fusion was quite solid and she had no neural deficits (Figs. 13-18, 13-19, and 13-20).

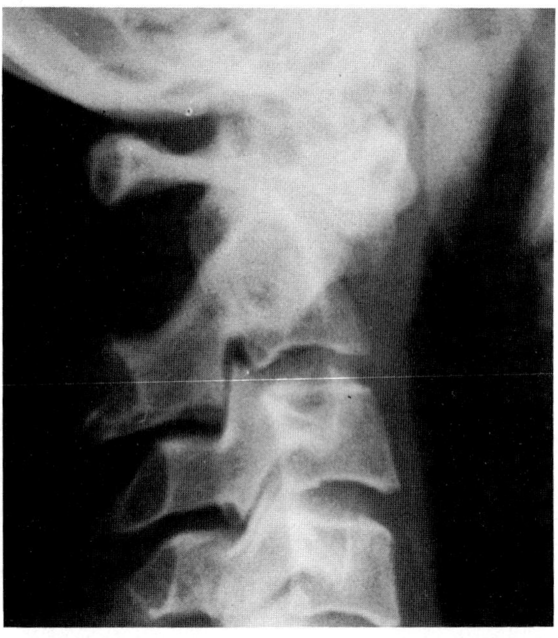

Fig. 13-18. Case 3. Lateral roentgenogram of a 30-year-old woman suffering long tract signs and medullary compression signs on ambulation.

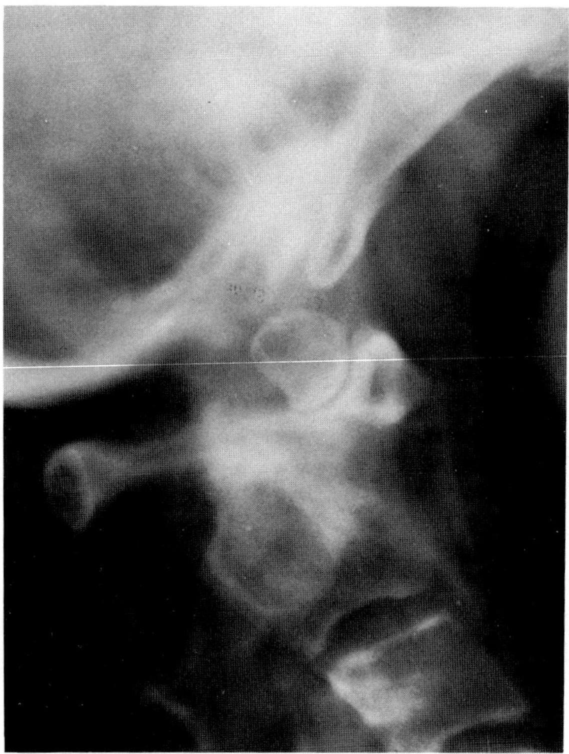

Fig. 13-19. Case 3. Lateral tomograms showing os odontoideum consistent with history of injury in childhood. Reduction was impossible despite prolonged halo traction. Anterior and posterior fusion were done in the same operative procedure and the patient was held for 3 months in a halo cast. Solid union resulted.

Case 4

A 47-year-old man was seen 3 months after initial therapy. He had suffered an upper cervical injury 20 years ago for which he received temporary external splintage and became asymptomatic. No records from that time are now available. He developed upper cervical pain without neural deficits, for which a posterior cervical fusion with wiring was done. He awoke from the operative procedure with continued pain but without neural deficit. He was placed into a soft cervical collar and within 10 days developed progressive quadriparesis. A repeat posterior wiring was carried out, using more and larger wires. He awoke from this operative procedure with more profound quadriparesis. Two months in cervical traction failed to relieve the situation or reduce the fixed dislocation. On transfer to a rehabilitation hospital he had severe quadriparesis with loss of bladder and sphincter function, and he was unable to lift his legs from the bed, feed himself, write, or carry out more than minor motions of the hand. A 5 cm × 7 cm decubitus ulcer was present over the occiput. He was then transferred from a distant city to my care.

The patient was placed into a halo cast and an attempt at reduction by posterior displacement with traction produced no change. The use of the halo cast allowed debridement of the occipital decubitus (which was down to the skull). A rotational flap was carried out with skin grafting of the defect and rapid closure of the wound. Then, under general anesthesia, the posterior aspect of the occipital cervical area was explored and the wires removed. The bone graft in place in this area was over the convexity of the displacement and under tension. Even at 3½ months following fusion, the graft was tenuous. The graft was augmented and, under the same anesthetic, an anterior fusion was carried out from C1 to C3; this procedure resulted in solid fusion in 3 months and progressive partial resolution of his neural deficits to the point that he can write, feed himself, and walk with external support secondary to moderate spasticity in the lower extremities; he has also had recovery of sphincter control and sexual function. Some ataxia in the upper extremities persists.

When there is irreducible anterior dislocation of C1 on C2, the spinal canal can be compromised even though the original space for the spinal cord is quite large. The compromise occurs between the posterosuperior border of the body of C2 and the anterior aspect of the posterior arch of C1. The compromise is possibly worsened by extension in C1–C2 articulations. Passage of wires beneath the arch of C1 and the arch of C2 encroaches upon this space even further; thus it is obviously extremely dangerous and should not be done in such irreducible states. I have not had success with posterior fusion alone in these irreducible states; however, in three such instances anterior fusion has been successful. In two, posterior fusion consolidated after the anterior fusion had consolidated, and in one (Case 3) the procedures were done simultaneously with success (Figs. 13-21, 13-22, and 13-23).

CONCLUSIONS

The lateral approach to the upper cervical spine has been useful in a variety of disease processes. Its performance demands expertise in the use of

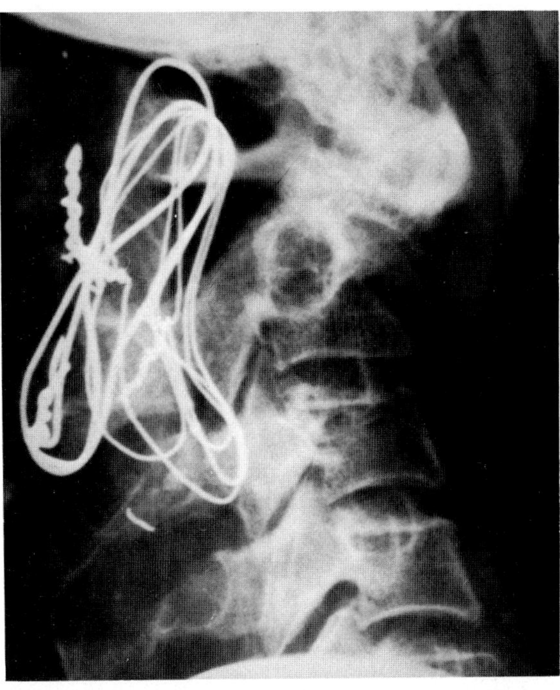

Fig. 13-21. Case 4. Roentgenogram of a 47-year-old man who suffered a cervical injury 20 years ago. A fixed anterior dislocation was present with an os odontoideum. Wire fixation had been carried out 3 months previously.

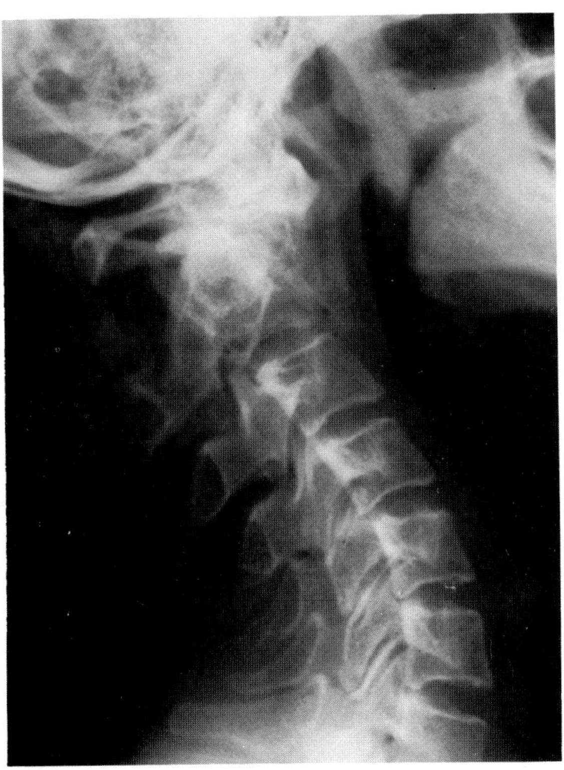

Fig. 13-20. Case 3. Lateral roentgenogram showing maturing anterior C1–C2 and posterior occiput–C2 fusion. Further maturation occurred. At surgery C1 was found to be fused to the occiput.

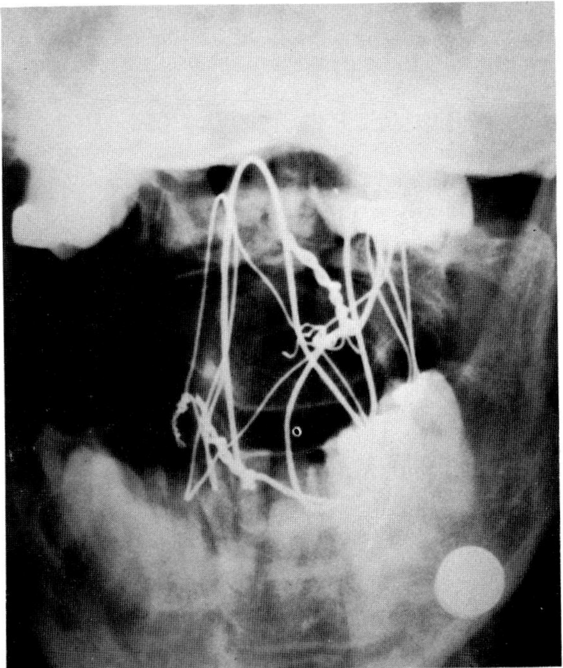

Fig. 13-22. Case 4. The patient suffered the rapid onset of neural deficits, which was treated by more and larger wire at a second operative procedure. Very severe quadriparesis resulted.

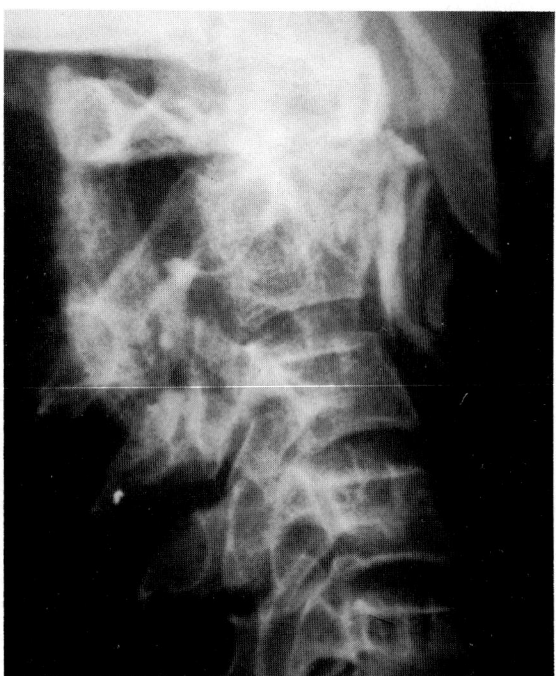

Fig. 13-23. Case 4. Wire removal and anterior fusion with augmentation of posterior fusion yielded rapid, significant recovery.

a number of techniques for upper cervical spine immobilization, varied and advanced diagnostic procedures, excellent anesthesia, high-quality postoperative nursing care, and the patience to carry out a very demanding operation through a somewhat limited exposure. I now also use cortical evoked potential monitoring. This exposure has been adequate in our experience to meet all the needs encountered in this area without resorting to a transoral approach. The depth of the wound, when measured from the side of the neck, is approximately half that from the incisors (as in a transoral approach). The reports of Hall and of Fang and Ong show an instance of infection of 50%.[4,5] In my series there has been a 2.5% incidence of infection. The incision can be extended distally to encompass the entire cervical and the upper thoracic spine when necessary. Tracheostomy should be done in all cases involving significant retropharyngeal dissection to avoid postoperative respiratory passage embarrassment. Considering the magnitude of the problems encountered, complications have been relatively few and rewarding results have been the rule.

REFERENCES

1. *Bailey RW, Badgley CE:* Stabilization of the cervical spine by anterior fusion. J Bone Joint Surg 42A:565, 1960
2. *Cloward RB:* Neurosurgery 15:602, 1958
3. *deAndrade JR, McNab I:* Anterior occipitocervical fusion using an extrapharyngeal approach. J Bone Joint Surg 51A:1621, 1969
4. *Fang HS, Ong GB:* Direct anterior approach to the upper cervical spine. J Bone Joint Surg 44A:1588, 1962
5. *Hall JE, Dennis F, Murray J:* Exposure of the upper cervical spine for spinal decompression by a mandible and tongue splitting approach. J Bone Joint Surg 59A:121, 1977
6. *Hartman JT, Palumbo DL, Hill BJ:* Cineradiography of the braced normal cervical spine. Clin Orthop 109:97, 1975
7. *Henry AK:* Extensile Exposure, 2nd ed. pp 53–80. Edinburgh, E & S Livingston, 1957
8. *Hodgson AR:* An approach to the cervical spine (C3–C7). Clin Orthop 39:129, 1965
9. *Ramsby GP, Southwick WO:* J Bone Joint Surg 59A:332, 1977
10. *Rothman RM, Simeone FA:* The Spine, pp 69–133. Philadelphia, WB Saunders, 1975
11. *Simmons E:* Bilateral screw fixation fusion C1–C2. Orthop Clin North Am 9(4):1978
12. *Southwick WO, Robinson RA:* Approaches to the vertebral bodies in the cervical and lumbar regions. J Bone Joint Surg 39A:631, 1957
13. *Whitesides TE Jr, Kelly RP:* Lateral approach to the upper cervical spine for anterior fusion. South Med J 59:879, 1966
14. *Whitesides TE Jr, McDonald P:* Lateral retropharyngeal approach to the upper cervical spine. Orthop Clin North Am 9(4): 1978

Direct Transoral Anterior Approaches to the Upper Cervical Spine

E. SHANNON STAUFFER

Surgical procedures for vertebral biopsy, disc excision, and fusion of the cervical vertebrae two, three, and four, up to the base of the odontoid can usually be achieved by the standard anterolateral approaches described elsewhere in this chapter. However, adequate exposure of the upper end of the anterolateral approach requires division of the superior thyroid and lingual and facial branches of the external carotid artery and places the superior laryngeal nerve in jeopardy.

Adequate exposure of the posterior aspects of the first, second and third cervical vertebral bodies and mass lesions dorsal to the vertebral bodies in the spinal canal may require a direct anterior transoral approach for adequate exposure and excision.

The transoral approach, retracting the mandible, as described by Fang and Ong,[4] provides direct anterior exposure of the first and second vertebrae. This is usually adequate for biopsy, aspiration, and excision and drainage of abscesses, but it provides limited access for reconstructive procedures due to the depth of the wound and the restricted space limited by the excursion of the temporal mandibular joint.[1,3]

Transoral approaches to the upper cervical spine have a reported higher risk of infection than retropharyngeal approaches.[2,9,10]

If wider exposure is necessary than can be achieved through the anterolateral or open-mouth approach, the mandibular-tongue-pharynx splitting approach offers direct anterior wide exposure of the cervical vertebral bodies from the clivus to C6. This allows adequate excision of the vertebral body, disc, tumor, or other pathologic tissue and reconstructive bone grafting. Although the original description by Fang and Ong reported a high incidence of postoperative infection problems, recent reports dealing with noninfected, clean surgical procedures with appropriate antibiotic coverage[5,9] indicate that the wider exposure with less tissue tension and tissue trauma results in a low risk of postoperative infection.

Frequently, the operation can be performed without removing a central lower incisor; however,

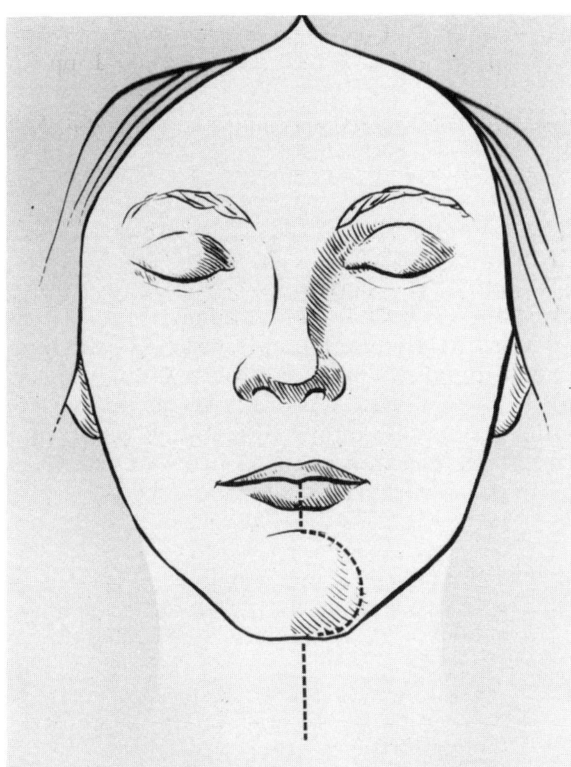

Fig. 13-24. Skin incision for mandible splitting approach.

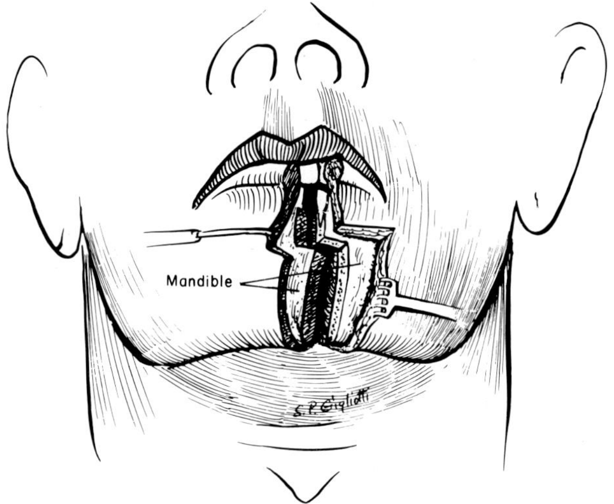

Fig. 13-25. The transoral mandible and tongue-splitting approach may require removal of a lower incisor. A step-cut osteotomy ensures correct realignment in closure. Tracheostomy is necessary in this procedure.

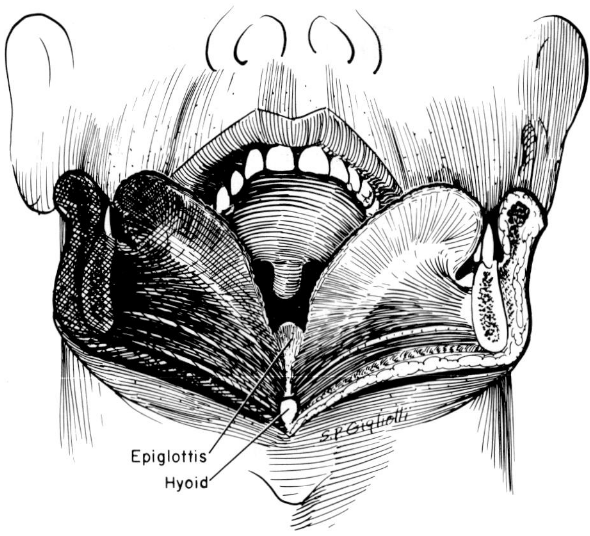

Fig. 13-26. Splitting the tongue after osteotomy of the mandible allows access to the posterior pharynx.

occasionally, a central lower incisor comes loose and must be removed.

The vertical incision is made from the center of the lower lip down to the prominence of the chin, which is circumscribed, and the incision is continued vertically to the back of the chin (Fig. 13-24). The mucous membrane is split, and the mandible is predrilled for closing sutures and cut in a step-cut fashion to facilitate accurate reapproximation (Fig. 13-25). The tongue is split longitudinally through its central raphe. The two halves of the mandible and tongue are retracted laterally on each side to expose the epiglottis and palate (Fig. 13-26). The vertebral prominences of the upper cervical spine can be palpated through the posterior pharyngeal wall, and the mucosa is split in the middle, creating a flap on either side, allowing exposure of the cervical vertebrae from the clivus to C6 (Fig. 13-27).

A preoperative tracheostomy is required for adequate anesthesia and postoperative management. The tongue is repaired with absorbable sutures. The mandible is repaired with wire sutures through predilled holes, and the skin with fine interrupted nonabsorbable sutures.

A halo jacket is usually necessary for postoperative immobilization to obviate the mandibular pressure inherent with a cervicothoracic orthosis. This also allows free visual access to the surgical incision and facilitates examination of pharyngeal healing.

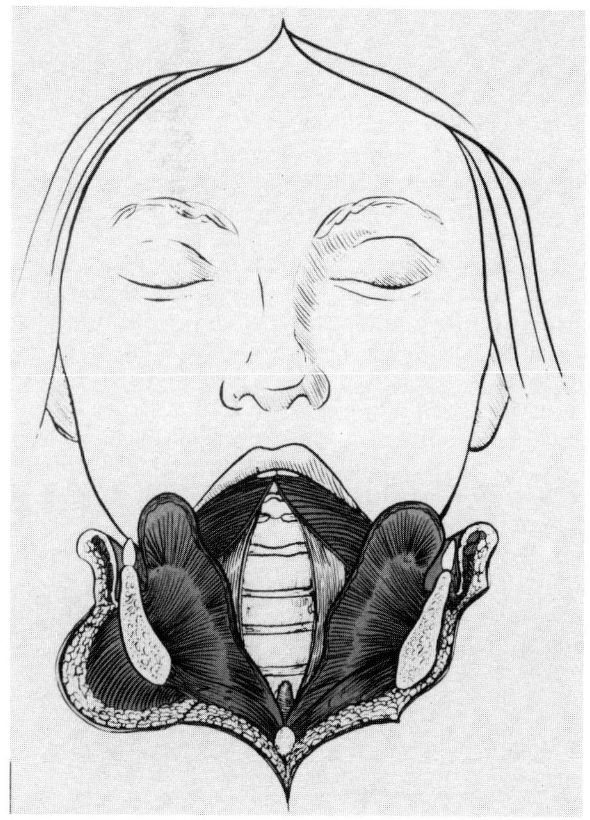

Fig. 13-27. Direct anterior exposure of C1 to C6.

The tracheostomy may be removed when the incision has healed and the airway is clear of swelling or obstruction.

Although the magnitude of the surgical procedure is greater than the standard anterolateral approach or the open-mouth approach, the mandibular-tongue splitting approach should be considered when wide exposure is necessary. The postoperative morbidity is minimal when compared with the safety of the improved exposure of the upper cervical spine and neural canal.

REFERENCES

1. *Apuzzo MLJ, Weiss HH, Heidon JS:* Transoral exposure of the atlantoaxial region. Neurosurgery 3:201, 1978
2. *deAndrade JR, MacNab I:* Anterior occipitocervical fusion using an extrapharyngeal approach. J Bone Joint Surg 51A:1621, 1969
3. *Estridge MN, Smith RA:* Transoral fusion of odontoid fracture. J Neurosurg 27:462, 1967
4. *Fang HS, Ong GB:* Direct anterior approach to

the upper cervical spine. J Bone Joint Surg 44A:1588, 1962

5. *Hall JE, Denis F, Murray J:* Exposure of the upper cervical spine for spinal decompression by a mandible and tongue-splitting approach. J Bone Joint Surg 59A:121, 1977
6. *Kocher T:* Surgery of the pharynx. In Kocher: Operative Surgery. London, Black, 1911
7. *Selman WR, Spetzler RF, Brown R:* The use of intraoperative fluoroscopy and spinal cord monitoring for transoral microsurgical odontoid resection. Clin Orthop 154:51, 1981
8. *Spetzler RF, Selman WR, Nash CL, et al:* Transoral microsurgical odontoid resection and spinal cord monitoring. Spine 4:506, 1979
9. *Stauffer ES:* Mandibular splitting approach to the upper anterior vertebral canal. In Kehr P, Weidner A (eds): Cervical Spine, Vol I, p 330. New York, Springer-Verlag, 1987
10. *Whitesides TE, Kelly RP:* Lateral approach to the upper cervical spine for anterior fusion. South Med J 59:879, 1966
11. *Whitesides TE, McDonald AP:* Lateral retropharyngeal approach to the upper cervical spine. Orthop Clin North Am 9:1115, 1978

Anterior Retropharyngeal Approach to the Upper Cervical Spine

PAUL C. MCAFEE, HENRY H. BOHLMAN, LEE H. RILEY, ROBERT A. ROBINSON, AND WAYNE O. SOUTHWICK

In a consecutive series of 15 patients, we utilized a superior extension of Robinson's anterior approach, which provided anterior access to the neural elements from the clivus to the C3 vertebral body without need of posterior dissection of the carotid sheath or entrance into the hypopharynx or oral cavity. The approach provided adequate exposure for iliac or fibular strut grafting. Because of its continuity with the conventional Robinson approach to the middle and lower cervical spine, it allowed exposure from the clivus superiorly to the lower cervical vertebra inferiorly.

The anterior surgery performed through the retropharyngeal approach was an anterior intralesional excision for tumor in eight patients, one marginal excision for an osteochondroma, two C2 corpectomies combined with removal of the odontoid, one C2 corpectomy for fixed atlantoaxial subluxation, one removal of a bullet anterior to the clivus, one anterior C2–C3 reduction and fusion of an unstable Hangman's fracture in a patient with Klippel-Feil syndrome, and one anterior débridement for pyogenic vertebral osteomyelitis. Thirteen patients had anterior strut fusions at the time of decompression.

In contrast to reports of the transmucosal approaches to the atlas and axis, there were no cases of infection among the total 17 cases. None of the patients had iatrogenic spinal neurologic deficits.

Twelve patients followed 2 or more years postoperatively had a solid anterior arthrodesis and no subsequent loss of cervical spine stability. Neck pain was relieved in all patients presenting with pathologic and traumatic fractures. Postoperative computed tomography (CT) was performed in four cases, and documented anatomically successful spinal cord decompressions in all four. In five additional patients, plain lateral tomography was obtained, which documented anatomically successful anterior decompression procedures. Plain roentgenograms at 10 years follow-up in the patient undergoing débridement for pyogenic vertebral osteomyelitis showed a successful decompression and fusion.

Four patients showed neurologic improvement postoperatively. One patient had a persisting Brown-Séquard syndrome but was ambulatory. The other five patients remained neurologically intact.

RETROPHARYNGEAL APPROACH

Anterior approaches and decompression of the cervical spinal cord are occasionally indicated superior to the C2–C3 intervertebral disc. Thus far, the previously described anterior approaches utilized (1) dislocation of the temporomandibular joint,[10] (2) osteotomy of the mandible and a tongue-splitting approach,[5] and (3) a transoral approach with an alarming 50% infection rate.[4] Whitesides described a lateral extrapharyngeal approach,[22,23] which does not readily allow strut grafting anteriorly in cases of instability and loss of bone stock.

The anterior retropharyngeal approach to the upper cervical spine achieves exposure sufficient for extirpation and stabilization of lesions involving the atlas and axis. This exposure is accomplished while remaining entirely extramucosal. It is a cranial extension of the anterior cervical approach described by Robinson and Smith in 1955,[11] and it can be used for spinal canal decompression as well as strut graft stabilization. We are reporting our experience with 17 patients who have undergone this procedure.

MATERIALS AND METHODS

Table 13-3 lists the information on 17 consecutive patients undergoing anterior retropharyngeal approaches to the upper cervical spine: 14 at The Johns Hopkins Hospital, two at the Yale New Haven Hospital, and one patient (Case 7) at Case Western Reserve University Hospitals. Robert A. Robinson, M.D. performed the first procedure on April 27, 1959 (Case 14), utilizing the anterior cervical approach described in 1955 without division of the stylohyoid or digastric tendons to permit rotation of the hyoid bone and hypopharynx. The extensile approach described here was first utilized for patient 3 and described in 1973 by Riley,[10] who included dislocation of one temporomandibular joint to increase exposure, a step necessary for only two patients in this series (Cases 2 and 3). We now believe sufficient exposure can be achieved without dislocation of the temporomandibular joint, except in patients in whom profound instability obviates extension of the spine and rotation of the skull to the contralateral side. In addition, we believe that adequate exposure can be achieved through a smaller skin incision than described by Riley in 1973.

The perioperative complications and technical considerations are known for all 15 patients. Twelve patients with 2 years or more follow-up are the basis for a review of the results—but we think a more accurate assessment of the difficulty of the procedure should be derived from analysis of the complications of all 17 cases.

There were 11 males and six females with a mean age of 44 years (range 14 to 66 years). The pathology of the upper cervical spine involved neoplasms in 11 patients (Cases 1 to 5, 10, 12 to 14 and 16, 17), trauma in three (Cases 6 to 8), basilar invagination of the odontoid in two patients (Cases 9 and 11), and one patient (Case 15) had a pyogenic vertebral osteomyelitis.

Seven patients presented with motor dysfunction: Cases 5, 9, and 17, quadriparesis; Case 11, cruciate paralysis of Bell; Case 7, Brown-Séquard syndrome; and Cases 8 to 10, spasticity. There were sensory problems only in Cases 14 and 17 and eight patients were neurologically intact (Cases 1 to 4, 6, 12, 13, and 15).

The anterior surgery performed through the retropharyngeal approach was an anterior intralesional excision in ten patients (Cases 2 to 5, 10, 12 to 14, 16, and 17), one marginal excision (Case 1), two C2 corpectomies combined with removal of the odontoid (Cases 9 and 11), one C2 corpectomy for fixed atlantoaxial subluxation (Case 7), one removal of a bullet anterior to the clivus (Case 6), one anterior C2–C3 reduction and fusion of an unstable Hangman's fracture in a patient with Klippel-Feil syndrome (Case 8), and one anterior débridement for a C2 to C4 pyogenic vertebral osteomyelitis. Fifteen patients had either tricortical iliac or fibular strut graft fusions combined with the anterior decompressions (Cases 2 to 5 and 7 to 17). In two instances (Cases 1 and 6) fusions were not necessary.

Due to the inherent instability of the pathologic processes at the axis or atlas, 11 patients required posterior stabilizations and fusions to augment the anterior procedures. In Cases 3, 7, 12, 14, and 16 the posterior fusion was performed first. Six patients (Cases 2, 4, 5, 9, 10, and 13) had the anterior surgery performed prior to the posterior stabilization and fusion procedure, with Cases 10 and 13 being combined into one anteroposterior operative procedure.

SURGICAL TECHNIQUE

The patient is transferred supine to an operative wedge turning frame, and a careful neurologic examination is repeated. Somatosensory evoked cortically recorded spinal cord monitoring is utilized from this point forward, throughout the operative procedure. Gardner-Wells tongs are utilized with 10 pounds of skeletal traction, rather than a head halter, which extends too far inferiorly around the mandible. The neck is extended maximally with the patient still awake, but only to a degree that does not cause L'Heurmitte's or other neurologic symptoms or spinal cord monitoring potential changes. This is designated as the maximal neck extension position and it is not exceeded at any time throughout the operative procedure. Fiberoptic nasotracheal intubation is performed under local anesthesia, and after the airway is secured the patient undergoes general anesthesia. The mouth is kept free of all tubes. No oral airways or esophageal stethoscopes are permitted in the mouth and all dentures are removed, as any depression of the mandible inferiorly increases the difficulty of the exposure.

A modified Schoebringer incision is used (Fig. 13-28). The vertical limb is extended inferiorly as needed, depending on the amount of cervical spine exposure required. The incision is made through the platysma muscle and the superomedial, inferomedial, and lateral flaps are elevated in the subplatysmal plane. The incision is made on the patient's right side, if the surgeon is right-handed. In contrast to the Robinson-Smith exposure in the midcervical levels, which we usually perform on the patient's left side, the extrapharyngeal exposure to the atlas and axis is sufficiently superior to the right recurrent laryngeal nerve, so that there is no increased morbidity with a right-sided exposure. The exposure is a superior extension of the standard Robinson-Smith exposure to the midcervical spine; therefore, only the specific modifications allowing visualization of the atlas and axis will be described. The surgeon should be thoroughly familiar with the fascial plains traversed by the Robinson-Smith anterior approach:[10–17] (1) the superficial fascia containing the platysma; (2) the superficial layer of the deep

Table 13-3. Anterior Retropharyngeal Approach (Clivus to Second Cervical Vertebra)

CASE	SEX, AGE (YRS.)	DIAGNOSIS	PRESENTING SYMPTOMS AND SIGNS	PREOPERATIVE NEUROLOGICAL FUNCTION	ANTERIOR PROCEDURES
1	F, 52	Osteochondroma	Stiff neck	Intact	Marginal excis., C2, without arthrodesis
2	M, 50	Chordoma	Neck pain	Intact	Ant. intralesional excis., C2, with arthrodesis
3	F, 55	Chordoma	Neck pain, path. C2 fract.	Intact	Ant. intralesional excis., C2, with arthrodesis
4	M, 58	Plasmacytoma	Neck pain, path. C2 fract.	Intact	Ant. intralesional excis., C2, with arthrodesis
5	M, 58	Chordoma	Neck pain	Quadriparesis	Ant. intralesional excis., C2, with arthrodesis
6	M, 26	Gunshot wound to clivus	Dysphagia	Intact	Removal of bullet from ant. aspect of clivus
7	M, 55	Malunion, odontoid fract., C1-C2 sublux.	Neck pain	Brown-Séquard syndrome	C2 corpect. and arthrodesis
8	F, 28	Non-union of hangman fract., C2-C3 sublux.	Neck pain	Lhermitte sign, spasticity	Ant. reduct., C2-C3 arthrodesis
9	F, 21	Basilar impression, dwarfism	Neck pain	Lhermitte sign, quadriparesis	Ant. C2 corpectomy, odontoid excision, and arthrodesis
10	F, 60	Metastatic breast carcinoma	Neck pain, path. C2 fract.	Spasticity	Ant. intralesional excis., C2, with arthrodesis
11	M, 53	Rheumatoid arthritis, basilar impression, atlanto-axial sublux.	Neck pain, ataxia, vertigo	Cruciate paralysis of Bell	Decompres. of pannus and C2, including odontoid, and arthrodesis
12	M, 56	Plasmacytoma	Neck pain, path. C2 fract.	Intact	Ant. intralesional excis., C2, with arthrodesis
13	F, 17	Osteogenic sarcoma	Neck pain, path. C2 fract.	Intact	Ant. intralesional excis., C2, with anthrodesis
14	M, 66	Plasmacytoma	Neck pain, first seen holding head in hands, path. odontoid fract.	C3 paresthesias bilat.	Ant. intralesional excis., C2 with arthrodesis
15	M, 14	*E. coli* vertebral osteomyelitis	Neck pain, numbness and tingling in fingers	Intact	Ant. débrid. and arthrodesis, C2-C4
16	M, 54	Adenocystic carcinoma of the salivary gland	Neck pain, weakness and numbness in arms, large lytic lesion at C1, C2, C3	Mild quadriparesis	Ant. intralesional excis. and arthrodesis, C1-C5
17	M, 23	Ependymoma, severe kyphosis and spinal cord compression after post. laminect. at age 11	Quadriparesis, dense numbness above C4	Quadriparesis	Excis. of vertebral bodies of C2, C3, C4, replacement with iliac graft

MANAGEMENT OF AIRWAY POSTOPERATIVELY	POSTERIOR PROCEDURES	LENGTH OF FOLLOW-UP (YRS.)	OPERATIVE COMPLICATIONS	RESULTS
Tracheostomy	None	2	None	Pain relieved, neurolog. intact
Extubation 24 hrs. postop.	2nd-stage post. intralesional excis. and arthrodesis	3	None	Died 3 yrs. postop.
Tracheostomy	Post. arthrodesis, C1-C4, before ant. procedure	8	Permanent unilat. hypoglossal nerve injury	Died 8 yrs. postop. from metastatic disease but had local recur. of tumor at C2; neurolog. changes never developed
Tracheostomy	Post. intralesional excis. and arthrodesis	3	None	Died 3 yrs. postop.
Tracheostomy	Post. intralesional excis. and arthrodesis	3	None	Died 3 yrs. postop.
Extubation 48 hrs. postop.	None	1	C-arm fluoroscopy necessary to localize metal foreign body	Neurolog. intact, without sequelae
Extubation 48 hrs. postop.	Prior C1-C2 arthrodesis	2	12th cranial nerve and 8th mandibular neuraprax., 0.05-cm entrance into hypophyarnx (repaired without sequelae)	Anatomically adequate decompression shown by comput. tomog. and magnetic res. imag., neuraprax. resolved, Brown-Séquard syndrome persisted
Extubation immed. postop.	None	2	Halo pin infect. with 2-mm ant. resublux.	Solid fusion with 2-mm malalign., neurolog. intact
Extubation immed. postop.	Post. occiput-C3 arthrodesis	4	None	Neurolog. intact
Extubation 72 hrs. postop.	Post. arthrodesis in same procedure	1	Ant. iliac strut graft dislodged on turning frame for post. procedure and was replaced, 12th nerve neuraprax.	Solid C1-C3 ant. and post. fusion at follow-up
Extubation 72 hrs. postop.	Prior occipital craniotomy and C1-C7 laminect. performed elsewhere	1	None	Solid fusion, clivus-C3
Tracheostomy	Prior occiput-C7 arthrodesis and stabilizat.	1	None	Solid fusion, C1-C3 ant., no loss of position despite progressive lysis post.
Extubation 72 hrs. postop.	Post. C1-C3 arthrodesis in same procedure	1	None	Path. fract. healed and solid fusion C1-C3 ant. and post., neurolog. intact
Extubation immed. postop.	Prior post. C1-C3 arthrodesis	2	None	Weakness of L arm due to enlargement of tumor at C2 before death from dissemin. disease
Extubation immed. postop.	None	10	None	Complete resolution of infect.
Extubation 48 hrs. postop.	Prev. post. iliac-bone grafts, C5-occiput	2.5	None	Excel. palliat., died of generalized metast., <2 mos. total hospital time
Tracheostomy preop. and postop.	None	8	None	Quadriparesis improved for 2 yrs., but still had weakness and spasticity of lower limbs

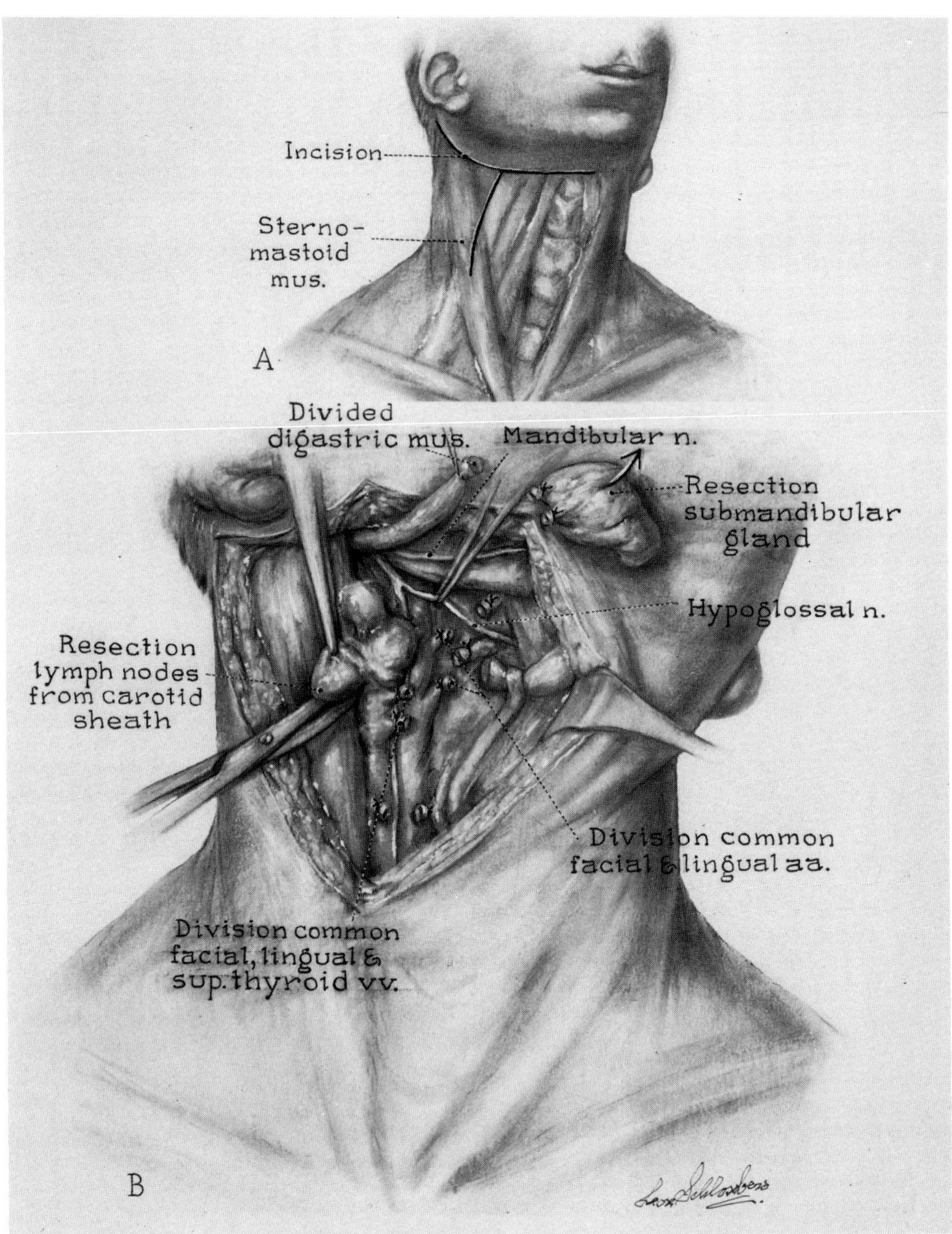

Fig. 13-28. Surgical technique of The Anterior Retropharyngeal approach. (*A* and *B*) The illustration shows the key features of the extramucosal anterior approach to the atlas and axis. From the right side through a modified Schoebringer incision the submandibular gland is resected and the digastric tendon is divided. (*C*) After the superficial layer of deep cervical fascia is incised along the anterior border of the sternocleidomastoid muscle, the superior thyroid artery and vein are divided. The hypoglossal and superior laryngeal nerves are mobilized. Additional branches of the carotid artery and internal jugular vein are ligated to allow mobilization of the carotid sheath contents laterally as the hypopharynx is mobilized medially. (*D* and *E*) The first step of the anterior spinal decompression is a meticulous removal of the C2–C3 intervertebral disc. The longus colli muscle is dissected in a lateral direction exposing the C2 vertebral body and the anterior C1 arch. The C2 corpectomy can then be performed with a high-speed bur.

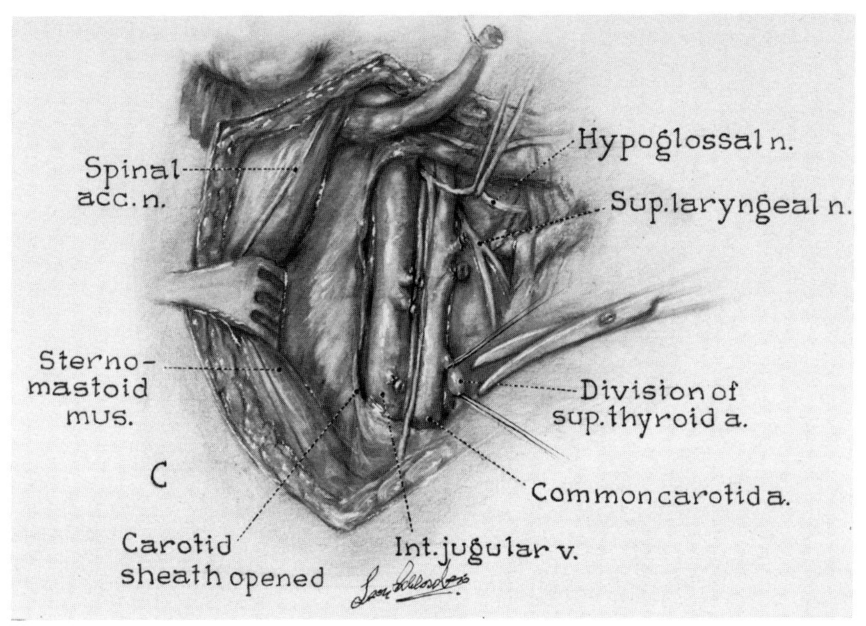

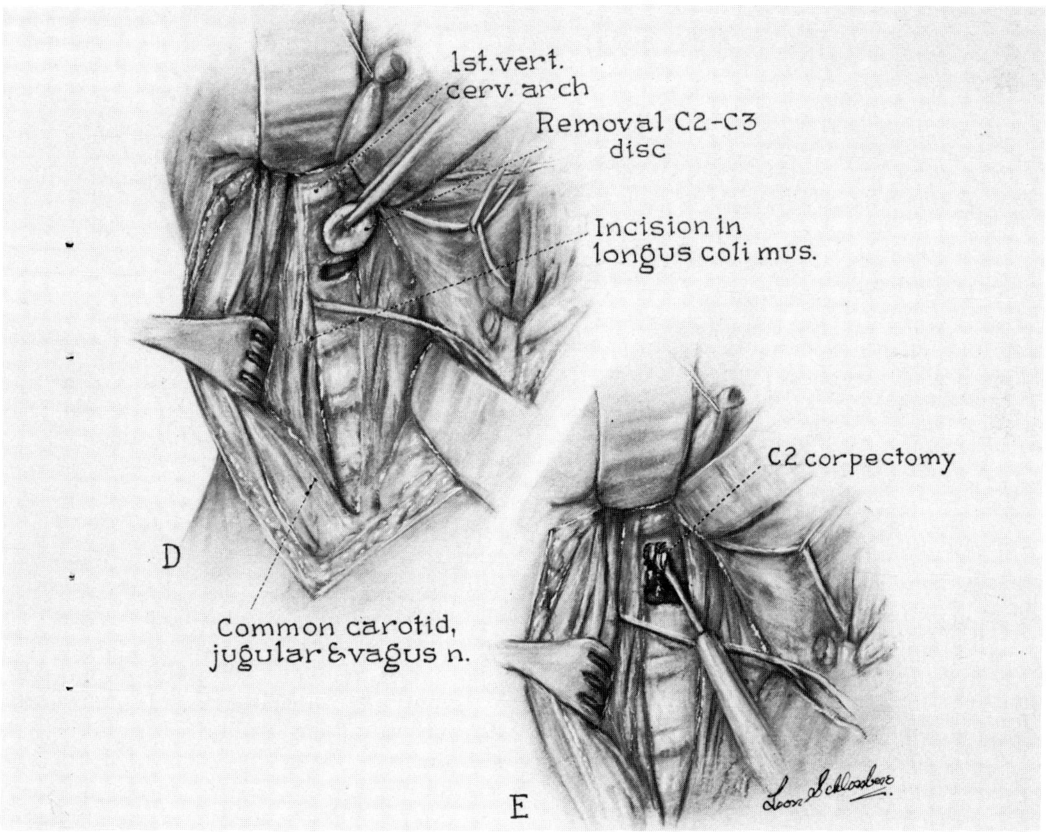

***Fig. 13-28,** cont'd.*

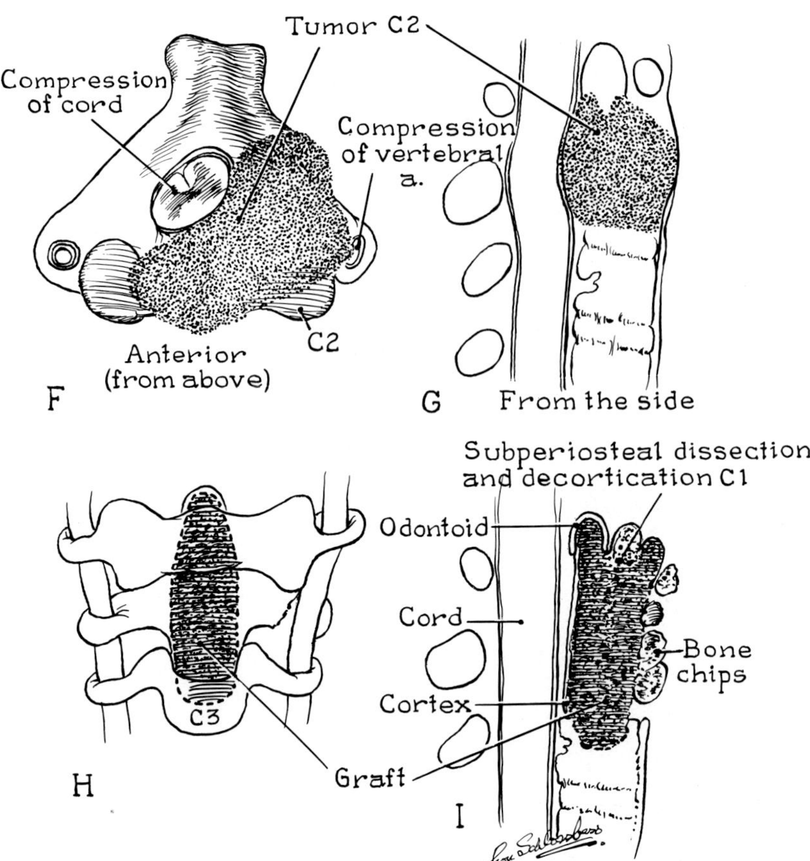

Fig. 13-28, cont'd.
(*F, G* and *H*) This illustration shows the typical involvement of tumors in the C2 vertebral body (aneurysmal bone cyst, cordoma, or metastasis). The anterior and posterior columns of spinal stability are affected, the spinal cord is compressed from an anterior direction, and the vertebral artery is occasionally involved. The lower figures show the insertion of a clothespin-shaped strut graft, which is wedged below the anterior C1 arch after subperiosteal dissection and decortication.

fascia surrounding the sternomastoid muscle; (3) the middle layer of the deep fascia that encloses the omohyoid, sternohyoid, sternothyroid, and thyrohyoid muscles and the visceral fascia enclosing the trachea, esophagus, and recurrent nerve; and (4) the deep layer of the deep cervical fascia, which is divided into the alar fascia connecting the two carotid sheaths and fused midline to the visceral fascia and the prevertebral fascia covering the longus colli and scalene muscles.

The marginal mandibular nerve (VII) is found by ligating and dissecting the retromandibular veins superiorly. The common facial vein is continuous with the retromandibular vein, and the branches of the marginal mandibular nerve usually cross the vein superficially and superiorly. By ligating the retromandibular vein as it joins the internal jugular vein, and by keeping the dissection deep and inferior to the vein as the exposure is extended superiorly to the mandible, the superficial branches of the facial nerve (VII) are thus protected.

The anterior border of the sternocleidomastoid muscle is mobilized by longitudinally transecting the superficial layer of deep cervical fascia. This allows location of the carotid sheath by palpation of the carotid arterial pulse. The submandibular gland is resected, with care taken to suture the duct in order to prevent a fistula. The jugular-digastric lymph nodes from the submandibular and carotid triangles can be resected and sent for frozen section histologic diagnosis at this point, if neoplasm is suspected. The posterior belly of the digastric muscle and the stylohyoid are identified. As mentioned by Whitesides, retraction superiorly at the base of the origin of the stylohyoid muscle can cause injury to the facial nerve (VII) as it exits the skull. The digastric tendon is divided and tagged for later repair. Division of the digastric and stylohyoid muscles allow mobilization of the hyoid bone and the hypopharynx medially. This maneuver helps keep the exposure out of the nasopharynx, hypopharynx, and esophagus, which are considered contaminated spaces with high con-

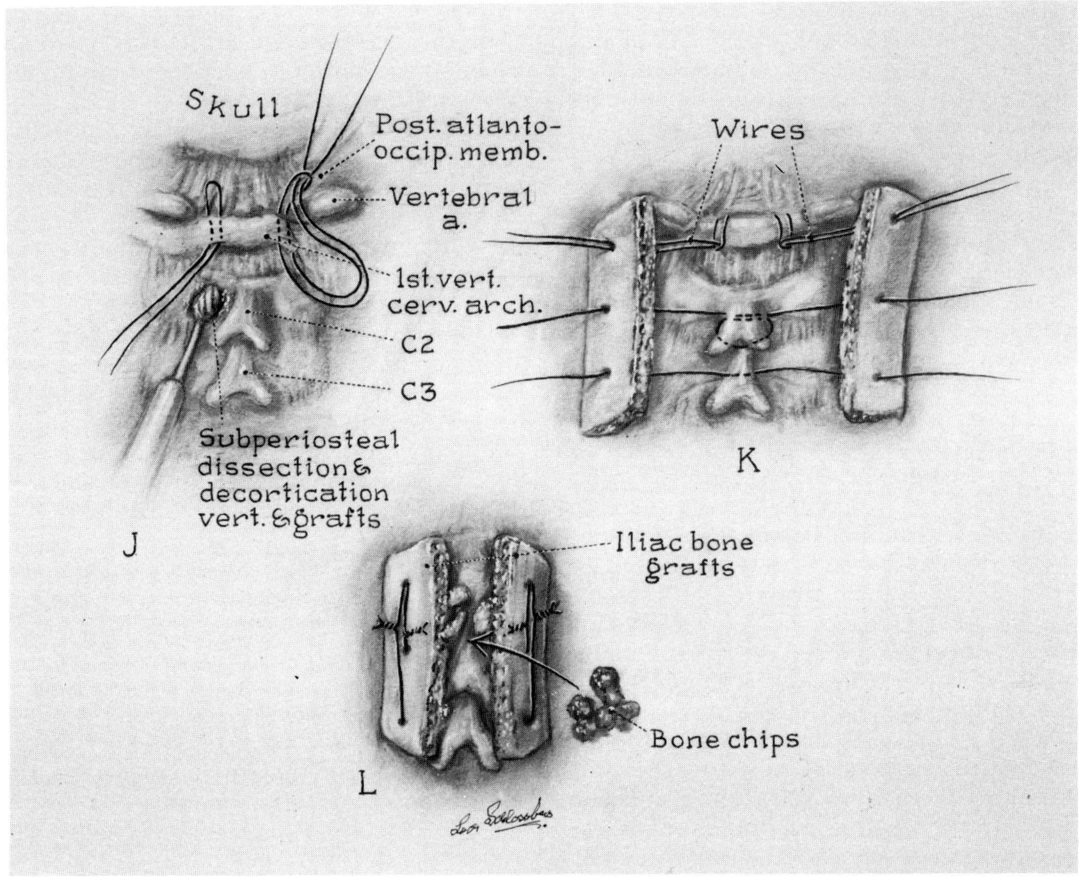

Fig. 13-28, *cont'd.*
(*J, K* and *L*) Following anterior decompression, a posterior wiring and fusion is performed from C1 to C3 to provide a circumferential spinal fusion, which was necessary in 11 of 17 patients.

centrations of anaerobic bacteria. If the hypopharynx is inadvertently entered, as it was in one of our patients (Case 12) a nasogastric tube should be passed immediately by an anesthetist while the surgeon visualizes the hole in the hypopharynx. The hypopharynx is closed in two layers with absorbable sutures. Parenteral antibiotics are added to the routine prophylactic antibiotic regimen with a spectrum against anaerobes. The nasogastric tube is left in place of 7 to 10 days postoperatively in this situation to help prevent eosphageal or hypopharyngeal leakage or fistula formation, which can lead to mediastinitis.

Complete mobilization of the hypoglossal nerve (XII) from the skull base to the anterior border of the hyoglossus muscle is performed. The nerve (XII) is retracted superiorly throughout the remainder of the procedure.

The dissection then proceeds to the retropharyngeal space, between the carotid sheath contents laterally, and the larynx and pharynx anteromedially. Superior exposure is facilitated by ligating the tethering branches of the carotid artery and internal jugular vein. Beginning inferiorly and progressing superiorly, ligating the following branches of these vessels will help mobilization of the carotid sheath laterally: (1) superior thyroid artery and vein, (2) lingual artery and vein, (3) ascending pharyngeal artery and vein, and (4) facial artery and vein. The superior laryngeal nerve is mobilized from its origin near the nodose ganglion to its entrance into the larynx. We have been able to preserve the superior laryngeal nerve, which was of particular importance in Case 10, a soprano singer, as the transection of the superior laryngeal nerve would have produced a loss of high-pitched phonation.

The prevertebral fascia is transected longitudinally, exposing the longus colli muscles, which course longitudinally. It is very important at this point to gain orientation to the midline by noting the attachment of the left and right longus colli muscles as they converge toward the anterior tubercle of the atlas. The amount of head rotation toward the side is gauged by palpating the anterior point of the jaw. If possible, head rotation is eliminated, as the fusion usually involves the anterior C1 arch. Orientation regarding the midline of the cervical spine is maintained as the longus colli muscles are detached from the anterior surface of the atlas and axis. This orientation is maintained throughout the anterior spinal cord decompression in order to extend the decompression laterally enough to decompress the spinal cord, yet not so far lateral as to enter the vertebral arteries. The anterior altantooccipital membrane is not violated, but the anterior longitudinal ligament is sacrificed. The anterior decompression is usually initiated by performing a thorough anterior C2–C3 discectomy. Visualization of the C2–C3 uncovertebral joints helps confirm the orientation of the midline and the discectomy provides visualization of the posterior longitudinal ligament with very minimal blood loss. A high-speed bur is utilized for the C2 corpectomy, if this is required. Histologic analysis is performed by frozen section as the anterior spinal decompression proceeds superiorly. The blood loss during this anterior C2 corpectomy can be minimized by generous use of thrombin-soaked Gelfoam, bone wax, and bipolar cauterization of feeding vessels (localized preoperatively by carotid and vertebral arteriography). The maximum blood loss for any of our 17 cases, including an aneurysmal bone cyst and a telangiectatic osteogenic sarcoma, was only 3 units (1200cc).

In patients without cranial settling (basilar invagination of the odontoid) the odontoid can be retained to help lock in the superior aspect of the strut graft (Figs. 13-28*F*, *G*, and *H*, and 13-29). A fibular or tricortical iliac strut graft is fashioned in the shape of a clothespin. The two prongs of the clothespin strut graft are placed to straddle the anterior arch of C1. The inferior edge of the graft is tamped into the superior aspect of the C3 vertebral body, which is undercut to help obtain stability. Closure is begun by the reapproximation of the digastric tendon. Suction drains are then placed in the retropharyngeal space and in the subcutaneous space. They are brought out through stab incisions beneath the cervical flap. The platysma and skin are sutured in the standard fashion. If spinal stability has been created by the pathologic process or anterior decompression, then the achievement of stability is dependent upon a good posterior cervical or posterior occipitocervical fusion. The anterior cervical strut graft should be thought of as conferring compressive stability only. The patient should be kept in skeletal traction until posterior stabilization is performed. Posterior stabilization may be performed during the same operative procedure under the same anesthetic in a one-stage combined anterior-posterior procedure (Fig. 13-28*J*, *K*, and *L*.).

The patient is awakened in the supine position, and a neurologic examination and spinal cord monitoring potentials are documented. The patient is carefully transferred to an intensive care unit bed with the head elevated 30 degrees to reduce hypopharyngeal edema. The patient is kept intubated for 48 hours postoperatively. Flexible nasopharyngoscopy is performed to ensure adequacy of the uppér airway prior to extubation. At the end of the surgical procedure, if it is anticipated, owing to the degree and duration of soft-tissue retraction, that extubation will not be probable within 48 to 72 hours postoperatively, then a tracheostomy is performed. Four to seven days postoperatively the patient's Gardner-Wells tongs are removed and the patient is placed in a halo vest for approximately 3 months.

RESULTS

In contrast to reports of transmucosal approaches to the atlas and axis, there were no cases of infection in our series of 17 patients.

No patients had respiratory arrest or required emergency tracheostomies. Five patients underwent prophylactic tracheostomies performed during the index operative procedure. Four patients were extubated immediately postoperatively, one was extubated 24 hours postoperatively, two at 48 hours (Fig. 13-30), and four at 72 hours postoperatively without complication.

In all 17 patients there were two cases with loss of position of anterior bone grafts. Case 8 was an unstable Hangman's fracture, which was reduced and fused at C2–C3 with a tricortical iliac strut graft. She had loosening of the halo pins by the fourth postoperative week and had 2-mm resubluxation of C2 anterior to C3. At 2 years follow-up she had a solid arthrodesis in this position and was neurologically intact. Case 10 had dislodgment of the inferior edge of the iliac C1 to C3 strut graft as she was being turned to undergo the posterior C1 to C3 stabilization and fusion procedure. This

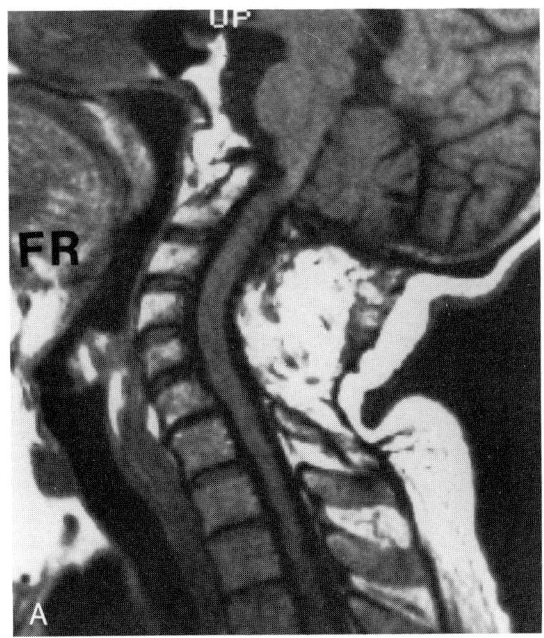

Fig. 13-29. (*A*) This magnetic resonance saggital image[9] shows anterior compression of the spinomedullary junction just inferior to the pons. The entire brainstem has been displaced posteriorly, evidenced by enlargement of the prepontine cistern. (*B*) The most frequent nonneoplastic cause of C2 compression is due to rheumatoid pannus associated with atlantoaxial subluxation and basilar invagination of the odontoid. The goal of the anterior decompression-stabilization is to provide an arthrodesis from the clivus to the subaxial spine.

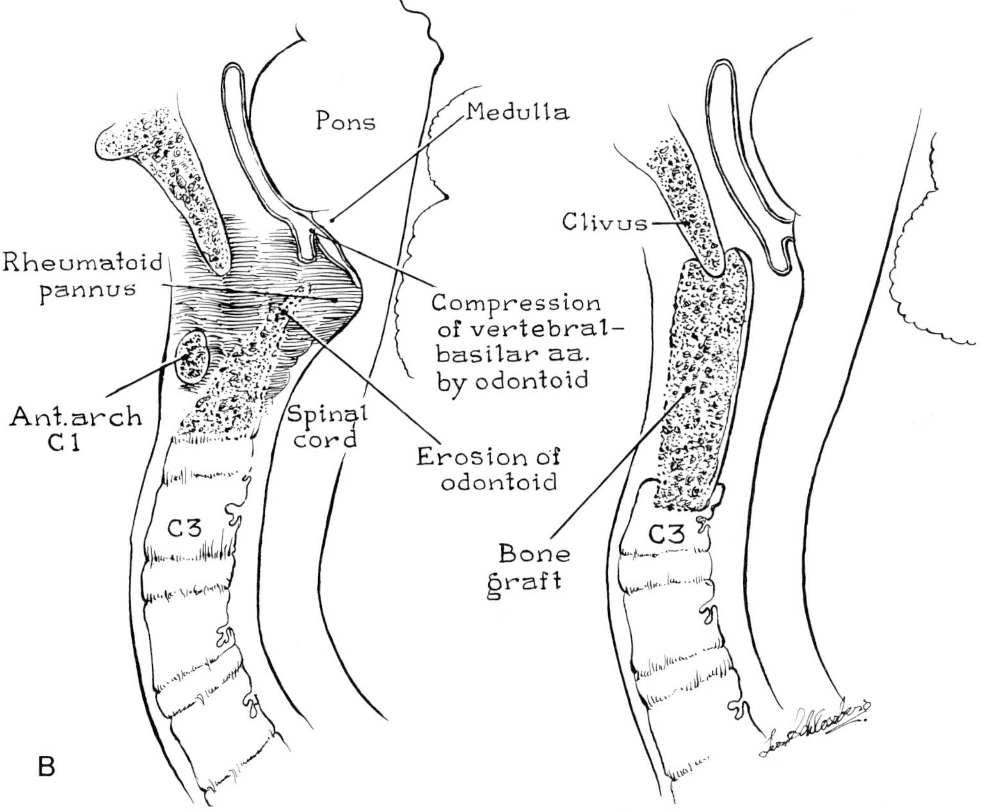

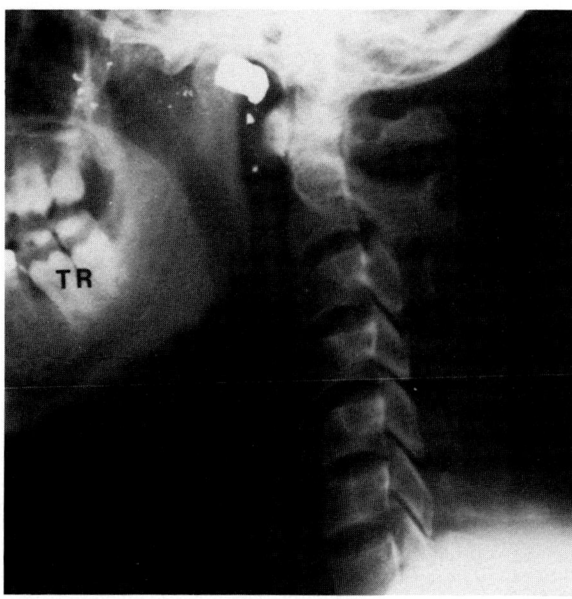

Fig. 13-30. This figure shows the superior limit of the anterior retropharyngeal approach. This patient sustained a gunshot wound to the clivus and C1 and had successful removal of the bullet through an extramucosal approach. Foreign bodies in this location are associated with a high incidence of hypopharyngeal erosion, esophagitis, and even mediastinitis.

occurred despite the use of a Stryker turning frame and 10 pounds of halo traction. Following the posterior procedure, the patient was turned supine on the frame and the graft was reinserted. The patient remained neurologically intact and went on to a solid arthrodesis.

Of the 17 patients, two had cranial nerve neuropraxias. Case 3 had a permanent unilateral hypoglossal nerve injury and was asymptomatic despite this deficit. Cases 7 and 10 had hypoglossal neuropraxias and Case 7 also had a mandibular branch of the facial nerve neuropraxia. All three neuropraxias resolved within 3 months postoperatively.

None of the 15 patients had an iatrogenic neurologic spinal cord deficit. Also, there were no cases of nonunion (Fig. 13-31).

Twelve patients were followed 2 or more years postoperatively (Cases 1 to 5, 7 to 9, 14, and 17), for an average of 3.9 years (range 2 to 10 years) (Fig. 13-32). All patients had a solid anterior fusion and no subsequent loss of cervical spine stability. Cases 5, 8, 9, 14 and 16, 17 improved neurologically postoperatively. Case 7 had a persisting Brown-Séquard syndrome but was ambulatory, and the other five cases remained neurologically intact (Cases 1 to 4, and 15). Neck pain was relieved in all cases with pathologic fractures (Fig. 13-33). Neck pain remained in one patient (Case 7); we believe this was due to chronic spinal cord compression prior to referral. Five patients died due to relentless progression of malignant tumors: Case 2, 3 years postoperatively; Case 3, 8 years postoperatively; Case 4, 3 years postoperatively; Case 5, 3 years postoperatively; and Case 14, 2 years and 1 month postoperatively. Two deaths were due to multiple myeloma, and three were due to cordomas. Case 14 developed left arm weakness 1 month prior to death due to enlargement of tumor at C2 2 years postoperatively, despite radiotherapy and an anatomically adequate anterior decompression.

The one case with a benign spine tumor (osteochondroma) treated by marginal resection remained disease-free at 2 years follow-up. The one case of pyogenic vertebral osteomyelitis also had complete resolution and was asymptomatic at 10 years and 1 month follow-up.

Computed tomography (CT) was not available at the time of treatment of Cases 2 to 5, 14, and 16. Postoperative CT was performed in five patients (Cases 1, 7 to 9, and 17), and it documented anatomically successful spinal cord decompressions in all four. Plain lateral tomography was obtained and documented anatomically successful anterior procedures in five (Cases 2, 3, 4, 5, and 14). Plain roentgenograms were thought to be adequate to document anterior success of the anterior procedures in the remaining patients with pyogenic vertebral osteomyelitis at 10 years and 1 month follow-up (Case 15).

DISCUSSION

The most popular, versatile, and complication-free anterior approach to the cervical spine has been described by Robinson and Smith in 1955.[2,6,7,10–18] Robinson and Smith developed the exposure from a general surgical approach originally described by Lahey and Warren[8] in 1954, designed for resection of esophageal diverticula.

The major concept of the approach is to develop the interval between the carotid sheath contents, which are retracted laterally, and the esophagus and trachea medially. When this approach is utilized for the midcervical spine it can be performed by blunt digital dissection. Many surgeons overlook the ability of the approach to provide access

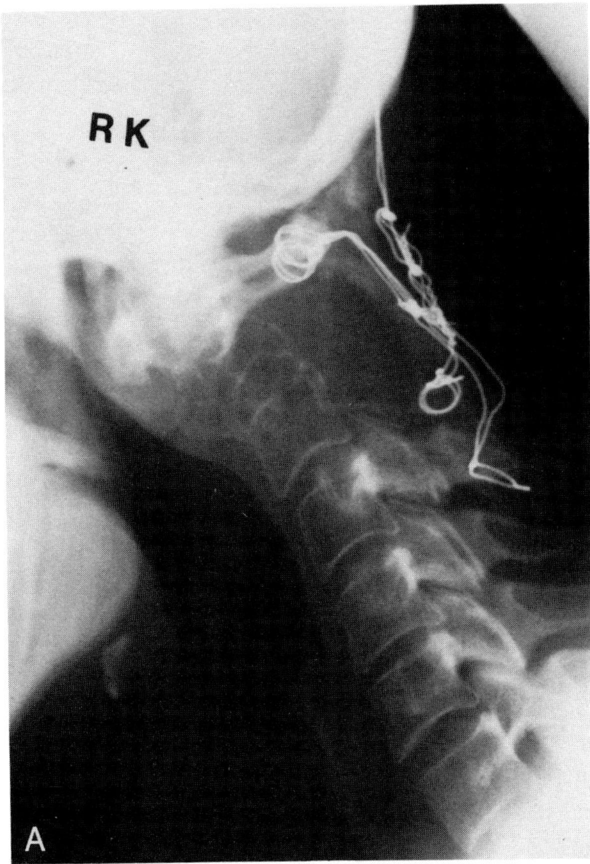

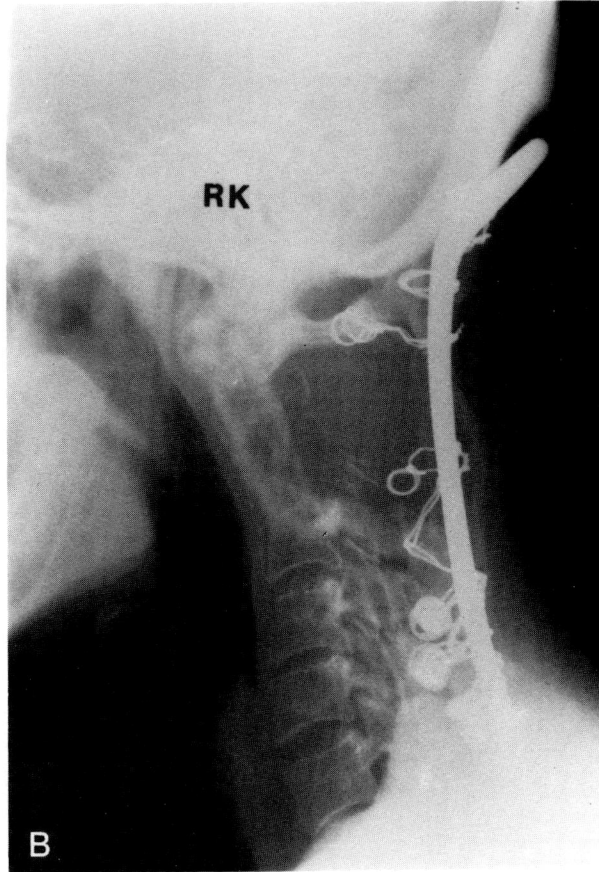

Fig. 13-31. Multiple myeloma. (*A*) This patient had a failed attempt at posterior stabilization and fusion from the occiput to C2, had failed radiotherapy and chemotherapy, and had spent the previous 2 years in a halo. (*B*) One week following posterior stabilization from the occiput to C4 he underwent anterior decompression of tumor and insertion of a fibular strut from C1 to C3. This case shows the ability of the anterior retropharyngeal approach to provide access to the upper cervical spine, even in patients in whom no cervical spine extension is possible. The radiograph demonstrates a solid fusion, and the patient is pain free without a neck brace, one year after surgery.

to the atlas and axis, because a more elaborate sharp dissection is required.

The transoral route to the atlas and axis is reserved in our judgment for biopsies and drainage of infections.[1,4,19,20] It provides very limited exposure for anterior spinal cord decompression. Because it necessitates contaminating the spine with oropharyngeal bacterial flora, it carries an attendant unacceptably high risk of infection (50%, according to Fang and Ong). The lateral retropharyngeal approach popularized and used extensively by Whitesides and Kelly[24] and recently updated by Whitesides[22] has the advantage of being extraoral. However, it involves a lateral dissection posterior to the carotid sheath. If an anterior spinal decompression is performed, the approach remains dangerously close to the ipsilateral vertebral artery, which is difficult to control in the case of the inadvertent laceration. On the other hand, the anterior approach allows visualization and control of the vertebral arteries. In Case 3, for example, L.H.R. was able to place temporary vascular ligatures around both left and right vertebral arteries between C1 and C2 in order to perform a safer excision of an extensive cordoma. Whitesides' experience is very impressive, with 27 procedures followed to a conclusive result. All but three of the procedures achieved solid fusion with pain relief,

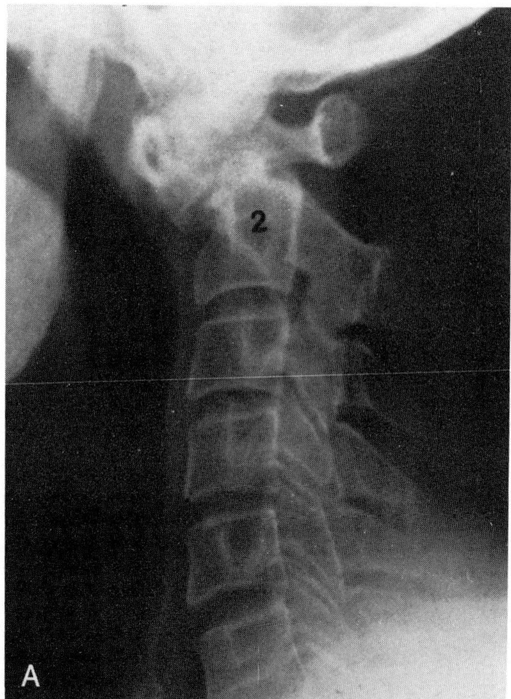

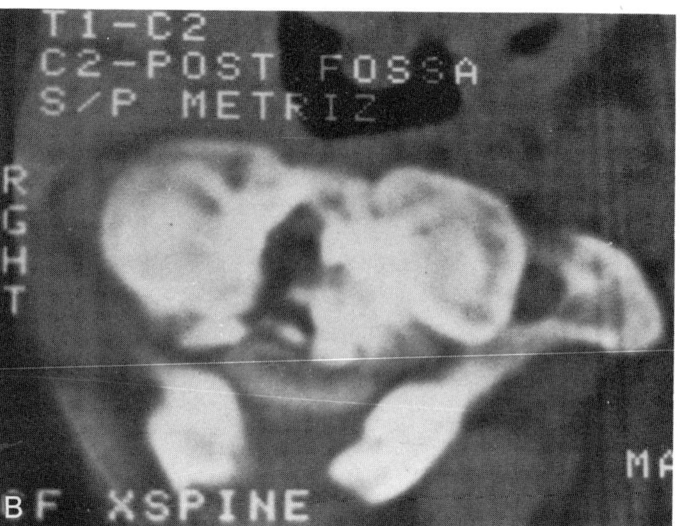

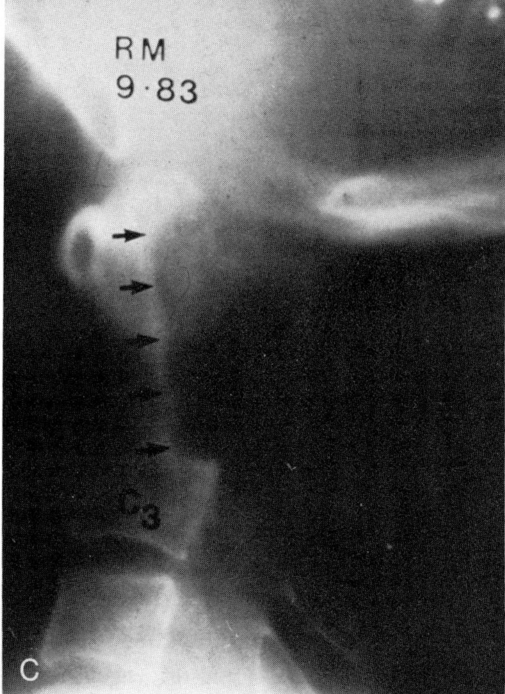

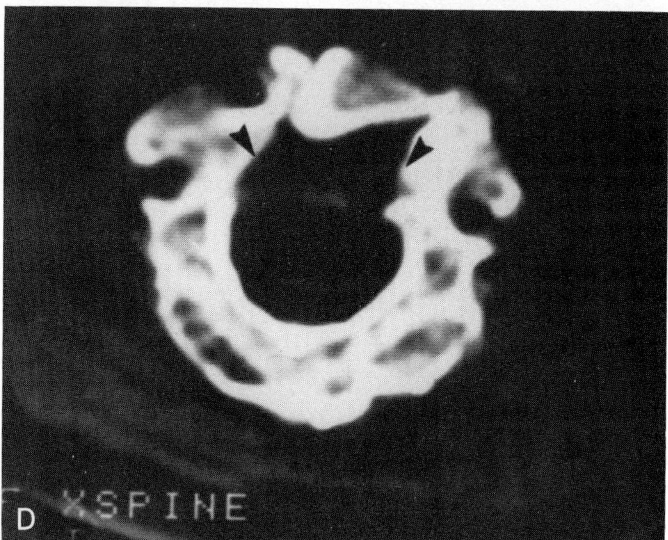

Fig. 13-32. (*A*) This 55-year-old male presented to us with fixed atlantoaxial subluxation following an odontoid fracture. (*B*) He had a Brown-Séquard syndrome with previous unsuccessful attempts at decompression through an anterior transoral approach and a posterior laminectomy. The CT shows that the previous attempt at anterior decompression was inadequate, as the spinal cord remained flattened. (*C*) The patient's neck became stable following anterior fusion from C1 to C3 performed through an anterior retropharyngeal approach. This lateral tomogram shows excellent decompression of the spinal canal. (*D*) This postoperative axial CT image documents successful anterior decompression of the spinal cord. The patient had relief of neck pain and spinal instability, but owing to the prolonged interval before referral, his Brown-Séquard syndrome persisted.

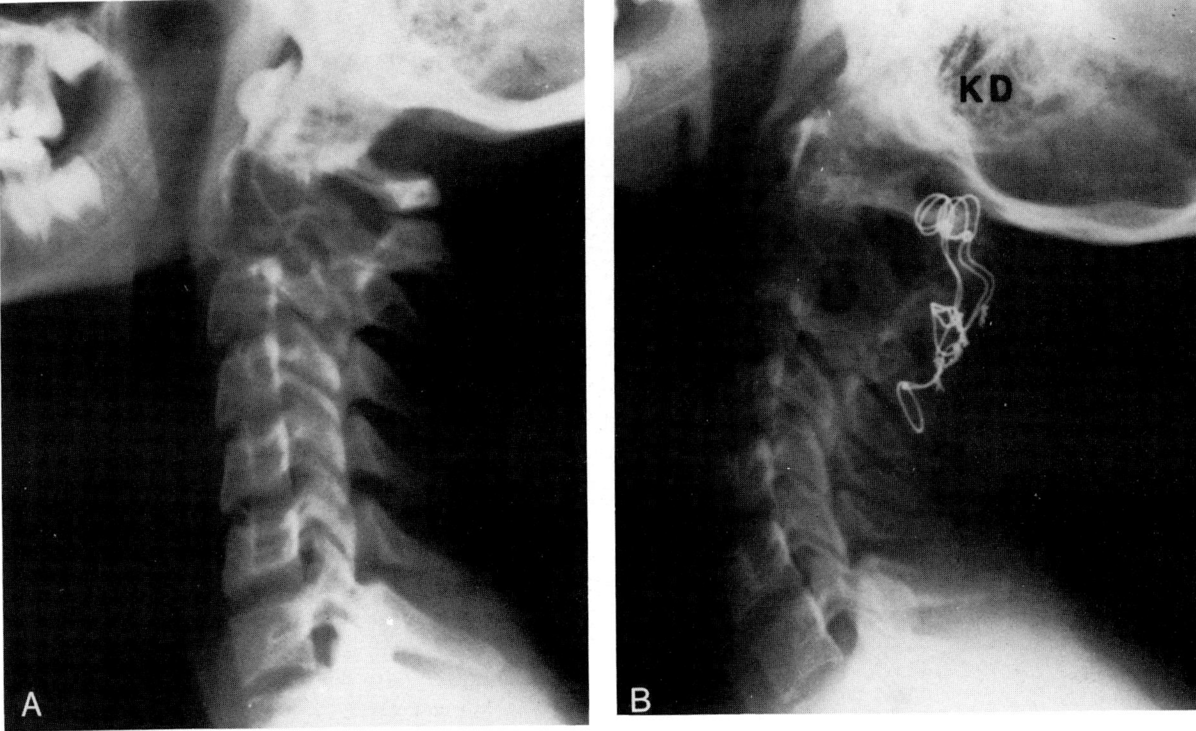

Fig. 13-33. Osteogenic sarcoma with pathologic fracture. (*A*) This 17-year-old girl presented with a pathologic fracture secondary to an osteogenic sarcoma of C2. (*B*) One year following anterior resection and strut grafting the patient is asymptomatic and remains neurologically intact. Although the chances of a permanent cure are small, she is currently able to enjoy athletic activities, including horseback riding and roller skating.

arrest of neurologic deterioration, or reversal of neurologic deficits. There were several major complications, including one failure of union, two early postoperative deaths, one infection in the anterior approach, and one infection in a distal wound associated with *Bacterioides* sepsis. Whitesides also emphasized the importance of not retracting superiorly near the origin of the posterior belly of the digastric muscle, as one case of temporary facial nerve palsy occurred. Two disadvantages of the lateral retropharyngeal approach, compared with the technique described in this series, are as follows: (1) the anterior spinal cord decompression is more difficult, because it does not afford a "straight shot" or direct anterior visualization—the visualization is from the side; (2) it is more difficult to insert a long strut graft in patients in whom the tumor spans several vertebral bodies. Verbiest has reported experience with lateral exposure to the upper and lower cervical spine (posterior to the carotid sheath) in 47 patients.[21] This requires mobilization of the vertebral artery, and most North American orthopedic surgeons are not familiar with the anterolateral approach posterior to the carotid sheath.

In 1969, De Andrade and MacNab[3] reported five patients undergoing anterior occipitocervical fusion using the same basic approach as used in our series. In their patients, however, anterior spinal canal decompressions were not performed. Mobilization and dissection of the superior laryngeal and lower cranial nerves was not necessary, and the muscles tethering the hyoid and hypopharynx were not divided. A more extensile exposure is needed if a formal anterior spinal cord decompression is necessary. Additionally, it is far easier to decorticate from C1 to C3 and apply strips of bone graft, rather than to lock in a tricortical strut graft as done in our patients. The inlay type of grafting did not confer compressive stability immediately postoperatively, as skeletal traction on a turning frame was required for 6 weeks in their patients. Hall and coworkers[5] described splitting the mandible in one patient, and Alonso and colleagues described division of the soft palate through transoral routes to facilitate exposure from the clivus to C2. We have not found these techniques to be necessary.

We have found that the anterior approach following mobilization of the marginal mandibular, hypoglossal, and superior laryngeal nerves with detachment of the hyoid bone and hypopharynx provides better anterior exposure, compared with the lateral approach. Furthermore, with flexible laryngoscopic techniques inspection of the airway may be performed postoperatively prior to extubation. In this way, tracheostomy should be avoided in most patients, and the infection rate should theoretically be decreased. The procedure can be performed expeditiously enough in some instances to allow posterior stabilization and fusion to be combined in the same operative procedure.

REFERENCES

1. *ALONSO WA, BLACK P, CONNOR GH, UEMATSU S:* Transoral, transpalatal approach for resection of clival chordoma. Laryngoscope 81:1626–1631, 1971
2. *BAILEY RW, BADGLEY CE:* Stabilization of the cervical spine by anterior fusion. J Bone Joint Surg 42A:565–594, 1960
3. *DEANDRADE JR, MACNAB I:* Anterior occipitocervical fusion using an extra-pharyngeal exposure. J Bone Joint Surg 51A:1621–1626, 1969
4. *FANG HSY, ONG GB:* Direct anterior approach to the upper cervical spine. J Bone Joint Surg 44A:1588–1604, 1962
5. *HALL JE, DENIS F, MURRAY J:* Exposure of the upper cervical spine for spinal decompression. J Bone Joint Surg 59A:121–123, 1977
6. *HENRY AK:* Extensile Exposure, 2nd ed, pp 53–80. Edinburg, E & S Livingstone, Ltd, 1957
7. *JOHNSON RN, SOUTHWICK WO:* Surgical approaches to the cervical spine. In Rothman RH, Simeone FA (eds): The Spine, pp 93–147. Philadelphia, WB Saunders, 1982
8. *LAHEY FH, WARREN KW:* Esophageal diverticula. Surg Gynecol Obstet 98:1–28, 1954
9. *MCAFEE PC, BOHLMAN HH, HAN JS, SALVAGNO RT:* Comparison of nuclear magnetic resonance imaging and computed tomography in the diagnosis of upper cervical spinal cord compression. Spine 11:295–304, 1986
10. *RILEY LH, JR:* Surgical approaches to the anterior structures of the cervical spine. Clin Orthop 91:16–20, 1973
11. *ROBINSON RA, SMITH GW:* Anterolateral cervical disc removal and interbody fusion for cervical disc syndrome. Bull Johns Hopkins Hosp 96:223–224, 1955
12. *ROBINSON RA:* Fusions of the cervical spine. J Bone Joint Surg 41A:1–6, 1959
13. *ROBINSON RA, SOUTHWICK WO:* Indications and techniques for early stabilization of the neck in some fracture dislocations of the cervical spine. South Med J 53:565–579, 1960
14. *ROBINSON RA, SOUTHWICK WO:* Surgical Approaches to the Cervical Spine. Instructional Course Lectures, The American Academy of Orthopaedic Surgeons, Vol 17, pp 299–330. St Louis, CV Mosby Co, 1960
15. *ROBINSON RA, RILEY LH:* Techniques of exposure and fusion of the cervical spine. Clin Orthop 109:78–84, 1975
16. *SMITH GW, ROBINSON RA:* The treatment of certain cervical spine disorders by anterior removal of the intervertebral disc and interbody fusion. J Bone Joint Surg 40A:607–624, 1958
17. *SOUTHWICK WO, ROBINSON RA:* Surgical approaches to the vertebral bodies in the cervical and lumbar regions. J Bone Joint Surg 39A:631–644, 1957
18. *SOUTHWICK WO, ROBINSON RA:* Recent advances in surgery of the cervical spine. Surg Clin North Am 41:1661–1683, 1961
19. *SPETZLER RF:* Transoral approach to the upper cervical spine. In Evants CM (ed): Surgery of the Musculoskeletal System, Vol 4, pp 19–24. New York, Churchill Livingstone, 1983
20. *SPETZLER RF, SELMAN WR, NASH C:* Transoral microsurgical odontoid resection and spinal cord monitoring. Spine 4:506–510, 1979
21. *VERBIEST H:* Anterolateral operations for fractures and dislocations in the middle and lower parts of the cervical spine. J Bone Joint Surg 51A:1489–1530, 1969
22. *WHITESIDES TE:* Lateral retropharyngeal approach to the upper cervical spine. In The Cervical Spine Research Society (eds): The Cervical Spine, pp 517–527. Philadelphia, JB Lippincott, 1983
23. *WHITESIDES TE:* Extrapharyngeal approach to the upper cervical spine. In Evants CM (ed): Surgery of the Musculoskeletal System, Vol 4, pp 13–18. New York, Churchill Livingstone, 1983
24. *WHITESIDES TE, JR, KELLY RP:* Lateral approach to the upper cervical spine for anterior fusion. South Med J 59:879–883, 1966

CHAPTER 14

Complications

Compensation Neck Pain

SAM W. WIESEL

Various types of trauma may result in neck pain. Although neck injuries occur in industry, the vast majority are associated with some type of traffic accident. The single most common diagnosis in such instances is a hyperextension injury. Because of the etiology (vehicle accidents), many neck injuries have both a compensation and a litigation component.[1–3] The topic can be an emotionally provocative one, because frequently a patient's subjective complaint is not substantiated by objective findings. This chapter defines the scope of neck injuries, presents a treatment approach for industry, and discusses impairment ratings for the cervical spine.

INCIDENCE

The precise number of neck injuries is difficult to determine. The most complete information comes primarily from the United States, although data are also available from Great Britain, Australia, and The Netherlands. The most accurate United States records are those of the National Accident Sampling System, which estimated that over 530,000 cases of hyperextension injury existed in 1979.[4]

These one-half million people represent 2.8% of all occupants in police-reported automobile accidents. In reviewing these figures, it is interesting to note that the gross number of hyperextension injuries to individuals in automobiles that did *not* require towing from the accident scene was much higher than the number to individuals in cars that did; in fact, the first figure was larger than the combined total of neck injuries to patients in towed vehicles and all other types of injuries in automobile accidents. Furthermore, there was no correlation between severity of damage to the vehicle and severity of the patient's complaints of neck pain.

The National Safety Council has stated that 20% of all automobile accidents are rear-end impacts. An estimated 85% of all neck injuries seen clinically result from automobile accidents. Of those that do result in neck injury, 85% are rear-end impacts, and the remaining 15% result from some other type of impact.[5–7]

Although acute neck injuries do not rank nearly as high as acute low back pain as a cause of lost work time, they must be considered a significant industrial problem. No reliable figures are available on hyperextension injuries in various categories of employment, but limited surveys of various work environments show that employees who drive on public highways (e.g., those in municipal transportation systems) have the highest incidence of hyperextension injuries, whereas those with less public vehicle contact have fewer such injuries.

LITIGATION IN ACUTE NECK INJURIES

The effect of litigation in acute neck injury cases has received much attention. Anecdotal incidents abound. A city bus, for example, filled with passengers is rear-ended by a Volkswagen "Beetle." No damage results to the Volkswagen or bus, but the bus driver suffers an acute whiplash injury. This and other such stories lead to speculation that litigation and compensation issues are the most important in incidence and severity of hyperextension injuries.

One characteristic of an accident that leads to hyperextension injury is that the striking vehicle is almost invariably held at fault; this removes the burden of proof of liability for the accident. Furthermore, the injured individual rarely presents an objective demonstrable abnormality and appears as a blameless victim incapacitated by subjective symptoms that are difficult to prove or to disprove. This combination of accident events and subjective symptoms has led many to view the accident victim as a ready candidate for legal intervention and disability remuneration.

How frequently do individuals with hyperextension injuries seek monetary remuneration? This question is difficult to answer because of the failure to report and follow up on minor injuries and because of the current trend toward settling out of court. However, in a few controlled studies, more than half of the accident victims eventually received some type of settlement.[8] Several studies have been undertaken to determine whether awarding monetary settlements has resulted in a significant lessening of symptoms. They showed that over 50% of patients with only subjective complaints improved significantly after litigation claims are settled. For patients with objective findings of injury, such as reduced range of cervical motion or objective neurologic loss, the percentage who improve after settlement drops below 25%.[1]

Finally, the possibility of emotional factors contributing to the symptoms and disability cannot be overlooked in these individuals. Such factors may be classified as malingering or conscious exaggeration of underlying complaints, or as subconscious exaggeration or modification of an acute neck injury. In studies of other types of back injuries, the malingerer is found much less frequently than the conscious exaggerator of an existing problem.

Although it is sometimes difficult to separate conscious from subconscious exaggeration, this differentiation can be made quite accurately by a careful examiner performing a detailed history and physical examination. We have found that the conscious manipulator is the patient who typically arrives at the doctor's office with extensive documentation of the accident or injury, demonstrates a persistently defensive attitude, is often overtly hostile, withholds information, actively involves an attorney (even to the point of refusing to answer simple questions without consulting the attorney), and shows variable and inconsistent hysterical symptoms.

The patient with a subconscious emotional overlay often demonstrates a significantly different pattern. This person is usually unconcerned with documentation, may start with a defensive attitude that later decreases (showing only transient episodes of anger), and does not knowingly withhold information. If hysterical symptoms are present, they usually are constant. Although this patient usually does have an attorney, the involvement is much more passive.

These are general descriptions and do not apply in all cases. Nevertheless, this differentiation has served us well in treatment management, particularly in our use of independent medical examiners to evaluate employees suffering acute neck injuries.

AN ORGANIZED APPROACH TO TREATMENT OF NECK PAIN IN INDUSTRY

Despite the prevalence of neck pain, industry has no standardized diagnostic and treatment protocols. Most episodes of neck pain are not medically serious, and most employees are able to return to work in a relatively short time, regardless of the treatment (provided it is not counterproductive). However, it has been shown that employees receive better care and return to work sooner if an organized, logical approach to evaluation, diagnosis, and treatment of their neck problems is used.[9]

A cervical spine algorithm was developed, computerized, and implemented in a public utility company, where an analysis indicated that 8% of all time lost from work was caused by neck injuries. The company has 5335 employees, of whom 3467 are blue-collar workers. The medical department has a full-time medical director, and all job-related injuries are evaluated by company medical personnel. An employee injured on the job may choose to see a private physician, but the medical department has the authority to follow the employee's care as they determine this is medically indicated.

This algorithm was applied to all cases of neck injury within 1 week of their occurrence. It was not intended to supplant the physician's judgments about an individual case or to suggest that all physicians should agree on all aspects of managing the pain. Rather, it included the generally accepted outer boundaries of treatment. Each work-related neck injury was monitored by the algorithm. If the patient's diagnosis, treatment, or clinical progress differed from that predicted by the algorithm, an unbiased independent medical examination was promptly obtained.

Results

The results were encouraging. Days lost from work were reduced 65%; light injury days were reduced 66%. The total number of acute neck accidents reported also was reduced more than 50%, compared with the number during the baseline period. No other significant changes took place in the company. The number and type of automobile accidents reported were unchanged.

One possible explanation for the reductions is that close monitoring of employee accidents became well known in the company, possibly resulting in fewer accident claims for individuals with minimal or nonexistent injuries. Another important factor in this study was the availability of light and limited duty work. The policy of this company is that, if an employee is ready to return to light or limited duty, every attempt is made to find work that fits the individual's specified limitations. In the past, there was some reluctance among managers to allow light- and limited-duty employees back on the job, because these people increase the complement of workers but do less work than full-time employees. This reluctance was partially overcome by including the managers' success in finding appropriate light- and limited-duty positions for returning employees as part of their performance evaluation.

The last factor in the success of algorithm has been careful follow-up of employees who have third-party suits. Those injured in automobile accidents involving third-party payments to the employee are followed carefully by the company. If the employee is reimbursed based on time off from work or medical costs, the company *insists* on being reimbursed, in turn, for these company-incurred expenses. This policy is made known to the employee in a nonthreatening way very early in the course of treatment in order to discourage the possible prolongation of a disability to justify a higher settlement payment.

Time Lost on Neck versus Low Back Cases

At the same time neck problems were being evaluated in this company, patients with low back pain also were being seen and evaluated with an algorithm. In comparing the two patient populations, neck cases were only 20% as frequent as low back cases, but the amounts of lost time and light-duty time per case were substantially higher for the neck patients. Low-back patients lost an average of 21.5 days per case, compared with 28.1 days for neck patients. Light duty days averaged 11.9 for low-back patients, 23.2 days for neck patients.

Summary of Benefits of the Algorithmic Approach

This type of program has been tried in other industries, with equally good results. It is a very attractive system because the program is automated and provides sophisticated medical guidance from the patient's first day of injury. This greatly expands the productivity of company doctors and nurses by supplementing their medical training. Also, the program uses carefully designed forms to facilitate the complete, accurate, and rapid collection of data. Thus, employers can obtain the information needed to review cases in a meaningful way.

ASSIGNING AN IMPAIRMENT RATING

Assigning a permanent partial impairment rating for neck injuries is a task fraught with inconsistencies. No official set of guidelines has been established. Each physician learns by trial and error. This section presents a brief overview of the problems inherent in determining impairment ratings, followed by a standardized rating system based on diagnosis.

Table 14-1. Work Restriction Classification of Compensable Neck Injuries.

WORK CATEGORY	WORK RESTRICTIONS	PPI*	RELEVANT DIAGNOSES
Very Heavy	Occasional lifting of over 100 lbs Frequent lifting of 50 lbs or more Overhead work	0%	Neck strain with complete recovery Hyperextension injury with complete recovery
Heavy	Occasional lifting of 100 lbs Frequent lifting of up to 50 lbs Overhead work	0%	Herniated nucleus pulposus, treated conservatively, with complete recovery Preexisting degenerative disease or cervical canal stenosis with secondary neck strain, with complete recovery
Medium	Occasional lifting of 50 lbs	5%	Chronic neck strain Degenerative cervical disc disease, under reasonable control
	Frequent lifting of 25 lbs		Herniated nucleus pulposus treated by surgical discectomy, with complete recovery Hyperextension injury with residual pain Healed odontoid/hangman's fracture treated nonoperatively
	Restricted overhead work		Preexisting, radiologically evident degenerative disease with secondary hyperextension injury, with moderate pain and restriction

Physical Disability versus Physical Impairment

Physical disability and physical impairment are not synonymous. A physical impairment rating is the objective assessment of body dysfunction. Physical disability, on the other hand, is very complex. It is affected by culture, socioeconomic background, education, experience, and the psychological makeup of the individual. A physician should be able to rate physical impairment objectively, and this rating should be reproducible from one physician to another. A physician may have a valid opinion about physical disability, but the full assessment of disability is not strictly a medical matter and is best calculated by nonmedical personnel.

In most cases, these nonmedical personnel are called rehabilitation specialists. They are trained, as vocational experts, to translate a physician's objective physical impairment rating into a disability rating. This assessment reflects an individual's ability to procure employment and is called "residual occupational access." It operates on the premise that all individuals, based on age, education, and previous work experience, qualify for a certain percentage of jobs found in the labor force. An injury that results in permanent impairment and functional restrictions reduces that percentage. Comparing an individual's preinjury access to the labor force with his or her postinjury access results in a measure of reduced employability (reduced occupational access) and, accordingly, a measure of loss of earning power. If these vocational experts can obtain reliable impairment ratings, they can calculate disability consistently.

The AMA Guides

Unfortunately, there are no standardized guidelines to aid physicians in determining physical impairment ratings for the neck.[10] The best available source is the American Medical Association's *Guide to the Evaluation of Permanent Impairment.* However, most physicians have stopped using this text because it uses loss of motion as the sole criteria for impairment and does not consider pain as a determinant except when it is associated with peripheral nerve injury or when "substantiated by clinical findings." In many instances, chronic neck pain is associated with few or no objective clinical signs, and even those present often are unrelated to the injury or disability in question. In effect, the factors considered by most physicians—motivation, age, education, personality, intelligence quotient, and social environment—strongly suggest that they are rating disability rather than impairment.

The AMA *Guides* do present one very useful

Table 14-1. (continued)

WORK CATEGORY	WORK RESTRICTIONS	PPPI*	RELEVANT DIAGNOSES
Light	Occasional lifting of no more than 20 lbs	10%	Degenerative cervical disc disease, with chronic pain and restriction
		to	Herinated nucleus pulposus treated conservatively or operatively, with residual
		15%	discomfort, restriction, and neurologic deficit
	Frequent lifting of up to 10 lbs		Hyperextension injury with chronic pain and restriction Cervical canal stenosis Moderately severe osteoarthritis accompanied by instability
	No overhead work		Hangman's fracture treated with fusion Odontoid fracture treated with fusion Burst/compression fracture of lower cervical spine with no neurologic deficit, treated with external fixation or fusion
Sedentary	Occasional lifting of 10 lbs	25%	Multiply operated neck (constant pain) Preexisting cervical stenosis with neck injury, treated by surgery, with patient subjectively and objectively worse

*PPPI = permanent partial physical impairment
Adapted from Social Security Administration Regulations

concept, that of the "whole man." Each part of the body is considered to represent only a part of the whole; the percentage each part contributes is based on its functional use. Since the spine (low back and neck) is important for many functions, it contributes a maximum of 60% of the whole man. Thus, once the impairment for a given part is assigned, the whole-man impairment can be determined easily.

STANDARDIZED GUIDELINES FOR NECK EVALUATION

In an attempt to create a standardized impairment rating system based on specific diagnoses rather than symptoms, a questionnaire was circulated among 53 American members of the Cervical Spine Research Society. Each respondent was asked to assign an impairment rating for 33 diagnostic entities. The responses were not consistent, but with statistical analysis, a medium range was obvious in most instances. Impairment ratings ranged from 0% for complete recovery from acute neck sprain to 20%, following a failed anterior neck fusion for herniated nucleus pulposus. The goal was to establish valid relationships among a specific diagnosis, the impairment rating, and physical exertion requirements.

Physical Exertion Requirements

Physical exertion requirements as defined by the Society Security Administration are simple and easy to use and can readily be adapted to conform to impairment ratings in a compensation or litigation setting.[11]

> *Very Heavy Work* is that which involves lifting objects weighing more than 100 pounds at a time, with frequent lifting or carrying of objects weighing fifty pounds or more.
> *Heavy Work* involves lifting no more than 100 pounds at a time, with frequent lifting or carrying of objects weighing up to 50 pounds.

No one with any neck-related permanent partial physical impairment can be expected to perform safely in either of these two categories. If the patient cannot be qualified to do any lighter work, that individual must be approved for total disability.

> *Medium Work* is defined as involving lifting no more than 50 pounds at a time, with fre-

Table 14-2. Disability Evaluation of the Cervical Spine

WORK ALLOWED	DIAGNOSIS AND COURSE	PPPI %
	*Acute neck sprain** → conservative care →	
Very Heavy	Complete recovery	0
Medium	Chronic neck strain (no x-ray findings)	5
	Preexisting, radiologically evident degenerative disease → *acute neck sprain* → conservative care →	
Heavy	Complete recovery	0
Medium	Acceptable level of discomfort and restriction	5
Light	Chronic pain and restriction	10
	Herniated nucleus pulposus → conservative care →	
Heavy	Complete recovery	0
Light	Acceptable level of discomfort and restriction, with or without neurologic deficit	10
	Herniated nucleus pulposus → surgical discectomy, with or without fusion →	
Medium	Complete recovery	5
Light	Acceptable level of discomfort, with or without neurologic deficit	10
Light	Pain and restriction, without neurologic deficit	15
Sedentary	Pain and restriction, with neurologic deficit	20
	Herniated nucleus pulposus → surgical discectomy (x times), with or without fusion →	
Medium	Complete recovery	10
Light	Moderate pain and restriction (employable)	15
Sedentary to None	Failed neck (constant pain)	20
	Hyperextension injury (no objective findings) → conservative care →	
Very Heavy	Complete recovery	0
Medium	Moderate pain and restriction (employable)	5
Light	Chronic pain and restriction	10
	Preexisting, radiologically evident degenerative disease → *hyperextension injury* → conservative care	
Heavy	Complete recovery	0
Medium	Moderate pain and restriction (employable)	5
Light	Chronic pain and restriction	10
	Preexisting cervical canal stenosis → *acute neck strain* → conservative care →	
Heavy	Status quo	0
Light	Subjectively worse	10
Light	Subjectively and objectively worse	15
	Preexisting cervical canal stenosis → *acute neck strain* → decompression, with or without fusion →	
Medium	Status quo	5
Light	Subjectively worse	15
Sedentary to None	Subjective and objectively worse	20
Medium	*Acute neck strain* → conservative care → no objective residuals → confirmed neurosis	0
Medium	*Odontoid fracture* → external fixation	10
Light	*Odontoid fracture* → fusion	20
Medium	*Hangman's fracture* → external fixation	10
Light	*Hangman's fracture* → fusion	15
Light	*Burst/compression fracture, lower cervical spine,* with no neurologic deficit → external fixation	15
Light	*Burst/compression fracture, lower cervical spine,* with no neurologic deficit → fusion	15

* Note: Compensable injuries are italicized.

quent lifting or carrying of objects weighing up to 25 pounds.

Only workers with 5% or less back-related permanent partial physical impairment can qualify in this category.

Light Work involves lifting no more than 20 pounds at a time, with frequent lifting or carrying of objects weighing up to 10 pounds.

Applicants with 10% to 15% permanent partial physical impairment ratings should be able to perform light work.

Sedentary Work involves lifting no more than 10 pounds at a time and occasional lifting or carrying of articles like docket files, ledgers, or small tools.

Persons with 20% neck-related permanent partial physical impairment will rarely qualify for any type of productive occupational activity, unless they have special sedentary qualifications that can be put to use at home or part time on the job. These work restrictions are summarized in Table 14-1.

Table 14-2 presents neck pain impairment ratings in a standardized set of diagnostic situations. It also matches physical exertion requirements with each diagnostic category. This Table can be referred to as patients are evaluated.

In Table 14-13, an acute neck sprain is defined as a soft-tissue injury of an otherwise normal neck. X-ray films are negative, and there is no radiating pain. In most such cases, patients should be able to return to their normal activities in 2 to 3 weeks.

Hyperextension injuries, also, are soft-tissue in nature, but their etiology is specific (vehicle accident). The return-to-work date for these patients depends on the severity of their symptoms and the type of work performed. Two weeks of treatment should yield enough improvement to permit nonmanual laborers to return to work. Very often, busy professional people return to work after 1 week. Patients employed in positions involving heavy manual labor may require 3 to 4 weeks of treatment. Generally, all patients are able to return to work by 6 weeks after injury and should be encouraged to do so, even if mild symptoms persist. Limitations at work generally include eliminating repeated episodes of stooping, bending, lifting, or carrying objects weighing over 50 pounds. These restrictions are often imposed for up to 3 weeks after the return to work. Depending on the severity of injury, patients generally make a complete recovery with no permanent disability.

Permanent partial impairment is often difficult to assess in these cases. A very small percentage of patients will have a persistent abnormal finding on physical examination—palpable muscle spasm, for example. However, the majority who remain symptomatic (only about 10% to 25%) will have continuing subjective complaints with no objective findings. Many of these workers are manual laborers and state they are fine as long as they are relatively inactive but complain of pain as soon as they resume work. In such cases, the physician's assessment of permanent partial impairment may depend on intuitive feelings about the patient, since objective signs are absent. If the physician believes the patient is honest and the patient is symptomatic, a 5% to 10% permanent partial impairment rating is reasonable. If the physician doubts the patient's honesty and objective signs are lacking, no permanent partial impairment should be assessed. Of course if would be preferable to have strict guidelines for use in this situation, but none are available.

Most patients who have a true radiculopathy (hard or soft disc damage) do not recover fully but have some residual physical impairment. It can be assumed that none ever go back to very heavy work, and a surgical procedure should not be expected to make this possible. Surgery is useful only to relieve an unacceptable level of pain or a deteriorating neurologic picture. As a rule, a patient who has had a disc removed may be expected to end up with a 10% to 20% permanent partial physical impairment. The patient with a perfect operative result will rate 10%, whereas the patient with continued symptoms will rate up to 20%.

Finally, some of the most difficult-to-evaluate situations involve on-the-job injuries to patients with preexisting osteoarthritis. Neck sprains suffered by such patients, for example, may be slow to respond, and the symptoms from the osteoarthritis tend to be perceived as more disabling than they were before the compensable injury. The spinal experts we surveyed were in favor of awarding a 5% permanent partial impairment to those who were subjectively worse, with light work as a permanent restriction.

REFERENCES

1. *Gotten N:* Survey of one hundred cases of whiplash injury after settlement of litigation. J Am Med Assoc 162:856–857, 1956
2. *Hohl M:* Soft-tissue injuries of the neck in automobile accidents: Factors influencing prognosis. J Bone Joint Surg 56A:1675–1682, 1974

3. *MACNAB I:* Acceleration injuries of the cervical spine. J Bone Joint Surg 46A:1797–1799, 1964
4. *PARTYKA S:* Whiplash and other inertial force neck injuries in traffic accidents. Paper for Mathematical Analysis Division, National Center for Statistics and Analysis, December, 1981
5. *JACKSON R:* The positive findings in alleged neck injuries. Am J Orthopaed 6:178–187, 1964
6. *JACKSON R:* Crashes cause most neck pain. Am Med News December 5, 1966
7. *STATES JD, KORN MW, MASENGILL JB:* The enigma of whiplash injuries. NY State J Med 70:2971–2978, 1970
8. *O'NEILL B, HADDON W, KELLEY AN, SORENSON W:* Automobile head restraint—frequency of neck injury claims in relation to the presence of head restraints. Am J Pub Health 62:399–406, 1972
9. *WIESEL SW, FEFFER HL, ROTHMAN RH:* The development of a cervical spine algorithm and its prospective application to industrial patients. J Occup Med 27:272–276, 1985
10. *ZIPORYN T:* Disability evaluation—a fledgling science? J Am Med Assoc 250:873–874, 879–880, 1983
11. *SOCIAL SECURITY RULINGS, TITLE 20:* Employees' Benefits, 404. 1567—Physical Exertion Requirements, 1968

Complications of Cervical Spine Surgery

JACOB J. GRAHAM

There are many traps in the path of the surgeon who approaches the cervical spine. A large number of vital neural, vascular, intestinal, and respiratory structures traverse this region. Only meticulous surgical exposure coupled with intimate knowledge of anatomy will help avoid complications. Of equal importance is proper patient selection, proper anatomic diagnosis correlating with the patient's complaints, and selection of the proper operation in order to avoid what Fager has described as the failed neck syndrome.[7] Most patients with complaints of neck and arm pain associated with restricted motion as a consequence of degenerative disc disease can be treated conservatively. Cervical spine trauma, when associated with instability, generally demands surgical stabilization. Incontrovertible evidence of cord and nerve root involvement usually requires operative intervention. Whether one approaches the cervical spine anteriorly or posteriorly is a matter of experience, individual judgment, and the need to "go where the money is." For example, disruption of the posterior tension members of the cervical spine (extensor muscles, interspinous ligaments, and ligamentum flavum) is appropriately treated by posterior stabilization and fusion, whereas the central herniated disc can best be approached from the front.

The ever-present risk of neural damage centers principally on the spinal cord. Often then is a cord whose physiologic reserve has already been partially compromised, either by trauma or spondylotic myelopathy, and, therefore, is highly susceptible to injury, even by minor indirect trauma or by vascular compromise. The patient with a cervical disc lesion or spondylosis associated with myelopathy, it has been stated, faces up to a 10% risk of deterioration of neurologic state when approached posteriorly, and quadriplegia has followed simple lateral disc excision at one level.[7] There is greater potential for more severe complications in anterior than in posterior approaches.[3] Tracheoesophageal problems are peculiar to the anterior approach, as are graft dislodgment and subsequent development of a kyphotic deformity. Late degenerative changes occurring above and below the fusion area are more apt to be seen with the anterior than with the posterior approach, whereas extension of the fusion area beyond the original intended limits is peculiar to the posterior approach.

The types of complications may be classified according to the approach used and whether they occur intraoperatively or postoperatively. The kind of condition, such as trauma, disc disease, tumor, or infection, also has a bearing on complication type and result (Table 14-3).

Much of what has been written about complications has been anecdotal with statistical results based on small series. Certain precaution maxims have been developed to forestall complications.

Perforation of pharynx, trachea, and esophagus can be avoided by careful retraction of these structures, while avoiding sharp blades and ensuring that in final placement the blades are under the longus colli muscles. Temporary dysphagia and hoarseness is a common complication due to edema secondary to retraction against an *in situ* endotracheal tube. This is usually mild edema, but serious forms must be recognized to guard against tracheal obstruction.

Vocal cord paresis is a result of injury to the recurrent laryngeal or vagus nerve. Hoarseness is usually temporary. A long follow-up of 85 cases by Heeneman[13] found 11% postoperative voice changes; of these, there were three cases with permanent vocal cord paralysis. Intraoperative injury to the recurrent laryngeal nerve can be avoided by staying in fascial planes and avoiding sharp dissection. The nerve is less vulnerable on the left side of the neck because of its longer course and more protected position in the tracheoeosphageal groove. The most likely cause of nerve injury is prolonged pressure against the trachea.

Injury to the cervical sympathetic with resultant Horner's syndrome is the result of trauma by dissection lateral to the longus colli muscles. If temperature gradient differences alone are the result, they are not of much clinical significance.

Tears in the vertebral artery may occur due to an inadvertent wandering by instrumentation with direct trauma. The problem can be repaired only by direct exposure of the vessel in the foramen transversarium and not by packing the interspace. Injury to the carotid artery or jugular vein with resultant thrombosis and cerebral ischemia is a rare lesion, usually the result of retractor injury.

Cerebrospinal fluid leak is usually referable to the use of a high-speed air drill and bone removal around the nerve root. Closure is not feasible, and the use of fascial graft beneath a bone plug has

Table 14-3. Classification of Types of Complications

Intraoperative complications

- I. Soft tissue
  - A. Anterior
    1. Esophageal or tracheal perforation
    2. Pneumothorax
    3. Injury to carotid artery, jugular vein, vertebral artery
    4. Hematoma
    5. Wound infection
    6. Injury to thoracic duct
  - B. Posterior
    1. Hematoma
    2. Wound infection
    3. Injury to vertebral artery
- II. Neural
  - A. Anterior
    1. Injury to spinal cord
    2. Injury to nerve roots
    3. Recurrent laryngeal nerve palsy
    4. Dural leak
    5. Injury to cervical sympathetic (Horner's syndrome)
  - B. Posterior
    1. Injury to spinal cord
    2. Injury to nerve roots
    3. Dural leak
- III. Osseous
  - A. Anterior
    1. Improper position of graft with compromise of neural canal
    2. Angulation of graft with loss of stability
    3. Improper positioning of screws in plate fixation
  - B. Posterior
    1. Wire pull-out
    2. Wrong level of fusion
  - C. Donor site problems
    1. Injury to lateral femoral cutaneous nerve
    2. Hematoma
    3. Infection

Postoperative complications

- I. Anterior
  - A. Soft tissue
    1. Tracheal and esophageal edema or fistulae
    2. Hoarseness
    3. Mediastinitis
  - B. Neural
    1. Spinal cord (monoparesis, paraparesis, Brown-Séquard, anterior cord syndrome, central cord syndrome, quadriparesis)
    2. Nerve root (motor and sensory)
    3. CSF fistulae
    4. Meningitis
  - C. Osseous
    1. Graft dislodgment (anteriorly or posteriorly into the canal)
    2. Angulation deformity
    3. Fractured bone graft
    4. Pseudarthrosis
    5. Aseptic necrosis and discitis
    6. Donor site problems (meralgia paresthetica, infection, neuroma cluneal nerve) and painful hip
- II. Posterior
  - A. Neural (spinal cord and/or nerve root)
  - B. Osseous (pseudarthrosis infection)
  - C. Wire breakage or pull-out

Halo Complications

- I. Pin Track (infection, penetration, loosening—pull-out)
- II. Dislodgment

been described. Any operation that enters the spinal canal, such as Cloward's drill and dowel technique for bony decompression, entails the risk of spinal cord or nerve root injury, particularly if there is a narrow canal. This need not always be the result of direct trauma, but could be indirect via injury to the anterior spinal artery system, an essentially independent arterial system without collateral circulation.[15]

Hematomas, which can lead to compressive tracheal and neurologic lesions, can easily be prevented by the use of a drain. Wound infection has no greater incidence in neck surgery than in other neurosurgical or orthopedic procedures in major hospitals (less than 1%).

Adequate illumination and magnification are the sine qua non of spinal surgery and go a long way toward reducing intraoperative trauma.

In posterior fusions associated with wire fixation, wire breakage and pull-out with painful pseudoarthrosis has been reported in a small number of cases.[3] However, many authors have reported a greater frequency of fusion and graft complications with anterior than with posterior procedures.[1,18,21–23]

Sugar,[19] in a review of spinal cord malfunction after anterior cervical discectomy, noted that risks of cord damage are calculated at less than 2 per 1000 and that the occurrence of myelopathy after laminectomy is well known, but supplied no figures. Disposition to trouble by preexisting myelopathy or stenosis was pointed out by cited cases of intraoperative trauma by dowel impaction or damage by osteotome or drill. Neck manipulation during anesthesia or position change, edema, hypertension, and other vascular disorders were also cited as causes. Cloward[4] reported the first case of intraoperative injury by an unguarded drill.

Scattered references in the literature have cited complications, some based on personal communication and many on relatively small numbers of cases. These are summarized in Tables 14-4, 14-5, 14-6, and 14-7.

Gregory,[12] in reporting on 61 anterior operations for fusion using the Robinson technique noted a 13% incidence of graft displacement and a 4.9% incidence of avascular necrosis of the vertebral body. Bohlman,[2] in a review of a 10-year experience with the Robinson anterior cervical disc and fusion in 1983, reported a 5% nonunion rate in single-level grafts to a 15% rate in multiple level grafts. He cited seven patients with increasing neurologic deficit, ranging from partial to complete quadraplegia following Cloward discectomy and fusion in which osteophytes were removed. There was one death in 103 patients from a coronary occlusion. He reported one instance of inadvertent section of the hypoglossal nerve mistaken for the superior laryngeal artery, which was successfully repaired.

Kraus and Stauffer[15] reviewed 10 patients with spinal cord injury in association with elective anterior cervical fusion and questioned the rationale for routinely entering the spinal canal for decompression, with the potential risk of either direct trauma of indirect compromise of vascular supply. They noted two of these cases of direct trauma, one due to posterior displacement of a circular dowel graft into the spinal canal and one due to a drill entering the canal. There was one transverse myelitis believed to be secondary to cautery on the posterior longitudinal ligament. Four cases were

Table 14-4. References to Complications in the Literature

AUTHOR	NUMBER OF CASES	NUMBER AND TYPE OF COMPLICATION
Connolly et al[5]	63	1 progressive myelopathy through Smith-Robinson approach
Galera & Tovi[12]	51	3 with Cloward 1 post-operative hemiplagia and brown sequard 1 impaired sphincter control 1 paraparesis with impaired sphincter control
Depalma[6]	281	1 brown séquard due to retropulsed disc material by neck hyperextension
Lunsford[18]	332	1 brown séquard

Table 14-5. Cervical Spine Research Society Data for 1982 to 1987.

	1982–83	*1983–84*	*1984–85*	*1985–86*	*1986–87*
# MAJORS	1054	833	1043	1265	1161
% COMPL.	4.40%	3.80%	3.90%	3.40%	2.93%
% NEURO	1.90%	0.24%	0.96%	1.42%	0.69%
DEATHS	0.95%	0.60%	0.60%	0.96%	0.34%

Table 14-6. Cervical Spine Research Society Data for 1982 to 1987

	1982–83	*1983–84*	*1984–85*	*1985–86*	*1986–87*
ANTER. PROC.	824(78%)	392(47%)	615(59%)	878(69%)	785(68%)
NEUR. CMPL. (ANTER.)	0.85%(7)	0.26%(1)	0.65%(4)	0.91%(8)	0.51%(4)
NEUR CMPL. (POSTER.)	5.65%(13)	0.23%(1)	1.40%(6)	2.58%(10)	1.06%(4)
GRFT. COMPL. (ANTER.)	2.10%	2.60%	1.60%	0.90%	1.02%
GRFT. COMPL. (POSTER.)	0.20%	0.00%	0.40%	0.00%	1.33%

Table 14-7. Cervical Spine Research Society Data for 1982 to 1987

	1982–83	*1983–84*	*1984–85*	*1985–86*	*1986–87*
# CORD CMPL. (ANTER.)	3	1	2	3	0
# CORD CMPL. (POSTER.)	12	1	5	8	2
# ROOT CMPL. (ANTER.)	3	0	2	4	4
# ROOT CMPL. (POSTER.)	1	0	1	2	2

attributable to vascular compromise of the anterior spinal artery system.

The most ambitious attempt to determine the magnitude of the neurologic problem by one individual can be attributed to Flynn,[10] who reported in 1974 on 704 replies to 1358 questionnaires on anterior cervical discectomy and fusion. There were 311 neurologic complications reported in replies for a total of 36,657 cases; no neurologic complications were reported in 45,457 cases (71% of replies). Thus, there was an incidence of 0.38% neurologic complications, in 82, 114 cases which included all types of myelopathy, radiculopathy, recurrent laryngeal nerve damage, Horner's syndrome, and even cerebral infarction. Of the cases of myelopathy, detail was sufficient to permit evaluation in 70 cases. Of these, 53 were immediate and 17 were delayed. Surgical exploration did not seem to make much difference in recovery (21% improved with surgery; 28% improved without it). Obvious exceptions to this observation would be the need to remove graft pressure on the cord or drain severe hematoma to relieve pressure.

In a follow-up questionnaire survey in 1984, to members of the Louisiana Neurosurgical Society in which 24 replies out of 49 were received, Flynn[9] noted 71% reported permanent or transient neurologic or soft-tissue complications, almost the reverse of his previous studies in which 71% stated that they were complication free. He subsequently presented 528 replies (134,246 cases) with a 1.26% incidence of neurologic complications.

Speculation about the etiology of spinal cord malfunction[15] has pointed to vascular causes. The anterior spinal artery system is an essentially independent vascular system dependent on contribution by the radicular arteries in the middle and lower cervical segments. It can be involved by cervical spondylosis. Removal of the posterior longitudinal ligament remains controversial. Excision of the ligament permits canal decompression; retention of the ligament protects against epidural bleeding and possible injury of the anterior spinal artery. The same controversy can apply to the question of whether or not to enter the spinal canal for osteophyte removal. Adequate visualization using intervertebral body spreaders, magnification, and light, as well as sufficient detachment of the longus colli muscles, are important. Hemostasis from bone with wax and Gelfoam are valuable, as

Table 14-8. Data

Operative Procedures / *Etiology*	Trauma	Fractures	Dislocations	HNP	Other	Congenital	Osseous	Soft-tissue	Other	Inflammatory	Infections	Rheumatoid	Other	Neoplastic	Soft tissue benign	Soft tissue malignant	Osseous benign	Osseous malignant	Other	Vascular	Soft tissue (AVM)	Osseous	Other	Degenerative	CSM	Stenosis	Hard Disc.	Other
Anterior discectomy																												
With interbody fusion																												
Robinson																												
Cloward																												
Bailey-Badgley																												
Cortical strut																												
Instrumentation																												
Other																												
Laminectomy without fusion																												
Two segments																												
Three or more segments																												
Other																												
Laminectomy with fusion																												
Two segments																												
Three or more segments																												
With acrylic																												
With instrumentation																												
Other																												
Posterior fusion only																												
Two segments																												
Three or more segments																												
With acrylic																												
With instrumentation																												
C1–C2																												
Occipitoatlantoaxial																												
Other																												
Vertebrectomy																												
Stabilization with bone																												
Stabilization with acrylic																												
With instrumentation																												
Other																												
Skeletal traction																												
Haloes																												
Crutchfield																												
Vinke																												
Other																												

is delicacy in instrumentation. The avoidance of unipolar coagulation around the posterior longitudinal ligament or the dura is to be emphasized. Only the bipolar current should be used. Accurate localization of the intraoperative level by x-ray monitor without a needle being placed too deeply in the interspace is important. Intraoperative verification of the graft position is essential.

Although complications appear to be more frequent and more grave in anterior than in posterior approaches, they unquestionably occur in posterior approaches. Fager,[8] emphasizing the efficacy of and better results obtained in posterior approaches for nerve root compression due to soft discs and/or osteophytes, cited 800 personal cases with two postoperative deaths and three additional recurrent nerve root deficits from surgical manipulation. There was no instance of significant spinal cord damage, but no mention is made of any spinal cord adverse effects, even temporary ones.

It is apparent that little is known concerning the true risks of cervical spine surgery, as most of the reports are of relatively small series and the larger ones have great variability. The need for a more accurate assessment of complications is self evident. An adequate knowledge helps in medicolegal issues, in informed consent and in assessing efficacy of surgical procedures. With this in mind, the Cervical Spine Research Society established in 1981 a Morbidity and Mortality Committee whose function has been to survey the membership annually and to provide ongoing statistics of morbidity and mortality. A printed data tabulation sheet has been prepared for the members to list the total number of surgical procedures performed annually, including halos, with cross reference to the disease for which it was done (Table 14-8). Complications were listed for each category, and separate sheets were filled out for each complication. To date, 5 year's experience has been accumulated. This has represented a total of 5,356 major operative procedures, not counting skeletal tractions—principally halos. The percentage of anterior procedures was 78% in 1982 to 1983, 47% in 1983 to 1984, 59% in 1984 to 1985, 69% in 1985 to 1986, and 68% in 1986-1987, average 64%. During the 5 years reported, the overall incidence of neurologic complications ranged from 0.24% in 1983 to 1984 to 1.90% in 1982 to 1983, with an average of 1.04%. The low of 0.24% may be a function of the small number of cases reported that year. Although the preponderant number of cases was anterior, there was a noticeably lower percentage of neurologic complications with anterior than with posterior approaches (an average of 0.64% versus 2.18%), which is the reverse of what literature experience would indicate. A small number of neurologic complications were referable to graft site (*e.g.*, lateral femoral cutaneous nerve complications) or to halos (*e.g.*, penetration with meningitis). Halo complications were a small but not significant number and usually represented pin loosening or infection. Many of the posterior complications occurred in posterior procedures for stenosis, where loss of cord function was established (actually or potentially). A small but definite number were due to iatrogenic trauma with an air drill. Cord complications appeared to be the preponderant neurologic complications in the posterior approach (a total of 28 compared with 9 for the anterior), while root complications predominated in the anterior approach (13 contrasted to 6).

Graft complications, on the other hand were largely in the anterior operative group, averaging 1.64% to be compared to an average of 0.39% with

Table 14-9.

	1985–1986	*1984–1985*	*1983–1984*	*1982–1983*
Total number of major operative procedures	1265	1043	833	1054
Incidence of complications	3.40%	3.90%	3.80%	4.40%
Incidence of neurologic complications	1.70%	1.05%	0.24%	2.18%
Mortalities	0.96%	0.60%	0.60%	0.95%
Anterior procedures	69.00% (878)	59.00% (615)	47.00% (392)	78.00% (824)
Graft complications, anterior	0.90%	1.60%	2.60%	2.10%
Graft complications, posterior	0.00%	0.40%	0.00%	0.20%
Neurologic complications, anterior	0.90% (8)	0.65% (4)	0.26% (1)	0.80% (7)
Neurologic complications, posterior	2.58% (10)	1.40% (6)	0.23% (1)	7.30% (13)

the posterior group. The significant results of 5 years experience are summarized in Table 14-9.

These statistics do not represent 100% of the membership, so their validity must be considered in this light. With the ongoing collection of future statistics, their validity will be determined.

REFERENCES

1. *Bailey RW, Badgley CE:* Stabilization of the cervical spine by anterior fusion. J Bone Joint Surg 42A:565, 1960
2. *Bohlman H:* Personal communication
3. *Capen DA, Garland DE, Waters RL:* Surgical stabilization of the cervical spine. Clin Orthop 196:1985
4. *Cloward RB:* New method of diagnosis and treatment of cervical disc disease. Clin Neurol 8:93–132, 1962
5. *Connolly ES, Seymour RJ, Adams JE:* Clinical evaluation of anterior cervical fusion for degenerative cervical disc disease. J Neurosurg 23:431–437, 1965
6. *DePalma A, Rothman R, Lewinnek G, Canale S:* Anterior interbody fusion for severe cervical disc degeneration. Surg Gyn Obs 134:755–758, 1972
7. *Fager CA:* Failed neck syndrome: An ounce of prevention. Clin Neurol 27:450–465, 1980
8. *Fager CA:* Management of cervical disc lesions and spondylosis by posterior approaches. Clin Neurol 24:488–507, 1977
9. *Flynn TB:* Neurologic complications of anterior cervical discectomy in Louisiana. J Louisiana State Med Soc 136(7):6-8, 1984
10. *Flynn TB:* Neurologic complications of anterior cervical interbody fusion. Spine 7:1982

10a. *Flynn TB:* Neurological complications of anterior cervical discectomy and interbody fusion: 1974 vs 1984. J. Neurosurg Abstracts 21:119, 1987

11. *Galera R, Tovi D:* Anterior disc excision with interbody fusion in cervical spondylotic myelopathy and rhizopathy. J Neurol 28:305–310, 1968
12. *Gregory CF:* Complications of anterior cervical fusion. J Bone Joint Surg 46B:715, 1964
13. *Heeneman H:* Vocal cord paralysis following approaches to anterior cervical spine. Laryngoscope 83:17–21, 1973
14. *Jacobs B:* Anterior cervical spine fusion. Surg Ann 8:413–446, 1976
15. *Kraus DR, Stauffer ES:* Spinal cord injury as a complication of elective anterior cervical fusion. Clin Orthop 112:1975
16. *Lunsford LD, Bissonette DJ, Janetta PJ, Sheptak PE, Zorub DS:* Anterior surgery for cervical disc disease. Part I: Treatment of lateral cervical disc herniation in 253 cases. J Neurol 43:1–11, 1980
17. *Lunsford LD, Bissonette JD, Zorub DS:* Anterior surgery for cervical disc disease. Part II: Treatment of cervical spondylotic myelopathy in 37 cases. J Neurol 53:12–19, 1980
18. *Pierce DS:* Spinal cord injury with anterior decompression, fusion, stabilization, and early rehabilitation. J Bone Joint Surg 51A:1675, 1969
19. *Sugar O:* Spinal cord malfunction after anterior cervical discectomy. Surg Neurol 15:4–8, 1981
20. *Tew JM, Mayfield FH:* Complications of surgery of anterior cervical spine. Clin Neurol 23, 1975
21. *VanPetegham PK, Schweigel JF:* The fractured cervical spine rendered unstable by anterior cervical fusion. Clin Trauma 19:110, 1979
22. *Verbiest A:* Anterolateral operations for fractures and dislocations in the middle and lower parts of the cervical spine. Report of a series of forty-seven cases. J Bone Joint Surg 51A:1489, 1969
23. *Whitecloud TS, LaRocca H:* Fibular strut graft in reconstructive surgery of the cervical spine. Spine 1:33, 1976

Failure of Methylmethacrylate Stabilization of the Spine. A Retrospective Analysis of 24 Cases

PAUL C. MCAFEE, HENRY H. BOHLMAN, THOMAS B. DUCKER, AND FRANK J. EISMONT

MATERIALS AND METHODS

We analyzed the complications from methylmethacrylate seen in 24 patients referred to the spine services at The Johns Hopkins and Case Western University Hospitals. The original spinal lesions were acute trauma in 15 and metastatic tumor in nine. No bone grafting had been performed in conjunction with the methylmethacrylate fixation in any of the 24 patients. As both institutions are tertiary referral centers, we have no way of determining the incidence of complications or the size of the population represented by these failures.

Spinal Instability Secondary to Acute Trauma

The average age of the 15 patients who had a spinal injury and an attempted stabilization with methylmethacrylate was 36.5 years (range 19 to 61 years). They had no concomitant diseases that would limit their life expectancy other than the traumatic spinal injury. The mean interval between injury and methylmethacrylate stabilization was 16.8 days (range 1 to 60 days). Their lesions included atlantoaxial subluxation in four, unstable fractures and dislocations at midcervical levels in 10, and a T9 compression fracture and ligament disruption in one. None of the spinal injuries involved more than two vertebral levels, but the average number of segments immobilized (including both anterior and posterior procedures) was 4.2 (range 2 to 8) levels. Many different metallic constructs were used to augment the methylmethacrylate fixation, most of them involving the use of 18- or 20-gauge wires. None of the metal implants were thought by the operating surgeon to have stabilized the injured vertebral segments prior to the insertion of the cement.

Of the 15 patients, four were neurologically intact, nine had incomplete spinal cord lesions, and two had complete spinal cord deficits immediately following their injuries.

Spinal Instability Secondary to Neoplasms

Nine patients had metastatic tumors, eight involving the cervical spine and one involving the seventh thoracic vertebra. Their average age was 51.3 years (range 27 to 72 years). Five patients had relatively slow-growing neoplasms, since they had been undergoing treatment for more than 2 years before their spinal metastasis was diagnosed; the other four patients' symptoms had been present for from 3 weeks to 8 months prior to attempted stabilization. (Cases 16, 19, 23, and 24). In all nine patients the methylmethacrylate was augmented with K wires, cancellous screws, or 18-gauge wire. Of these nine patients, two were neurologically intact when the methylmethacrylate was inserted, two had nerve root involvement only, four had incomplete spinal cord lesions but were ambulatory with the aid of a cane, and one (Case 23) was quadriparetic and nonambulatory before treatment.

RESULTS AFTER METHACRYLATE FIXATION

Loss of Fixation

Loss of fixation was the most common complication. It occurred in 12 of the 15 patients treated for posttraumatic lesions (Cases 2 and 4 to 14), and in eight of the nine with spinal neoplasms (Cases 16 through 22, and 24).

In the 15 patients with traumatic lesions, the average time between operation and failure of fixation was 208.3 days (range, less than 1 day to 730 days) excluding Case 14, in which loss of fixation at the atlantoaxial joint was probably not recognized for 9 years.

It is of interest that all of the failures of fixation in trauma were failures of attempted *posterior* stabilization techniques. There were no cases of failed anterior fixation in trauma referred to either of our institutions—we believe this probably reflects a lack of indications for anterior methylmethacrylate in trauma rather than the existence of anteriorly stabilized cases elsewhere, having done well.

In the nine patients with spinal metastases, the average time until failure was 193.7 days (range, 4 to 730 days). This is comparable to the length of time elapsing before failure of fixation in trauma cases. These findings, relative to loss of fixation, are not surprising, since all of the failures of fixation appeared to be due to biomechanical factors and not to local recurrence of the neoplasms.

In eight of the nine tumor cases, failure of methylmethacrylate fixation occurred in all instances at

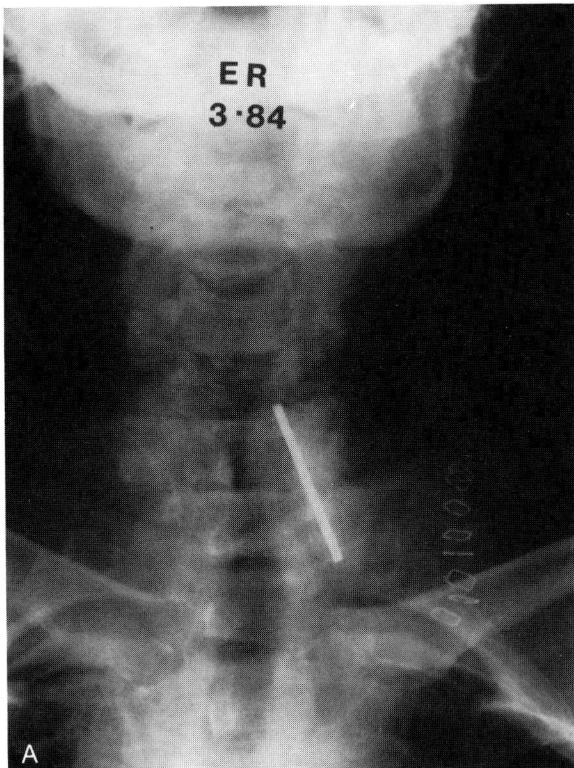

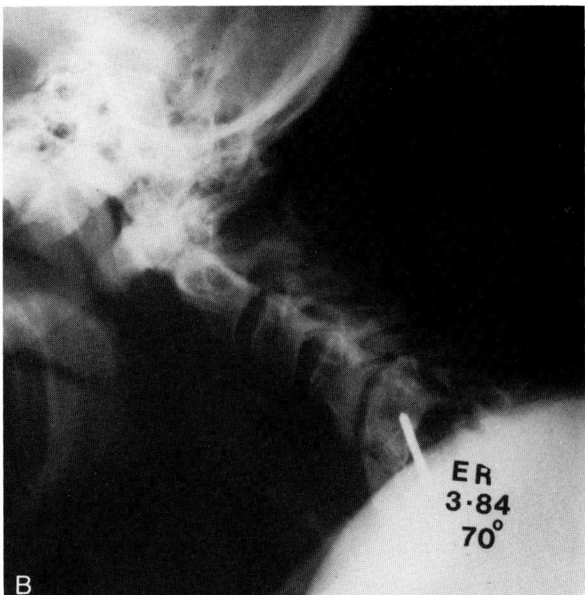

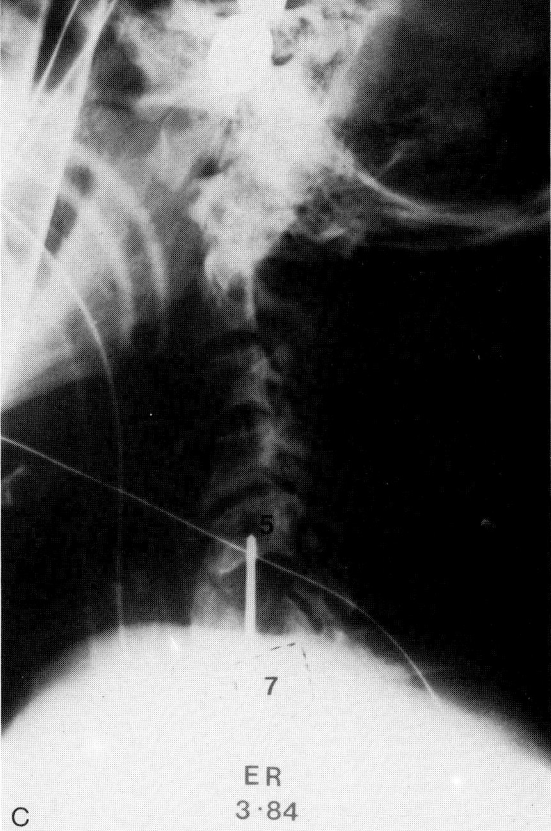

Fig. 14-1. Case 19. A 72-year-old man in whom metastatic adenocarcinoma to C6 was treated by corpectomy and attempted stabilization with a Kirschner wire and methylmethacrylate. (*A* and *B*) Twelve days postoperatively a 70-degree acute gibbus developed with lateral displacement of the cement mass. (*C*) Just prior to surgical exploration, the cervical spine was so unstable that it was realigned with just 10 pounds of skeletal traction. Stability was restored by a one-stage anterior and posterior grafting and stabilization. The patient was free of deformity and neck pain until he died 6 months later from his underlying disease.

the bone–cement interface. Five cases represented a failure of fixation of anterior vertebral body replacement with methylmethacrylate (Fig. 14-1). Three of four patients undergoing posterior methylmethacrylate insertion had loss of fixation. One patient (Case 23) died 18 months after posterior methylmethacrylate; although the posterior wound dehisced and he was bed-ridden, he did not experience biomechanical failure of the implant.

It has been implied by other investigators[2,8] that methylmethacrylate might be more resistant to fatigue failure when inserted anteriorly due to the inherent ability of the material to resist compression loads better than tension loads. In tumor cases the failures of fixation were fairly evenly distributed between failure of anterior and posterior constructs. Some investigators have stated that PMMA might be appropriate for anterior fixation, because the anterior column is subjected to pure compression loads and PMMA is more resistant to compression than tension. Vertebral motion data of White and Panjabi show that the anterior and posterior spinal columns are subject to large rotational, tensile, and lateral sheer stresses. Stabilization of both anterior and posterior spinal columns was important in restoring stability in tumor reconstruction (Fig. 14-2).

Neural Deficits After Methylmethacrylate Fixation of Acute Fractures

In 11 of the 24 patients in this series, a progressive neural deficit developed secondary to failure of the methylmethacrylate fixation. Of these 11, five

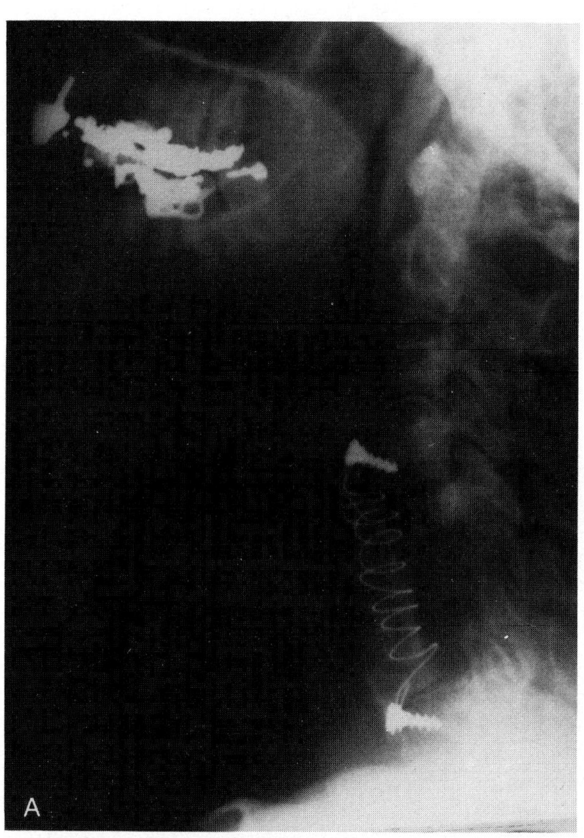

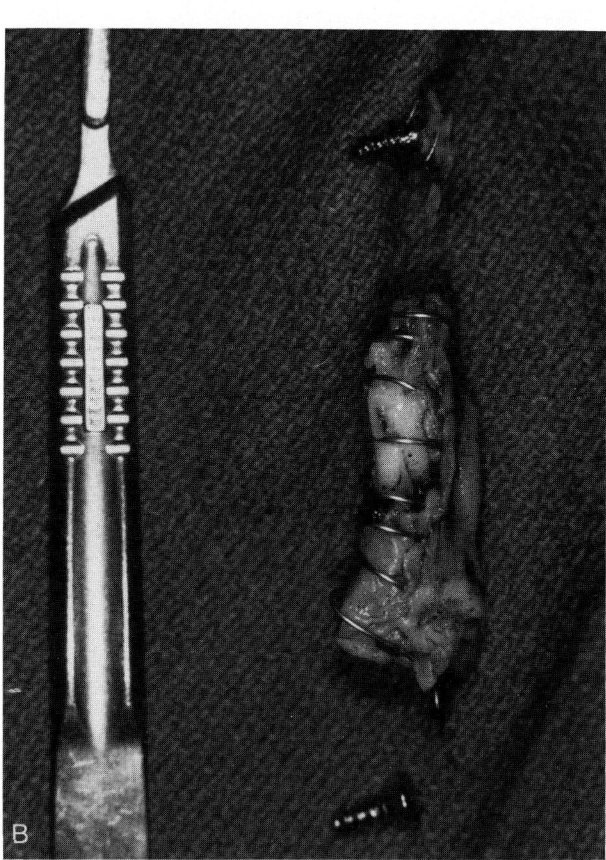

Fig. 14-2. Case 22. Anterior extrusion of methylmethacrylate. (*A*) This 42-year-old female with metastatic breast carcinoma to C5 through C7 had anterior dislodgment of PMMA within 4 days. She had no neurologic deterioration, but she developed dysphagia. The PMMA construct was successfully débrided and revised in one stage with posterior wiring and iliac fusion from C4 to T1. (*B*) The appearance of the dislodged PMMA construct at the time of débridement.

had acute traumatic lesions and six had spinal neoplasms. Of the 11 patients with iatrogenic neurologic progression, eight occurred following posterior procedures and three occurred following anterior reconstructions.

In the five with acute traumatic deficits and postoperative neural deficits, the findings were as follows.

CASE 6. A 55-year-old woman lost the use of her left upper extremity 6 months after methylmethacrylate fixation from C1 to C3 for a minimally displaced subluxation of C1 on C2. Six months after fixation she had 6 mm of anterior displacement of C1 on C2, which was significantly more than the initial displacement.

CASE 11. A 19-year-old boy with a T9 compression fracture had disruption of the posterior ligaments. After fixation using methylmethacrylate and wiring with circumferential sublaminar wires, the fracture was incompletely reduced and the thoracic spine was fixed with a 42-degree kyphotic deformity. Fifteen months later, the kyphosis had progressed to 68 degrees, and spinal cord function had deteriorated from a Frankel level C to a Frankel level B. After surgical revision, removal of the cement, reduction of the kyphosis with bilateral Harrington compression instrumentation and posterior fusion, the patient did not regain motor function in his lower extremities (Frankel level B).

CASE 12. A 42-year-old construction worker sustained a C5–C6 facet fracture and dislocation in a motor vehicle accident. Initial examination in the emergency room showed a complete C6 quadriplegia with bilateral normal deltoid (Grade 5/5) and good bicep (Grade 4/5) strength bilaterally. Within 24 hours, reduction of a bilateral facet dislocation and stabilization with a wire–methylmethacrylate construct was carried out. The patient had complete return of C6 sensory and motor function in the early postoperative period. Eight months later, after he had finished his rehabilitation, he noticed increasing neck pain and increasing difficulty when transferring from bed to wheelchair. Radiographs showed redisplacement of the C5–C6 fracture–dislocation, and objective testing showed complete loss of C6 nerve root function bilaterally. At surgical exploration, the acrylic on the left side was in three pieces, and on the right side the wires had pulled through the posterior elements. The patient's spine was realigned on the operating frame, and a Southwick facet wiring and iliac fusion were performed. Postoperatively, he was treated with skeletal traction for 5 weeks, followed by a two-post orthosis. Neck pain resolved over the next 6 months, and solid fusion occurred at C5–C6, but C6 nerve root function was not regained.

CASE 14. A 52-year-old man was seen 9 years after a C1–C2 subluxation with rupture of the transverse ligament, which had been treated by occiput-to-C2 fixation using methylmethacrylate and sublaminar wires. Nine years later when he came to our attention, he gave a long history of neck pain, and it was presumed that disruption of the fixation had occurred long before he was seen by us. However, right deltoid, biceps, and intrinsic muscle weakness had developed *only recently* due to cord compression caused by fragments of cement and granulation tissue in the neural canal. Presumably PMMA fragmentation had occurred with proliferation of granulation tissue, until cervical stenosis with neurologic deficit resulted. The patient had been neurologically intact originally. Decompression and fusion wire were recommended, but the patient refused further treatment.

CASE 15. A 22-year-old girl had had a unilateral C5–C6 facet subluxation with a Brown-Séquard syndrome at the C5 level. Immediately following posterior fixation with methylmethacrylate and wiring from C3 to C7, a complete C4 quadriplegia had developed. Emergency myelography showed complete blockage of the intrathecal contrast medium due to a posterior epidural mass of cement at the C3 level. Emergency removal of the wires and methylmethacrylate did not result in any neurologic recovery, and the patient remained a complete C4 quadriplegic with no useful extremity function.

In addition to the five patients with frank iatrogenic progressive neural deficits after fixation of acute spinal fractures with methylmethacrylate, there were six others (Cases 2, 3, 5, and 7 to 9) similarly treated whose recovery of neural function may have been impaired by their methylmethacrylate fixation (Fig. 14-3). Ordinarily after fractures and dislocations of the spine with incomplete neural deficits some improvement in function occurs. In these 6 cases, however, there was no further improvement after fixation with methylmethacrylate. In Case 9 neural function rapidly improved after removal of the methylmethacrylate, and postoperative myelography showed im-

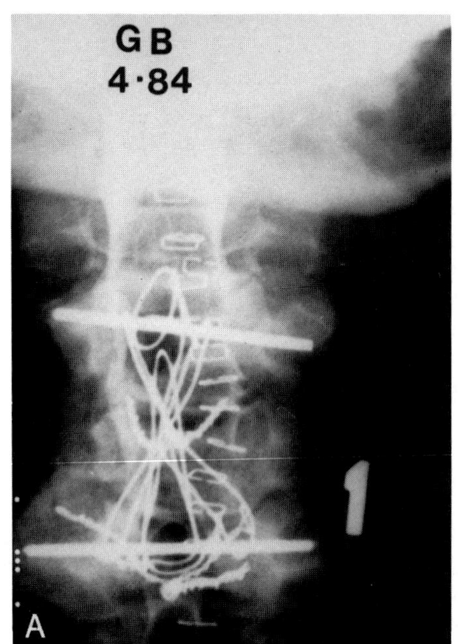
GB
4·84
1
A

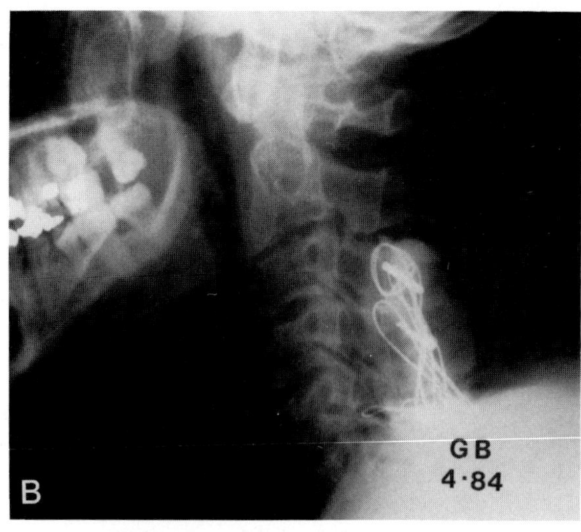
GB
4·84
B

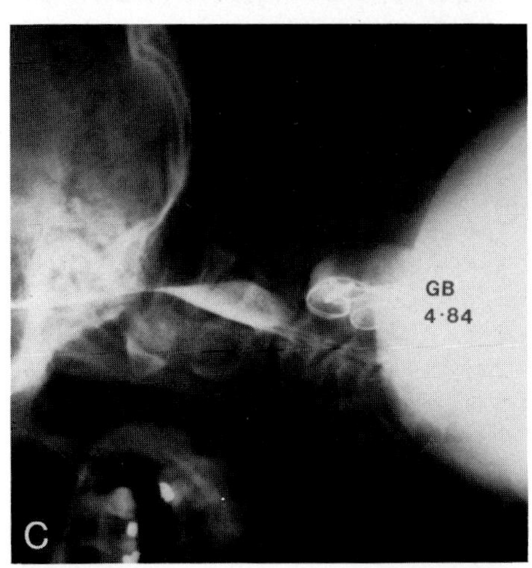
GB
4·84
C

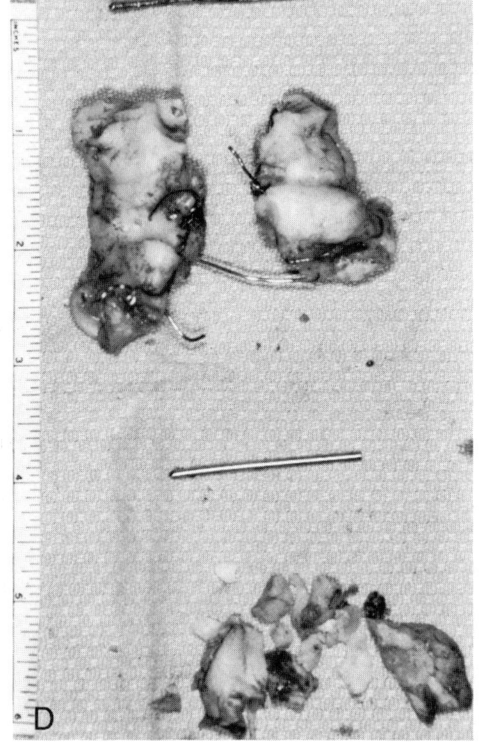
D

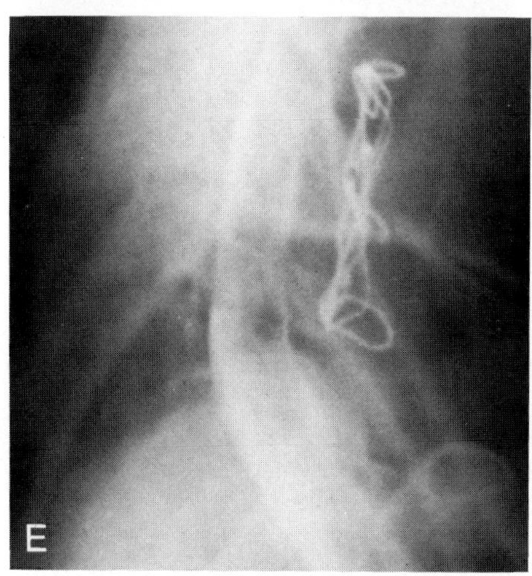
E

provement in the flow of metrizamide dye past the level of injury.

Neural Deficit after Methylmethacrylate Reconstruction for Spinal Neoplasms

Of the nine patients with methylmethacrylate reconstructions for tumor, six had progressive loss of neural function (Cases 16–18, 20, 21, and 24) and three (Cases 19, 22, and 23) showed no deterioration. The pertinent findings in the five with loss of function were as follows.

Case 16. A 55-year-old man with a pathologic fracture of the odontoid due to metastatic squamous cell carcinoma presented with a paraparesis of the central cord pattern (Grade 3/5 strength upper extremities, Grade 4+/5 lower extremities). He was treated by C1 to C3 fixation with sublaminar wires and methylmethacrylate. Five days postoperatively, while he was sitting in a chair wearing a Philadelphia collar, he felt a "pop" in his neck and 5 days later he became quadriplegic due to complete loss of fixation. Halo traction was instituted, but he died less then 1 month postoperatively due to pulmonary complications associated with prolonged recumbency rather than to progressive tumor involvement.

Case 20. A 53-year-old woman with carcinoma of the breast and a metastasis to C6 was treated by a C6 corpectomy and reconstruction with longitudinal Kirschner wires and methylmethacrylate. One month later C5 and C6 radiculopathies developed (right deltoid Grade 3/5 and right biceps Grade 4/5) when the methylmethacrylate–Kirschner wire construct separated from the C7 vertebral body. At reoperation the cervical spine was stabilized by posterior wiring and fusion of C4 to C7, but neural function remained unchanged.

Case 17. A 27-year-old woman with a metastasis to T7 from a chemodectoma was treated by a transthoracic T7 corpectomy in reconstruction of postlaminectomy instability. Anterior stabilization was attempted with three longitudinal K wires extending into the T6 and T8 vertebral bodies and methylmethacrylate. Postoperatively, her condition deteriorated from a mild T6 paraparesis (Grade 4/5 lower extremity strength and able to walk with a cane) to a Frankel level B T3 paraplegia (no lower extremity motor function and loss of bowel and bladder function) (Fig. 14-4). Within 4 months of her surgery, her spine became unstable and collapsed into a 87-degree gibbus deformity. Unfortunately, the patient became pregnant and carried a fetus to full-term delivery, preventing any spinal reconstructive procedure. Two years following her attempted stabilization with methylmethacrylate, an exploration was performed and two of the anteriorly placed longitudinal K wires had migrated superiorly into the spinal canal. One wire was completely buried within the substance of the spinal cord, accounting for a ascending sensory dysesthesias that had moved up from T6 to T3. The patient died from anesthesia-related adult respiratory distress syndrome and pulmonary fibro-

Fig. 14-3. Case 9. A 47-year-old man with a C5–C6 fracture–dislocation in whom subsequent neurologic recovery was impaired by the use of methylmethacrylate. (*A* and *B*) After injury anteroposterior and lateral radiographs show the four-level methylmethacrylate and wire construct, which had been inserted 6 days after injury. (*C*) A metrizamide myelogram in the prone position showing complete blockage of contrast at the C3 level due to posterior compression. The patient had a severe incomplete quadriparesis with very little biceps function as well as neck pain associated with loosening at the bone–cement interface. (*D*) Cement and wire removed at surgical revision. The operative findings included loosening at the bone–cement interface and PMMA in the spinal canal that had come through the laminotomy sites. (*E*) After débridement of the PMMA and stabilization from C4 to C6, using iliac struts and wires kept outside the spinal canal, the postreconstruction metrizamide myelogram showed free flow of contrast material through the vertebral levels of injury. The night after the surgery the patient recovered bilateral C6 nerve root function, and within 1 week had lower-extremity movement for the first time since injury.

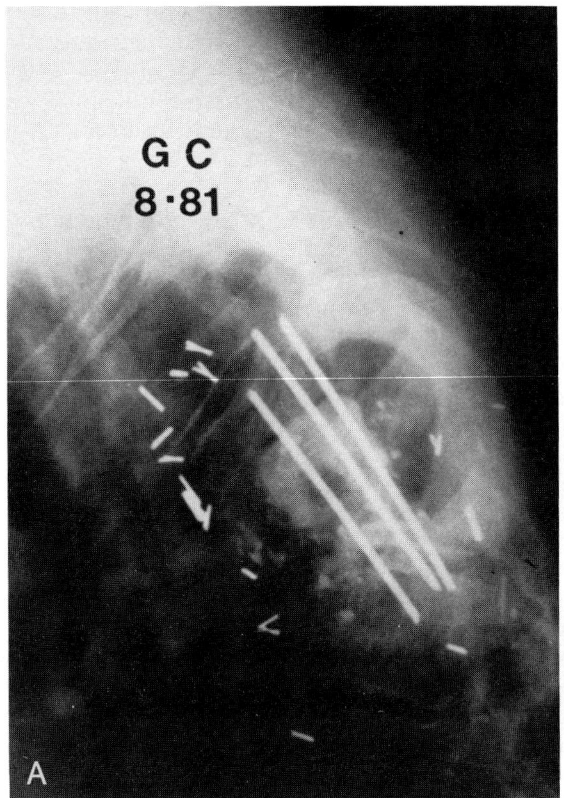

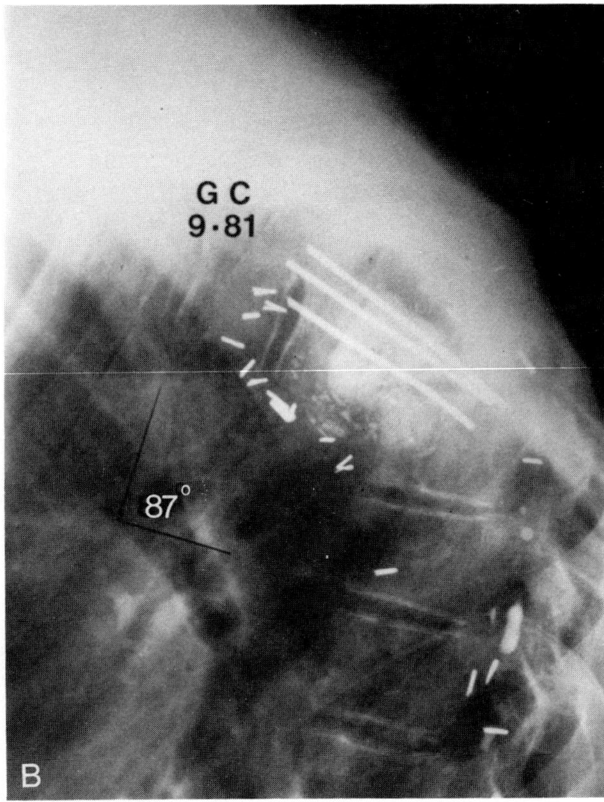

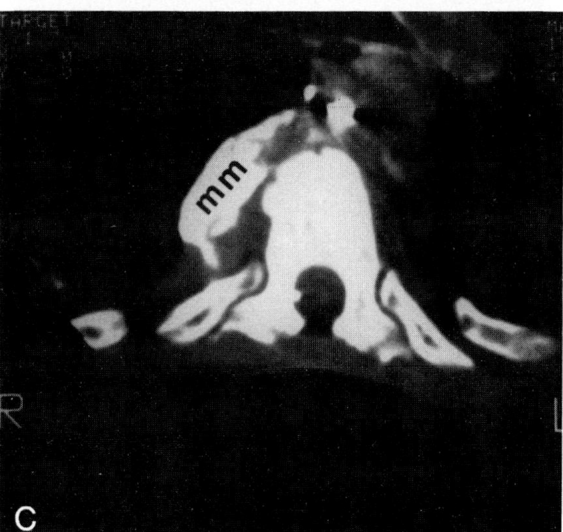

Fig. 14-4. Case 17. Neurologic deficit resulting from PMMA in tumor reconstruction. (*A*) This is a lateral radiograph of a 27-year-old woman stabilized with three longitudinal K wires and PMMA following transthoracic T7 corpectomy. The patient had a mild T6 paraparesis upon original presentation. (*B*) Within the next 9 months the patient's wire–PMMA construct further disrupted, with superior migration of two of the three wires into the spinal canal. The patient's neurologic function deteriorated to a dense ascending T3 paraplegia, she became wheelchair dependent, and she required narcotics for relief of severe mechanical thoracic pain. (*C*) This CT transaxial image shows a large radiolucent line between the methylmethacrylate mass (*mm*) and the vertebral body. There is also a K wire visible within the spinal canal.

sis, as secondary complications of the failed stabilization.

CASE 18. A 47-year-old woman with Hodgkin's disease and destruction of the C4, C5, and C7 vertebral bodies was treated by posterior methacrylate and wire stabilization from C2 to T1. She had no neural deficit prior to stabilization. Postoperatively, however, C6 and C7 nerve root involvement developed when a 68-degree angulation of the spine occurred at the C7 level due to separation of the cement from the bone. After reoperation that included anterior and posterior stabilization and bone grafting, weakness in the left upper extremity improved to Grade 4/5, while the right upper extremity regained normal strength.

CASE 21. A 68-year-old woman with carcinoma of the breast and metastasis to C2 was treated with a posterior stabilization from C1 to C3 using methacrylate and 18-gauge wire. Two years later, collapse of the fixation and subluxation occurred at the C2–C3 level. Originally she had L'hermitte's syndrome and upper-extremity paresthesias. After failure of the fixation and the C2–C3 subluxation, she became quadriparetic with a central-cord pattern. She improved following removal of the PMMA, reduction of the subluxation with halo traction, and stabilization by an occiput-to-C4 fusion. She recovered to 4+/5 lower-extremity strength and 4/5 left upper-extremity strength.

CASE 24. A 53-year-old woman underwent anterior reconstruction of C6 and C7 vertebral body destruction from a mestastatic carcinoma of unknown primary origin. She presented with a C6 myelopathy, lower-extremity hyperreflexia, and spasticity, but she was ambulatory without aid. Four days postoperatively she experienced neck pain while being treated in bed, and radiographs showed anterior dislodgment of the cement construct at C7–T1. The patient had anterior revision and posterior stabilization and fusion but did not regain her premethylmethacrylate level of function.

Surgical revision after failure of the methylmethacrylate stabilization was performed in all but two patients. The first of these (Case 7) had a spontaneous fusion from C5 to C6, and the second (Case 14) refused operation. In all 19 patients who had revision for failure of fixation, the methylmethacrylate was separated from the underlying vertebrae by a fibrous membrane. Except in Case 9, in which the cement had separated from the posterior elements as a single mass, the cement had fragmented into several pieces (Fig. 14-1).

Revision procedures using autogenous bone grafts restored spinal stability in all of the 11 patients with posttraumatic conditions who were so treated, and in six of the eight patients who had tumors. The other two patients with tumors and loss of stability died before their fusions consolidated.

Infections

Severe deep wound infections (Fig. 14-5) developed in six patients (Cases 2, 4, 5, 13, 16, and 23). Four of these (Cases 2, 4, 5, and 13) were late infections recognized at 4, 4.5, and 11 months, and at 7 weeks postoperatively. In five of six cases, extensive débridement, including removal of all cement and restabilization using autogenous iliac bone grafts, was required to control the infection. In Case 23 the infection was never resolved and the patient died. Of special interest was a 61-year-oldhousewife (Case 13) who had been treated by methylmethacrylate fixation at C1–C2 for a displaced Type II odontoid fracture. In this woman there was no evidence of infection until 7 weeks postoperatively when she had some dental surgery. Four days later a deep wound infection developed. To control this, complete débridement of the posterior cervical cement mass was required, after which the wound was packed open for 3 weeks.

A disturbing aspect of these infections was their time of occurrence—three of them more than 4 months after stabilization. Cervical fractures treated by autogenous iliac grafts and conventional techniques are usually fused within 4 months. Once fused by conventional techniques, patients are no longer susceptible to deep wound infections. Late hematogenous infections of autogenous cervical fusions without methylmethacrylate (in contrast to Cases 2, 4, 5, and 13) have not been reported, to our knowledge. Following revision, solid fusions and spinal stability were demonstrated after follow-ups of more than 2 years, attesting to the fact that it would have been possible to achieve spinal stability using traditional bone grafting methods originally.

Because the patients included in this study were referred from a wide geographic area, the incidence of infection or loosening after methylmethacrylate stabilization of the spine could not be determined. However, once these complications developed, the magnitude of the surgical procedures necessary for their management far exceeded what would have been required to manage

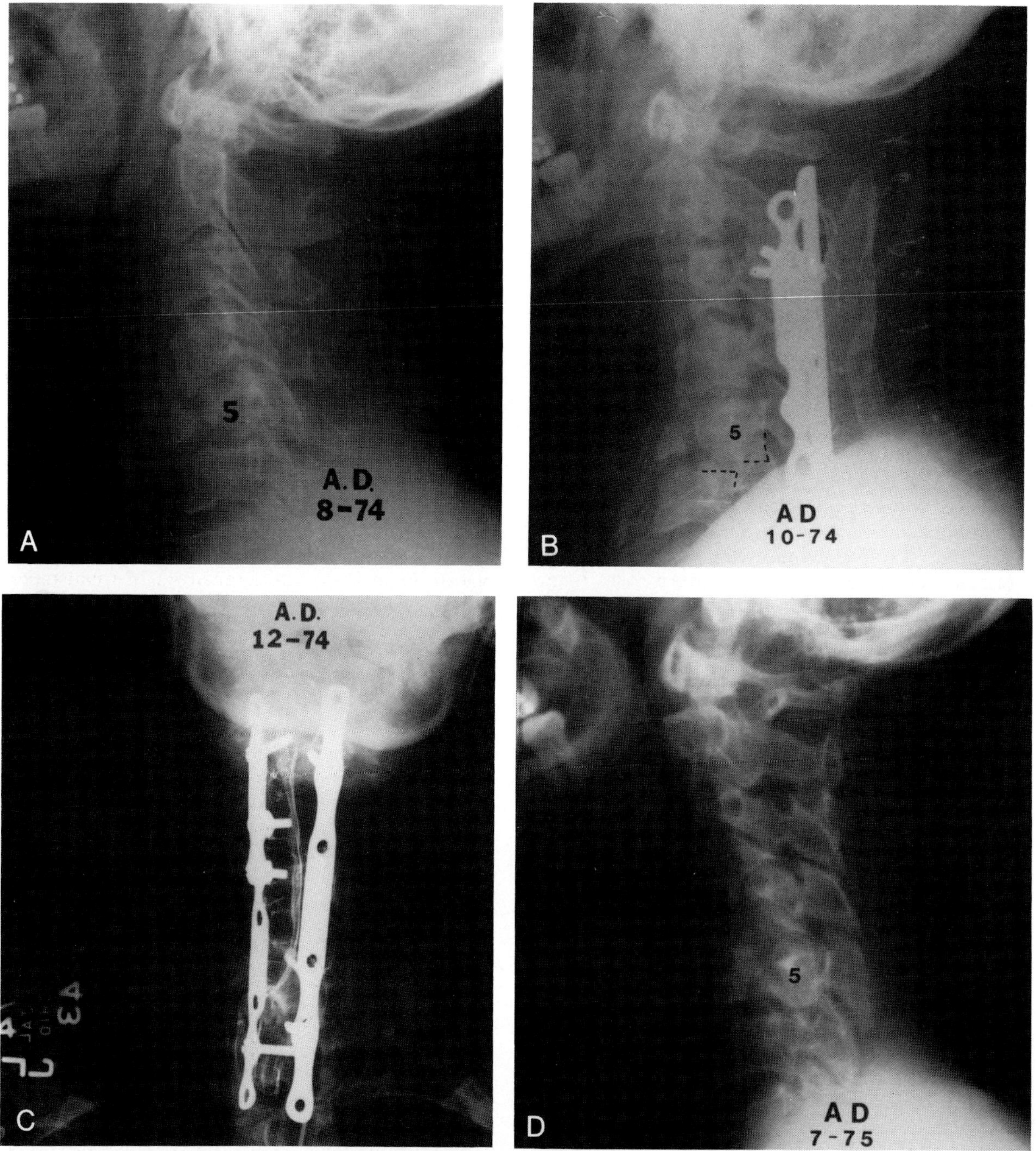

Fig. 14-5. Case 4. A 32-year-old man in whom a deep wound infection developed after attempted stabilization of a C5 burst fracture with complete C4 quadriplegia using a construct composed of cement, plates, screws, and wire mesh, and extending from C2 to T2. (*A*) Lateral radiograph after injury. (*B*) Two months after injury, stabilization of the fracture was attempted elsewhere. (*C*) After a deep wound infection developed with a *Staphylococcus aureus* abscess, the plates and PMMA became loose and the spine was grossly unstable. The wound failed to respond to local débridement, and septic meningitis resulted. (*D*) After removal of the cement and metal the wound healed completely. Eleven months after injury, the spine became stable due to a spontaneous anterior C4 to C6 fusion.

these complications in patients treated with traditional bone grafting techniques.

DISCUSSION

There are some theoretical disadvantages related to the use of methylmethacrylate for the fixation of the spine. These include (1) increased risk of infection due to decreased chemotaxis of leukocytes,[11] impairment of bacterial phagocytosis,[6] and killing by polymorphonuclear leukocytes,[12] and (2) decreasing mechanical stability of PMMA implants with time under cyclical loading conditions.[15] In the present study, six of the 24 patients had deep wound infections. Although the incidence of infections when methacrylate spinal constructs are used cannot be proved to be higher than when traditional methods are used, the management of infections after spinal surgery in which acrylic is used is certainly more difficult.

Petty and coworkers[13] performed experiments on 187 dogs in order to evaluate the effect of methylmethacrylate polymerized *in vivo,* prepolymerized methylmethacrylate, stainless steel, high-density polyethylene and cobalt-chromium alloys. Of all these commonly used orthopedic implants, the one that was associated with the highest incidence of infection (*S. aureus, S. epidermidis,* and *E. coli*) was methylmethacrylate polymerized *in vivo.*

In all 19 patients who had a revision for failure of the methylmethacrylate fixation, a synovium-like fibrous membrane was found between the cement and the underlying vertebral bone. The tissue in this membrane seemed histologically similar to that described by Goldring and coworkers,[5] who retrieved tissue from 20 patients with loose total hip replacements. These authors found that the membrane at the bone–cement interface had histochemical characteristics of synovium, including synovium-like cells adjacent to the cement and a deeper layer of macrophages. This membrane had the capacity to produce prostaglandin E_2 and collagenase, both of which can cause progressive lysis of bone. In our patients a radiolucent zone at the bone–cement interface often preceded evidence of instability on flexion–extension radiographs.

Of the patients in this series who had posterior PMMA constructs in place for more than 1 year, all six demonstrated a radiolucent line at the bone–cement interface on flexion–extension radiographs at 1 year. In patients who have been referred from elsewhere with posterior PMMA constructs that have not yet failed, we have observed increasing radiolucency occurring by 12 months postoperatively.

This is the first study of which we are aware that reports on clinical failures after methylmethacrylate stabilization of the spine. However, even in the published preliminary studies of methylmethacrylate, complications in the spine were rather common.[2–8,10]

Harrington[8] reported on 14 patients with spinal instability due to tumor destruction who were treated with anterior and posterior methylmethacrylate constructs. One patient had failure of fixation, and another had a massive 12 × 25–cm full-thickness skin and muscle slough posteriorly. The anterior construct of methylmethacrylate and Harrington compression rods remained unexposed.

Clark and coworkers[2] reported on 52 patients whose spines were stabilized with methylmethacrylate: 18 for malignant disease, 17 for fractures, 12 for rheumatoid arthritis, and five for osteoarthritis. Iliac crest grafts were used whenever possible, so that this study includes the results of PMMA when used to augment conventional fusion methods. Four patients died during the first postoperative month because of their primary underlying disease; two with anterior PMMA constructs only (no grafts) had postoperative dislocations of their anterior interbody strut, and one patient had a fracture of the methylmethacrylate mass but was asymptomatic with no gross instability.

Bryan and coworkers[1] reported on the results in 11 patients who were treated for rheumatoid arthritis by cervical spine fusion using autogenous iliac bone grafts augmented with stainless steel wire, titanium mesh, perforated titanium sheets, and methylmethacrylate for rheumatoid arthritis. Six of these patients had superior migration of the dens necessitating fusion to the occiput, and five had atlantoaxial subluxation treated by fusions below the occiput. Four of the 11 patients had wound dehiscences, two of which were infected. In one patient, rapidly progressive quadraparesis at the C5 level developed 3 months postoperatively, owing to complete dislocation of the fifth on the sixth cervical vertebra.

These authors concluded that methylmethacrylate-reinforced constructs should be used when traditional techniques have failed and a pseudarthrosis is to be repaired. In this series, the PMMA composites were supplemented with iliac bone grafts. The main advantage of using methylmethacrylate and iliac crest grafts was the elimination of the need for external fixation devices such as a halo cast.

In another study under the auspices of the Cervical Spine Research Society, 24 patients who had methylmethacrylate stabilization for spinal tumors were analyzed in an attempt to establish indications for the use of cement in stabilization of the spine.[3] Ten patients had corpectomy and replacement of the vertebral body by methylmethacrylate, and 14 had posterior stabilization. During the first postoperative month, five patients had died with widespread metastatic disease and four showed gross radiographic and clinical loss of fixation. Two patients had loss of anterior fixation, and two had failure of posterior constructs.

Anterior versus Posterior

In reviewing our series and the literature, we found a definite increased complication rate when PMMA is used for posterior rather than anterior stabilization. In our series of 24 complications, only five occurred with anterior reconstruction (and Case 17 had a prior laminectomy). Of 11 patients with iatrogenic neurologic progression, eight developed this problem after undergoing posterior procedures, and these occurred following anterior PMMA insertion. Five of the six deep wound infections occurred with posterior PMMA.

As a general rule it is not appropriate to apply the biomechanics of tumor stabilization to fracture–dislocations, as the latter have widespread ligamentous instability and no intact surrounding soft-tissue envelope. As we have previously stated, PMMA should not be used in the primary treatment of traumatic conditions, because conventional bone grafting and posterior stabilization methods show predictably good results.

However, in a patient with limited life expectancy with loss of anterior vertebral bone stock due to neoplastic destruction, anterior PMMA has merit. Harrington[8] and Siegal and coworkers[14] have experience with vertebral body replacement for malignant epidural tumors. Siegal and coworkers reported dislodgment of the construct in three cases, owing to faulty anchorage to adjacent vertebrae. None has occurred since introduction of anterior instrumentation using two sacral hooks on a heavy threaded compression rod. Harrington's experience had extended to only five failures of fixation in a total of 94 consecutive cases often using anterior Harrington or Knodt rods. Our experience with 10 cases of multiple-level corpectomy deficits treated successfully with anterior Caspar plates and methylmethacrylate leads to similar conclusions. Improved results of PMMA can be expected if rigid fixation is present between a metal surgical implant and the adjacent vertebrae prior to cement insertion. The anterior role of PMMA is then to increase the surface area of fixation between the implant and the bone. To further provide long-term stability, autogenous bone graft should also supplement the fixation.

We reiterate the conclusions reached from Dunn's multicenter study:

> There has been almost unanimous agreement on the indications for methylmethacrylate stabilization of the cervical spine—a patient with a metastatic or unresectable primary tumor with a limited life span, yet who could be expected to withstand surgery and who is troubled by severe neck pain and/or progressive deformity or instability likely to lead to or already producing a neurological deficit.[3]

It was also concluded that most patients with metastatic lesions of the cervical spine do not meet these criteria and are better managed with radiotherapy, chemotherapy, and conservative nonoperative methods of stabilization, such as an orthosis. Finally, there were clear reservations as to the use of methylmethacrylate in patients without tumors or in patients with normal longevity.

Based on the findings in this study and information available in the literature, we would make the following recommendations.

1. Methylmethacrylate for spinal fixation should be used only as a salvage technique.
2. Only patients with a life expectancy of less than 1 year should be considered candidates for methylmethacrylate.
3. When methylmethacrylate is used, it should be supplemented with autogenous bone grafts whenever possible. If the patient is to have postoperative radiotherapy for an anterior lesion, it may be advisable to defer posterior bone grafting and formal fusion until completion of the radiotherapy.
4. Methylmethacrylate is not indicated for stabilization of the spine for traumatic lesions, osteoarthritis, or rheumatoid arthritis in its early stages—all conditions in which conventional iliac bone grafting gives excellent long-term results.
5. When a deep wound infection develops, all of the methylmethacrylate must be débrided. Any patient who has methylmethacrylate augmentation of a spine fusion should have antibiotic coverage during dental procedures or any procedures that may produce a transient bacteremia. Whenever possible, a metal fixation device such as Harrington instrumenta-

tion or an anterior cervical plate and screws should be used with the methylmethacrylate. The methylmethacrylate should be used for augmentation, rather than for primary stabilization. The purpose of the methylmethacrylate is to increase the surface area between the metal construct and the surface of the vertebrae. Longitudinal K wires or small transverse pins tend to loosen within the methylmethacrylate, migrate, and cause neural injury.

ACKNOWLEDGMENTS

The authors gratefully acknowledge the assistance of Ms. Cathi Connelly, Ms. Shari Tate, and Charles Mick, M.D., formerly at The Johns Hopkins Hospital, in preparing this manuscript.

REFERENCES

1. *Bryan WJ, Inglis AE, Scuko TP, Ranawat CS:* Methylmethacrylate stabilization for enhancement of posterior cervical arthrodesis in rheumatoid arthritis. J Bone Joint Surg 64A:1045–1050, 1982
2. *Clark CC, Keggi KJ, Panjabi MM:* Methylmethacrylate stabilization of the cervical spine. J Bone Joint Surg 66A:40–46, 1984
3. *Dunn EJ:* The role of methylmethacrylate in the stabilization and replacement of tumors of the cervical spine—a project of The Cervical Spine Research Society. Spine 2:15–24, 1977
4. *Eismont FJ, Bohlman HH:* Posterior methylmethacrylate fixation for cervical trauma. Spine 6:347–353, 1981
5. *Goldring SR, Schiller AL, Roelke M, Rourke CM, O'Neil PA, Harris WH:* The synoviac-like membrane at the bone–cement interface in loose total hip replacements and its proposed role in bone lysis. J Bone Joint Surg 65A:575–589, 1983
6. *Green SA:* The effect of methylmethacrylate on phagocytosis. Proceedings of the Orthopaedic Research Society. J Bone Joint Surg 57A:583, 1975
7. *Gristina AG, Kolkin JW:* Current concepts review. Total joint replacement and sepsis. J Bone Joint Surg 65A:128–134, 1983
8. *Harrington KD:* The use of methylmethacrylate for vertebral body replacement and anterior stabilization of pathologic fracture—dislocation of the spine due to metastatic malignant disease. J Bone Joint Surg 63A:36–46, 1981
9. *Harrington KD:* Personal communication
10. *Panjabi MM, Hopper W, White AA, Keggi KJ:* Posterior stabilization with methylmethacrylate. Biomechanical testing of a surgical specimen. Spine 2:241–247, 1977
11. *Petty W:* The effect of methylmethacrylate on chemotaxis of polymorphonuclear leukocytes. J Bone Joint Surg 60A:492–498, 1978
12. *Petty W:* The effect of methylmethacrylate on bacterial phagocytosis and killing by human polymorphonuclear leukocytes. J Bone Joint Surg 60A:752–757, 1978
13. *Petty W, Spanier S, Shuster JJ, Silverthorne C:* The influence of skeletal implants on incidence of infection. Experiments in a canine model. J Bone Joint Surg 67A:375–382, 1985
14. *Siegal T, Tiqva P, Siegal T:* Vertebral body resection for epidural compression by malignant tumors. Results of forty-seven consecutive operative procedures. J Bone Joint Surg 67A:375–382, 1985
15. *White AA III, Panjabi MM:* Surgical constructs employing methylmethacrylate in clinical biomechanics of the spine, pp 423–431. Philadelphia, JB Lippincott, 1978
16. *Whitehill R, Barry JC:* The evolution of stability in cervical spinal constructs using either autogenous bone graft or methylmethacrylate cement. A follow up report on a canine *in vivo* model. Spine 10:32–41, 1985
17. *Whitehill R, Roger SI, Fox E, Payne R, Barry J, Cole C, Richman J, Bruce J:* The use of methylmethacrylate cement as an instantaneous fusion mass in posterior cervical fusions: A canine *in vivo* experimental model. Spine 9:246–252, 1984

Index

A

E

J

K

L

M

O

Q

U

V

ISBN 0-397-50827-1